Clinical Ophthalmology

A Systematic Approach

Second Edition

Clinical Ophthalmology

A Systematic Approach

Second Edition

Jack J. Kanski, MD, FRCS
Consultant Surgeon, Prince Charles Eye Unit, King Edward VII Hospital, Windsor

Butterworths
London Boston Singapore Sydney Toronto Wellington

First published 1984
Second edition 1989

Butterworths International Edition, 1989
ISBN 0 407 01021 1

British Library Cataloguing in Publication Data

Kanski, Jack J.
Clinical Ophthalmology: a systematic approach.
1. Ophthalmology
I. Title
617.7 RE46

ISBN 0-407-01020-3

Library of Congress Cataloging in Publication Data

Kanski, Jack J.
Clinical Ophthalmology.

Includes bibliographies and index.
1. Ophthalmology. I. Title.
[DNLM: 1. Eye Diseases. WW140 K16c]
RE46.K35 1988 617.7 87-33529
ISBN 0-407-01020-3

Photoset by Butterworths Litho Preparation Department
Printed by Toppan Printing Company (H.K.) Ltd, Hong Kong

Preface to the Second Edition

This book is intended mainly for the trainee ophthalmologist. It should also prove to be useful to those wishing to update their knowledge in this rapidly advancing branch of medicine. The main emphasis is on the clinical interpretation of clinical signs which still form the mainstay of diagnosis of eye disorders. It is hoped that the systematic outlay of the text will enable those preparing for examinations to assimilate the subject matter more easily. Although this is not intended to be a textbook of eye surgery, detailed descriptions of surgical techniques and complications of the more commonly performed procedures have been included. The bibliography will provide the reader with key references from which to pursue a particular topic in depth.

Because of the significant advances made in ophthalmology during the last few years it has been necessary to update and reorganize the second edition of *Clinical Ophthalmology* substantially. Although the number of chapters has been reduced from seventeen to fifteen, the number of illustrations has increased and some of the older ones have been replaced. The descriptions of the surgical procedures have been updated and expanded and some of the older and now obsolete procedures and investigations have been omitted.

I am extremely grateful to the following colleagues for taking the time and care to review the manuscript and for making many helpful suggestions: Mr A. Bron, Miss P. Burgess, Mr I. Chisholm, Dr P. Cibelli, Mr R. Collin, Miss A. Crisp, Professor D. Easty, Mrs L. Frost, Mr B. Holland, Mrs D. Marshall, Mr J. McAllister, Mr C. Migdal, Professor P. Morse, Mr C. O'Brien, Mr N. Strong, Mr D. Taylor, Dr D. Thomas, Mr R. Welham, Mr R. Whitelocke and Mr J. Wright. The new artwork has been provided by Mr T. Tarrant and new photographs by Miss D. Bannister. I would also like to thank Professor M. Spitznas for allowing me to use some of the illustrations from the German translation of the book. Last but not least I would like to convey my gratitude to my publishers.

Windsor 1988

Contents

1 The Eyelids 1
2 The Orbit 21
3 The Lacrimal System 45
4 The Conjunctiva 61
5 The Cornea and Sclera 87
6 Uveitis 135
7 Glaucoma 181
8 The Lens 233
9 Retinal Detachment 261
10 Retinal Vascular Disorders 299
11 Acquired Maculopathies 339
12 Hereditary Disorders of the Retina and Choroid 369
13 Tumours of the Uvea and Retina 389
14 Strabismus 411
15 Neuro-ophthalmology 439
Index 481

1

The Eyelids

Common cysts

Applied anatomy of eyelid margin
External hordeolum (stye)
Meibomian cyst (chalazion)
Internal hordeolum
Cyst of Moll
Cyst of Zeis
Sebaceous cyst

Benign tumours

Molluscum contagiosum
Squamous papilloma
Verruca vulgaris
Seborrhoeic keratosis
Senile keratosis
Xanthelasma
Keratoacanthoma
Cutaneous horn
Haemangioma

Malignant tumours

Classification
Clinical features
Treatment

Disorders of eyelashes

Trichiasis
Distichiasis

Entropion

Classification
Involutional (senile)
Cicatricial
Congenital
Acute spastic

Ectropion

Classification
Involutional (senile)
Ciactricial
Congenital
Paralytic

Ptosis

Applied anatomy
Classification
Neurogenic
Aponeurotic
Mechanical
Myogenic
Clinical evaluation
Treatment

Miscellaneous congenital disorders

Dermatitis

Contact
Atopic

Common cysts

Applied anatomy of eyelid margin

The lid margin is divided into anterior and posterior parts by the grey line (*Figure 1.1*). The eyelashes (cilia) originate anterior to the grey line and the ducts of the meibomian glands are located posterior to the grey line at the mucocutaneous junction. Each tarsus contains about 30 modified sebaceous (meibomian) glands that secrete sebum. Each meibomian gland consists of a large central excretory canal and between 10 and 50 glandular lobules.

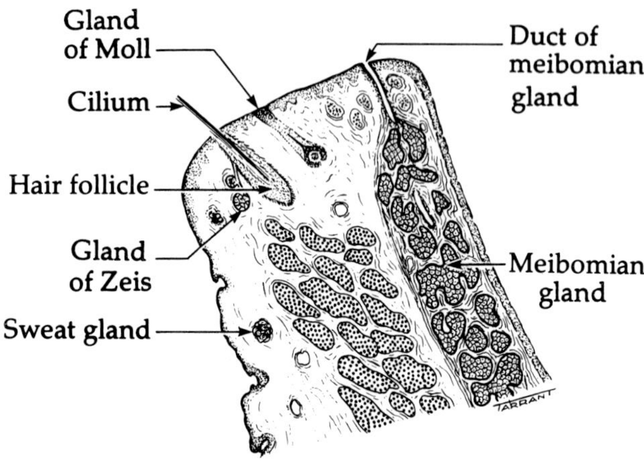

Figure 1.1 Cross-section of lower eyelid

The glands of Zeis are also modified sebaceous glands which are associated with the lash follicles. The function of the oily secretions of the meibomian glands and the glands of Zeis is to lubricate the lid margin and prevent the overflow of tears, and also to form the outer lipid layer of the precorneal tear film which prevents the evaporation of tears. The ducts of the glands of Moll (modified sweat glands) open either into a lash follicle or directly onto the anterior lid margin between the lashes.

External hordeolum (stye)

This is a small abscess caused by an acute staphylococcal infection of a lash follicle and its associated gland of Zeis or Moll. Styes are common in patients with staphylococcal blepharitis.

Clinical features

A stye presents as a tender inflamed swelling in the lid margin which points anteriorly through the skin. Frequently, more than one lesion is present and, occasionally, multiple minute abscesses may involve virtually the entire eyelid.

Treatment

Most styes either resolve spontaneously or discharge anteriorly close to the lash roots. Resolution may be promoted by removing the eyelash associated with the infected follicle followed by hot compresses or hot spoon bathing. Application of an antibiotic ointment to the lid margin may prevent spread of the infection to adjacent lash follicles. Surgical incision is required only in the rare event of a large abscess.

Meibomian cyst (chalazion)

This is a chronic lipogranulomatous inflammation secondary to retention of sebum caused by obstruction of a duct of a meibomian gland. Strictly speaking, a chalazion is not a true cyst because its walls consist of granulomatous tissue and are not lined by epithelium. Chalazia are common in patients with meibomian gland dysfunction (*see* Chapter 4).

Clinical features

A chalazion presents as a painless, slowly enlarging, roundish, firm lesion in the tarsal plate (*Figure 1.2*). Eversion of the lid may show the presence of an external conjunctival granuloma in the region of the cyst. Occasionally, a cyst of the upper lid presses on the cornea and causes blurred vision from induced astigmatism.

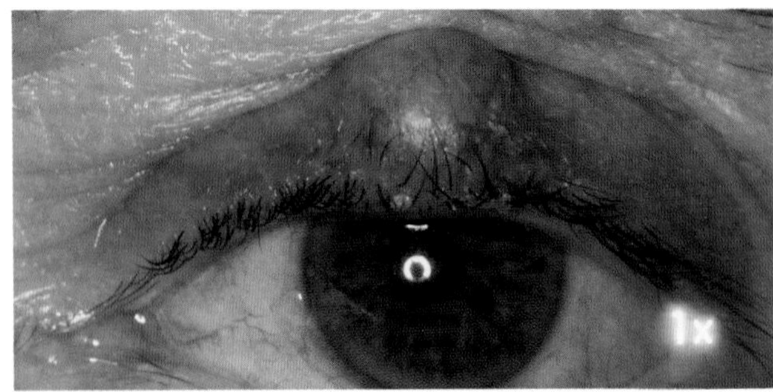

Figure 1.2 Meibomian cyst

Treatment

Although small chalazia occasionally disappear spontaneously, the majority require incision and curettage. The eyelid in the region of the cyst is infiltrated with anaesthetic. The lid is then everted with a special chalazion clamp. An incision is then made through the conjunctiva into the cyst, the contents are curetted and any associated external conjunctival granulomatous tissue excised with scissors. An antibiotic ointment is instilled and the eye padded for about 2 hours. An alternative method is to inject triamcinolone directly into the cyst.

Recurrences are common in patients with seborrheic dermatitis and acne rosacea. It is, however, extremely important not to mistake a meibomian gland carcinoma or a basal cell carcinoma for a 'recurrent chalazion'. In cases of doubt, the lesion should be biopsied and examined histologically.

Internal hordeolum

This is a small abscess caused by an acute staphylococcal infection of meibomian glands.

Clinical features

An internal hordeolum presents as a tender inflamed swelling within the tarsal plate, which is usually more painful than a stye. The lesion may enlarge and discharge either posteriorly through the conjunctiva or anteriorly through the skin. In some cases, it gradually diminishes in size without discharging and leaves a small hard nodule.

Treatment

Treatment is the same as for a stye although surgical intervention is more frequently required.

Cyst of Moll

This is a cyst of one of the modified sweat glands which is caused by a blockage of its duct (*Figure 1.3*). It contains clear fluid and presents as a small, round, non-tender, translucent lesion on the anterior lid margin. Treatment is by puncture with hyperdermic needle, or by cauterization.

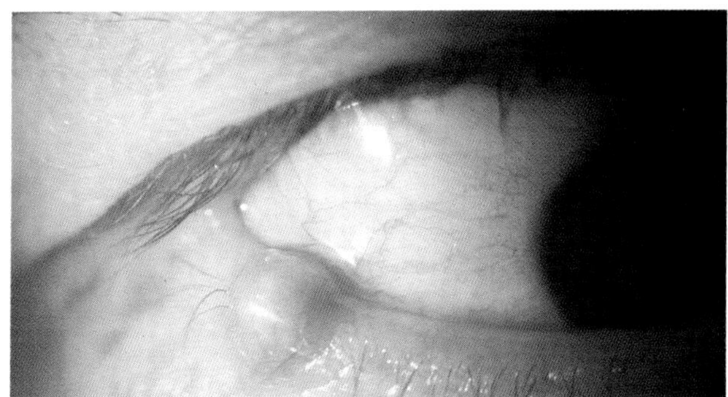

Figure 1.3 *Cyst of Moll*

Cyst of Zeis

This is a cyst of one of the modified sebaceous glands which is caused by blockage of its duct and the cyst contains sebum. Its appearance is similar to that of a cyst of Moll but it is less translucent. Treatment is the same as for a cyst of Moll.

Sebaceous cyst

This is a cyst of one of the ordinary sebaceous glands in the lid which is caused by a blockage of its duct (*Figure 1.4*). It contains a central punctum, and the retained cheesy secretions give it a yellowish-white colour. Treatment is by simple excision.

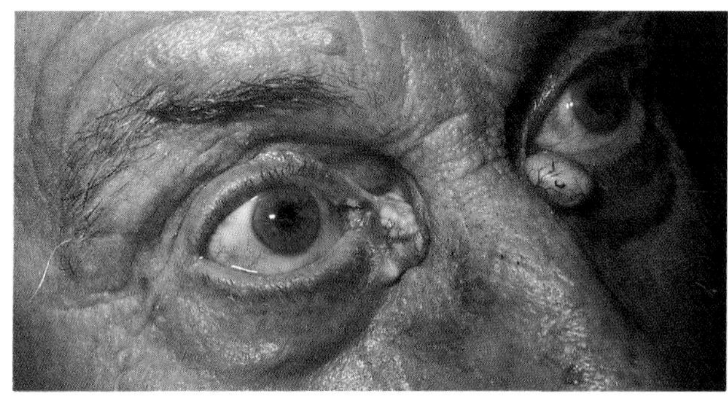

Figure 1.4 *Sebaceous cysts*

Benign tumours

Molluscum contagiosum

This is caused by a viral infection which most commonly affects children. The typical lesion is a pale, waxy, umbilicated, elevated nodule which disappears spontaneously within 6–9 months. The chronic shedding of cells laden with viral particles can produce a chronic follicular conjunctivitis and, occasionally, also a superficial keratitis. Treatment of the skin lesion is by expression or cauterization.

Squamous papilloma

This is the most common benign tumour of the eyelids (*Figure 1.5*). The lesion may have a broad base (sessile) or it may be pedunculated.

Verruca vulgaris

This is caused by a virus infection and it typically appears as a filiform wart. Occasionally a crop of lesions appears simultaneously.

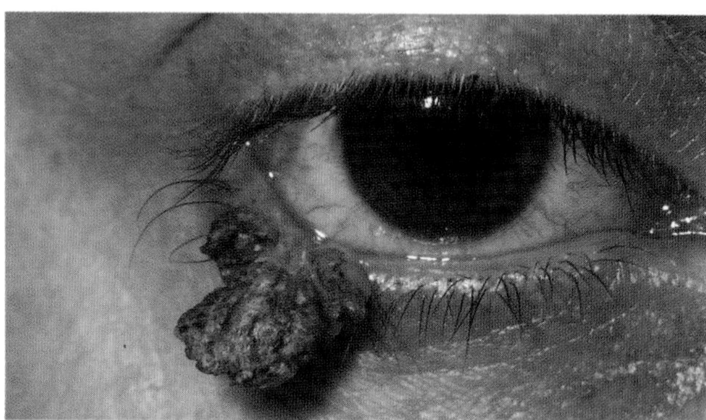

Figure 1.5 Papilloma

Seborrhoeic keratosis

This is extremely common in the elderly and appears as a slow-growing, discrete, greasy, brown, round or oval lesion with a friable verrucose surface (*Figure 1.6*).

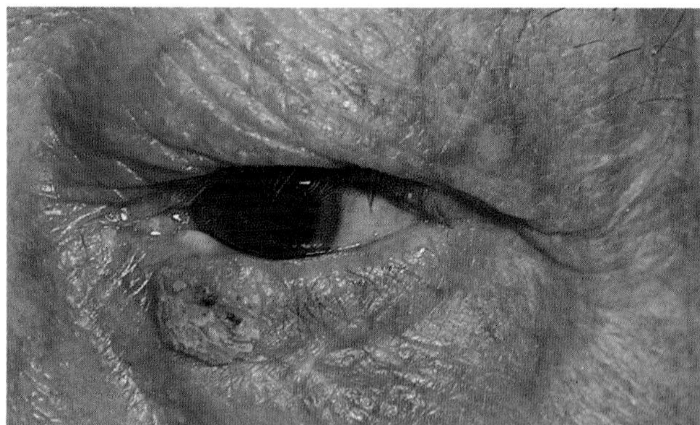

Figure 1.6 Seborrhoeic keratosis

Senile keratosis

This consists of flat, multiple, scaly lesions which may assume a papillomatous configuration. Occasionally, senile keratosis undergoes transformation into a squamous cell carcinoma.

Xanthelasma

These are very common yellowish, slightly elevated lipid deposits, most frequently located in the medial aspects of both eyelids (*Figure 1.7*).

Keratoacanthoma

This rare tumour typically starts as an erythematous papule. Within a few weeks it grows into a firm, raised, pinkish, indurated nodule with a keratin-filled crater and it then undergoes spontaneous regression. If it does not disappear within 3 months, it should be excised and examined histologically.

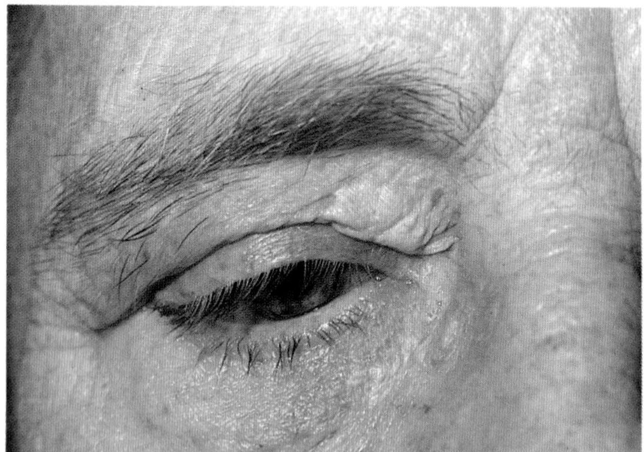

Figure 1.7 Xanthelasma

Cutaneous horn

This is a fairly common lesion which consists of a firm projecting keratinized mass. Occasionally, a cutaneous horn overlies a senile keratosis or a basal cell carcinoma.

Haemangioma

Haemangiomas of the strawberry type are rare, flat, red lesions which are usually either noted at birth or within the first 6 months of life (*Figure 1.8*). After an initial period of growth, they resolve spontaneously by the age of about 5 years. In some cases, haemangiomas of the eyelids are associated with intraorbital extension (*see* Chapter 2).

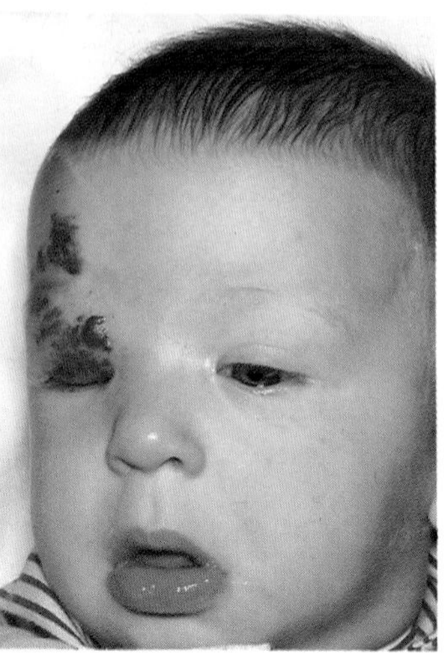

Figure 1.8 Haemangioma (courtesy of Miss P. Burgess)

Malignant tumours

Clinical features

Basal cell carcinoma

Basal cell carcinoma (BCC) is the most common primary malignant tumour of the eyelid with a peak incidence in the seventh and eighth decades. The tumour most frequently arises from the lower eyelid or medial canthus. It is slow growing, locally invasive, but it does not metastasize. Tumours located near the medial canthus are more prone to invade the orbit and are more difficult to manage than those arising elsewhere.

The clinical appearance of the tumour is variable and the correct diagnosis from external inspection alone may be unreliable. Two main forms of BCC are recognized.

Noduloulcerative (rodent ulcer) BCC (*Figure 1.9*)

This starts as an asymptomatic well-defined nodule. Associated hyperkeratosis gives the lesion a pearly appearance. The margins are well defined and rolled. Fine vessels frequently course over its surface. Its centre becomes ulcerated and crusted and the lesion may bleed following relatively trivial trauma.

Sclerosing (*Figure 1.10*)

This originates in the epidermis but may invade the dermis and then spread radially beneath normal epidermis. It has no telangiectatic vessels over its surface and its margins are impossible to delineate. Occasionally, the tumour is multifocal. Because of its flat scar-like appearance, this type of BCC is also described as being of the morphea (scleroderma) type.

In between these two main types, BCCs have many variations in appearance.

Squamous cell carcinoma

This is the second most common malignancy of the eyelid. However, it is much less common than BCC and accounts for only 5% of malignant lid tumours. It may appear as a nodule, an ulcerated lesion, or a 'papilloma'. The growth rate is faster than that of a BCC and it may metastasize to the regional lymph nodes. Tumours arising from the lateral two-thirds of the upper lid or the lateral third of the lower lid metastasize to the preauricular nodes, whereas those elsewhere on the lid metastasize to the submandibular nodes.

Sebaceous gland carcinoma

This arises from the meibomian glands and is even less common than squamous cell carcinoma. Clinically, the tumour appears as a discrete, yellow, firm, nodule which is sometimes incorrectly diagnosed as 'recurrent chalazion'.

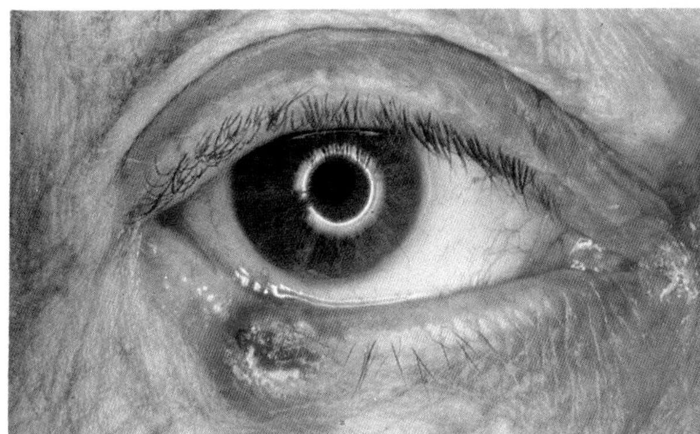

Figure 1.9 *Noduloulcerative basal cell carcinoma*

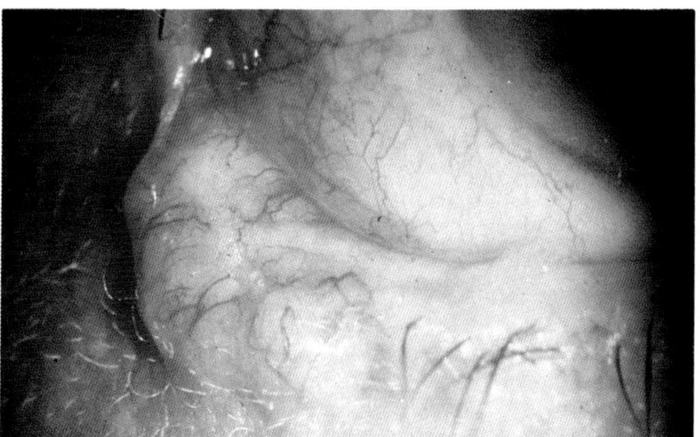

Figure 1.10 *Sclerosing basal cell carcinoma*

In some cases, the tumour is multicentric and causes diffusely inflamed areas along the eyelid margin which may be mistaken as 'chronic blepharitis'. These difficulties in diagnosis, and the infrequent occurrence of the tumour, may delay treatment and are responsible for a 5-year mortality rare of about 30%, due to widespread metastases.

Treatment

Local surgical excision

Local surgical excision with a 3-mm margin outside obvious tumour is the treatment of choice, with the lowest rate of recurrence for BCC. Because the margins of eyelid tumours may be difficult to define in some cases, the resected specimen should be examined histologically to ensure that the margins are free of tumour cells. The extent of surgical excision should be larger for squamous and sebaceous gland carcinoma than for BCC, as the first two are more aggressive.

Radiotherapy

This should probably be reserved for patients who are either unsuitable for or refuse surgery. There is a higher recurrence rate than with surgical excision, particularly in patients with sebaceous gland carcinoma. Radiotherapy should also be avoided in medial canthus tumours as these frequently infiltrate deeply and are difficult to eliminate by this method alone. Complications of radiotherapy include loss of eyelashes, keratinization of the conjunctiva, dry eye and damage to the skin.

Cryotherapy

This relies on exceedingly cold temperatures (−30 °C) to cause tissue death using a freeze–thaw–freeze technique. This method is effective in curing relatively small and superficial basal cell carcinomas and has the same recurrence rate as radiotherapy. Complications of cryotherapy include skin depigmentation and loss of eyelashes.

Mohs' micrographic technique (chemosurgery)

This has revolutionized the management of difficult eyelid tumours such as recurrences and those that grow diffusely and have indefinite margins. The technique consists of excising the affected tissue in successive layers and microscopically scanning the entire underside of each layer by the systematic use of frozen sections. The purpose of total microscopic control is to locate slender tumour outgrowths which may extend beyond the clinically visible and palpable borders of the tumour. This method, although slow and tedious, assures optimal eradication of the tumour as well as maximal sparing of adjacent normal tissue.

Exenteration

This procedure, in which the globe and orbital contents are excised, is occasionally required for extensive tumours that have invaded the orbit. *Radical neck dissection* may be required in patients with involvement of the preauricular or anterior cervical glands.

Disorders of eyelashes

Trichiasis

Trichiasis is an inward misdirection of the lashes. It should be differentiated from pseudotriachiasis in which the misdirection is secondary to entropion. In both cases, however, irritation of the cornea by the lashes causes punctate epithelial erosions and, in severe long-standing cases, a pannus may develop (*Figure 1.11*).

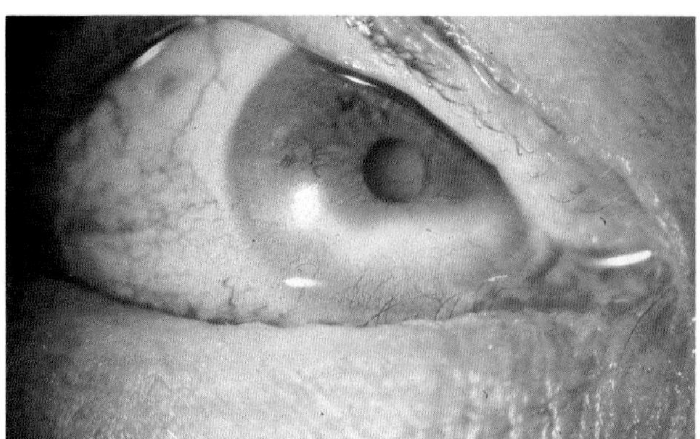

Figure 1.11 *Inferior corneal pannus from trichiasis*

Treatment

1. *Epilation* (mechanical removal with forceps) is simple and effective. Unfortunately, recurrences within 4–6 weeks are common and the procedure has to be repeated.
2. *Electrolysis* consists of destroying the lash follicle by the passage of an electric current through a fine needle inserted into the lash root. The procedure is tedious, and frequently multiple treatments are required to obtain a satisfactory result.
3. *Cryotherapy* is very effective in eliminating a large number of ingrowing lashes simultaneously by using a special nitrous oxide cryoprobe. First, the eyelid is infiltrated with anaesthetic and then the cryoprobe is applied to the external lid margin (20 seconds for the lower lid and 25 seconds for the upper lid). This freezes the lash follicles to −20 °C. The frozen tissue is then allowed to thaw spontaneously and the cycle is repeated once. Within a few hours of treatment, the eyelid becomes temporarily oedematous and occasionally blistered. The main disadvantage of cryotherapy is skin depigmentation which may be cosmetically undesirable in darkly pigmented individuals.
4. *Irradiation* is effective in severe and persistent cases, although since the advent of cryotherapy it is now seldom used.
5. *Contact lenses* to protect the cornea are useful as a temporary measure in patients with severe trichiasis.

Distichiasis

Clinical features

In this condition an accessory row of lashes is situated in or near to the openings of the meibomian glands (*Figure 1.12*). The two types are: congenital, which is rare and frequently familial, and acquired, which is secondary to scarring as from ocular cicatricial pemphigoid and chemical burns.

Treatment

Treatment is by cryotherapy. The eyelid is first divided along the grey line into an anterior and a posterior lamella. The posterior lamella is then treated by cryotherapy and the two lamellae are reapposed. This procedure avoids depigmentation of the skin and ensures that the aberrant lashes are eliminated without damaging the normal lashes in the anterior lamella.

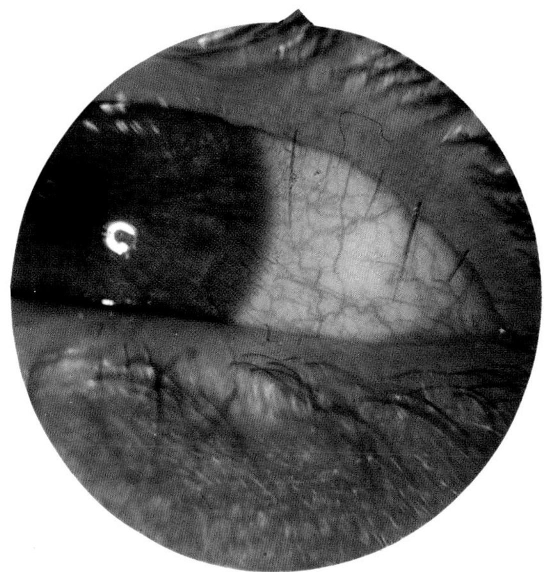

Figure 1.12 *Distichiasis*

Entropion

Entropion is an inversion of the eyelid (*Figure 1.13*). It usually causes discomfort due to the rubbing of the eyelashes on the cornea.

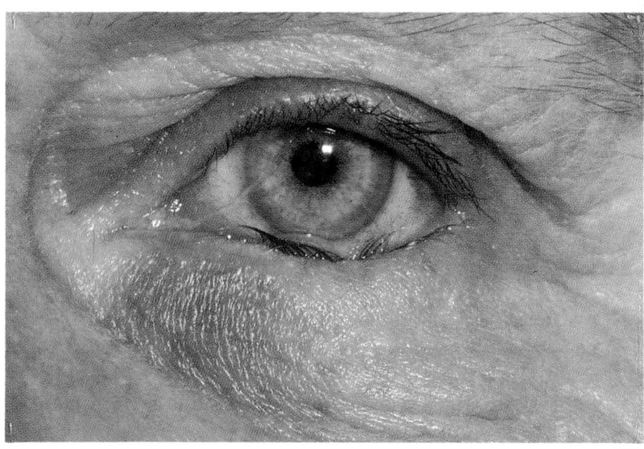

Figure 1.13 *Entropion of lower eyelid*

Classification

Involutional (senile)
Cicatricial
Congenital
Acute spastic

Involutional (senile) entropion

This is by far the most common type of entropion and only affects the lower lid. In order to understand its aetiology and the principles of treatment, a knowledge of the anatomy and pathophysiology of the lower lid is essential.

Orbicularis muscle

Anatomy

The palpebral orbicularis is divided into pretarsal and preseptal portions. The preseptal orbicularis is attached less firmly to the orbital septum than is the pretarsal portion to the tarsus.

Pathophysiology

With age, the subcutaneous tissues and overlying skin become atonic, redundant and less adherent to the orbicularis. During lid closure, the lower lid rises and the preseptal orbicularis tends to override the pretarsal portion (*Figure 1.14*). This tends to move the lower tarsal border away from the globe and the upper border towards the globe. In certain cases, the whole lid will roll in and entropion results.

Tarsal sling

Anatomy

The tarsal sling consists of the tarsus and the medial and lateral canthal tendons. It gives the lower lid horizontal stability by keeping it in its normal position against the globe.

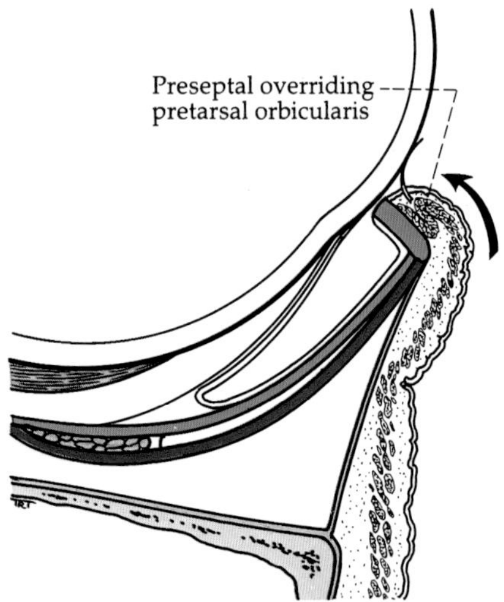

Figure 1.14 *Involutional entropion*

Pathophysiology

With age the tarsus becomes thinned and atrophic. This allows it to bend so that the upper border inverts more than the lower border. There is also stretching of the canthal tendons and the orbicularis muscle. All these factors give rise to horizontal lid laxity, which is frequently aggravated by enophthalmos due to atrophy of orbital fat. The tarsal sling becomes unstable and is able to swing like a hammock. Clinically, horizontal lid laxity is detected by the ability to pull the central part of the lower lid 6 mm or more from the globe and failure of the lid to snap back snugly into its normal position on release. Horizontal lid laxity is corrected surgically by a full-thickness lid shortening procedure.

Lower lid retractors

Anatomy

The inferior rectus is the only extraocular muscle with a dual function. In down-gaze it depresses the globe and also retracts the lower lid. The latter is a function of its capsulopalpebral expansion which consists of the inferior tarsal aponeurosis (analogous to the levator aponeurosis in the upper lid) and the inferior tarsal muscle (analogous to the superior tarsal (Müller's) muscle in the upper lid). Both parts of the capsulopalpebral expansion are attached to the inferior border of the lower tarsus and, together with the orbital septum which is also attached to the inferior tarsal border, they give the lower lid vertical stability.

Pathophysiology

With age the orbital septum becomes thin and stretched and the lower lid retractors weak. This is either due to a dehiscence in the aponeurosis or a disinsertion in its attachment to the tarsus. These changes decrease the vertical stability of the lower lid and allow the lower border of the tarsus to become more mobile with a tendency to rotate outwards. Clinically, weakness of the lower lid retractors is recognized by the decreased excursion of the lower lid in down-gaze. It can be corrected surgically by inferior aponeurosis tucking or plication.

Treatment

The treatment of involutional entropion is aimed at correcting three aetiological factors:

1. Prevention of upward movement of the preseptal orbicularis.
2. Correction of horizontal lid laxity.
3. Strengthening of lower lid retractors.

Cautery (*Figure 1.15*)

Cautery through the skin below the lashes may create a scar and temporarily correct factor 1.

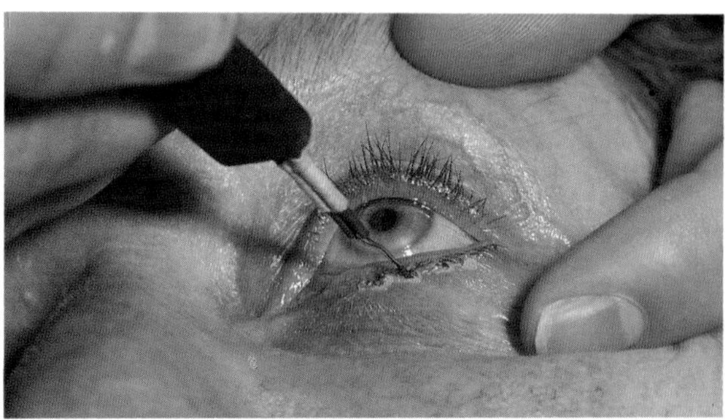

Figure 1.15 *Treatment of entropion by cautery*

Transverse lid-everting sutures

These will also correct factor 1 and are useful as a temporary measure when more extensive procedures cannot be tolerated by the patient.

Wies procedure

This is a full-thickness horizontal lid-splitting and a marginal rotation procedure (*Figure 1.16*). The scar creates a barrier between the preseptal and pretarsal orbicularis (factor 1), and the everting suture transfers the pull of the lower lid retractors from the tarsus to the skin and orbicularis (factor 3).

Horizontal lid shortening

Excision of a full-thickness trapezoid of lid at the lateral canthus is necessary in cases of marked horizontal lid laxity (factor 2) and it can be combined with the Wies procedure.

Inferior aponeurosis tucking or plication (*Figure 1.17*)

This is necessary in cases of marked weakness of lower lid retractors (factor 3). It also creates a barrier between the preseptal and pretarsal orbicularis (factor 1). Although it can be performed as a primary procedure, some authorities reserve this operation for cases of recurrence following a Wies procedure and horizontal lid shortening.

Fox procedure

This consists of excising a base-down triangle of tarsus and conjunctiva (*Figure 1.18*). Although it is an easy operation, it has a high rate of recurrence.

Cicatricial entropion

Cicatricial entropion is usually caused by scarring of the palpebral conjunctiva, which pulls the lid margin towards the globe. Important causes include ocular cicatricial pemphigoid, Stevens–Johnson syndrome, trachoma, and chemical burns. It can involve both upper and lower lids. Management is aimed at keeping the lashes away from the cornea (contact lenses, epilation) and surgical correction of

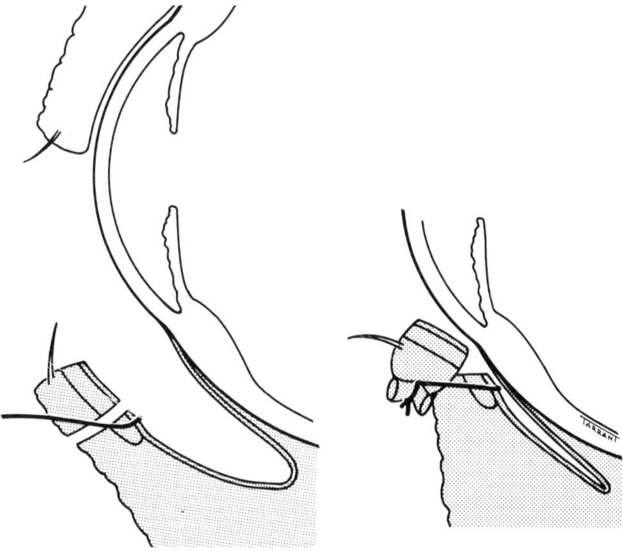

Figure 1.16 *Wies procedure for entropion*

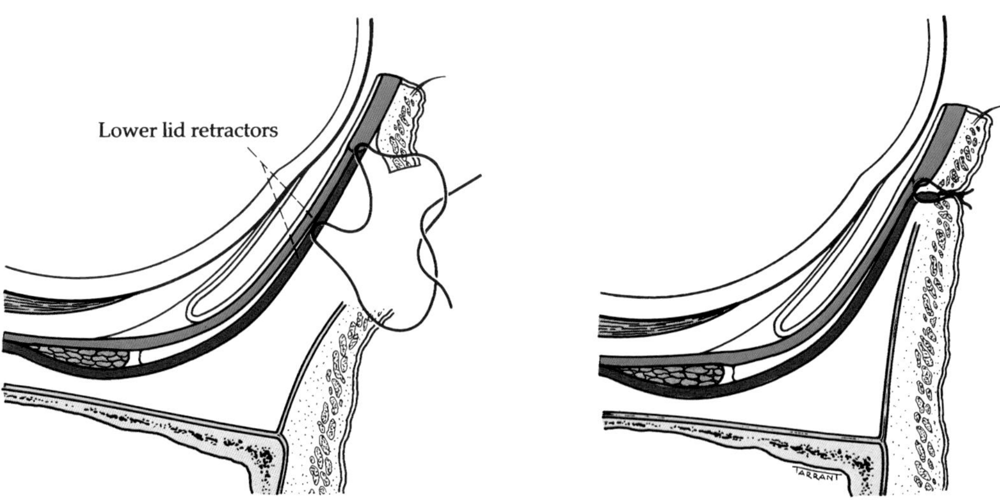

Figure 1.17 *Shortening of lower eyelid retractors*

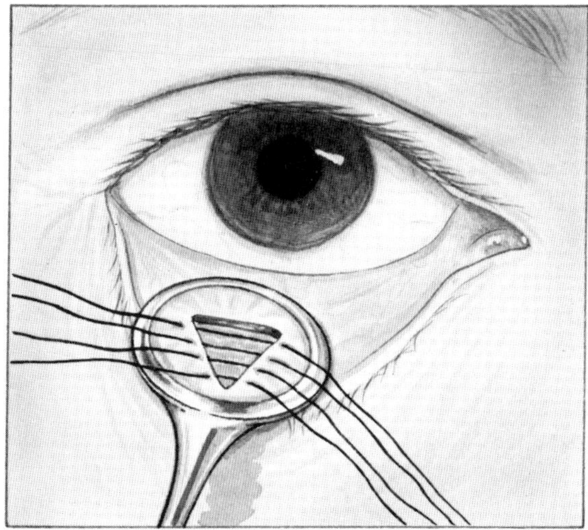

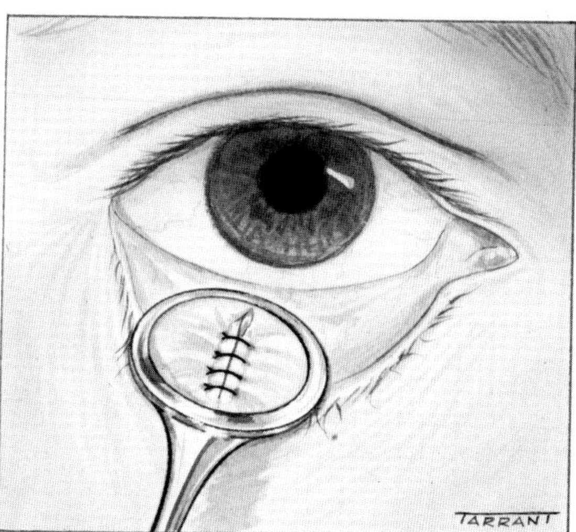

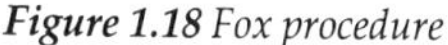

Figure 1.18 *Fox procedure*

the deformity. In mild cases involving the lower lid, a Wies procedure will suffice. However, in more severe cases, replacement of contracted conjunctival tissue with mucous membrane grafts is necessary.

Congenital entropion

Congenital entropion (*Figure 1.19, right*), which is rare, is characterized by an inward turning of the entire lower eyelid and lashes with absence of the lower lid crease. The condition usually persists and most cases require surgical correction. It is important not to confuse congenital entropion with the more common epiblepharon. The latter is characterized by the presence of a horizontal fold of skin adjacent to the lower lid margin.

Epiblepharon (*Figure 1.19, left*) typically involves only the medial aspect of the lower lid although, in some cases, the entire lid may be affected. The lid crease is either absent or positioned very close to the lid margin. The lashes assume a vertical direction and may traumatize the cornea, particularly in down-gaze. In some patients the condition resolves spontaneously by the age of 1 or 2 years. However, in the presence of corneal irritation, surgical correction should not be delayed.

Acute spastic entropion

Acute spastic entropion is due to spasm of the orbicularis as a result of ocular irritation or essential blepharospasm. It usually resolves spontaneously once the cause has been eliminated. In the meantime, the lid can be everted by taping it to the skin of the cheek or by a lid-everting suture. Not infrequently, the constant irritation of the lashes against the globe in cases of involutional entropion causes an additional spastic element to the disorder.

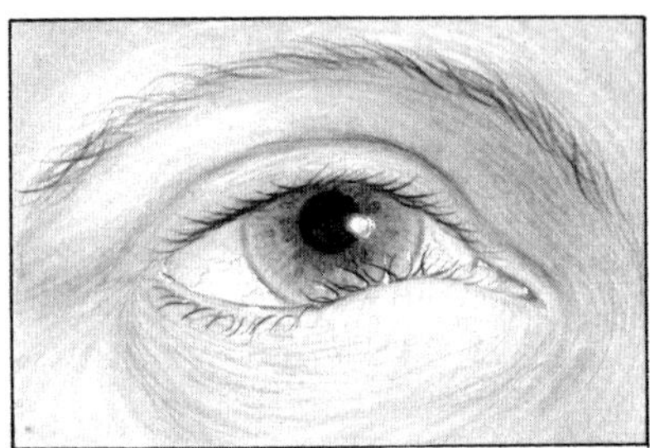

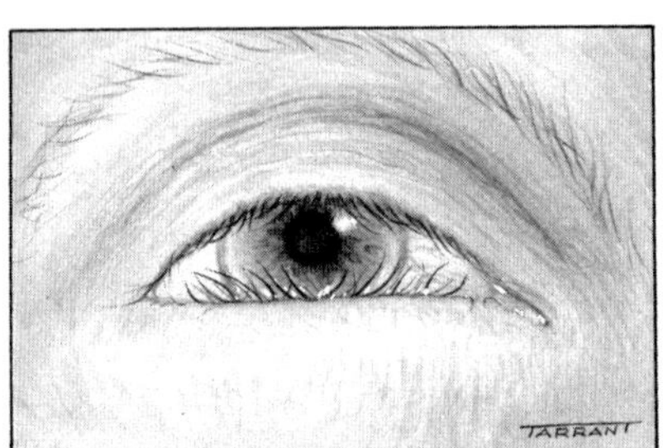

Figure 1.19 *Left: epiblepharon; right: congenital entropion*

Ectropion

Ectropion is an outward turning of the eyelid from the globe. It is frequently associated with epiphora and chronic conjunctivitis. Long-standing advanced cases may give rise to conjunctival hypertrophy and keratinization as a result of exposure (*Figure 1.20*).

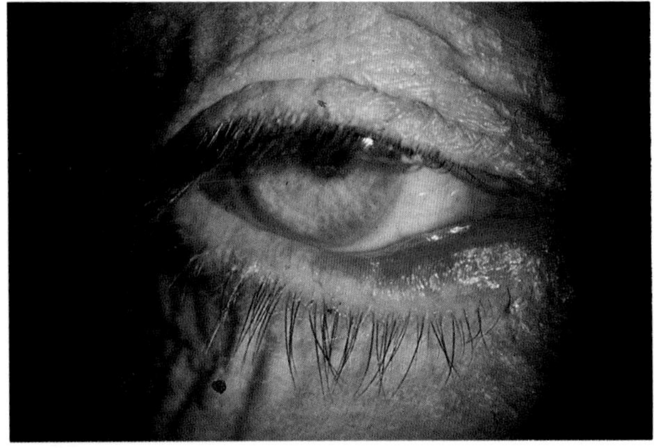

Figure 1.20 *Ectropion with conjunctival keratinization*

Classification

Involutional (senile)
Cicatricial
Congenital
Paralytic

The first three types of ectropion and entropion have similar aetiologies and it is only the fourth type in each classification that is different (i.e. acute spastic or paralytic).

Involutional (senile)

Clinical features

This has many features in common with involutional entropion:

1. It affects the lower lid in elderly patients.
2. The ageing changes responsible for both are similar.

Involutional ectropion is characterized by excessive horizontal eyelid length coupled with weakness of the pretarsal portion of the orbicularis. This is also frequently accompanied by laxity of the medial and lateral canthal tendons, which can be demonstrated clinically by a marked temporal displacement of the lower punctum when the lid is pulled laterally.

Treatment

The management of ectropion is governed mainly by the amount of horizontal lid laxity.

Ziegler cautery

Punctures placed 5 mm below the punctum are effective in correcting mild medial laxity with punctal eversion.

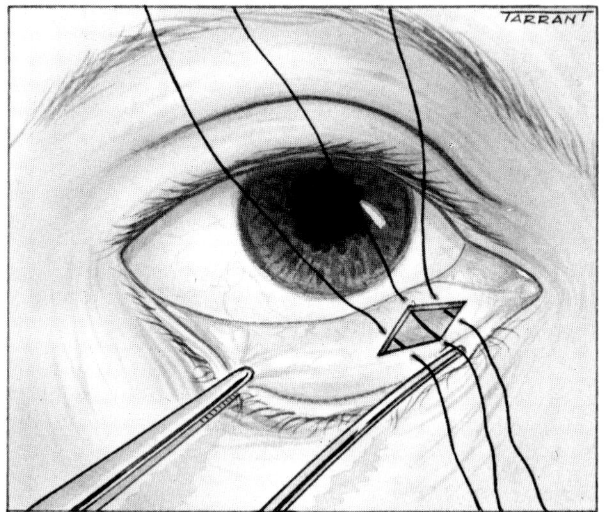

Figure 1.21 *Surgical correction of medial ectropion*

Medial conjunctivoplasty

This is also useful for mild cases of medial ectropion. It consists of excising a diamond-shaped piece of tissue about 4 mm high and 8 mm long, parallel with and inferior to the canaliculus and punctum (*Figure 1.21*).

Horizontal lid shortening

This is required to correct ectropion involving the entire lid. The three most commonly used operations are:

1. *Bick's procedure* which consists of excising a full-thickness wedge of lid at the outer canthus (*Figure 1.22*).
2. *Fox procedure* which consists of excising a base-up triangle of tarsus and conjunctiva.
3. *Modified Kuhnt–Szymanowski* (*Figure 1.23*). The problem with any procedure that relies on a simple base-up triangular resection is that, although the lid is shortened, it may still sag, especially medially in the punctal area. For this reason it is usually necessary to elevate the lid by excising a triangle of skin laterally and combining this with the excision of a base-up pentagon from the lateral third of the lid (Byron Smith modification). If excessive laxity of the medial canthal tendon is present, as indicated by a marked temporal displacement of the lower punctum when the lid is pulled laterally, the medial canthal tendon should be imbricated or shortened prior to estimating how much lateral tissue should be excised.

Cicatricial

Cicatricial ectropion is caused by scarring or contracture of skin and underlying tissues which pulls the eyelid away from the globe. Important causes include tumours, trauma, and burns. Severe cases are treated by excising the

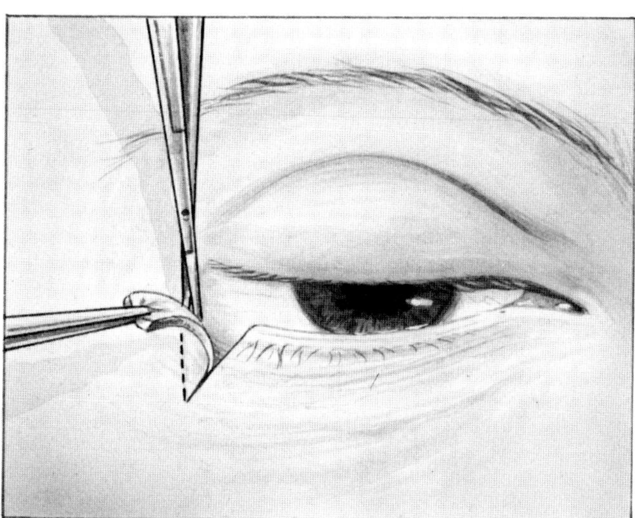

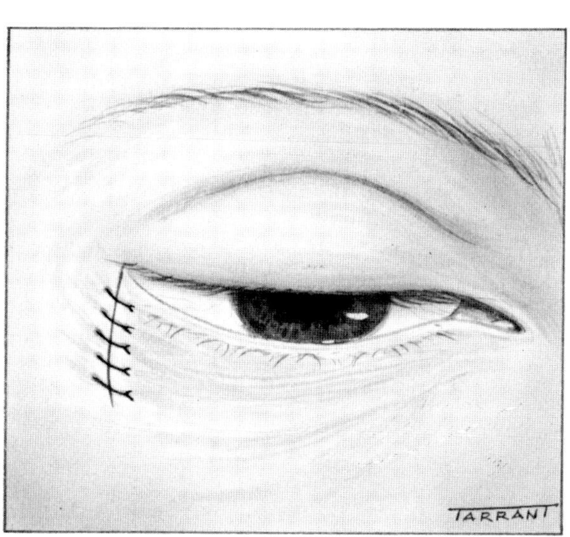

Figure 1.22 *Horizontal eyelid shortening (Bick's procedure)*

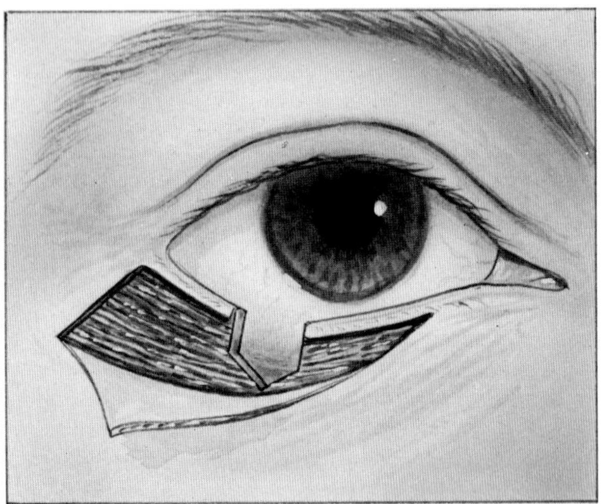

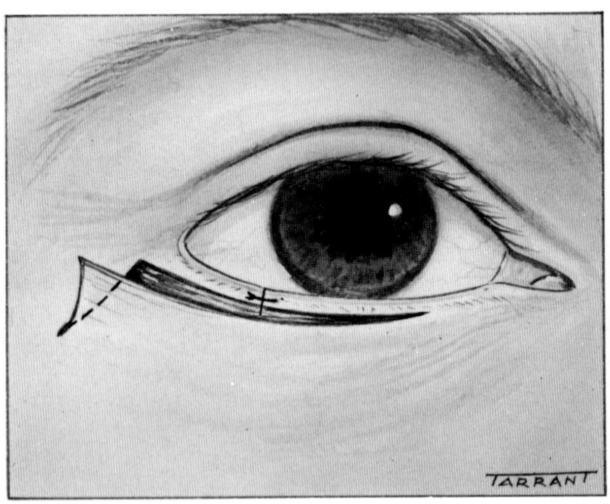

Figure 1.23 *Modified Kuhnt–Szymanowski procedure*

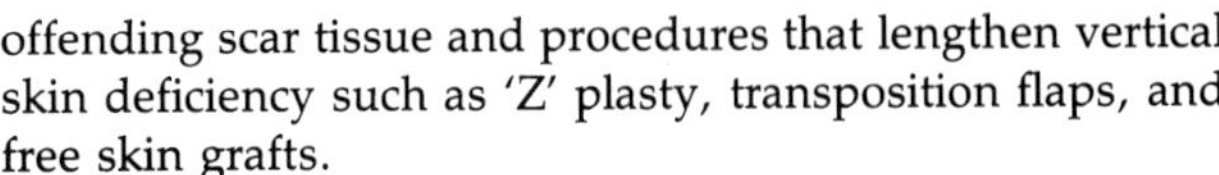

offending scar tissue and procedures that lengthen vertical skin deficiency such as 'Z' plasty, transposition flaps, and free skin grafts.

Congenital

Congenital ectropion is rare and may be associated with blepharophimosis (*see Figure 1.30*). In severe cases, replacement of a vertical skin defect with full-thickness skin grafts is necessary.

Paralytic

Paralytic ectropion is caused by a facial nerve palsy. It is usually not severe unless there is associated pre-existing horizontal lid laxity.

Clinical features of facial nerve palsy

Weakness of the orbicularis causes incomplete blinking, inability to close the lids (lagophthalmos), and watering of the eye due to failure of the lacrimal pump mechanism (*see* Chapter 3). Weakness of other facial muscles causes inability to elevate the brow normally, less well-defined forehead furrow on attempted brow elevation, less well-defined nasolabial fold, and decreased ability to pucker the mouth.

Treatment

The main aim is to prevent exposure keratopathy. The treatment is different for mild temporary cases (e.g. Bell's palsy) as opposed to severe and permanent cases.

Temporary

1. *Prevention of corneal drying*, due to the inability of the eyelids to resurface the cornea by the tear film, is by the frequent instillation of artificial tears.
2. *Prevention of corneal exposure* during sleep is by the instillation of ointment and strapping of the lids.

Permanent

1. *Tarsorrhaphy*, in which the upper lid is stitched to the lower lid, is effective in preventing exposure keratopathy. However, the operation is cosmetically disfiguring.
2. *Canthoplasty* is much more acceptable cosmetically. If muscle tone is relatively good, a lateral canthoplasty and shortening of the lateral canthal tendon places the lower lid in apposition to the globe. A medial canthoplasty inverts the punctum and shortens the eyelid fissure between the inner canthus and the lower punctum.
3. *Silicone slings* are positioned so that they encircle the eyelid. This is a most useful technique for patients with permanent facial paralysis, as it provides dynamic function to the eyelids so that opening and closure of the lids are possible.

Ptosis

Ptosis is an abnormally low position (drooping) of the upper eyelid.

Applied anatomy

The anatomy of the upper lid is analogous to that of the lower lid (*Figure 1.24*). The two elevators of the upper lid are the levator aponeurosis and Müller's muscle. Both originate from the levator muscle proper, at or just below Whitnall's ligament.

The levator aponeurosis

This fuses with the orbital septum about 4 mm above the upper border of the tarsus. Its posterior fibres are inserted into the lower third of the anterior surface of the tarsus. The anterior fibrous elements pass through the orbicularis and subcutaneous tissues to be attached to the skin where they are responsible for the lid crease. The medial and lateral horns of the aponeurosis are expansions which act as check ligaments.

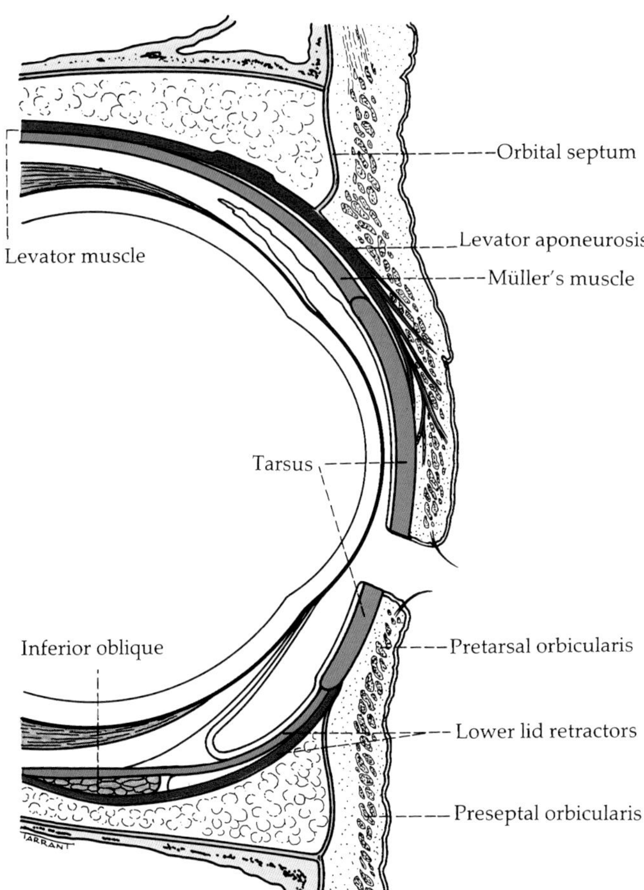

Figure 1.24 *Anatomy of levator and lower eyelid retractors*

The superior tarsal (Müller's) muscle

This is inserted into the upper border of the tarsus and is sympathetically innervated. It can be approached transconjunctivally.

Classification

- Neurogenic
  - third nerve palsy
  - Horner's syndrome
  - synkinetic
    - Marcus Gunn
    - misdirection of third nerve
- Aponeurotic
  - involutional (senile)
  - postoperative
  - blepharochalasis
- Mechanical
  - excess weight
    - oedema
    - tumours
    - dermatochalasis
  - conjunctival scarring
- Myogenic
  - congenital
    - simple
    - blepharophimosis syndrome
  - acquired
    - myasthenia gravis
    - dystrophia myotonica
    - ocular myopathy
    - oculopharyngeal muscular dystrophy

Neurogenic

Neurogenic ptosis is caused by an acquired or congenital innervational defect. Important causes include:

Third nerve palsy

See Chapter 15.

Oculosympathetic palsy (Horner's syndrome)

See Chapter 15.

Synkinetic ptosis

This consists of two disorders:

1. *Marcus Gunn jaw-winking phenomenon* is characterized by a unilateral congenital ptosis in which there is a retraction of the affected eyelid in conjunction with stimulation of the ipsilateral pterygoid muscles. The

eyelid retraction or 'wink' commonly results from opening the mouth, chewing, sucking, or movement of the jaw towards the contralateral side. Other less common stimuli to winking include jaw protrusion, smiling, swallowing and clenching the teeth. About 5% of all cases of congenital ptosis belong to this category.
2. *Misdirection of the third nerve* may be congenital or it may follow an acquired third nerve palsy. It is characterized by the presence of bizarre movements of the upper lid that accompany various eye movements.

In neurogenic ptosis the amount of levator function is inversely proportional to the innervational defect.

Aponeurotic

Aponeurotic ptosis is caused by a defect in the transmission of force from a functioning levator to the upper lid. The aponeurotic defect may be a localized dehiscence or disinsertion, or a generalized attenuation or stretching.

Involutional (senile) (*Figure 1.25*)

This is due to a degenerative process involving the levator aponeurosis analogous to that involving the lower lid retractors in involutional entropion. Clinically, involutional

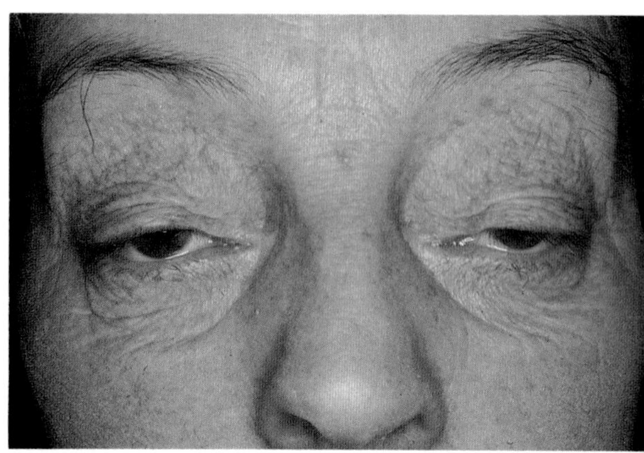

Figure 1.25 *Involutional ptosis (courtesy of Photographic Department, Wexham Park Hospital)*

ptosis is characterized by a high or absent eyelid crease, thinning of the eyelid above the tarsal plate, good levator function, a palpable defect in the levator aponeurosis, and a tendency to occur bilaterally.

Postoperative

This occurs following surgery for cataract or retinal detachment. Although the exact cause is unknown, it is thought to result from a dehiscence or disinsertion of the levator aponeurosis secondary to manipulation of the eyelids or the superior levator complex by a bridle suture.

Blepharochalasis

This is a rare disorder characterized by recurrent episodes of oedema of the upper eyelids. The condition usually starts before the age of 20 years and affects both sexes equally. The swelling is generally non-pitting and usually resolves after several days. With time, the episodes become less frequent but leave the skin of the upper lids thinned and atrophic, giving rise to a wrinkled redundant appearance (*Figure 1.26*). In some cases, thinning or dehiscence of the levator aponeurosis gives rise to ptosis.

In patients with aponeurotic ptosis, levator function is usually normal although the degree of ptosis is variable.

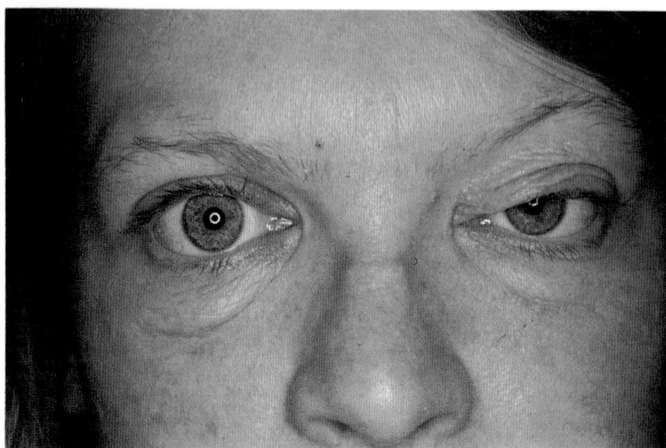

Figure 1.26 *Left aponeurotic ptosis due to blepharochalasis (courtesy of Photographic Department, Wexham Park Hospital)*

Mechanical

Mechanical ptosis is due to two main causes: excessive weight and conjunctival scarring.

Excessive weight

Excessive weight on the upper lid which may be caused by:

1. *Lid oedema.*
2. *Tumours* such as neurofibromas (*Figure 1.27*).
3. *Dermatochalasis* in which there is a redundancy of upper lid skin (*Figure 1.28*). This invariably occurs in elderly individuals and may be associated with protrusion of fat through a weakened orbital septum giving the lids a baggy appearance. The ptotic lid has an indistinct lid crease. Symptoms include a heavy feeling around the eyes, browache, and obstruction of vision in severe cases.

Conjunctival scarring

This may cause ptosis by interfering with the mobility of the upper lid.

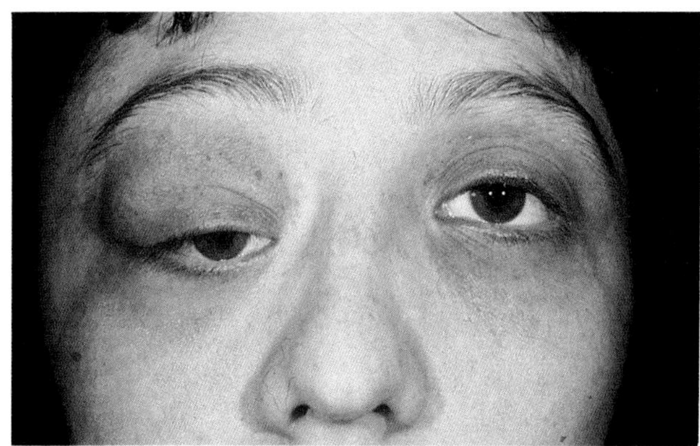

Figure 1.27 Right mechanical ptosis due to neurofibroma (courtesy of Mr D. Taylor)

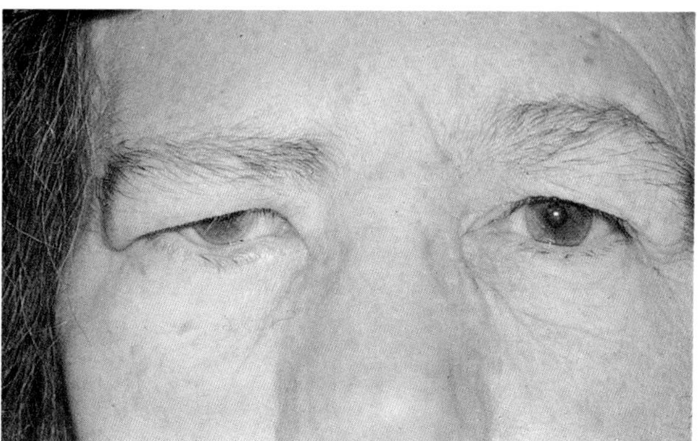

Figure 1.28 Dermatochalasis

Myogenic

Myogenic ptosis is caused by a disorder of the levator muscle itself or of the myoneural junction (myasthenia gravis).

Congenital

Important causes of congenital myogenic ptosis include: simple ptosis and blepharophimosis syndrome.

Simple

This is due to dystrophy of the levator (*Figure 1.29*) and is characterized by poor contraction as well as incomplete relaxation of the muscle. Owing to the close embryological association between the superior rectus and levator muscles, some patients also have a weakness of the superior rectus.

Blepharophimosis syndrome (*Figure 1.30*)

This is inherited as an autosomal dominant trait. It is characterized by a wide intercanthal distance, epicanthus inversus (lower lid fold larger than upper lid fold), and congenital ectropion of the lower lid.

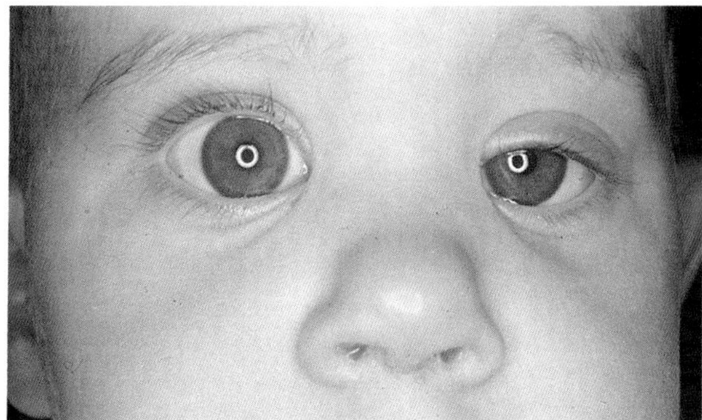

Figure 1.29 Left congenital ptosis (courtesy of Photographic Department, Wexham Park Hospital)

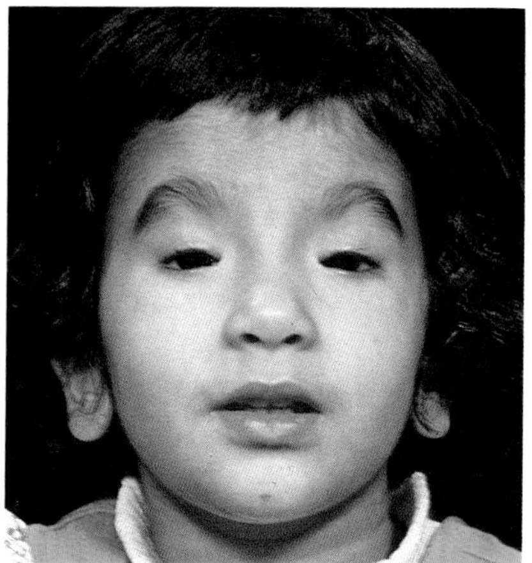

Figure 1.30 Blepharophimosis syndrome (courtesy of Dr P. Malleson)

Acquired

Important causes of acquired myogenic ptosis include myasthenia gravis, dystrophia myotonica, ocular myopathy, and oculopharyngeal muscular dystrophy. They are discussed in detail in Chapter 15.

It is important to realize that some cases of ptosis are caused by two factors. The most common combination is a defect in the aponeurosis secondary to long-standing mechanical ptosis. Trauma may cause a myogenic, neurogenic, or an aponeurotic ptosis.

Clinical evaluation

The following steps should be taken in the evaluation of a patient with ptosis.

History

This includes the age of onset, family history, symptoms of systemic disease, presence of associated diplopia, variability of ptosis, and any contributing factors.

Examination

Exclude a pseudoptosis

This can be due either to a small globe (microphthalmos, phthisis bulbi) or lid retraction of the opposite eye.

Levator function

This is determined by placing the thumb firmly against the patient's brow to negate the action of the frontalis muscle. The patient is then asked to look down as far as possible and then to look up. The amount of excursion is then measured with a rule (*Figure 1.31*). Levator function is then graded as normal, good, fair, or poor:

Normal	15 mm
Good	8 mm or more
Fair	5–7 mm
Poor	4 mm or less

These measurements are important as they indicate the feasibility of using a levator resection procedure to correct the ptosis. It is important to emphasize that, in simple congenital ptosis, the ptotic lid is slightly higher in down-gaze as the levator is unable to relax. In acquired ptosis, however, the ptotic lid is usually slightly lower than the normal lid in down-gaze.

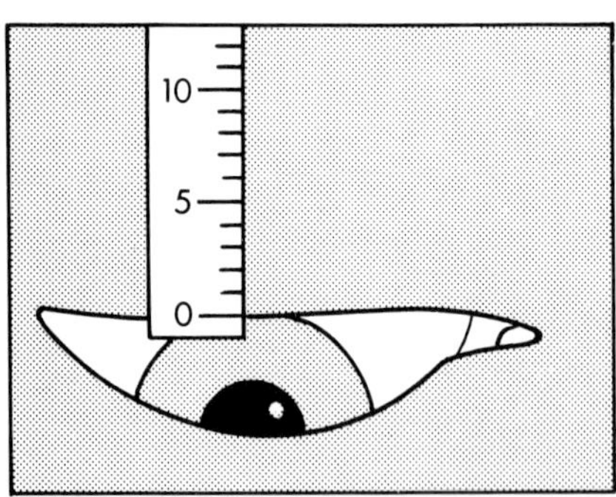

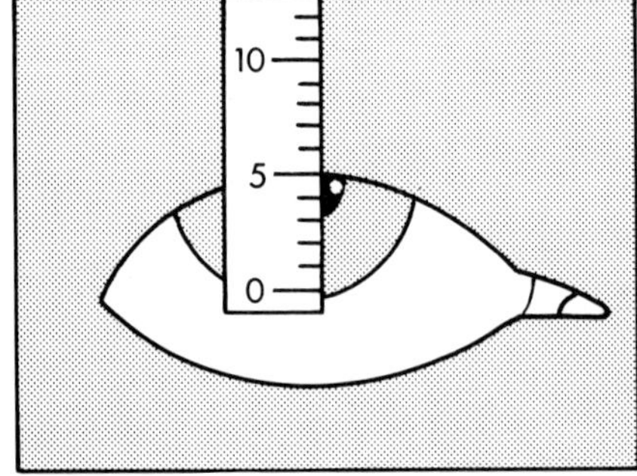

Figure 1.31 *Elevation of levator function*

Amount of ptosis

In unilateral cases this is determined by measuring the vertical fissures on both sides. The difference in measurement indicates the degree of ptosis. However, in bilateral cases, the amount of ptosis can only be determined against an arbitrary determination of normality. Because the average vertical diameter of the cornea is about 11 mm, and in the primary position of gaze the upper lid usually covers about 2 mm of the cornea, the amount of ptosis can be determined by measuring the amount of cornea covered by the upper lid and then subtracting 2 mm (*Figure 1.32*).

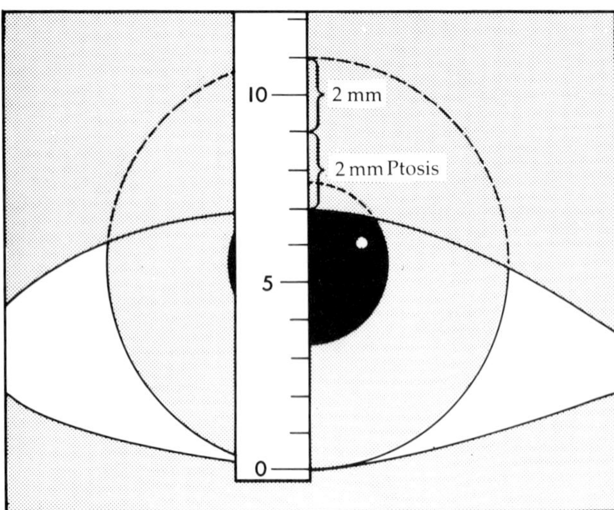

Figure 1.32 *Evaluation of amount of ptosis*

However, with practice the amount of ptosis can be estimated by inspection:

Mild ptosis measures 2 mm.
Moderate ptosis measures 3 mm.
Severe ptosis measures 4 mm or more.

A drawing should be made of the eyelid relative to the limbus and, ideally, photographs should be taken in the primary position, as well as in up-gaze and down-gaze.

The height of the upper lid crease and its configuration should be noted in both eyes. Usually, the presence of the crease is indicative of some levator function.

Other criteria

1. Evaluation of *ocular motility*.
2. *Jaw-winking phenomenon* in congenital ptosis by making the child chew and move his jaws from side to side.
3. *Bell's phenomenon*—if absent, postoperative exposure keratopathy may occur.
4. *Dry eye*—if present, ptosis surgery is usually contraindicated.
5. *Corneal sensitivity* should be tested in acquired neurogenic ptosis.

Special investigations

Special investigations, that may be required if a systemic disorder is suspected, include the Tensilon test, and neurological investigations (*see* Chapter 15).

Treatment

Levator resection (*Figure 1.33*)

This is usually necessary for correction of congenital myogenic ptosis. It is not a useful procedure unless some levator function is present. Small to moderate resections can be performed either through the skin or transconjunctivally, but large resections should only be performed through the skin.

In cases of moderate congenital ptosis (3 mm) with good levator function, a moderate levator resection (between 14 mm and 17 mm) either through the skin or conjunctiva is usually adequate. If levator function is only fair, a larger resection (between 18 mm and 22 mm) through a skin approach is necessary.

In cases of severe ptosis, levator function is usually only fair or poor. If levator function is fair a maximal resection consisting of 23 mm or even more through the skin is necessary. In cases of severe ptosis associated with poor levator function, the results of levator resection are poor even when this is combined with an advancement of the aponeurosis onto the tarsal plate. In these cases a sling procedure gives superior results.

Frontalis (brow) suspension (*Figure 1.34*)

This is necessary when there is essentially no levator function. In this operation the tarsus is attached to the frontalis via a sling (fascia lata or non-absorbable materials). In patients with the jaw-winking phenomenon, a bilateral suspension is performed in order to obtain a symmetrical result (*Figure 1.35*).

Tarsoconjunctival resection (Fasanella–Servat operation; *Figure 1.36*)

This is a very useful and simple procedure for the correction of relatively mild ptosis associated with fairly good levator function (Horner's syndrome).

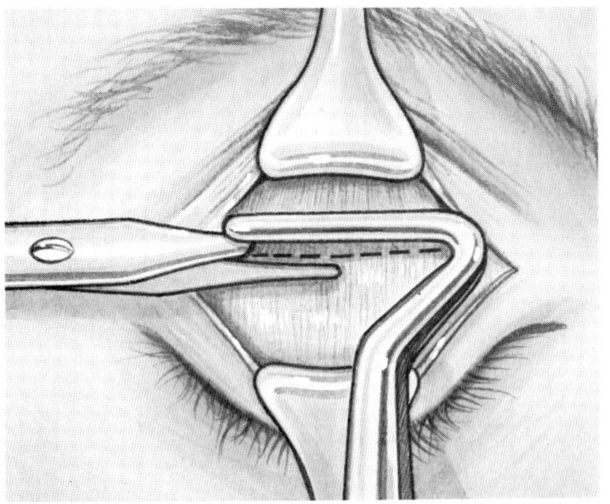

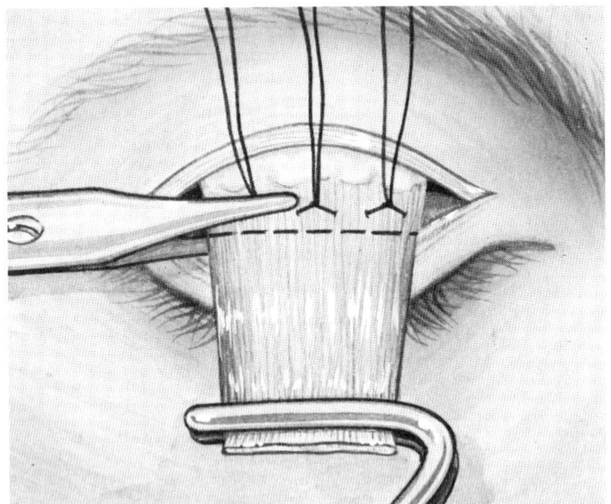

Figure 1.33 *Levator resection*

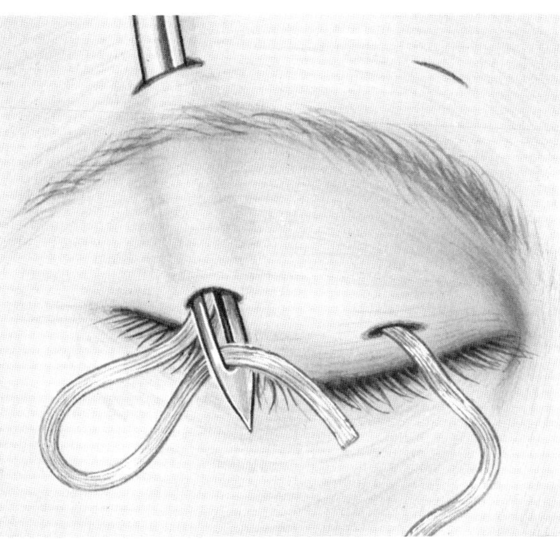

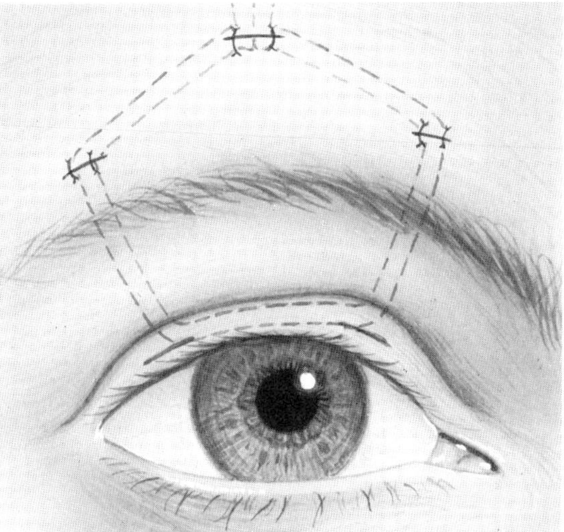

Figure 1.34 *Frontalis (brow) suspension*

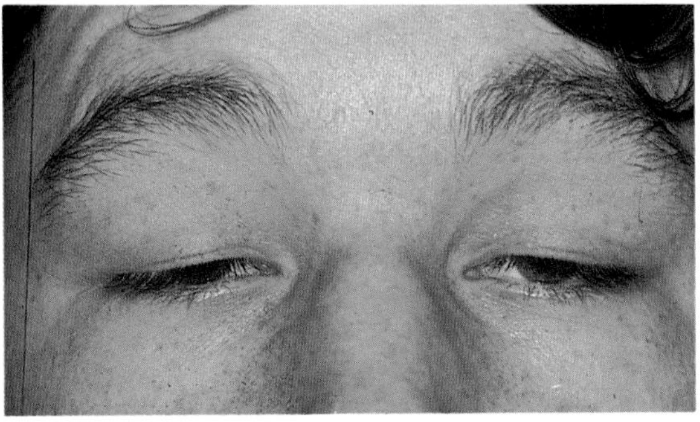

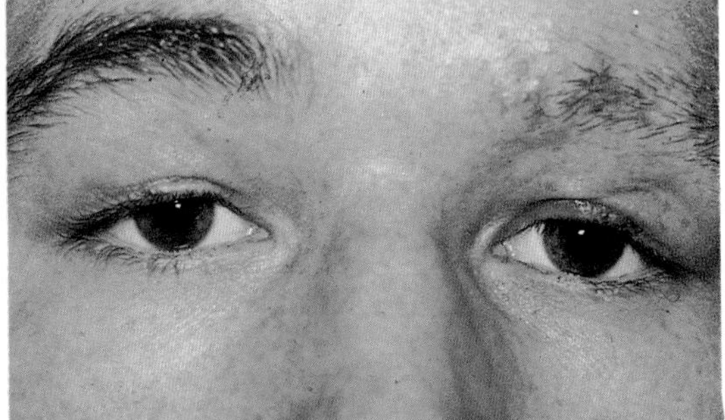

Figure 1.35 *Frontalis suspension. Left: preoperative; right: postoperative*

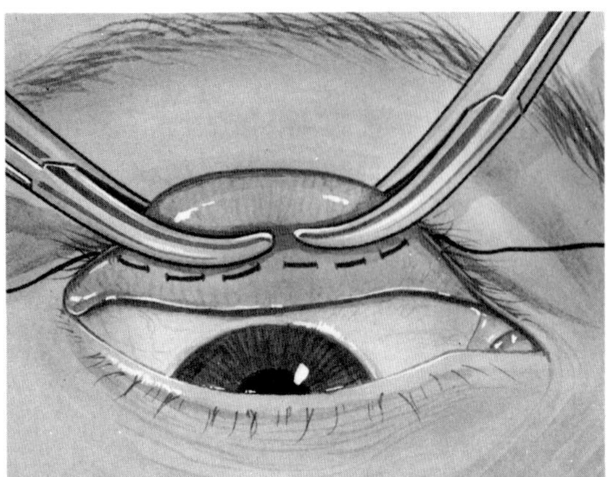

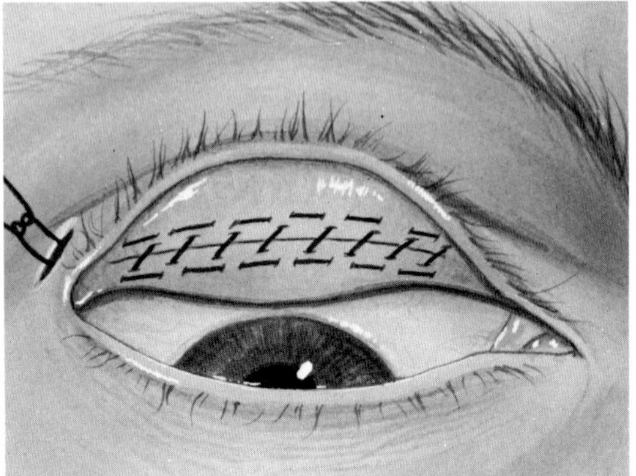

Figure 1.36 *Fasanella–Servat procedure*

Aponeurosis strengthening

This procedure is performed either by an advancement or a tucking with or without repair of a dehiscence of disinsertion, and is useful for cases of acquired ptosis with good levator function. The operation can usually be performed under local anaesthesia through the skin.

Timing of surgery for congenital ptosis

Mild to moderate congenital ptosis can be corrected between the ages of 3 and 4 years when accurate measurements can be obtained. However, surgical intervention should be considered earlier in cases of severe ptosis if there is a danger of vision deprivation amblyopia.

Miscellaneous congenital disorders

Coloboma

This is an embryological defect in the lid which may be an isolated finding or it may be associated with other congenital defects, such as cleft lip, mandibulofacial dysostoses, or small dermoids. Large defects should be corrected surgically without delay.

Epicanthus

This is a fold of skin that stretches from the upper to lower eyelid and covers the medial canthal angle. In infants it is very common due to immature facial bones and may give the appearance of a pseudoesotropia. In some cases the upper fold is larger than the lower (epicanthus tarsalis), or vice versa (epicanthus inversus).

Dermatitis

The skin covering the eyelids is one of the most easily extensible and thinnest areas of the cutaneous surface. For this reason it may be affected by dermatitis on exposure to irritants and sensitizers in much lower concentration than that required to cause dermatitis elsewhere.

Acute dermatitis is characterized by erythema, oedema, vesiculation, and crusting. Symptoms of burning or itching are common.

Chronic dermatitis is characterized by thickening of the skin with only minimal erythema. Pruritis is a common symptom.

Contact

Clinical features

Contact dermatitis involving the eyelids is very common. In most cases it is caused by the transmission of irritating substances to the lids on the fingers. Failure to rinse the hands adequately following washing and transfer of irritating chemicals in soaps is the most common cause. Various aerosols and perfumes may also be responsible. An allergic eczematous contact lid dermatitis is also commonly related to the use of cosmetics. Nail-lacquer, as well as nail-care products, can also be irritating to the skin. Sensitization due to medications used in and about the eyes is usually associated with a conjunctivitis.

Treatment

Management involves patch testing in order to identify the irritant and then its withdrawal. Acute dermatitis is best treated first with cool compresses followed by a non-fluorinated corticosteroid cream such as hydrocortisone 1%. Long-term corticosteroid use is contraindicated as it may aggravate the dermatitis.

Atopic

Patients with atopic dermatitis have a skin that is intolerant to irritants to a much greater degree than normal skin. They frequently have a personal or family history of other 'atopic' diseases such as asthma and hay fever. Some patients have increased levels of serum IgE. Apart from the eyelids, other classic atopic skin areas are the lateral neck folds, and the antecubital and popliteal fossae.

Other ocular manifestations include chronic keratoconjunctivitis, posterior or occasionally anterior stellate subcapsular cataracts, and keratoconus.

Further reading

Malignant tumours

Anderson, R.L. (1986) (Editorial) Mohs' micrographic technique. *Archives of Ophthalmology,* **104,** 818–819

Beard, C. (1981) Management of malignancy of the eyelids. *American Journal of Ophthalmology,* **92,** 1–6

Collin, J.R.O. (1976) Basal cell carcinoma of the eyelid region. *British Journal of Ophthalmology,* **60,** 806–809

Doxanas, M.T. and Green, W.R. (1984) Sebaceous gland carcinoma. *Archives of Ophthalmology,* **102,** 245–249

Mohs, F.E. (1986) Micrographic surgery for the microscopically controlled excision of eyelid cancers. *Archives of Ophthalmology,* **104,** 901–909

Trichiasis

Anderson, R.L. and Harvey, J.T. (1981) Lid splitting and posterior lamella cryosurgery for congenital and acquired distichiasis. *Archives of Ophthalmology,* **99,** 631–634

Johnson, B.L.C. and Collin, J.R.O. (1985) Treatment of trichiasis with a lid cryoprobe. *British Journal of Ophthalmology,* **69,** 267–270

Entropion

Collin, J.R.O. and Rathbun, J.E. (1978) Involutional entropion: a review with evaluation of a procedure. *Archives of Ophthalmology,* **96,** 1058–1064

Dryden, R.M., Leibsohn, J. and Wobig, J. (1978) Senile entropion: pathogenesis and treatment. *Archives of Ophthalmology,* **96,** 1883–1885

Gavaris, P.T. and Kaplan, L.J. (1983) Management of entropion and ectropion. *Clinical Modules for Ophthalmologists,* Vol. 1, Module 12

Hargiss, J.L. (1980) Inferior aponeurosis tucking revisited. *Ophthalmology,* **87,** 1001–1004

Schaefer, A.J. (1981) Involutional entropion. *Perspectives in Ophthalmology,* **5,** 137–144

Ectropion

Buerger, G.F. Jr (1981) Plastic repair of ectropion: involutional and cicatricial. *Perspectives in Ophthalmology,* **5,** 217–219

Crawford, G.J., Collin, J.R.O. and Moriarty, P.A.J. (1985) The correction of medial paralytic ectropion. *British Journal of Ophthalmology,* **68,** 639–641

Freuh, B.R. and Schoengarth, L.D. (1982) Evaluation and treatment of the patient with ectropion. *Ophthalmology,* **89,** 1049–1054

Liu, D. and Stasior, O.G. (1983) Lower eyelid laxity and ocular symptoms. *American Journal of Ophthalmology,* **95,** 545–551

Ptosis

Anderson, R.L. (1981) Acquired ptosis and its surgical correction. *Perspectives in Ophthalmology,* **5,** 145–155

Collin, J.R.O., Beard, C. and Stern, W.H. (1979) Blepharochalasis. *British Journal of Ophthalmology,* **63,** 542–546

Custer, P.L., Tenzel, R.R. and Kowalczyk, A. P. (1985) Blepharochalasis syndrome. *American Journal of Ophthalmology,* **99,** 424–428

Freuh, B.R. (1980) The mechanical classification of ptosis. *Ophthalmology,* **87,** 1019–1021

Kaplan, J., Jaffe, N.S. and Clayman, H.M. (1985) Ptosis and cataract surgery. *Ophthalmology,* **92,** 237–242

Miller, N.R. (1979) Myasthenia gravis: systemic and ocular considerations. *Ophthalmology,* **86,** 2165–2174

Pratt, S.G., Beyer, C.K. and Johnson, C.C. (1984) The Marcus Gunn phenomenon. *Ophthalmology,* **91,** 27–30

Van Dyk, H.J.L. and Florence, L. (1980) The Tensilon test. *Ophthalmology,* **87,** 210–212

2

The Orbit

Introduction

Applied anatomy

Clinical evaluation

Special investigations

Thyroid ophthalmopathy

Introduction

Clinical features

Management

Fractures

Blow-out fractures of the orbital floor

Blow-out fractures of the medial floor

Roof fractures

Vascular abnormalities

Varix

Arteriovenous communications

Infections

Cellulitis

Mucormycosis

Inflammatory disease (pseudotumour)

Tumours

Classification

Vascular

Lacrimal gland

Lymphoproliferative disorders

Rhabdomyosarcoma

Histiocytic

Cystic lesions

Metastases

Invasion from adjacent structures

Introduction

Applied anatomy

The orbit is a pear-shaped bony cavity whose stalk is the optic canal. It is surrounded by the paranasal sinuses inferiorly and medially, by the temporal fossa laterally, and the cranial cavity superiorly. The orbit lies behind the orbital septum and has a roof, a floor, a medial wall, and a lateral wall. The two medial walls are parallel and the two lateral walls form a 90° angle with each other. The intraorbital portion of the optic nerve is much longer (25 mm) than the distance between the back of the globe to the optic foramen (18 mm). This allows for significant forward displacement of the globe without causing excessive stretching of the optic nerve.

The orbit is made up of seven bones (*Figure 2.1*): (1) sphenoid, (2) frontal, (3) zygomatic, (4) maxillary, (5) palatine, (6) lacrimal and (7) ethmoid. A part of the sphenoid bone is involved in making up the roof, lateral wall, medial wall but *not* the floor.

The roof

This consists of two bones: lesser wing of the sphenoid and the frontal. It is located adjacent to the anterior cranial fossa and frontal sinus. The lacrimal gland fossa is located in the superotemporal aspect of the roof. A lacrimal gland tumour would therefore displace the globe inferonasally.

The lateral wall

This consists of two bones: greater wing of the sphenoid and the zygomatic. The anterior half of the globe is vulnerable to lateral trauma because the lateral wall only protects the posterior half of the globe.

The floor

This is made of three bones: zygomatic, maxillary, and palatine. The posteromedial portion of the maxillary bone is relatively weak and may be involved in a 'blow-out' fracture. The floor of the orbit also forms the roof of the maxillary sinus so that a maxillary carcinoma invading the orbit would displace the globe upwards.

The medial wall

This consists of four bones: maxillary, lacrimal, ethmoid and sphenoid. The lamina papyracea, which covers the ethmoid sinuses along the medial wall, is extremely thin. In children, spread of infection from the ethmoidal sinuses into the orbit is the commonest cause of orbital cellulitis.

The following bony landmarks of the orbital rim can be palpated:

1. *The anterior lacrimal crest* nasally as it blends with the inferior orbital margin.
2. *The zygomatic–maxillary suture* which lies approximately in the middle of the infraorbital margin. The infraorbital foramen which contains the infraorbital nerve is situated just inferiorly. Damage to this nerve from a 'blow-out' fracture of the orbit may cause numbness of the lower lid, cheek, side of nose, upper lip, and upper teeth.
3. *The supraorbital notch* which lies at the junction of the nasal and middle third of the superior orbital rim.
4. *The trochlea* which may be palpated about 5 mm back from the orbital rim where the roof blends with the medial wall.

Clinical evaluation

Careful history and examination should precede radiological and laboratory investigations.

The main features of orbital disease are: proptosis, pain, diplopia, visual impairment, and occasionally enophthalmos. Proptosis is defined as a forward displacement of the

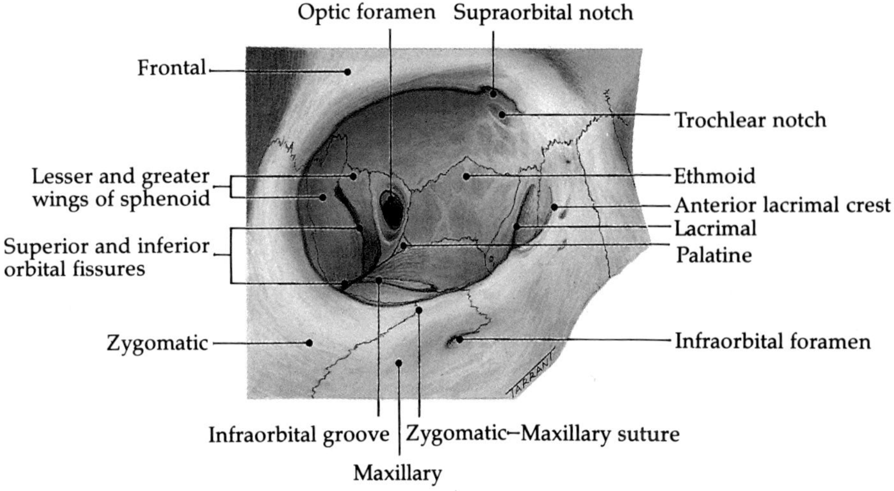

Figure 2.1 *Anatomy of orbital cavity*

globe beyond the orbital margin with the patient looking straight ahead—the term is synonymous with exophthalmos. Space-occupying lesions within the muscle cone usually cause an axial proptosis, whereas those outside the muscle cone will cause the proptosis to be eccentric with the displacement of the globe away from the location of the lesion.

History

In the history, the two most helpful symptoms are the presence of pain and the mode of onset of proptosis. For example, a benign tumour is usually slow growing and painless. On the other hand, a rapidly progressive proptosis in a child might point to orbital cellulitis or a rhabdomyosarcoma, whereas in an adult an acute onset of painful proptosis would be more suggestive of a pseudotumour. When taking past history, it is also important to enquire about malignancies, thyroid dysfunction, orbital trauma, and sinus disease.

Clinical examination

In a patient with suspected proptosis it is important to first rule out the possibility of pseudoproptosis and enophthalmos of the opposite eye.

Pseudoproptosis

The most important causes are:

1. *Enlargement of the ipsilateral eye* from buphthalmos or more commonly high axial myopia (4 D of myopia are approximately equal to 1 mm of axial enlargement) (*Figure 2.2*).
2. *Enophthalmos* of the opposite eye.
3. *Retraction of the upper eyelid* on the ipsilateral side.
4. *Shallow orbit* as from craniofacial dysostosis or facial asymmetry.

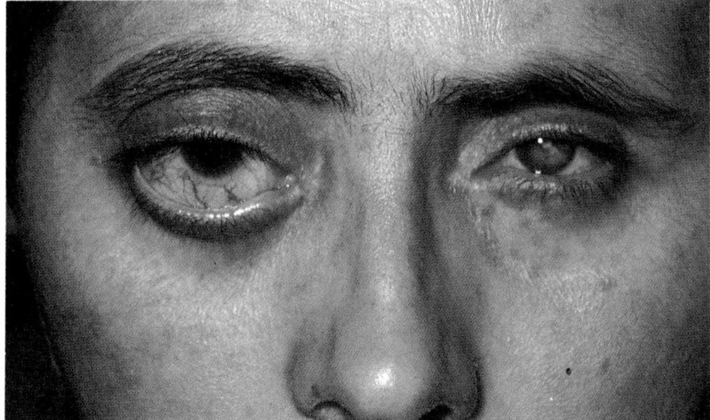

Figure 2.2 *Pseudoproptosis. Right eye is highly myopic and left is phthisical*

Enophthalmos

This is an important and frequently subtle clinical sign which is easily overlooked. In fact, about 50% of patients with enophthalmos are initially misdiagnosed as having ipsilateral ptosis or contralateral proptosis. There are basically three mechanisms which alone, or in combination, may lead to enophthalmos (*Table 2.1*).

Table 2.1 Causes of enophthalmos

Structural abnormalities
Post-traumatic as from a blow-out fracture of the orbital floor
Microphthalmos
Congenital defects such as maxillary hypoplasia, orbital asymmetry, and absence of the greater wing of the sphenoid in neurofibromatosis
Atrophy of orbital contents
Postirradiation for malignant tumours
Orbital varices
Scleroderma
Traction
Cicatrizing metastatic carcinoma – most frequently from the breast
Postinflammatory cicatrization of extraocular muscles as in the pseudotumour syndrome
Postsurgical shortening of extraocular muscles following excessive resections

Measurement of proptosis

The normal distance between the apex of the cornea and the lateral orbital rim is usually less than 20 mm and a reading of 21 mm or more is regarded as abnormal. In comparing the two eyes, a difference of 2 mm is suspect and a difference of over 2 mm warrants further investigation. It is important to measure, not only the amount of proptosis, but also the extent of vertical or horizontal displacement of the globe, and the size of the interpalpebral fissures.

The amount of proptosis is measured with a Hertel exophthalmometer (*Figure 2.3*) or a plastic rule placed at the lateral canthus and resting on bone (*Figure 2.4*). The measurements should be made both in the erect and the supine positions. The extent of vertical or horizontal deviation is measured by placing a plastic rule over the bridge of the nose.

Palpation of the orbital rim

This may reveal bony erosion or a mass. The clinician should be familiar with normal anatomical landmarks.

Orbital compression

This is performed by first pushing the normal and then the proptosed eye gently back into the orbit with the index fingers of both hands. Increased resistance to retropulsion is suggestive of a tumour, but may also be present in thyroid ophthalmopathy.

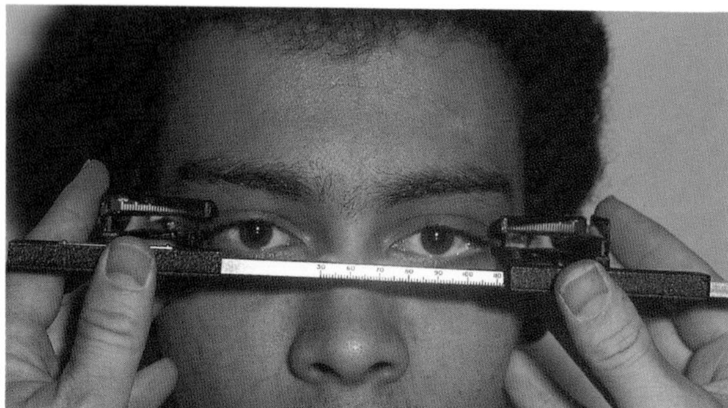

Figure 2.3 Hertel exophthalmometer

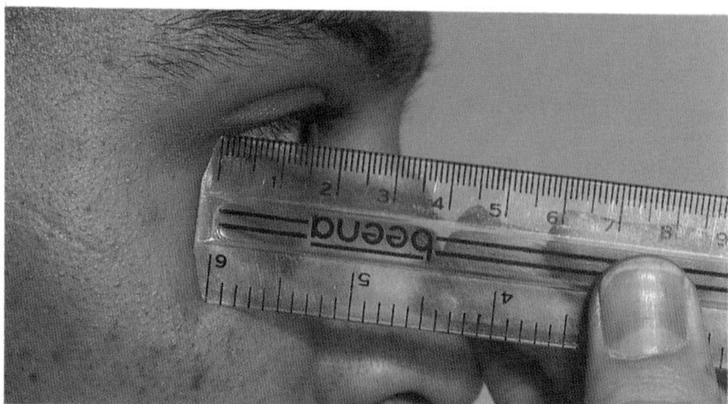

Figure 2.4 Measurement of proptosis with a plastic rule

Ocular movements

Defective movements may be caused by a restrictive myopathy, splinting of the optic nerve as in optic nerve sheath meningioma, a neurological lesion, or blow-out fracture.

Visual acuity

Orbital lesions may impair visual acuity by three mechanisms: optic nerve compression, exposure keratopathy, and choroidal folds involving the posterior pole. In general, orbital tumours cause a considerable amount of proptosis before interfering with optic nerve function. However, occasionally a granuloma or a cavernous haemangioma at the orbital apex may compress the optic nerve in the absence of significant proptosis. In children, the finding of a marked impairment of vision with only a minimal amount of proptosis is suggestive of an optic nerve glioma. In thyroid ophthalmopathy, involvement of the optic nerve has no direct relationship to the amount of proptosis.

Pupillary reactions

The presence of a Marcus Gunn pupil is suggestive of optic nerve compression and is an indication for plotting the visual fields in both eyes.

Ophthalmoscopy

The optic disc may show pallor, swelling, or opticociliary shunt vessels (*see Figure 15.20*). Choroidal folds (*see Figure 11.48*) may occur in patients with orbital tumours as well as in thyroid ophthalmopathy.

Dynamic properties

Certain orbital lesions may rapidly change in size, pulsate or be associated with a bruit. These dynamic properties should be evaluated as follows:

1. Try to precipitate the proptosis by: dependent head position, a Valsalva manoeuvre, and jugular compression. In patients with orbital varices or infants with capillary orbital haemangiomas, these manoeuvres may induce or exacerbate the proptosis.
2. Look for pulsation which, if mild, may be missed unless the patient is examined with the slitlamp. Two main causes of pulsation are: a defect in the orbital roof through which CSF pulsation is transmitted to the orbit (*Figure 2.5*)—this will not be associated with a bruit; and an arteriovenous communication. Defects in the roof of the orbit may be congenital (neurofibromatosis) or acquired (traumatic or iatrogenic).
3. A bruit is detected by auscultating the orbit with the bell of the stethoscope. A bruit may be heard in patients with carotid–cavernous fistulae and occasionally with an extremely vascular orbital tumour. In carotid–cavernous fistula, the bruit will be associated with pulsation and both can be diminished or abolished by gentle compression of the ipsilateral carotid artery in the neck.

Slitlamp biomicroscopy

This may reveal pulsation that is not apparent on gross examination. In addition, the presence of tortuous vessels over hypertrophied lateral recti, especially if associated with superior limbic keratoconjunctivitis, is strongly suggestive of dysthyroid ophthalmopathy.

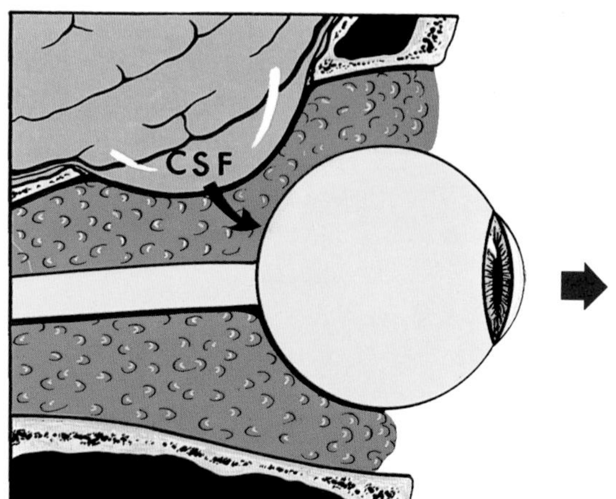

Figure 2.5 Pulsatile proptosis from defect in orbital roof

Forced duction test

This test is used to differentiate defective ocular movements due to a fibrotic contracture from a neurological lesion. It is performed as follows:

1. Instil cocaine drops into the conjunctiva and place a cotton pledget soaked in cocaine over the insertion of the muscle to be tested into *both* eyes. Leave the pledget for about 5 minutes.
2. Grasp the insertion of the muscle in the involved eye with toothed forceps and gently attempt to rotate the eye in the field of action of the weak muscle. Then repeat the test in the unaffected eye.

Positive test. If the muscle is involved by a fibrotic contracture (thyroid myopathy) or trapped in an orbital floor fracture it will be difficult or impossible to move the globe with the forceps. In the opposite eye, no such resistance will be encountered.

Negative test. If the muscle is paretic due to a neurological lesion (third nerve palsy), no resistance will be encountered in either eye.

Differential intraocular pressure test

This, like the forced duction test, differentiates neurological from restrictive defects in ocular motility. It is performed by first measuring the intraocular pressure in the primary position of gaze and then with the patient attempting to look in the field of action of the involved muscle. An increase in the intraocular pressure of 6 mmHg or more denotes resistance transmitted to the globe due to muscle restriction. No change in intraocular pressure suggests a neurological lesion. The advantage of this test over the forced duction test is less pain for the patient, the end point is objective rather than subjective, and results are easier to interpret.

The various clinical findings in orbital disease are summarized in *Table 2.2*.

Table 2.2 Clinical findings in orbital disease

Finding	*Causes*
Reduced visual acuity	Optic nerve compression Exposure keratopathy Choroidal folds
Marcus Gunn pupil	Optic nerve compression
Lid retraction and lag	Thyroid ophthalmopathy
Increased resistance to retropulsion	Tumour Thyroid ophthalmopathy
Defective ocular movements	Restrictive myopathy Optic nerve sheath meningioma Blow-out fracture Neurological lesion
Abnormal optic disc	
Optic atrophy	Optic nerve compression
Disc swelling	Raised intraorbital pressure
Opticociliary shunt vessels	Optic nerve sheath meningioma
Dynamic properties	
Rapid change in size	Capillary haemangioma (infants) Orbital varices
Pulsation + bruit	Carotid–cavernous fistula
Pulsation − bruit	Orbital roof defect
Slitlamp examination	
Hypertrophied rectus muscles	Thyroid ophthalmopathy
Superior limbic keratoconjunctivitis	Thyroid ophthalmopathy
Positive forced duction test	Fibrotic contracture of muscles Blow-out fracture

Special investigations

Plain X-rays

The Caldwell view (*Figure 2.6*)

This view taken with the patient's nose and forehead touching the film, is most useful in the detection of orbital lesions. The beam is angled at about 25° so that the petrous pyramids are projected inferiorly and do not obscure orbital details.

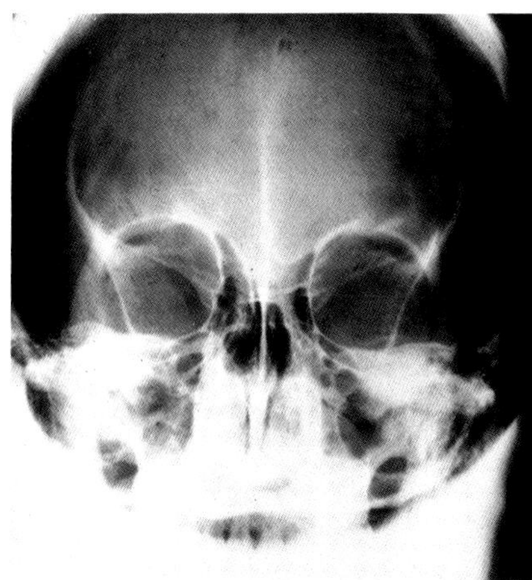

Figure 2.6 *Caldwell view of orbit (courtesy of Dr I. Yentis)*

The Waters' view (*Figure 2.7*)

This view is particularly useful in detecting orbital floor fractures. The film is taken with the patient's chin slightly elevated (similar to the position adopted when drinking water).

The Rhese view

This view is a special projection used to visualize the optic foramina. In normal subjects the diameters of the two canals should not differ by more than 1 mm.

The lateral view is useful in studying the nasopharynx and the *axial basal views* will show up the ethmoidal sinuses and sphenoid bones.

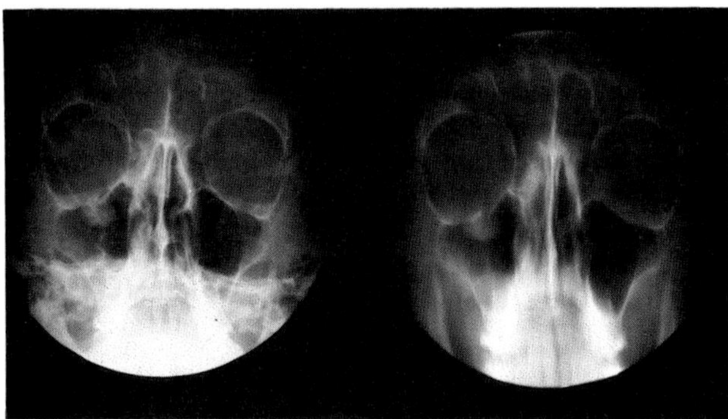

Figure 2.7 Waters' view of orbit. Left: plain X-ray; right: laminogram

Five X-ray signs of orbital disease

See Table 2.3.

Table 2.3 X-ray signs in orbital disease

Signs	*Causes*
Orbital enlargement	
Diffuse	Intraconal tumour (usually benign)
Asymmetrical	Extraconal tumour
Changes in bone density	
Decreased localized	Benign tumour
Diffuse destruction	Malignant tumour
Increased	Meningioma
	Paget's disease
	Osteoblastic metastases
	Fibrous dysplasia
Calcification	Orbital varix (phlebolith)
	Optic nerve sheath meningioma
	Lacrimal gland carcinoma
	Retinoblastoma
Enlargement of superior orbital fissure	Infraclinoid aneurysm
	Intracavernous aneurysm
	Orbital tumour (posterior extension)
Enlargement of optic canal	Optic nerve glioma

Enlargement

In adults, orbital enlargement is a sign of long-standing raised intraorbital pressure, usually due to a benign tumour. In children, however, the response of the orbit to a space-occupying lesion may be more rapid, so that enlargement may occur in association with a rapidly growing malignant tumour (rhabdomyosarcoma). A diffuse enlargement of the orbit is usually indicative of an intraconal tumour, whereas asymmetrical enlargement occurs with extraconal tumours.

Bone density

Localized indentation of the orbital wall is characteristic of benign lesions, such as dermoids or mixed-cell lacrimal gland tumours. Ill-defined or diffuse bony destruction is usually indicative of malignancy (lacrimal gland carcinoma, spread of tumour from paranasal sinuses). Increased density occurs in meningioma, osteoblastic secondaries, fibrous dysplasia, and Paget's disease.

Intraorbital calcification

Calcification within the soft tissues of the orbit may indicate the presence and nature of the tumour. Calcification is associated with optic nerve sheath meningioma, lacrimal gland carcinoma, and retinoblastoma (fine stippled calcification). The identification of phleboliths is virtually pathognomonic of orbital varices.

Enlargement of the superior orbital fissure

The superior orbital fissure appears as a dark space which separates the lesser from the greater wing of the sphenoid. Widening of the fissure is a classic sign of infraclinoid carotid aneurysm or intracavernous aneurysm and it may also occur from a backward extension of an orbital tumour.

Enlargement of the optic canals

It is important to emphasize that the optic canals cannot be seen on a Caldwell view. A uniform concentric widening is seen in children with optic nerve gliomas. A localized defect in the walls of the canals is caused by extrinsic lesions in adjacent structures. The optic strut, which is formed by the lateral and medial wall, is generally affected by those conditions that also cause an enlargement of the superior orbital fissure. Erosions of the medial wall occurs in conditions which also affect the sphenoidal sinus (tumours, mucoceles).

Computerized tomography scanning

The advent of computerized tomography (CT) scanning in the 1970s has transformed the investigation of orbital disorders. CT scanning is a non-invasive method which uses thin X-ray beams to obtain tissue density values from which detailed cross-sectional images are formed by a computer.

Axial scanning forms images in a plane parallel to the course of the optic nerves (*Figure 2.8, bottom*).

Coronal scanning forms vertical images in a plane parallel to the globe (analogous to the Caldwell view) (*Figure 2.8, top*).

A combination of axial and coronal cuts enables a space-occupying lesion within the orbit to be visualized in three dimensions. CT scanning is, therefore, extremely useful at determining the location and size of a space-occupying orbital lesion. In some cases, lesions with an intrinsic vasculature, such as arteriovenous malformations, may be better visualized by contrast-enhanced CT. Its main disadvantage is its inability to distinguish between pathological soft tissue masses which are radiologically isodense. The test is also relatively expensive.

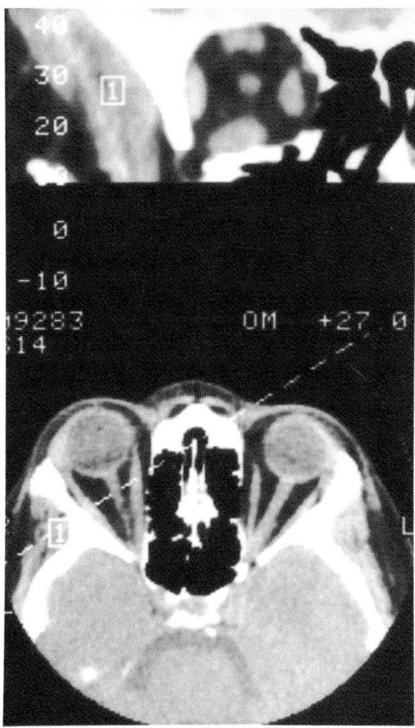

Figure 2.8 CT scan of orbit. Top: coronal scan; bottom: axial scan

Ultrasonography

Ultrasonography uses high frequency sound waves to produce echoes as they strike interfaces between acoustically different structures (*Figure 2.9*).

The A-scan

This scan is a time–amplitude evaluation. The more sound that is reflected, the greater the vertical deflection. The greater the distance to the right, the greater the distance from the source of the sound and the reflecting surface. The A-scan therefore produces a one-dimensional image.

The B-scan

This scan produces a two-dimensional picture of orbital structures. The amount of reflected sound is portrayed as a dot of light. The more sound that has been reflected, the brighter the dot. The B-scan gives an anatomical display which is much easier for the non-expert to interpret than the A-scan.

Ultrasonography is complementary to CT scanning in the diagnosis of orbital lesions and is of particular value as an initial screening procedure. The ultrasonographic patterns of pathological lesions depend mainly on the displacement of orbital fat. When the scan passes through the plane of the optic nerve, the normal echo pattern appears as a W-shaped acoustically opaque area. The optic nerve itself appears as an acoustically empty area forming a black notch in the retrobulbar fat.

Ultrasound is useful in the diagnosis of thyroid ophthalmopathy where clinical and laboratory tests are equivocal. Even in patients without proptosis, ultrasound may show up large extraocular muscles and specific echoes from the orbital fat (*Figure 2.10*). Ultrasound is superior to CT scanning in actual tissue diagnosis and can usually differentiate a vascular lesion from a metastasis or an inflammatory pseudotumour. It is, however, less useful in the evaluation of lesions against bony structures and at the apex of the orbit.

Magnetic resonance imaging

This new technique depends on the rearrangement of hydrogen nuclei when the tissues are exposed to a short electromagnetic pulse. When the pulse subsides the nuclei return to their normal position re-radiating in the process some of the energy they have absorbed. Sensitive receivers pick up this electromagnetic echo. The information about the characteristics of the tissue comes from the timing and the intensity of the signal which is analysed by computers and displayed as a cross-sectional image of the area under study.

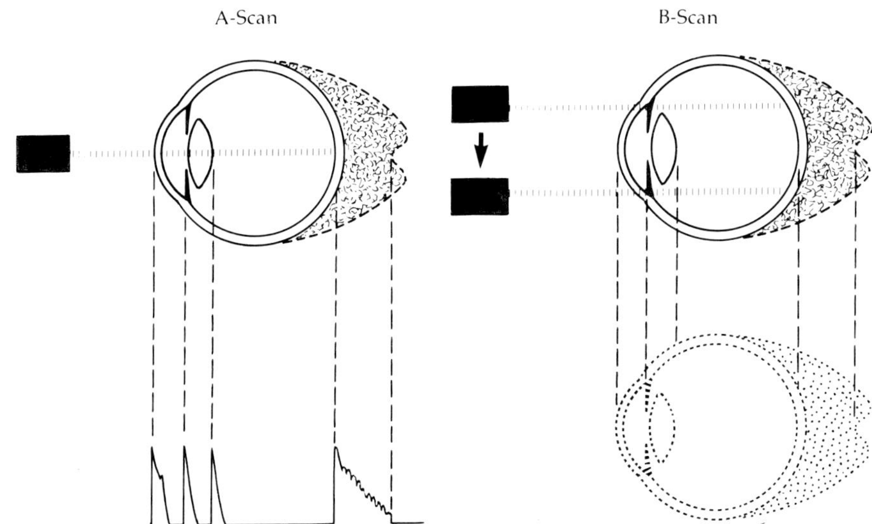

Figure 2.9 Principles of A and B ultrasonography

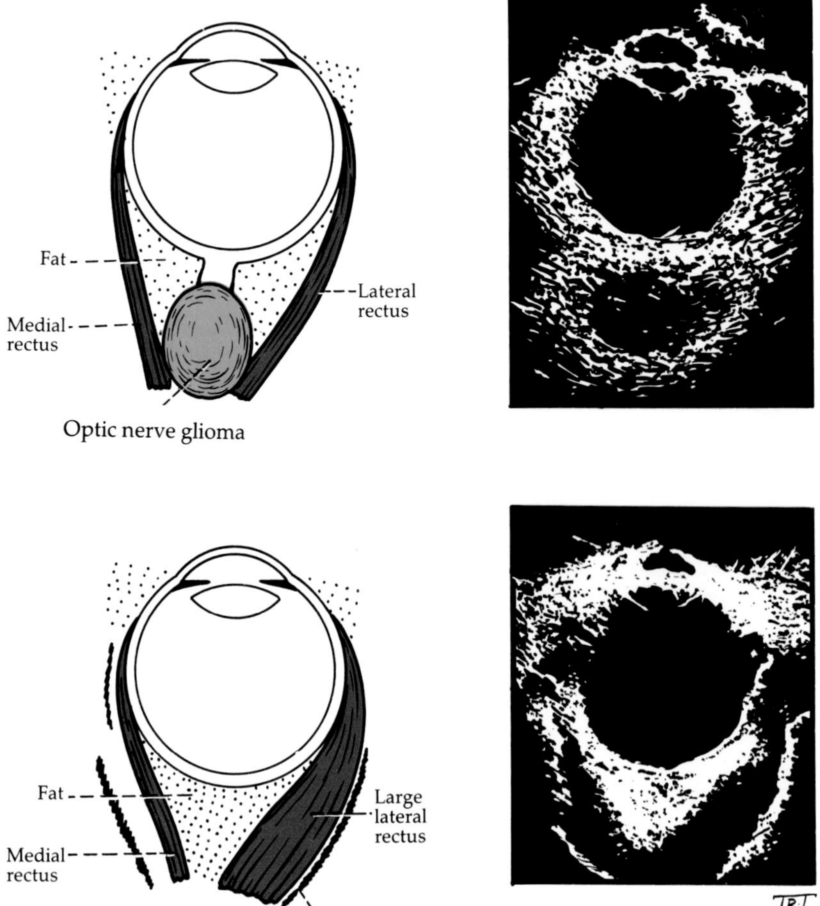

Figure 2.10 *Ultrasound appearance of optic nerve glioma (above) and enlargement of lateral rectus muscle (below)*

Although magnetic resonance imaging (MRI) is still in its infancy, it promises to distinguish between lesions based not only on location and tissue structure but also on metabolic profile. It has the added advantage of not being hampered by bone and, unlike conventional radiography and CT scanning, does not subject the patient to ionizing irradiation.

Fine needle aspiration biopsy

The biopsy material is obtained under CT and ultrasound guidance using a 23-gauge needle. This technique is particularly valuable in patients with strongly suspected orbital metastases and in those with secondary neoplasms from contiguous orbital structures.

Thyroid ophthalmopathy

Introduction

Basic thyroid physiology

The two hormones secreted by the thyroid gland are thyroxine (T_4) and triiodothyronine (T_3). The complicated enzymatic reactions in which iodine is trapped and converted into these two hormones is under the control of the anterior pituitary gland through thyrotrophin (thyroid stimulating hormone—TSH). The anterior pituitary is, in turn, under the control of the hypothalamus through the thyrotrophin-releasing hormone (TRH). TRH passes down from the hypothalamus to the anterior pituitary in the portal venous system. Both the anterior pituitary and the hypothalamus are under feedback control so that their levels of secretion vary inversely with the levels of circulating T_3 and T_4 (*Figure 2.11*).

In the plasma, over 99.9% of both T_3 and T_4 are bound to protein and only a very small fraction of both hormones exists in an unbound or free form. However, despite their exceedingly low concentrations, these free fractions are

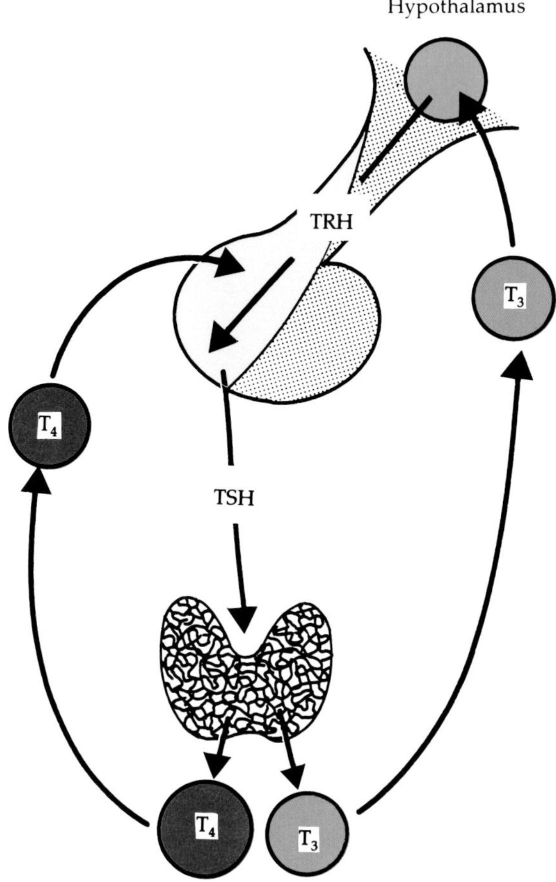

Figure 2.11 Thyroid physiology

very important because they are able to diffuse out of the circulation and enter cells where they exert their biological actions. T_3 is thought to be as important as T_4 in total metabolic activity despite the fact that its concentration is very much lower.

Graves' disease

Hyperthyroidism occurs in a number of diseases, including Graves' disease, toxic goitre, thyroiditis, and ingestion of excessive amounts of thyroid hormones. Excessive levels of T_4 give rise to weight loss, tachycardia, tremor, sweating, and changes in the nails, skin, and hair. Subjectively, the patient notices nervousness, heat intolerance, and palpitations.

Graves' disease is a term used to describe the commonest variety of hyperthyroidism, which is regarded as having an autoimmune basis. It typically affects women between the ages of 20 years and 45 years and is characterized by goitre, infiltrative ophthalmopathy, clubbing (thyroid acropathy), and pretibial myxoedema. When the eye signs of Graves' disease occur in a patient who is not clinically hyperthyroid, or who gives no past history of thyroid dysfunction, the condition is referred to as euthyroid or ophthalmic Graves' disease (OGD). Although the usual tests for thyroid function may be normal in patients with OGD, more sophisticated investigations usually reveal some abnormality in the majority of patients. In patients with Graves' disease, the ophthalmopathy may precede, be coincident with, or follow the hyperthyroidism. The therapeutic control of hyperthyroidism tends not to improve the exophthalmos. In general the ocular features of Graves' disease and OGD are similar, although they tend to be more asymmetrical in OGD than in Graves' disease (*Figure 2.12*).

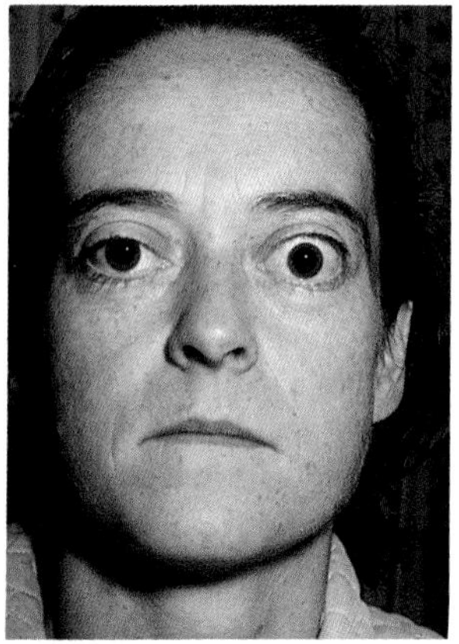
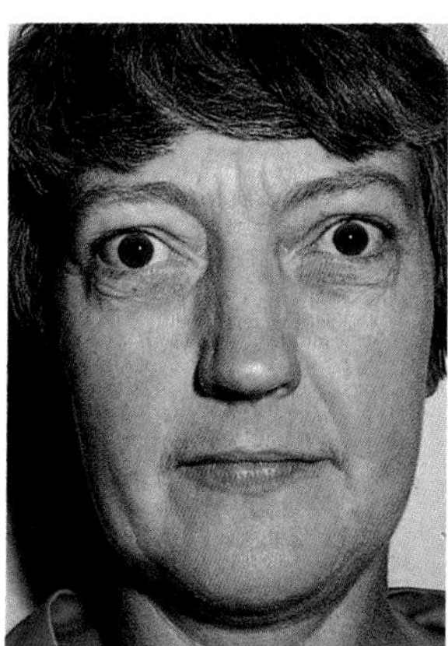

Figure 2.12 Left: asymmetrical features of ophthalmic Graves' disease; right: symmetrical signs of Graves' disease

Clinical features

Eyelid retraction
Infiltrative ophthalmopathy
- soft tissue involvement
  - conjunctival injection
  - chemosis
  - lid oedema
  - superior limbic keratoconjunctivitis
- proptosis
- optic neuropathy
- restrictive myopathy

Eyelid retraction

Retraction of both upper and lower lids has long been recognized as one of the cardinal signs of Graves' disease and is responsible for functional and cosmetic problems. In many patients there is both true lid retraction as well as pseudo-lid retraction due to associated proptosis.

Mechanism

Although the cause of lid retraction is still incompletely understood, several factors seem to be contributory:

1. *Müller's muscle overaction* due to sympathetic overstimulation. (Pupillary signs are, however, absent.)

2. *Overaction of the levator–superior rectus complex* in response to the hypophoria produced by fibrosis and contraction of the inferior rectus muscle.
3. *Contraction of the levator* as a result of infiltration.

In the lower lid, sympathetic overstimulation also seems to play some part, but more important is the fibrosis of the inferior rectus muscle exerting a retracting action on the lower lid via its capsulopalpebral head.

Signs

In the normal patient, when the eye is in the primary position, the upper lid covers about 2 mm of the superior part of the cornea (*Figure 2.13, top*). Lid retraction is recognized by elevation of the upper lid so that its margin is either level with or above the superior limbus, allowing sclera to be visible (*Figure 2.13, bottom*). The occurrence of lid retraction has led to the description of several clinical signs:

1. *Dalrymple's sign* refers to the lid retraction itself.
2. *Von Graefe's sign* consists of the retarded descent of the upper lid in down-gaze. When the patient changes from down-gaze to up-gaze, the position of the globe lags behind the upper lid.
3. *Kocher's sign* is a staring and frightened appearance of the eyes which is particularly marked on attentive fixation. Other lid signs include a fine tremor of the closed lids, jerky spasmodic lid movements when the lids are open, and infrequent blinking.

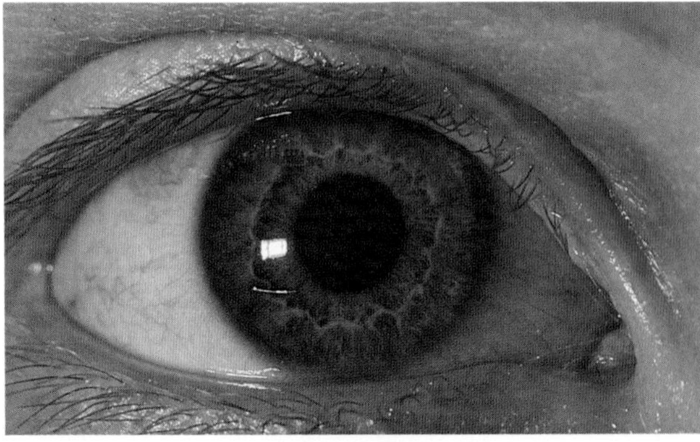

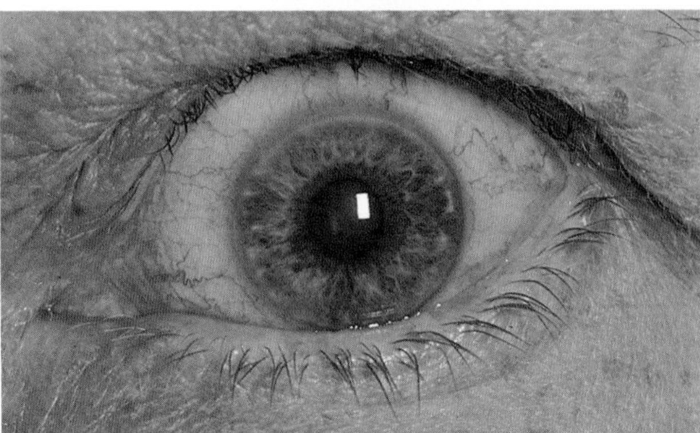

Figure 2.13 *Top: normal position of upper eyelid; bottom: lid retracted*

Other causes of lid retraction

Apart from thyroid ophthalmopathy other causes of lid retraction are:

1. Aberrant regeneration of the third nerve (*see* Chapter 15).
2. Unilateral ptosis with contralateral overaction of the levator muscle.
3. Collier's sign (*see* Chapter 15) of the dorsal midbrain (Parinaud's syndrome).

Infiltrative ophthalmopathy

It seems likely that a humoral agent is responsible for the orbital changes in thyroid ophthalmopathy (*Figure 2.14*). The two main characteristics are:

1. *Enlargement of extraocular muscles* due to an increase in their mucopolysaccharide content. This accumulation of hydrophilic macromolecules in turn results in marked oedema. In some cases, the muscles may be enlarged up to eight times their normal size and may mimic an orbital tumour. The muscle enlargement can be demonstrated by ultrasonography (*see Figure 2.10*) and CT scanning (*Figure 2.15*). The congestive phase is followed by round cell infiltration of interstitial tissues. Subsequent degeneration of muscle fibres eventually leads to fibrosis which exerts a tethering effect on the involved muscle and results in restrictive myopathy.
2. *Proliferation of orbital fat and connective tissue* with retention of fluid and accumulation of mucopolysaccharides as well as infiltration of the orbital tissue by plasma cells and lymphocytes.

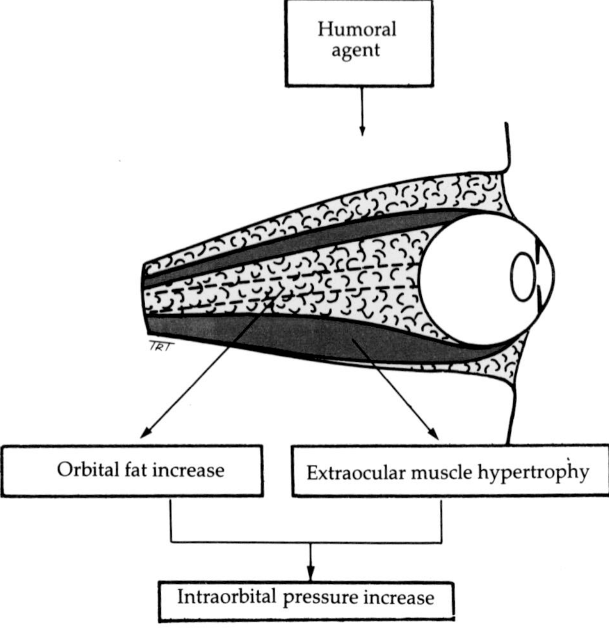

Figure 2.14 *Infiltrative thyroid ophthalmopathy*

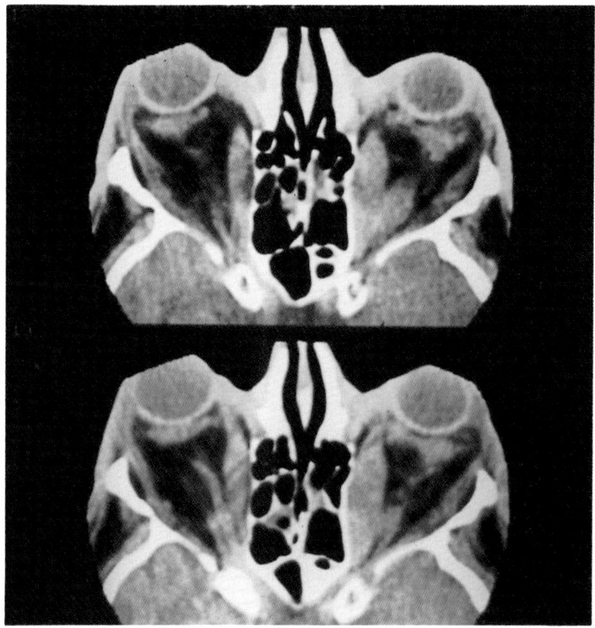

Figure 2.15 *CT scan showing large extraocular muscles in thyroid ophthalmopathy (courtesy of Mr P. Rosen)*

This increase in size of the intraorbital contents causes a rise in the intraorbital pressure which may itself cause further retention of fluid within the orbit.

On *CT scanning*, the four cardinal signs of orbital involvement are proptosis, muscle swelling, thickening of the optic nerve, and anterior prolapse of the orbital septum due to excessive orbital fat and/or muscle swelling.

Clinical features

Soft tissue involvement

The symptoms of soft tissue involvement include excessive lacrimation, a 'sandy' sensation, retrobulbar discomfort, and photophobia.

The signs include:

1. *Injection* of the conjunctiva (which is a sensitive sign of disease activity). An intense focal hyperaemia may be seen outlining and overlying the horizontal rectus tendons.
2. *Chemosis* refers to oedema of the conjunctiva and caruncle. If minimal it is manifest as a small fold of redundant conjunctiva overhanging the mucocutaneous junction of the lower lid. In severe cases the conjunctiva prolapses across the lower lid (*Figure 2.16*).
3. *Oedema and fullness of the lids* often coexist although oedema may occasionally be present without fullness. It appears that lid fullness reflects oedema and infiltration behind the orbital septum, whereas lid oedema alone is due to fluid anterior to the orbital septum, just under the skin and orbicularis muscle.
4. *Superior limbic keratoconjunctivitis*—*see* Chapter 4.

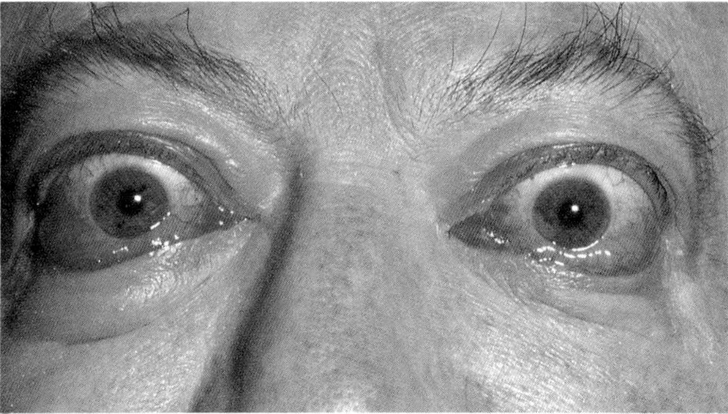

Figure 2.16 *Severe chemosis in thyroid ophthalmopathy*

Proptosis

Thyroid ophthalmopathy is the most common cause of both bilateral and unilateral proptosis in adults. It has been estimated that about 80% of cases of unilateral proptosis are of endocrine origin. It is useful to think of proptosis as being a safety mechanism which protects the optic nerve from the potentially dangerous effects of raised intraorbital pressure. However, in some eyes a strong orbital septum enables the intraorbital pressure to rise to dangerous levels without causing proptosis. In the majority of cases the proptosis is self-limiting and uninfluenced by treatment for hyperthyroidism.

Dysthyroid optic neuropathy

The prevalence of this serious complication is probably less than 5%. Although all the mechanisms responsible are not clear, it seems likely that it is caused mainly by a direct compression of the optic nerve or its blood supply at the orbital apex by the congested and enlarged recti. This compression, which often occurs in the absence of significant proptosis, may lead to severe but preventable visual impairment. The symptom of optic nerve involvement is a slowly progressive impairment of central vision. The fundus may be normal or show varying degrees of vascular congestion, swelling or atrophy of the optic nerve head, and chorioretinal folds. It is important not to attribute a disproportionate visual loss to minor corneal complications and to miss the presence of optic neuropathy. Visual field examination usually demonstrates a central or paracentral scotoma which may be combined with nerve fibre bundle defects. These findings combined with a slightly increased intraocular pressure may be confused with primary open-angle glaucoma. Two other important signs of optic nerve involvement are impairment of colour vision and an afferent pupillary conduction defect. In order to detect early involvement of the optic nerve, patients should be encouraged to monitor their own vision at home by alternatively occluding each eye and reading small print as well as assessing the intensity of colours on a television screen.

Restrictive thyroid myopathy

The single most common ocular motility defect is a unilateral elevator palsy caused by a fibrotic contraction of the inferior rectus muscle. The restriction of upward gaze mimics a superior rectus palsy (*Figure 2.17*). The next most frequent motility disturbance is a contracture of the medial rectus which will result in a failure of abduction and can simulate a sixth nerve palsy (*Figure 2.18*). Involvement of the superior rectus is relatively uncommon and causes impairment of downward gaze. The least commonly involved muscle is the lateral rectus, involvement of which will cause failure of adduction.

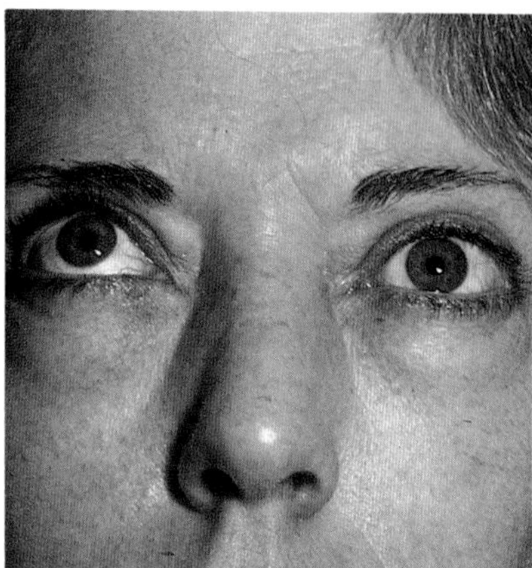

Figure 2.17 *Defective elevation of left eye due to involvement of the inferior rectus muscle*

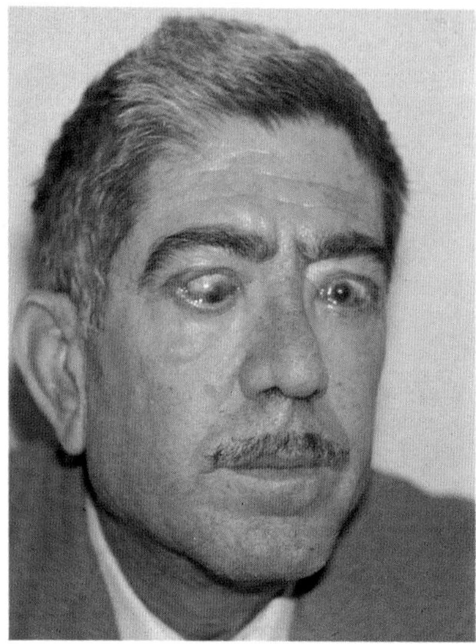

Figure 2.18 *Bilateral contracture of medial recti simulating sixth nerve paresis (courtesy of Mr B. Mathalone)*

Management

The management of patients with thyroid ophthalmopathy may be difficult and complex and may range from merely reassurance to the use of orbital decompression for vision-threatening complications. Therapy should therefore be tailored to the nature and severity of involvement, so that any or all of the following forms of treatment may be required (*Table 2.4*).

Table 2.4 Management of thyroid ophthalmopathy

Non-specific
Reassurance
Head elevation
Taping of eyelids
Prisms
Topical therapy
Lubricants
Guanethidine drops
Systemic therapy
Diuretics
Steroids
Cytotoxic agents
Radiotherapy
Surgery
Orbital decompression
On extraocular muscles
On eyelids

Non-specific

Reassurance

Many patients have relatively mild involvement which resolves spontaneously within months or a few years and which only causes a mild nuisance. All that these patients require is reassurance every 6–9 months that they are not developing any vision-threatening complications.

Head elevation

Periorbital oedema may be reduced by the use of three pillows during sleep to elevate the head.

Taping of eyelids

Patients with corneal exposure during sleep should have their eyes taped.

Prisms

Mild diplopia may be controlled by using prisms.

Topical therapy

Lubricants

Chronic ocular irritation in patients with thyroid ophthalmopathy may be caused by conjunctival inflammation, corneal exposure, and keratoconjunctivitis sicca caused by infiltration of the lacrimal gland by inflammatory cells. Lubricants in the form of artificial tears and ointment at bedtime are useful in obtaining symptomatic relief.

Guanethidine 5%

Lid retraction due to overaction of Müller's muscle may be lessened by the use of the α-adrenergic blocking agent guanethidine 5% drops two or three times a day.

Systemic therapy

At present three groups of drugs are available:

Diuretics

These may be tried to reduce the amount of periorbital oedema but their efficacy is usually disappointing.

Steroids

These are indicated for the following reasons:

1. *Optic neuropathy.*
2. *Rapidly progressive* chemosis and proptosis and pain during the *early* course of the disease.

An initial high dose of prednisolone 80–100 mg/day should be administered and a favourable response expected within 48 hours with a reduction of discomfort, chemosis and periorbital oedema. The dose should then be tapered and a maximal response is usually achieved within 2–8 weeks. If possible, steroid therapy should be withdrawn after about 3 months. Prolonged steroid administration should be reserved only for the few patients who are unresponsive to other forms of therapy. However, it should be emphasized that steroids will have little or no effect on the degree of myopathy or lid retraction.

Cytotoxic agents

Agents such as azathioprine and cyclophosphamide have been tried but their benefits are still uncertain.

Radiotherapy

The indications for radiotherapy are essentially the same as for steroid therapy in patients who: have contraindications to steroids; refuse steroids; are unresponsive to steroids despite an *adequate* dose; and are developing steroid side-effects.

The dose is 20 Gy to the posterior orbit given over a 10-day period of 2 Gy per day. A positive response is usually evident within 6 weeks with maximal improvement evident by 4 months. It should be emphasized that patients unresponsive to steroids may benefit from radiotherapy which, just like steroid therapy, does not influence the degree of myopathy. Complications of radiotherapy include: cataract formation, keratitis, localized erythema and mild loss of hair.

Surgical management

Shorr and Seiff (1986) have recommended the following rational and systematic 'four-stage' surgical rehabilitation of patients with thyroid ophthalmopathy. Of course, not every patient will necessarily require all four procedures:

Stage 1—orbital decompression.
Stage 2—surgery on extraocular muscles.
Stage 3—lid surgery.
Stage 4—blepharoplasty.

It is important that surgery be performed in the correct order. For example if lid surgery is performed before orbital decompression, eyelid position may change after decompression so that lid surgery may have to be repeated.

Stage 1—orbital decompression

Indications

In general, orbital decompression should only be considered when non-invasive methods (i.e. systemic steroids and/or radiotherapy) have been tried and proved to be ineffective. The three main indications for orbital decompression are:

1. *Severe exposure keratopathy* secondary to proptosis and lid retraction.
2. *Compressive optic neuropathy* with imminent danger of permanent visual damage.
3. *Cosmetically unacceptable proptosis.* Because of the potential complications of surgical decompression, this indication applies only to a few carefully selected patients in whom the proptosis has been stable for at least 9 months.

Types

The four main operations used for orbital decompression are:

1. *'One-wall' decompression* can be of two types:
   a. *Lateral wall decompression* is seldom used alone as it achieves only about 2 mm of retroplacement of the globe.
   b. *Medial wall decompression* is also seldom used alone except in the rare event of optic neuropathy with minimal proptosis and marked enlargement of a medial rectus muscle.
2. *'Two-wall' (antral–ethmoidal) decompression* (*Figure 2.19*) in which part of the floor and the posterior portion of the medial wall are removed either via a translid, a forniceal or an antral approach. This is the most commonly used type of orbital decompression which achieves between 3 and 16 mm of retroplacement.
3. *'Three-wall' decompression* in which an antral–ethmoidal decompression is combined with removal of the lateral wall. The amount of retroplacement by this method is between 6 and 10 mm.
4. *'Four-wall' decompression* is a 'three-wall' decompression combined with removal of a large portion of the

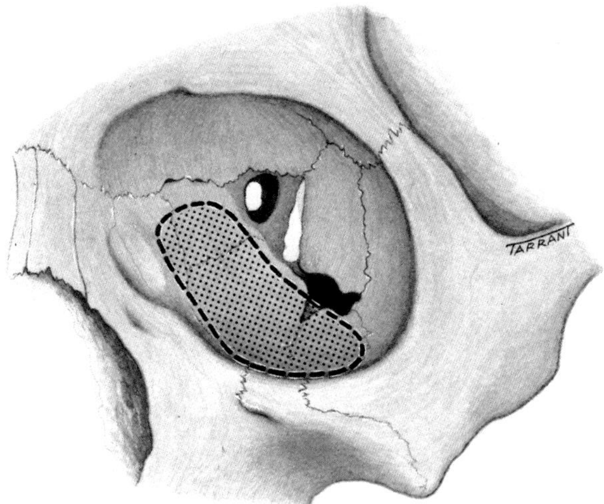

Figure 2.19 *Two-wall orbital decompression*

sphenoid bone at the apex of the orbit and the lateral half of the orbital roof. This achieves between 10 and 16 mm of retroplacement of the globe and is, therefore, reserved for the very rare cases of extremely severe proptosis.

Stage 2—extraocular muscle surgery

When to operate

Operation should only be performed when diplopia is present in the primary or reading positions of gaze or in both and the angle of deviation has been shown to be stable by performing regular Hess tests for at least 6 months; also when there is little or no evidence of congestive ophthalmopathy indicative of active disease.

Goals of surgery

The goals are to achieve binocular single vision in the primary position of gaze and when reading. Because restrictive thyroid myopathy causes an incomitant strabismus, the patient should be warned not to expect binocular single vision in all positions of gaze. However, with the passage of time the field of binocular single vision will probably enlarge due to increasing vergences.

Techniques

Surgery should be tailored to the individual muscle with most patients requiring surgery on the inferior recti and/or the medial recti. Recessions of the involved muscles using an adjustable suture are most effective (*see* Chapter 14). The suture is adjusted on the first postoperative day to obtain the optimal alignment, and the patient is encouraged to practice achieving single vision with a distant target such as a television. A recent study has reported promising results by injecting botulinum toxin into the involved muscles.

Stage 3—eyelid surgery

Lateral canthus surgery

This involves joining of the lateral aspect of the upper and lower eyelids. The two main indications are:

1. *Exposure keratopathy* uncontrolled by lubricants.
2. *Increase in vertical fissure* which is mild to moderate and cosmetically unacceptable.

Surgical techniques include:

1. *Lateral tarsorrhaphy* involving the stripping of the mucosa from the lid margin to create two raw edges and making a vertical incision 5 mm into the grey line. The raw edges are then united with a suture. The tarsorrhaphy can be further opened or closed as necessary.
2. *Lateral canthorrhaphy* is similar to a tarsorrhaphy except that the anterior lid margin including the eyelashes is excised. This causes a permanent inward of the lateral canthus so that a canthorrhaphy is very difficult to open.

Surgery on lid retractors

This involves weakening of the lid retractors in order to decrease the vertical palpebral fissure.

1. *Excision of Müller's muscle* reduces the palpebral fissure by about 2 mm.
2. *Levator and Müller's muscle recession* is necessary if a reduction of more than 2 mm is required (*Figure 2.20*).

Stage 4—blepharoplasty

This involves the removal of excess fatty tissue and redundant skin from around the eyelids.

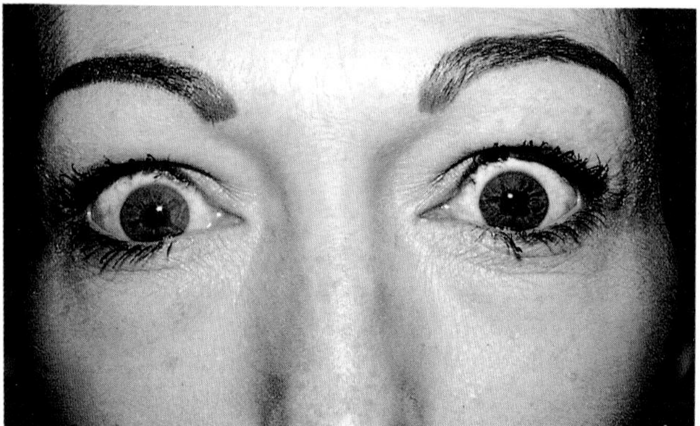

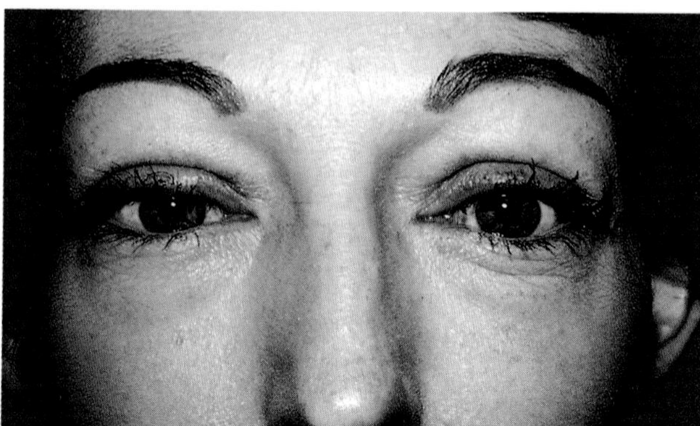

Figure 2.20 *Left: preoperative appearance; right: appearance following recession of levator and Müller's muscle*

Fractures

Blow-out fractures of orbital floor

The term 'pure blow-out fracture of the orbit' is used to describe a specific type of orbital fracture which is not associated with involvement of the orbital rim. It is typically caused by a sudden increase in the orbital pressure by a striking object which is greater than 5 cm in diameter, such as a fist or a tennis ball (*Figure 2.21*). Because the bones of the lateral wall and the roof are usually able to withstand raised intraorbital pressure, the fracture usually involves the floor of the orbit along the thin bone covering the infraorbital canal. Occasionally, the medial orbital floor may be fractured.

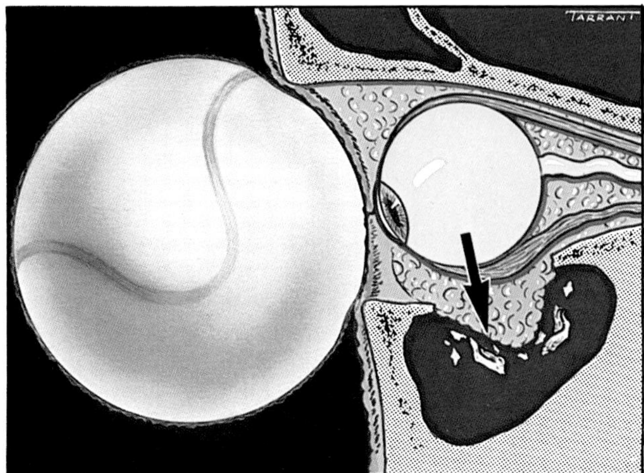

Figure 2.21 *Blow-out fracture of orbital floor*

Clinical features

The clinical features of a blow-out fracture vary according to the severity of trauma and the time interval between the fracture and the examination.

1. *Periocular ecchymosis and oedema* are common initial findings.
2. *Enophthalmos* is usually initially absent because of associated orbital oedema or haemorrhage and, in fact, occasionally the globe may be slightly proptotic. In significant fractures, enophthalmos may develop after about 10 days to 2 weeks as the oedema subsides. Its progression should be evaluated by taking regular readings with an exophthalmometer. In the absence of surgical intervention, the severity of enophthalmos may then continue to increase for about 6 months as post-traumatic orbital degeneration and fibrosis develop.
3. *Infraorbital nerve anaesthesia* (lower lid, cheek, side of nose, upper lip and upper teeth) is very common because a blow-out fracture typically begins along the medial edge of the infraorbital canal and extends nasally.
4. *Diplopia* due to mechanical tethering of either the muscle or adjacent orbital connective tissue along the fracture line is common except in very small fractures. The diplopia typically occurs in both up- and down-gaze (double diplopia). The presence of muscle restriction can be confirmed by positive forced duction and differential intraocular pressure tests. The extent and progression of diplopia can be followed by performing the Hess or Lees test (*see* Chapter 14). The field of binocular single vision can be assessed on the Lister or Goldmann perimenter (*see* Chapter 7).
5. *Nasal bleeding* may initially be present as a result of haemorrhage from the maxillary sinus into the nose.
6. *Periocular subcutaneous emphysema* occurs more frequently with medial wall than with floor fractures. It may be made worse by blowing the nose.
7. *Ocular damage.* Although subconjunctival haemorrhage is frequent, severe ocular damage is rare. This is because a blow-out fracture is nature's way of protecting the globe from injury. Nevertheless the eye should be carefully examined to exclude the possibility of intraocular damage (e.g. hyphaema, angle recession, retinal dialysis).

Special investigations

1. *Plain X-rays.* The most useful projection for detecting an orbital floor fracture is a Waters' view (*see Figure 2.7*). However, in some cases a plain X-ray may show a soft tissue density in the antrum in the absence of a fracture.
2. *CT scanning* permits visualization of the soft tissue structures in more detail than a plain X-ray. Coronal sections are particularly useful in evaluating the extent of the fracture, as well as determining the nature of antral soft tissue densities which may represent prolapsed orbital fat, extraocular muscles, haematoma, or unrelated antral polyps.

Treatment

The two main aims of treatment are: to prevent permanent vertical diplopia and/or cosmetically unacceptable enophthalmos. The three factors that determine the risk of these late complications are: fracture size, herniation of orbital contents into the maxillary sinus, and muscle entrapment. Although there may be some overlap, most fractures will fall into one of the following categories:

1. Small cracks in the floor unassociated with herniation. These do not require treatment as the risk of permanent complications is negligible.
2. Fracture involving less than half of the orbital floor, with little or no herniation, and rapidly improving diplopia. Here again surgery is unnecessary unless more than 2 mm of enophthalmos develops.
3. Fractures involving half or more of the orbital floor with entrapment of orbital contents and persistent and

significant diplopia. These are associated with a high risk of permanent complications and should be repaired within 2 weeks. If surgery is delayed, the results are less satisfactory because of the development of secondary fibrotic changes in the orbit.

Surgical technique

The periosteum is elevated from the floor of the orbit and all entrapped orbital contents are removed from the antrum. The defect in the floor is then repaired by using bone grafts or synthetic material.

Blow-out fracture of medial wall

This may occur in isolation. Surgical intervention is seldom necessary unless the medial rectus is entrapped.

Roof fractures

These are usually caused by the patient falling on a sharp object. They are characterized by ipsilateral periocular ecchymosis which later spreads to the opposite side. Occasionally, leakage of CSF may occur and the fracture may be complicated by meningitis.

Vascular abnormalities

Varix

The most common orbital vascular lesion is a varix, which is a pathological enlargement of one or more pre-existing venous channels (*Figure 2.22*). A varix typically presents with intermittent proptosis which is non-pulsatile and not associated with a bruit. Not infrequently, the proptosis can be precipitated by the Valsalva manoeuvre or compression of the jugular veins. Plain X-rays may show phleboliths.

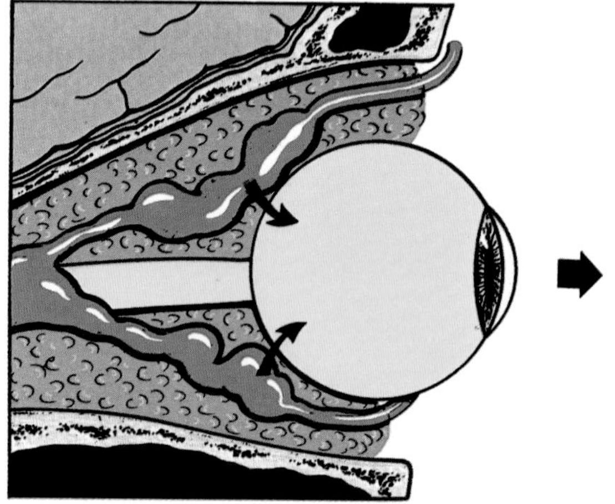

Figure 2.22 *Proptosis from orbital varices*

Arteriovenous communications

See Chapter 15.

Infections

Cellulitis

Preseptal

This is frequently preceded by dental or sinus infection, or a history of sharp or blunt trauma, and is characterized by periorbital swelling and tenderness (*Figure 2.23*). The infection does not penetrate the orbital septum which separates the anterior structures from the orbit.

Treatment is with oral antibiotics on an outpatient basis.

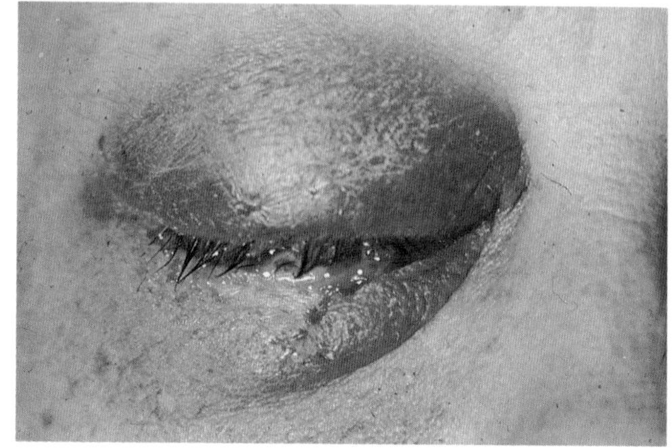

Figure 2.23 *Preseptal cellulitis*

Orbital

Orbital cellulitis is much less common but potentially very much more serious than preseptal cellulitis. The infection most frequently spreads to the orbit from the nasopharynx or from the frontal, maxillary or ethmoidal sinus. Sphenoidal sinusitis is, however, uncommon. The most common causative organisms are *Streptococcus pneumoniae, Staphylococcus aureus, Streptococcus pyogenes* and, in children under the age of 5 years, *Haemophilus influenzae.*

Clinical features

The patient is usually a child or a young adult who presents with a relatively sudden onset of unilateral chemosis, pain, lid oedema, reduction of ocular movements and proptosis, which is most frequently laterally and downwards. Unless treated promptly with appropriate antibiotics, the potentially lethal systemic complications are meningitis, brain abscess, and cavernous sinus thrombosis. The most serious ocular complication is blindness from occlusion of the central retinal artery and contiguous inflammation of the optic nerve.

Management

The patient should be admitted to hospital immediately.

Investigations

The patient is frequently pyrexial but may have a normal erythrocyte sedimentation rate and white blood cell count. Nasal and conjunctival cultures are seldom helpful and are rarely positive for the offending organism. About 70% of patients show X-ray evidence of sinusitis. In adults the frontal, maxillary and ethmoidal sinuses show equal involvement, in contradistinction to the ethmoidal sinus in younger children. Ultrasound may be useful in detecting the development of an orbital abscess.

Antibiotic therapy

1. *In children* under the age of 5 years the antibiotics should cover *Haemophilus influenzae.* Ampicillin 200 mg/kg per day in divided doses combined with a penicillinase-resistant antibiotic (nafcillin or oxacillin 100 mg/kg per day) administered parenterally.
2. *In adults* the treatment is with a high intravenous dose of penicillin (2000 000 units) alternating with nafcillin or oxacillin 1.5 mg every 4 hours. This should be given so that the patient receives the antibiotics every 2 hours.

If the patient has a history of non-anaphylactic reaction to penicillin, cefotaxime 1–2 g every 6 hours should be substituted. In the case of previous anaphylactic reaction to penicillin or its derivatives, the patient should be treated with clindamycin, chloramphenicol or vancomycin.

Surgery

Indications for surgical intervention include unresponsiveness to antibiotics, decreasing vision, presence of an orbital (*Figure 2.24*) or subperiosteal abscess, and the need for a diagnostic biopsy in atypical cases. In most cases, it is necessary to drain the orbit as well as the infected sinuses.

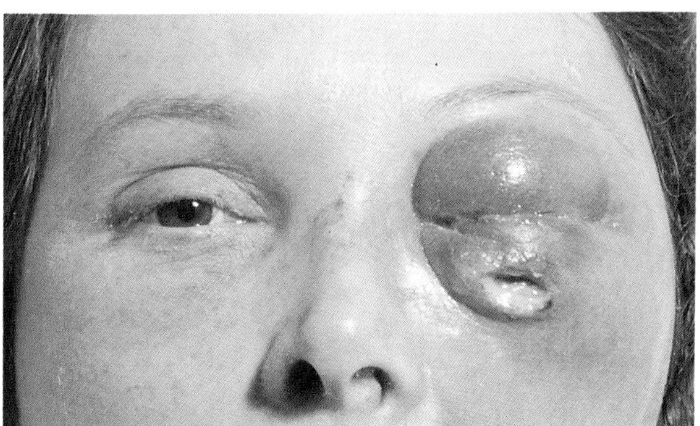

Figure 2.24 *Discharging orbital abscess*

Mucormycosis

Rhino-orbital mucormycosis is a very rare opportunistic infection caused by fungi of the order Mucorales. Mucormycosis has a very high morbidity and mortality, and typically affects patients with diabetic ketoacidosis or severely debilitating diseases (e.g. carcinomatosis, lymphoma etc.).

Clinical features

The inhalation of spores causes an oropharyngitis and nasopharyngitis. The fungus then may spread to contiguous structures, such as the paranasal sinuses, and subsequently to the orbit, meninges and brain by direct extension. The infection preferentially invades the walls of blood vessels resulting in vascular occlusion, thrombosis, and infarction. Ischaemic infarction superimposed upon septic necrosis is responsible for the black eschar, an important diagnostic sign, which may develop on the palate, turbinate, nasal septum or skin. Orbital invasion, which is usually unilateral, is characterized by the development of cellulitis, chemosis, proptosis, ophthalmoplegia, headache, and acute visual loss. The fungi may grow into the brain, either via the ophthalmic vessels or across the infarcted walls of the paranasal air sinuses. This may give rise to convulsions, contralateral hemiplegia, multiple cranial nerve palsies, and coma.

Management

This consists of the following:

1. Correction of the underlying metabolic derangement.
2. Intravenous amphotericin B.
3. Wide excision of devitalized and necrotic tissues.
4. Daily packing and irrigation of the involved areas with amphotericin B.
5. Orbital exenteration may be necessary in very severe and unresponsive cases.

Inflammatory disease (pseudotumour)

Inflammatory orbital disease (IOD) is a general term for relatively rare, idiopathic, non-neoplastic, space-occupying periocular lesions. The inflammatory process may involve any or all of the soft tissue components of the orbit. Because, on occasion, IOD may simulate an orbital neoplasm, the condition is also referred to as the orbital 'pseudotumour syndrome'. Histopathological analyses have so far failed to show any correlation between clinical and pathological features and the subsequent course of the disease.

Clinical features

IOD typically affects middle-aged individuals. Most cases are unilateral, although both sides may be involved at different times (*Figure 2.25*). The onset is usually abrupt with pain, lid oedema, chemosis, conjunctival injection, limitation of gaze and proptosis. Dependent on the site of primary involvement, a palpable mass may be present or absent. This clinical presentation differs from thyroid ophthalmopathy which has a more gradual onset and is usually associated with eyelid retraction and lag. IOD may, on occasion, be confused with orbital cellulitis. The latter, however, usually affects children and IOD typically affects middle-aged individuals.

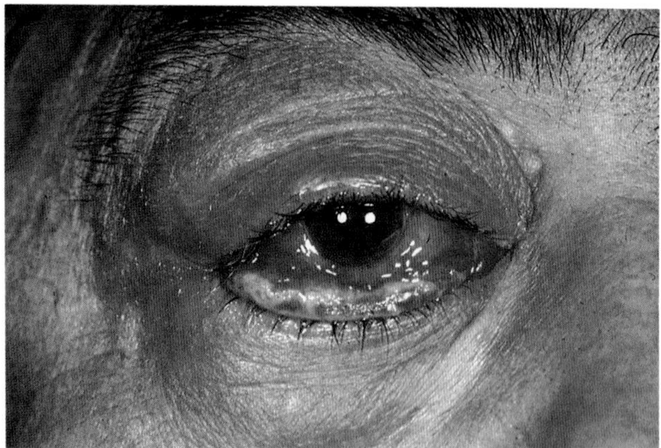

Figure 2.25 *Orbital pseudotumour (courtesy of Mr A. Shun-Shin)*

Special investigations

CT scanning may show muscle enlargement and scleral thickening. Ultrasound may demonstrate sonolucency (oedema) posterior to the globe, a squaring-off of the posterior normal W-shaped optic nerve area, and thickening of the extraocular muscles.

Clinical course

IOD may follow one of the following clinical courses:

1. Spontaneous remission after a few weeks without sequelae.
2. Prolonged and intermittent episodes of activity with eventual remission.
3. Severe prolonged inflammation eventually leading to progressive fibrosis of orbital tissues resulting in a 'frozen orbit' which may be associated with visual impairment and ptosis.

Treatment

The following therapeutic options should be considered.

Observation

Some cases are relatively mild and remit spontaneously within a few weeks and require no specific treatment.

Systemic corticosteroids

These should be used in patients with moderate to severe involvement. The initial dose is between 60 and 80 mg/day for about 2 weeks. If there is a good response, the dose is gradually tapered and reintroduced in the event of recurrence. Between 50 and 75% of patients will show a favourable response to steroids.

Radiotherapy

This should be considered if there has been no improvement after 2 weeks of *adequate* steroid therapy. However, prior to the initiation of orbital irradiation, a biopsy should be performed to rule out a tumour. About 75% of patients respond to 25 Gy given in 12 fractions. Even a low dose of 10 Gy may produce long-term and sometimes permanent remission in patients who are steroid resistant. Lesions initially responsive to steroids are also likely to be responsive to radiotherapy.

Cytotoxic agents

Agents such as cyclophosphamide 200 mg/day may be necessary in the relatively few cases who are resistant to both steroids and radiotherapy.

Variants of the pseudotumour syndrome

Bilateral pseudotumour

In children, about one in three idiopathic pseudotumours is bilateral. In adults, however, the presence of bilateral involvement should raise suspicion of a coexisting systemic disease such as polyarteritis nodosa, Wegener's granulomatosis, tuberculosis, sarcoidosis, or Waldenström's macroglobulinaemia.

Orbital myositis

This is an immunologically induced inflammation which usually affects one extraocular muscle. Two forms are recognized.

Acute

This is characterized by a sudden onset of redness and pain over the involved muscle. When the patient attempts to move the eye in the field of action of the involved muscle, the pain is worsened and he experiences diplopia due to its underaction. The clinical course is usually short and the response to systemic steroids good. Recurrences may occur in certain patients.

Chronic

This is characterized by less prominent pain and, on cursory examination, it may be mistaken for thyroid ophthalmopathy. However, in myositis the eye cannot move in the direction of the involved muscle, whereas in thyroid ophthalmopathy the reverse is true. Patients with chronic myositis do not usually respond well to systemic corticosteroids and may require radiotherapy to the involved muscle.

Tolosa–Hunt syndrome

This rare condition is characterized by unilateral ocular cranial nerve palsies with ipsilateral periorbital or hemicranial pain, pupillomotor dysfunction, and sensory loss along the distribution of the first and second divisions of the trigeminal nerve. The syndrome is thought to be caused by a non-specific granulomatous inflammation of the cavernous sinus and should be differentiated from a variety of other diseases that involve the orbital apex, the superior orbital fissure, or the cavernous sinus, such as specific inflammatory processes, vascular and traumatic lesions, and tumours. The clinical course of the Tolosa–Hunt syndrome is characterized by spontaneous remissions and recurrences and an excellent response to systemic steroid therapy.

Orbital and sinus pseudotumour

Simultaneous orbital and sinus involvement by pseudotumour seems to be a distinct clinicopathological entity.

Tumours

Classification

- Vascular
  - capillary haemangioma
  - cavernous haemangioma
  - lymphangioma
- Lacrimal gland
  - mixed cell
  - malignant
- Lymphoproliferative
- Rhabdomyosarcoma
- Histiocytic
  - Letterer–Siwe
  - Hand–Schüller–Christian
  - eosinophilic granuloma
- Cystic lesions
  - dermoid cyst
  - blood cyst
  - mucocele
- Neural
  - optic nerve glioma
  - optic nerve sheath meningioma
- Metastases
- Invasion from adjacent structures

Vascular

Vascular tumours are the most common primary benign tumours of the orbit.

Capillary haemangioma

Clinical features

This tumour typically presents at birth, or soon after, as a periocular swelling which is usually situated in the anterior part of the orbit (*Figure 2.26*). It typically increases in size during crying or straining, but is not associated with either pulsation or a bruit. Not infrequently, haemangiomatous tissue can be seen in the fornices on everting the lids. The lesion may also involve the surrounding subcutaneous tissues giving the eyelids a darkish red or bluish discolouration. Superficial 'strawberry' naevi may also be found on the eyelids (*see Figure 1.8*) or other parts of the body in about one out of three patients. The natural course of the tumour is similar to that of a capillary haemangioma in other parts of the body. During the first year of life, it may undergo periods of growth, followed by stabilization and then eventual regression and disappearance by the age of about 5 years.

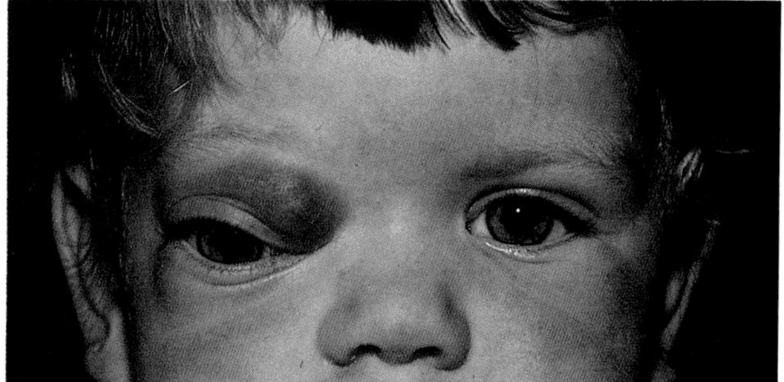

Figure 2.26 *Capillary haemangioma (courtesy of Mr A. Fielder)*

Management

Indications for treatment include the possibility of amblyopia (vision deprivation, or anisometropic), optic nerve compression, and exposure keratopathy, and if the lesion causes a significant blemish. Methods of treatment include systemic corticosteroids, injection of steroids into the tumour, radiation therapy and, occasionally, surgical excision using a cutting diathermy. The injection of sclerosing solutions and cryotherapy are of limited value and should be avoided.

Cavernous haemangioma

Clinical features

This is the most common benign orbital tumour in adults, typically presenting during the second to fourth decades of life as a slowly progressive unilateral proptosis. In women the growth rate may be accelerated by pregnancy. The tumour is usually located within the muscle cone behind the globe and gives rise to an axial proptosis. Occasionally, a cavernous haemangioma situated at the orbital apex may compress the optic nerve without causing much proptosis.

Special investigations

1. *Ultrasound* shows a characteristic pattern with a hard surface and high internal reflectivity.
2. *CT scan* shows a well circumscribed lesion without bony erosion.

Treatment

Unlike the capillary haemangioma, the cavernous variety is usually well encapsulated and easy to remove. Because the tumour is commonly situated within the muscle cone, a lateral orbitotomy is required.

Lymphangioma

Clinical features

This histologically benign but potentially 'aggressive' tumour typically presents with a slowly progressive proptosis in a young person. Occasionally, the proptosis becomes rapidly progressive and is associated with pain due to bleeding from the tumour. The blood subsequently becomes encysted with the formation of so-called 'chocolate cysts', which may regress spontaneously with the passage of time.

Management

Because the tumour is not encapsulated and is friable, surgical excision may be difficult. If the 'chocolate cysts' persist and threaten the patient's vision, they should be drained.

Lacrimal gland

About 50% of all lacrimal gland tumours consist of inflammations and lymphoid proliferations, and the remainder are of epithelial origin. About half of the latter are benign mixed-cell tumours and half are carcinomas.

Of all patients whose tumours are derived from epithelial elements, 75% present with proptosis and 50% have a palpable mass in the lacrimal gland fossa. A careful palpation of the fossa is therefore crucial in the evaluation of all patients with proptosis.

Mixed-cell tumour

This tumour exhibits a broad spectrum of histological patterns and its clinical course is not always benign, as recurrences following incomplete surgical excision are common.

Clinical features

A benign mixed-cell tumour presents as a painless, slowly progressive swelling in the lacrimal fossa, with or without proptosis. The swelling is smooth, firm, non-tender, and confined to the region of the lacrimal gland. The slow growth rate and the initially benign nature of the tumour can be confirmed by X-ray findings of a pressure indentation of the lacrimal fossa without evidence of bony destruction.

Special investigations

CT scanning is very useful in confirming the diagnosis. It shows the tumour to be round or oval, encapsulated, and located within the lacrimal fossa. Dacryoadenitis has a more oblong appearance on CT. Malignant tumours characteristically show bony involvement, consisting of hyperostosis, sclerosis, or erosion.

Treatment

This is by an *en-bloc* excision through a lateral orbitotomy. It is extremely important to preserve the capsule of the tumour in order to prevent recurrence and, for this reason, a biopsy of a mixed-cell tumour is contraindicated.

Malignant tumours

Clinical features

Adenoid cystic carcinoma ('cylindroma'), adenocarcinoma, mucoepidermoid carcinoma and, occasionally, malignant mixed-cell tumours have a more rapid rate of growth than benign mixed-cell tumours. In early cases, X-ray findings may be negative, but as the tumour grows it destroys bone and causes pain.

Management

A biopsy should be performed first, followed by exenteration and removal of bone that is suspected of being involved. Unfortunately, the tumour is frequently beyond surgical excision when the diagnosis is made, and the only treatment that can be offered to the patient is palliative radiotherapy.

Lymphoproliferative disorders

Clinical features

Lymphoproliferative disorders of the orbit (*Figure 2.27*) usually affect patients over the age of 60 years and can involve any part of the orbit. Occasionally, they may be localized to the conjunctiva or lacrimal gland.

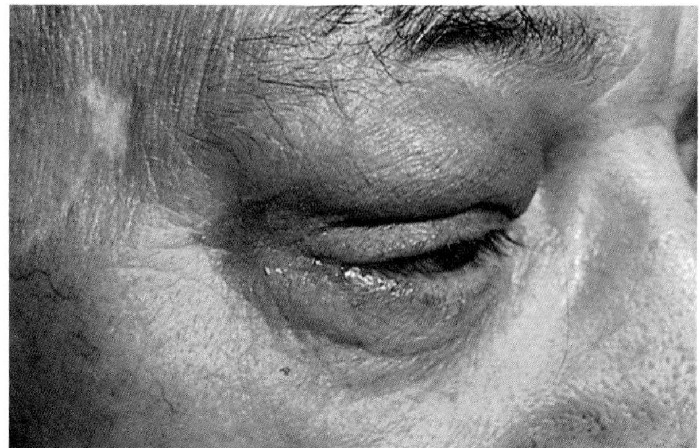

Figure 2.27 *Orbital lymphoma*

Bilateral involvement is an occasional feature. Although histological studies will usually allow an unequivocal distinction to be made between inflammatory lesions and frank malignant lymphomas, in some cases the histological features raise suspicion of malignancy and yet the lesion resolves spontaneously or with the help of systemic corticosteroid therapy. In other patients, what looks like a benign reactive lymphoid hyperplasia may be followed several years later by the development of a systemic lymphoma. For this reason, all patients with both benign and malignant hypercellular lymphoid lesions of the orbit should have a thorough systemic evaluation including chest X-ray, serum immunoprotein electrophoresis (and if necessary bone marrow aspiration), and lymphangiography for the detection of retroperitoneal involvement.

It therefore appears that some lesions occupy an intermediate position, making an accurate histological differentiation impossible, so that the true diagnosis can only be made in retrospect when a long-term follow-up fails to show any evidence of multifocal dissemination.

Management

Radiotherapy is the only method of treatment. Benign lesions are treated by 10–30 Gy, while malignant lesions need higher doses. Disseminated disease is treated by chemotherapy.

Rhabdomyosarcoma

Clinical features

The rhabdomyosarcoma is the most common primary malignant orbital tumour in children (*Figure 2.28*). It typically presents at about the age of 7 years as a rapidly progressive proptosis. Occasionally, this mode of presentation may be mistaken for an inflammatory process. Although the tumour can involve any part of the orbit, it typically presents with a mass in the superonasal quadrant. The three histological types of rhabdomyosarcoma are:

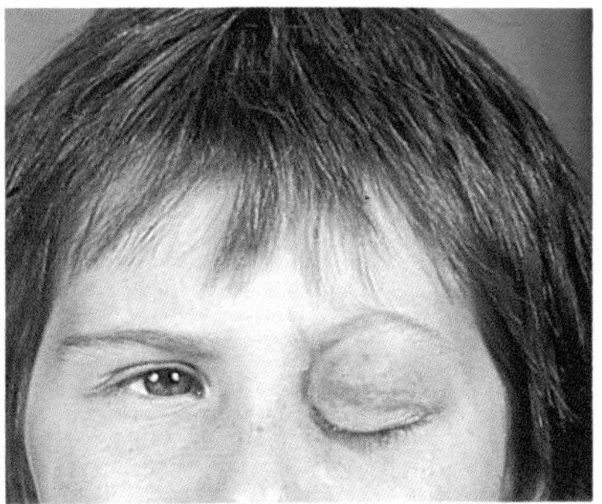

Figure 2.28 *Rhabdomyosarcoma (courtesy of Mr C. Migdal)*

1. *Embryonal.*
2. *Alveolar*—this is the most malignant.
3. *Pleomorphic*—this has the best prognosis but is the rarest.

Special investigations

CT scan. The tumour appears to arise from an extraocular muscle and the presence of bony involvement implies a poor prognosis for life.

Treatment

After the diagnosis has been confirmed by biopsy, treatment is by combined radiotherapy and chemotherapy. The survival rate is 90% when the tumour is confined to the orbit and 65% in the presence of bony destruction and extension. In unresponsive cases death usually occurs within 18 months. Exenteration is now seldom used.

Histiocytic

Histiocytosis X refers to a group of very rare diseases that primarily affect children. They have a variable clinical course, but share a common histopathological abnormality which consists of abnormal proliferations of histiocytes with granuloma formation. The orbital bones are involved in about 20% of cases. The ophthalmologist may see a patient with known disseminated involvement who develops proptosis during the course of the disease, or less frequently with proptosis as the presenting feature. The three diseases which are grouped together as histiocytosis X are given below.

Letterer–Siwe disease

This is a disease in which orbital involvement is relatively rare. It typically affects infants and has a subacute and sometimes fatal course with widespread soft tissue and visceral involvement with or without bony changes.

Hand–Schüller–Christian disease

This disease consists of a triad of proptosis, diabetes insipidus and bony defects in the skull. The disease has a slower rate of progression than Letterer–Siwe disease, although occasionally the eponym is used to describe the chronic disseminated form of histiocytosis X involving both soft tissues and bone.

Eosinophilic granuloma

This frequently involves the orbital bones. Although initially this subgroup was used to describe a single histiocytic lesion in bone, it is now used to describe a condition where the lesions, which may be multiple, are confined to bone.

Management

1. Nil as some patients with mild involvement may have a spontaneous regression.
2. Surgery to curette or excise a single bony lesion.
3. Radiotherapy for advanced bony lesions.
4. Systemic steroids may be beneficial in some patients.
5. Chemotherapy (vincristine or vinblastine) for patients with disseminated disease.

Cystic lesions

Dermoid cysts

Dermoids are common developmental choristomas believed to result from an embryonic displacement of epidermis to a subcutaneous location. They are characteristically lined by keratinizing epithelium and may contain sebaceous glands and hair follicles. Dermoids may occur in two clinical settings:

Simple

These typically present in infancy as an asymptomatic firm, round localized lesion in the upper temporal or upper nasal aspect of the orbit. They have easily palpable posterior margins denoting lack of deeper origin or extension. They are not associated with bony defects and neither displace the globe nor give rise to proptosis because they are located anterior to the orbital septum.

Complicated

These typically present in adolescence or adult life with proptosis or a mass lesion with indistinct posterior margins. They arise from deeper sites and are frequently misdiagnosed as to extent and complexity. Some deep dermoids may extend beyond the orbit into the temporalis fossa or intracranially, and they may be associated with bony defects.

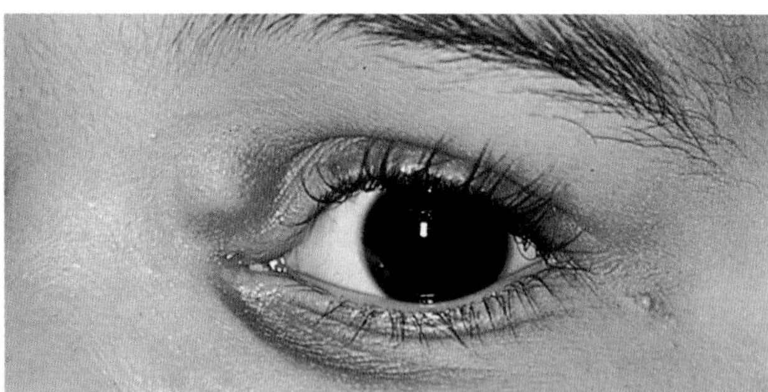

Figure 2.29 *Dermoid cyst*

Blood cysts

Haematic (blood) cysts of the orbit are relatively rare and may be associated with blunt orbital trauma, lymphangioma, blood dyscrasia, and cavernous haemangioma. Clinically, they appear as progressive, non-tender space-occupying lesions which enlarge by absorbing fluid into the cyst cavity due to an osmotic pressure gradient caused by haematogenous debris within the cyst cavity. Rarely, they may be mistaken for malignant tumours because they may cause proptosis and erosion of orbital bones.

Mucoceles

A mucocele is a slowly expanding cystic accumulation of mucoid secretions and epithelial debris which gradually erodes the bony walls of the sinuses and causes symptoms by encroaching on surrounding tissues. A mucocele develops when the drainage of normal sinus secretions is obstructed, from scarring, infection or tumour. Orbital invasion usually occurs from either frontal or ethmoidal mucoceles and only very rarely from those arising in the maxillary sinus.

Metastases

In children

Neuroblastoma. About 40% of children with neuroblastoma will have orbital metastases at some time during the course of the disease. The deposits may be bilateral and typically present with an abrupt onset of proptosis accompanied by lid ecchymosis.

Ewing's sarcoma is a malignant tumour of bone which can also cause an abrupt haemorrhagic proptosis. Unlike those in neuroblastoma, the deposits are usually unilateral.

Others. In children, other causes of secondary deposits include leukaemia and Wilms' tumour.

In adults

In adults, the most common primary sites for tumours that metastatize to the orbit are the bronchus, the breast, the prostate, the kidney, and the gastrointestinal tract.

Treatment of orbital metastases is usually palliative local radiotherapy. CT scanning may be helpful in following the response to treatment.

Invasion from adjacent structures

Orbital invasion by malignant tumours of the paranasal and nasal sinuses occurs in about 50% of patients. Although these tumours are rare, they carry a poor prognosis unless diagnosed early. It is therefore important for the ophthalmologist to be aware of the otolaryngological as well as the ophthalmic features of these tumours. By far the most common tumour to invade the orbit is squamous carcinoma of the maxillary antrum (*Figure 2.30*).

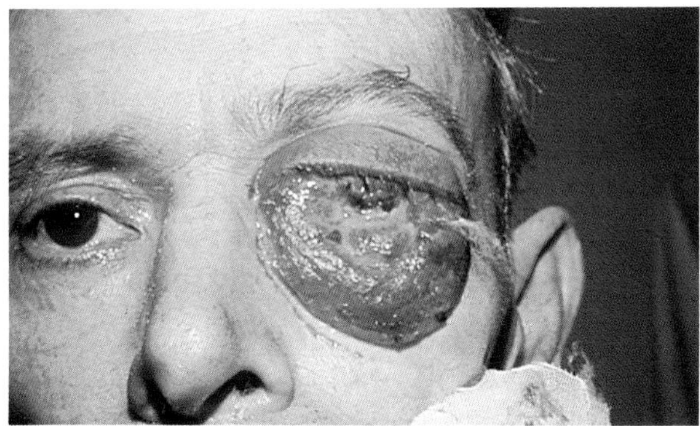

Figure 2.30 *Carcinoma of maxillary antrum invading orbit (courtesy of Mr R. Packard)*

Otolaryngological features in order of importance include:

1. Facial pain.
2. Facial congestion and swelling.
3. Epistaxis.
4. Nasal discharge.

Ophthalmic features in order of importance include:

1. Proptosis in which the globe is usually displaced upwards and anteriorly.
2. Diplopia.
3. Visual loss.
4. Ocular pain.
5. Epiphora.

Carcinoma arising from the ethmoid sinuses may displace the globe laterally. Frontal and sphenoidal carcinomas are rare. Nasopharyngeal carcinomas may spread into the orbit through the inferior orbital fissure. Proptosis is invariably a late finding.

Neural tumours

Neural tumours (optic nerve glioma, optic nerve sheath meningioma) are discussed in Chapter 15.

Further reading

Evaluation of orbital disease

Bullock, J.D. and Bartley, G.B. (1986) Dynamic proptosis. *American Journal of Ophthalmology,* **102,** 104–110

Char, D.H., Sobel, D., Kelly, W.M. *et al.* (1985) Magnetic resonance scanning in orbital tumour diagnosis. *Ophthalmology,* **92,** 1305–1310

Cline, R.A. and Rootman, J. (1984) Enophthalmos: A clinical review. *Ophthalmology,* **91,** 229–237

Kincaid, M.C. and Green, W.R. (1984) Diagnostic methods in orbital disease. *Ophthalmology,* **91,** 719–725

Kline, L.B. (1985) Computed tomography in ophthalmology. *Clinical Modules in Ophthalmology,* Vol. 3, Module 9

Thyroid eye disease

Dixon, R. (1982) The surgical management of thyroid related upper eyelid retraction. *Ophthalmology,* **89,** 52–57

Evans, D. and Kennerdell, J.S. (1983) Extraocular muscle surgery for thyroid myopathy. *American Journal of Ophthalmology,* **95,** 767–771

Hurbli, T., Char, D.H., Harris, J. *et al.* (1985) Radiation therapy for thyroid eye disease. *American Journal of Ophthalmology,* **99,** 633–637

Leone, C.R. Jr (1984) The management of ophthalmic Graves' disease. *Ophthalmology,* **91,** 770–779

McCord, C.D. Jr (1985) Current trends in orbital decompression. *Ophthalmology,* **92,** 21–33

Panzo, G.J. and Tomsak, R.L. (1983) A retrospective review of 26 cases of dysthyroid optic neuropathy. *American Journal of Ophthalmology,* **96,** 190–194

Shorr, N. and Sieff, S.R. (1986) The four stages of surgical rehabilitation of the patient with dysthyroid ophthalmopathy. *Ophthalmology,* **88,** 479–483

Orbital fractures

Hawes, M.J. and Dortzbach, R.K. (1983) Surgery on orbital floor fractures. *Ophthalmology,* **90,** 1066–1070

Nunery, W.R. (1986) Diagnosis and management of blunt ocular trauma. *Clinical Modules for Ophthalmologists,* Vol. 4, Module 11

Wilkins, R.B. and Havins, W.E. (1982) Current treatment of blow-out fractures. *Ophthalmology,* **89,** 464–466

Orbital infections

Bergin, D.J. and Wright, J.E. (1986) Orbital cellulitis. *British Journal of Ophthalmology,* **70,** 174–178

Ferry, A.P. and Abedi, S. (1983) Diagnosis and management of rhino-orbitocerebral mucormycosis. *Ophthalmology,* **90,** 1096–1104

Krohel, G.B., Krauss, H.R. and Winnick, J. (1982) Orbital abscess—presentation, diagnosis, therapy, and sequelae. *Ophthalmology,* **89,** 492–498

Macy, J.I., Mandelbaum, S.H. and Minckler, D.S. (1980) Orbital cellulitis. *Ophthalmology,* **87,** 1309–1313

Weiss, A., Friendly, D., Eglin, K. *et al.* (1983) Bacterial periorbital and orbital cellulitis in childhood. *Ophthalmology,* **90,** 195–203

Inflammatory orbital disease

Leone, C.R. Jr and Lloyd, W.C. (1985) Treatment protocol for orbital inflammatory disease. *Ophthalmology,* **92,** 1325–1331

Orcutt, J.C., Garner, A., Henk, J.M. *et al.* (1983) Treatment of idiopathic inflammatory orbital tumours by radiotherapy. *British Journal of Ophthalmology,* **67,** 570–574

Rootman, J. and Nugent, R. (1982) The classification and management of acute orbital pseudotumours. *Ophthalmology,* **89,** 1040–1048

Slavin, M.L. and Glaser, J.S. (1982) Idiopathic orbital myositis. *Archives of Ophthalmology,* **100,** 1261–1265

Weinstein, G.S., Dresner, S.C., Slamovits, T.L. *et al.* (1983) Acute and subacute orbital myositis. *Ophthalmology,* **96,** 209–217

Orbital tumours

Garner, A., Rahi, A.H.S. and Wright, J.E. (1983) Lymphoproliferative disorders of the orbit: an immunological approach to diagnosis and pathogenesis. *British Journal of Ophthalmology*, **67**, 561–569

Ghafoor, S.Y.A. and Dudgeon, J. (1985) Orbital rhabdomyosarcoma: improved survival with combined chemotherapy and irradiation. *British Journal of Ophthalmology*, **69**, 557–561

Johnson, L.N., Krohel, G.B., Yeon, E.B. *et al.* (1984) Sinus tumours invading the orbit. *Ophthalmology*, **91**, 209–271

Kushner, B.J. (1982) Intralesional corticosteroid injection for infantile adnexal hemangioma. *American Journal of Ophthalmology*, **93**, 496–506

Moore, A.T., Pritchard, J. and Taylor, D.S.I. (1985) Histiocytosis X: an ophthalmological review. *British Journal of Ophthalmology*, **69**, 7–14

Ruchman, M.C. and Flanagan, J. (1983) Cavernous haemangioma of the orbit. *Ophthalmology*, **90**, 1328–1336

Sherman, R.P., Rootman, J. and Lapointe, J.S. (1984) Orbital dermoids: clinical presentation and management. *British Journal of Ophthalmology*, **68**, 642–652

Shields, J.A., Bakewell, B., Augsburger, J.J. *et al.* (1984) Classification and incidence of space-occupying lesions of the orbit. *Archives of Ophthalmology*, **102**, 1606–1611

Wright, J.E., Stewart, W.B. and Krohel, G.B. (1979) Clinical presentation and management of lacrimal gland tumours. *British Journal of Ophthalmology*, **63**, 600–606

3

The Lacrimal System

The dry eye

Applied anatomy

Applied physiology

Causes of aqueous tear deficiency (keratoconjunctivitis sicca)

Causes of mucin deficiency

Clinical evaluation

Special tests

Treatment

The watering eye

Applied anatomy

Applied physiology

Causes

Clinical evaluation

Special investigations

Treatment

Surgical techniques

Infection of lacrimal passages

Canaliculitis

Dacryocystitis

Tumours of the lacrimal sac

The dry eye

Applied anatomy

Main lacrimal gland

About 95% of the aqueous component of tears is produced by the main lacrimal gland which consists of two portions: the *orbital* portion which lies in a fossa on the frontal bone and a smaller *palpebral* portion. The palpebral portion may be prolapsed by asking the patient to look down and in, while the outer part of the upper lid is elevated and the lateral canthus pulled temporally (*Figure 3.1*). The secretions of the lobular acini of the lacrimal gland pass first into fine interlobular ductules and finally into about 12 definitive secretory ducts which open into the upper fornix approximately 5 mm above the upper border of the tarsal plate.

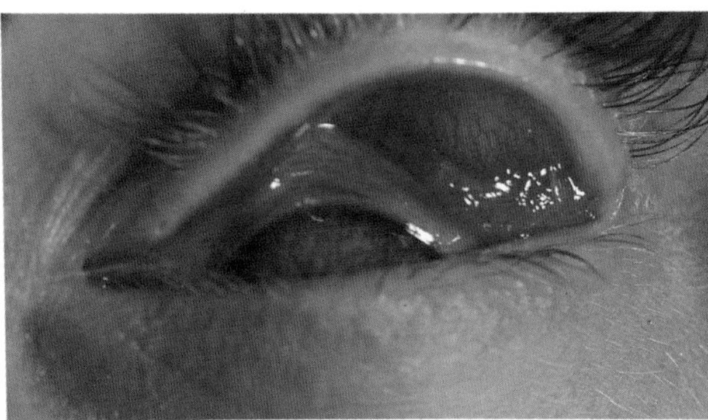

Figure 3.1 *Palpebral portion of lacrimal gland*

Accessory lacrimal glands

About 5% of the aqueous component of tears is produced by the accessory lacrimal glands of Krause and Wolfring. About 40 accessory glands of Krause are located in the substantia propria of the lateral aspect of the upper forniceal conjunctiva, while a further six to eight open into the lower fornix. Two to five accessory glands of Wolfring are found at the centre of the superior border of the upper tarsal plate, and two in the inferior border of the lower tarsal plate.

Applied physiology

Basic and reflex secretion

Reflex secretion of tears is many hundreds of times greater than basic or resting secretion. The stimulus to reflex secretion appears to be derived from the superficial corneal and conjunctival sensory stimulation, probably as a result of tear break up and dry spot formation. The secretory stimulus to the lacrimal gland is purely parasympathetic with reflex secretion occurring in both eyes following superficial stimulation of one eye. Reflex secretion is reduced by topical corneal and conjunctival anaesthesia. Although in the past basic secretion has been ascribed to the accessory lacrimal glands and reflex secretion to the main lacrimal gland, it now seems probable that the whole mass of lacrimal tissue responds as one unit.

Functions of precorneal tear film

The precorneal tear film consists of three layers, each of which has separate functions (*Figure 3.2*).

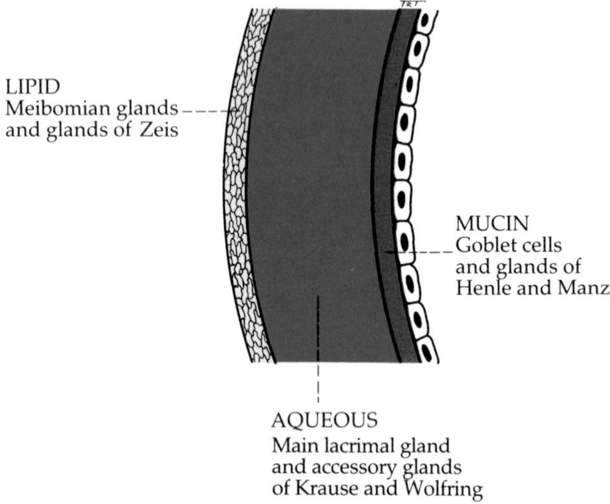

Figure 3.2 *Three layers of the precorneal tear film*

The outer lipid layer

This is secreted by the meibomian glands and has three main functions:

1. To retard the evaporation of the aqueous layer of the tear film.
2. To increase surface tension and thereby assist in the vertical stability of the tear film so that tears do not overflow the lower lid margin.
3. To lubricate the eyelids as they pass over the surface of the globe.

The middle aqueous layer

This is secreted by the main lacrimal gland and the accessory lacrimal glands, and has four main functions:

1. Most importantly, it supplies atmospheric oxygen to the corneal epithelium.
2. It has antibacterial substances, such as lactoferrin and lysozyme. A dry eye is therefore more susceptible to infection than a normal eye.
3. It provides a smooth optical surface by abolishing any minute irregularities of the cornea.
4. It washes away debris from the conjunctiva and cornea.

Keratoconjunctivitis sicca (KCS) is a dry eye due to aqueous tear deficiency.

The inner mucin layer

This is very thin and is secreted by the goblet cells in the conjunctiva and also by the crypts of Henle and glands of Manz. The exact location of these glands is described in Chapter 4. Its main function is to convert the corneal epithelium from a hydro*phobic* to a hydro*philic* surface (*Figure 3.3*). An aqueous solution will form a smooth and

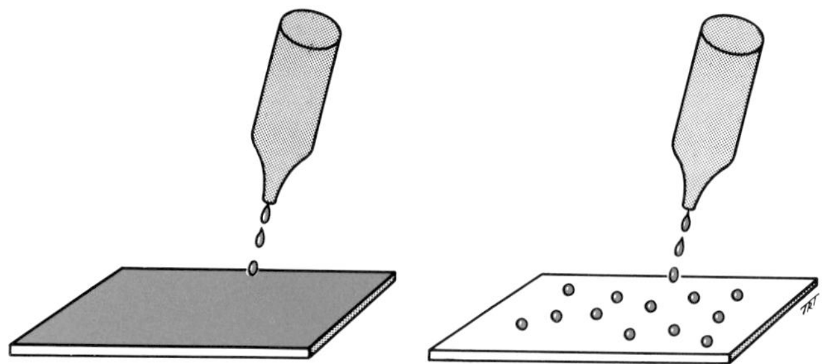

Figure 3.3 *Left: hydrophilic surface; right: hydrophobic surface*

even layer when dropped onto a hydrophilic surface, whereas when dropped onto a hydrophobic surface the aqueous solution will contract into small droplets (like on a greasy windscreen). In the absence of mucin, the corneal epithelial cells are hydrophobic and therefore cannot be wetted by aqueous tears. Mucin, which is a glycoprotein, becomes adsorbed onto the cell membranes of the epithelial cells and anchored by their microvilli. In this way it converts a hydrophobic surface into a hydrophilic surface and enables the corneal epithelium to be adequately wetted (*Figure 3.4*).

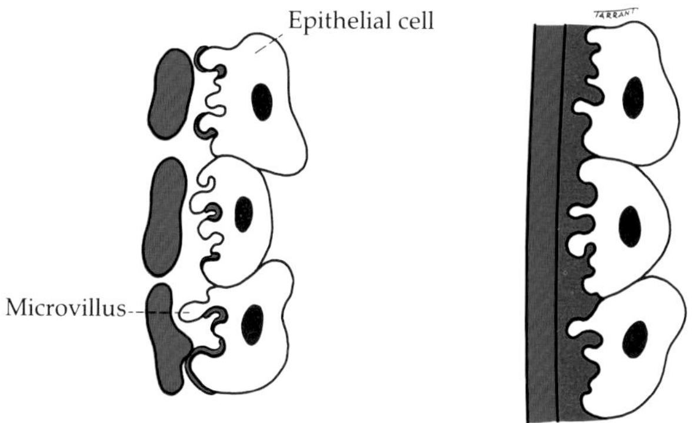

Figure 3.4 *Function of mucin layer. Left: mucin deficiency; right: normal*

Corneal resurfacing

In addition to adequate amounts of aqueous tears and mucin, three other factors are necessary for effective resurfacing of the cornea by the precorneal tear film.

1. *A normal blink reflex* which will ensure that the mucin is brought from the inferior conjunctiva and rubbed into the corneal epithelium. Patients with facial palsy and lagophthalmos (inability to close eyelids) will therefore develop corneal drying (*Figure 3.5, left*).

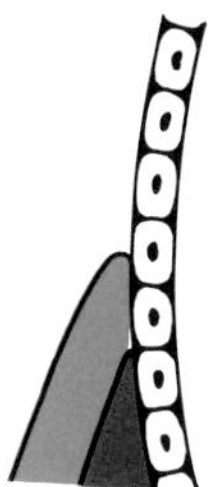

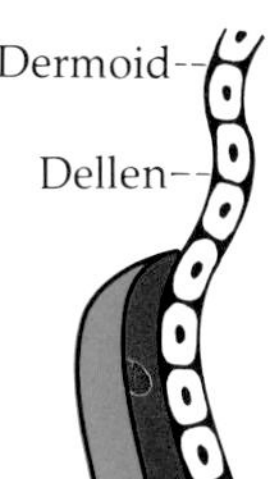

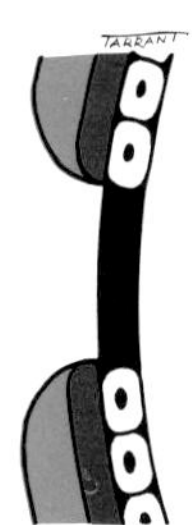

Figure 3.5 *Three causes of inadequate resurfacing of the cornea*

2. *Congruity* between the external ocular surface and the eyelids ensures that the precorneal tear film will be spread evenly over the entire cornea. Limbal lesions such as dellen or dermoids may interfere with the apposition of the lids to the globe and give rise to local areas of drying (*Figure 3.5, centre*).
3. *Normal epithelium* is necessary for the adsorption of mucin onto its surface cells. Corneal scars, keratinization, and various epitheliopathies will interfere with corneal wetting (*Figure 3.5, right*).

Causes of aqueous tear deficiency (keratoconjunctivitis sicca)

Atrophy and fibrosis

Atrophy and fibrosis of lacrimal tissue due to a destructive infiltration by mononuclear cells may occur in two different clinical settings:

1. *Pure KCS* is characterized by involvement of the lacrimal glands alone.
2. *Sjögren's syndrome* is an autoimmune disease characterized by the frequent presence of hypergammaglobulinaemia (50% of cases), rheumatoid factor (70–90% of cases), and antinuclear antibody (up to 80% of cases). Less common findings include the presence of antibodies to DNA, salivary duct tissue, smooth muscle, and gastric parietal cells. Involvement of the salivary glands causes a dry mouth (xerostomia) so that the patient complains of sticking of food and may require liquid for mastication and swallowing. Occasionally, other mucous membranes such as the bronchial epithelium and vagina become involved. When these features occur alone the condition is referred to as 'primary Sjögren's syndrome' or the 'sicca complex'. When they are associated with a connective tissue disorder, most commonly seropositive rheumatoid arthritis, the condition is called 'secondary Sjögren's syndrome'. Other systemic associations of Sjögren's syndrome include: systemic lupus erythematosus, systemic sclerosis, psoriatic arthritis, juvenile chronic arthritis, polymyositis, Hashimoto's thyroiditis and primary biliary cirrhosis.

Miscellaneous

1. *Damage or destruction of lacrimal tissue* by granulomatous (sarcoidosis), chronic inflammatory (pseudotumour) or neoplastic lesions.

2. *Absence of the lacrimal gland* which may be congenital or acquired.
3. *Blockage of excretory ducts* of the lacrimal gland as a result of severe conjunctival scarring.
4. *Neurogenic lesions* (such as familial dysautonomia).
5. *Meibomian gland dysfunction*—the exact mechanism is not well understood.

Causes of mucin deficiency

Mucin deficiency occurs when the goblet cells are damaged. This is usually due to one of two causes:

1. *Hypovitaminosis A* (xerophthalmia).
2. *Conjunctival scarring* which may be due to the Stevens–Johnson syndrome, cicatricial ocular pemphigoid, chemical burns, irradiation, and trachoma (*see* Chapter 4). The associated scarring of the excretory ducts of the lacrimal gland will also cause KCS.

Clinical evaluation

Symptoms

The most common symptoms are irritation, a foreign body sensation, presence of a stringy mucus, and transient blurring of vision. Some patients may complain of a burning sensation in the eyes, particularly when exposed to conditions associated with increased evaporation of tears (e.g. heat, air-conditioning), or prolonged reading (when the blink reflex may be reduced). Less frequent symptoms include: itching, photophobia, and a tired or heavy feeling to the eyelids. A history of resistant 'conjunctivitis' is not infrequent. It is important to point out that patients seldom complain that their eyes are dry, although some may report a lack of emotional tears or a deficient response when peeling onions.

Signs

Frequently the diagnosis of KCS can be suspected by examining the precorneal tear film, the marginal tear strip, and the cornea itself.

Precorneal tear film

One of the earlist signs of KCS is the presence of an increased amount of mucus strands and debris in the precorneal tear film. This material has a characteristic viscous appearance and tends to move *en masse* with each blink. In the healthy eye, as the tear film breaks down the mucin layer becomes contaminated with lipid but is washed away. In the dry eye, the lipid-contaminated mucin accumulates in the precorneal tear film.

Marginal tear strip

In eyes with KCS the marginal tear strip is reduced in height, is concave and contains mucus and debris. In severe cases it may be absent altogether.

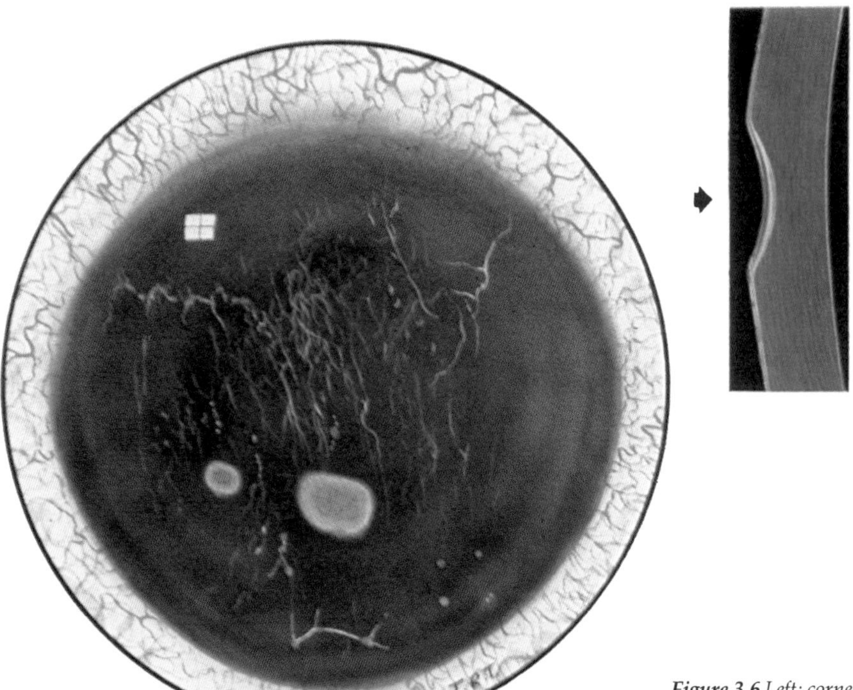

Figure 3.6 *Left: corneal filaments and plaques; right: localized areas of thinning*

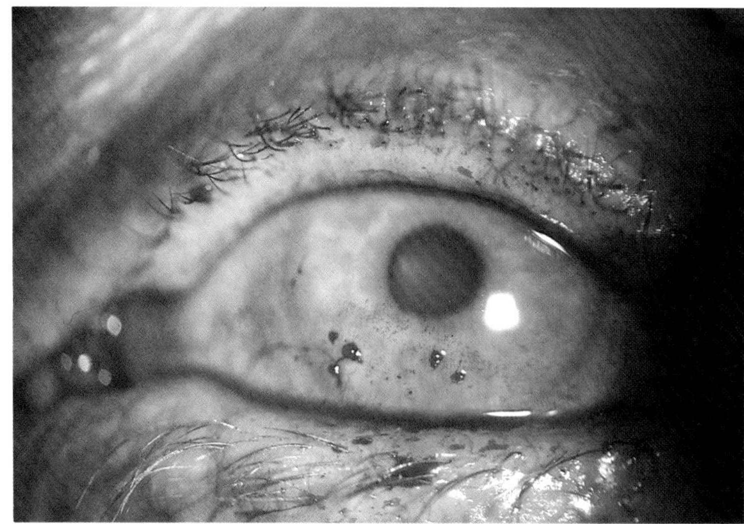

Figure 3.7 Mucous threads and corneal filaments stained with rose bengal in eye with keratoconjunctivitis sicca

Cornea

In moderate to severe cases the following corneal changes may be present:

1. *Punctate epithelial erosions* involving the inferior cornea which are best detected following the instillation of fluorescein into the inferior conjunctival fornix.
2. *Filaments* appear as small comma-shaped opacities with the unattached end hanging over the cornea and moving with each blink (*Figure 3.6, left*). They are composed of a central mucus core encased by epithelial cells and show up best following the instillation of rose bengal dye (*Figure 3.7*).
3. *Mucus plaques* appear as semi-translucent, white-to-grey, slightly elevated lesions of varying size and shape (*Figure 3.6, left*). They consist of mucus, epithelial cells, and proteinaceous and lipoidal material. They are usually seen in association with corneal filaments and they also take up rose bengal.
4. *Dellen* unassociated with limbal elevations may be seen in eyes with severe KCS (*see* Chapter 5).
5. *Thinning* and rarely perforation may occur in eyes with very severely dry eye (*Figure 3.6, right*).

Tear film break-up time

The tear film break-up time (BUT) is a simple test which assesses the stability of the precorneal tear film. It is performed by instilling fluorescein into the lower fornix, taking great care not to touch the cornea. The patient is then instructed to blink several times and then to refrain from blinking. The tear film is scanned with a broad beam and a cobalt blue filter. After an interval of time, black spots or lines, which indicate the formation of dry spots, will appear in the tear film. The BUT is the interval between the last blink and the appearance of the first randomly distributed dry spot. Ideally, the average of three measurements should be taken. The appearance of dry spots in the same location should be ignored as this is indicative of a local epithelial defect or a corneal surface abnormality and not an intrinsic instability of the precorneal tear film. A normal BUT is more than 10 seconds and a BUT of less than 10 seconds is considered abnormal. Although in most eyes with KCS, the BUT is accelerated, the test may also be abnormal in eyes with mucin or lipid deficiency.

Special tests

Vital dye staining

1. *Rose bengal 1%* has an affinity for devitalized epithelial cells and mucus in contrast to fluorescein which remains extracellular and which is more useful in showing up epithelial defects. Rose bengal is very useful in detecting even mild cases of KCS by staining the interpalpebral conjunctiva in the form of two triangles with their bases at the limbus (*Figure 3.8*). As already mentioned, corneal

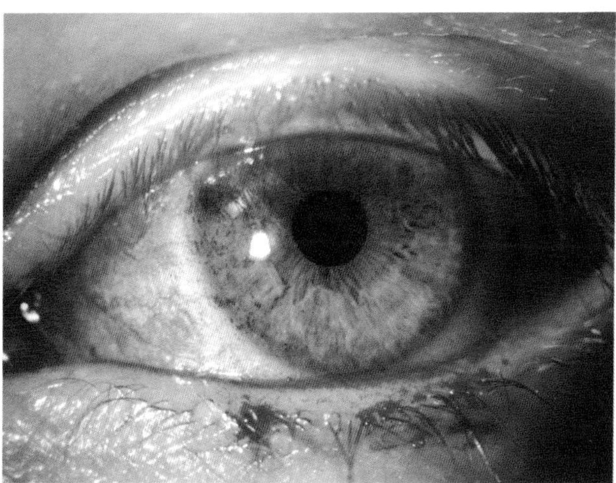

Figure 3.8 Staining of conjunctiva with rose bengal

filaments and plaques are also shown up more clearly by the dye. One disadvantage of rose bengal is that it may cause ocular irritation which can last for up to one day following its use, particularly in eyes with severe KCS. In order to reduce the amount of irritation, only a very small drop should be instilled. A topical anaesthetic should not be used prior to the instillation of rose bengal as it may induce a false positive result.
2. *Alcian blue,* although not generally available, has the same properties as rose bengal but is less irritant.

Schirmer's test

Although subject to many variables this test is clinically useful when obvious slitlamp signs of KCS are not present and yet there is suspicion of inadequate tear production. The test is performed by measuring the amount of wetting of a special filter paper which is 5 mm wide and 35 mm long.

Schirmer's test 1 is performed as follows: the filter paper is folded 5 mm from one end and inserted between the middle and outer third of the lower lid (*Figure 3.9, left*). The patient is asked to keep his eyes open and to blink as necessary. After 5 minutes, the filter strip is removed and the amount of wetting from the fold is measured. A normal eye will wet between 10 mm and 25 mm during that period. Measurements between 5 mm and 10 mm are considered borderline, and values of less than 5 mm indicative of impaired secretion, particularly if obtained on several consecutive occasions. In theory, when the test is performed without the prior instillation of a topical anaesthetic, it measures total secretion (i.e. basic and reflex), whereas with an anaesthetic it is believed to measure only basic secretion. In practice, however, although the use of topical anaesthesia will reduce the amount of reflex secretion it will not abolish it completely.

Schirmer's test 2 measures reflex tear secretion. It is performed by instilling a topical anaesthetic in the eye and irritating the unanaesthetized ipsilateral nasal mucosa with a cotton swab. The amount of wetting is measured after 2 minutes. Less than 15 mm indicates failure of reflex secretion. However, this test is seldom used because reflex secretion is usually intact.

Research tests

1. *Lysozyme assay* (*Figure 3.9, right*) is a test based on the fact that, in KCS, there may be a reduction in the concentration of lysozyme in tears. The test is performed by placing the wetted filter strip into an agar plate containing certain bacteria. The plate is then incubated for 24 hours and the zone of lysis is measured. The zone will be reduced if the concentration of lysozyme in the tears is decreased.
2. *Tear osmolarity* is increased in KCS.
3. *Biopsy of the conjunctiva* and an estimation of the number of goblet cells is an investigation that is only performed in research projects. In mucin deficiency states, the number of goblet cells will be diminished.

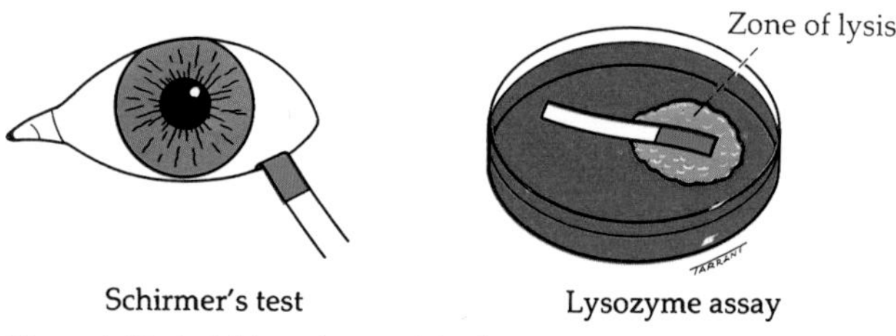

Figure 3.9 *Left: Schirmer's test; right: lysozyme assay*

Treatment

Although at present there is no cure for KCS, there are a number of therapeutic options available to relieve symptoms (*Table 3.1*). Before starting treatment, it is extremely important to explain to the patient the chronic nature of the condition while reassuring him that with appropriate treatment permanent damage to vision is unlikely.

Table 3.1 Treatment of dry eye

Tear conservation
- Reduction of room temperature
- Humidifiers
- Protective spectacles
- Tarsorrhapy

Tear substitution
- Drops
  - Cellulose derivatives
  - Polyvinyl alcohol
  - Mucomimetics
- Ointments
- Slow-release inserts
- Sodium hyaluronate
- Gel tears

Mucolytics

Reduction of tear drainage
- Temporary
- Permanent

Systemic therapy
- Steroids
- Bromhexine

Treatment of associated disease
- Blepharitis
- Infection

Tear conservation

Evaporation of tears is dependent on the following factors: temperature of air at the air–tear interface; humidity of air at the air–tear interface; air flow over the surface of the eye; surface area of the interpalpebral fissure; and integrity of the lipid layer of the precorneal tear film. Although, at present, there is no substitute available to correct the last factor, the following measures may be helpful in correcting the other factors:

1. *Reduction of room temperature.* The patient should be told to avoid a warm room with central heating.

2. *Humidifiers.* Although in theory the use of a room humidifier may be useful, in practice the results are usually disappointing because the apparatus is incapable of significantly increasing the relatively humidity of an average sized room. However, a temporary *local* increase in humidity can be achieved by the use of moist chamber goggles.
3. *Protective spectacles.* The eye can be protected from the effect of wind in an outdoor setting by the use of protective spectacles with side pieces.
4. *Tarsorrhaphy.* Although a partial tarsorrhaphy will decrease the surface area of the interpalpebral fissure, this is seldom used except in patients with incomplete lid closure or localized corneal thinning in association with severe KCS.

Tear substitutes

Drops

Tear-substitute drops still form the mainstay of treatment of mild to moderate KCS. It is crucial that the patient uses the drops regularly and frequently. The frequency of instillation is governed by the patient's symptoms and severity of KCS. In severe cases, the drops have to be instilled at half-hourly or hourly intervals, while in milder cases four times a day may be sufficient. The main disadvantages of drops are a short duration of action and the development of sensitivity to the preservative (e.g. benzalkonium, thiomersal).

The three main groups of drop tear substitutes are: cellulose derivatives, polyvinyl alcohol, and mucomimetics. In theory the latter create a stable hydrophilic corneal surface and enhance corneal wetting. Unfortunately, in practice they do not appear to be superior to either of the first two, so that the patient selects the most suitable and least irritating preparation by trial and error. The preparations of drop tear substitutes available are given in *Table 3.2*.

Table 3.2 Preparations of drop tear substitutes

Trade name	*Manufacturers*	*Constituents*
Cellulose derivatives		
BJ6	MacCarthy; Thornton & Ross	Hypromellose 0.25%
Isopto Plain	Alcon	Hypromellose 0.5%
Isopto Alkaline	Alcon	Hypromellose 1.0%
Polyvinyl alcohol		
Liquifilm Tears	Allergan	Polyvinyl alcohol 1.4%
SNO Tears	S & N Pharmaceuticals	Polyvinyl alcohol 1.4%
Hypotears	Cooper Vision	Polyvinyl alcohol 1.4% + polyethylene glycol 2.0%
Mucomimetics		
Tears Naturale	Alcon	Hypromellose 0.3% + Dextran 70

Ointments

Lacri-Lube is an ointment containing petrolatum mineral oil which can be used at bedtime.

Slow-release inserts

The insert consists of a 5 mg rod (1 mm × 3 mm) of hydroxypropylcellulose which is placed into the inferior fornix. The insert swells to several times its original volume by absorbing available tears or added substitutes. The pellet then dissolves slowly and releases the polymer into the tear film. Day-long relief of symptoms may be achieved by a single insert placed in the eye early in the morning. Although the inserts do not contain a preservative, they may cause blurring of vision, ocular irritation, and they may cause problems with insertion and retention.

Sodium hyaluronate 0.1%

This has properties akin to those of normal tears. Preliminary reports suggest that this substance could have a role in the management of KCS.

Gel tears

These consist of a clear, semisolid formulation of synthetic, high-molecular-weight polymers of acrylic acid. The gel persists in the conjunctiva for several hours after instillation and dissolves very slowly.

Mucolytics

Acetylcysteine 5% (Ilube)

Acetylcysteine drops instilled four times a day are useful in eyes with excess mucus, because acetylcysteine is a mucolytic agent which lessens ocular irritation by dispersing mucous threads and decreasing tear viscosity.

Reduction of tear drainage

Punctal occlusion is of the greatest value in patients with severe KCS, particularly when associated with toxicity from preservatives in frequently instilled drops. Punctal occlusion may be temporary or permanent.

Temporary

Temporary punctal occlusion can be performed by inserting either commercially available plugs or silicone rods, or a 2-0 catgut suture into the canaliculus. The main aim of temporary occlusion is to ensure that excessive wetness does not occur following permanent occlusion. Initially, all four puncta are occluded and the patient is reviewed in 1 week. If this causes epiphora, the upper plugs are removed and the patient is re-examined 1 week later. If the patient is now asymptomatic, the plugs are removed and the lower canaliculi can be permanently occluded.

Permanent

Permanent punctal occlusion should be undertaken only in patients with severe KCS and repeated Schirmer's test values of 2 mm or less of wetting in 5 minutes. It should not be performed in patients who develop epiphora following temporary occlusion of only the inferior puncta. Permanent occlusion should also be avoided in young patients as their tear production tends to fluctuate more than in the elderly. A permanent occlusion is achieved by first dilating the punctum vigorously and then gently heating the mucosal lining of the proximal canaliculus with electric cautery at black heat. Following successful punctal occlusion it is important to watch for signs of recanalization. Argon laser canaliculoplasty is another new method of permanent occlusion which can be easily reversed.

Systemic therapy

Corticosteroids

Treatment of an underlying systemic disease in patients with secondary syndrome with corticosteroids and/or non-steroidal anti-inflammatory agents may ameliorate the symptoms of KCS.

Bromhexine

This drug given orally (32 mg/day) may be beneficial in the treatment of both KCS and xerostomia.

Treatment of associated disorders

Blepharitis

Because dry eye patients frequently suffer from chronic blepharitis or meibomian gland dysfunction, it is important not to overlook these conditions and not to misinterpret the symptoms of chronic blepharitis for an exacerbation of KCS.

Infection

Because patients with KCS have an increased susceptibility to infection, special precautions should be taken when cataract surgery is contemplated on a dry eye. An anterior sub-Tenon's injection of gentamicin should be given prophylactically after the completion of surgery. Corneal grafting is also difficult in patients with severe KCS, as is the wearing of contact lenses.

The watering eye

Applied anatomy

The lacrimal drainage system consists of the puncta, ampullae, canaliculi, lacrimal sac, and nasolacrimal duct (*Figure 3.10*).

1. *The puncta* are located near the medial end of each eyelid. Normally they face slightly posteriorly and can be inspected by everting the medial aspect of the lids. Treatment of excessive watering due to punctal stenosis or malposition is relatively straghtforward.
2. *The ampullae* (vertical canaliculi) are about 2 mm long and form the most proximal part of the drainage system. In a one-snip procedure, the ampulla is slit vertically with scissors.
3. *The horizontal canaliculi* are about 8 mm long. In about 90% of cases, the upper and lower canaliculi form a common canaliculus which opens into the lateral wall of the lacrimal sac. In the remainder, each canaliculus opens separately. A small flap of mucosa (valve of Rosenmüller) overhangs the entrance of the common canaliculus and prevents reflux of tears from the sac into the canaliculi. Reflux of mucopurulent material on pressure over the sac implies a patent canalicular system.
4. *The lacrimal sac* is about 10 mm long and lies in the lacrimal fossa between the anterior and posterior lacrimal crests. The lacrimal bone and the frontal process of the maxilla separate the lacrimal sac from the middle meatus of the nasal cavity. In a dacryocystorhinostomy an anastomosis is made between the sac and nasal mucosa in order to bypass an obstruction in the nasolacrimal duct.
5. *The nasolacrimal duct* is about 12 mm long and is the continuation of the lacrimal sac. It passes downwards and angles slightly medially and posteriorly to open into the inferior nasal meatus lateral to and below the inferior turbinate. The opening of the duct is partially covered by a mucosal fold (valve of Hasner). Obstruction of the duct may cause a secondary distension of the sac.

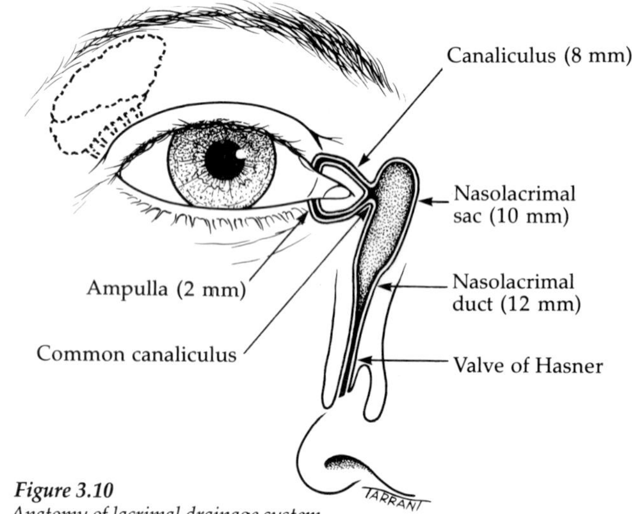

Figure 3.10
Anatomy of lacrimal drainage system

Applied physiology

Tears flow along the upper and lower marginal strips and enter the upper and lower canaliculi by capillarity and possibly also by suction. About 70% of tear drainage is via the lower canaliculus and the remainder through the upper canaliculus (*Figure 3.11a*). With each blink, the superficial and deep heads of the pretarsal orbicularis muscle compress the ampullae, shorten the horizontal canaliculi and move the puncta medially (*Figure 3.11b*). Simultaneously, the deep heads of the preseptal orbicularis muscle, which are attached to the fascia of the lacrimal sac, contract and expand the sac. This creates a negative pressure which sucks the tears from the canaliculi into the sac. When the eyes are opened the muscles relax, the sac collapses and a positive pressure is created which forces the tears down the duct into the nose (*Figure 3.11c*). Gravity also plays an important role in sac emptying. The puncta move laterally, the canaliculi lengthen and become filled with tears.

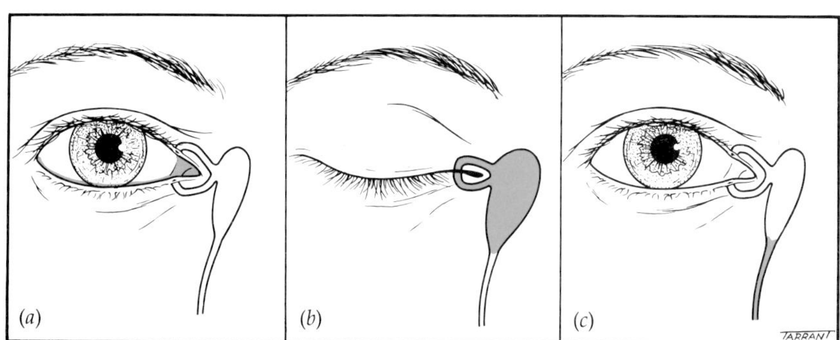

Figure 3.11 *Lacrimal pump mechanism*

Causes

The two causes of excessive watering of the eye are:

1. *Lacrimation* from reflex hypersecretion, due to irritation of the cornea or conjunctiva.
2. *Obstructive epiphora* as a result of failure of tear drainage. The two main causes are lacrimal pump failure due to lower lid laxity or weakness of the orbicularis muscle and, more frequently, mechanical obstruction to the drainage system.

Clinical evaluation

History

1. *Present.* A careful history is helpful in differentiating lacrimation from epiphora. The watering due to obstructive epiphora is usually unilateral and not associated with ocular irritation. It is worst outdoors, particularly when it is cold and windy, and least in a warm dry room. On the other hand, excessive bilateral watering in association with itching, irritation, photophobia or a foreign body sensation would be more suggestive of lacrimation.
2. *Past.* A past history of Bell's palsy is important as it would suggest lacrimal pump failure due to an orbicularis weakness.
3. *Medication* with topical idoxuridine, Phospholine Iodide, and systemic 5-fluorouracil may cause punctal stenosis.

External inspection

1. *Inspect the eyelids* for evidence of ectropion, trichiasis, eversion of the lower punctum, and lower lid laxity.
2. *Inspect the medial canthal area* below the medial canthal tendon for enlargement of the lacrimal sac which may occur from acute dacryocystitis, mucocele and, very rarely, a tumour.
3. *Palpate and then apply pressure over the lacrimal sac.* Reflux of mucopurulent material is indicative of a mucocele with a patent canalicular system, by an obstruction either at the lower end of the lacrimal sac or in the lacrimal duct. In this case no further investigations are required. In acute dacryocystitis, pressure over the sac will cause pain. Occasionally palpation of the sac will reveal a stone or a tumour.

Slitlamp biomicroscopy

1. *Inspect the puncta* for malposition, stenosis, or obstruction due to a foreign body or eyelash. Pouting of the punctum is suggestive of canaliculitis.
2. *Apply pressure over the canaliculi* with a glass rod. In the presence of canaliculitis, pus or fungal concretions may be expressed from the puncta.
3. *Inspect the marginal tear strip.* Many patients with epiphora do not show an obvious overflow of tears onto the face, but merely show a high marginal tear strip.
4. *Assess the dynamics of lid closure.* Normally, the lid margins approximate and the puncta are apposed when the lids are closed. In patients with lower lid laxity, one lid may override the other or the puncta may evert.
5. *Instil fluorescein drops* into both conjunctival sacs. Normally, in the absence of obstruction to lacrimal drainage, very little or no dye will remain after 2 minutes. A prolonged retention of dye is indicative of inadequate lacrimal drainage and can be graded from +1 to +4.

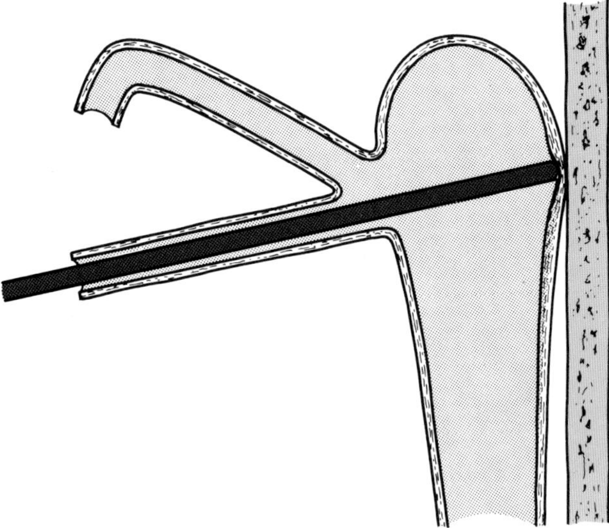

Figure 3.12 *Left: hard stop; right: soft stop*

Irrigation

A drop of topical anaesthetic is instilled into the conjunctival sac and a straight lacrimal cannula on a 3-ml saline-filled syringe is inserted into the lower canaliculus (*Figure 3.12*). As the cannula is inserted deeper an attempt is made to touch the medial wall of the lacrimal sac and the lacrimal bone. The cannula can come either to a 'hard stop' or to a 'soft stop'.

Hard stop

This is a firm feeling caused by the cannula touching the medial wall of the lacrimal sac and the lacrimal bone. This usually indicates that the lacrimal sac has been entered and excludes a complete obstruction to the canalicular system. The examiner then places one finger over the lacrimal fossa and starts to irrigate. If the saline passes into the nose the patient may have no obstruction (and the cause of watering is either hypersecretion or failure of the lacrimal pump system), or he may have a partial obstruction. If no saline reaches the nose then there is a total obstruction of the nasolacrimal duct. In this situation, the lacrimal sac will become distended during irrigation and there will also be reflux through the upper punctum. In the presence of infection the saline may be purulent.

Soft stop

This is a spongy feeling as the lacrimal cannula presses the common canaliculus and the lateral wall against the medial wall of the sac. This indicates that the cannula has been prevented from entering the lacrimal sac by an obstruction in the canalicular system. Irrigation will therefore not cause the sac to distend. In the case of lower canalicular obstruction there will be reflex of saline through the lower canaliculus. Reflux through the upper canaliculus indicates patency of both upper and lower canaliculi, but a total obstruction of the common canaliculus.

Dye testing

These tests (*Figure 3.13*) are only indicated in patients with suspected partial obstruction to the drainage system through which few or no tears can normally pass, but one that can be successfully syringe irrigated. If a total obstruction is present then dye testing is of no value.

Jones primary test

This is a physiological test which differentiates a watering due to a partial obstruction of the lacrimal passages from primary hypersecretion of tears.

First, fluorescein 2% drops are instilled into the conjunctival sac. After about 5 minutes a cotton-tipped bud (moistened in cocaine 4%) is inserted under the inferior turbinate at the nasolacrimal duct opening. One must remember that this is situated about 3 cm from the external nares.

The results are interpreted as follows:

1. *Positive.* If fluorescein is recovered from the nose the excretory system is patent and the cause of watering is primary hypersecretion. No further tests are necessary.
2. *Negative.* If no dye is recovered from the nose a partial obstruction (site unknown) is present or there is failure of the lacrimal pump mechanism. In this situation the secondary dye test is performed.

Jones secondary (irrigation) test

This is a non-physiological test which helps to identify the probable site of partial obstruction.

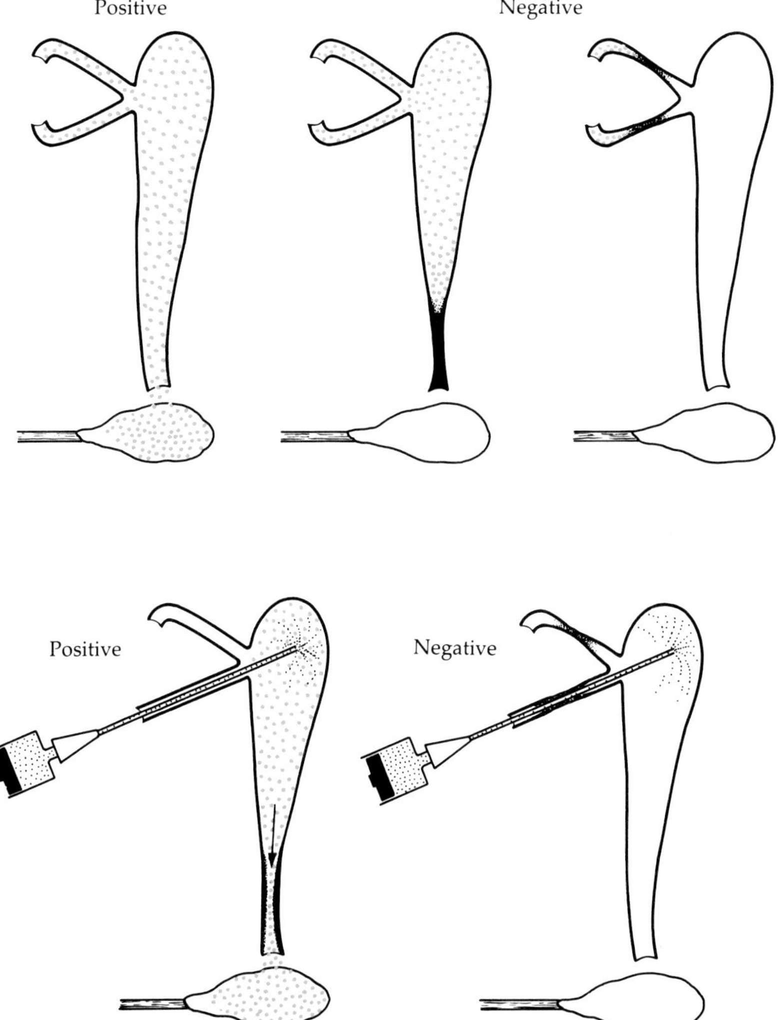

Figure 3.13 *Dye testing. Top: Jones primary test; bottom: Jones secondary test*

Topical anaesthetic is instilled into the conjunctival sac and any residual fluorescein is washed out. The nasolacrimal system is then irrigated using clear saline. The patient is positioned with his head down by about 45° so that the saline runs out of the nose into white paper tissues and not into the pharynx.

The results are interpreted as follows:

1. *Positive.* If fluorescein-stained saline is recovered from the nose, the dye must have reached the lacrimal sac during the primary dye test but was prevented from entering the nose by a partial obstruction in the nasolacrimal duct. However, the syringing of the lacrimal system had forced the dye past the obstruction into the nose. A positive secondary dye test indicates a partial obstruction to the nasolacrimal duct which can be treated by a dacryocystorhinostomy (DCR) in which the lacrimal sac is anastomosed to the nose.
2. *Negative.* If unstained saline is recovered from the nose it means that no dye had entered the lacrimal sac during the primary dye test. This implies a partial obstruction in the upper drainage system (punctum, canaliculi, or common canaliculus) or a defective lacrimal pump mechanism. In this situation, a DCR would fail and some other procedure will be necessary. Previous probing and irrigation of the canalicular system will have excluded canalicular disease, thereby confirming the presence of lacrimal pump failure.

Examination of the nose

This examination should be performed in order to determine the position of normal nasal structures, particularly the position of the anterior end of the middle turbinate when surgery is contemplated. It will also detect the presence of polyps or tumours.

Special investigations

Intubation dacryocystography

The conventional method of dacryocystography consists of injecting contrast medium into one of the canaliculi followed by the taking of posteroanterior and lateral X-rays. However, much superior definition of the canalicular system can be obtained by using a technique that combines injection of Lipiodol Ultra-Fluid through a catheter with macrography. In common canalicular lesions, subtraction macrodacryocystography may provide even more sophisticated information. These special investigations are not only extremely valuable in demonstrating the exact location of the obstruction but they are also of help in the diagnosis of diverticula, fistulae, filling defects, due to stones or tumours, and infections by *Streptothrix* sp.

Radionucleotide testing (scintillography)

This involves the labelling of tears with a gamma-emitting substance such as technetium-99m and monitoring their progress through the drainage system.

Treatment

The correct management of lacrimal obstruction depends on its cause and location.

Punctal obstruction

This may be primary, or secondary to eversion of the punctum.

Primary stenosis

The initial procedure is dilatation of the punctum with a Nettleship dilator. If repeated dilatation fails to cure the condition, then one of the following procedures is available:

1. *One-snip ampullotomy* in which a vertical 2-mm snip is made in the posterior wall of the ampulla with sharp pointed scissors.
2. *Two-snip procedure* consisting of both a vertical and a small horizontal cut in the ampulla (*Figure 3.14*). This yields larger and more permanent opening than a one-snip procedure.
3. *Three-snip procedure* in which a triangle consisting of the posterior wall of the ampulla together with a small portion of the posterior part of the horizontal canaliculus is excised. If possible this procedure should be avoided as it may interfere with the lacrimal pump mechanism.
4. *Laser punctoplasty* in which the punctum is opened using an argon laser. This method is particularly useful in elderly patients in whom the punctum is occluded by an overgrowth of conjunctival epithelium.

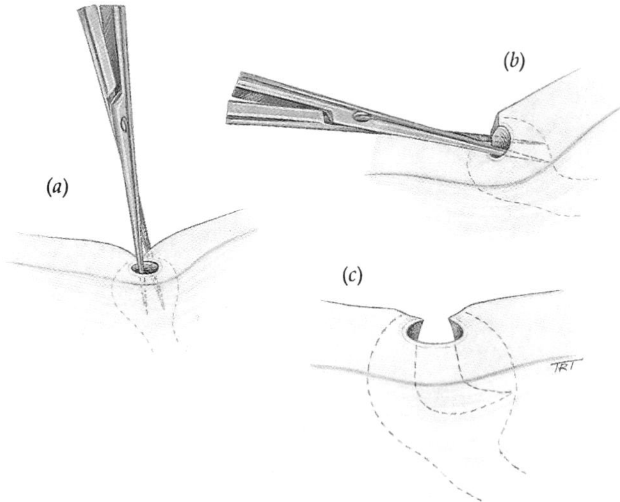

Figure 3.14 *Two-snip procedure for punctal stenosis*

Stenosis secondary to punctal eversion

The treatment of punctal eversion unassociated with significant involutional ectropion can be treated by one of the following procedures:

1. *Retropunctal cautery* in which two horizontal rows of six burns each are applied to the conjunctiva and tarsus 3 mm below the punctum. Subsequent shrinkage of the cauterized tissue will invert the punctum.
2. *Excision of a full-thickness wedge* of the lower eyelid just lateral to the punctum with retroplacement of the punctum by an obliquely placed suture.
3. *Medial conjunctivoplasty* as described in Chapter 1.

Once the punctum is restored to its normal position, it is dilated in the hope that it will remain open once normal tear flow is established. If the punctum remains stenosed then the treatment is the same as for primary stenosis.

Canalicular obstruction

The management of canalicular obstruction depends on its severity and extent.

Total

1. *Common canalicular medial end obstruction* is usually due to a thin membrane which probably develops as a result of long-standing sac obstruction. Treatment is by dacryocystorhinostomy (DCR) and excision of the membrane from its sac aspect. The lacrimal system is then intubated for 3 months.
2. *Common canalicular lateral end obstruction with more than 7 mm of healthy canaliculi.* Treatment is by canaliculodacryocystorhinostomy (CDCR) in which the obstructed common canaliculus is resected and the patent canaliculi

are anastomosed to the lacrimal sac which, in turn, is anastomosed into the nose. The lacrimal system is intubated for 3 months.

3. *Total common canalicular lateral end obstruction with less than 7 mm of healthy canaliculi.* The success rate of CDCR depends to a large extent on the length of healthy and patent canaliculi. When there is less than 7 mm of healthy canaliculus, the results of CDCR are disappointing. In these circumstances the creation of an artificial tear drainage system by means of a thin glass tube (Lester Jones tube) offers the best hope of cure. The tube is inserted between the inner canthus and the nose through a DCR.
4. *Obstruction of individual canaliculi.* Treatment depends on the length of patent canaliculus. If at least 8 mm of patent canaliculus is present between the punctum and the obstruction, treatment is by CDCR and intubation. When the block is less than 8 mm from the punctum, a CDCR is impossible and the insertion of a Lester Jones tube has the highest likelihood of success.

Partial

Partial obstruction of the common or individual canaliculi can be managed by either *Quickert* or *Crawford tubes.* The canalicular system is intubated and the tubes are passed through the nasolacrimal sac into the nose. They are then tied in the nose and left in place for at least 6 months. Another solution to partial obstruction to the canaliculi is the insertion of *Veirs' canalicular rods.* These are inserted past the obstruction into the sac and are kept in place for at least 6 weeks.

Nasolacrimal duct obstruction

Acquired

Acquired causes of nasolacrimal duct obstruction include involutional stenosis in the elderly (probably the most common cause), naso-orbital trauma, chronic sinus disease, and dacryocystitis. The management depends on the completeness of obstruction.

1. *Complete obstruction* is managed by DCR (*see* later).
2. *Incomplete obstruction* may sometimes respond to intubation of the entire lacrimal system with silicone tubes or stents. This should only be performed if the tubes or stents can be passed easily, otherwise a DCR should be done.

Congenital

The nasolacrimal duct is the last portion of the lacrimal drainage system to canalize. At birth the lower end of the nasolacrimal duct is frequently non-canalized (usually near the valve of Hasner), but this is usually of no clinical significance as it becomes spontaneously patent during the first few weeks of life and before the onset of the formation of tears. Failure of canalization within a few weeks of birth presents as epiphora and mattering of the eye. The diagnosis can be confirmed by gently pressing over the lacrimal sac and observing the reflux of purulent material from the puncta.

Controversy still exists regarding the correct management.

1. *'Hydrostatic' massage.* A recent study has shown that massaging the nasolacrimal duct in a manner that increases the hydrostatic pressure and ruptures the membranous obstruction is more effective than simple massage or no massage at all. In performing this manoeuvre, the index finger is placed over the common canaliculus to block the exit of material through the puncta and then stroked downwards firmly to increase the hydrostatic pressure within the lacrimal sac. Ten strokes should be applied four times a day. Sulphacetamide drops are also prescribed four times a day.
2. *Probing.* There are differences of opinion as to the optimal age for probing. It is generally agreed that it should not be performed until the age of 6 months and many authorities like to wait for 12 months as they feel that, with conservative treatment, canalization will occur in about 95% of cases. If probing is carried out within the first year of life, the success rate is very high. After the age of about 4 years the success rate decreases. Probing should be carried out under a general anaesthetic. Some advise probing through the upper punctum while others probe through the lower punctum. A Bowman's probe with a diameter of 1.10 mm is used and the nature and location of the obstruction is determined.

   Postoperatively the child is placed on antibiotic drops, four times a day for 1 week; phenylephrine 0.125% nose drops three times a day may also be helpful. If after 4 weeks there is no improvement, the probing should be repeated. About 90% of patients are cured by the first probing and a further 6% by the second probing. Failure are usually due to altered nasolacrimal duct anatomy. This can usually be recognized at the time of the initial probing by difficulty in passing the probe and subsequent inability to irrigate saline through the nasolacrimal duct into the nose.
3. *Intubation.* If two probings fail to cure the obstruction, intubation with silicone tubes (Crawford, or Quickert and Dryden) may be performed and the tube should remain *in situ* for 6 months.
4. *Dacryocystorhinostomy* may be necessary in exceptional circumstances.

Canalicular laceration

The management of canalicular laceration is controversial. Some authorities merely repair the eyelid while others locate and approximate the ends of the laceration using an operating microscope. The defect is then bridged with a stent (Veirs' rod or silicone tubing) which is left *in situ* for about 6 months.

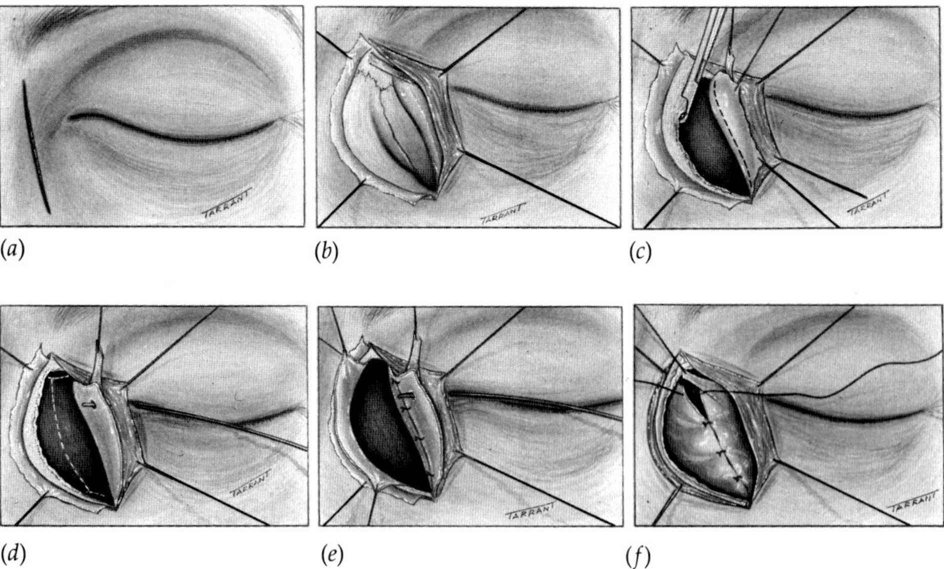

Figure 3.15 *Dacryocystorhinostomy*

Surgical techniques

Dacryocystorhinostomy

1. A straight incision is made 8 mm medial to the inner canthus (*Figure 3.15a*).
2. The anterior lacrimal crest is exposed and the superficial portion of the medial palpebral ligament is divided.
3. The periosteum is divided from the spine on the anterior lacrimal crest to the fundus of the sac and reflected forwards. The sac is reflected laterally from the lacrimal fossa (*Figure 3.15b*).
4. The anterior lacrimal crest and the bone from the lacrimal fossa are removed (*Figure 3.15c*).
5. A probe is introduced into the lacrimal sac through the lower canaliculus and the sac is incised vertically to create two flaps.
6. A vertical incision is made in the nasal mucosa to create anterior and posterior flaps (*Figure 3.15d*).
7. The posterior flaps are sutured with four 6-0 collagen sutures (*Figure 3.15e*).
8. The anterior flaps are sutured (*Figure 3.15f*).
9. The two heads of the orbicularis muscle are re-apposed with 6-0 catgut and the skin incision is closed with interrupted silk sutures.

Insertion of Lester Jones tube

1. A DCR is performed as far as suturing the posterior flaps.
2. The caruncle is excised.
3. A stab incision is made with a Graefe knife from a point about 2 mm behind the internal commissure so that the tip of the knife emerges just behind the anterior tear sac flap and anterior to the body of the middle turbinate (*Figure 3.16a*).
4. The tract is enlarged sufficiently to allow the introduction of a polythene tube (*Figure 3.16b*).
5. The incision is sutured as for a DCR.
6. After about 2 weeks, the polythene tube is replaced by a Pyrex tube.

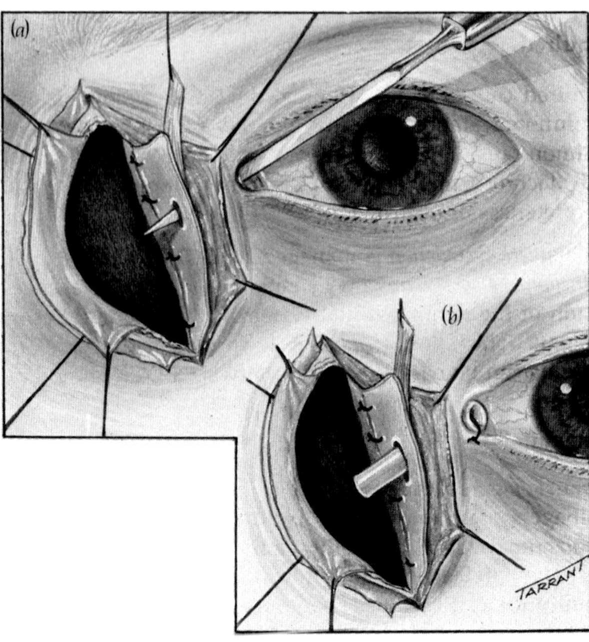

Figure 3.16 *Insertion of Lester Jones tube*

Infections of lacrimal passages

Canaliculitis

Chronic canaliculitis is frequently caused by *Actinomyces israelii* (*Streptothrix*). Acute canaliculitis is usually due to herpes simplex infection. A chronic infection causes discharge and a pouting punctum and concretions within the canaliculus (*Figure 3.17*) which have to be removed by performing a linear section into the conjunctival side of the canaliculus (canaliculotomy). Occasionally, streptothrix infection may cause a cast or stone (dacryolith) to form in the lacrimal sac.

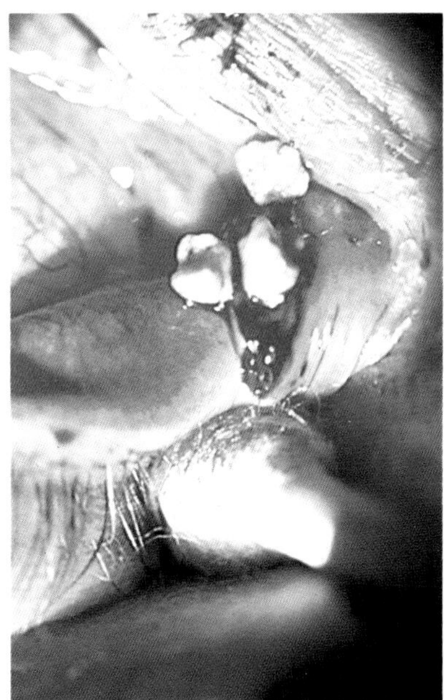

Figure 3.17 *Large concretions due to streptothrix canaliculitis (courtesy of Mr J. Kennerley Bankes)*

Dacryocystitis

Infection of the lacrimal sac is now fairly rare. It usually occurs when there is a blockage of the nasolacrimal duct. An acute infection is treated by broad-spectrum antibiotics and warm compresses. Irrigation and probing should not be carried out. If the sac is distended and filled with pus (*Figure 3.18*), a stab incision through the skin may be necessary. Although fistulae may develop following this procedure, they are relatively rare. After the acute infection has been controlled, a DCR is carried out to relieve any obstruction.

It is important to distinguish between an acute dacryocystitis in which the sac is full of pus and a mucocele in which the sac is filled with mucoid material in the absence of infection. A mucocele should not be drained through the skin but is an indication for a DCR.

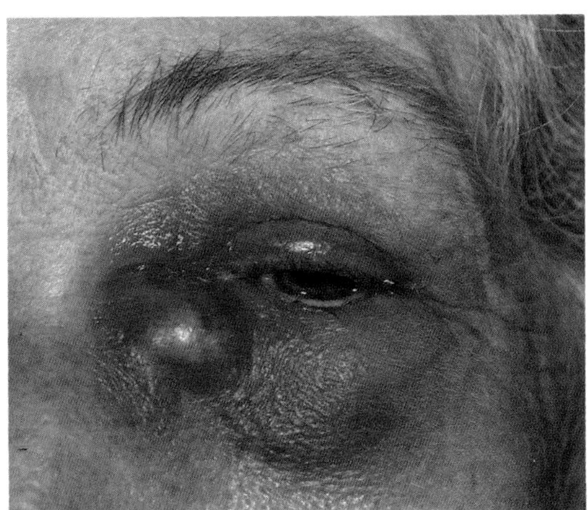

Figure 3.18 *Abscess of lacrimal sac*

Tumours of the lacrimal sac

Clinical features

Tumours of the lacrimal sac, although rare, represent a potentially life-threatening situation which can be easily overlooked. A high index of suspicion is important. The triad of a mass below the medial canthal tendon, chronic dacryocystitis that irrigates freely, and bloody reflux on irrigation should alert the ophthalmologist to this possibility. Tumours of epithelial cell origin are the most common. They can be classified into transitional cell papilloma, transitional cell carcinoma, and an intermediate type.

Treatment

This is by complete excision followed by irradiation.

Further reading

The dry eye

Bron, A.J. (1985) Duke-Elder Lecture. Perspectives for the dry eye. *Transactions of the Ophthalmological Society of the United Kingdom*, **104**, 801–826

Clinch, T.E., Benedetto, D.A., Felberg, N.T. *et al.* (1983) Schirmer's test. A closer look. *Archives of Ophthalmology*, **101**, 1383–1386

Doane, M.G. (1980) Interaction of eyelids and tears in corneal wetting and the dynamics of the normal human eyeblink. *American Journal of Ophthalmology*, **89**, 507–516

Farris, R.L., Stuchell, R.N. and Mandel, I.D. (1981) Basal and reflex human tear analysis. *Ophthalmology*, **88**, 852–861

Jordan, A. and Baum, J. (1980) Basic tear flow—does it exist? *Ophthalmology*, **87**, 920–930

Leibowitz, H.M., Chang, R.K. and Mandell, A.I. (1984) Gel tears. A new medication for the treatment of dry eyes. *Ophthalmology*, **91**, 1199–1204

Mackie, I.A. and Seal, D.V. (1981) The questionable dry eye. *British Journal of Ophthalmology*, **65**, 2–9

Mengher, L.S., Pandher, K.S., Bron, A.J. *et al.* (1986) Effect of sodium hyaluronate (0.1%) on tear break-up time (NIBUT) in patients with dry eyes. *British Journal of Ophthalmology*, **70**, 442–447

Tuberville, A.W., Frederick, W.R. and Wood, T.O. (1982) Punctal occlusion in tear deficiency syndromes. *Ophthalmology*, **89**, 1170–1172

Wright, P. (1985) Normal tear production and drainage. *Transactions of the Ophthalmological Society of the United Kingdom*, **104**, 351–354

Wright, P. and Vogel, R. (1983) Slow release artificial tears in the treatment of dry eyes resulting from oculocutaneous disorders. *British Journal of Ophthalmology*, **67**, 393–397

The watering eye

Awan, K.J. (1985) Laser punctoplasty for the treatment of punctal stenosis. *American Journal of Ophthalmology*, **100**, 341–342

Doane, M.G. (1981) Blinking and the mechanism of the lacrimal drainage system. *Ophthalmology*, **88**, 844–850

Dortzbach, R.K., France, T.D., Kushner, B.J. *et al.* (1982) Silicone intubation for obstruction of the nasolacrimal duct in children. *American Journal of Ophthalmology*, **94**, 585–590

Dryden, R.M. and Wulc, A.E. (1986) Diagnosis and management of tearing in adults. *Clinical Modules for Ophthalmologists*, Vol. 4, Module 12

English, F.P. and Kearney, R.J. (1983) Ectropion of the lower punctum. *American Journal of Ophthalmology*, **96**, 805–806

Kushner, B.J. (1982) Congenital nasolacrimal system obstruction. *Archives of Ophthalmology*, **100**, 597–600

Katowitz, J.A. (1983) Management of lacrimal disorders. *Clinical Modules for Ophthalmologists*, Vol. 1, Module 3

Nelson, L.B., Calhoun, J.H. and Menduke, H. (1985) Medical management of congenital nasolacrimal duct obstruction. *Ophthalmology*, **92**, 1187–1190

Robb, R.M. (1986) Probing and irrigation for congenital nasolacrimal duct obstruction. *Archives of Ophthalmology*, **104**, 378–379

Welham, R.A.N. (1982) Immediate management of injuries to the lacrimal drainage system. *Transactions of the Ophthalmological Society of the United Kingdom*, **102**, 216–217

Welham, R.A.N. and Hughes, S.M. (1985) Lacrimal surgery in children. *American Journal of Ophthalmology*, **99**, 27–34

Wobig, J.L. (1981) Epiphora, causes and treatment. *Perspectives in Ophthalmology*, **5**, 177–181

4

The Conjunctiva

Introduction

Applied anatomy

Evaluation of conjunctival inflammation

Bacterial infections

Chronic blepharoconjunctivitis

Simple acute conjunctivitis

Gonococcal conjunctivitis

Viral infections

Adenoviral keratoconjunctivitis

Acute haemorrhagic conjunctivitis

Herpes simplex conjunctivitis

Molluscum contagiosum conjunctivitis

Chlamydial infections

Adult inclusion conjunctivitis

Trachoma

Ophthalmia neonatorum

Allergic disorders

Classification

Hay fever (seasonal) conjunctivitis

Acute 'allergic' conjunctivitis

Chronic allergic conjunctivitis

Vernal keratoconjunctivitis (spring catarrh)

Atopic keratoconjunctivitis

Giant papillary conjunctivitis

Cicatricial pemphigoid

Stevens–Johnson syndrome (erythema multiforme major)

Chemical burns

Miscellaneous

Superior limbic keratoconjunctivitis of Theodore

Parinaud's oculoglandular conjunctivitis

Mucus fishing syndrome

Floppy eyelid syndrome

Reiter's syndrome

Degenerations

Pinguecula

Pterygium

Concretions

Retention cyst

Pigmented lesions

Classification

Melanocytic

Non-melanocytic

Non-pigmented tumours

Classification

Papilloma

Intraepithelial epithelioma (carcinoma *in situ*)

Invasive squamous carcinoma

Choristoma

Introduction

Applied anatomy of conjunctiva

The conjunctiva (*Figure 4.1*), like all mucous membranes, consists of two layers: the epithelium and the stroma.

The epithelium

This varies from two to five layers in thickness. The basal cells are cuboidal and evolve into flattened polyhedral cells as they reach the surface. With chronic exposure and drying, the epithelium may assume some of the characteristics of skin and become keratinized.

The stroma (substantia propria)

This consists of richly vascularized connective tissue which is separated from the epithelium by a basement membrane. The adenoid superficial layer contains lymphoid tissue which does not develop until 2–3 months postnatally. For this reason, conjunctival inflammation in the newborn cannot produce a follicular reaction. The deep thicker fibrous layer belongs to the subconjunctival tissues rather than to the conjunctiva. It is continuous with the tarsal plates.

The conjunctiva contains two types of glands: mucin secretors and accessory lacrimal glands.

Mucin secretors

1. *Goblet cells* are unicellular mucus glands located within the epithelium. Because they are most dense in the inferonasal part of the conjunctiva, this is the best site for diagnostic biopsy.

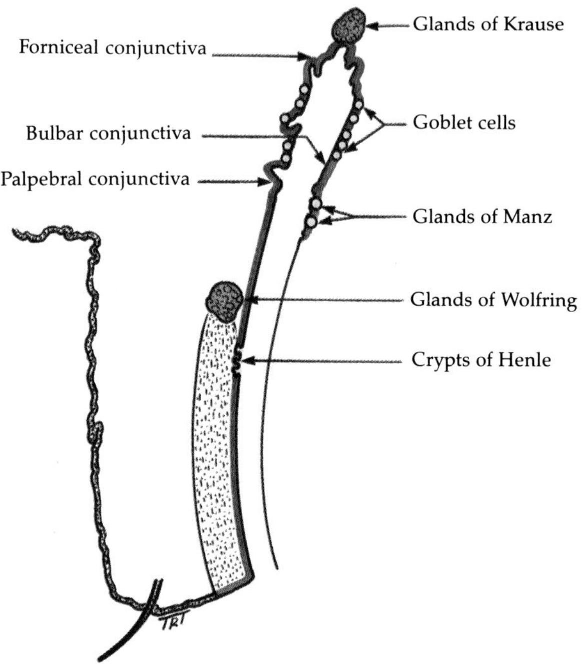

Figure 4.1 *Anatomy of conjunctiva*

2. *The crypts of Henle* are located along the upper third of the superior tarsal conjunctiva and along the lower third of the inferior tarsal conjunctiva.
3. *Glands of Manz* are found in a circumferential ring of limbal conjunctiva.

Destructive disorders of the conjunctiva (cicatricial pemphigoid) frequently damage the mucin secretors and cause a dry eye due to mucin deficiency. On the other hand, chronic inflammatory disorders may be associated with an increase in goblet cells.

Accessory lacrimal glands

In contrast to the mucin secretors, the accessory lacrimal glands are located in the stroma.

Clinical divisions

Clinically it is convenient to divide the conjunctiva into three parts:

1. *The palpebral* part starts at the mucocutaneous junction and lines the inside of the eyelids. It is firmly adherent to the tarsus.
2. *The forniceal* conjunctiva is loose and redundant so that it swells easily and becomes thrown into folds.
3. *The bulbar* conjunctiva lines the anterior part of the sclera, becoming continuous with the cornea at the limbus. The stroma of the bulbar conjunctiva is loosely attached to the underlying Tenon's capsule, except at the limbus where the attachment is firm.

Lymphatic drainage is to the preauricular and submandibular nodes.

Evaluation of conjunctival inflammation

Clinical features

The three main clinical features that should be considered in the differential diagnosis of conjunctival inflammation are:

1. The type of discharge.
2. The characteristics of the conjunctival reaction.
3. The presence or absence of lymphadenopathy.

Discharge

The discharge is composed of the exudate that has filtered through the conjunctival epithelium from dilated blood vessels. On the surface of the conjunctiva, variable amounts of epithelial debris, mucus and tears are added.

1. *A watery discharge* composed of a serous exudate and a variable amount of reflexly secreted tears is typical of viral and toxic inflammations.
2. *A mucinous discharge* is typical of vernal conjunctivitis and keratoconjunctivitis sicca.

3. *A purulent discharge* occurs in severe acute bacterial infections.
4. *A mucopurulent discharge* occurs in mild bacterial as well as chlamydial infections. It characteristically gives rise to glueing up of the eyelids in the mornings.

Reaction

A careful slitlamp examination of the conjunctiva may provide valuable clues as to the likely aetiology of the inflammation.

Hyperaemia

This is a non-specific reaction occurring in all types of conjunctivitis. It is characteristically most intense in the fornices and least at the limbus.

Oedema

This occurs whenever the conjunctiva is inflamed and hyperaemic. The transudation of fibrin and protein-rich fluid through the walls of damaged blood vessels produces a translucent swelling of the conjunctiva. In the tightly adherent tarsal conjunctiva, this causes enlargement of papillae. In the forniceal conjunctiva, large redundant folds form. In the bulbar conjunctiva, where the attachments to the globe are lax, large quantities of transudate may cause the conjunctiva to balloon away from the sclera (chemosis; *Figure 4.2*). In particularly severe cases, the chemotic conjunctiva may protrude through the closed eyelids.

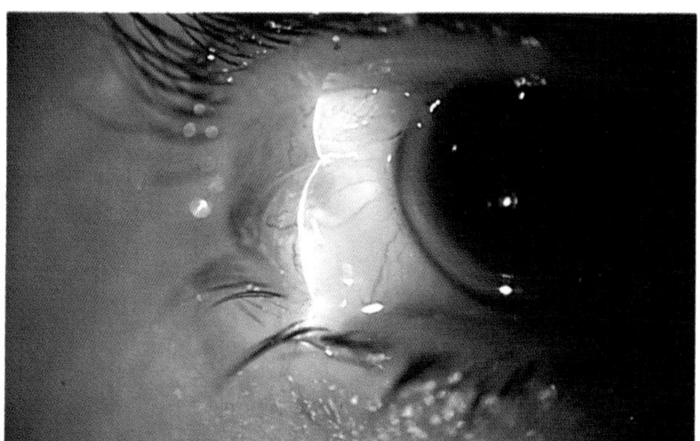

Figure 4.2 *Chemosis*

Follicles

These are minute lymph follicles with accessory vascularization that are usually most prominent in the inferior forniceal conjunctiva. Clinically, they appear as multiple, discrete, slightly elevated lesions reminiscent of small grains of rice (*Figure 4.3*). Each follicle is encircled by a tiny blood vessel and the size of each lesion, which can vary from 0.5 to 5 mm, is related to the severity and duration of the inflammation. As the follicle increases in size, the accompanying vessels are displaced peripherally, eventually appearing as a vascular capsule enclosing the base of the

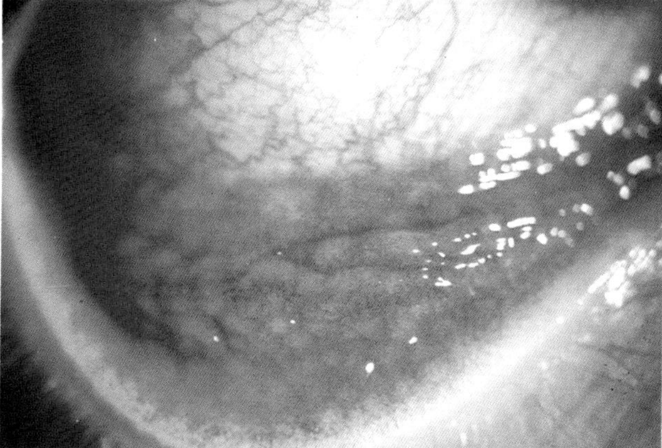

Figure 4.3 *Follicular conjunctivitis*

follicle. In the infant, follicles cannot develop until about 2–3 months after birth. In asymptomatic children and young adults, their presence is usually of no clinical significance. However, a follicular conjunctivitis is usually of viral, chlamydial, or toxic origin.

Papillae

These are essentially vascular structures that have been invaded by inflammatory cells. They are most frequently seen in the upper palpebral conjunctiva; on slitlamp examination a fine mosaic-like pattern of elevated polygonal hyperaemic areas separated by paler channels is seen. The central fibrovascular core produces a glomerulus-like appearance on reaching the surface. Occasionally, an intense papillary reaction may mask an underlying follicular response. A papillary reaction is more non-specific, being of less diagnostic importance than a follicular response. With prolonged inflammation, the fibrous septa which anchor the papillae to the underlying tissues may rupture, leading either to papillary confluence, as in bacterial infections, or to the formation of giant papillae typical of vernal conjunctivitis(*see Figure 4.19*).

Membranes

1. *Pseudomembranes* (*Figure 4.4*) consist of coagulated exudate adherent to the inflamed conjunctival epithelium. Characteristically they can be easily peeled off, leaving the epithelium intact. Causes include adenoviral, vernal, and gonococcal conjunctivitis.
2. *True membranes* form when the inflammatory exudate permeates the superficial layers of the conjunctival epithelium. Attempts to remove the membrane may be accompanied by tearing of the epithelium and bleeding. True membrane formation occurs in certain bacterial infections, particularly diphtheria.

Subconjunctival haemorrhages

These occur in acute haemorrhagic conjunctivitis due to picornaviruses, adenoviral conjunctivitis, and certain bacterial conjunctivitides (*Pneumococcus* and *Haemophilus* spp.).

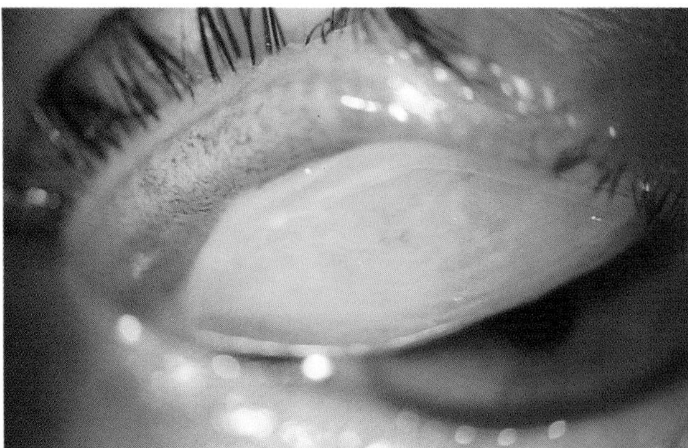

Figure 4.4 Pseudomembrane

Lymphadenopathy

Enlargement of the preauricular nodes is a feature of viral and chlamydial infections but is seldom present in bacterial conjunctivitis.

Laboratory investigations

Indications

The main indications for laboratory investigations are:

1. Severe purulent conjunctivitis—in order to identify the pathogens and decide on appropriate antimicrobial therapy based on sensitivity data.
2. Follicular conjunctivitis—to differentiate viral from chlamydial disease because the early appearance of the follicular reaction can be very similar.
3. Conjunctival inflammations in which the clinical picture is not sufficiently distinctive to suggest an aetiological diagnosis (i.e. chronic or recurrent conjunctivitis).
4. Ophthalmia neonatorum.

Scrapings

Conjunctival scrapings should be taken with a Kimura spatula from the site of maximal disease, preferably during the active stage. The specimens are placed on glass slides for Gram and Giemsa staining:

1. *Gram staining* is used to identify and differentiate Gram-positive from Gram-negative bacteria. Fungi may be identified by the Gram-positive staining of their protoplasm. However, Gram staining is useless for detecting the cytological response.
2. *Giemsa staining* is used to identify the type of inflammatory and epithelial cells. Because all bacteria are stained uniformly, it does not differentiate Gram-positive from Gram-negative species.

Acute bacterial conjunctivitis causes a predominantly neutrophilic cellular reaction.

Viral conjunctivitis is typically characterized by a mononuclear cellular response with predominance of lymphocytes and monocytes. Viral inclusion bodies are not seen with Giemsa stain, being better identified with the Papanicolaou (PAP) technique.

Inclusion conjunctivitis caused by *Chlamydia* sp. is characterized by an intense mixed neutrophilic and mononuclear response, with the former cell type usually predominating. However, the pathognomonic cytological finding is the basophilic cytoplasmic inclusion body of Halberstaedter–Prowazek, typically seen capping the epithelial cell nucleus.

Acute allergic conjunctivitis is characterized by the presense of eosinophils and eosinophilic granules.

Cultures

Cultures from the lid margins and conjunctival sac are taken with sterile cotton-tipped applicators.

Bacterial infections

Chronic blepharoconjunctivitis

Although chronic blepharitis (blepharoconjunctivitis) is the most common external eye disorder encountered in clinical practice, its exact aetiology is still unclear and its management frequently unsatisfactory. It is thought that staphylococcal infection and seborrhoea are its most important causes. Because many patients also have tear film instability, they are frequently described as suffering from the triple-S syndrome (*Staphylococcus*, seborrhoea, and sicca). In order to understand the classification and clinical features of chronic blepharitis, a knowledge of the anatomy of the lid margin is essential (*see* Chapter 1).

Classification

Anterior
- staphylococcal
- seborrhoeic
- mixed

Posterior

Mixed anterior and posterior

The three main types of blepharitis are anterior, posterior, and mixed. Anterior blepharitis affects the lid margin anterior to the grey line. It can be staphylococcal, seborrhoeic, or mixed (most common). Posterior blepharitis affects the meibomian glands. This condition is also frequently referred to as 'meibomitis', 'meibomianitis', or 'meibomian gland dysfunction'. It may be primary or it may be associated with anterior blepharitis.

Clinical features

Staphylococcal blepharitis

This is caused by chronic staphylococcal infection of the bases of the lashes. Although pure staphylococcal blepharitis is now relatively uncommon, the condition is frequently seen in patients with dry eyes and atopic eczema. The disorder usually starts in childhood and may continue throughout life.

Symptoms

In the early stages, the patient is frequently asymptomatic but, as the disease progresses, it causes chronic irritation, burning, itching and mild photophobia which are characteristically worse in the morning.

Signs

The anterior lid margin shows dilated blood vessels (rosettes), and hard, brittle, fibrinous scales. The scales are centred around the bases of the lashes (collarettes) (*Figure 4.5*) and they may leave a small bleeding ulcer when removed. In long-standing cases, the lashes become

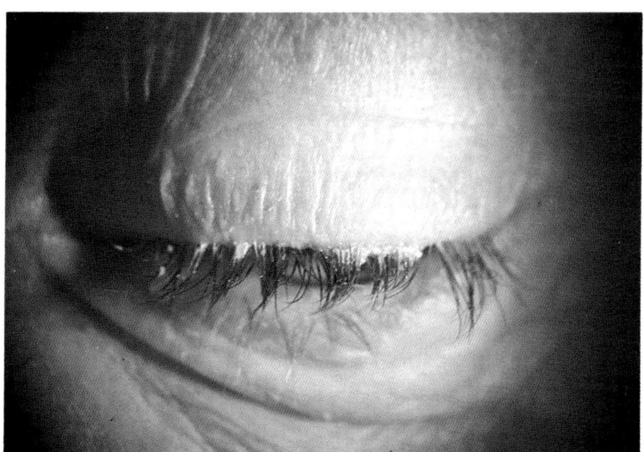

Figure 4.5 *Staphylococcal blepharitis*

misdirected and inverted (trichiasis), fewer in number (madarosis) (*Figure 4.6*), and occasionally white in colour (poliosis). The anterior lid margin may show scarring, notching, and hypertrophy. Recurrent styes (external hordeolum) and recurrent attacks of acute bacterial conjunctivitis are common.

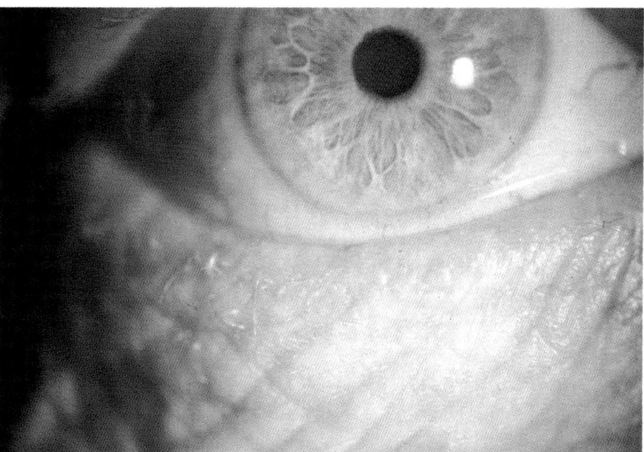

Figure 4.6 *Madarosis due to blepharitis*

Secondary changes

These are caused by hypersensitivity reactions to staphylococcal exotoxins and include: mild papillary conjunctivitis involving the inferior tarsal and forniceal conjunctiva, punctate epithelial erosions (epitheliopathy) involving primarily the inferior third of the cornea, marginal keratitis (catarrhal ulcer), and occasionally phlyctenulosis and pannus (*Figure 4.7*).

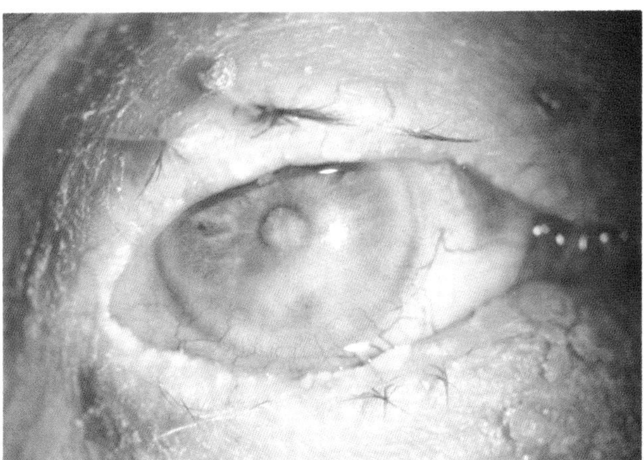

Figure 4.7 *Very severe staphylococcal blepharitis with inferior corneal pannus*

Seborrhoeic blepharitis

This is disorder of the glands of Zeis which is frequently associated with seborrhoeic dermatitis. The skin changes, which are usually fairly mild, may involve the scalp, eyebrows, nasolabial folds, retroauricular areas, and sternum. The two main forms of seborrhoea are the oily type in which the scaly eruptions are greasy, and the dry type (pityriasis capitis or dandruff). It has been postulated that the excessive amounts of neutral lipids in patients with seborrhoea are broken down by *Corynebacterium acnes* into irritating free fatty acids.

Symptoms

These are similar but less severe than in staphylococcal blepharitis.

Signs

The anterior lid margin has a shiny waxy appearance and the lashes are greasy and stuck together. The scales are soft, located anywhere along the lid margin and they do not leave an ulcer when removed.

Secondary changes

These are uncommon and include papillary conjunctivitis, and punctate epithelial erosions involving the middle third of the cornea. When present, they are less severe than in staphylococcal blepharitis.

Posterior blepharitis (meibomian gland dysfunction)

This is a disorder of the meibomian glands and can be thought of as a posterior form of seborrhoeic blepharitis. Meibomian gland dysfunction may occur in isolation or it can be seen in combination with seborrhoeic blepharitis in patients with seborrhoeic dermatitis or acne rosacea.

Symptoms

The irritating lipid in the tear film gives rise to stinging similar to that caused by soap in the eyes. The excess amount of oil in the precorneal tear film may also cause mild blurring of vision, particularly in contact lens wearers.

Signs

Careful slitlamp examination may show minute oil globules at the orifices of the meibomian glands (*Figure 4.8*). Patients frequently mistake these globules for small 'ulcers'. The excess lipid in the tear film gives rise to foam (meibomian serborrhoea) in the lower lid tear meniscus. In some cases, the lipid within the meibomian glands solidifies and plugs the duct orifices giving rise to secondary dilatation and distortion of the glands and the formation of microliths and chalazia.

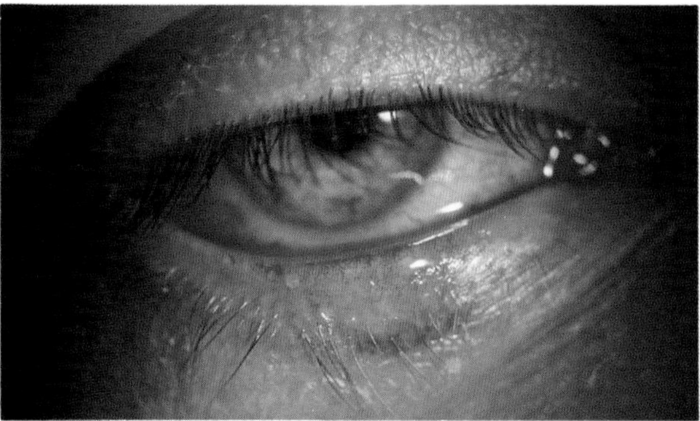

Figure 4.8 *Posterior blepharitis with oil globules at orifices of meibomian glands*

Secondary changes

These are caused by direct toxicity and include mild conjunctivitis and punctate epithelial erosions. Associated destabilization of the precorneal tear film causes a shortening of the tear film break-up time.

Treatment

It is important to emphasize that, although blepharitis is an extremely common disease, it is frequently undiagnosed because the severity of the patient's symptoms may be out of proportion to the clinical findings. The clinician should first classify the blepharitis into anterior, posterior, or mixed, and then examine the patient for evidence of an associated skin disorder such as seborrhoeic dermatitis or acne rosacea. Crucial in the treatment is the patient's motivation and ability to correctly comply with instructions. The patient should be informed at the outset that complete eradication may not be possible but elimination of annoying symptoms is usually effective. In severe long-standing cases, several weeks of intensive treatment may be necessary before improvement is achieved.

Lid hygiene

This is aimed at removing crusts and toxic products from the lid margins. This can be achieved by scrubbing the lid margins twice a day with a cotton-tipped bud dipped in a weak baby shampoo. A clean face-cloth can be used as an alternative to a cotton-tipped bud. Gradually, lid hygiene can be performed less frequently as the disease is brought under control.

Antibiotics

If possible, the organisms should be identified and their sensitivities to various antibiotics tested. Patients with staphylococcal blepharitis usually respond to bacitracin, gentamicin, erythromycin, or sulphacetamide ointment which is rubbed into the lid margins with a clean finger after all crusts have been removed. Systemic antibiotics such as tetracycline may be useful in patients with seborrhoeic blepharitis associated with seborrhoeic dermatitis. It is thought that they may act by reducing the bacteria that are responsible for splitting neutral lipids into irritating fatty acids. Systemic tetracycline is also useful in patients with blepharitis and acne rosacea. Its mode of action in this clinical setting is unclear.

Corticosteroids

These should be avoided in pure and uncomplicated staphylococcal blepharitis. However, topical corticosteroids are extremely useful in the treatment of secondary effects (papillary conjunctivitis, toxic epitheliopathy, marginal keratitis, and phlyctenulosis) associated with hypersensitivity reactions to staphylococcal exotoxins. Short courses of topical corticosteroids may also be required in severe cases of seborrhoeic blepharitis.

Other measures

1. *Warm compresses* may be helpful in melting solidified sebum in patients with meibomitis.
2. *Mechanical expression* of the meibomian glands may reduce the amount of irritating lipids within the glands in patients with meibomian gland dysfunction.
3. *Treatment of seborrhoeic dermatitis and dandruff* with special medicated shampoos may be beneficial.
4. *Artificial tears.* It must be remembered that the last letter *S* in the triple-S syndrome stands for *sicca.* This is particularly common in patients with staphylococcal blepharitis and can be recognized by a rapid tear film break-up time. Unless this aspect of the disease is recognized and treated, the relief of symptoms will be incomplete.

Simple acute conjunctivitis

Acute bacterial conjunctivitis is a very common and usually self-limiting condition. In order of frequency the most common causative organisms are *Staphylococcus epidermidis, Staphylococcus aureus, Haemophilus* and *Streptococcus* spp.

Clinical features

Symptoms

There is a subacute onset of redness, grittiness, discharge and crusting. On waking, the eyelids are frequently stuck together and may have to be bathed open. Both eyes are usually involved although one may become affected before the other by a day or so.

Signs

Examination shows conjunctival hyperaemia which is maximal in the fornices (*Figure 4.9*), a mild papillary reaction, a purulent or mucopurulent discharge, and lid crusting. Visual acuity is usually normal unless a secondary superficial punctate epitheliopathy involving the entire cornea is also present. Preauricular lymphadenopathy is usually absent.

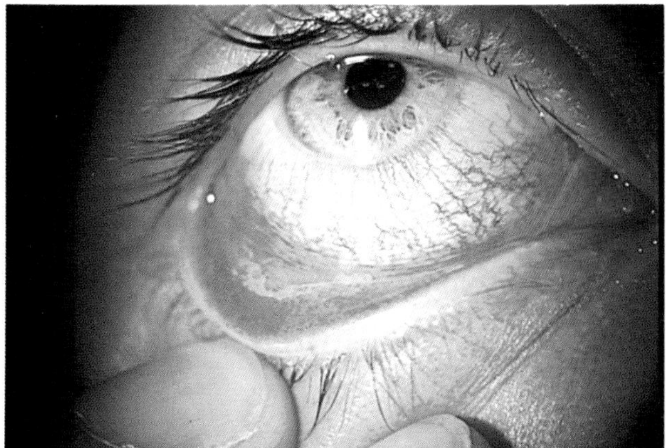

Figure 4.9 *Acute bacterial conjunctivitis*

Treatment

Even without treatment, the inflammation usually resolves within 10–14 days. Laboratory tests are not routinely performed. The initial treatment is with chloramphenicol drops at frequent intervals during the day and ointment at night. Neomycin should be avoided as it causes topical sensitivity in about 8% of the population. This may in fact be worse than the initial infection and may occasionally lead to confusion with an escalation of medication in the belief that the infection is getting worse. Gentamicin is a useful standby as it has a very broad spectrum. However, it should not be used routinely in order to prevent the development of resistant strains.

Causes of chronic or recurrent conjunctivitis

The following associated conditions should be considered if the conjunctivitis become chronic or recurs at frequent intervals:

1. *Resistant organisms*—perform conjunctival cultures and change antibiotics according to results.
2. *Obstruction or infection (dacryocystitis, canaliculitis) of the lacrimal drainage system.*
3. *Chronic blepharitis.*
4. *Rosacea keratoconjunctivitis*—easy to miss as skin changes may be mild.
5. *Chlamydial infection*—may require systemic therapy.
6. *Self inflicted*—mucus fishing syndrome (*see* later).
7. *Floppy eyelid syndrome* (*see* later).

Gonoccal conjunctivitis

This rare disease is characterized by an acute purulent conjunctivitis (*Figure 4.10*) with lid oedema, marked conjunctival hyperaemia, chemosis with or without membrane formation, and prominent preauricular adenopathy. If inadequately treated, corneal ulceration and perforation may result.Treatment is with systemic and topical antibiotics.

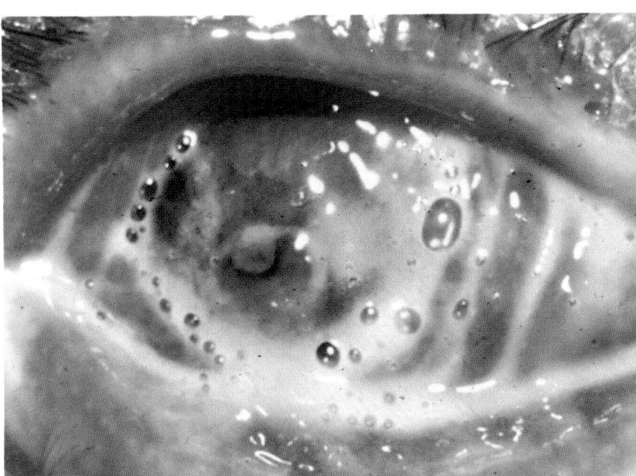

Figure 4.10 *Gonococcal conjunctivitis in an adult*

Viral infections

Adenoviral keratoconjunctivitis

Ten of the 31 serotypes of adenoviruses have been implicated in causing eye infection. The spectrum of disease varies from mild and almost inapparent, to full-blown cases characterized by the two syndromes of adenoviral infection: pharyngoconjunctival fever (PCF) and epidemic keratoconjunctivitis (EKC), both of which are epidemic in nature and highly contagious for up to 2 weeks (*Table 4.1*).

Table 4.1 Comparison between PCF and EKC

	EKC	*PCF*
Virus serotypes	8 and 19	3 and 7
Age	Any age	Usually children
Systemic symptoms	–	+++
Keratitis incidence	80% (may be severe)	30% (mild)

Because the virus can be spread by finger-to-eye contact, it is important for ophthalmologists to wash their hands after being in contact with an acute red eye. The virus can also be spread by contaminated instruments such as applanation tonometers.

PCF is associated with adenovirus types 3 and 7. It typically affects children, and causes an upper respiratory tract infection. Keratitis develops in 30% of cases.

EKC is most frequently caused by adenovirus types 8 and 19, and is usually unassociated with systemic symptoms. Keratitis occurs in about 80% of cases.

Conjunctivitis

Clinical features

This (*see Figure 4.3*) is follicular and is frequently associated with preauricular adenopathy, and usually develops acutely with symptoms of watering, redness, discomfort, and photophobia. In severe cases, subconjunctival haemorrhages, chemosis, and pseudomembranes may develop. Involvement is bilateral in two-thirds of cases and the conjunctivitis resolves after about 2 weeks without residua.

Treatment

This is mainly supportive. Antiviral agents are ineffective and corticosteroids should not be used during the acute stage unless the inflammation is very severe and the possibility of herpes simplex infection has been excluded.

Keratitis

Clinical features

Keratitis (*Figure 4.11*) is rarely a problem in PCF, but it may be severe in patients with EKC. When present it tends to progress through three stages in an orderly sequence.

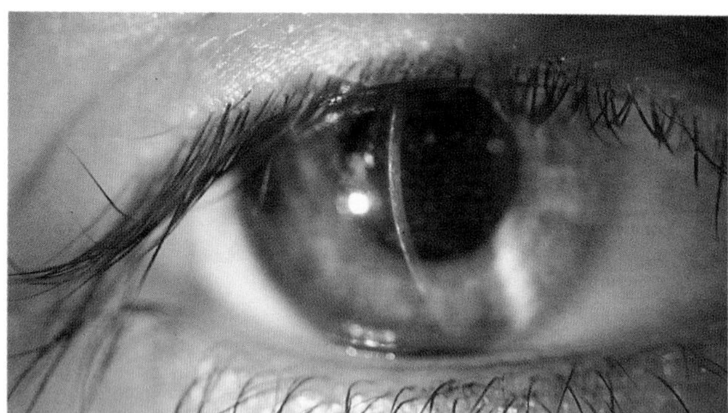

Figure 4.11 *Adenoviral keratitis*

1. *Stage 1* occurs within 7–10 days of the onset of ocular symptoms. It is characterized by a diffuse punctate epithelial keratitis (*Figure 4.12, left*). Like the conjunctivitis, it may resolve within 2 weeks, or it may go on to stage 2.
2. *Stage 2* is characterized by focal white subepithelial opacities which develop beneath the epithelial lesions. They are thought to represent immune responses to the adenovirus and, on occasion, they may be associated with a transient mild anterior uveitis.
3. *Stage 3* is characterized by anterior stromal infiltrates which may very occasionally persist for months and even years (*Figure 4.12, right*).

Treatment

Although the keratitis responds well to topical corticosteroids, treatment is only indicated if the eye is uncomfortable or visual acuity diminished. It is important to realize that corticosteroids will not shorten the natural course of the disease but merely suppress the corneal inflammation.

Acute haemorrhagic conjunctivitis

This fairly rare disease is usually caused by enterovirus 70. It typically affects individuals of low socioeconomic status, crowded living conditions, and poor handwashing practices. The disease is highly contagious but self-limiting.

Clinical features

The onset is characterized by bilateral conjunctival injection, lid oedema, a profuse watery discharge, palpebral follicles, and subconjunctival haemorrhages that vary in severity (*Figure 4.13*). The infection usually resolves without sequelae within 7 days.

Treatment

There is no effective treatment.

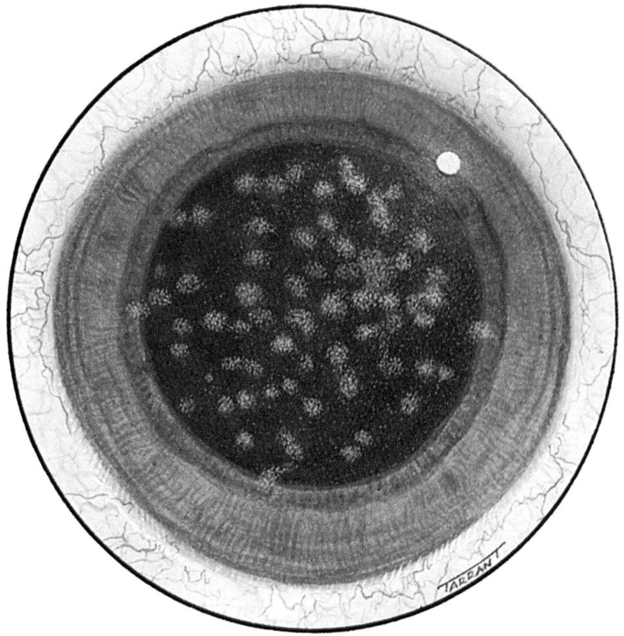

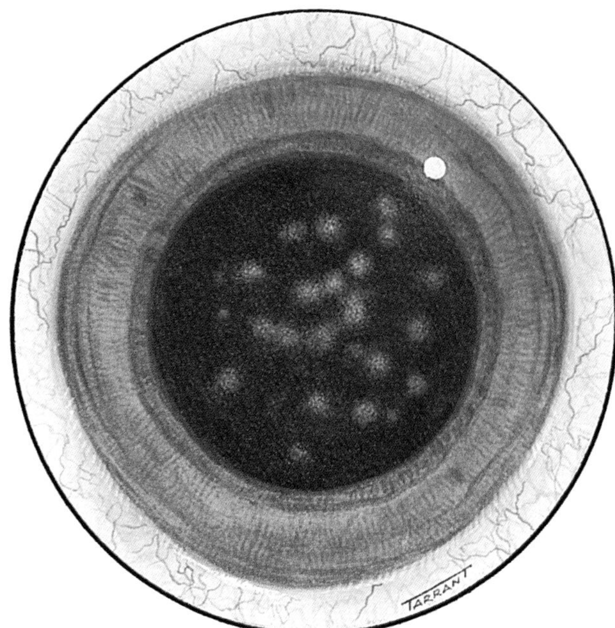

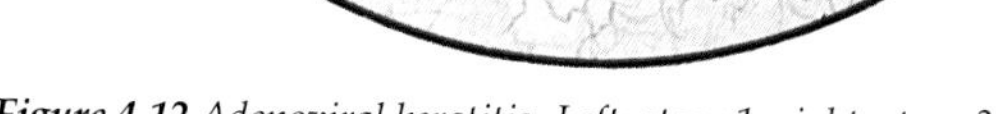
Figure 4.12 *Adenoviral keratitis. Left: stage 1; right: stage 3*

Herpes simplex conjunctivitis

See Chapter 5.

Molluscum contagiosum conjunctivitis

See Chapter 1.

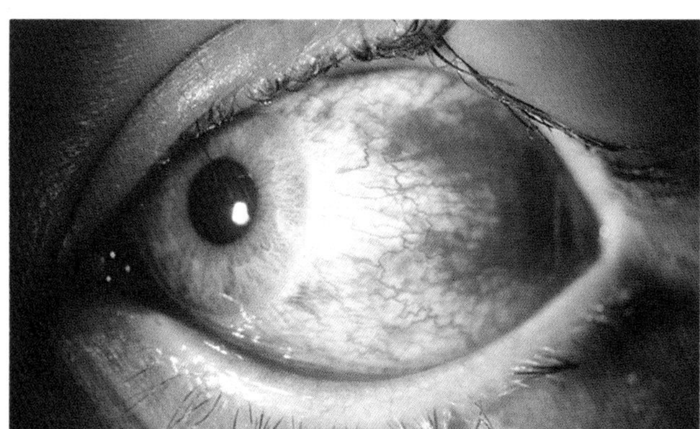
Figure 4.13 *Acute haemorrhagic conjunctivitis*

Chlamydial infections

Adult inclusion conjunctivitis

Adult inclusion conjunctivitis (TRIC) typically affects young adults during their sexually active years. The infection is almost invariably venereal in nature and is caused by the serotypes D to K of *Chlamydia trachomatis*. The eye lesions present about 1 week following sexual exposure and may be associated with a non-specific urethritis or cervicitis.

Clinical features

Conjunctivitis

This is bilateral, acute, and mucopurulent. Large opalescent follicles are seen in the fornices and in severe cases upper tarsal involvement predominates. As the disease progresses, follicles may also develop in the limbal region and over the bulbar conjunctiva. Oedema of the plica and chemosis may also be present. *Preauricular adenopathy* is a common finding but fever and pharyngitis are absent.

Keratitis

Epithelial keratitis of the upper half of the cornea is the most frequent corneal finding (*Figure 4.14*). *Marginal infiltrates* and a *superior micropannus* may also occur.

If untreated, the disease has a prolonged remittent course. The conjunctivitis becomes chronic with worsening of the keratitis and occasional development of anterior

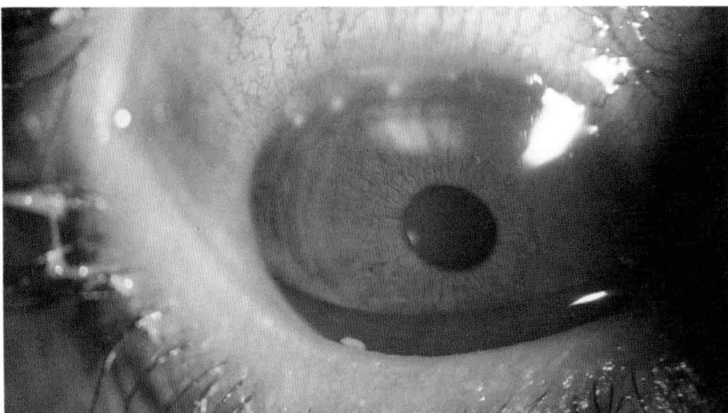

Figure 4.14 *Superior epithelial keratitis in TRIC*

uveitis. (*See Table 4.2* for a comparison with viral follicular conjunctivitis.)

Table 4.2 Comparison between chlamydial and viral follicular conjunctivitis

	Inclusion	*Viral*
Incubation	4–19 days	3–7 days
Age	Young adults	All ages
Systemic findings	Genitourinary	Respiratory
Discharge	Mucopurulent	Watery
Course	Chronic	Self-limiting
Adenopathy	++	+++
Follicles	+++	+++
bulbar and limbal	++	–
Keratitis	Common	Common
	Upper half	Diffuse
	Epithelial and subepithelial	Early–epithelial Late–subepithelial
Cytology	Inclusion bodies	
	Polymorphs	Mononuclear cells
Response to tetracycline	+	–
Response to steroids	–	+

Special investigations

Reliable differentiation between a chlamydial and viral infection can only be made through culture, serological and cytological studies. The diagnosis of chlamydial infection is usually made by finding basophilic cytoplasmic inclusion bodies of Halberstaedter–Prowazek in Giemsa-stained conjunctival scrapings. In view of the venereal nature of the disease, tests for syphilis and gonorrhoea should be done.

Treatment

Topical

This is with tetracycline ointment four times a day for 6 weeks.

Systemic

This can be with one of the following antibiotics all of which are administered orally:

1. *Tetracycline* 250 mg four times a day for 6 weeks.
2. *Erythromycin* 250 mg four times a day for 6 weeks. This is a useful alternative if tetracycline cannot be given as in pregnant women or nursing mothers, for fear of causing discolouration of teeth in the infant, as well as in patients who are allergic to tetracycline.
3. *Doxycycline* 300 mg weekly for 3 weeks or 100 mg daily for 1–2 weeks. This long-acting derivative of tetracycline is very effective in curing both the ocular and genital infection. Its use enhances patient compliance and it is also better absorbed than tetracycline from the gut as it is not affected by diet.

Trachoma

Trachoma is due to serotypes A, B, Ba, and C of *Chlamydia trachomatis.* It is a disease of underprivileged populations with poor hygienic conditions; the common fly is probably the major vector in the infection–reinfection cycle. Currently, trachoma is the leading cause of preventable blindness in the world. The natural course of the disease is characterized by an acute inflammation which appears at some time during the first decade of life, slowly progressing until the disease becomes inactive during the second decade. However, late sequelae may not appear for many years.

The MacCallan classification is based entirely on the conjunctival findings and describes the progression of structural changes. Although, in general, corneal complications increase in severity with each stage of the disease it may be highly variable from patient to patient.

Stage 1 (incipient trachoma)	Immature follicles on upper tarsus
Stage 2 (established trachoma) *Stage 2a* follicles predominant *Stage 2b* papillae predominant	Mature follicles on upper tarsus, keratitis, limbal follicles, intense activity with mature follicles buried within papillary hypertrophy
Stage 3 (cicatrizing trachoma)	Scarring of upper tarsus (*Figure 4.15*) with early trichiasis and entropion

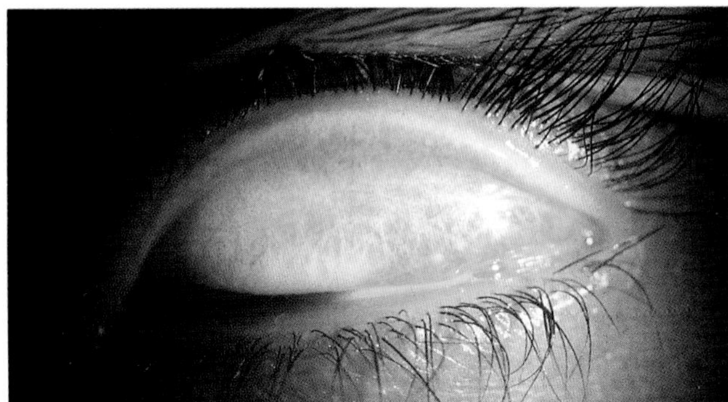

Figure 4.15 *Scarring of tarsal conjunctiva in trachoma*

Stage 4 (healed trachoma) — Inactive, varying degrees of scarring, no follicles or papillae

Corneal changes — These include epithelial keratitis, peripheral and central infiltrates, superficial fibrovascular pannus predominantly at the superior limbus (*Figure 4.16*), and limbal follicular swellings which cicatrize to form depressions called Herbert's pits (*Figure 4.17*).

Treatment of active disease is similar to that for adult inclusion conjunctivitis.

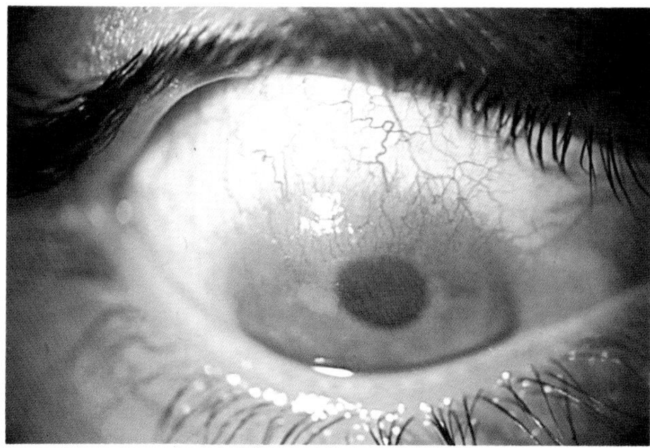

Figure 4.16 *Superior trachomatous pannus*

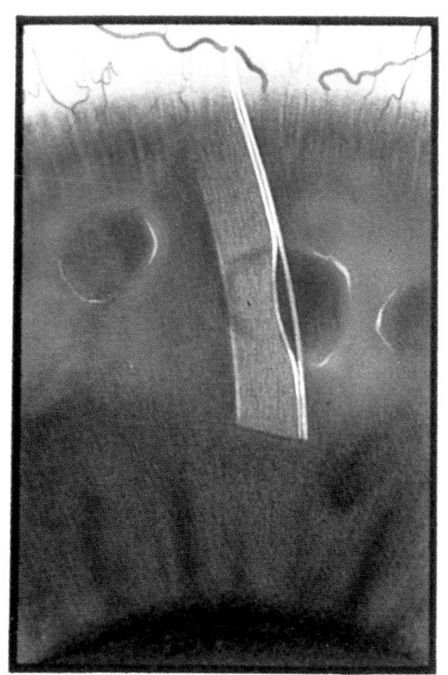

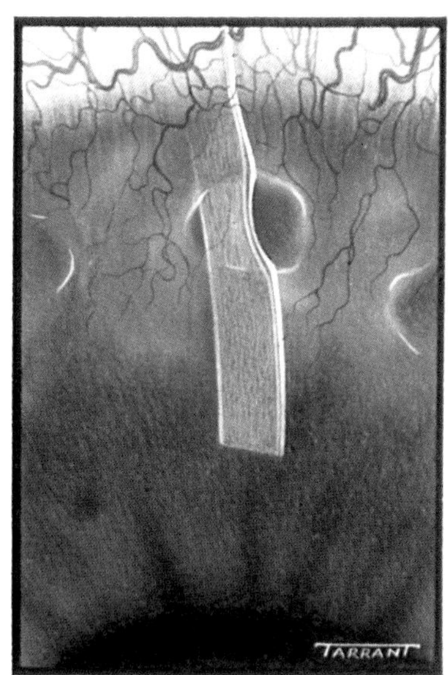

Figure 4.17 *Herbert's pits from trachoma*

Ophthalmia neonatorum

Ophthalmia neonatorum is a conjunctival inflammation (*Figure 4.18*) occurring during the first month of life. It is a notifiable condition.

Differential diagnosis

The traditional teachings concerning the time of onset of the inflammation are not always helpful in differential diagnosis (*Table 4.3*).

Chemical

This is usually evident a few hours after delivery and lasts no longer than 24 hours. It may be caused by silver nitrate or antibiotics used as prophylaxis against gonorrhoeal infection. The clinical picture is that of a transient mild hyperaemia.

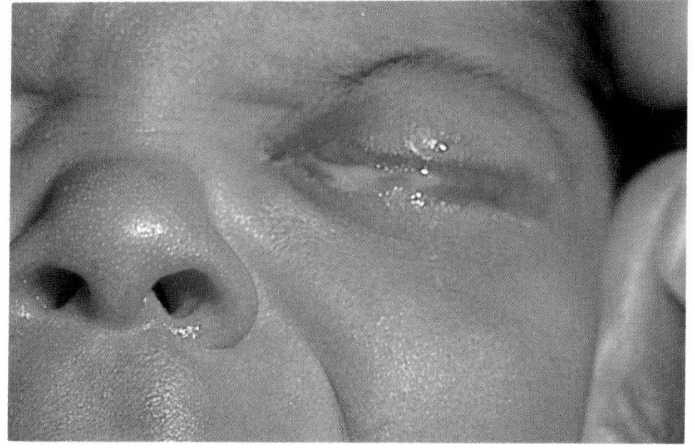

Figure 4.18 *Ophthalmia neonatorum*

Table 4.3 Ophthalmia neonatorum

Cause	*Manifestation*
Chemical	Hours
Gonococcal	2–4 days
Bacterial	4–5 days
Herpes simplex	5–7 days
Inclusion	5–14 days

Gonococcal

This is now a rare cause of ophthalmia neonatorum. It usually presents between 2 and 4 days after birth with a hyperacute purulent conjunctivitis associated with chemosis and sometimes membrane or pseudomembrane formation. If treatment with topical and systemic penicillin is delayed, corneal ulceration and even perforation may occur. The dose of systemic benzylpenicillin is 50 000 units/kg in two divided daily doses given for 7 days.

Bacterial

This is said to develop typically between the fourth and fifth days after birth, but it may occur at any time.

Herpes simplex

This usually develops between the fifth and seventh days of life. It is due to type 2 herpes virus in the majority of cases and is characterized by blepharoconjunctivitis which may be complicated by keratitis.

Inclusion

Chlamydia trachomatis is the most common cause of ophthalmia neonatorum. It has an incubation period of 5–14 days and is characterized by an acute mucopurulent conjunctivitis, although it may be frankly purulent and hyperacute. The conjunctival reaction is papillary as the infant cannot form follicles until about the third month of life. The correct diagnosis and treatment is important as occasionally it may give rise to a superior corneal pannus, conjunctival scarring and, very rarely, a corneal opacity. It is also important to be aware that systemic complications such as otitis, rhinitis, and even pneumonitis may develop.

Treatment is with topical tetracycline and oral erythromycin 50 mg/kg in four divided doses for 3 weeks. As in infants with gonococcal conjunctivitis, the infection is transmitted from the mother during delivery. It is therefore important that both parents are examined for evidence of genital infection.

Allergic disorders

Classification

Hay fever conjunctivitis
Acute allergic conjunctivitis
Chronic 'allergic' conjunctivitis
Vernal keratoconjunctivitis
Atopic keratoconjunctivitis
Giant papillary conjunctivitis
Cicatricial pemphigoid
Stevens–Johnson syndrome

Hay fever (seasonal allergic) conjunctivitis

This very common and innocuous condition is usually managed by a non-ophthalmologist.

Clinical features

The symptoms are transient attacks of itching, lacrimation, and redness during the hay fever season. The conjunctiva shows mild chemosis and a diffuse papillary reaction. In severe cases, the eyelids may be slightly oedematous but the cornea is uninvolved.

Treatment

This is with either sodium cromoglycate or Vasocon-A drops four times a day. The latter consists of a combination of a vasoconstrictor (naphazoline) and an antihistamine (antazoline). Although systemic antihistamines are effective in suppressing other symptoms of hay fever, they are of limited benefit in the eye.

Acute allergic conjunctivitis

This is an urticarial reaction due to a large amount of allergen reaching the conjunctival sac. It frequently affects young children after playing in grass or stroking pet animals.

Clinical features

The condition is characterized by a sudden onset of severe chemosis and swelling of the eyelids.

Treatment

The majority of cases resolve spontaneously within a few hours and apart from reassurance require no specific treatment.

Chronic 'allergic' conjunctivitis

This is a broad term which includes hypersensitivity or toxic reaction to a variety of substances such as preservatives (thiomersal), antiviral agents (idoxuridine), antibiotics (neomycin), and the prolonged use of antiglaucoma drops (pilocarpine and adrenaline). Frequently, however, the actual allergen is impossible to identify.

Clinical features

The symptoms of this extremely common disorder include non-specific chronic ocular irritation, itching and redness. Soft contact lens wearers with preservative-related problems may notice a progressive loss of lens tolerance. The conjunctiva shows mild hyperaemia with a generalized fine papillary or follicular response and the cornea may develop a mild punctate epithelial keratopathy. The lids and the surrounding skin may show evidence of contact dermatitis.

Treatment

If the allergen can be identified it should be withdrawn. If this is not possible, treatment with Vasocon-A or sodium cromoglycate may give symptomatic relief.

Vernal keratoconjunctivitis (spring catarrh)

Vernal keratoconjunctivitis (VKC) is an uncommon recurrent, bilateral external ocular inflammation, affecting children and commonly showing exacerbations during spring. Recent studies have suggested that it is an allergic disorder in which IgE-mediated mechanisms play an important role. Two populations with VKC probably exist:

1. *Atopic patients* with a history of hay fever, asthma, and eczema. Their peripheral blood shows eosinophilia and increased serum IgE levels. Treatment with sodium cromoglycate is most useful in this group.
2. *Non-atopic patients.*

Clinical features

The predominant symptom is intense ocular itching which may be associated with lacrimation, photophobia, foreign body sensation, and burning. Thick mucus discharge from the eyes and ptosis also occur. The disease can be divided into palpebral and the less common limbal types.

Palpebral

The initial conjunctival reaction consists of hyperaemia and chemosis, followed by a diffuse papillary hypertrophy, most marked on the superior tarsus. The papillae then become larger and have a flat-topped 'cobblestone' appearance (*Figure 4.19*). In severe cases, the connective tissue septa rupture, giving rise to giant papillae. The conjunctival changes are associated with a sticky exudate.

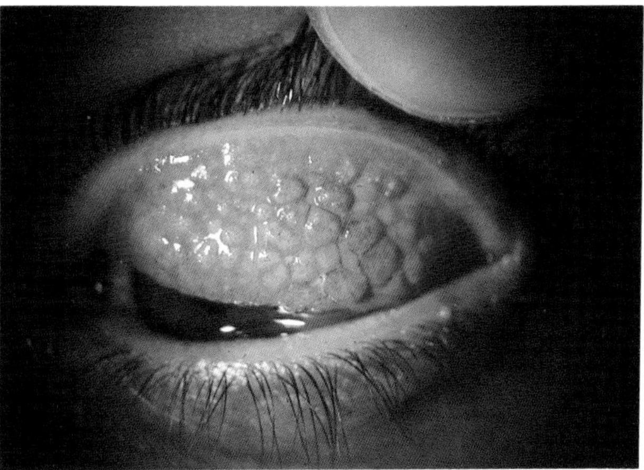

Figure 4.19 *Vernal conjunctivitis*

Limbal

The limbitis is characterized by hyperaemic, oedematous, and thickened conjunctiva. As the disease progresses, the thickening becomes irregular and assumes the appearance of mucoid nodules (*Figure 4.20*). Discrete white superficial spots (Trantas' dots) composed predominantly of eosinophils are found scattered around the limbus at the apices of the vegetations. Limbal vernal is more common in black patients.

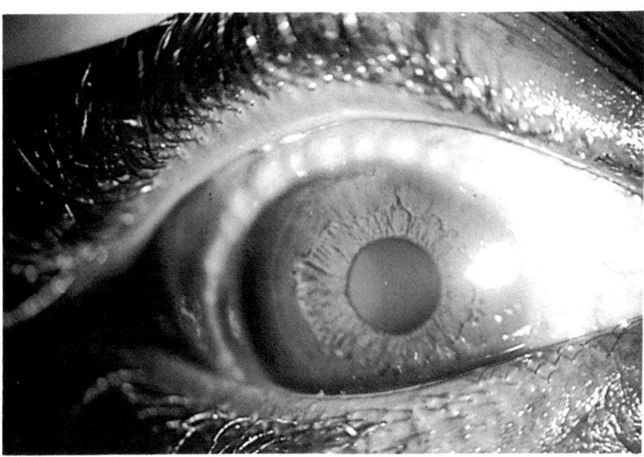

Figure 4.20 *Vernal limbitis*

Keratopathy

Buckley has classified vernal corneal changes into five types:

1. *Punctate epithelial keratitis* is the most benign form. It begins as discrete microerosions which coalesce and are usually more concentrated in the upper cornea, sparing the narrow strip adjacent to the limbus. Tiny particles of adherent desquamated epithelial cells and flecks of mucus may also be seen.
2. *Epithelial macroerosions* are caused by continued epithelial loss and result in ulceration.

3. *Plaque* is usually caused by epithelial macroerosions in which the bare area becomes coated with layers of altered exudate which cannot be wetted by tears and resists re-epithelialization (*Figure 4.21*).

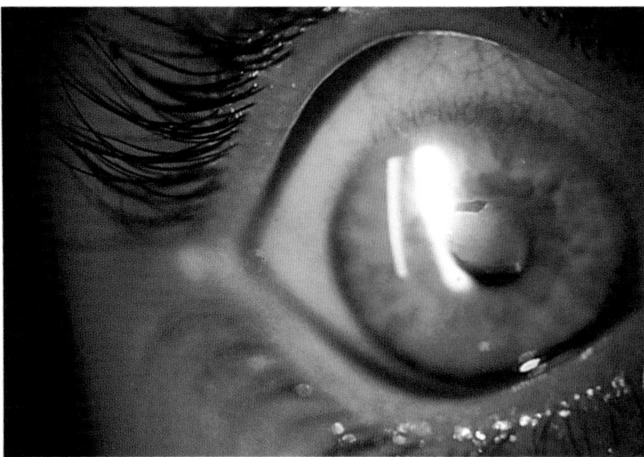

Figure 4.21 *Corneal plaque in vernal disease*

4. *Subepithelial scarring*, usually in the form of a 'ring scar', is a sign of severe corneal involvement.
5. *Pseudogerontoxon* resembles an arcus senilis and is usually characterized by a 'cupid's bow' outline in a previously inflamed segment of the limbus (*Figure 4.22*).

Patients with vernal disease also have a higher incidence of keratoconus.

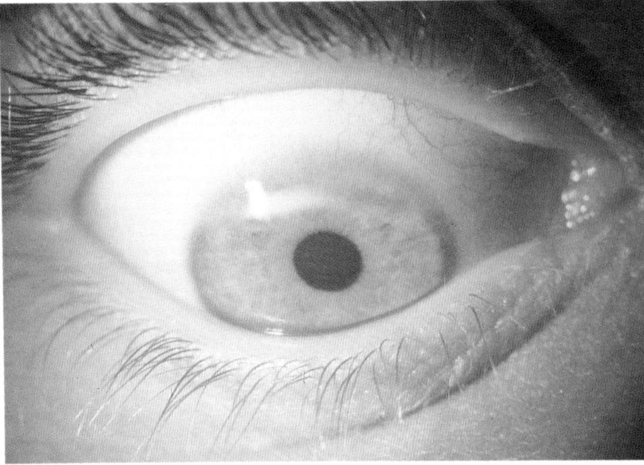

Figure 4.22 *'Cupid's bow' pseudogerontoxon in vernal disease*

Treatment

Topical steroids

Until recently corticosteroids have provided the main form of therapy. They are usually effective but may not achieve complete control of the disease in all cases. Because a prolonged course of treatment is usually required, corticosteroid-induced complications are high and corticosteroids must be used with great caution. Frequently, it is possible to discontinue medication completely between attacks and treat exacerbations vigorously with high doses, tapering to a relatively small dose as quickly as possible.

Sodium cromoglycate 2% drops (Opticrom)

This, instilled four times a day, is very useful in enabling patients to reduce or even discontinue steroid medication. Cromoglycate does not have any of the side-effects of corticosteroids and can therefore be used for prolonged periods as a prophylactic measure. It is not, however, as effective as corticosteroids in controlling an acute exacerbation.

Atopic keratoconjunctivitis

This relatively rare but potentially serious condition typically affects young adult atopic males. It can be considered as the adult equivalent of vernal disease.

Clinical features

The eyelids are thickened, crusted, and fissured. Apart from the eyelids, other classic atopic skin areas are the lateral neck folds, and the antecubital and antepopliteal fossae. Patients with atopic dermatitis are also predisposed to skin infections and chronic staphylococcal blepharitis. The conjunctiva shows hyperaemic infiltration and papillae. The main causes of visual impairment is progressive corneal scarring and neovascularization which may occasionally be associated with mucus plaques. Other occasional complications are keratoconus and subcapsular cataracts.

Treatment

This can be extremely difficult and prolonged. Topical steroids are the mainstay of treatment, although sodium cromoglycate may also be useful. It is also very important to treat associated blepharitis.

Giant papillary conjunctivitis

This is a foreign body associated conjunctivitis typically affecting three groups of patients:

1. Contact lens wearers.
2. Artificial eye wearers.
3. Patients with protruding ends of monofilament sutures following cataract extraction or keratoplasty.

The clinical features and treatment are discussed in Chapter 5.

Cicatricial pemphigoid

This rare chronic progressive autoimmune disease is characterized by recurrent blisters and bullae of the skin and mucous membranes. It usually occurs late in life (the average age at onset is 58 years) and affects women more commonly than men. It is associated with an increased prevalence of the HLA-B12 histocompatibility antigen.

Systemic features

Skin

Skin lesions occur in about 25% of cases and can be of two types:

1. A recurrent, vesiculobullous, non-scarring eruption that may involve the inguinal areas and/or extremities and which occasionally becomes generalized.
2. Localized erythematous plaques with recurrent vesicles and bullae appearing on the scalp and face near the affected mucous membranes. The lesions eventually heal leaving smooth atrophic scars.

Mucous membranes

Mucous membrane involvement includes the nose, oral cavity, pharynx, larynx, oesophagus, anus, and vagina. The oral mucosa eventually becomes involved in about 80% of all cases. The rupture of submucous blisters leaves erosions which often heal with scarring and the subsequent formation of strictures.

Ocular features

Ocular cicatricial pemphigoid (essential shrinkage of the conjunctiva) is a bilateral disease, although it is frequently asymmetrical with regard to the time of onset, severity of involvement, and rate of progression. The presenting feature is a subacute papillary conjunctivitis with diffuse conjunctival hyperaemia and a mucoid discharge. This is followed by the formation of subconjunctival bullae which, on bursting, give rise to conjunctival ulceration and the formation of pseudomembranes. The healing process is accompanied by chronic inflammation, subepithelial fibrosis and conjunctival shrinkage. The chronic and usually progressive course of the disease may be interrupted by episodes of subacute activity characterized by diffuse conjunctival hyperaemic and oedema or the appearance of fresh conjunctival bullae.

The disease may give rise to the following complications:

1. *Keratoconjunctivitis sicca* is caused by the fibrous occlusion of the ductules of the lacrimal and accessory lacrimal glands.
2. *Xerophthalmia* is caused by destruction of the mucin-secreting goblet cells in the conjunctiva. The tear film becomes unstable and the tear film break-up time markedly reduced.
3. *Symblepharon* is a serious complication in which adhesions form between the palpebral and bulbar conjunctiva (*Figure 4.23*). The adhesions typically involve the canthi and result in a flattening of the contour of the plica and the caruncle.
4. *Ankyloblepharon* is a condition in which adhesions form between the eyelids (*Figure 4.24*).
5. *Entropion, trichiasis, and lagophthalmos* are due to conjunctival scarring and symblepharon.
6. *Corneal involvement* is due to a combination of entropion, trichiasis, lagophthalmos and dryness. Eventually, corneal opacification occurs due to secondary bacterial infection, ulceration and neovascularization (*Figure 4.25*). Occasionally, corneal perforation may also occur.

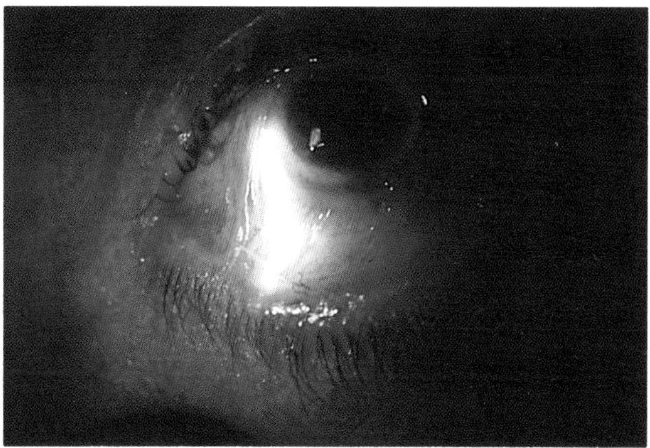

Figure 4.23 *Symblepharon in ocular cicatricial pemphigoid*

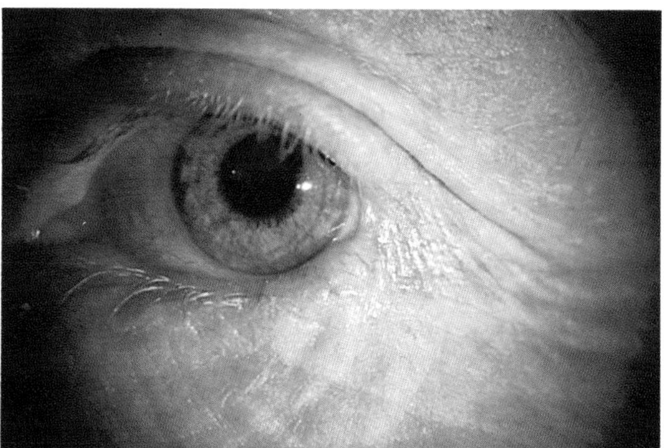

Figure 4.24 *Ankyloblepharon in ocular pemphigoid*

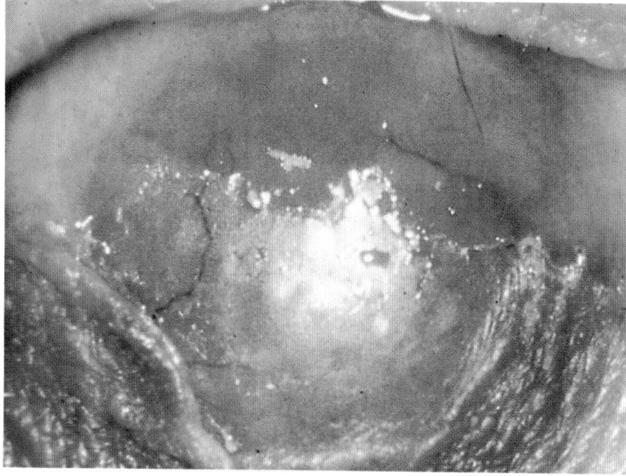

Figure 4.25 *Severe corneal scarring in ocular cicatricial pemphigoid*

Treatment

1. *Artificial tears* may alleviate the aqueous tear deficiency.
2. *Antibiotics* should be prescribed after cultures of the conjunctiva and lids have been taken.
3. *Corticosteroids*, both systemic and topical, are of definite benefit in the acute manifestations of the disease.
4. *Immunusuppressive agents* are at present being evaluated, but their effect is not yet established.
5. *Surgery* for entropion and trichiasis should be performed as early as possible.
6. *Soft contact lenses* may be used with caution to protect the cornea from trichiasis and drying. It may be necessary to use artificial tears frequently to prevent the lenses themselves from drying. Because the risk of infection is high when contact lenses are used in a dry eye, the patient should be seen frequently.
7. *Keratoprosthesis* may be useful in restoring a limited amount of sight in the final stages of the disease with ankyloblepharon and extensive keratinization of the ocular surface.

Stevens–Johnson syndrome (erythema multiforme major)

This is a mucocutaneous vesiculobullous disease, probably caused by a hypersensitivity reaction to antibiotics, sulphonamides (including acetazolamide), bacteria and viruses. The basic lesion is thought to be an acute vasculitis affecting skin and conjunctiva.

Systemic features

The disease begins with a fever, malaise, sore throat, cough, and arthralgia. These symptoms last for between 1 and 14 days. A rapidly developing, symmetrical, erythematous, vesiculocutaneous eruption then occurs, affecting any part of the body (*Figure 4.26*) although the scalp is usually spared. Haemorrhage into the vesicles results in a characteristic target lesion. Healing occurs within days or weeks, sometimes leaving a scar. The disease may recur in about one in four cases after re-exposure to the inciting antigen.

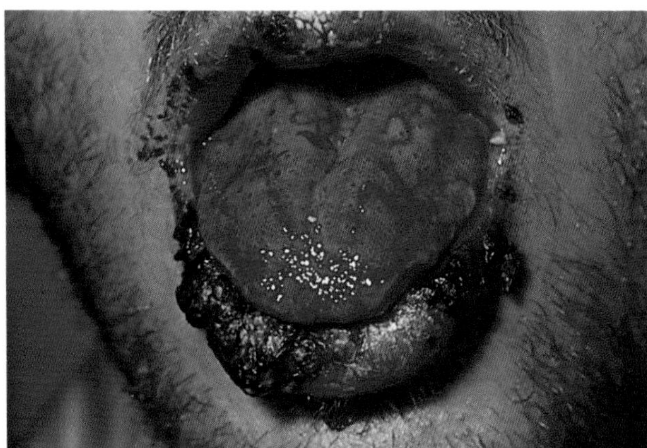

Figure 4.26 *Stevens–Johnson syndrome*

Ocular features

The conjunctiva is involved in about 50% of patients (*Figure 4.27*). The presenting finding is a mucopurulent conjunctivitis with engorged and inflamed papillae. This is followed by the development of red focal infarcts in ischaemic conjunctiva and the formation of white-yellow membranes, which, on shedding, reveal focal fibrotic patches. These fibrotic changes, which vary in size and distribution, are usually localized rather than diffuse and, according to their location, may lead to severe visual loss from corneal damage as a result of a combination of cicatricial entropion, aberrant eyelashes and abnormal keratinization of the conjunctiva. The metaplastic eyelashes are very fine and arise from the openings of damaged meibomian glands (acquired distichiasis). Although occasional involvement of the lacrimal ductules produces a dry eye, more often the eye is wet because of lacrimal drainage obstruction. Following the acute phase of the disease no further scarring occurs.

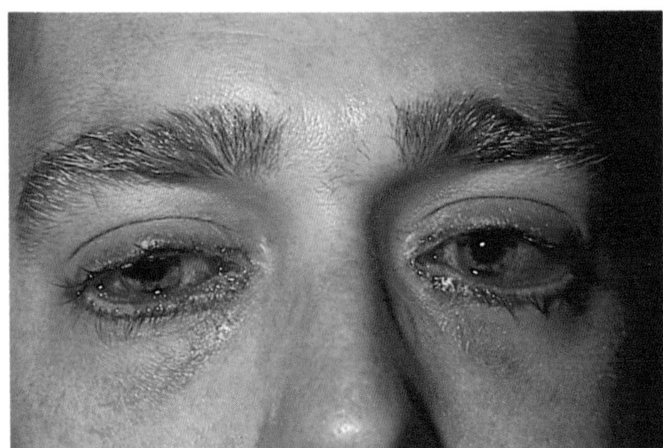

Figure 4.27 *Stevens–Johnson syndrome*

Treatment

1. *Medical*—topical steroids administered early during the course of the disease may control the vasculitis and prevent conjunctival infarction.
2. *Surgical* treatment is aimed at correcting entropion and abnormal eyelashes.

Chemical burns

A chemical burn is the only type of ocular injury that requires immediate treatment without first taking a history and performing a careful examination.

Acid

These are usually less serious than those caused by alkalis. This is because acids tend to precipitate tissue proteins which coagulate and form a barrier that prevents deep penetration. The main damage is therefore restricted to the lids, conjunctiva, and cornea.

Alkaline

Alkalis saponify lipids in the corneal epithelium and bind to the mucoproteins and collagen in the corneal stroma. They therefore disrupt the normal barriers of the cornea and gain rapid access to the anterior chamber, the lens, and anterior uvea. The complications of alkali burns not only involve the external ocular structures but they can also give rise to severe intraocular complications such as cataract, uveitis, and secondary glaucoma. In severe cases phthisis bulbi is the tragic end result.

Treatment

Immediate

Immediate treatment of all chemical burns is copious irrigation with bland sterile fluid and removal of all particulate matter. Because alkalis bind to the corneal stroma, they may continue to injure ocular structures after initial irrigation has removed all free alkali. For this reason, prolonged irrigation for several hours is necessary in eyes with alkali burns. The pH of the conjunctiva and, if possible, also of the offending chemical should be tested.

Subsequent

Subsequent treatment of alkali burns is aimed at preventing the complications that occur 2–3 weeks after the initial insult (failure of corneal re-epithelialization, melting, and descemetocele formation).

1. *Corticosteroids* together with mydriatics can be used safely during the first week to combat uveitis without increasing the risk of corneal melting. They are also useful in reducing the amount of symblepharon formation. However, during the second and third weeks, fibroblasts, presumably derived from surrounding keratocytes, repopulate the acellular burned areas. Topical corticosteroids should be avoided during this period as they may inhibit collagen synthesis and thereby enhance corneal ulceration and melting. After the third week, fibrocytic repopulation of the cornea has occurred and corticosteroids can once again be used if required.
2. *Vitamin C.* Hourly administration of sodium ascorbate 10% drops and a daily oral dose of ascorbic acid 1 g has a favourable influence on the prognosis of eyes with significant alkali burns. Once the epithelium has healed the drops are given less frequently for the remaining 4–6 weeks. At present the exact mechanism of action of ascorbate is unknown.
3. *Collagenase inhibitors.* It has been suggested that proteolytic enzymes (collagenases) may be responsible for the persistent epithelial defects, stromal melting, and corneal perforation. Peter Wright feels that 'collagenase inhibitors' in the form of L-cysteine and penicillamine applied topically are helpful but not universally successful in preventing corneal perforation.
4. *Tear substitutes* and, if necessary, punctal occlusion should be used to prevent the effects of xerophthalmia.
5. *Contact lenses* are useful in the prevention of symblepharon formation.

Late

1. *Division of bands* or adhesions of the conjunctiva.
2. *Grafting* of conjunctiva or mucous membrane.
3. *Eyelid surgery* to correct any associated deformity.
4. *Keratoplasty* should be delayed for at least 6 months and preferably for 12 months in order to allow maximal resolution of inflammation. The results of grafting are relatively poor because of a high rate of complications.

Miscellaneous syndromes

Superior limbic keratoconjunctivitis of Theodore

This uncommon chronic inflammatory disorder typically affects middle-aged women with thyroid dysfunction. The condition is frequently misdiagnosed because symptoms are more severe than clinical findings would suggest. At the time of presentation, the patient has invariably already been treated by various medications including corticosteroids and antibiotics without obtaining relief.

Clinical features

Symptoms

This disease is usually bilateral, although the severity of involvement may be asymmetrical. The symptoms consist of a foreign body sensation, burning, photophobia, and varying amounts of mucoid discharge. The condition is characterized by remissions and exacerbations and eventual resolution without sequelae.

Signs

On cursory examination the eye may look strikingly normal. However, examination of the superior conjunctiva and cornea will show the following changes (*Figure 4.28*):

1. *Superior tarsus* shows papillary hypertrophy which, in severe cases, gives rise to a diffuse velvety appearance.
2. *Superior bulbar conjunctiva* is hyperaemic with the injection being most intense at the limbus and fading as it approaches the superior fornix. The epithelial cells may become keratinized and the affected area may lack lustre (*Figure 4.29*).
3. *Limbus* may also show papillary hypertrophy and a grey thickening in its superior aspect.
4. *Superior cornea* frequently shows punctate epithelial erosions and a third of patients also have corneal filaments which may or may not be associated with diminished tear secretion.

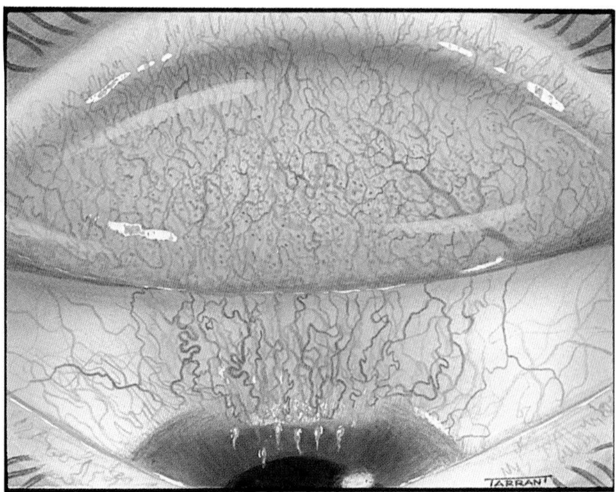

Figure 4.28 *Superior limbic keratoconjunctivitis*

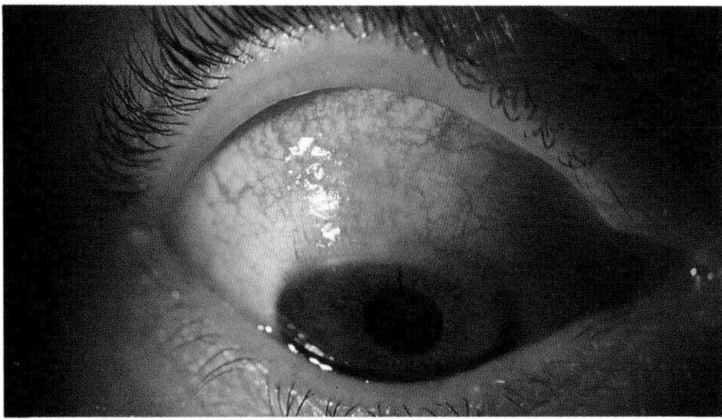

Figure 4.29 *Superior limbic keratoconjunctivitis*

Treatment

Although there is no cure for superior limbic keratoconjunctivitis of Theodore (SLK), the following therapeutic options are available:

1. *Topical medication*—adrenaline 1% drops may give symptomatic relief in mild cases. The number of corneal filaments can be reduced with acetylcysteine 5% drops. Patients with associated keratoconjunctivitis sicca should have tear substitutes.
2. *Silver nitrate 1%* applied to the superior tarsal and/or bulbar conjunctiva with a cotton-tipped applicator is effective in obtaining temporary symptomatic relief in many patients.
3. *Soft bandage contact lenses* are useful in some patients, although they should be used with caution because they have recently been implicated in causing a syndrome similar to SLK.
4. *Recession or resection of the superior bulbar conjunctiva.*
5. *Thermocauterization* of the superior bulbar conjunctiva is a recently described approach which appears to be safe and effective in a high proportion of cases.

Parinaud's oculoglandular conjunctivitis

This rare condition is characterized by the following:

1. *Unilateral granulomatous conjunctivitis* with nodular elevations surrounded by follicles and occasionally accompanied by ulceration.
2. *Lymphadenopathy* involving the preauricular and/or submandibular glands on the affected side.
3. *Systemic features* such as fever and malaise.

The most common causes are cat-scratch fever, tularaemia, and sporotrichosis. Less frequent causes are tuberculosis, syphilis and lymphogranuloma venereum. Treatment varies according to the cause.

Mucus fishing syndrome

The most frequent underlying disease that initiates the cycle of mucus fishing is keratoconjunctivitis sicca, although any condition that causes excess mucus production may be responsible. While trying to remove the excess mucus from the conjunctival sac, the patient traumatizes the conjunctival epithelium. This further increases mucus secretion, creating a vicious cycle.

Clinical features

This condition should be suspected when appropriate treatment of an external ocular disease does not produce the expected result. On direct questioning, the patient may deny mucus fishing. The characteristic traumatic conjunctival lesions are isolated, well-circumscribed areas that stain heavily with rose bengal. They are most commonly situated over the caruncle, plica, nasal and inferior bulbar conjunctivae, and inferior tarsal conjunctiva.

Treatment

The patient must be instructed not to touch or to attempt directly to remove mucus from the eye. It is also very important to adequately treat the underlying disorder responsible for excess mucus production.

Floppy eyelid syndrome

This is an uncommon and frequently misdiagnosed condition that typically affects obese men in whom a rubbery tarsus and loose upper eyelid everts during sleep and exposes the upper tarsal conjunctiva and cornea to trauma.

Clinical features

The exposure of the tarsal conjunctiva gives rise to a bilateral or unilateral chronic papillary conjunctivitis. The upper eyelids are extremely loose and readily evert when elevated.

Treatment

Treatment consists of either protecting the eye with a shield or by taping the lids shut during sleep to prevent lid eversion. A permanent cure can be achieved by horizontal lid shortening. It may, however, take several months for the conjunctival changes to resolve completely.

Reiter's syndrome

See Chapter 6.

Degenerations

Pinguecula

This extremely common lesion consists of a yellow-white deposit on the bulbar conjunctiva adjacent to the nasal or temporal aspect of the limbus. Histological examination shows degeneration of the collagen fibres of the conjunctival stroma, thinning of the overlying epithelium, and occasionally calcification. Some pingueculae may enlarge very slowly but surgical excision is seldom required.

Pterygium

Clinical features

Pterygia typically develop in patients who have been living in hot climates and may represent a response to chronic dryness and exposure to the sun. The lesion commences with the development of small grey corneal opacities near the nasal limbus. The conjunctiva then overgrows the opacities and encroaches onto the cornea in a triangular fashion (*Figure 4.30*). Beneath the body of the lesion there is destruction of Bowman's membrane and the superficial corneal lamellae. A deposit of iron (Stocker's line) may be seen in the corneal epithelium anterior to the advancing head of the pterygium. The conjunctival portion of the pterygium shows histological changes similar to a pinguecula but with more neovascularization and epithelial thickening.

A true pterygium is adherent to the underlying structures throughout, but a pseudopterygium (caused by the adhesion of a fold of conjunctiva to a peripheral corneal ulcer) is fixed only at its apex to the cornea.

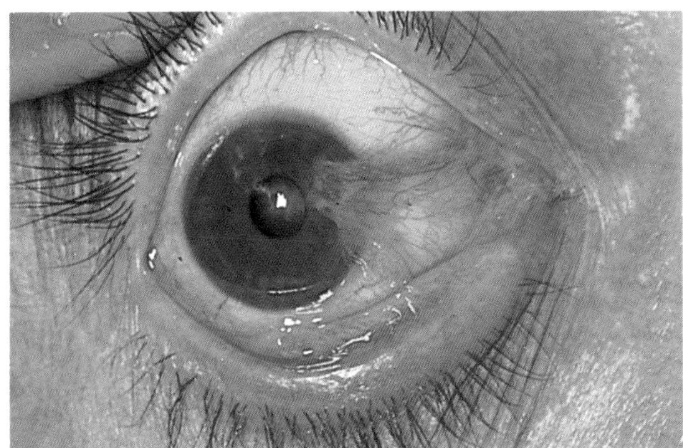

Figure 4.30 *Pterygium (courtesy of Mr B. Mathalone)*

Treatment

Surgical excision is indicated either for cosmetic reasons or in cases of progression towards the visual axis. Some surgeons prefer to use the bare sclera technique in order to prevent recurrences. In this operation, after excision of the conjunctival component of the lesion, the conjunctiva is sutured directly to the episclera, leaving a triangular area of sclera exposed. The postoperative use of beta-radiation and/or topical thiotepa drops may also be effective in the prevention of recurrence. Early argon laser treatment of recurrences may be helpful in preventing progression.

Concretions

These are small deposits of calcium commonly present in the palpebral conjunctiva of older individuals (*Figure 4.31*). They are usually asymptomatic, but may occasionally erode through the epithelium and give rise to a foreign body sensation. They can be easily removed with a needle.

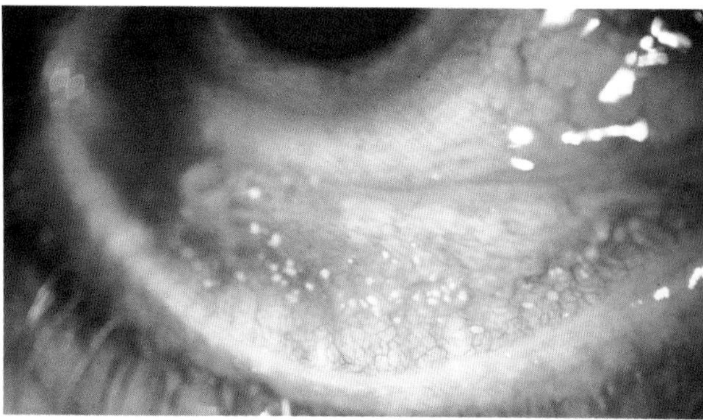

Figure 4.31 *Conjunctival concretions*

Retention cyst

This very common lesion usually presents as an asymptomatic thin-walled lesion which contains clear fluid (*Figure 4.32*). Excision of a cyst is unnecessary unless a large cyst causes ocular irritation or interferes with the wearing of a contact lens.

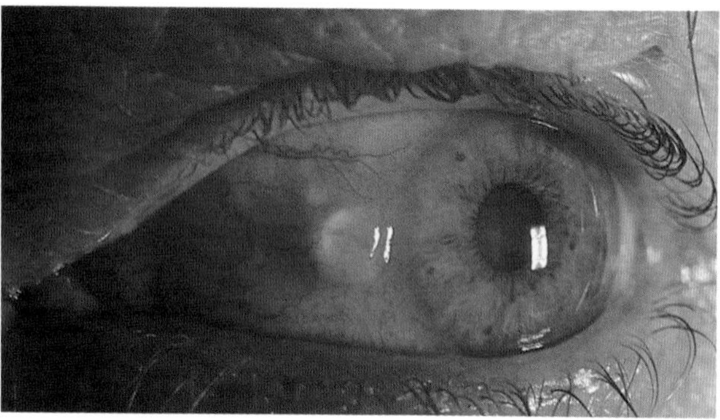

Figure 4.32 *Conjunctival retention cyst*

Pigmented lesions

Classification

Melanocytic pigmentation
- conjunctival epithelial melanosis
- subepithelial melanosis
- naevus
- precancerous melanosis
  - superficial spreading melanoma
  - lentigo maligna (Hutchinson's freckle)
- primary melanoma

Non-melanocytic pigmentation
- pseudopigmentation
- endogenous
- exogenous

Definitions

1. *Melanocytes* are cells derived from the neural crest which have migrated to the skin and mucous membranes. They synthesize a special organelle called a melanosome which is responsible for the characteristic colour of the skin in different races. The production of melanin requires the enzymatic oxidation of tyrosine. In albinism, the number of melanocytes is normal but melanin cannot be produced because of an enzyme deficiency.
2. *Melanosis* is a term used to describe increased pigmentation due to hyperplasia or hypertrophy of melanocytes.
3. *Naevus* is a benign tumour composed of naevus cells or naevocytes. Like melanocytes these cells contain melanosomes and are therefore capable of producing melanin.
4. *Melanoma* is a malignant tumour resulting from a transformation of melanocytes or naevus cells. It may be pigmented or non-pigmented.

Melanocytic pigmentation

Conjunctival epithelial melanosis

This is found in about 90% of blacks and 10% of whites. It usually develops during the first few years of life and becomes static by early adulthood. It typically appears as areas of flat, patchy, brownish pigmentation which are scattered throughout the conjunctiva, but it is usually most marked at the limbus and around the perforating branches of the anterior ciliary nerves as they enter the sclera (*Figure 4.33*). With the slitlamp, the pigment is seen to be within the epithelium, and the conjunctiva moves freely over the sclera. This type of pigmentary change has no malignant potential and requires no treatment.

Subepithelial melanosis

This may occur as an isolated congenital anomaly which is referred to as congenital melanosis oculi, or it may be associated with an ipsilateral hyperpigmentation of the skin of the face in the distribution of the first and second divisions of the trigeminal nerve. In this context it is referred to as oculodermal melanosis or the naevus of Ota. When seen on the slitlamp, subepithelial melanosis consists of pigmentation which lies beneath the epithelium and, because of this, it usually appears bluish-black in colour (*Figure 4.34*). The condition may occasionally be associated with hyperpigmentation of other ocular structures such as the sclera and uveal tract (*Figure 4.35*). Although it is usually benign it may rarely be associated with malignant melanomas of the choroid and orbit.

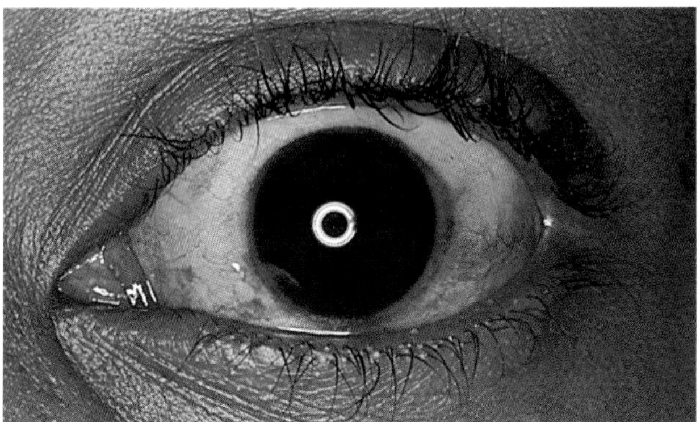

Figure 4.33 *Conjunctival epithelial melanosis (courtesy of Photographic Department, Wexham Park Hospital)*

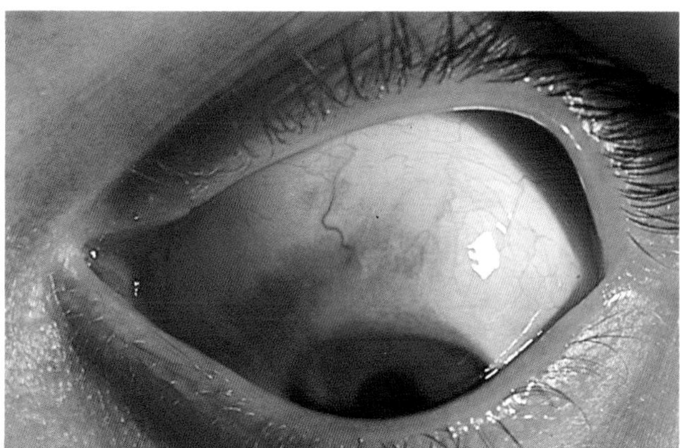

Figure 4.34 *Subepithelial melanosis*

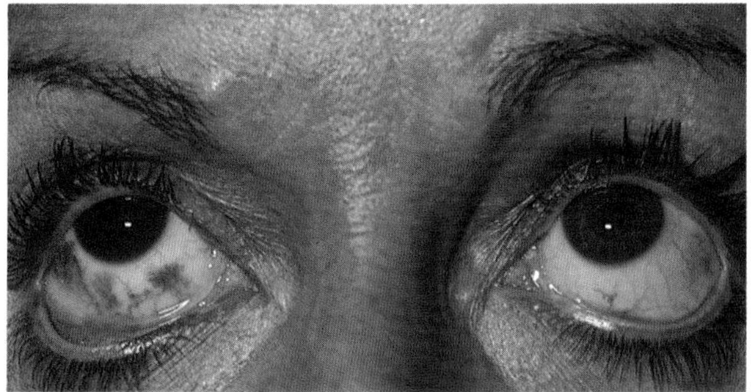

Figure 4.35 *Naevus of Ota; note hyperpigmentation of right iris*

Naevi

Naevi of the conjunctiva are common. They usually appear first during childhood as single, sharply demarcated, flat or slightly elevated lesions, most commonly located near the limbus. On slitlamp examination, cystic spaces are frequently seen within their substance. The amount of pigment within a naevus varies; about one-third show little or no pigmentation (*Figure 4.36*). However, both the amount of pigment and also the size of the lesion may increase at puberty or occasionally during pregnancy. It is generally agreed that the vast majority of naevi do not undergo malignant transformation and excision is indicated only for cosmetic reasons or if the lesion causes constant irritation. In these circumstances, the entire lesion should be excised using the bare sclera technique.

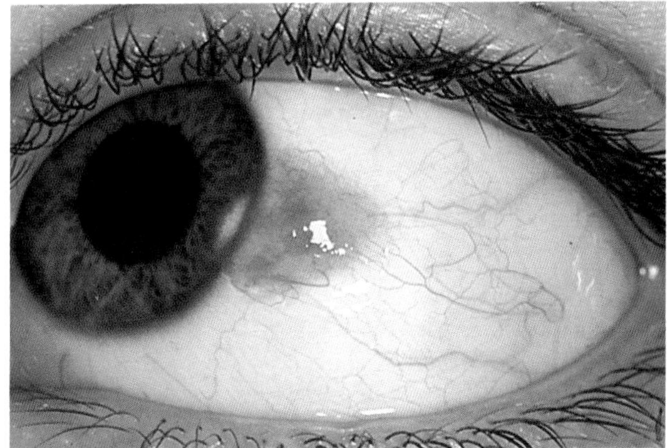

Figure 4.36 *Conjunctival naevus*

Precancerous melanosis

Two clinically and histologically different types of intraepithelial melanoma are recognized, although frequently they are both 'lumped together' as precancerous melanosis.

Superficial spreading melanoma

This typically develops during middle or old age, although occasionally it may affect young adults. It is characterized by the presence of one or more areas of pigmentation involving the conjunctiva and occasionally the eyelids. Although the lesion may occasionally be stationary, it usually progresses very slowly. As long as it maintains its radial growth, it does not metastasize, although ultimately it starts to invade the subepithelial tissues and turns into a frank malignant melanoma which may metastasize widely.

Management depends on the extent of the lesion. If the patient has multicentric flat lesions which have developed during later life, they should be photographed at 6-monthly intervals. If the patches become thicker or nodular (*Figure 4.37*), local excision should be carried out.

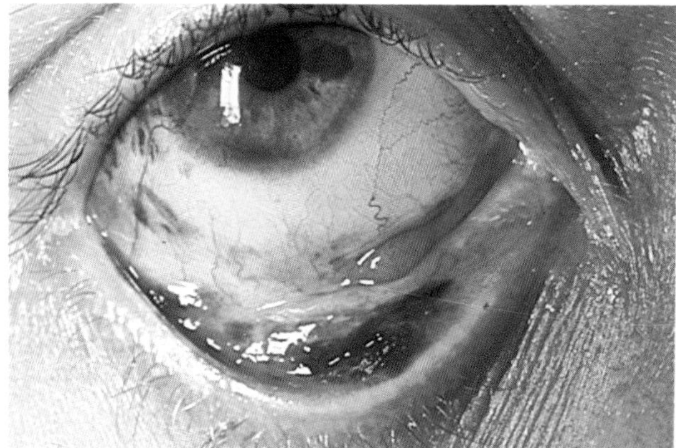

Figure 4.37 Superficial spreading melanoma (courtesy of Mr C. Migdal)

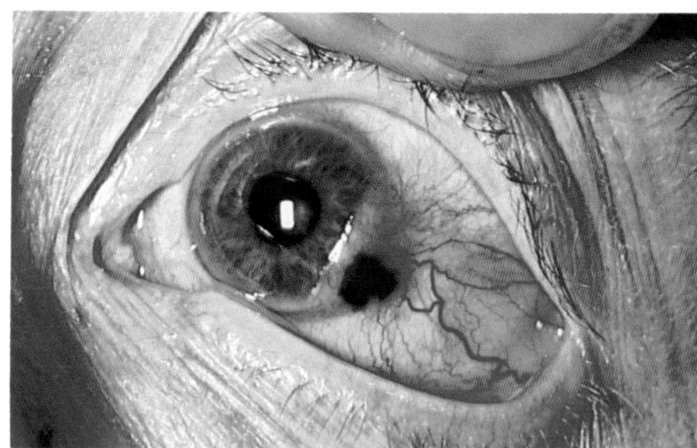

Figure 4.39 Conjunctival malignant melanoma

Lentigo maligna (Hutchinson's freckle)

This typically occurs on the faces of elderly patients (*Figure 4.38*). It usually has a much slower radial growth rate than superficial spreading melanoma and it may be present for many years or even decades before subepithelial invasion occurs. It seems to have a better prognosis than superficial spreading melanoma.

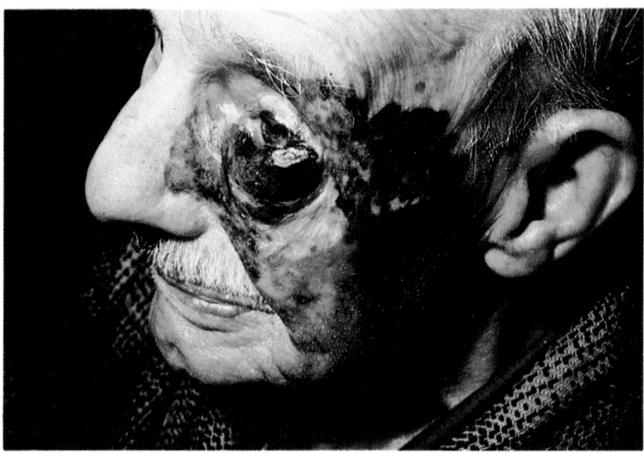

Figure 4.38 Lentigo maligna

Primary melanoma

A primary nodular form of malignant conjunctival melanoma may arise *de novo*, most commonly at the limbus (*Figure 4.39*) and may be pigmented or non-pigmented. It appears to have a better prognosis than malignant melanoma arising from pre-existing lesions. Tumours arising from the bulbar conjunctiva have a 100% 5-year survival rate, those arising at the limbus have an 83% 5-year survival rate, and those arising from the palpebral areas a 50% 5-year survival rate. The unfavourable prognosis in the latter may be related in part to delay in diagnosis. Treatment consists of local excision, enucleation if the tumour has invaded deeper structures such as the sclera, and exenteration if the tumour has arisen from the palpebral conjunctiva and has spread to the lids or orbit. Other therapeutic modalities have been advocated from time to time in selected cases, including radiation, cryotherapy, regional lymph node dissection, and chemotherapy for metastatic disease.

Non-melanocytic pigmentation

1. *Pseudopigmentation* may occur in patients with blue sclera and scleromalacia perforans.
2. *Endogenous pigmentation* occurs in patients with Addison's disease, jaundice, and ochronosis.
3. *Exogenous pigmentation* may develop from the long-term use of topical adrenaline in the treatment of glaucoma (*Figure 4.40*). Occasionally, the pigmentation may be so extensive that it is mistaken for a malignant melanoma. Mascara may also cause black pigmentation of the superior border of the upper tarsus. Argyrosis is another form of exogenous pigmentation.

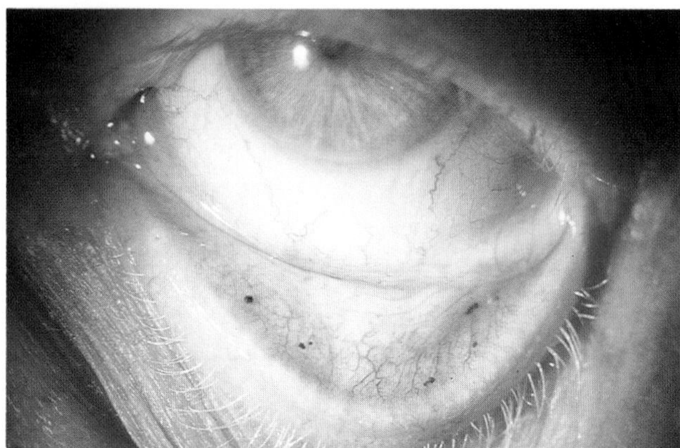

Figure 4.40 Conjunctival pigment deposits from use of topical adrenaline for glaucoma

Non-pigmented tumours

Classification

Papilloma
Intraepithelial epithelioma
Invasive squamous cell carcinoma
Choristomas
  dermoid
  lipodermoid

Papilloma

Just like those occurring on the eyelids, conjunctival papillomas can be sessile or pedunculated. It is likely that some of these tumours are caused by infection with papillomaviruses. Occasionally they are very large and may simulate malignant tumours (*Figure 4.41*). Following surgical excision the recurrence rate is high.

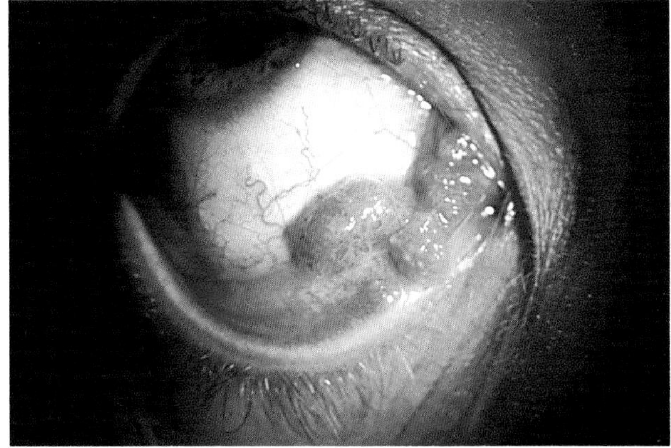

Figure 4.41 *Conjunctival papilloma*

Intraepithelial epithelioma (carcinoma *in situ*)

This premalignant tumour of the conjunctival epithelium usually begins near the limbus (*Figure 4.42*) and spreads to involve the fornices and cornea. It most commonly appears as a slightly elevated fleshy mass with tufted blood vessels, although occasionally it may appear as a gelatinous avascular tumour. Because the lesion is superficial to the basement membrane, the conjunctiva is freely movable over the underlying episcleral tissue. Treatment can be by surgical excision, cryotherapy or both.

Invasive squamous cell carcinoma

This is characterized by deep invasion of the stroma with fixation to underlying tissues. If untreated, the tumour may penetrate deeply to reach the inside of the eye where it may show rapid growth.

Treatment of early cases is the same as for intraepithelial epithelioma, although enucleation or even exenteration may be necessary for advanced cases.

Choristoma

Choristomas are congenital overgrowths of normal tissue in abnormal locations. They are the commonest type of epibulbar tumour in children. The two main types are dermoids and lipodermoids (dermolipomas).

Dermoids consist of collagenous connective tissue covered by epidermoid epithelium. They appear as solid white masses most frequently located at the limbus (*Figure 4.43*).

Lipodermoids consist of adipose tissue with surrounding dermis-like connective tissue. They appear as soft, yellow, movable subconjunctival masses located most commonly at the limbus or outer canthus (*Figure 4.44*).

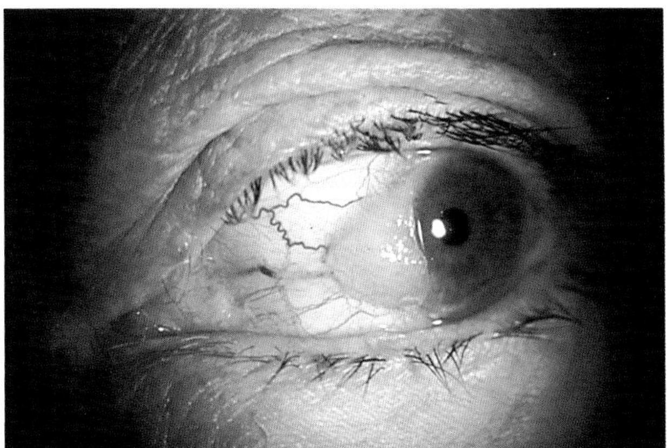

Figure 4.42 *Intraepithelial epithelioma of conjunctiva*

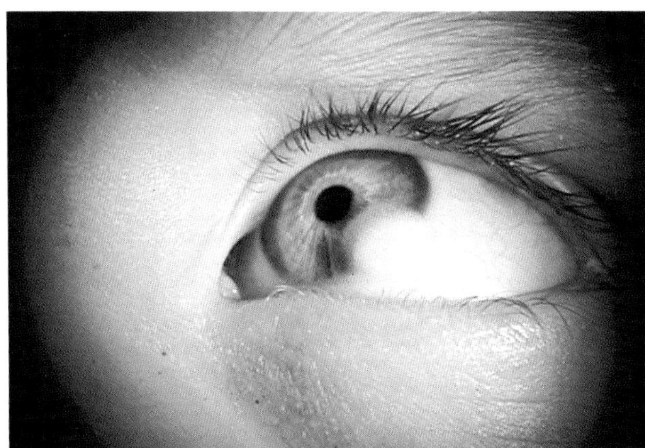

Figure 4.43 *Limbal dermoid*

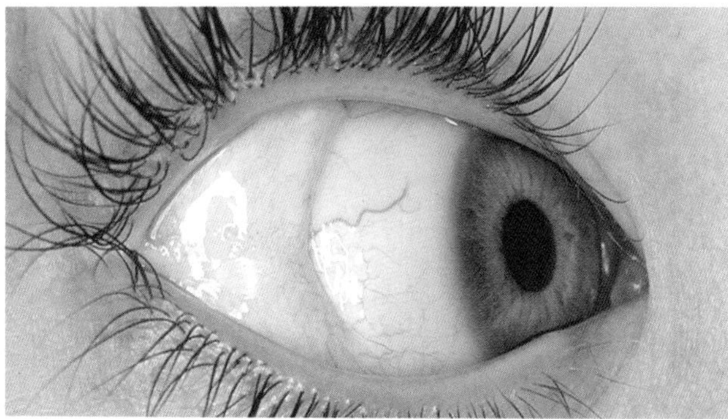

Figure 4.44 Conjunctival lipodermoid

Patients with Goldenhar's syndrome frequently have epibulbar choristomas in association with preauricular skin tags, vertebral anomalies, and hemifacial hypoplasia. Other ocular anomalies that have been reported in some patients with this syndrome include microphthalmos, anophthalmos, tilted disc, optic nerve hypoplasia, macular hypoplasia, and strabismus.

Further reading

Bacterial infections

Dougherty, J.M. and McCulley, J.P. (1984) Comparative bacteriology of chronic blepharitis. *British Journal of Ophthalmology*, **68,** 524–528

Gutscell, V.J., Stern, G.A. and Hood, C.I. (1980) Histopathology of meibomian gland dysfunction. *American Journal of Ophthalmology*, **94,** 383–387

Leibowitz, H.W., Pratt, M.V., Flagstad, I.J. *et al.* (1976) Human conjunctivitis: 1. Diagnostic evaluation: 2. Treatment. *Archives of Ophthalmology*, **94,** 1747–1749, 1752–1756

Lempert, S.L., Jenkins, M.S. and Brown, S.I. (1979) Chalazia and rosacea. *Archives of Opthalmology*, **97,** 1652–1653

McCulley, J.P., Dougherty, J.M. and Deneau, D. G. (1982) Classification of chronic blepharitis. *Ophthalmology*, **89,** 1173–1180

McGill, J.I. (1986) Bacterial conjunctivitis. *Transactions of the Ophthalmological Society of the United Kingdom*, **105,** 37–40

Perry, H.D. and Serniuk, R.A. (1980) Conservative treatment of chalazia. *Ophthalmology*, **87,** 218–221

Seal, D.V., Barrett, S.P. and McGill, J.I. (1982) Aetiology and treatment of acute bacterial infection of the external eye. *British Journal of Ophthalmology*, **66,** 357–360

Smolin, G. and Okamoto, M. (1977) Staphylococcal blepharitis. *Archives of Ophthalmology*, **95,** 812–816

Stenson, S., Newman, R. and Fedukowicz, H. (1982) Laboratory studies in acute conjunctivitis. *Archives of Ophthalmology*, **100,** 1275–1277

Viral infections

Darougar, S., Grey, R.H.B., Thaker, U. *et al.* (1983) Clinical and epidemiological features of adenovirus keratoconjunctivitis in London. *British Journal of Ophthalmology*, **76,** 1–7

Schwartz, H. and Sugar, J. (1979) Adenovirus conjunctivitis in children. *Perspectives in Ophthalmology*, **3,** 285–290

Chlamydial infections

Stenson, S. (1981) Adult inclusion conjunctivitis: clinical characteristics and corneal changes. *Archives of Ophthalmology*, **99,** 605–608

Viswalingam, N.D., Darougar, S. and Yearsley, P. (1986) Oral doxycycline in the treatment of adult chlamydial ophthalmia. *British Journal of Ophthalmology*, **70,** 301–304

Ophthalmia neonatorum

Forstot, S.L. (1979) Ophthalmia neonatorum: neonatal ocular syndromes. *Perspectives in Ophthalmology*, **3,** 243–248

Perry, D. and Brinser, J.H. (1978) Diagnosis and management of ophthalmia neonatorum. *Perspectives in Ophthalmology*, **2,** 163–170

Pierce, J.W., Ward, M.E. and Seal, D.V. (1982) Ophthalmia neonatorum in the 1980's: incidence, aetiology and treatment. *British Journal of Ophthalmology*, **66,** 728–731

Rapoza, P.A., Quinn, T.C., Kiessling, L.A. *et al.* (1986) Epidemiology of neonatal conjunctivitis. *Ophthalmology*, **93,** 456–461

Ridgway, G.L. (1986) A fresh look at ophthalmia neonatorum. *Transactions of the Ophthalmological Society of the United Kingdom*, **105,** 41–42

Allergic disorders

Abelson, M.B., Butrus, S.I. and Weston, J.H. (1983) Asprin therapy in vernal conjunctivitis. *American Journal of Ophthalmology*, **95,** 502–505

Allansmith, M.R., Korb, D.R., Greiner, J.V. *et al.* (1977) Giant papillary conjunctivitis in contact lens wearers. *American Journal of Ophthalmology*, **83,** 697–708

Buckley, R.J. (1981) Vernal keratopathy and its management. *Transactions of the Ophthalmological Society of the United Kingdom*, **101,** 234–238

Foster, C.S. and Duncan, J. (1980) Randomised clinical trial of topical administration of Cromylyn in vernal keratoconjunctivitis. *American Journal of Ophthalmology*, **90,** 175–181

Foster, C.S., Wilson, L.A. and Ekins, M.B. (1982) Immunosuppressive therapy for progressive ocular cicatricial pemphigoid. *Ophthalmology*, **89,** 340–353

Mondino, B.J. and Brown, S.I. (1981) Ocular cicatricial pemphigoid. *Ophthalmology*, **88,** 95–100

Mondino, B.J. and Brown, S.I. (1983) Immunosuppressive therapy in ocular cicatricial pemphigoid. *American Journal of Ophthalmology*, **96,** 453–459

Wright, P. (1979) Enigma of ocular cicatricial pemphigoid. *Transactions of the Ophthalmological Society of the United Kingdom*, **99,** 141–145

Wright, P. (1986) Cicatrizing conjunctivitis. Doyne Lecture. *Transactions of the Ophthalmological Society of the United Kingdom*, **105,** 1–17

Wright, P. and Collin, J.R.O. (1983) The ocular complications of erythema multiforme (Stevens Johnson Syndrome) and their management. *Transactions of the Ophthalmological Society of the United Kingdom*, **103,** 338–341

Chemical burns

Pfister, R.R. and Paterson, C.A. (1980) Ascorbic acid in the treatment of alkali burns of the eye. *Ophthalmology*, **87,** 1050–1057

Wright, P. (1982) The chemically injured eye. *Transactions of the Ophthalmological Society of the United Kingdom*, **102,** 85–87

Miscellaneous syndromes

Chin, G.N. (1980) Diagnosis and treatment of Parinaud's (oculoglandular) conjunctivitis. *Perspectives in Ophthalmology*, **4,** 39–44

Culbertson, W.W. and Ostler, H.B. (1981) The floppy eyelid syndrome. *American Journal of Ophthalmology*, **92,** 568–575

Martin, X., Uffer, S. and Gailloud, C. (1986) Ophthalmia nodosa and the oculoglandular syndrome of Parinaud. *British Journal of Ophthalmology*, **70**, 536–542

McCulley, J.P., Moore, B. and Matoba, A.Y. (1985) Mucus fishing syndrome. *Ophthalmology*, **92**, 1262–1265

Moore, M.B., Harrington, J. and McCulley, J.P. (1986) Floppy eyelid syndrome. Management including surgery. *Ophthalmology*, **93**, 184–188

Passons, G.A. and Wood, T.O. (1984) Conjunctival resection for superior limbic keratoconjunctivitis. *Ophthalmology*, **91**, 966–968

Udell, I.J., Kenyon, K.R., Sawa, M. *et al.* (1986) Treatment of superior limbic keratoconjunctivitis by thermocauterization of the superior bulbar conjunctiva. *Ophthalmology*, **93**, 162–166

Wear, D.J., Malaty, R.H., Zimmerman, L.E. *et al.* (1985) Cat scratch disease bacilli in the conjunctiva of patients with Parinaud's oculoglandular syndrome. *Ophthalmology*, **92**, 1282–1287

Pigmented lesions

Dutton, J.J., Anderson, R.L., Schelper, R.L. *et al.* (1984) Orbital malignant melanoma and oculodermal melanocytosis. *Ophthalmology*, **91**, 497–507

Folberg, R., McLean, I.W. and Zimmerman, L.E. (1984) Conjunctival melanosis and melanoma. *Ophthalmology*, **91**, 673–678

Henkind, P. and Benjamin, J.V. (1977) Conjunctival melanocytic lesions: natural history. *Transactions of the Ophthalmological Society of the United Kingdom*, **97**, 373–377

Jakobiec, F.A. (1980) (Editorial) Conjunctival melanoma: unfinished business. *Archives of Ophthalmology*, **98**, 1378–1484

Jakobiec, F.A., Brownstein, S., Wilkinson, R.D. *et al.* (1980) Combined surgery and cryotherapy for diffuse malignant melanoma of the conjunctiva. *Archives of Ophthalmology*, **98**, 1390–1396

Valazquez, N. and Jones, I.S. (1983) Ocular and oculodermal melanocytosis associated with uveal melanoma. *Ophthalmology*, **90**, 1472–1476

Non-pigmented tumours

Divine R.D. and Anderson, R.L. (1983) Nitrous oxide cryotherapy for intraepithelial epithelioma of the conjunctiva. *Archives of Ophthalmology*, **101**, 782–786

Fraunfelder, F.T. and Wingfield, D. (1983) Management of intraepithelial conjunctival tumors and squamous carcinoma. *American Journal of Ophthalmology*, **95**, 359–363

Lass, J.H., Jenson, A.B., Papale, J.J. *et al.* (1983) Papillomavirus in human conjunctival papilloma. *American Journal of Ophthalmology*, **95**, 364–368

Mansour, A.M., Wang, F., Henkind, P. *et al.* (1985) Ocular findings in the facioauriculovertebral sequence (Goldehar–Gorlin syndrome). *American Journal of Ophthalmology*, **100**, 555–559

Nicholson, D.H. and Herschler, J. (1977) Intraocular invasion of squamous cell carcinoma of the conjunctiva. *Archives of Ophthalmology*, **95**, 843–846

5

The Cornea and Sclera

Introduction

Applied anatomy
Evaluation of corneal disease
Principles of management of corneal disease

Microbial keratitis

Bacterial
Fungal
Acanthamoeba
Interstitial

Viral keratitis

Herpes simplex
Herpes zoster
Vaccinia
Thygeson's superficial punctate

Exposure keratopathy

Neurotrophic keratopathy

Peripheral ulceration and thinning

Classification
Dellen
Marginal keratitis (catarrhal ulcer)
Rosacea keratitis
Phlyctenulosis
Terrien's marginal degeneration
Mooren's ulcer
Systemic collagen vascular disorders

Degenerations

Arcus senilis
Vogt's white limbal girdle
Lipid keratopathy
Band keratopathy
Spheroidal
Salzmann's nodular

Dystrophies

Classification
Anterior
Stromal
Posterior
Ectatic

Changes in metabolic and toxic disorders

Wilson's disease (hepatolenticular degeneration)
Corneal crystalline deposits
Cornea verticillata (vortex keratopathy)
Mucopolysaccharidoses

Contact lenses

Forms
Principles of fitting
Medical indications
Complications

Principles of keratoplasty

Penetrating
Lamellar

Principles of refractive corneal surgery

Radial keratotomy
Epikeratophakia

Episcleritis and scleritis

Applied anatomy
Episcleritis
Scleritis

Introduction

Applied anatomy

The cornea consists of five layers (*Figure 5.1*):

1. The epithelium.
2. Bowman's layer.
3. The stroma.
4. Descemet's membrane.
5. The endothelium.

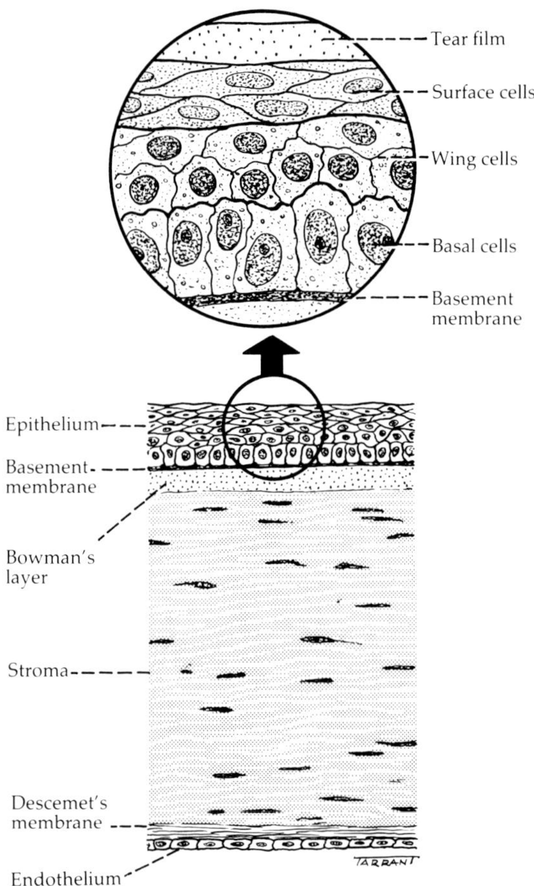

Figure 5.1 *Anatomy of cornea*

The epithelium

This accounts for about one-tenth of total corneal thickness and is made up of three cell types:

1. *The basal columnar* cells from a single layer which is attached to the basement membrane (basal lamina) by hemidesmosomes. It has been suggested that a lack of hemidesmosomes may be responsible for recurrent corneal erosions. The nucleus of each basal cell is displaced towards its apex. The wing cells and surface cells are derived from the basal cells.
2. *The wing cells* are arranged in two or three rows and have thin 'wing-like' extensions.
3. *The surface cells* are long and thin with flat nuclei. They are arranged in two layers and are joined by bridges. The surface area of the outermost cells is increased by microplicae and microvilli in order to facilitate the adsorption of mucin which is essential for corneal wetting. After a lifespan of a few days the superficial cells are shed into the tears. Because of its excellent ability to regenerate, the epithelium does not scar as a result of inflammation. However, scarring in the form of pannus can develop immediately beneath the epithelium.

Bowman's layer

This is an acellular structure that merely represents the superficial layer of the corneal stroma. It does not regenerate when damaged.

The stroma

This makes up 90% of corneal thickness. It is composed of collagen-producing fibroblasts (keratocytes), collagen fibrils, and ground substance. The fibrils are of uniform size and extend across the entire length of the cornea as bundles (lamellae) which criss-cross at approximate right angles but interlace infrequently. The ground substance which occupies the space in between the lamellae is composed of mucoprotein and glycoprotein. A few wandering cells (leucocytes and macrophages) are also present in the stroma.

Descemet's membrane

This is the basal lamina of the corneal endothelium. It is composed of a fine lattice-work of collagen fibrils consisting of an interior banded zone, which develops *in utero*, and a posterior non-banded zone which is laid down throughout life by the corneal endothelium.

The endothelium

This consists of a single layer of hexagonal cells. It plays a vital role in maintaining the deturgescence of the cornea. With age, the number of endothelial cells gradually decreases. Because the endothelium is incapable of regeneration, neighbouring cells have to spread in order to fill any vacant gaps.

Evaluation of corneal disease

Symptoms

The five main symptoms of corneal disease are:

1. *Pain.* The cornea is richly supplied by sensory nerve endings via the first division of the trigeminal nerve. It has a subepithelial plexus and a stromal plexus. In eyes with corneal abrasions or bullous keratopathy, the direct stimulation of bare nerve endings causes severe pain. Patients with mild punctate erosions may complain only of slight irritation which is made worse by blinking.

2. *Impairment of visual acuity* is caused by loss of central corneal transparency.
3. *Haloes* are due to the diffraction of light as a result of epithelial oedema. The blue end of the spectrum is nearest to the light source.
4. *Photophobia* is undue sensitivity to light of normal luminosity. It is caused by an abnormally strong light-induced miosis of an inflamed iris.
5. *Lacrimation* (excessive tear production) is due to reflex stimulation of corneal nerves. Its degree frequently parallels the severity of photophobia.

Slitlamp biomicroscopy

Essentially, three techniques are used to examine the cornea (*Figure 5.2*): direct illumination, scleral scatter, and retroillumination.

Direct illumination

First, diffuse illumination is used to detect gross lesions and then the beam is narrowed and directed obliquely, allowing a quadrilateral cross-section of the cornea to be visualized. On narrowing the beam still more, a very thin optical section of the cornea is seen. Then, by passing the beam across the entire cornea, the thickness and depth of corneal lesions can be determined.

When the next two methods of examination are used, it is necessary to dissociate the light source from the angle of the microscope. This is done by unlocking the centre-locking screw, allowing the beam to be decentred.

Scleral scatter

The slit beam is displaced laterally so that the light falls onto the limbus while the microscope is focused centrally on the cornea. In this way, light is transmitted within the cornea by total internal reflection and exits at the opposite limbus. If the cornea is normal no light is seen. If the light is obstructed by an opacity the lesion will become illuminated because it alters the path of the internally reflected light beam. This technique is especially useful in the detection of subtle opacities and mild corneal oedema.

Retroillumination

This technique utilizes the reflection from the iris in order to illuminate the cornea from behind. This allows the detection of fine epithelial and endothelial changes, keratic precipitates, and small blood vessels.

Clinical interpretation of corneal lesions

Epithelium

Punctate epithelial erosions (epitheliopathy)

These erosions (*PEEs; Table 5.1*) are slightly depressed grey-white spots that stain brilliantly with fluorescein (*Figure 5.3*) but poorly with rose bengal. They are non-specific changes that may be seen during the early stages of a wide variety of keratopathies. Frequently their location may serve as a clue to the aetiology of the keratopathy.

Table 5.1 Punctate epitheliopathy

Location	*Causes*
Superior	Subtarsal foreign body Vernal disease Superior limbic keratoconjunctivitis
Inferior	Staphylococcal blepharitis Trichiasis Entropion Lagophthalmos Drug toxicity
Interpalpebral	Seborrhoeic blepharitis Sicca Neurotrophic Ultraviolet light exposure

Superior PEEs occur in subtarsal foreign bodies, vernal keratoconjunctivitis, and superior limbic keratoconjunctivitis.

Inferior PEEs may be seen in staphylococcal blepharitis, trichiasis, entropion, corneal exposure due to lagophthalmos, and drug toxicity.

Interpalpebral PEEs are associated with seborrhoeic blepharitis, keratoconjunctivitis sicca, neurotrophic keratopathy, and following exposure to ultraviolet light.

Oedema

This is characterized by loss of normal corneal lustre and the presence of optically empty vacuoles within the epithelium. In severe cases vesicles and bullae may develop (*Figure 5.4*). Epithelial oedema occurs in acute angle-closure glaucoma as well as in eyes with endothelial decompensation due to surgical trauma, Fuchs' dystrophy, stromal inflammation (disciform keratitis), and keratoconus.

Filaments

These are composed of mucous threads and hypertrophied epithelial cells attached to abnormal receptor sites. On slitlamp biomicroscopy they appear as comma-shaped opacities with the unattached end hanging down over the cornea and moving with each blink. Beneath their attachments to the epithelium, grey subepithelial opacities may be seen. Some of the many causes of filamentary keratitis are keratoconjunctivitis sicca, superior limbic keratoconjunctivitis, neurotrophic keratopathy, herpes zoster keratitis, recurrent corneal erosion syndrome, and prolonged patching of the eye.

Punctate epithelial keratitis

This is the hallmark of viral infections of the cornea. The lesions consist of granular, opalescent epithelial cells that stain brilliantly with rose bengal but poorly with fluorescein.

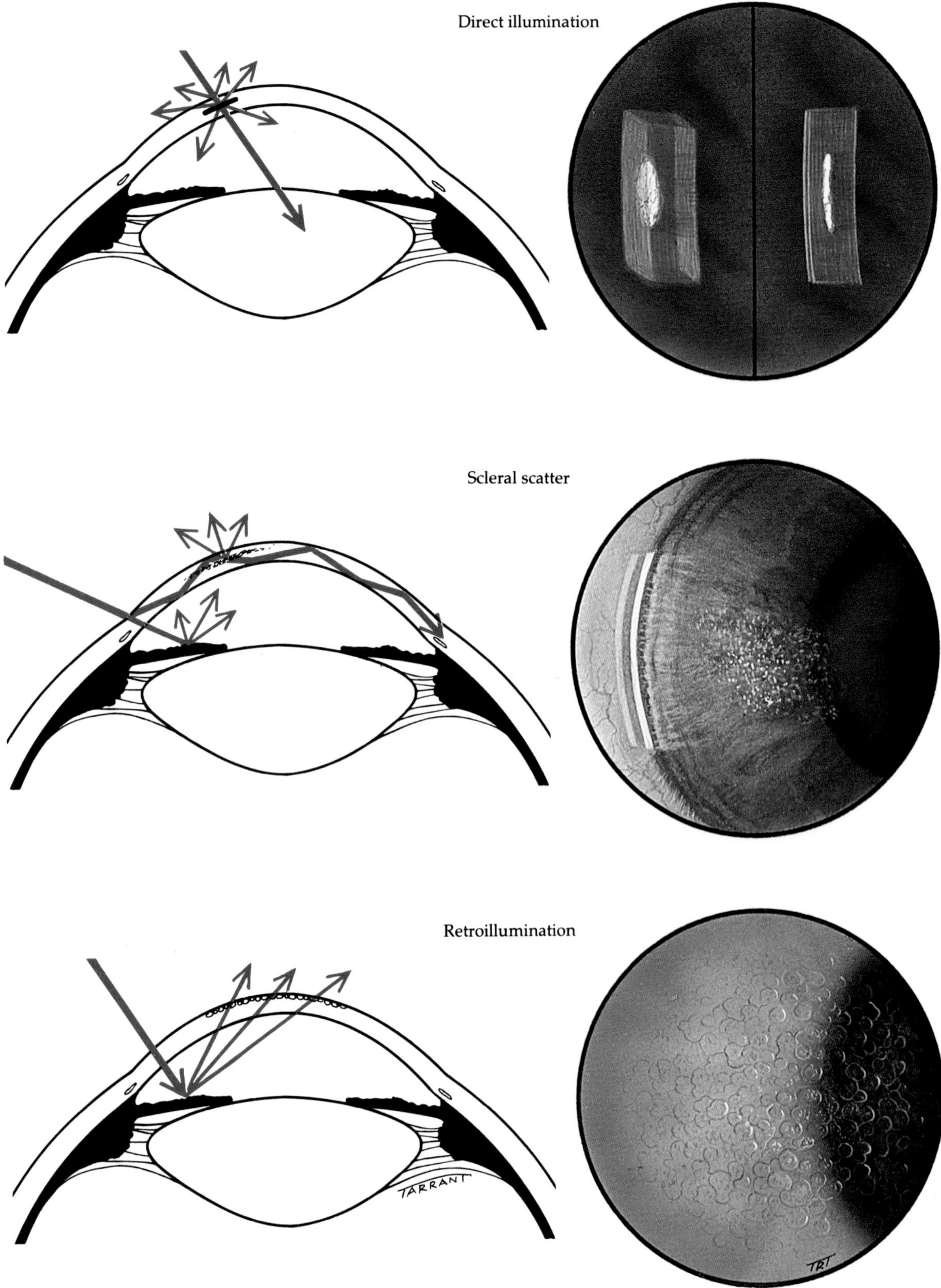

Figure 5.2 *Slitlamp biomicroscopy of cornea*

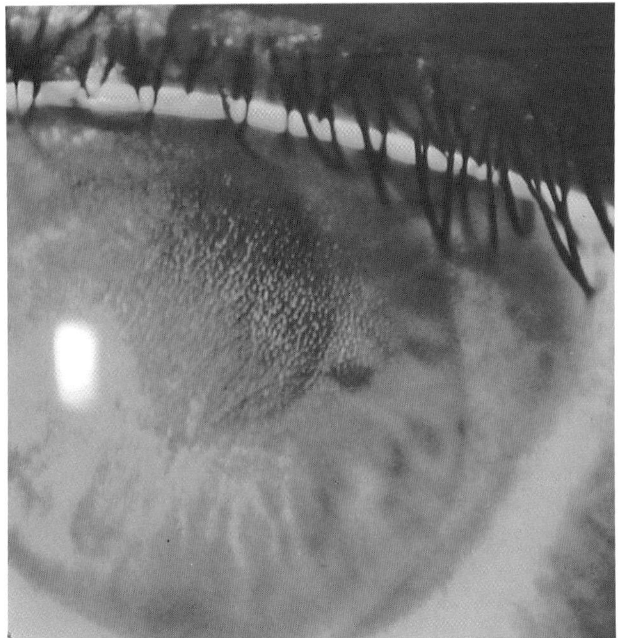

Figure 5.3 Punctate epithelial erosions stained with fluorescein (courtesy of Dr M. Guillon, Hydron Europe Ltd)

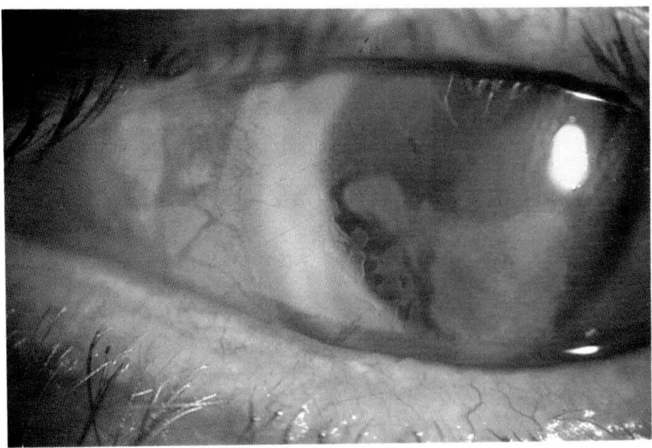

Figure 5.4 Bullous keratopathy

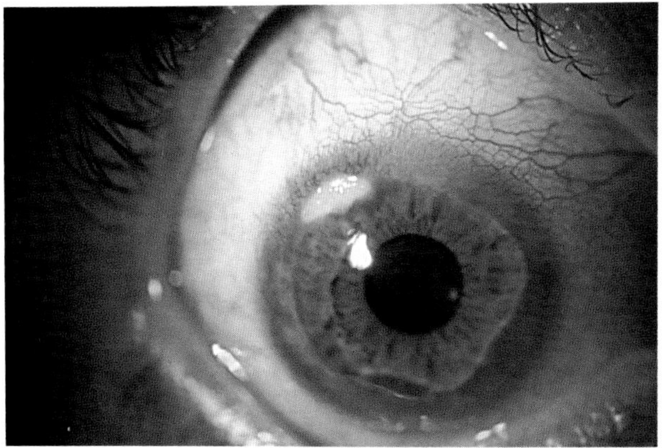

Figure 5.5 Corneal infiltrate at 11 o'clock and circumferential thinning

Superficial punctate keratitis

This is a term used to describe a specific type of keratitis originally described by Thygeson (*see* later).

Stroma

Infiltrates

Infiltrates composed of leucocytes are indicative of active inflammation (*Figure 5.5*). On slitlamp examination they appear as focal granular opacities that may be located at any level within the stroma. The cellular elements comprising infiltrates may originate from the limbal vascular arcades and migrate to the site of injury. If the cornea contains new vessels the cells merely make their way along the vascular channels. In the presence of an epithelial defect they may enter the stroma from the tear film.

Oedema

This usually coexists with inflammatory infiltration. Clinically, it is recognized as optically empty spaces between stromal lamellae. It is associated with increased corneal thickness and variable decrease in transparency due to disruption of the regular arrangement of corneal lamellae. Three important causes of central corneal oedema are disciform keratitis, Fuchs' dystrophy, and keratoconus.

Neovascularization

This occurs in a wide variety of corneal disorders. The new vessels may be superficial or deep.

A pannus is an ingrowth of fibrovascular tissue from the limbus onto the superficial cornea (usually between the epithelium and Bowman's layer). Superior pannus is associated with contact lens wear and trachoma (*see Figure 4.16*). Inferior pannus occurs in exposure keratopathy, rosacea, and long-standing irritation of the cornea from trichiasis. Generalized pannus may develop in cicatricial pemphigoid, Stevens–Johnson syndrome, Mooren's ulcer, and following chemical burns.

Localized superficial vascularization (fascicle) is usually associated with one specific corneal lesion. Deep vascularization is derived from the anterior ciliary vessels. The deep vessels usually run a fairly straight course (unlike superficial vessels which are wavy) and disappear at the limbus. When non-perfused they appear as 'ghost vessels' which are best detected by retroillumination.

Deposits

Deposits of lipid, calcium, and proteinaceous material may occur in association with long-standing inflammation. Band-shaped keratopathy refers to a characteristic deposition of calcium in the subepithelial space and Bowman's layer.

Scarring

This is usually associated with corneal thinning due to the contraction of newly formed collagen (*Figure 5.6*).

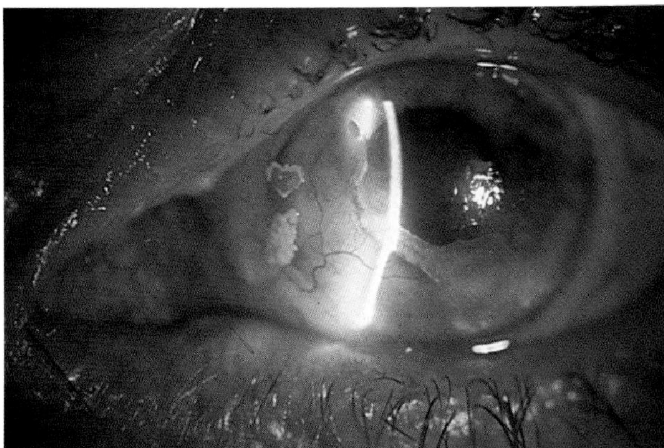

Figure 5.6 Severe corneal stromal thinning and scarring

Descemet's membrane

1. *Posterior embryotoxon* refers to an unusual prominence of Schwalbe's line which is the peripheral termination of Descemet's membrane. It is present to some extent in about 15% of normal eyes.
2. *Hassall–Henle warts* are peripheral excrescences in Descemet's membrane that are frequently seen in elderly individuals. Similar centrally located lesions are referred to as cornea guttata. In Fuchs' dystrophy, many such lesions are found in association with endothelial cell decompensation.
3. *Breaks* in Descemet's membrane occur from corneal enlargement in patients with congenital glaucoma. They can also be caused by birth trauma and keratoconus.
4. *Folds* in Descemet's membrane are usually secondary to ocular hypotony or stromal inflammation (*Figure 5.7*).

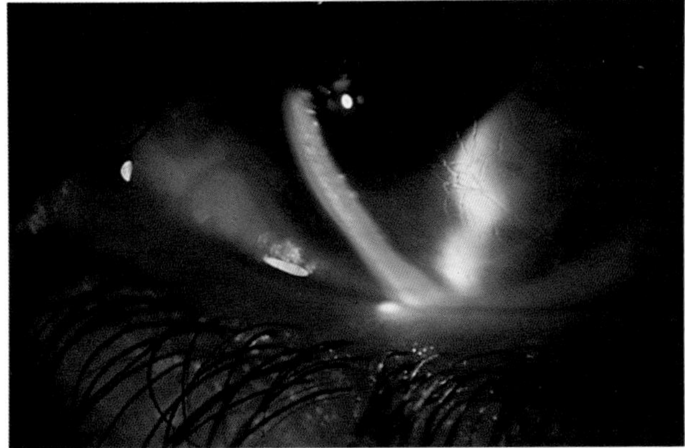

Figure 5.7 Folds in Descemet's membrane

Pigmentation

Corneal pigment deposition is very common and is associated with a great variety of disorders (*Table 5.2*).

Iron pigment is found in the following conditions:

1. Blood staining due to hyphaema and secondary glaucoma mainly affects the stroma.

Table 5.2 Corneal pigmentation

Type of pigment	*Causes*	*Location*
Iron	Keratoconus (Fleischer's ring)	Epithelium
	Old age (Hudson–Stähli line)	Epithelium
	Pterygium (Stocker's line)	Epithelium
	Filtering bleb (Ferry's line)	Epithelium
	Hyphaema–blood staining	Mainly stroma
	Siderosis	Mainly stroma
Silver	Argyrosis	Stroma and Descemet's
Gold	Chrysiasis	Mainly epithelium
Copper	Wilson's disease (Kayser–Fleischer ring)	Descement's
Melanin	Pigment dispersion syndrome (Krukenberg's spindle)	Endothelium

2. Siderosis affects chiefly the stroma and occasionally also the epithelium.
3. Fleischer's ring develops in the epithelium and surrounds the base of the cone in keratoconus.
4. Hudson–Stähli line is a common finding in elderly individuals. It is located at the junction of the upper two-thirds with the lower two-thirds of the epithelium, alone the line of lid closure.
5. Stocker's line develops in front of the head of a pterygium and is located within the epithelium.
6. Ferry's line develops in the epithelium anterior to a filtering bleb.

Silver is found in the stroma and Descemet's membrane in argyrosis.

Gold is present in the stroma in patients with chrysiasis.

Copper is deposited in the periphery of Descemet's membrane in patients with Wilson's disease.

Melanin in the form of Krukenberg's spindle is deposited on the endothelium.

Drawing corneal abnormalities

First the major outlines are sketched, and then the details are filled in, both in frontal and slit views (*Figure 5.8*).

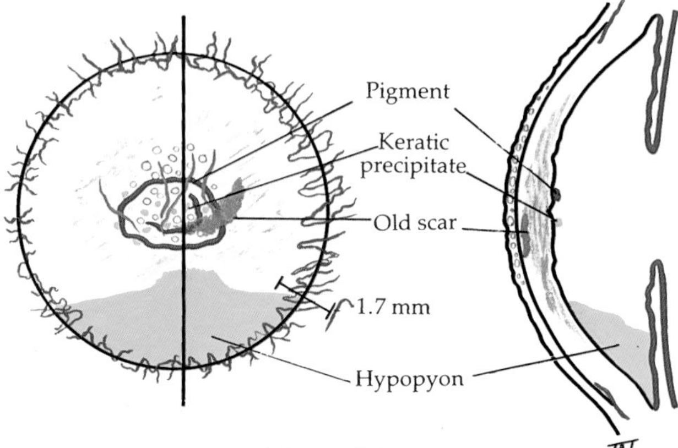

Figure 5.8 Drawing corneal abnormalities

Frontal view

1. Scars and degenerations are drawn *in black*.
2. Epithelial oedema is represented by *fine blue circles*, stromal oedema as *blue shading*, and folds in Descemet's membrane as *wavy blue lines*.
3. Leucocytes, keratic precipitates, and hypopyon are shown in *orange*.
4. Superficial vessels are *wavy red lines* that begin outside the limbus.
5. Deep vessels are *straight red lines* that begin at the limbus.
6. *Pigment* is shown in *brown*.

Slit view

The slit view is drawn with the location of the slit beam indicated on the frontal view by a vertical line. The exact location and depth of the lesion is indicated and, if necessary, changes in the anterior chamber such as vitreocorneal touch are added.

Vital staining

Vital staining is important in the evaluation of corneal and conjunctival disease. It should be performed before corneal sensation is tested and also prior to the measurement of intraocular pressure.

Fluorescein

This is a dye which remains extracellular and does not stain mucus. However, because it stains the tear film, it shows up epithelial corneal defects when examined under a cobalt blue filter (*see Figure 5.3*). The dye will also enter the microcysts in eyes with epithelial oedema.

Rose bengal

This stains mucus as well as dead and damaged cells but not epithelial defects. In a geographical herpetic ulcer, rose bengal will stain the peripheral virus-infected cells whereas fluorescein will stain the base of the ulcer. Rose bengal is particularly useful in the diagnosis of keratoconjunctivitis sicca. Prior to instillation the patient should be warned that it will cause stinging.

Slitlamp examination of the corneal endothelium using specular reflection

A simple subjective quantitative evaluation of the endothelium can be performed with a slitlamp. It is necessary to use high magnification (e.g. 1.6 × objective magnification and 25 × eyepiece) and keep the angle between the light source and the microscope between 40° and 60°. By observing the cornea adjacent to the illuminating beam and altering the angle of the beam, a point will be reached at which the reflection of the posterior corneal surface will enable visualization of the corneal endothelial cells. A special mosaic matcher (McIntyre, Karickoff) can be used to compare the mosaic of the endothelium with varying artificial patterns of endothelial density.

Pachometry

This measures corneal thickness which is an indirect function of the integrity of the corneal endothelium. The normal corneal thickness increases irregularly towards the limbus where it ranges from 0.7 to 0.9 mm. The central corneal thickness is between 0.49 mm and 0.56 mm and readings of 0.6 mm or more are suggestive of endothelial disease. The two types of pachometers in current use are:

1. *Optical pachometry* which measures corneal thickness using an image-splitting device in the Haag–Streit slitlamp with a Mishima–Hedbys attachment.
2. *Ultrasonic pachometry* is a rapid test which is performed with a portable instrument. It is particularly useful when performing radial keratotomy.

Specular microscopy

This method photographs the corneal endothelium delineating various cellular characteristics such as size, shape, density, and distribution. Specular microscopes are of two types: contact and non-contact. The former contacts the corneal surface directly whereas, in the latter, the observer finds the zone of specular reflection.

Laboratory investigations

Material for laboratory analysis can be obtained either with a special Kimura spatula or by simply using the bent tip of a 21-gauge 1.5 inch (3.8 cm) hyperdermic needle. Following the instillation of a topical anaesthetic, the base and margins of the ulcer are gently scraped under slitlamp visualization. The material is then plated onto glass slides for Gram staining and onto the following culture media:

1. *Blood agar* promotes the growth of aerobic organisms. It is useful for both bacteria and fungi.
2. *Thyoglycolate broth* is used for facultative anaerobic organisms.
3. *Chocolate agar* is used to isolate *Neisseria* and *Haemophilus* spp.
4. *Sabouraud's agar* promotes growth of fungi. It is incubated at room temperature as well as 37 °C.
5. *Brain–heart infusion broth* is useful for fungi that fail to grow on Sabouraud's agar.

Principles of management of corneal disease

Primary therapy

1. *Antimicrobials.* Corneal infections should be treated with the appropriate agents as soon as preliminary investigations have been completed. However, the prolonged topical use of potentially toxic agents, such as idoxuridine and gentamicin, may delay epithelial healing.

2. *Corticosteroids.* Although steroids are the primary treatment of certain forms of non-infected keratitis (e.g. marginal keratitis, chemical burns), their injudicious use may promote bacterial, fungal, and viral growth. Steroids may also suppress corneal repair and promote ulceration and perforation.

Promotion of re-epithelialization

In eyes with stromal thinning, it is important to encourage healing of any associated epithelial defects. This is because stromal thinning seldom progresses in the presence of an intact epithelium. The three main ways in which epithelial healing can be encouraged are:

1. *Lubrication* with artificial tears and ointments is useful irrespective of the presence or absence of keratoconjunctivitis sicca. If possible, tear substitutes containing toxic (benzalkonium chloride) or sensitizing (thiomersal) preservatives should be avoided.
2. *Lid closure.* Although this is particularly useful in eyes with exposure and neurotrophic keratopathy, it is also beneficial in eyes with persistent epithelial defects from other causes. The lids can be temporarily closed with a piece of tape extending horizontally. Patients with corneal anaesthesia or exposure keratopathy due to facial nerve palsy may require a tarsorrhaphy.
3. *Bandage soft contact lenses* protect the regenerating corneal epithelium from the constant rubbing action of the eyelids and are a useful alternative to continuous taping.

Prevention of perforation

1. *Tissue adhesive glue,* such as isobutyl cyanoacrylate, is useful in limiting stromal ulceration and preventing perforation. It can also be used to seal small perforations.
2. *Conjunctival flap.* The cornea may be completely or partially covered by a conjunctival flap if corneal ulceration is progressive and unresponsive to other measures. This procedure is particularly suitable in cases of chronic unilateral disease in which the prognosis for useful vision is poor due to associated vascularization or scarring.
3. *Ascorbate,* both systemic and topical, may be helpful in reducing stromal ulceration in eyes with severe alkali burns.
4. *Immunosuppressive agents* (cyclophosphamide, azathioprine, methotrexate) may be beneficial in patients with certain forms of severe peripheral corneal ulceration, such as Mooren's ulcer, and those associated with a systemic connective tissue disorder (rheumatoid arthritis, Wegener's granulomatosis).

Restoration of transparency

Eyes with reduced visual acuity due to permanent corneal scarring may require corneal grafting (keratoplasty) in which the diseased host tissue is excised and replaced by transparent donor tissue.

Microbial keratitis

Bacterial

Predisposing factors

The three pathogens reputed to be able to produce corneal infection in the presence of an intact epithelium include *Neisseria gonorrhoea, N. meningitidis* and *Corynebacterium diphtheriae.* In these cases, suppurative keratitis is always associated with a purulent conjunctivitis. With other bacteria, keratitis is invariably associated with one or more of the following predisposing factors:

1. Chronic infection of the ocular adnexa.
2. Underlying corneal disease (herpetic keratitis, bullous keratopathy, trauma).
3. Dry eyes.
4. Contact lens wear—particularly extended wear soft lenses.
5. Neurotrophic or exposure keratopathy.
6. Administration of topical or systemic immunosuppressive agents.

Bacterial keratitis is particularly prevalent in elderly patients and is frequently preceded by trauma.

Clinical features

Although there is no reliable method of identifying the causative organism by slitlamp biomicroscopy, certain bacteria produce characteristic corneal responses.

1. *Staphylococcus aureus* and *Streptococcus pneumoniae* tend to produce oval, yellow-white, densely opaque stromal suppuration surrounded by relatively clear cornea (*Figure 5.9*).
2. *Pseudomonas* sp. usually causes irregularly sharp ulceration, thick mucopurulent exudate, diffuse liquefactive necrosis, and semi-opaque 'ground-glass' appearance of adjacent stroma (*Figure 5.10*). The infection may progress rapidly and result in corneal perforation within 48 hours.
3. *Enterobacteriaceae* (*Escherichia coli, Proteus* sp., *Klebsiella* sp., *Serratia marcescens*) usually cause a shallow ulceration, grey-white pleomorphic suppuration, and diffuse stromal opalescence. The endotoxins present in Gram-negative bacteria may induce ring-shaped corneal infiltrates ('corneal rings').

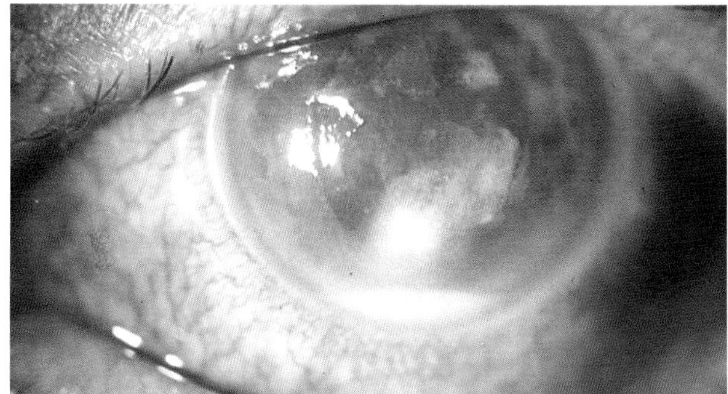

Figure 5.9 Pneumococcal keratitis with hypopyon

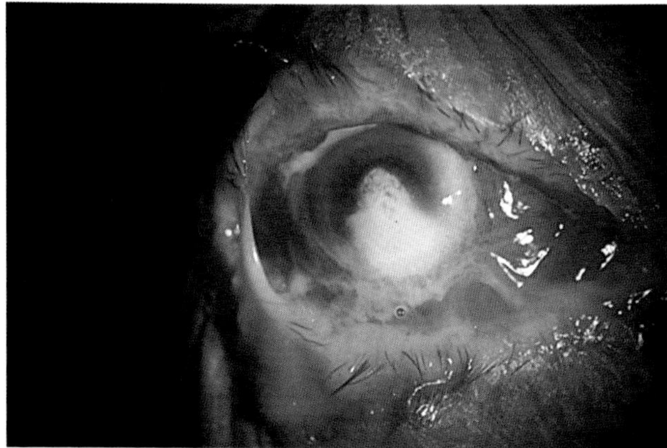

Figure 5.10 Pseudomonas keratitis

Management

A bacterial corneal ulcer is a sight-threatening condition that demands urgent identification and eradication of the causative organism. This is best performed with the patient hospitalized.

Identification of organisms

Scrapings should be taken from the base of the ulcer as already described.

Antibiotics

Most strains of *Pseudomonas* are sensitive to gentamicin, although this is not always the case for other Gram-negative bacteria. Cephazolin is indicated for Gram-positive infections. Unfortunately, there is frequently poor correlation between the initial Gram stain results and subsequent culture identification of the organism. For this reason, the initial therapy should be with a combination of gentamicin and cephazolin. The frequent use of fortified (high concentration) drops is the most effective way of maintaining a high and sustained level of antibiotics at the site of infection and is therefore the delivery system of choice.

Preparation of fortified drops

1. *Gentamicin*—add 2 ml (40 mg) of parenteral gentamicin into a 5-ml bottle of commercially available gentamicin eye drops. The resultant solution contains 14 mg/ml and is stable for up to 30 days.
2. *Cephazolin*—add 2 ml of sterile saline to an ampoule of 500 mg of cephazolin and dissolve the powder. Remove 2 ml from a 15-ml bottle containing artificial tears. Inject the reconstituted cephazolin into the bottle containing artificial tears. The resultant solution contains 33 mg/ml and is stable for up to 48 hours.

Frequency of instillation

For the first few days the drops are instilled at half-hourly intervals around the clock. If two different antibiotics are used, one can be given on the hour and the other on the half hour. If the response to therapy is favourable, the frequency of instillation can be reduced to hourly and then 2-hourly during waking hours. The patient can then be discharged from hospital and followed closely in the out-patient clinic. If progress is maintained, the fortified drops can be substituted for the more diluted commercial preparations which are gradually tapered and eventually discontinued. It is, however, important to note that the frequent instillation of drops may cause corneal toxicity and delay epithelialization.

Subconjunctival injections

Subconjunctival injections provide a high but transient peak of antibiotic at the site of infection and must be used in conjunction with topical therapy. In relatively mild cases, they are unnecessary, but their use should be considered for moderate-to-severe infections, particularly when the visual axis is threatened. The injections are given at 24-hourly intervals for about 5 days. The doses are gentamicin 40 mg, cephazolin 125 mg.

Technique of subconjunctival injection

It is extremely important to have the conjunctiva well anaesthetized prior to attempting a subconjunctival injection. If this is done correctly, the injection can be given with minimal discomfort to the patient. The conjunctiva is anaesthetized as follows:

1. Instil a topical anaesthetic such as amethocaine at 1-min intervals for 10 min.
2. Place a small cotton pledget impregnated with cocaine into the conjunctival sac at the site of injection and leave it there for 5 min.
3. Ask the patient to look away from the site of injection.
4. With toothed (St Martin's) forceps grasp the conjunctiva.
5. Inject the antibiotic using a 25-gauge 3/8 inch (10 mm) disposable needle bevel up.

When to change antibiotics

The initial regimen of gentamicin and cephazolin should be changed only if a resistant pathogen is grown and the ulcer is progressing. In these cases, pseudomonas corneal ulcers can be treated with both topical and subconjunctival tobramycin, and those caused by penicillin-resistant staphylococci with topical bacitracin and subconjunctival oxacillin. There is no need to change the initial therapy if this has induced a favourable response, even if subsequent cultures show a resistant organism. It is, however, very important not to confuse failure of re-epithelialization due to drug toxicity from overtreatment, with persistent infection.

Cycloplegics and corticosteroids

1. *Cycloplegics* such as atropine should be used in all eyes with bacterial keratitis to prevent the formation of posterior synechiae from secondary anterior uveitis, and to reduce pain from ciliary spasm.
2. *Corticosteroids.* The use of topical steroids in the management of active bacterial keratitis is still controversial. The potential benefits of topical steroids in reducing the extent of stromal necrosis should be weighed against their effects in decreasing fibroblastic activity and inhibiting wound healing, thereby increasing the danger of perforation. Steroids also have the potential for prolonging infection, particularly pseudomonal, and ideally they should be initiated only when cultures become sterile.

Fungal

Although fungal corneal infection is rare, it should always be considered if the differential diagnosis is suspected of suppurative bacterial keratitis and herpetic stromal necrotic keratitis.

Clinical features

Filamentous

This is usually caused by *Aspergillus* or *Fusarium* spp. It is most prevalent in agricultural areas and is typically preceded by ocular trauma, most frequently involving vegetable matter.

It typically presents as a greyish-white lesion with indistinct margins and delicate feathery finger-like projections into adjacent stroma. It may be ringed by a greyish halo and multiple satellite small foci may also be present. The overlying epithelium is elevated but intact.

Yeast

This is most commonly due to *Candida albicans* and frequently affects a compromised host (*Figure 5.11*). A typical lesion has a yellow-white colour and is associated with dense suppuration similar to a bacterial keratitis.

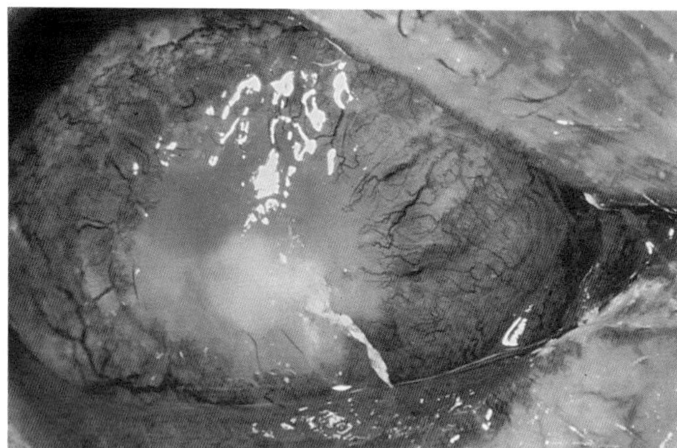

Figure 5.11 *Fungal keratitis (courtesy of Mr T. A. Casey)*

Treatment

Filamentous fungi are treated with oral and topical ketoconazole. Yeast infections are treated with topical and oral flucytosine.

Acanthamoeba

Acanthamoeba is a genus of free-living amoeba that may cause a chronic stromal keratitis after minor trauma. Contact lens wearers who use distilled water and salt tablets instead of commercially prepared saline solutions for their lens care are at particular risk.

Clinical features

The condition may be misdiagnosed for many weeks or months and confused with herpetic or fungal keratitis. Acanthamoeba keratitis is characterized by recurrent breakdown of the corneal epithelium and a chronic deep inflammation of the cornea which frequently consists of a paracentral ring-shaped infiltrate or abscess. A diffuse or nodular scleritis is also a frequent finding. Characteristically, pain is severe and out of all proportion to the degree of ocular inflammation. Other clues to the diagnosis are negative cultures for bacteria, fungi, and viruses, together with a lack of response to conventional antimicrobial therapy.

Treatment

The diagnosis can be confirmed by staining corneal scrapings with calcofluor white which is a chemifluorescent dye with an affinity for amoebic cysts. Medical treatment with a combination of dibromopropamidine and propamidine isethionate (Brolene) ointment and drops, and neomycin drops. Penetrating keratoplasy may be required in resistant cases.

Interstitial

Interstitial keratitis (IK) is a rare inflammation of the corneal stroma without primary involvement of the epithelium or endothelium. It has been associated with a wide variety of causes, most notably congenital syphilis, tuberculosis, and Cogan's syndrome.

Luetic

IK is a late manifestation of congenital syphilis which usually develops between the ages of 5 and 25 years. Acute IK is characterized by bilateral diffuse midstromal corneal clouding due to cellular infiltration. The effect on vision is usually profound. Within a few weeks deep vascularization develops and, when the vessels meet in the centre of the cornea, they give rise to the so-called 'salmon patch'. After several months, the cornea begins to clear and the vessels become non-perfused (ghost vessels). If the cornea becomes re-inflamed the vessels may refill with blood. Treatment of luetic IK is with systemic penicillin, topical steroids and cycloplegics.

Tuberculous

This is similar to luetic IK but is more frequently unilateral and sectorial. Treatment is with systemic antituberculous drugs, topical steroids and cycloplegics.

Cogan's syndrome

This very rare disorder is characterized by non-luetic IK, in association with acute tinnitus, vertigo, and deafness. Cogan's syndrome typically affects middle-aged adults some of whom also suffer from polyarteritis nodosa. The early corneal lesions consist of anterior stromal infiltrates similar to those seen in chlamydial and adenoviral keratitis. If these early lesions are treated with topical steroids progression to classic IK with deep corneal vascularization is rare. Early diagnosis of Cogan's syndrome is important because prompt treatment of the cochlear symptoms with systemic steroids may prevent permanent and profound deafness.

Viral keratitis

Herpes simplex

Introduction

Infection with the herpes simplex virus (HSV) is extremely common although in the majority of cases it is subclinical. In fact about 90% of the adult population are seropositive for HSV antibodies, indicating a prior infection. According to different clinical and immunological properties, HSV is subdivided into two types: type 1 and type 2.

HSV-1

This causes infection above the waist (skin, lips and eyes) and is usually acquired by kissing or coming into close contact with a person who either has active herpetic vesicles on the lips (herpes labialis) or is shedding the virus asymptomatically.

HSV-2

This typically causes infection below the waist (genital herpes) and is acquired venereally. Very occasionally, HSV-2 is transmitted to the eye through infected genital secretions, particularly in neonates during passage through the birth canal. It is important to distinguish primary from secondary infection.

Primary infection occurs in a non-immune subject through infected secretions and is usually acquired early in life. Because of the protection bestowed by maternal antibodies, it is uncommon during the first 6 months of life. Primary infection may be subclinical or it may cause a mild fever and malaise. Rarely in immunodeficient patients, the infection becomes generalized and even life threatening. Following the primary infection, the virus travels up the axon of a sensory nerve to its ganglion (trigeminal ganglion for HVS-1, and spinal ganglia for HVS-2) where it lies in a latent state. In some patients, this latent state is subsequently reversed and the virus travels down the axon of the sensory nerve to its target tissue and causes recurrent infection (genital herpes, herpes labialis, and herpetic keratitis). Frequently one of the following stress stimuli is associated with recurrences:

1. Poor general health.
2. Exposure to the sun.
3. Fever.
4. Menstruation.
5. Mild trauma.
6. Psychiatric disturbances.
7. Topical corticosteroid administration (which may provoke recurrences as well as enhance replication of established lesions).
8. Systemic corticosteroids.
9. Immunosuppressive agents.

Primary ocular infection

Primary ocular infection typically occurs in children between the ages of 6 months and 5 years.

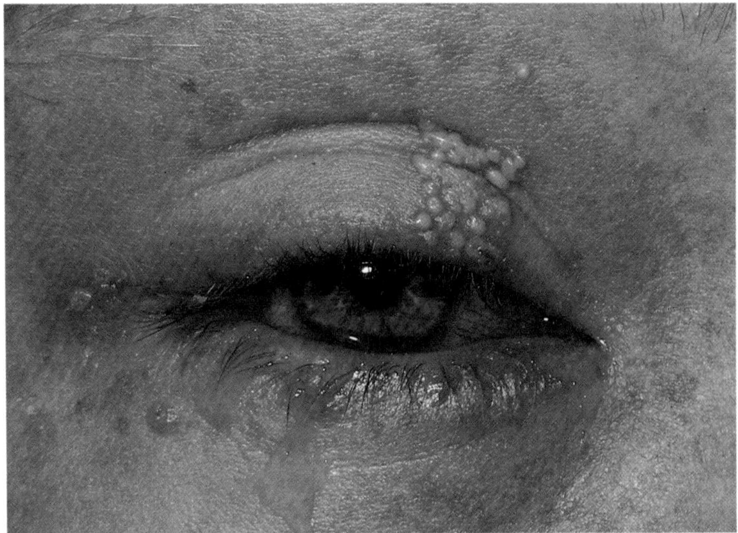

Figure 5.12 *Herpes simplex of eyelid*

Clinical features

Skin lesions

These typically involve the lids and periorbital area. Initially they consist of vesicles which rapidly form superficial crusts and then heal without scarring (*Figure 5.12*).

Acute follicular conjunctivitis

This is unilateral and associated with a watery discharge and preauricular adenopathy. In children this may be the only ocular manifestation of primary herpetic infection.

Keratitis

This develops within a few days in about 50% of patients with blepharoconjunctivitis. *Fine epithelial punctate keratitis* may be a transient finding. *Coarse epithelial punctate keratitis* may give rise to a variety of epithelial lesions that subsequently progress to dendritic figures. Within 2–3 weeks, subepithelial infiltrates appear and these may persist for several weeks before healing. Rarely, the stromal lesions may progress to form a disciform keratitis, but in the vast majority of cases most of the lesions heal without residua. Severe conjunctival reaction with pseudomembrane formation and subsequent scarring is rare.

Treatment

Antiviral ointment should be applied to the eye five times a day for about 21 days. Fortunately, primary herpetic infection is usually self-limiting and seldom presents serious problems. However, recurrent infection occurring in the presence of host antibody is a very much more serious threat to vision.

Classification of recurrent keratitis

- Active epithelial
  - dendritic ulcer
  - geographical ulcer
- Stromal
  - necrotic
  - disciform
- Trophic

Clinical features of active epithelial keratitis

These are of two types: dendritic and geographical ulcers.

Dendritic ulcer

Dendritic ulceration which may be single or multiple is the hallmark of epithelial disease. The initial lesions consist of opaque cells arranged in a dendritic, coarse punctate, or stellate pattern (*Figure 5.13*). Following central desquamation a linear-branching ulcer begins to form (*Figure 5.14*). The bed of the ulcer stains with fluorescein and the virus-laden cells at the margin of the ulcer take up rose bengal. The lesion is associated with diminished corneal sensitivity. After a few days, the anterior stromal infiltrates begin to appear under the ulcer but usually resolve rapidly once the epithelium has healed.

It is very important not to mistake the stromal infiltrates associated with a peripheral dendritic ulcer for a marginal (catarrhal) ulcer. The differentiation is extremely important because topical steroid therapy, which is extremely effective for marginal keratitis, may exacerbate an herpetic infection. As compared with a central dendritic ulcer, a peripheral lesion tends to result in more severe stromal

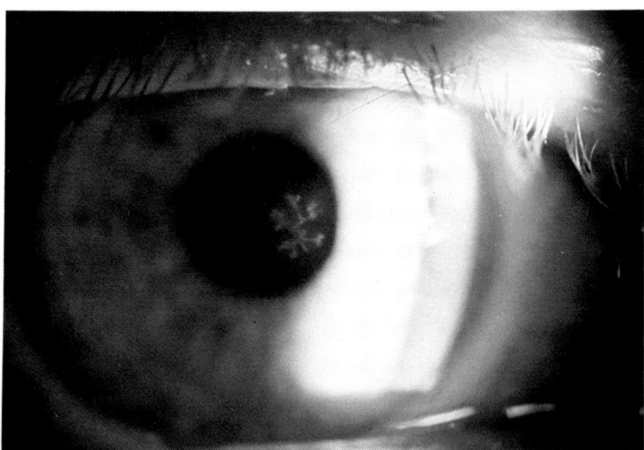

Figure 5.13 Small dendritic ulcer

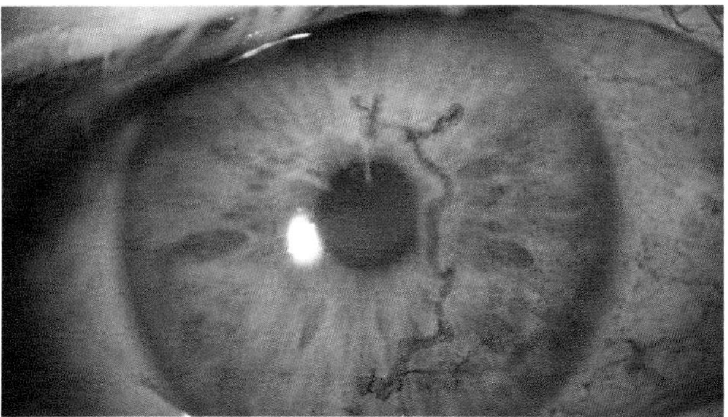

Figure 5.14 Dendritic ulcer stained with rose bengal

reaction, is more frequently accompanied by anterior uveitis and keratic precipitates, and tends to run a more prolonged course.

Following the healing of a dendritic ulcer, the corneal epithelium may continue to show the presence of linear, and sometimes branching, figures which represent one or more waves of healing epithelium. These pseudodendrites will eventually disappear spontaneously and should not be mistaken for persistent active infection.

Other causes of non-herpetic dendritic ulceration include:

1. *Herpes zoster keratitis* (*see* later).
2. *A healing corneal abrasion.*
3. *Thygeson's superficial punctate keratitis,* which is not infrequently confused with herpetic keratitis (*see* later).
4. *Soft contact lenses* which may rarely give rise to a pseudodendrite in the midperipheral cornea.

Geographical ulcer

Occasionally, the continued enlargement of a dendritic ulcer leads to a much larger epithelial lesion which has a geographical or 'amoeboid' configuration. This is particularly likely to occur when the rate of virus replication has been enhanced by the inadvertent use of topical corticosteroids.

Treatment

Even without treatment, about 50% of active epithelial lesions heal without residua. The cure rate is in the order of 95% with treatment which, ideally, should promote rapid uneventful healing with minimal adverse effects, and is best achieved by the use of antiviral agents.

Antiviral agents

Antivirals are usually the first line of treatment, especially in eyes with geographical ulcers. In general, initial treatment is with drops or ointment. By day 4, the lesion should start to diminish in size and by day 10 it should have healed. After healing has occurred, medication should be quickly tapered and discontinued by day 14. If by day 7 there is no response, resistance to the antiviral agent should be assumed and either another agent substituted or debridement carried out. Four antiviral agents are currently available:

Acycloguanosine (acyclovir, Zovirax) 3% ointment

This is administered five times a day. It is more potent than both idoxuridine and adenine arabinoside and as effective as trifluorothymidine. Acyclovir differs from the other antiviral agents in that it acts preferentially on virus-infected cells. Because the drug is relatively non-toxic, even when given for up to 60 days, it is particularly suitable as an antiviral cover to steroids in the management of disciform keratitis which requires more prolonged treatment than simple dendritic ulceration (*see* later). Acyclovir is able to penetrate the intact corneal epithelium and stroma, achieving therapeutic levels in the aqueous humour, unlike other currently available antiviral agents, and therefore probably also has a role in the treatment of stromal herpetic keratitis (*see* later).

Trifluorothymidine 1% drops

This is administered every 2 hours during the day. Like acyclovir, it heals about 95% of dendritic ulcers within 2 weeks. It shows no cross-resistance with older drugs and has little tendency to produce resistant strains. It is however, more toxic than acyclovir.

Adenine arabinoside 3% ointment, 0.1% drops

This is administered five times a day. It is as potent as idoxuridine but less toxic than both idoxuridine and trifluorothymidine.

Idoxuridine 0.5% ointment, 0.1% drops

The ointment is administered five times a day and the drops every hour during the day and every 2 hours during the night. Like adenine arabinoside it cures about 80% of dendritic ulcers within 2 weeks. Its main disadvantages are poor solubility, the emergence of resistant strains, and toxicity.

Because of their limitations, both idoxuridine and adenine arabinoside are now used mainly in the rare event of resistance to acyclovir or trifluorothymidine.

Side-effects of antiviral agents

The following toxic effects may be encountered particularly with idoxuridine:

1. *Corneal punctate erosions*, superficial pannus, epithelial opacification, and delayed wound healing.
2. *Conjunctival cicatrization* and follicular conjunctivitis.
3. *Lacrimal obstruction.*
4. *Contact dermatitis.*

Debridement

Debridement is an effective way of treating dendritic ulcers, but is not appropriate for geographical ulcers. Since the advent of antiviral agents this mode of treatment has generally been relegated to:

1. Resistant cases.
2. Non-compliance.
3. Allergy to antiviral agents.
4. Unavailability of antiviral agents.

The removal of the virus-containing cells protects adjacent healthy cells from infection and eliminates the antigenic stimulus to stromal inflammation. The corneal surface is wiped with a sterile cotton-tipped bud and the visibly abnormal cells at the edge of the ulcer are removed. Although the ulcer usually heals rapidly, focal microscopic lesions recur in up to 60% of cases within 7 days. Chemical debridement with alcohol or iodine can damage the corneal stroma and delay epithelial healing, and is now obsolete.

Risk of recurrence

There is a one in four chance of a second attack of herpes within 5 years of the initial episode. If a second attack occurs, the risk of further recurrence within the next 2 years is increased to about 50%.

Stromal necrotic keratitis

Clinical features

Stromal necrotic (infiltrative) keratitis is caused by active viral invasion and destruction. Fortunately it is fairly rare. It may be associated with an intact epithelium or it may follow epithelial disease. On examination, the stroma may have a cheesy, necrotic appearance, reminiscent of a bacterial or fungal infection, or it may show a profound interstitial opacification. There may be an associated anterior uveitis with keratic precipitates underlying the area of active stromal infiltration. Pain, photophobia, and ciliary injection are common findings. If the condition is inappropriately treated, vascularization, scarring, and even perforation may result.

Treatment

Treatment of stromal keratitis is controversial, difficult, and frequently unsatisfactory. The first aim is to heal any active epithelial lesions with antiviral agents. If after 14 days there is no evidence of active epithelial disease but the epithelium is still not healed, treatment is similar to that for trophic keratitis (i.e. lubricant ointments, pressure patching, or a bandage contact lens). Once the epithelium has been healed the stromal reaction may diminish. However, in resistant cases with incapacitating symptoms and severe anterior uveitis, the cautious use of corticosteroids combined with topical antiviral and antibiotic cover will be necessary to relieve symptoms and prevent severe corneal scarring.

Disciform keratitis

Clinical features

Disciform keratitis (oedema) is probably caused by a hypersensitivity reaction which may or may not be associated with a past history of dendritic ulceration. The oedema may be due to a low-grade stromal inflammation and/or damage to the underlying endothelium, which allows the passage of aqueous into the corneal stroma.

A typical disciform keratitis consists of a central zone of epithelial oedema overlying an area of oedematous stromal thickening (*Figure 5.15*). Occasionally, the lesion may be eccentric. There is usually little stromal infiltration, although a surrounding (Wessely) ring of infiltrates may sometimes be present. Other features include folds in Descemet's membrane, a mild to moderate anterior uveitis, and keratic precipitates. The latter are concentrated beneath the involved area of the cornea, presumably due to the increased 'stickiness' of the diseased endothelium.

Occasionally, the intraocular pressure may be elevated despite the presence of only a mild anterior uveitis. Although in some cases the disciform oedema becomes more diffuse, in the majority of cases it resolves over a period of months. Frequently, the diagnosis of old healed disciform keratitis may be made by finding a faint ring of

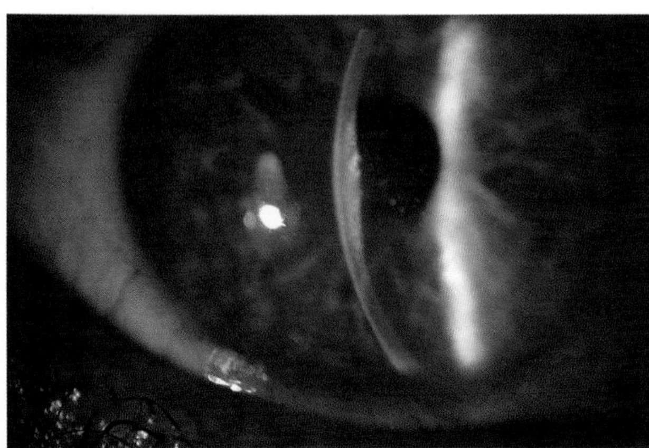

Figure 5.15 *Disciform keratitis with stromal oedema and keratic precipitates*

stromal opacification that permanently marks the periphery of the previously oedematous area.

During the active stage, the presence of reduced corneal sensation and keratic precipitates helps to differentiate herpetic disciform keratitis from other causes of stromal corneal oedema such as the hydrops of keratoconus, trauma, and Fuchs' dystrophy (*see* later).

Treatment

This is much more satisfactory than that of stromal necrotic keratitis. The first aim is to heal any associated epithelial lesion. Because disciform keratitis is usually unassociated with severe discomfort, small lesions away from the visual axis may be treated conservatively with cycloplegics alone. However, if the visual axis is involved topical corticosteroids combined with an antiviral cover (acyclovir, trifluorothymidine) are required. The steroid drops are initially given three to five times a day and the antiviral agent twice a day. The use of diluted solutions of prednisolone (0.25%, 0.125%, 0.025% and 0.0025%) reduces the incidence of complications. Corticosteroids should be tapered over a period of several weeks, although some patients will need one drop of a weak concentration once a day for a prolonged period of time in order to prevent rebound. Periodic attempts to taper the dose further or to stop medication altogether should be made.

Trophic keratitis

Clinical features

Trophic keratitis, sometimes referred to as 'metaherpetic keratitis', is not caused by active viral disease but is due to persistent defects in the basement membrane. It is therefore similar to recurrent corneal erosions of traumatic origin. When trying to differentiate a geographical from a trophic ulcer it should be noted that a geographical ulcer will have linear 'foot-like' extensions, which stain with rose bengal, branching from its margin; these findings are absent in a trophic ulcer.

Treatment

This is with lubricants, patching, and bandage contact lenses in order to promote epithelial healing (*see* later).

Herpes zoster

Introduction

Herpes zoster is a common infection caused by the varicella-zoster virus which is morphologically identical to the herpes simplex virus but different both antigenically and clinically. Although the infection mainly affects elderly patients it can occur at any age. It tends to be more common and more severe in patients with lymphomas and in those being treated by radiotherapy or immunosuppressives.

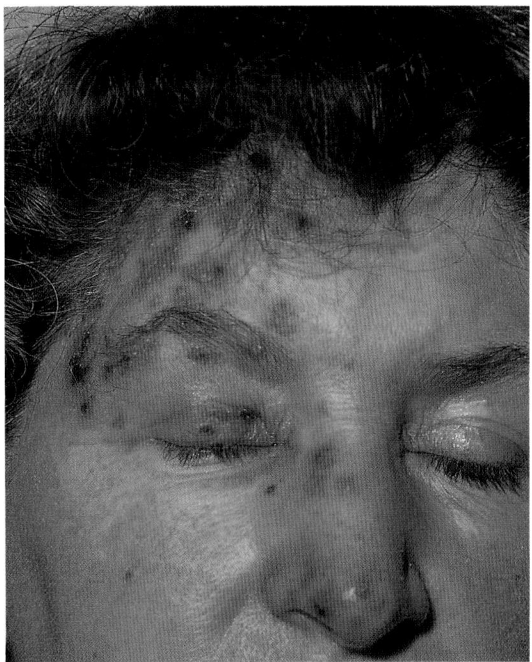

Figure 5.16 *Hutchinson's sign*

It is thought that, after initial exposure, the virus remains latent in a sensory ganglion (like the herpes simplex virus). It then becomes reactivated, replicates, and migrates down a sensory nerve to reach the skin.

Approximately 10% of all cases of herpes zoster affect the ophthalmic division of the trigeminal nerve. Half of these will develop ocular complications. Very rarely, the eye may become involved when the disease affects the maxillary nerve. The old rule that cutaneous involvement of the nasociliary nerve, Hutchinson's sign (*Figure 5.16*), heralds ocular complications is useful but not infallible. It is important to remember that severe ocular complications may occur even in patients with only a slight rash anywhere on the forehead. There are three stages to the disease.

Stage one

This consists of acute lesions which develop within 3 weeks of the rash.

Skin lesions

Clinical features

The rash may involve one or all three branches of the ophthalmic nerve (frontal, lacrimal, and nasociliary). Initially it is maculopapular and then becomes pustular. The pustules subsequently burst to form crusting ulcers. Because, during the initial stage of the disease, the virus can be isolated from the skin lesions, close contacts who have not suffered from chickenpox are at risk of acquiring the infection. Initially the rash is accompanied by periorbital oedema. In severe cases, it may close the eyelids and spread to the opposite side, giving the erroneous impression that the condition is bilateral.

Treatment

This is aimed at promoting rapid healing of the skin without the formation of massive crusts which result in scarring of the nerves and postherpetic neuralgia (*Figure 5.17*).

1. *Acyclovir (Zovirax)* two 400 mg tablets administered five times daily for 7 days significantly curtails vesiculation, accelerates healing and reduces pain during the eruptive phase. In order to be effective, treatment should start as early as possible after the onset of the rash. The drug may also reduce both the incidence and the duration of anterior uveitis but so far no benefit has been demonstrated on postherpetic neuralgia.
2. *Antibiotic–corticosteroid* preparations (Neo-Cortef ointment or Terra-Cortril spray) should be used three times a day until all crusts have separated. Calamine and starch powder promote crust formation and should therefore be avoided.
3. *Systemic corticosteroid* administered may have a beneficial effect on the severity of postherpetic neuralgia.

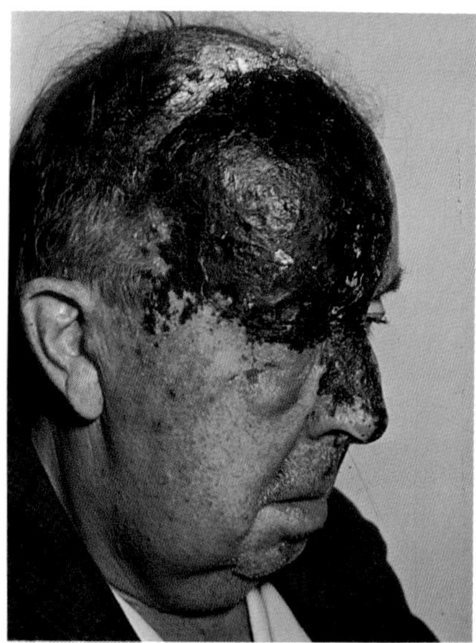

Figure 5.17 *Severe skin crusting in herpes zoster*

Ocular lesions

Mucopurulent conjunctivitis

This is one of the most common complications of herpes zoster. It is always associated with vesicles on the lid margin, and usually resolves within 1 week.

Episcleritis

This occurs in about one-third of cases. It usually appears at the onset of the rash and is frequently concealed by the overlying conjunctivitis.

Scleritis

This is much less common. It usually develops after 1 week and also involves the cornea (sclerokeratitis).

Keratitis

Corneal lesions in order of chronological clinical occurrence are:

1. *Punctate epithelial*—these develop in about 50% of patients and are the initial corneal manifestation, typically appearing within 2 days of the onset of the rash. The foci are thought to consist of swollen epithelial cells containing replicating virus. The lesions, which stain with rose bengal, are usually peripheral, multiple, raised, small, and occasionally coated with mucus (filamentary keratitis). They are either transient in about 50% of cases or they subsequently coalesce to form pseudodendrites.
2. *Microdendrites* (*Figure 5.18*) consisting of small, fine, multiple dendritic or stellate lesions of swollen, raised epithelial cells appear most commonly at 4–6 days. They stain moderately well with rose bengal. Unlike the dendritic ulcers of HSV, they are usually peripheral, broader, more plaque-like, without central ulceration and more frequently stellate rather than dendritic in shape. The lesions are usually transient, although about half are associated with the subsequent development of anterior stromal infiltrates.

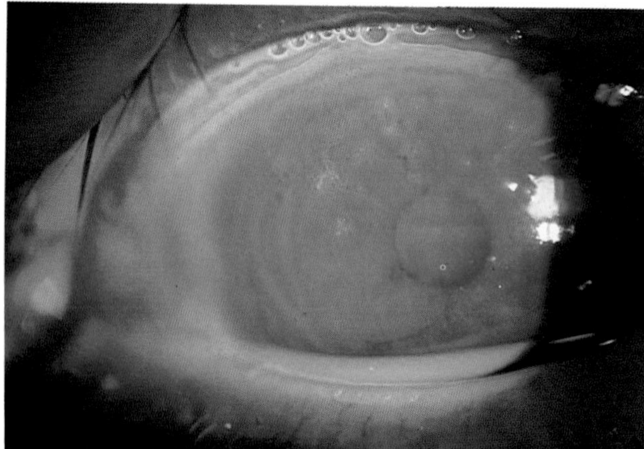

Figure 5.18 *Corneal microdendrites due to herpes zoster*

3. *Nummular* (seen in about one in three cases)— typically these appear about 10 days following the onset of the disease, and are characterized by multiple fine granular deposits (just beneath Bowman's membrane), which are surrounded by a halo of stromal haze (*Figure 5.19*). At first they are white but later become brown. The lesions fluctuate in density and can become chronic. The nummular keratitis due to herpes zoster behaves in a similar way to the stromal infiltrates seen in adenovirus infection when treated with topical corticosteroids. Both fade initially but recur if treatment is discontinued prematurely.

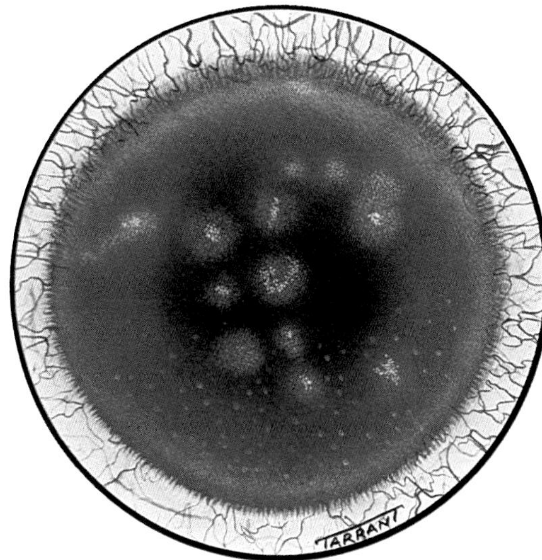

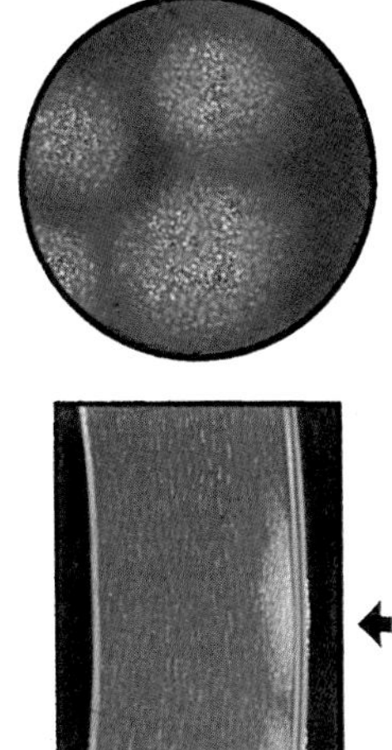

Figure 5.19
Nummular keratitis due to herpes zoster

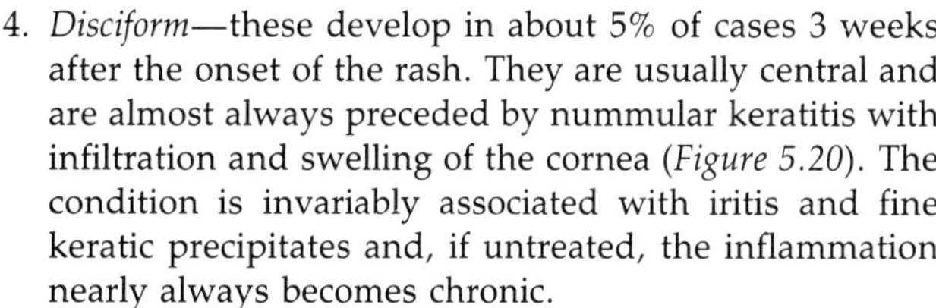

4. *Disciform*—these develop in about 5% of cases 3 weeks after the onset of the rash. They are usually central and are almost always preceded by nummular keratitis with infiltration and swelling of the cornea (*Figure 5.20*). The condition is invariably associated with iritis and fine keratic precipitates and, if untreated, the inflammation nearly always becomes chronic.

The corneal lesions are insensitive to antiviral agents but usually respond well to topical corticosteroids. The dose should be very slowly reduced, as an abrupt stoppage may precipitate a relapse.

Anterior uveitis

See Chapter 6.

Neurological complications

1. *Cranial nerve palsies* affecting the third (most common), fourth and sixth nerves are fairly frequent. Spontaneous recovery occurs within 6 months.
2. *Optic neuritis* occurs in about 1 in 100 cases.
3. *Encephalitis* is very rare and only occurs with severe infection.
4. *Contralateral hemiplegia* is also rare and usually mild, typically developing 2 months after the rash.

Stage two

Stage two consists of chronic lesions that may persist for up to 10 years.

Skin lesions

These are typical 'punched-out' scars associated with varying degrees of hyperpigmentation and hypopigmentation. *Ptosis* may occur as a result of scarring of the lids. It may be associated with trichiasis, loss of lashes, ectropion, entropion, and lid-notching.

Ocular lesions

Mucus-secreting conjunctivitis

This is a common chronic lesion, which may be accompanied by lipid-filled granulomas under the tarsal conjunctiva and submucosal conjunctival scarring (*Figure 5.21*).

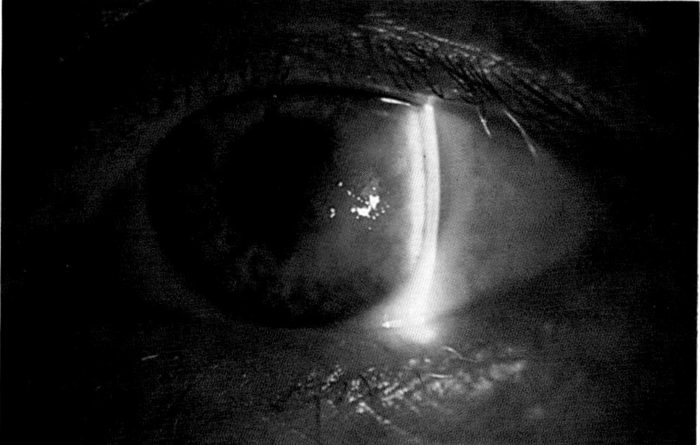

Figure 5.20 *Eccentric disciform keratitis due to herpes zoster*

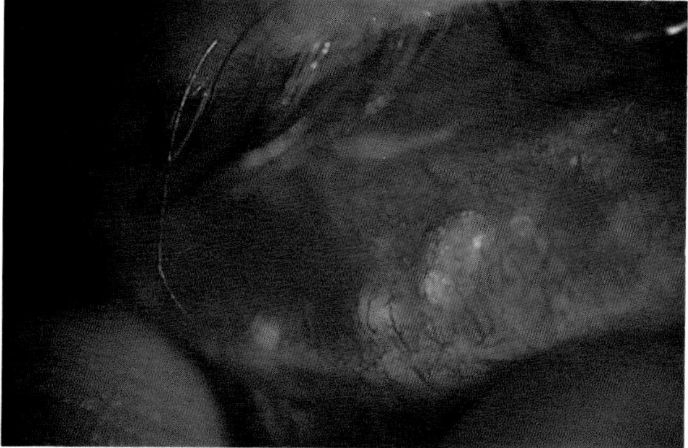

Figure 5.21 *Mucus-secreting conjunctivitis due to herpes zoster*

Scleritis

This frequently becomes chronic and leads to patches of scleral atrophy. Neglected sclerokeratitis may lead to a progressive scarring of the cornea.

Keratitis

1. *Nummular* may persist for many months, the peripheral lesions sometimes forming facets which later become vascularized and infiltrated by lipid.
2. *Disciform*, if neglected, gives rise to scarring, vascularization, and lipid deposition.
3. *Neurotrophic* may lead to severe ulceration and even perforation.
4. *Mucous plaque* develops in about 5% of cases at any time between 1 week and 4 years after the onset of the rash, but most commonly between the third and sixth months. It is characterized by a sudden onset of ciliary injection and the production of mucous plaque deposits on the surface of a diffusely swollen corneal epithelium. The lesions may resemble pieces of white blotting paper and can be easily removed without damaging the underlying epithelium. From day to day the plaques vary in size, shape and number. They are accompanied by diffuse stromal haze and when they assume a dendritiform configuration they may be confused with the dendritic ulcers caused by herpes simplex. They stain brilliantly with rose bengal and moderately well with fluorescein. After about 3 months, the plaques disappear, leaving a faint diffuse corneal haze.

Neuralgia

Neuralgia which is severe and chronic affects about 7% of patients. It may be constant or intermittently severe and stabbing as in tic douloureux. The pain may be worse at night and aggravated by touch and heat. It generally improves slowly with time although it may lead to depression, sometimes of sufficient severity to present the danger of suicide. Unfortunately treatment may be extremely difficult.

Stage three

Stage three consists of recurrent lesions that may reappear as long as 10 years after the acute lesions. They are frequently precipitated by the sudden withdrawal or reduction of topical corticosteroids. The most commonly occurring lesions are episcleritis, scleritis, nummular, disciform and mucous plaque keratitis, iritis, and glaucoma. It must be remembered that all these complications may appear as isolated lesions because the initial attack of zoster may have been forgotten by the patient or have been so mild that it passed undiagnosed.

Vaccinia

Vaccinia is usually caused by autoinoculation from an arm pustule to the eye.

Clinical features

1. *Keratitis* is characterized by small dendritic figures or geographical ulceration. Occasionally a disciform keratitis may develop.
2. *Blepharoconjunctivitis* consists of a papillary conjunctival reaction with chemosis and hyperaemia.

Treatment

Adenine arabinoside may be effective in some cases.

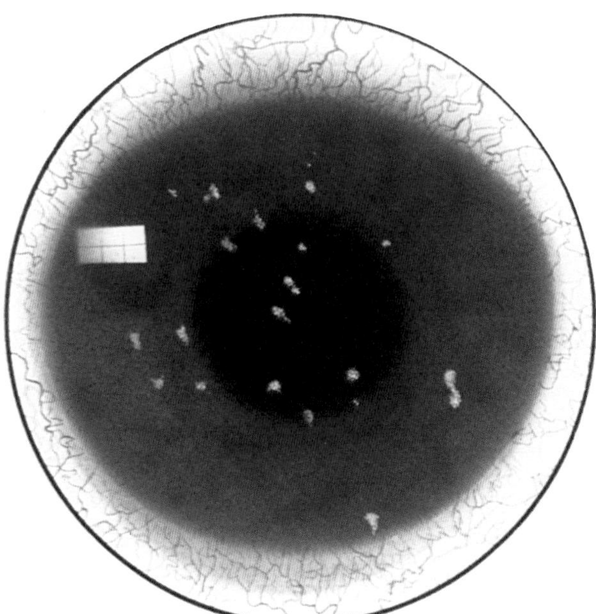

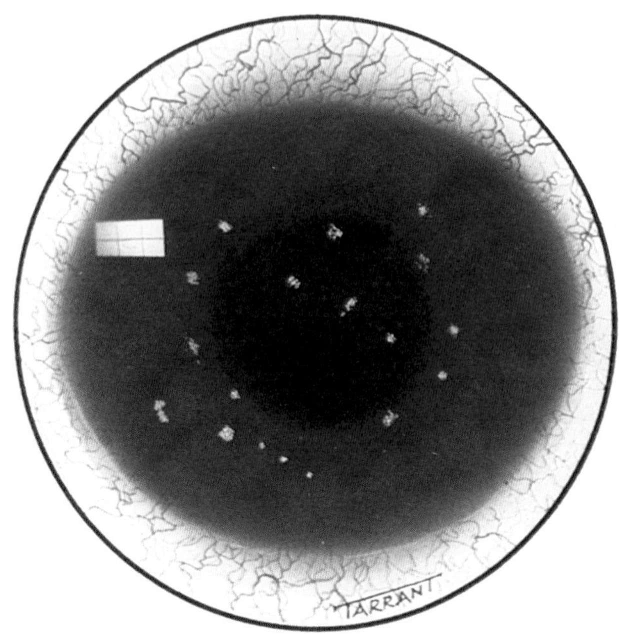

Figure 5.22 *Thygeson's superficial punctate keratitis*

Thygeson's superficial punctate

Thygeson's superficial punctate keratitis (SPK) is a rare, usually bilateral, non-contagious, chronic keratitis characterized by remissions and exacerbations. A viral aetiology is suspected but unproven.

Clinical features

The conjunctiva is uninflamed. The characteristic finding is a superficial keratitis consisting of stellate, round or oval conglomerates of distinct granular, greyish-white intraepithelial dots some of which may be associated with a mild subepithelial haze (*Figure 5.22*).

Treatment

The condition disappears spontaneously after several years without serious sequelae. The main aim of treatment is to relieve symptoms during exacerbations. Some patients with relatively mild involvement may be treated with simple lubricants. Topical steroids are usually effective in suppressing the keratitis although they may prolong the course of the disease. The few steroid-resistant patients can be treated with soft contact lenses. Although the use of the antiviral agent idoxuridine is said to make SPK worse with more severe subepithelial infiltrates, a recent report has shown a favourable response to trifluorothymidine drops.

Exposure keratopathy

This condition is caused by improper wetting of the corneal surface by the precorneal tear film from an ability of the lids to resurface the cornea at each blink. This occurs despite the presence of normal lacrimal secretions.

Aetiology

Important causes include facial nerve palsy (neuroparalytic keratitis), severe proptosis, and cicatricial lid disorders. Occasionally corneal exposure during sleep may occur in normal healthy individuals in the absence of any of the other factors.

Clinical features

The spectrum of clinical findings ranges from minimal inferior punctate epithelial erosions to severe ulceration with neovascularization, infection, and even perforation. Corneal exposure during sleep is now considered to be a relatively common cause of previously undiagnosed chronic keratitis. The diagnosis can be made by asking the patient to gently close his lids, and usually within a minute or two a small crack will be seen between the lids on shining a light on the interpalpebral area. In these patients symptoms may be similar to recurrent corneal erosions.

Treatment

If possible, the cause should be corrected (i.e. proptosis or lid abnormalities). If recovery is anticipated, conservative measures such as frequent instillation of artificial tears, with or without soft contact lenses, may be sufficient to prevent complications. At night ointment should be instilled and the lids kept closed with a piece of tape extending from the upper lid to the lower lid and cheek. If the condition is likely to be permanent, lid surgery is usually necessary.

Neurotrophic keratopathy

Neurotrophic keratopathy occurs in an anaesthetic cornea. The exact pathological process responsible is unclear. It appears that the corneal sensory nerves are very important in maintaining the health of the corneal epithelium. The loss of neural influences causes oedema and exfoliation of the epithelial cells, presumably by altering their metabolic activity. Corneal changes can occur in the presence of a normal blink reflex and normal lacrimal secretions.

Aetiology

1. *Acquired* causes include section of the fifth nerve, herpes simplex and herpes zoster keratitis, diabetes, leprosy, and certain corneal dystrophies.
2. *Congenital* causes are very rare. They include familial dysautonomia (Riley–Day syndrome), anhidrotic ectodermal dysplasia, and congenital insensitivity to pain.

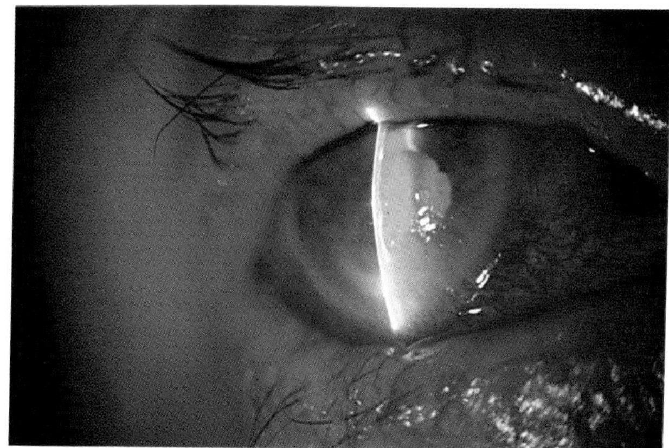

Figure 5.23 *Neurotrophic keratopathy due to herpes zoster with secondary bacterial infection*

Clinical features

The corneal changes are characterized by the development of punctate epithelial erosions involving primarily the interpalpebral area of the cornea. The epithelial cells then become grey, slightly opaque, and oedematous. Exfoliation of the epithelium is followed by ulceration (*Figure 5.23*).

Treatment

If keratopathy can be predicted prior to neurosurgical procedures involving the trigeminal nerve, then tarsorrhaphy is the best preventive measure. Once ulceration develops, healing is slow since the epithelial mitotic rate is diminished. Treatment is with ointments and patching.

Peripheral ulceration and thinning

This is a miscellaneous group of conditions characterized by ulceration and/or melting of the corneal periphery.

Classification

Dellen
Marginal keratitis (catarrhal ulcer)
Rosacea keratitis
Phlyctenulosis
Terrien's marginal degeneration
Mooren's ulcer
Associated with systemic collagen vascular diseases

Dellen

Clinical features

Dellen are common saucer-like thinnings of the peripheral cornea (*Figure 5.24*) occurring in areas of tear film instability. They are caused by a local dehydration of the corneal stroma leading to compaction of its lamellae. If normal hydration is not restored within a few days, the stroma may undergo secondary degeneration leading to localized scarring and vascularization. However, in the vast majority of cases, the condition is completely innocuous and transient.

Aetiology

1. *Raised limbal lesions*—dermoids, episcleritis, pterygia, large subconjunctival haemorrhage, and glaucoma-filtering blebs.
2. *Squint surgery* and postoperative chemosis is a common cause.
3. *Senility* may cause transient dellen.

Treatment

This involves elimination of the cause, and promoting corneal rehydration by patching and the use of lubricants.

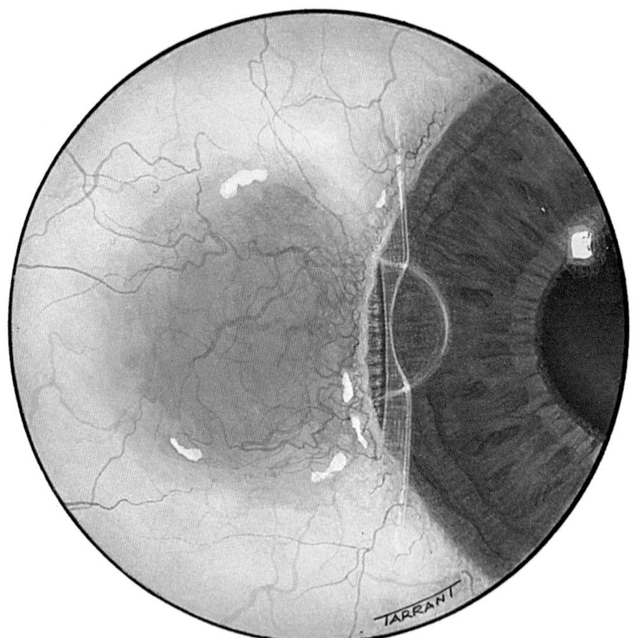

Figure 5.24 Dellen

Marginal keratitis (catarrhal ulcer)

This extremely common condition is thought to be caused by a hypersensitivity reaction to staphylococcal exotoxins. It is particularly prevalent in patients suffering from chronic staphylococcal blepharitis.

Clinical features

The ulcer presents with symptoms of mild ocular irritation, which may be accompanied by watering and photophobia. It starts as a subepithelial infiltrate which is separated from the limbus by a clear zone of cornea. The 10, 2, 4, or 8 o'clock positions are most commonly affected first. The lesion then spreads circumferentially and is accompanied by a breakdown of the overlying epithelium, giving rise to a fluorescein-staining ulcer. Within a few days blood vessels bridge the clear corneal zone and resolution occurs.

Differential diagnosis

It is important not to confuse marginal keratitis with a peripheral ulcer due to herpes simplex because the treatment of the two is entirely different. A herpetic ulcer *starts* as an epithelial defect and is *followed* by subepithelial infiltration. Corneal sensation may be diminished in herpetic ulceration but is unaffected in marginal keratitis.

Treatment

A short course of topical corticosteroid drops is extremely effective in promoting resolution. In order to prevent recurrence, it is also important to treat any associated blepharitis.

Rosacea keratitis

Acne rosacea is a common, yet frequently undiagnosed, skin disease of unknown aetiology which typically affects women between the ages of 30 and 50 years.

Skin manifestations

Ocular complications occur in about 20% of cases prior to the onset of skin changes. The skin lesions consist of a chronic hyperaemia of the face, usually involving the nose, central forehead, and upper cheeks (*Figure 5.25*). Flushing

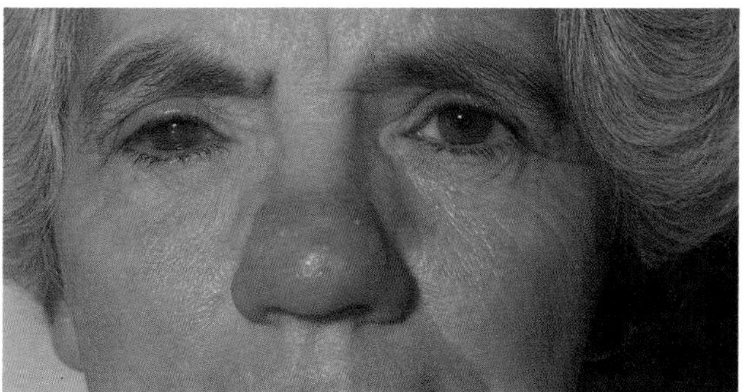

Figure 5.25 *Advanced acne rosacea showing keratitis of right eye and early rhinophyma*

of these areas may be precipitated by ingestion of alcohol or spicy foods. Other features include variable degrees of telangiectasia, papules, pustules, and hypertrophic sebaceous glands leading to increased sebum production. Rhinophyma is the most advanced form of the disease. The term 'acne rosacea' is, in a way, misleading because it implies the presence of pustules, which are not necessary for the diagnosis. If pustules form they resolve without scarring, unlike those associated with acne vulgaris. There is no association between the severity of skin manifestations and the extent of ocular involvement.

Ocular manifestations

Keratitis

This is seen in about 5% of cases and may take several forms:

1. *Peripheral vascularization,* especially involving the inferotemporal and inferonasal quadrants, is followed by subepithelial infiltrates central to the vessels (*Figure 5.26*). Pannus formation may obscure the visual axis, and wedge-shaped scarring may occur (*Figure 5.27*).

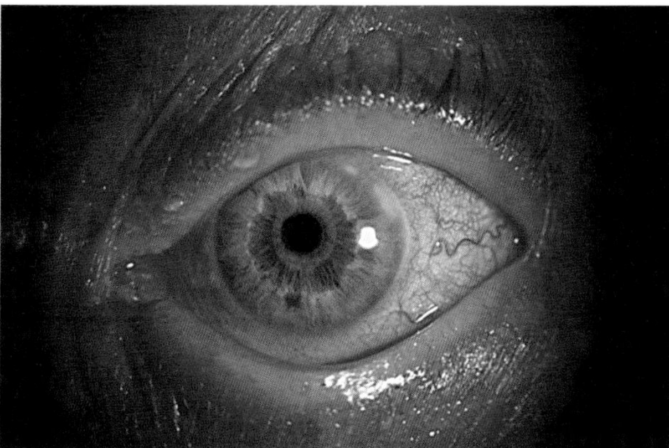

Figure 5.26 *Peripheral keratitis between 1 and 2 o'clock (left eye)*

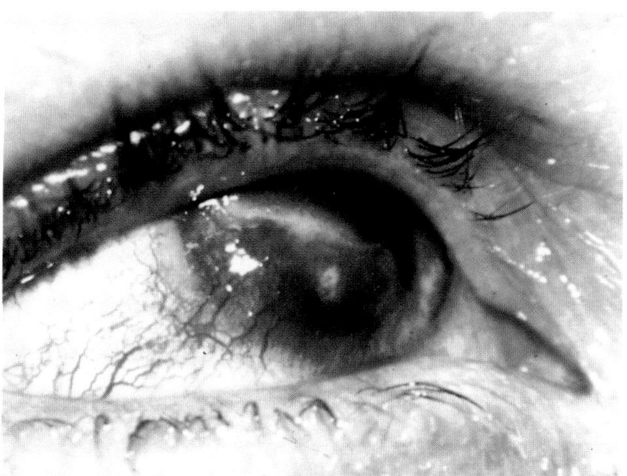

Figure 5.27 *Corneal pannus in rosacea keratitis*

2. *Thinning* of the cornea occurs either by resolution of the infiltrates or by gross ulceration. Perforation may occasionally occur as a result of severe peripheral or central melting which may be precipitated by the excessive use of topical steroids.
3. *Punctate epithelial keratopathy* involving the lower two-thirds of the cornea.

If left untreated, rosacea keratitis can progress steadily to corneal melting with neovascularization, finally resulting in stromal scarring (*Figure 5.28*).

Blepharoconjunctivitis

Chronic blepharitis and meibomitis are very common in patients with acne rosacea. The interpalpebral bulbar conjunctiva commonly shows hyperaemia. Recurrent chalazia are almost twice as common in patients with rosacea as in those without and styes are also a frequent complication (*see* Chapter 4).

Treatment

1. *Topical corticosteroids* are a very effective short-term measure for the treatment of keratitis and conjunctivitis.

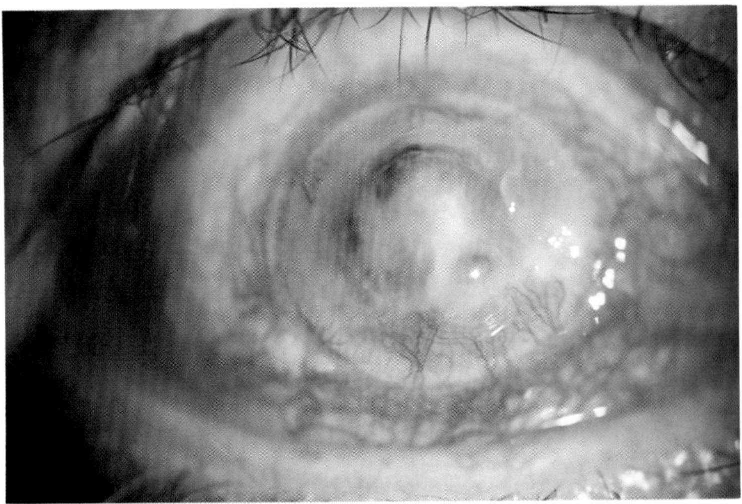

Figure 5.28 Advanced rosacea keratitis

2. *Systemic tetracycline* 250 mg four times a day for 1 month followed by 250 mg daily for at least 6 months (or twice a day throughout) is usually extremely successful in alleviating both the ocular and skin lesions. The antibiotic should be taken before meals but should not be administered to pregnant women for fear of inducing discolouration of teeth in the offspring. The therapeutic effect of tetracycline does not appear to be related to the antibacterial action of the drug. It is important to remember that tetracycline suppresses but does not cure the disease, although improvement usually lasts for 6 months after cessation of therapy. A more gradual tapering may be required for ocular lesions than for skin lesions.

Phlyctenulosis

This fairly rare disease predominantly affects children. Although in the past tuberculosis was considered to be a common aetiological factor, it is now thought that phlyctenulosis is probably caused by a non-specific delayed hypersensitivity reaction to staphylococci or other bacterial antigens.

Clinical features

Although most cases are self-limiting, very occasionally the disease is severe and may even be blinding. Even in relatively mild cases, photophobia, lacrimation, and blepharospasm may be very distressing. A conjunctival phlycten starts as a small pinkish-white nodule near the limbus, surrounded by hyperaemia (*Figure 5.29*). It is usually transient and resolves spontaneously. A corneal phlycten starts astride the limbus. Just like the conjunctival lesion it may resolve spontaneously or it may extend radially onto the cornea and, very occasionally, it may give rise to severe ulceration and even perforation. A healed corneal phlycten usually leaves a triangular limbal-based scar.

Treatment

A short course of topical corticosteroids is usually very effective in promoting resolution. In the rare resistant case, systemic tetracycline may be necessary. Any associated chronic staphylococcal blepharitis should also be treated.

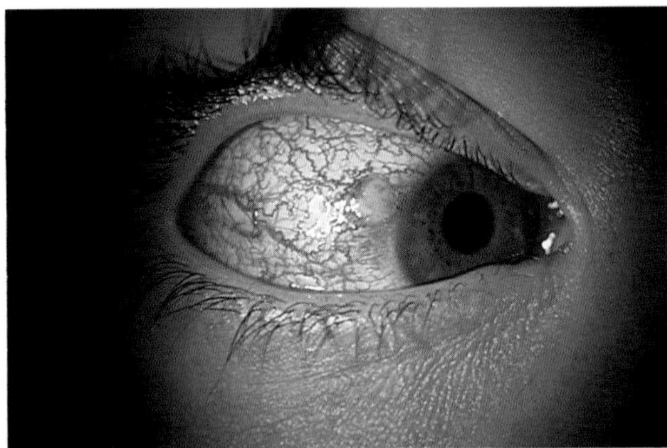

Figure 5.29 Conjunctival phlycten

Terrien's marginal degeneration

This is an uncommon thinning of the peripheral cornea. About 75% of affected patients are males, two-thirds of whom are over the age of 40 years. The condition is usually bilateral although the severity of involvement may be asymmetrical.

Clinical features

Early

Early features consist of fine, yellow-white, punctate stromal opacities which are frequently associated with mild superficial vascularization. These changes usually start in the upper part of the cornea and are separated from the limbus by a clear zone. On cursory examination they may resemble arcus senilis. This stage is usually asymptomatic.

Late

Progression of the disease is extremely slow. Eventually thinning leads to the formation of a peripheral gutter, the outer slope of which 'shelves' gradually while the central part rises sharply (*Figure 5.30*). The sharp edge may become demarcated by a white-grey line or show dense yellow-white lipid deposits. Although the floor of the gutter becomes thin and vascularized, the overlying epithelium remains intact and does not stain with fluorescein. The thinning slowly spreads circumferentially, often resulting in ectasia superiorly and a furrow below. Occasionally, there are localized ectasias along the course of the furrow. Vision gradually deteriorates due to increasing corneal astigmatism. A few patients develop recurrent episodes of disabling pain and inflammation.

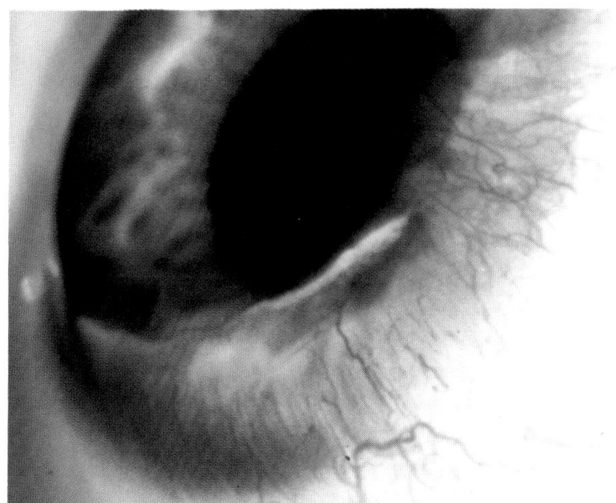

Figure 5.30 *Terrien's marginal degeneration*

Complications

1. *Pseudopterygia* develop in about 20% of cases at positions other than 9 and 3 o'clock meridians. They grow onto the cornea at an oblique angle, and may occur early in the disease when thinning is subtle
2. *Perforation* occurs in about 15% of cases. In these, keratoplasty, either full-thickness or deep lamellar sector, is necessary.
3. *Severe astigmatism* can also be treated by a crescent-shaped excision of the gutter with suturing of the 'healthier' margins.

Mooren's ulcer

Mooren's ulcer is a very rare peripheral ulcerative keratitis. Although its exact aetiology is unknown, it has been suggested that it may be due to an ischaemic necrosis resulting from a vasculitis of limbal vessels. The conjunctiva adjacent to the ulcer has been shown to produce enzymes such as collagenase and proteoglyconase which may also be important in its causation. Occasionally it may occur following cataract surgery.

It has been suggested by some authorities that two types of Mooren's ulcer exist:

1. *A limited* form which is usually unilateral, mostly affecting old people.
2. *The progressive* form is bilateral, affecting relatively young individuals, and is relentlessly progressive.

Clinical features

Early

The presenting symptom is usually blurred vision due to irregular astigmatism. The ulceration begins as patches of grey infiltrate near the margin of the cornea, which spreads by slowly undermining the corneal epithelium and superficial corneal lamellae at its advancing border, forming an overhanging edge (*Figure 5.31*). The spread may be self-limiting or progressive.

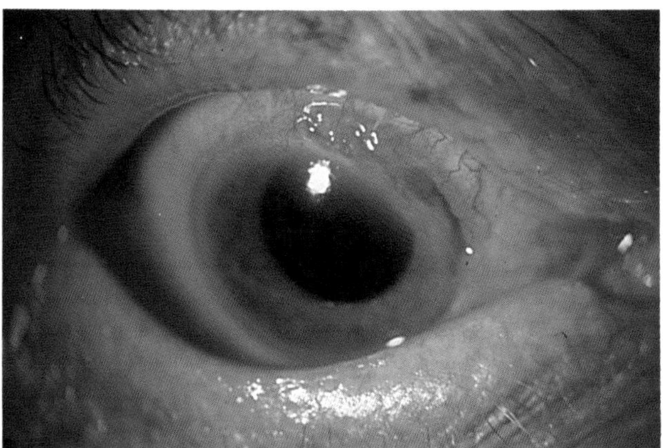

Figure 5.31 *Early Mooren's ulcer*

Late

In severe cases the ulceration spreads to involve the entire circumference of the cornea. It also spreads towards the centre of the cornea and may even invade the sclera (*Figure 5.32*). Behind the active margin of the ulcer, healing takes place from the periphery but the healed area remains thin, vascularized, and opaque. At this stage the patient experiences severe pain, photophobia, and lacrimation. Vision is lost when the visual axis becomes involved. Secondary cataract may form but perforation is rare.

Treatment

At present three options are available for the treatment of Mooren's ulcer.

1. *Topical corticosteroids.* The initial approach is the use of strong topical steroids applied at hourly intervals.
2. *Conjunctival excision.* Ulcers that fail to respond to topical steroids are treated by excision of conjunctiva approximately 3 mm from the limbus and parallel to the ulcer.

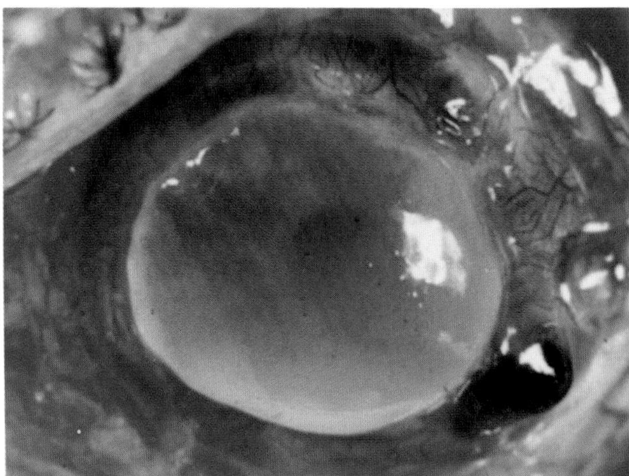

Figure 5.32 *Advanced Mooren's ulcer*

In general, patients with unilateral or bilateral non-simultaneous ulcers behave similarly and respond favourably to topical steroids or conjunctival resection.

3. *Immunosuppressive therapy.* Patients with bilateral simultaneous ulceration have the worst prognosis and are the most difficult to treat. If conjunctival excision is unsuccessful, the use of immunosuppressive agents such as systemic steroids and cytotoxic drugs (cyclophosphamide, azathioprine, methotrexate) should be considered. The success rate is less than 50%.

Systemic collagen vascular disorders

The presence of severe persistent peripheral corneal ulceration or thinning unexplained by coexistent ocular disease should prompt a search for an associated systemic collagen vascular disease. The four main diseases that should be considered are rheumatoid arthritis, systemic lupus erythematosus, polyarteritis nodosa, and Wegener's granulomatosis. It should be remembered that, on occasion, the ocular lesions may preceed the clinical manifestation of the systemic disease.

Rheumatoid arthritis

Systemic features

Rheumatoid arthritis (RA) is a common idiopathic multisystem disorder characterized by symmetrical and predominantly peripheral inflammatory arthritis. It typically affects women between the ages of 35 and 40 years. Most patients are positive for rheumatoid factor (seropositive). Important extra-articular manifestations of RA are subcutaneous nodules, vasculitis, and occasionally heart and lung disease. Ocular complications are keratoconjunctivitis sicca, scleritis, and keratitis. In fact, RA is the most common collagen vascular disorder to affect the peripheral cornea.

Peripheral keratitis

The four types of peripheral corneal changes which may be primary or secondary to scleritis are:

Sclerosing keratitis

This is characterized by gradual peripheral thickening and opacification of the stroma adjacent to the site of scleritis. The process may progress centrally and be complicated by scarring, vascularization, and lipid deposition.

Acute stromal keratitis

This is characterized by superficial and/or midstromal peripheral infiltrates associated with non-necrotizing scleritis. Late complications include diffuse peripheral opacification and vascularization, and occasionally epithelial breakdown and stromal melting.

Peripheral corneal guttering ('contact lens cornea')

This may be secondary to scleritis or occur in isolation. The thinning may spread circumferentially to involve the entire corneal periphery. Because the central part of the cornea remains of normal thickness, the appearance resembles a contact lens placed on the eye—hence the term 'contact lens cornea' (*Figure 5.33, right*). Secondary changes include vascularization and deposition of lipid within the gutter. The corneal epithelium, however, remains intact.

Keratolysis

This is characterized by acute and severe melting of clear cornea. In some cases, the entire corneal stroma melts within a few days resulting in descemetocele formation (*Figure 5.33, left*).

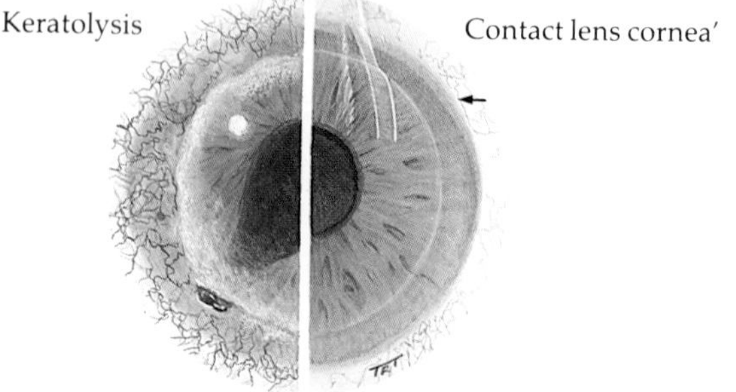

Figure 5.33 *Peripheral keratitis in rheumatoid arthritis*

Treatment

1. Active scleral inflammation should be treated with *systemic steroids and/or immunosuppressive agents (see later)*.
2. *Topical steroids* may be useful in acute stromal keratitis, but they should be avoided in peripheral corneal guttering and keratolysis for fear of inducing further corneal thinning and eventual perforation.

3. *Tissue adhesive glue* (isobutyl cyanoacrylate) and bandage soft contact lenses may be useful in treating descemetoceles and preventing corneal perforation.
4. *Conjunctival excision* may halt the progression of corneal furrowing in refractory cases. The technique is the same as already described for Mooren's ulcer.
5. *Keratoplasty* may be required either as an emergency measure to prevent perforation or, electively, to restore visual acuity.

Systemic lupus erythematosus

Systemic features

Systemic lupus erythematosus (SLE) is a relatively common, idiopathic, multisystem disorder which may affect articular, cutaneous, renal, blood, pulmonary, cardiovascular, and CNS systems. SLE is much more common in females than in males and patients are invariably positive for antinuclear antibody. The prognosis for life is good, with a 98% 5-year survival, even in those with severe disease. The most common ocular complication of SLE is punctate epithelial keratopathy. Other less frequent manifestations are keratoconjunctivitis sicca, scleritis, retinal vasculitis, anterior ischaemic optic neuropathy and peripheral keratitis.

Peripheral keratitis

The two types of peripheral corneal change in SLE are:

1. Asymptomatic non-infiltrative marginal thinning.
2. Marginal ulceration with infiltration and vascularization.

Polyarteritis nodosa

Systemic features

Polyarteritis nodosa (PAN) is a rare, chronic, idiopathic, necrotizing systemic vasculitis which affects medium-sized and small arteries. PAN is more common in males than females by a 2:1 ratio. Arteries throughout the body may be involved, leading to widespread changes in many organs such as skin ulceration which is slow to heal, renal disease with secondary hypertension, mesenteric infarction, lung disease, arthritis, as well as involvement of peripheral nerves (mononeuritis multiplex), the heart, and the CNS. Ocular manifestations of PAN include: scleritis, choroidal vasculitis, retinal vasculitis, anterior ischaemic optic neuropathy, and peripheral keratitis.

Peripheral keratitis

Keratitis may occasionally be the presenting feature of PAN. It usually begins with the appearance of bilateral marginal stromal infiltrates. The overlying epithelium then breaks down and the anterior stroma begins to ulcerate. The ulceration spreads circumferentially, and may also extend centrally similar to a Mooren's ulcer. The keratitis is unresponsive to topical steroid therapy although systemic treatment of PAN with a combination of steroids and cyclophosphamide may be beneficial.

Wegener's granulomatosis

Systemic features

Wegener's granulomatosis is a very rare, idiopathic, multisystem disease characterized by necrotizing granulomatous inflammation of the upper and lower respiratory tract, focal necrotizing glomerulonephritis, and varying degrees of diffuse systemic granulomatous vasculitis. Ocular complications include orbital involvement which may be primary or secondary to sinus disease, retinal vasculitis, uveitis, scleritis, conjunctivitis, and peripheral keratitis.

Peripheral keratitis

The clinical features and management of peripheral corneal ulceration are essentially the same as in PAN.

Degenerations

Classification

Arcus senilis
Vogt's white limbal girdle
Lipid keratopathy
Band keratopathy
Spheroidal
Salzmann's nodular

Arcus senilis

This is an innocuous age-related change which is present in 60% of patients between the ages of 40 and 60 years and in nearly all patients over the age of 80. In children and young adults, it may occasionally be a feature of systemic hyperlipidaemias, particularly those associated with raised blood cholesterol levels. Arcus senilis consists of bilateral lipid deposition which starts in the superior and inferior

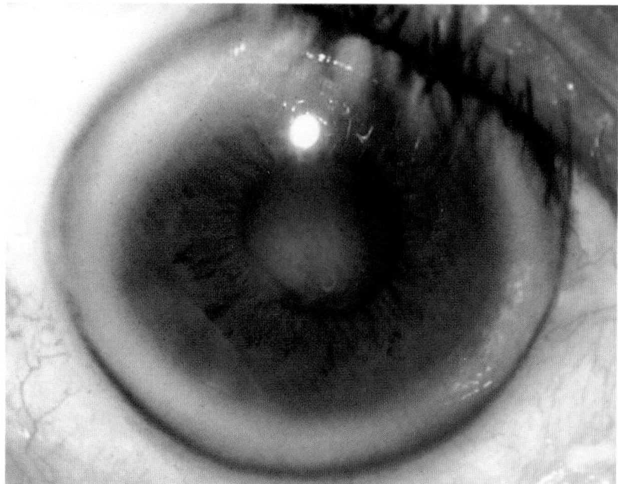

Figure 5.34 Arcus senilis

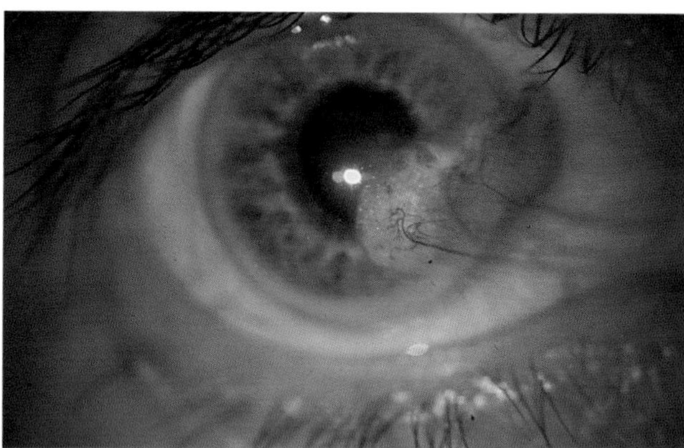

Figure 5.35 Lipid keratopathy

perilimbal cornea and then progresses circumferentially to form a band which is about 1 mm wide (*Figure 5.34*). The central border of the band is diffuse while the sharp peripheral edge is separated from the limbus by a clear zone of cornea. This clear interval may occasionally undergo a mild thinning (senile furrow). Histological studies have shown that the lipid is first deposited in the anterior half of Descemet's membrane and then in the anterior stroma, just beneath Bowman's layer.

Vogt's white limbal girdle

This is also a very common and innocuous age-related degeneration characterized by bilateral chalky white opacities involving the temporal and nasal peripheral cornea. Two clinical types are described: type 1 contains multiple holes and has a perilimbal clear zone similar to arcus senilis; type 2 on the other hand has neither a clear zone nor holes but has central prolongations.

Lipid keratopathy

This is a lipid degeneration of the cornea manifest by the presence of white or yellowish corneal stromal deposits consisting of cholesterol, fats, and phospholipids. Lipid keratopathy can be primary or secondary. The primary form occurs spontaneously in an avascular cornea. The secondary type, which is much more common, is associated with previous ocular injury or disease that has resulted in a corneal vascularization (*Figure 5.35*). In some cases slow resorption of the lipid infiltrate can be induced by argon laser photocoagulation to the new blood vessels.

Band keratopathy

This fairly common condition is caused by a deposition of calcium salts in the subepithelial space and anterior part of Bowman's layer. Its distribution is quite chararacteristically interpalpebral with a clear space separating the sharp margin of the band from the limbus (*see Figure 6.18*). Slitlamp examination reveals holes in the calcium plaques which are thought to represent nerve canals in Bowman's layer. Transparent clefts secondary to cracks or tears in the calcium may also be seen. As the band progresses, the epithelium becomes irregular and subsequent corneal breakdown may be painful.

Aetiology

1. Chronic iridocyclitis in childhood.
2. Phthisis bulbi.
3. Idiopathic in the elderly.
4. Hypercalcaemia.

Management

Treatment is indicated for visual or cosmetic reasons.

1. The corneal epithelium overlying the opacity is scraped off with a knife.
2. A 0.01 M solution of sodium versenate is then applied to the denuded cornea with a cotton-tipped bud until all calcium has been removed. This usually takes about 10 minutes. The eye is then padded until the epithelium has regenerated.

Spheroidal

This condition is also known under many eponyms including corneal elastosis, Labrador keratopathy, climatic droplet keratopathy, and Bietti's nodular dystrophy. Spheroidal degeneration typically occurs in men who work outdoors. It is characterized by the presence of small amber-coloured spheroidal granules seen in the anterior stroma of the interpalpebral area of the cornea. The disease varies in severity from a localized mistiness to the development of large nodules and corneal opacification.

Salzmann's nodular

This is a non-inflammatory condition that may develop following chronic keratitis, trachoma, or phlyctenulosis. It is characterized by elevated subepithelial nodules in either scarred cornea (*Figure 5.36*) or at the edge of transparent cornea. The base of a nodule may be surrounded by epithelial iron deposits. Bowman's layer is usually replaced by scar tissue and the epithelium is irregular.

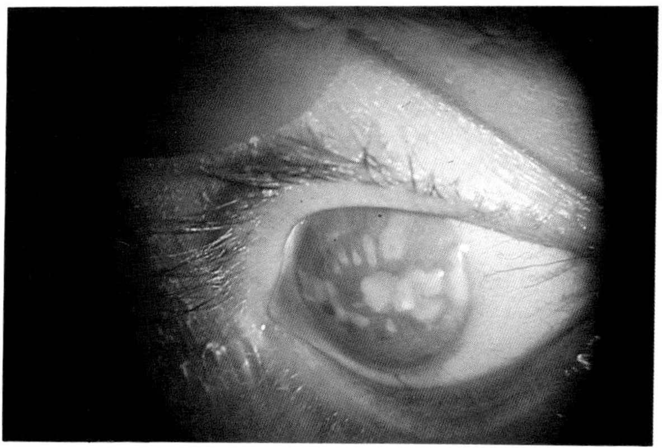

Figure 5.36 *Salzmann's nodular degeneration*

Dystrophies

Classification

Anterior dystrophies affecting the corneal epithelium and Bowman's layer
- microcystic (Cogan's)
- recurrent corneal erosion syndrome
- Reis–Bücklers'
- Meesmann's

Stromal dystrophies
- lattice
- macular
- granular

Posterior dystrophies affecting the corneal endothelium and Descemet's membrane
- cornea guttata
- Fuchs' endothelial
- posterior polymorphous

Ectatic dystrophies
- keratoconus
- posterior keratoconus
- keratoglobus
- pellucid marginal degeneration

Anterior

Microcystic (Cogan's)

This is probably the most common of all corneal dystrophies seen in clinical practice. Despite this, it is frequently misdiagnosed, mainly due to its variable appearance. In the literature it is reported under a wide variety of names, including Cogan's microcystic dystrophy, map–dot–fingerprint dystrophy, bleb-like dystrophy, and epithelial basement membrane dystrophy.

Clinical features

Microcystic dystrophy is characterized by bilateral dot-like, cystic, or linear fingerprint-like lesions, limited to the corneal epithelium (*Figure 5.37*). When the patient is observed over a prolonged period of time, one pattern will often change to another and the distribution of the lesions may also vary. Most patients with this condition remain asymptomatic throughout life, but about 10% develop the recurrent corneal erosion syndrome, usually after the age of 30 years. The simultaneous occurrence of bilateral recurrent erosions is strongly suggestive of microcystic dystrophy.

Recurrent corneal erosion syndrome

Apart from microcystic dystrophy, this condition may also be associated with other corneal dystrophies. However, the most important and common cause is trauma, especially from a scratch. Recent studies have suggested that a deficiency in the basement membrane, or lack of hemidesmosomes attaching the basal cell layer of the corneal epithelium to the basement membrane, plays a role in the development of this condition. It is seen with increased prevalence in diabetics.

Clinical features

The recurrent corneal erosion syndrome typically presents with pain, lacrimation, photophobia, and blurred vision involving one eye when the patient awakes from sleep. Although these symptoms usually resolve rapidly, those that experience recurrences are often plagued for months, or even years, until normal attachment of the basal cell layer of the epithelium is finally restored. The condition appears to be particularly troublesome in diabetic patients.

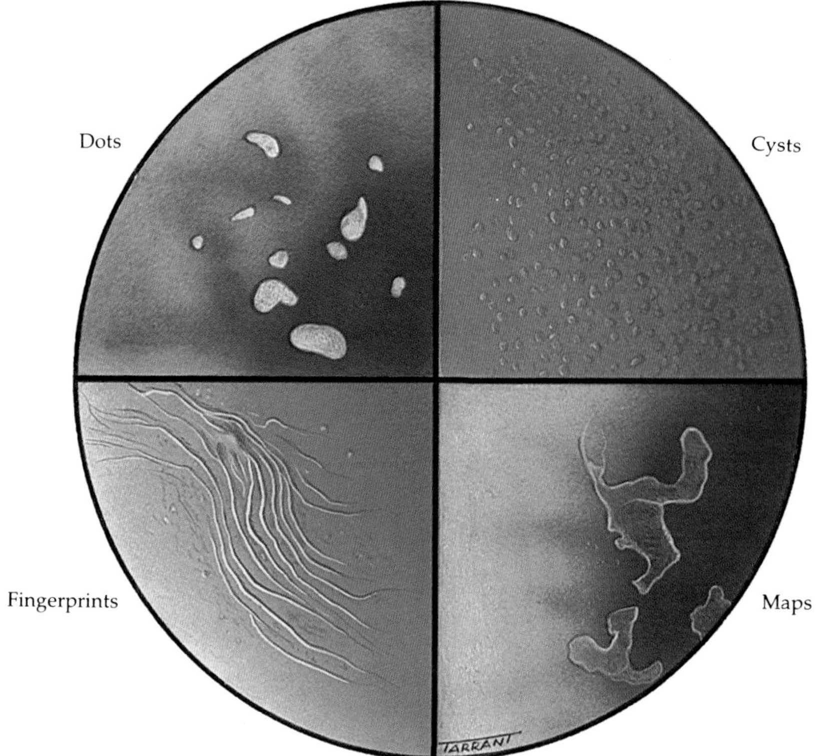

Figure 5.37 *Microcystic dystrophy*

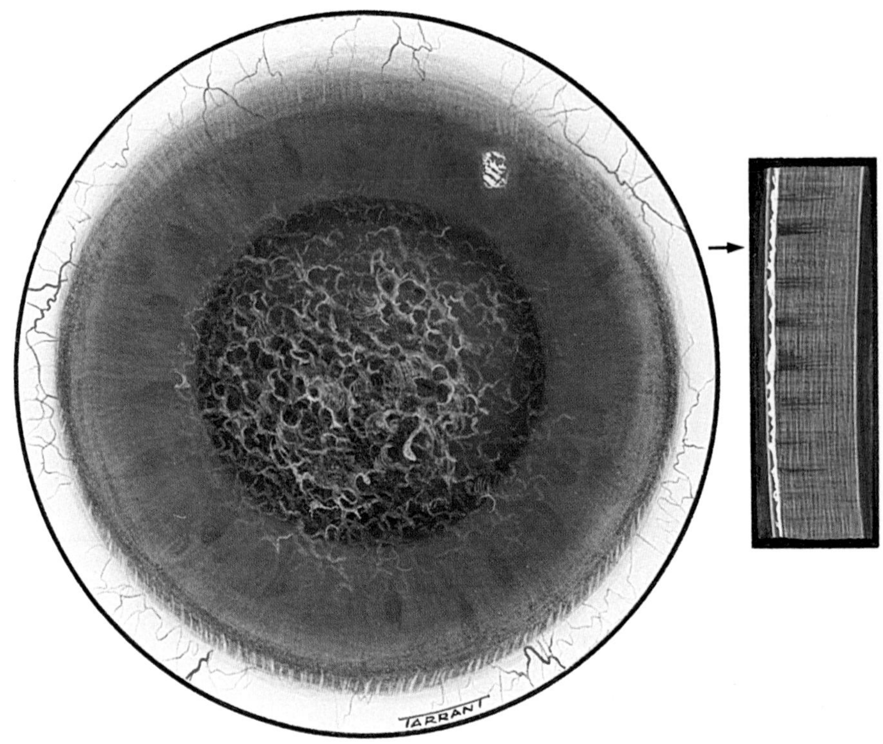

Figure 5.38 *Reis–Bücklers' dystrophy*

Treatment

It is important to reassure the patient that, although the condition may be extremely uncomfortable, it is relatively innocuous and long-term vision-threatening complications are extremely rare. The form of management depends on the severity of the erosions.

1. *Mild cases* are treated with topical artificial tears four times a day and instillation of a simple lubricating ointment (Lacri-Lube) at night.
2. *Severe cases* with large areas of epithelial loss are treated by mechanical removal of all loose epithelium followed by the instillation of a cycloplegic agent (homatropine 1% or cyclopentolate 1%) and an antibiotic ointment. The eye should then be patched until the epithelium has healed.
3. *Recurrent severe cases* which fail to respond to conventional conservative therapy may be treated by removing the entire corneal epithelium. The total removal of epithelium and abnormal basement membrane apparently allows for the regeneration of a new and stable epithelium and adequate hemidesmosomes.

Reis–Bücklers' dystrophy

Inheritance

This is autosomal dominant.

Clinical features

This relatively common progressive dystrophy usually presents during early childhood. It is characterized by superficial, ring-shaped opacities, most dense in the centre, which give the cornea a 'honeycomb' appearance (*Figure 5.38*). Most patients develop severe attacks of recurrent erosions. Eventually, keratoplasty (lamellar or penetrating) may be necessary if visual acuity is significantly impaired. Recurrence of the dystrophy in the graft is common.

Meesmann's dystrophy

Inheritance

This is autosomal dominant.

Clinical features

This very rare dystrophy appears during early life. It is characterized by tiny epithelial cysts which are best detected on corneal retroillumination (*Figure 5.39*). The lesions extend to the limbus and are most numerous in the interpalpebral area. The condition is usually visually inconsequential although some patients develop mild ocular irritation.

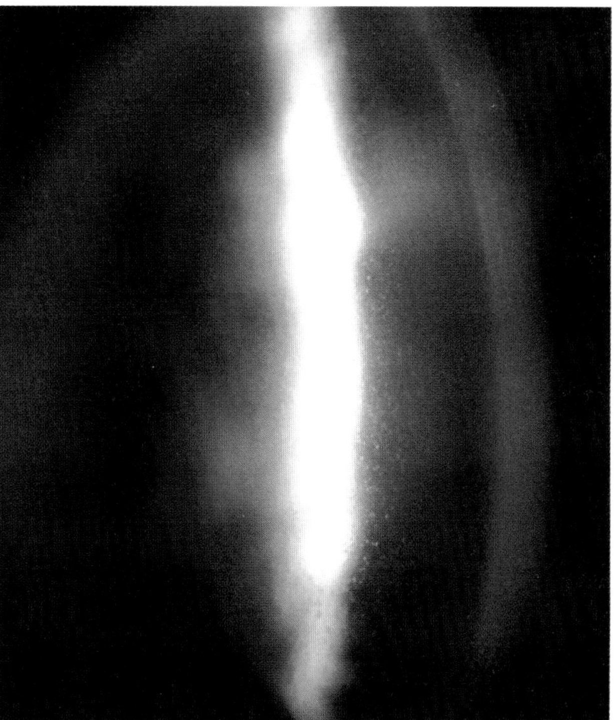

Figure 5.39 *Meesmann's dystrophy*

Stromal

Lattice

Inheritance

This is autosomal dominant with variable expressivity.

Clinical features

This progressive dystrophy usually presents during the end of the first decade of life with recurrent corneal erosions. It is characterized by branching spider-like deposits of amyloid which interlace and overlap at different levels within the stroma, but spare the corneal periphery (*Figures 5.40* and *5.41*). On cursory examination they may be mistaken for prominent corneal nerves. Microscopically the deposits stain with Congo red. As the condition progresses, a diffuse corneal haze develops and corneal sensation is diminished. By the age of about 30 years, visual acuity may become significantly impaired and penetrating keratoplasty may be necessary. Recurrence of the dystrophy in the graft may occur.

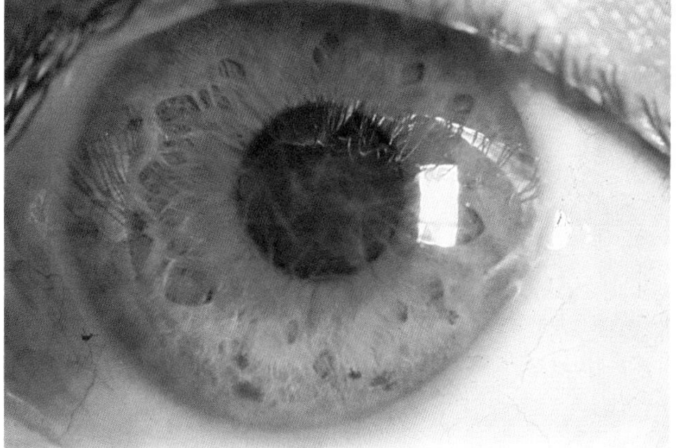

Figure 5.40 *Lattice dystrophy (courtesy of Mr T. A. Casey)*

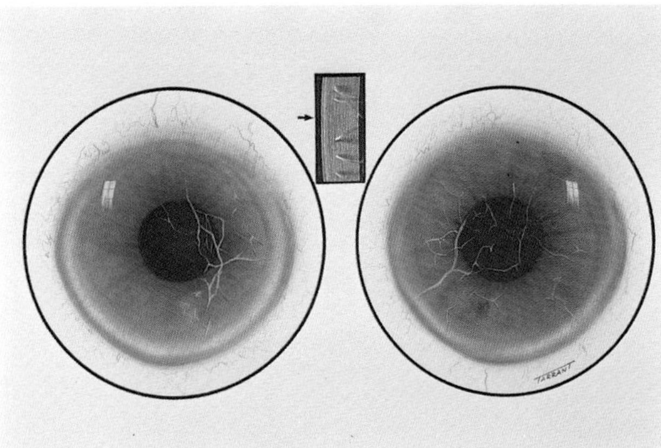

Figure 5.41 Lattice dystrophy

Granular

Inheritance

This is autosomal dominant.

Clinical features

This slowly progressive dystrophy usually develops during the first decade of life with the appearance of discrete, crumb-like, white granules of hyaline within the anterior stroma of the axial cornea. In between the lesions the stroma is clear (*Figure 5.42*). With time the lesions spread deeper and extend outwards but never involve the peripheral cornea. Microscopically the deposits stain bright red with Masson trichome. The stroma in between the lesions remains clear. Granular dystrophy usually remains asymptomatic for many years, although a few patients develop recurrent corneal erosions. Some patients may also complain of light scattering which is particularly troublesome during night driving. Visual acuity, however, usually remains good and keratoplasty is seldom required.

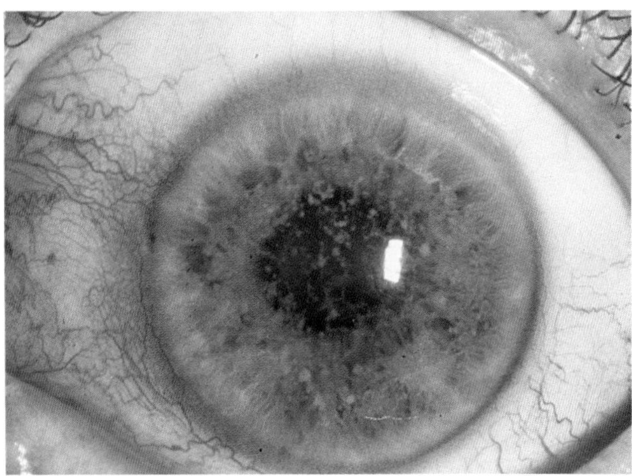

Figure 5.42 Granular dystrophy

Macular

Inheritance

This is autosomal recessive.

Clinical features

This is the least common but most serious of the three classic stromal dystrophies. It is characterized by focal, grey-white, poorly delineated opacities consisting of glycosaminoglycan. The stroma in between the lesions is diffusely cloudy. Although initially the opacities involve the superficial stroma, with the passage of time the entire stromal thickness including the peripheral cornea becomes involved (*Figure 5.43*). Microscopically the deposits stain with alcian blue. Symptoms of recurrent erosions are infrequent but most patients require penetrating keratoplasty during early life to improve visual acuity. Recurrence of the dystrophy in the graft is less frequent than in lattice dystrophy.

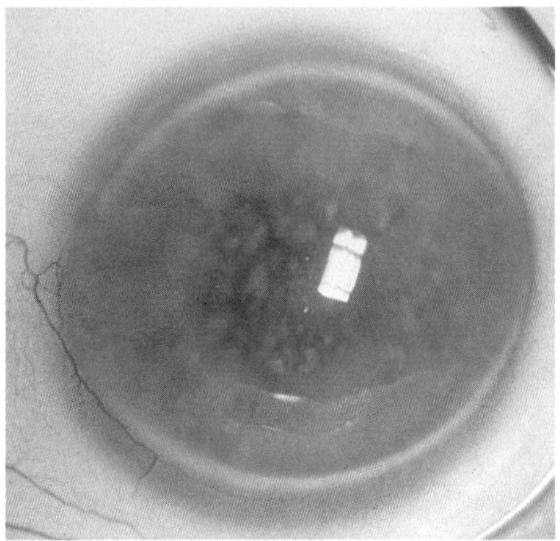

Figure 5.43 Macular dystrophy

The main differences between macular and the other two stromal dystrophies are:

1. *Inheritance is autosomal recessive.*
2. *The peripheral cornea is involved.*
3. *Significant impairment of vision occurs during early life.*

Posterior

Cornea guttata

This common condition consists of focal accumulations of collagen on the posterior surface of Descemet's membrane. They are apparently formed by stressed or abnormal endothelial cells and appear as warts or excresences of Descemet's membrane. When the lesions disrupt the regular endothelial mosaic, specular reflection reveals dark spots. In more advanced cases, these have a 'beaten metal' appearance or associated melanin pigment deposits on the endothelium.

When the lesions involve the corneal periphery they are referred to as Hassall–Henle bodies and are of no particular significance except as an indication of age. The term 'cornea guttata' is reserved for the same lesions involving the central cornea, which may occur as a result of ageing, or as part of the early stages of Fuchs' endothelial dystrophy.

Fuchs' endothelial

Inheritance

This is occasionally autosomal dominant.

Clinical features

This slowly progressive, usually bilateral, disease typically affects elderly patients and is more common in females than in males.

Early

These changes consist of cornea guttata without apparent alterations in the other corneal layers. During an interval of time that may span many years, the central endothelial protuberances become more numerous and begin to spread towards the corneal periphery (*Figure 5.44, left*).

Endothelial decompensation

This causes the stroma to become slowly oedematous. This is because of malfunction of the corneal endothelial cells, which in the healthy cornea constantly pump fluid from the stroma into the aqueous.

Bullous keratopathy

Epithelial oedema usually develops when the oedematous stroma thickness has increased by about 30%. At this stage, visual acuity is usually impaired. The persistence of epithelial oedema leads to the formation of bullae which cause pain and discomfort on rupturing (*Figure 5.44, right*).

Complications

As the condition progresses, the stroma gradually develops opacities and may become vascularized. Bowman's layer is replaced by a degenerative pannus. It is important to remember that primary open-angle glaucoma has an increased prevalence in patients with Fuchs' dystrophy.

Treatment

1. *Hypertonic agents* such as sodium chloride 5% drops or ointment may occasionally be effective in the treatment of early epithelial oedema.

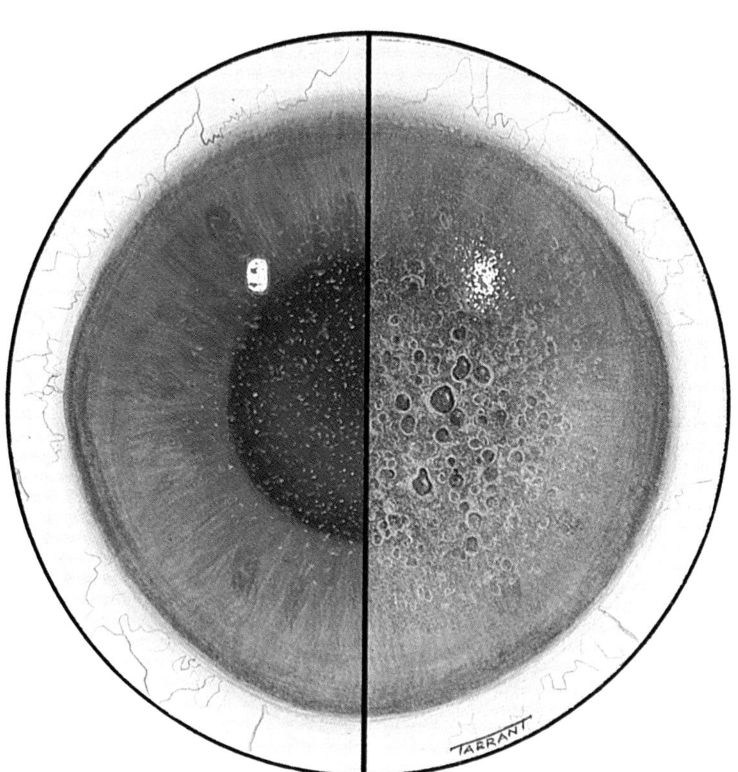

Cornea guttata → bullous keratopathy

Figure 5.44 *Fuchs' dystrophy*

2. *Reduction of intraocular pressure* may cause a reduction of both stromal and epithelial oedema.
3. *Soft bandage contact lens* may make the eye more comfortable by protecting the exposed corneal nerve endings and also by flattening the bullae.
4. *Keratoplasty*. The success rate of penetrating keratoplasty is now in the order of 80%.

Posterior polymorphous

Inheritance

This is usually autosomal dominant but may be autosomal recessive.

Clinical features

This rare congenital dystrophy is characterized by the presence of vesicular, geographical, or band-like opacities on the posterior corneal surface. The condition is usually asymptomatic and innocuous, although some patients eventually require keratoplasty when endothelial dysfunction results in stromal and epithelial oedema. A few patients develop glaucoma which may be either of the open-angle or angle-closure type. Those with angle-closure glaucoma have extensive iridocorneal adhesions with corectopia.

Ectatic dystrophies

Keratoconus

Keratoconus (conical cornea) is a condition in which the symmetrical curvature of the cornea is distorted by an abnormal thinning of its central and inferior paracentral areas. It usually starts at around puberty and progresses slowly thereafter, although it may become stationary at any time. Both eyes are affected in about 85% of cases although the severity of involvement may be extremely asymmetrical. Most patients do not have a positive family history.

Clinical features

Early

The presenting symptom is impaired vision in one eye due to irregular astigmatism. Due to the asymmetrical nature of the condition, the fellow eye usually has normal vision with negligible astigmatism. As the condition progresses, the amount of astigmatism in the fellow eye also increases and vision can only be improved by contact lenses. Unfortunately, the wearing of contact lenses does not affect progression of the disease. The astigmatism can be noted by obtaining irregular reflex on retinoscopy. This can be confirmed by keratometry and also by using Placido's disc. In early cases, slitlamp biomicroscopy will show very fine vertical folds (Vogt's lines) at the level of deep stroma and Descemet's membrane (*Figure 5.45*) and also prominent corneal nerves.

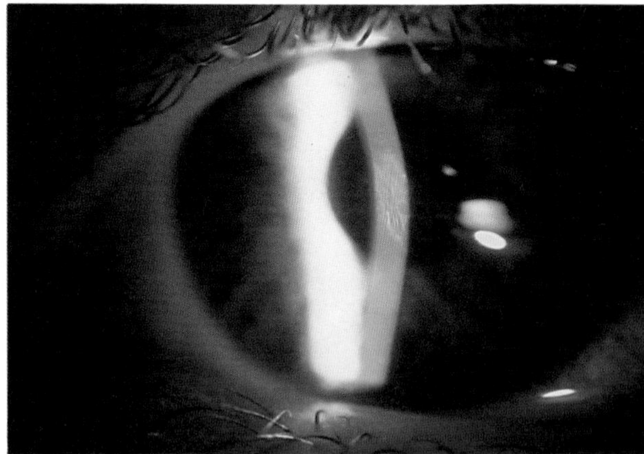

Figure 5.45 *Vogt's striae in keratoconus*

Late

Progression occurs with thinning of the central cornea and further impairment of vision (*Figure 5.46*). This may cause a bulging of the lower lid when the patient looks down (Munson's sign; *Figure 5.47*). In some cases, epithelial iron deposits (Fleischer's ring) may surround the base of the cone.

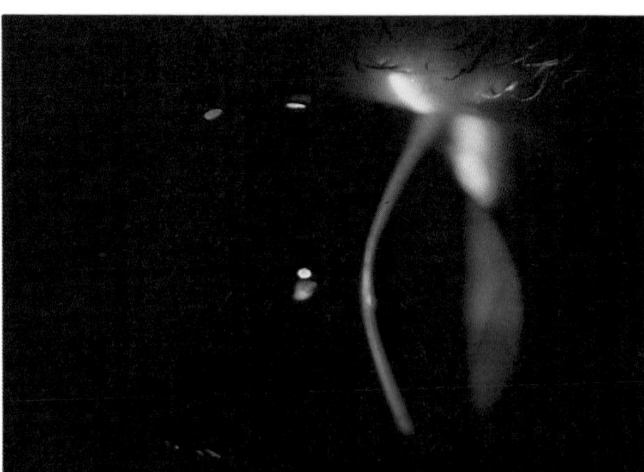

Figure 5.46 *Keratoconus*

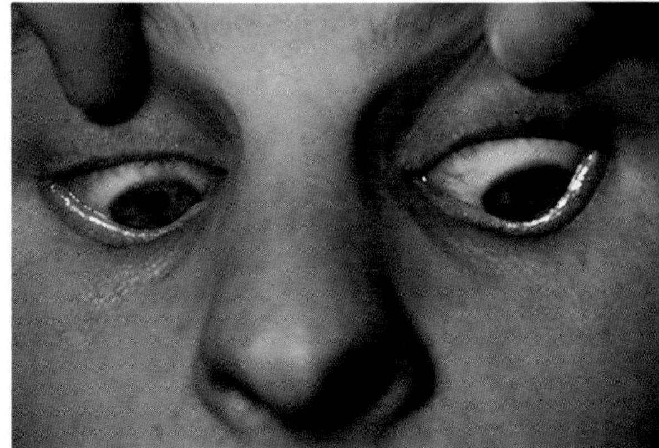

Figure 5.47 *Munson's sign (left eye)*

Complications

Acute hydrops is due to ruptures in Descemet's membrane and acute leakage of fluid into the corneal stroma and epithelium. Although the break usually heals within 6–10 weeks and the corneal oedema clears, a variable amount of stromal scarring may develop.

Treatment

1. *Contact lenses* when spectacles become inefficient.
2. *Hypertonic saline* and patching or a soft bandage contact lens for acute hydrops.
3. *Keratoplasty* is indicated when contact lenses no longer correct the irregular astigmatism, or when the visual axis is permanently scarred or oedematous. The prognosis is excellent.
4. *Epikeratophakia*—*see* later.

Associations

The many ocular and systemic associations of keratoconus include Down's syndrome, Turner's syndrome, Marfan's syndrome, Ehlers–Danlos syndrome, Leber's congenital amaurosis, blue sclera, atopic dermatitis, vernal catarrh, aniridia, retinitis pigmentosa, osteogenesis imperfecta, and ectopia lentis.

Posterior keratoconus

This is a very rare disorder in which the posterior cornea contains one or more variably sized excavation(s) and the anterior cornea does not protrude. Associated stromal scarring is sometimes seen, along with iron rings and mild irregular astigmatism. Stress lines do not occur and the condition is non-progressive.

Keratoglobus

This extremely rare condition is characterized by thinning and protrusion of the entire cornea. Astigmatism is not usually very irregular unless scarring has occurred following hydrops. Families have been reported in which keratoconus has occurred in one member and keratoglobus in another.

Pellucid marginal degeneration

This very rare bilateral, slowly progressive, peripheral thinning disorder usually presents between the ages of 20 and 40 years. It differs from keratoconus because the thinning involves only the inferior cornea and the protrusion is located above rather than within the area of thinning (*Figure 5.48*). Fleischer's ring does not occur but the condition may be complicated by acute hydrops. There is no evidence that the condition is hereditary.

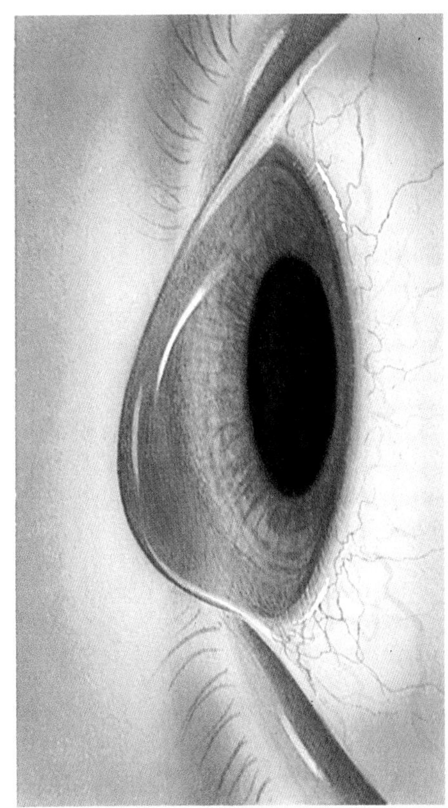

Figure 5.48 *Pellucid marginal degeneration*

Changes in metabolic and toxic disorders

Wilson's disease (hepatolenticular degeneration)

This rare condition is due to a deficiency of the alpha-2-globulin ceruloplasmin and is characterized by a widespread deposition of copper in the tissues.

Systemic features

Five types of presentation are described:

1. During early childhood with jaundice and hepatosplenomegaly.
2. During infancy with a flapping tremor of the wrists and shoulders, and normal liver function.
3. Juvenile cerebral degeneration with spasticity, dysarthria, and dysphagia.
4. Cirrhosis as the initial presentation without CNS signs.
5. Mental changes and emotional instability without CNS signs.

Ocular features

The classic Kayser–Fleischer ring is present in nearly all cases. It is located at the peripheral part of Descemet's membrane and appears as a zone of granules that change colour under different types of illumination (*Figure 5.49*). The copper appears to be deposited preferentially in the vertical meridian of the cornea and may disappear with penicillamine therapy. Some patients also have a green 'sunflower' cataract.

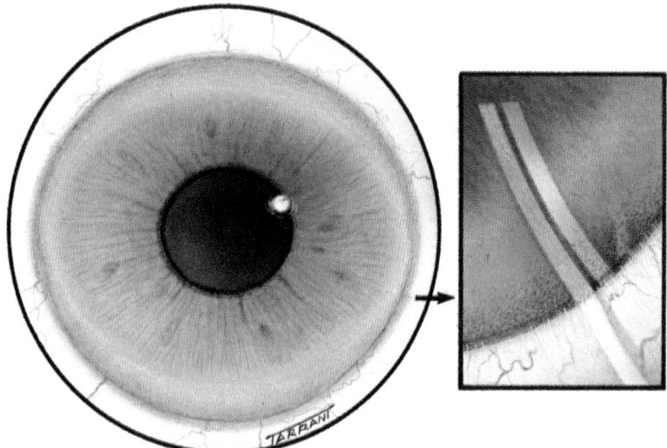

Figure 5.49 *Kayser–Fleischer ring in Wilson's disease*

Corneal crystalline deposits

The following systemic conditions may be associated with crystalline corneal deposits.

Chrysotherapy

Chrysiasis is the deposition of gold in living tissue, occurring after prolonged administration of gold, usually in the treatment of rheumatoid arthritis. Virtually all patients on continuous chrysotherapy who have received a total dose of gold compound exceeding 1000 mg develop corneal deposits and about half also develop lenticular deposits. Corneal chrysiasis is seen biomicroscopically as fine purple or reddish particles suspended in the posterior half of the stroma which tend to be more concentrated inferiorly and to spare the superior and peripheral cornea. These findings are entirely innocuous and are therefore not an indication for cessation of therapy. Visually inconsequential lens deposits develop in about 50% of patients treated for 3 or more years.

Cystinosis

This is a rare autosomal recessively inherited disorder characterized by widespread tissue deposition of cysteine crystals. Patients with the most severe nephropathic form usually die from renal failure before the second decade. Crystal deposition may occur in the conjunctiva, cornea (*Figure 5.50*) and retina. Peripherally, the corneal crystals involve the entire stromal thickness while centrally only the anterior two-thirds is affected.

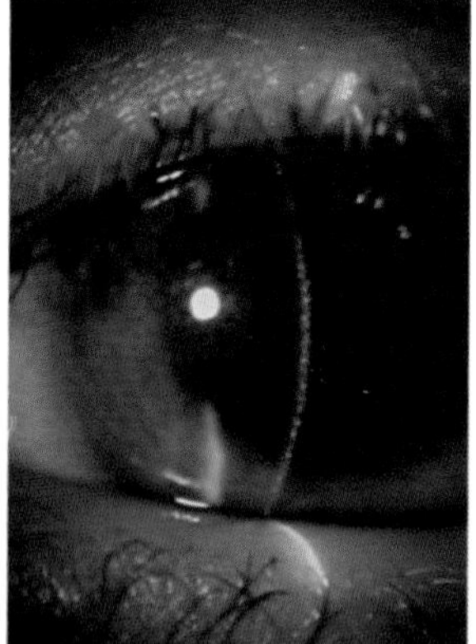

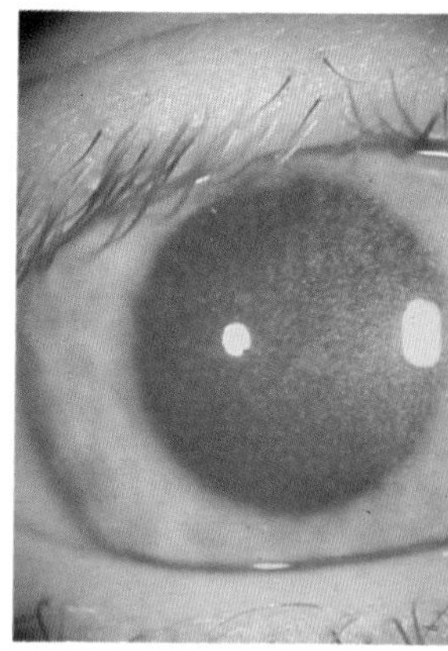

Figure 5.50 *Corneal crystals in cystinosis (courtesy of Mr D. Taylor)*

Monoclonal gammopathy

In monoclonal gammopathy which occurs in association with multiple myeloma, Waldenström's macroglobulinaemia and lymphoma, the corneal crystals may be the earliest sign of systemic disease. They are usually diffusely distributed in the corneal stroma, although epithelial involvement alone may occur occasionally.

Cornea verticillata (vortex keratopathy)

This condition is characterized by symmetrical, bilateral, greyish or golden corneal epithelial deposits that appear in a vortex fashion from a point below the pupil and swirl outwards sparing the limbus (*Figure 5.51*). The early

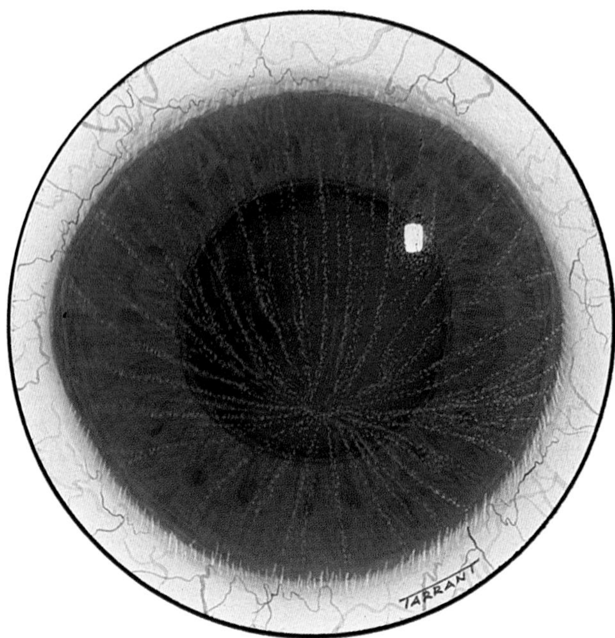

Figure 5.51 *Cornea verticillata*

changes may be confused with the more common Hudson–Stähli line. Cornea verticillata has been described in Fabry's disease and in patients being treated with a variety of drugs including chloroquine, amodiaquine, meperidine, amiodarone, indomethacin, chlorpromazine, tamoxifen and perhexilene maleate.

Chloroquine

This keratopathy is probably due to actual drug deposition in the corneal epithelium. Interestingly, unlike chloroquine retinopathy, it bears no relationship to dosage or duration of treatment. The changes are usually reversible on cessation of therapy, although occasionally they may clear despite continued administration. Rarely, severe deposition of the drug may give rise to symptoms of haloes and impaired vision.

Amiodarone

This keratopathy, unlike chloroquine keratopathy, is related to dosage and duration of administration. The drug is used in the treatment of a variety of cardiac arrhythmias. On low doses of 100–200 mg/day, patients show clear corneas or only very mild changes. However, on doses of 400–1400 mg/day a moderate to severe keratopathy develops, depending on the duration of treatment. Visually inconsequential anterior subcapsular lens opacities develop in about 50% of patients using moderate to high doses.

Fabry's disease

This is a glycolipidosis due to a deficiency in the enzyme α-galactosidase A. Systemic features include angiokeratomas (purple telangiectatic skin lesions), cardiovascular and renal lesions, and episodes of excruciating pain involving the toes and fingers. The ocular lesions include cornea verticillata and spoke-like lens opacities.

Mucopolysaccharidoses

These represent a group of inborn errors of metabolism consisting of at least six well-defined entities. The ocular features include corneal stromal infiltration, retinal pigmentary degeneration, and optic atrophy. The systemic features include skeletal anomalies, mental retardation, and facial coarseness.

Classification

		Corneal deposition	*Retinal degeneration*	*Optic atrophy*
MPS 1-H	= Hurler	+++	+	+
MPS 1-S	= Scheie	+++	+	+
MPS 2	= Hunter	–	+	+
MPS 3	= Sanfilippo	–	+	+
MPS 4	= Morquio	+	–	+
MPS 5	= vacant			
MPS 6	= Maroteaux–Lamy	+	–	+

Corneal deposition occurs in all of the mucopolysaccharidoses except Hunter's and Sanfilippo's. It is most severe in Hurler's and Scheie's and causes corneal clouding which is present at birth. This should be differentiated from corneal oedema in congenital glaucoma, rubella keratopathy, and birth trauma. In general, corneal deposition is associated with skeletal anomalies.

Pigmentary retinopathy, reported in all but Morquio's and Maroteaux–Lamy's, is generally associated with mental retardation.

Optic atrophy has been reported in all six mucopolysaccharidoses.

Contact lenses

Forms of contact lenses

Hard lenses

Hard lenses are made from plastic non-toxic material called polymethylmethacrylate (PMMA) or Perspex. This substance has reproducible physical properties which enable it to be fenestrated and moulded into any size or shape to give good optical and cosmetic results.

Hard lenses are of three types:

1. *Corneal* lenses with a diameter of between 8.5 and 10 mm.
2. *Scleral* (haptic) lenses which override the cornea and rest on the sclera. Their use is now limited to certain specific conditions such as advanced keratoconus or severe lid disorders.
3. *Hybrid* lenses which are the same diameter as the cornea. These are used mainly as cosmetic lenses to hide an unsightly eye.

Disadvantages

These lenses are only suitable for daily wear. This is because oxygen does not permeate PMMA so that the cornea depends on the tear pump to obtain its oxygen. If the lens is worn for too long or during sleep, corneal hypoxia may cause blurring of vision due to epithelial oedema. In order to supplement the tear pump, the PMMA lens must be made small and steep. Although this allows more oxygen to reach the cornea, it results in a small optic zone. This may give rise to annoying glare at night from oncoming headlights when the pupil becomes as large as the optic zone of the lens and light enters the pupil around the optic zone.

Advantages

Because hard lenses are very durable they are particularly suitable for children who might handle a contact lens more roughly than an adult.

Gas permeable

These are made from a mixture of a hard and a soft material. They may be adjusted and polished, similar to PMMA lenses, and are treated in the same way, with regard to handling and aftercare. They are often used in patients who are unable to wear soft lenses owing to allergies or other associated pathology. Because they are usually more comfortable than hard PMMA lenses, they are a good choice for more sensitive eyes.

Disadvantages

The material from which the lenses are made is softer and more brittle than PMMA so that it tends to scratch and fracture more easily.

Advantages

Since these lenses are permeable to oxygen, they can be made with a larger optic zone than a hard PMMA lens, providing optimal vision both day and night. The larger size of the gas-permeable lens also makes it more comfortable than a PMMA lens. Because the upper eyelid does not engage the upper edge of a gas-permeable lens, it is less likely to pop out of the eye than a PMMA lens.

Soft (hydrophilic)

The basic plastic used in the manufacture of soft hydrophilic contact lenses is hydroxymethylmethacrylate (HEMA). Depending on other chemical refinements, the degree of hydration of these lenses varies between 25 and 85%. The water-absorbing property increases the weight of the lens and they are, therefore, made larger than hard lenses in order to offset this problem. Soft lenses overlap the limbus. In general, the physiological performance of a soft lens is related to its thickness and its water content. The greater the water content the greater the oxygen permeability. In a very thin soft lens, adequate oxygen can diffuse through the lens to supply the corneal epithelium making the lens suitable for extended wear.

Disadvantages

When compared with a hard contact lens, a soft lens is more delicate, more easily damaged and has a shorter lifespan. Visual acuity may not be as crisp and it is associated with a higher incidence of potential complications.

Advantages

Soft lenses are more comfortable to wear and are more stable in the eye than hard lenses. They do not require either the prolonged adaptation period or the rigid wearing schedule for successful wear.

Principles of fitting

Curvatures

The essential feature of most contact lenses is that the posterior surface must conform to the shape of the cornea (*Figure 5.52*). The axial region of the cornea has a largely spherical curvature, peripheral to which there is a band of progressively decreased curvature. The central portion of the posterior surface of a contact lens must therefore be the most steeply curved. This so-called 'back optic zone' thus

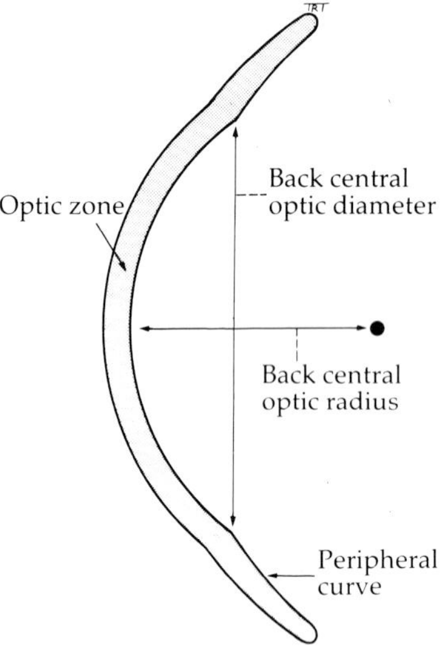

Figure 5.52 *Contact lens curvatures*

has a spherical curvature measured as 'the back central optic radius'. The diameter of the back optic zone is the 'back central optic diameter'. The peripheral part of the posterior surface of a contact lens also has to follow the shape of the cornea so that it is less curved than the axial region and, in its simplest form, it has a single peripheral curvature, the radius of which is greater than that of the optic zone.

Dimensions

The aim of fitting a contact lens is to choose the smallest and thinnest lens that gives optimum vision and comfort, without interfering with corneal physiology. The combination of keratometry and trial lenses is probably the best method of fitting. Keratometry is taken as a preliminary guide and the refraction to be ordered is then simply determined by the spectacle correction. A suitable modification should be made for the back vertex distance of particularly powerful prescriptions. The overall diameter of the contact lens is determined by the diameter and radius of the cornea, and the tension and position of the eyelids. The extent of the back central optic diameter of the contact lens is determined by the average size of the pupil and the radius of curvature of the cornea.

Fluorescein pattern

Much experience is required to correctly interpret the fluorescein patterns as these vary with the technique of examination and parameters of the lens. In principle, loose areas are seen as pools of fluorescein and areas of corneal touch as dark areas (*Figure 5.53*). The bearing relationship that is generally favoured is that of minimal apical clearance.

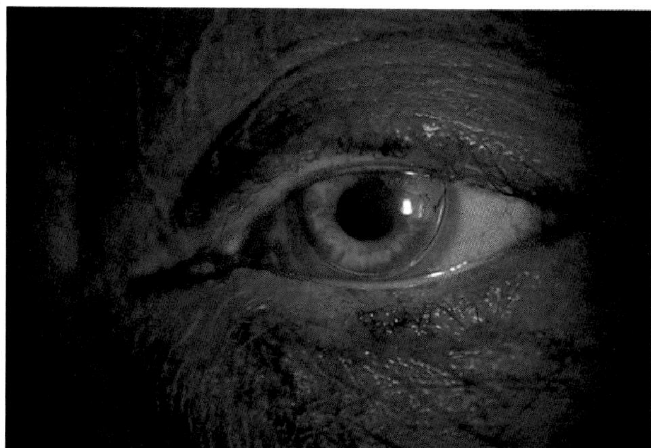

Figure 5.53 *Fluorescein pattern*

Centring

Ideally, the contact lens should be well centred so that the optical axes of the eye and contact lens coincide. Whenever a contact lens is significantly decentred its optical function suffers, particularly in cases of high refractive errors.

Mobility

The mobility of the contact lens during blinking is important. A correctly fitted contact lens moves downwards relative to the cornea with the descent of the upper eyelid (*Figure 5.54b*) and is then taken rapidly upwards at a level above its static position as the upper eyelid ascends (*Figure 5.54c*). Finally it settles slowly to its initial position (*Figure 5.54a*). Any undue delay in this resettling may give rise to temporary blurring of vision. In addition, this mobility during blinking is believed to be of importance for the continued health of the cornea as it creates a satisfactory tear film which is vital to corneal integrity.

Insertion and removal

When inserting a contact lens (hard or soft) it is first moistened and then placed on the tip of the index finger

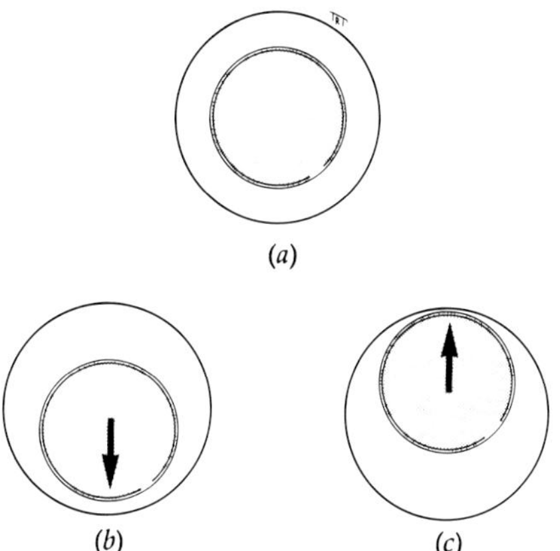

Figure 5.54 *Normal contact lens mobility during blinking*

(*Figure 5.55, left*). The lids are then retracted and the eye gazes steadily at the approaching lens until it is applied gently to the cornea. When it is in position, the upper eyelid is released before the lower eyelid.

When removing a hard contact lens, the eye is opened widely so that the lid margins are beyond the edges of the lens. The index finger is then placed at the outer canthus and, with firm pressure, the skin and lids are stretched laterally (*Figure 5.55, right*). This causes the lens to become dislocated from the eye, either onto the lashes or into the waiting hand. A soft contact lens can be removed by simply pinching it out between the thumb and index finger.

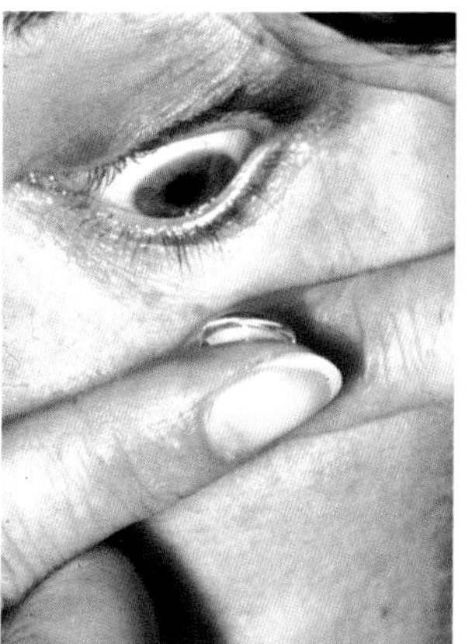

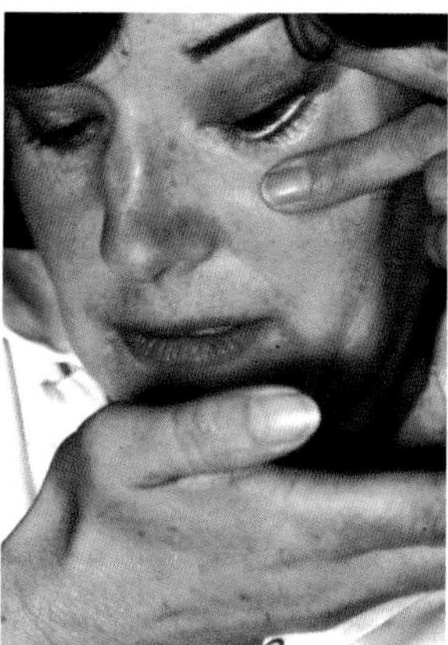

Figure 5.55 *Left: insertion of contact lens; right: removal*

Medical indications

The medical indications for contact lenses can be divided into three main groups:

1. Aphakia and astigmatism.
2. Corneal disorders.
3. Miscellaneous.

Aphakia and astigmatism

This group consists of patients who are unable to obtain satisfactory vision with the use of spectacles.

1. *Unilateral aphakics* with good vision in the fellow eye can only achieve fusion with either a contact lens or an intraocular implant.
2. *High myopes* with macular degeneration are particularly suitable for contact lenses. This is because the aberrations associated with a high power lens are abolished and the concomitant increased magnification may improve visual acuity.
3. *Irregular astigmatism* associated with keratoconus can be corrected with a hard contact lens long after spectacles have failed and long before corneal grafting becomes necessary.

Corneal disorders

Soft bandage contact lenses may be beneficial in certain corneal disorders. The lenses are made afocal so that they do not impair vision. They can be used as short- or long-term treatment in the following conditions (*Figure 5.56*).

1. *Corneal irregularities.* A contact lens can replace a superficial irregular corneal surface by a smoother and optically more perfect surface. In this way visual acuity can be improved, provided the irregularities are not too severe.
2. *Epithelial healing defects* can be healed more quickly by protecting the regenerating corneal epithelium from the constant rubbing action of the lids and thus allowing the development of hemidesmosomal attachments to the epithelial basement membrane.
3. *Recurrent corneal erosion syndrome.* If the syndrome is associated with a corneal dystrophy (microcystic, Reis–Bücklers' or lattice), long-standing lens wear is usually necessary. In traumatic cases lens wear can usually be discontinued after a few weeks.
4. *Bullous keratopathy* can be managed by soft contact lenses which relieve pain by protecting the denuded corneal nerve endings from trauma by the eyelids. The lens may also flatten the bullae and convert them into diffuse fine epithelial oedema. The additional instillation of hypertonic (5%) saline may be beneficial in further reducing the amount of oedema and improving vision.
5. *Filamentary keratitis* can be treated by soft lenses in combination with artificial tears. It is hoped that the lens will reduce evaporation of any existing tears. The main problems that can occur are infection, drying of the lens, and deposition of mucus on the lens. This form of treatment should only be undertaken by an expert who is able to provide an adequate and speedy follow-up should complications occur.
6. *Wound leaks* can be covered with a contact lens as a temporary measure to allow sufficient time for natural healing to occur.

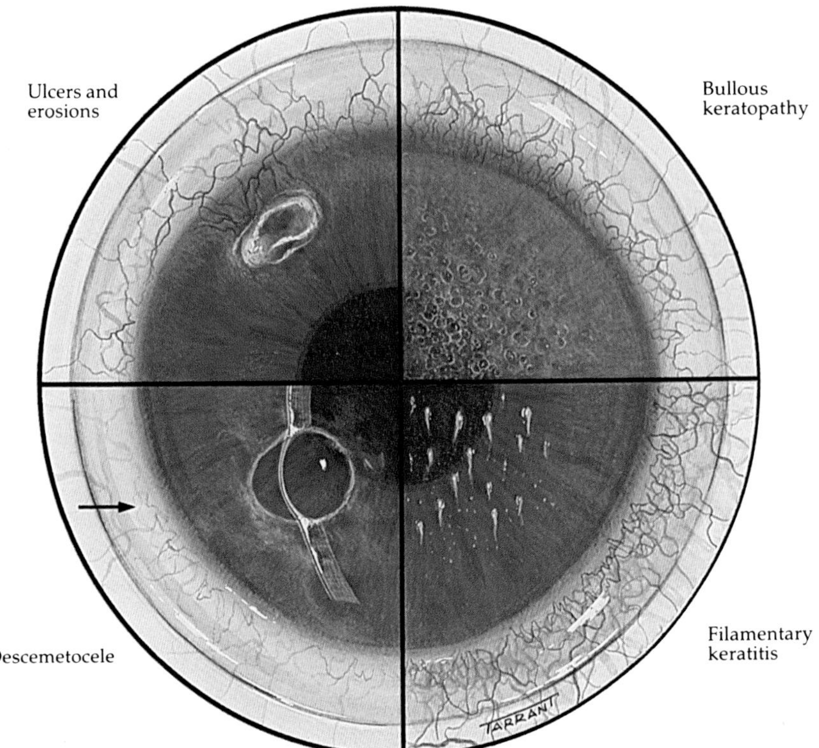

Figure 5.56 *Indication for soft contact lenses in corneal disorders*

Miscellaneous

1. *Ptosis*. Haptic contact lenses can be used in the management of ptosis in patients with no Bell's phenomenon in whom surgical correction is contraindicated because of the risk of postoperative exposure keratopathy during sleep.
2. *Cosmetic reasons* to hide an unsightly eye.
3. *Occluders*. Contact lenses can be used as occluders in the treatment of amblyopia in children who will not tolerate conventional patch occlusion.
4. *Vehicle for drug delivery*. Because a high concentration of a drug can be obtained by soaking a soft contact lens and then applying it to the cornea, it can be used as a vehicle for drug delivery.
5. *Protection of normal corneal epithelium* in eyes with trichiasis or threatened exposure keratopathy.
6. *Prevention of symblepharon* during the acute phase of destructive conjunctival disorders, especially those due to chemical burns.

Complications

Although any type of contact lens may give rise to complications, serious complications are more common with extended wear lenses that extend beyond the limbus.

Allergic conjunctivitis

The most common cause of problems with soft contact lenses is allergy to the preservatives in contact lens cleansing solutions. It is now apparent that at least 10% of soft contact lens wearers are allergic or sensitized to thiomersal and are unable to use solutions containing this preservative.

Clinical features

The main symptoms are redness, burning, and itching soon after lens insertion. These symptoms may develop within days to months following the initial exposure to thiomersal. Examination shows mild perilimbal injection following the edge of the contact lens and a fine papillary conjunctival reaction.

Management

Solutions containing thiomersal should be avoided and the lenses should be disinfected with heat and non-preserved saline. The thiomersal can be extracted from the lens by soaking it in hydrogen peroxide 3% for 10 minutes.

Giant papillary conjunctivitis

Giant papillary conjunctivitis (GPC) is a relatively rare complication. The most commonly fitted lenses in patients with GPC are ultrathin, low water content, soft lenses. Patients with asthma, hay fever, or animal allergies appear to be at increased risk. It has been postulated that GPC has an immunological origin in which contact lens deposits, especially proteins, act as allergens. Thiomersal has been implicated in altering lens proteins and predisposing patients to GPC.

Clinical features

The patient may present months or years after beginning lens wear with ocular irritation, itching, photophobia, increased mucus production, and decreased lens tolerance. Eversion of the upper lid is necessary to make the diagnosis. The spectrum of changes on the upper tarsal conjunctiva ranges from a mild papillary response to the full blown picture of GPC characterized by giant papillae (*Figure 5.57*). Excessive mucus in the eye and on the contact lens is also noted. In some cases, Tranta's dots and limbitis similar to that seen in vernal disease are present.

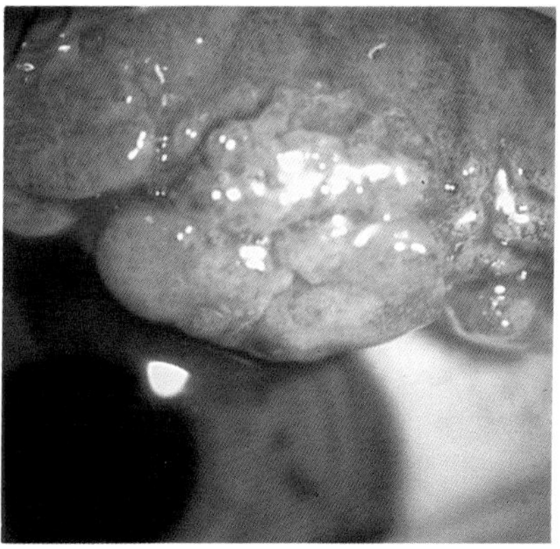

Figure 5.57 *Giant papillary conjunctivitis due to soft contact lens wear (courtesy of Dr M. Guillon, Hydron Europe Ltd)*

Management

Contact lens wear should be discontinued for 3 months. In patients with severe GPC treatment with topical sodium cromoglycate (Opticrom) or a weak steroid such as fluoromethalone may be helpful. After 3 months, an attempt can be made to refit the patient either with a soft lens of a different polymer or a hard lens and preservative-containing disinfecting solutions should be eliminated. If these measures fail it may be necessary to discontinue contact lens wear permanently.

Corneal complications (*Figure 5.58*)

1. *Epithelial oedema* due to hypoxia is usually reversible.
2. *Peripheral corneal vascularization* occurs in some eyes with prolonged wear lenses and occasionally with daily wear lenses. Although the new vessels usually regress once contact lens wear is discontinued, a small number of eyes develop extensive deep vascularization.

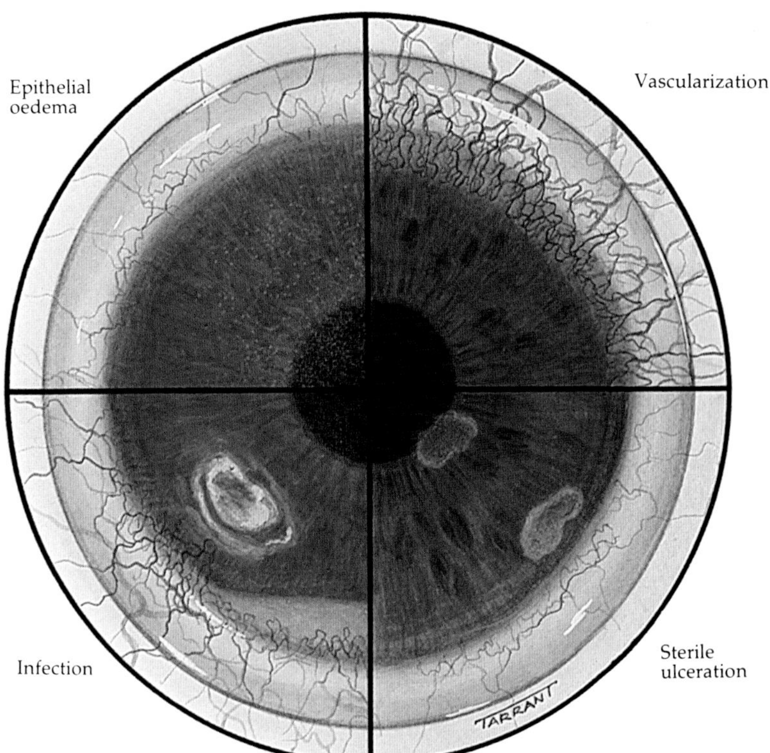

Figure 5.58 *Corneal complications of contact lens wear*

3. *Sterile corneal ulceration,* either in the centre or periphery of the cornea, may occur. Fortunately it usually heals once wear has been discontinued.
4. *Infection* is the most serious, but fortunately, a very rare complication.
5. *Warping of the cornea* resulting in severe and permanent astigmatism may occur in some eyes with extended wear lenses.

Changes within the contact lens

1. *Deposits of mucoproteins* can adhere to the lens surface making the eye uncomfortable. The deposits generally develop in an unpredictable manner and some patients can only wear a lens for a few weeks before it becomes covered with deposits. Sometimes the deposits can be removed by cleaning, but those with chronic deposit formation may not be able to wear contact lenses on a long-term basis.
2. *Calcium deposits,* which appear as small round hard opacities, can also accumulate on the lens surface.
3. *Lens digestion.* Although the lens pore size is generally too small for microbial organisms to enter, it has been shown that organisms such as fungi can attach themselves to the surface of the lens and digest the lens material while growing into it.

Principles of keratoplasty

Keratoplasty (corneal transplantation or grafting) is an operation in which abnormal host tissue is replaced by donor corneal tissue. The graft may be partial thickness (lamellar) or full thickness (penetrating).

Penetrating

Indications

The four indications for this operation are:

1. *Optical* is performed primarily to improve visual acuity by replacing opaque corneal tissue with clear donor tissue.
2. *Tectonic* is aimed at restoring or preserving corneal anatomy in eyes with severe structural changes such as stromal thinning and descemetoceles.
3. *Therapeutic* removes inflamed corneal tissue in eyes unresponsive to conventional antimicrobial or antiviral therapy.
4. *Cosmetic,* to improve the appearance of the eye, is a relatively rare indication.

Prognostic factors

Donor tissue

Ideally, the eyes should be removed less than 6 hours following death. Young patients are preferred because of the denser population of endothelial cells. HIV-positive patients should not be used as donors for fear of transferring the virus to the recipient (HIV = human immunodeficiency virus).

Recipient cornea

Adverse prognostic factors include severe stromal vascularization, absence of corneal sensation, extreme thinning at the proposed host–graft junction, and active corneal inflammation. In general, the most favourable cases are localized corneal scars, keratoconus, and corneal dystrophies.

Associated anterior segment disease

Associated factors involving the anterior segment that may diminish the prognosis of obtaining a clear graft postoperatively include uncontrolled glaucoma, anterior synechiae, uveitis, and recurrent or progressive forms of conjunctival inflammation such as acne rosacea and ocular cicatricial pemphigoid.

Associated adnexal disorders

Tear film dysfunction and abnormalities of the eyelids such as ectropion, entropion, and trichiasis should be corrected prior to surgery.

Age of patient

The prognosis is less favourable in very young patients.

Surgical procedure

Determination of graft size

The diameter of diseased corneal tissue can be measured preoperatively using a variable slit beam and also at the time of surgery by trial placement of trephines with different diameters. In general, grafts greater than 8.5 mm in diameter have an increased incidence of postoperative anterior synechiae formation, vascularization, and increased intraocular pressure. An ideal size is 7.5 mm; grafts smaller than this may give rise to astigmatism.

Excision of donor cornea

This should always precede excision of host cornea. Great care should be taken not to damage the endothelium.

Excision of diseased host tissue

Care must be taken not to damage the iris and lens with the trephine. The lens can be protected to some extent by ensuring that the pupil is miosed before the operation is started. Too rapid decompression of the eye can be avoided by first performing a partial-thickness trephination (*Figure 5.59a*) and then entering the anterior chamber with a knife. The excision is then completed with scissors (*Figure 5.59b*).

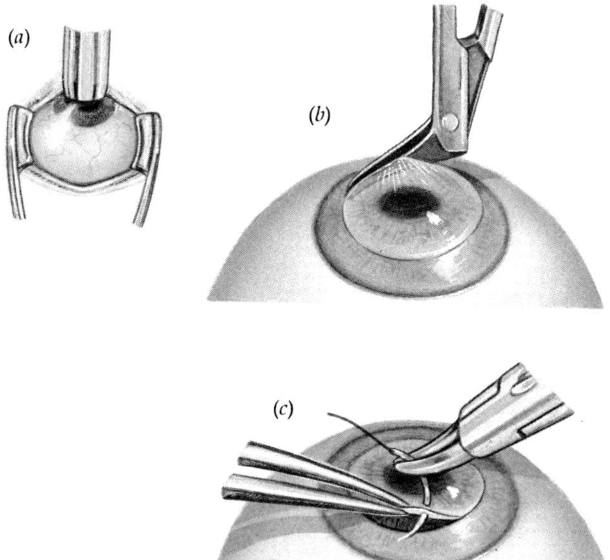

Figure 5.59 *Technique of penetrating keratoplasty*

Fixation of donor tissue

This is done with either interrupted or continuous running sutures (*Figure 5.59c*). The anterior chamber should be reformed with balanced salt solution.

Postoperative management

The eye can be left uncovered after 24 hours. Topical corticosteroids are instilled four times a day and mydriatics twice daily for 2 weeks. The mydriatics can then be discontinued but the corticosteroids should be used for 12 months (once daily for 6 months and then on alternate days). Suture removal in non-vascularized cornea is performed 1 year after keratoplasty.

Complications

Early

These postoperative complications include flat anterior chamber, iris prolapse, persistent epithelial defects, and infection.

Late

These postoperative complications include glaucoma, astigmatism, retrocorneal membrane formation, late wound separation, cystoid macular oedema, and recurrence of the initial disease process on the graft.

Graft failure

Early

Early failure is characterized by cloudiness of the graft from the first postoperative day. It is caused by endothelial dysfunction due to defective donor endothelium or surgical trauma at the time of operation or it may be secondary to glaucoma, intraocular inflammation, or vitreo-endothelial adhesion.

Late

Late failure is most frequently due to allograft reaction. About 50% of cases occur within the first 6 months postoperatively, and the vast majority within 1 year. The earliest clinical sign is the occurrence of keratic precipitates on the graft endothelium. This is followed by a ciliary flush, an increase in the number of keratic precipitates, an endothelial rejection line, and graft oedema. Occasionally an increase in graft thickness due to endothelial dysfunction is the earliest feature. Graft rejection should be treated by the prompt administration of hourly topical corticosteroids and also periocular corticosteroid injections. In severe resistant cases systemic immunosuppressive agents may have to be used.

Lamellar

Indications

1. Opacification of the superficial one-third of the corneal stroma not due to potentially recurrent disease.
2. Marginal corneal thinning or infiltration as in recurrent pterygium, Terrien's marginal degeneration, and limbal dermoids or other tumours.
3. Localized thinning or descemetocele formation.

Principles of refractive corneal surgery

Radial keratotomy

Radial keratotomy (RK) decreases myopia by flattening the cornea by making a series of deep radial incisions.

Indications

RK may be considered for adults with stable myopia of between 2 and 8 D, preferably with minimal astigmatism, who for various reasons are not satisfied with spectacle or contact lens wear.

Contraindications

Patients with more than 8 D of myopia are unusuitable because their final refractive correction is unpredictable. RK should also be avoided in patients with pre-existing corneal disease because of the increased risk of perforation and also of worsening their corneal disease. Because the myopia must be stable before RK is performed, patients younger than 21 years are unsuitable.

Surgical technique

First, the visual axis and a surrounding clear optical zone about 4 mm in diameter are marked and the corneal thickness is then measured with an ultrasonic pachymeter. Then, with a specially calibrated diamond knife, 16 very deep radial incisions are made from the edge of the optical clear zone to the limbus (*Figure 5.60*). It has been suggested that this weakens the cornea causing the midperiphery to bulge out and the centre to flatten.

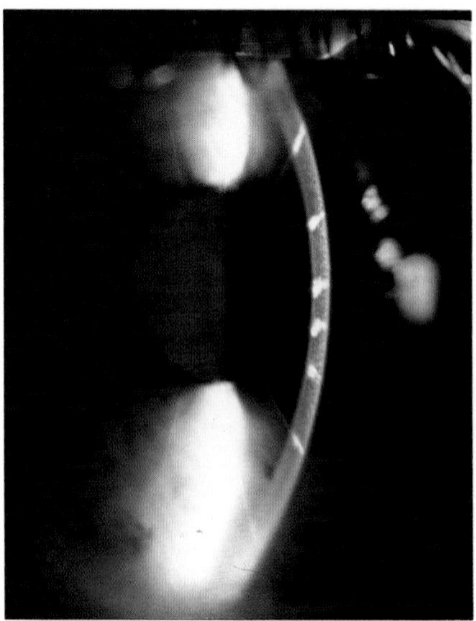

Figure 5.60 *Appearance of cornea following radial keratotomy*

Results

Although RK can correct between 2 and 8 D of myopia the final correction cannot be predicted with certainty. Sixty per cent of patients are within ±1 D of emmetropia, 30% are undercorrected by more than 1 D, and 10% are overcorrected by more than 1 D. The final correction is more accurate in patients with less than 5 D of myopia, and becomes less accurate between 5 and 8 D. Older patients also seem to obtain better visual results than younger patients.

Complications

The main postoperative problems and complications are:

1. Loss of one to two Snellen lines of best corrected visual acuity in about 10% of eyes.
2. Diurnal fluctuations in visual acuity.
3. Difficulties with driving at night due to glare.
4. Intrastromal epithelial inclusion cysts.

Epikeratophakia

Epikeratophakia is a procedure in which a lenticule of donor tissue is used to alter the surface topography of the cornea.

Indications

Epikeratophakia can be used to correct any degree of myopia, as well as aphakia up to 27 D, in both adults and children in whom spectacles or contact lenses are unsatisfactory. The procedure is particularly useful in preventing vision-deprivation amblyopia in young child with monocular aphakia. It can also be used to treat keratoconus. A plus lenticule is used to correct aphakia (*Figure 5.61b*), a minus lenticule to correct myopia (*Figure 5.61c*), and a plano lens for keratoconus.

Contraindications

Because epikeratophakia involves removal of the corneal epithelium, the procedure is unsuitable for patients with severe dry eyes or lagophthalmos. The procedure is also contraindicated in patients with less than 4 D of myopia in whom RK is preferred.

Surgical technique

The donor lenticule of the desired power is kept in a freeze-dried (lyophilized) state until required. The visual axis is marked on the cornea and most of the surrounding epithelium removed. With the trephine centred over the visual axis mark, a circular cut is made about 8 mm in diameter and 3 mm deep. An annular keratectomy is then made by resecting the inner wall of the trephine cut and removing a wedge of tissue (*Figure 5.61a*). The edge of the lenticule is then sutured into the keratotectomy with 10-0 interrupted nylon sutures.

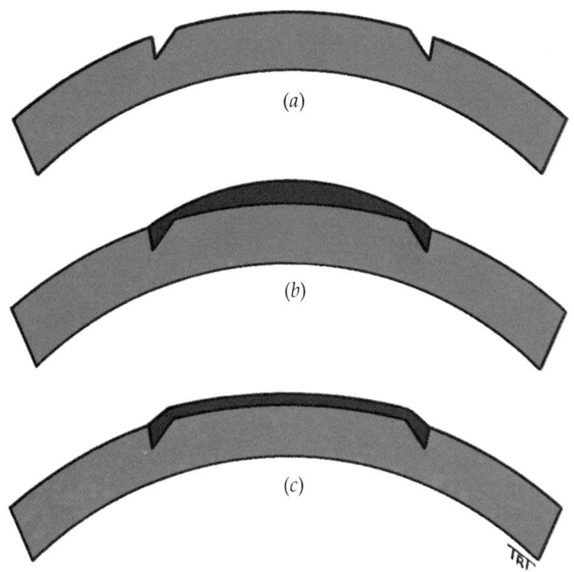

Figure 5.61 *Epikeratophakia*

Results

Although this technique is still in its infancy, recent short-term reports have shown a satisfactory level of visual acuity in a high proportion of patients.

Complications

Occasional complications include glare and chronic epithelial defects.

Episcleritis and scleritis

Applied anatomy

The scleral stroma is composed of collagen bundles of varying size and shape that are not as uniformly orientated as in the cornea. The inner layer of the sclera (lamina fusca) blends with the suprachoroidal and supraciliary lamellae of the uveal tract. Anteriorly the episclera consists of a dense, vascular connective tissue which merges with the superficial sclera stroma and Tenon's capsule.

Three vascular layers cover the anterior segment (*Figure 5.62*):

1. *Conjunctival vessels* are the most superficial.
2. *Superficial episcleral vessels* within Tenon's capsule that have a radial configuration (*Figure 5.62a*). In eyes with episcleritis maximal congestion occurs within this vascular plexus (*Figure 5.62b*). Tenon's capsule and the episclera are infiltrated with inflammatory cells but the sclera itself is not swollen. Topical phenylephrine drops will cause blanching of the conjunctival vessels and, to a certain extent also, of the superficial episcleral plexus.
3. *Deep vascular plexus* lies adjacent to the sclera and shows maximal congestion in eyes with scleritis (*Figure 5.62c*). There is also inevitably some engorgement of the superficial episcleral vessels but this should be ignored

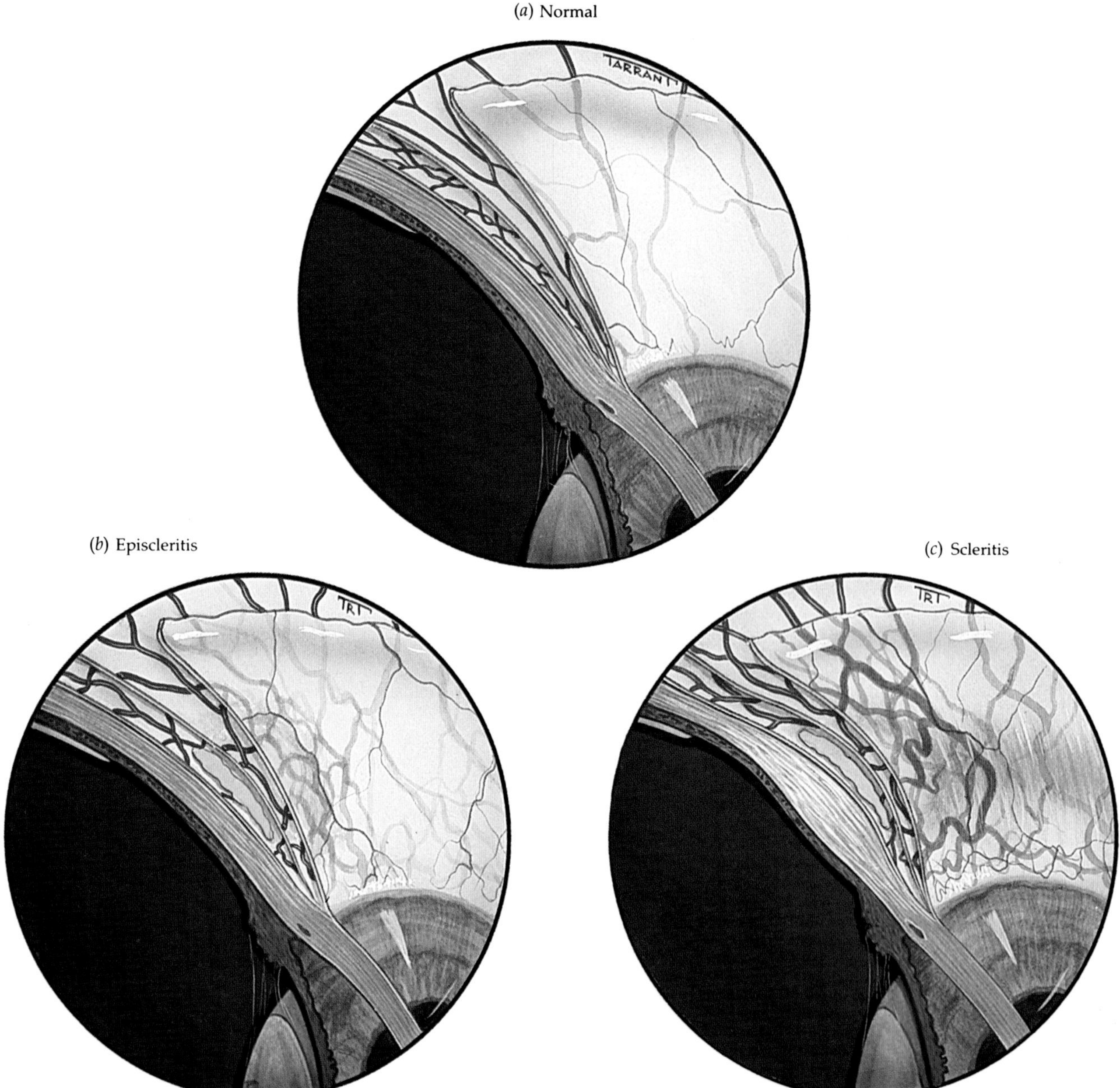

Figure 5.62 *Applied anatomy of anterior vascular coats*

when making the diagnosis of scleritis. The instillation of phenylephrine will have no effect on the degree of engorgement of the deep vascular plexus. External examination in daylight is extremely important in localizing the level of maximal injection.

Episcleritis

Episcleritis is a common, benign, self-limiting, frequently recurrent disorder that typically affects young adults. It is seldom associated with a systemic disorder and never progresses to a true scleritis.

Clinical features

Two clinical types of episcleritis are recognized: simple and nodular (*Figure 5.63*). In both types the patient may be asymptomatic and may merely notice redness of the eye. Occasionally the onset of the inflammation (which may be very acute) is associated with mild discomfort, tenderness to touch, and watering. In simple episcleritis the redness may be sectoral or rarely diffuse. By contrast, nodular episcleritis is localized to one area of the globe, forming a nodule with surrounding injection. A slitlamp section will show that the deep scleral part of the beam is not displaced.

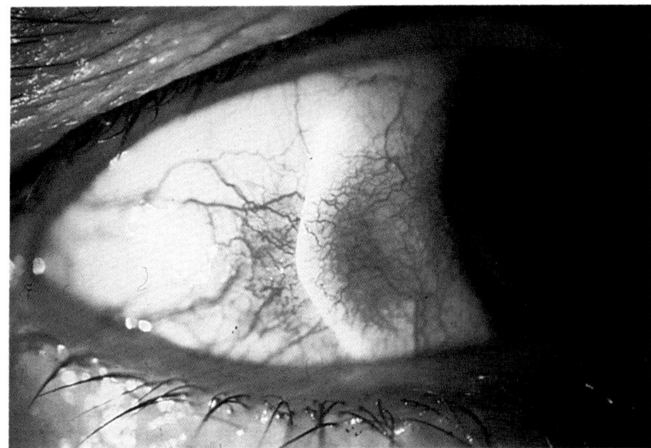

Figure 5.63 Nodular episcleritis (courtesy of Mr A. Shun-Shin)

Following recurrent attacks of nodular episcleritis, the superficial scleral lamellae may become rearranged into more parallel rows, making the sclera appear more translucent. It is important not to mistake this increased scleral translucency for actual scleral thinning caused by necrotizing scleritis.

Treatment

Usually simple episcleritis resolves spontaneously within 1–2 weeks although the nodular type may take longer to clear. Mild cases may need no specific therapy but, if discomfort is annoying, topical corticosteroids and/or oxyphenbutazone (Tanderil) may be helpful. In the rare unresponsive recurrent disease, systemic indomethacin (50 mg twice daily) taken at the first symptom of recurrence may be successful in aborting the attack.

Scleritis

In contrast to episcleritis, scleritis is very much less common. It occurs in an older age group affecting women more commonly than men. It is characterized by pain, potentially blinding complications, and a high incidence of associated systemic disease.

Aetiology

1. *Herpes zoster* is the most important local cause of scleritis.
2. *Connective tissue disorders* are the most important systemic associations. Rheumatoid arthritis is by far the most frequent and it has been estimated that about 1 in 200 patients with seropositive rheumatoid arthritis develop scleritis. Other diseases in this group include systemic lupus erythematosus, polyarteritis nodosa and Wegener's granulomatosis.
3. *Miscellaneous* systemic associations include sarcoidosis and tuberculosis.

Classification

- Anterior
  - non-necrotizing
    - nodular
    - diffuse
  - necrotizing
    - with inflammation
    - without inflammation
- Posterior

Anterior non-necrotizing scleritis

Clinical features

Nodular *(Figure 5.64, left)*

Although on cursory examination this may resemble nodular episcleritis, it will be evident on a more detailed evaluation that the nodule consists of oedematous sclera and cannot be moved over the underlying scleral tissue.

Diffuse *(Figure 5.64, right)*

In this form, the inflammation is more widespread involving either a segment of the globe or the entire anterior sclera (brawny scleritis). Distortion of the pattern of the vascular plexuses is characteristic with loss of the normal radial pattern.

Treatment

Treatment is with indomethacin 100 mg daily for 4 days reducing to 75 mg daily unitl the inflammation resolves.

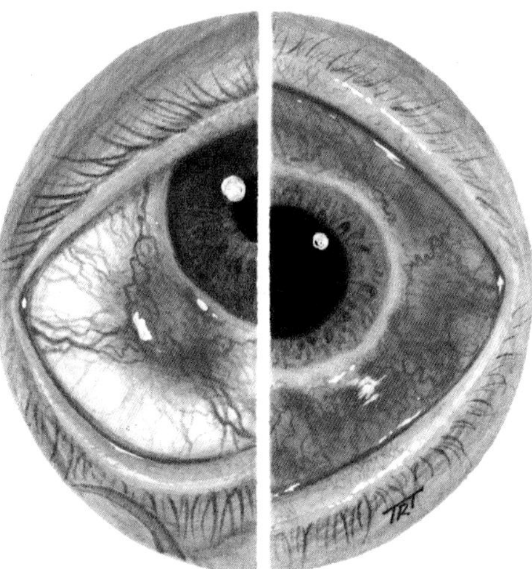

Figure 5.64 Non-necrotizing scleritis. Left: nodular; right: diffuse

Anterior necrotizing scleritis with inflammation

Clinical features

This most severe form of scleritis presents with a gradual onset of pain and localized redness. The blood vessels in the affected area may appear distorted or occluded with avascular patches appearing in the episcleral tissue. Eventually, the sclera becomes transparent and the underlying uvea shows through. The inflamed area gradually spreads around the globe often from the primary sites of involvement and may join up with other separate foci. An associated anterior uveitis is universally present and, unless the disease process is halted, severe vision-threatening complications may develop (cataract, keratitis, keratolysis, and secondary glaucoma). About a quarter of patients with this type of necrotizing scleritis are dead within 5 years from associated systemic disease.

Treatment

Initial treatment is with 60–80 mg of systemic prednisolone. This usually has a dramatic effect on the severity of pain which is a very important indicator of active disease. The dose can then be tapered accordingly, as the pain subsides. In patients intolerant or unresponsive to corticosterids, immunosuppressive agents may be necessary.

Anterior necrotizing scleritis without inflammation (scleromalacia perforans)

This specific form of scleritis typically occurs in female patients with long-standing seropositive rheumatoid arthritis. The condition is asymptomatic and starts with a yellow necrotic scleral patch in normal sclera. Eventually large areas of the underlying uvea become exposed due to scleral thinning (*Figure 5.65*). However, unless the intraocular pressure is elevated, spontaneous perforation is extremely rare. There is no effective treatment.

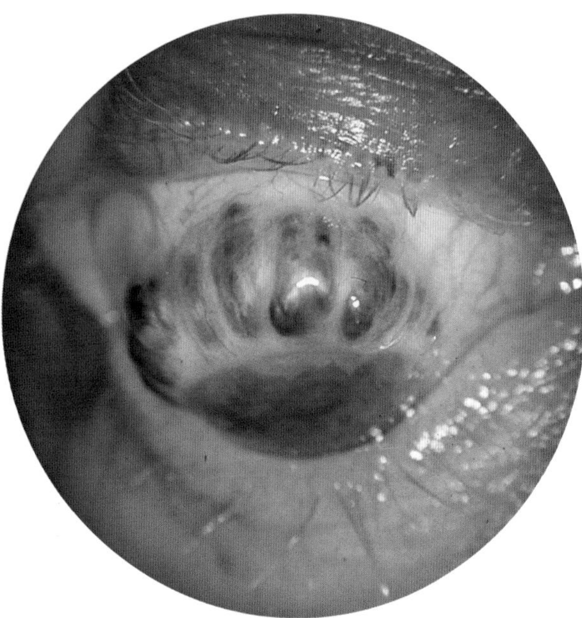

Figure 5.65 *Scleromalacia perforans (courtesy of Mr B. Mathalone)*

Posterior scleritis

This type of scleritis is frequently misdiagnosed, although it probably represents about 20% of all cases. It is usually unassociated with any specific systemic disorder.

Clinical features

Extension of the inflammatory process inwards may give rise to a uveal effusion syndrome, exudative retinal detachment, and choroidal detachment which may be mistaken for a choroidal tumour; macular and optic disc oedema are also frequent findings. Outward extension into the orbit may give rise to proptosis, and involvement of the extraocular muscles may cause defective ocular motility.

Treatment

This is similar to that of anterior scleritis.

Further reading

Introduction

Barraquer-Somers, H., Chan, C.C. and Green, W.R. (1983) Corneal epithelial iron deposition. *Ophthalmology*, **90**, 729–734

Hirst, L.W. (1986) Clinical evaluation of the corneal endothelium. *Clinical Modules for Ophthalmologists*, Vol. 4, Module 8

Smith, S.G., Herman, W.K., Lindstrom, R.L. *et al.* (1984) A method of collecting material from corneal ulcers. *American Journal of Ophthalmology*, **97**, 105–106

Wagoner, M.D. and Kenyon, K.R. (1985) Diagnosis and treatment of noninfected corneal ulcers. *Clinical Modules for Ophthalmologists*, Vol. 3, Module 7

Waring, G.O. and Laibson, P.R. (1977) A systematic method of drawing corneal pathologic conditions. *Archives of Ophthalmology*, **95**, 1540–1542

Microbial keratitis

Adams, C.P. Jr, Cohen, E.J., Laibson, P.R. *et al.* (1983) Corneal ulcers in patients with cosmetic extended-wear contact lenses. *American Journal of Ophthalmology*, **96**, 705–709

Baum, J. (1986) Therapy of ocular bacterial infection. *Transactions of the Ophthalmological Society of the United Kingdom*, **105**, 69–77

Baum, J. and Barza, M. (1983) Topical vs subconjunctival treatment of bacterial corneal ulcers. *Ophthalmology*, **90**, 162–168

Chalupa, E., Swarbrick, H.A., Holden, B.A. *et al.* (1987) Severe corneal infections associated with contact lens wear. *Ophthalmology*, **94**, 17–22

Jones, D.B. (1978) Pathogenesis of bacterial and fungal keratitis. *Transactions of the Ophthalmological Society of the United Kingdom*, **98**, 367–371

Jones, D.B. (1981) Decision making in the management of microbial keratitis. *Ophthalmology*, **88**, 814–820

Mannis, M.J., Tamaru, R., Roth, A.M. *et al.* (1986) Acanthamoeba sclerokeratitis. Determining diagnostic criteria. *Archives of Ophthalmology*, **104**, 1313–1317

Musch, D.C., Sugar, A. and Mayer, R.F. (1983) Demographic and predisposing factors in corneal ulceration. *Archives of Ophthalmology*, **101**, 1545–1548

Stenson, S. (1986) (Editorial) Soft contact lenses and corneal infection. *Archives of Ophthalmology*, **104**, 1287–1289

Torres, M.A., Mohamed, J., Cavazos-Adame, H. *et al.* (1985) Topical ketoconazole for fungal keratitis. *American Journal of Ophthalmology*, **100**, 293–298

Wilson, L.A. (1986) Acute bacterial infection of the eye: Bacterial keratitis and endophthalmitis. *Transactions of the Ophthalmological Society of the United Kingdom*, **105**, 43–60

Wright, P., Warhurst, D. and Jones, B.R. (1985) Acanthamoeba keratitis successfully treated medically. *British Journal of Ophthalmology*, **69**, 778–782

Viral keratitis

Collum, L.M.T., Logan, P., McAuliffe-Curtin, D. *et al.* (1985) Randomised double-blind trial of acyclovir (Zovirax) and adenine arabinoside in herpes simplex amoeboid corneal ulceration. *British Journal of Ophthalmology*, **69**, 847–850

Collum L.T.M., Logan, P. and Ravenscroft, T. (1983) Acyclovir (Zovirax) in herpetic disciform keratitis. *British Journal of Ophthalmology*, **67**, 115–118

Kaufman, H.E. (1985) Update on antiviral agents. *Ophthalmology*, **92**, 533–536

Kaufman, H.E., Centifanto-Fitzgerald, Y.M. and Yarnell, E.D. (1983) Herpes simplex keratitis. *Ophthalmology*, **90**, 700–706

Liesegang, T.J. (1985) Corneal complications from herpes zoster ophthalmicus. *Ophthalmology*, **92**, 316–324

Lightman, S., Marsh, R.J. and Powell, D. (1981) Herpes zoster ophthalmicus: a medical review. *British Journal of Ophthalmology*, **65**, 539–541

Nesburn, A.B., Lowe, G.H., Lepoff, N.J. *et al.* (1984) Effects of topical trifluridine on Thygeson's superficial punctate keratitis. *Ophthalmology*, **91**, 1188–1192

Sanitato, J.J., Asbell, P.A., Varnell, E.D. *et al.* (1984) Acyclovir in the treatment of herpetic stromal disease. *American Journal of Ophthalmology*, **98**, 537–547

Peripheral ulceration and thinning

Austin, P. and Brown, S.I. (1981) Inflammatory Terrien's marginal corneal disease. *American Journal of Ophthalmology*, **92**, 189–192

Brown, S.I. and Mondino, B.J. (1984) Therapy of Mooren's ulcer. *American Journal of Ophthalmology*, **98**, 1–6

Browning, D.J. and Proia, A.D. (1986) Ocular rosacea. *Survey of Ophthalmology*, **31**, 145–158

Feder, R.S. and Krachmer, J.H. (1984) Conjunctival resection for the treatment of rheumatoid corneal ulceration. *Ophthalmology*, **91**, 111–115

Foster, C.S. and Mondino, B.J. (1984) Systemic immunosuppressive therapy for progressive Mooren's ulcer. *Ophthalmology*, **92**, 1436–1439

Jenkins, M.S., Brown, S.I., Lempert, S.L. *et al.* (1979) Ocular rosacea. *American Journal of Ophthalmology*, **88**, 618–622

Kenyon, K.R. (1982) Decision-making in the therapy of external eye disease-noninfected corneal ulcers. *Ophthalmology*, **89**, 44–51

Lemp, M.A., Mahmood, M.A. and Weiler, H.H. (1984) Association of rosacea and keratoconjunctivitis sicca. *Archives of Ophthalmology*, **102**, 556–557

Mondino, B.J. (1980) Peripheral corneal ulcers and thinning. *Perspectives in Ophthalmology*, **4**, 9–16

Robin, J.B., Schanzlin, D.J., Verity, S.M. *et al.* (1986) Peripheral corneal disorders. *Survey of Ophthalmology*, **31**, 1–36

Soong, H.K. and Quigley, H.A. (1983) Dellen associated with filtering blebs. *Archives of Ophthalmology*, **101**, 385–387

Winder, A.F. (1983) Relationship between corneal arcus and hyperlipidaemia is clarified by studies in familial hypercholesterolaemia. *British Journal of Ophthalmology*, **67**, 789–794

Zaidman, G.W. and Brown, S.I. (1981) Orally administered tetracycline for phlyctenular keratoconjunctivitis. *American Journal of Ophthalmology*, **92**, 173–182

Degenerations

Lembach, R.G. and Keates, R.H. (1977) Band keratopathy: its significance and treatment. *Perspectives in Ophthalmology*, **1**, 13–16

Marsh, R.J. and Marshall, J. (1982) Treatment of lipid keratopathy with the argon laser. *British Journal of Ophthalmology*, **66**, 127–135

Dystrophies

Bourgeois, J., Shields, M.B. and Thresher, R. (1984) Open-angle glaucoma associated with posterior polymorphous dystrophy. *Ophthalmology*, **91**, 420–423

Bron, A.J. and Burgess, S.E.P. (1981) Inherited recurrent corneal erosions. *Transactions of the Ophthalmological Society of the United Kingdom*, **101**, 239–243

Cibis, G.W., Krachmer, J.H., Phelps, C.D. *et al.* (1977) The clinical spectrum of posterior polymorphous dystrophy. *Archives of Ophthalmology*, **95**, 1529–1537

Krachmer, J.H. (1978) Pellucid marginal corneal degeneration. *Archives of Ophthalmology*, **96**, 1217–1221

Krachmer, J.H. and Rodrigues, M.M. (1978) Posterior keratoconus. *Archives of Ophthalmology*, **96**, 1867–1873

Perry, H.D., Fine, B.S. and Caldwell, D.R. (1979) Reis–Bücklers' dystrophy. *Archives of Ophthalmology*, **97**, 664–671

Sturrock, G.D. (1983) Lattice corneal dystrophy: a source of confusion. *British Journal of Ophthalmology*, **67**, 629–634

Werblin, T.P., Hirst, L.W., Stark, W.J. *et al.* (1981) Prevalence of map–dot–fingerprint changes in the cornea. *British Journal of Ophthalmology*, **65**, 401–409

Williams, R. and Buckley, R.J. (1985) Pathogenesis and treatment of recurrent erosion. *British Journal of Ophthalmology*, **69**, 435–437

Changes in metabolic and toxic disorders

Fraunfelder, F.T. and Myer, S.M. (1983) Ocular toxicity of antineoplastic agents. *Ophthalmology*, **90**, 1–3

Kaplan, L.J. and Cappaert, W.E. (1982) Amiodarone keratopathy. *Archives of Ophthalmology*, **100**, 601–602

Kincaid, M.C., Green, W.R., Hoover, R.W. *et al.* (1982) Ocular chrysiasis. *Archives of Ophthalmology*, **100**, 1791–1794

McCormick, S.A., DiBartolomeo, A.G., Raju, V.K. *et al.* (1985) Ocular chrysiasis. *Ophthalmology*, **92**, 1432–1435

Orlando, R.G., Dangel, M.E. and Scaal, S.F. (1984) Clinical experience and grading of amiodarone keratopathy. *Ophthalmology*, **91**, 1184–1187

Contact lenses

Aquavella, J.V. and Rao, G.N. (1980) Which lens: contact lenses currently available for extended wear in aphakia. *Ophalmology*, **87**, 1151–1154

Driebe, W.T., Rabell, C.G. and Houde, W.L. (1983) Solving soft contact lens problems. *Survey of Ophthalmology*, **27**, 259–263

Fowler, S.A., Korb, D.R., Finnemore, V.M. *et al.* (1984) Surface deposits on worn hard contact lenses. *Archives of Ophthalmology*, **102**, 757–759

Korb, D.R., Allansmith, M.R., Greiner, J.V. *et al.* (1980) Prevalence of conjunctival changes in wearers of hard contact lenses. *American Journal of Ophthalmology*, **90**, 336–341

Lembach, R.G. (1984) Aphakic and myopic extender-wear contact lenses. *Clinical Modules for Ophthalmologists*, Vol. 2, Module 6

Spoor, T.C., Hartel, W.C., Wynn, P. *et al.* (1984) Complications of continuous-wear soft contact lenses in a non-referred population. *Archives of Ophthalmology*, **102**, 1312–1313

Wright, P. and Mackie, I. (1982) Preservative-related problems in soft contact lens wearers. *Ophthalmological Society of the United Kingdom*, **102**, 3–6

Principles of refractive corneal surgery

Arrowsmith, P.N. and Marks, R.G. (1984) Visual, refractive, and keratometric results of radial keratotomy: One-year, follow-up. *Archives of Ophthalmology*, **10**, 1612–1617

Deitz, M.R., Sanders, D.R. and Marks, R.G. (1984) Radial keratotomy: An overview of the Kansas City study. *Ophthalmology*, **91**, 467–478

McDonald, M.B., Koenig, S.B., Safir, A. *et al.* (1983) Epikeratophakia: The surgical correction of aphakia, update, 1982. *Ophthalmology*, **90**, 668–672

McDonald, M.B., Koenig, S.B., Safir, A. *et al.* (1983) On-lay lamellar keratoplasty for the treatment of keratoconus. *British Journal of Ophthalmology*, **67**, 615–618

McDonald, M.B. and Kaufman, H.E. (1984) Refractive corneal surgery. *Clinical Modules for Ophthalmologists*, Vol. 2, Module 11

Morgan, K.S., McDonald, M.B., Hiles, D.A. *et al.* (1987) The nationwide study of epikeratophakia for aphakia in children. *American Journal of Ophthalmology*, **103**, 366–374

Episcleritis and scleritis

Barr, C.C., Davis, H. and Culbertson, W.W. (1981) Rheumatoid scleritis. *Ophthalmology*, **88**, 1269–1273

Benson, W.E., Shields, J.A. and Tasman, W. (1979) Posterior scleritis: a cause of diagnostic confusion. *Ophthalmology*, **97**, 1482–1486

Foster, C.S., Forstot, S.L. and Wilson, L.A. (1984) Mortality rate in rheumatoid arthritis patients developing necrotizing scleritis or peripheral ulcerative keratitis. *Ophthalmology*, **91**, 1253–1263

Rao, N.A., Marak, G.E. and Hidayat, A.A. (1985) Necrotizing scleritis. *Ophthalmology*, **92**, 1542–1549

Singh, G., Guthoff, R. and Foster, C.S. (1986) Observation on long-term follow-up of posterior scleritis. *American Journal of Ophthalmology*, **101**, 570–575

Watson, P.G. (1980) The diagnosis and management of scleritis. *Ophthalmology*, **97**, 1482–1486

Watson, P.G. (1982) The nature and treatment of scleral inflammation. *Transactions of the Ophthalmological Society of the United Kingdom*, **102**, 257–281

6

Uveitis

Introduction

Definitions

Classifications

Clinical features

Differential diagnosis

Arthritis

Ankylosing spondylitis

Reiter's syndrome

Psoriatic arthritis

Juvenile chronic arthritis

Non-infectious systemic diseases

Sarcoidosis

Behçet's disease

Vogt–Koyanagi–Harada syndrome

Chronic systemic infections

Acquired syphilis

Tuberculosis

Leprosy

Parasitic infestations

Toxoplasmosis

Toxocariasis

Viral infections

Herpes zoster

Herpes simplex

Acquired cytomegalovirus

Acquired immune deficiency syndrome

Other viruses

Fungal infections

Presumed ocular histoplasmosis syndrome

Candidiasis

Common idiopathic specific uveitis syndromes

Fuchs' uveitis syndrome

Intermediate uveitis

Juvenile chronic iridocyclitis

Acute anterior uveitis in young adults

Rare idiopathic specific uveitis syndromes

Sympathetic uveitis

Eales' disease

Acute posterior multifocal placoid pigment epitheliopathy

Serpiginous choroidopathy

Birdshot retinochoroidopathy

Acute retinal necrosis

Glaucomatocyclitic crisis

Management of uveitis

Mydriatics

Steroids

Cytotoxic agents

Cyclosporin

Introduction

Definitions

Uveitis

Although by strict definition uveitis is an inflammation of the uveal tract, the term is now used to describe many forms of intraocular inflammation which may involve, not only the uvea, but also adjacent structures.

Endophthalmitis

This is a severe form of intraocular inflammation involving the ocular cavities and their immediate adjacent structures without extension of the inflammatory process beyond the sclera.

Panophthalmitis

This is similar to endophthalmitis except that the inflammatory process also involves the outer ocular coats as well as Tenon's capsule. In very severe cases, the orbital tissues may also be affected.

Vitritis

This is an infiltration of the vitreous cavity by inflammatory cells either due to uveitis or endophthalmitis.

Vasculitis

This is an inflammation of the retinal blood vessels.

Keratic precipitates

These are cellular deposits on the corneal endothelium.

Classifications

Many classifications of uveitis have been proposed, none of which is perfect. The four most useful classifications are:

Anatomical
Clinical
Aetiological
Pathological

Anatomical classification

Classified anatomically, uveitis can be anterior, intermediate, posterior, or diffuse (*Figure 6.1*).

Anterior uveitis

Anterior uveitis is subdivided into *iritis* in which the inflammation predominantly affects the iris and *iridocyclitis* in which both the iris and the anterior part of the ciliary body (pars plicata) are equally involved.

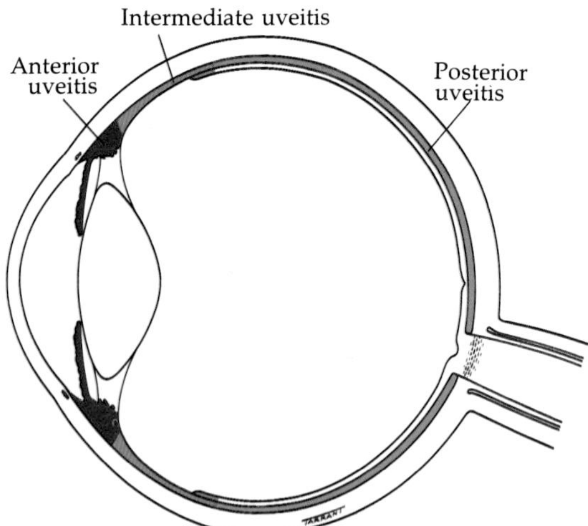

Figure 6.1 *Anatomical classification of uveitis*

Intermediate uveitis

Intermediate uveitis (pars planitis, chronic cyclitis) is characterized by predominant involvement of the posterior part of the ciliary body (pars plana) and the extreme periphery of the retina.

Posterior uveitis

In posterior uveitis, the inflammation is located behind the posterior border of the vitreous base. According to the site of primary involvement, posterior uveitis is subdivided into choroiditis, retinitis, chorioretinitis, and retinochoroiditis.

Diffuse or panuveitis

Diffuse or panuveitis is characterized by involvement of the entire uveal tract.

Anterior uveitis is the most common type followed by intermediate, posterior, and diffuse.

Clinical classification

Classified according to the mode of onset and duration, uveitis can be acute or chronic.

Acute uveitis

Acute uveitis usually has a sudden symptomatic onset and persists for 6 weeks or less. If the inflammation recurs following the initial attack it is referred to as acute recurrent.

Chronic uveitis

Chronic uveitis persists for months or years. Its onset is frequently insidious and asymptomatic although occasionally acute or subacute exacerbations of inflammation may occur during the course of a chronic uveitis.

Classified according to severity, uveitis may be *mild* or *severe*.

Aetiological classification

Classified aetiologically, uveitis can be exogenous or endogenous.

Exogenous uveitis

Exogenous uveitis is caused by either external injury to the uvea or by the invasion of micro-organisms or other agents from outside.

Endogenous uveitis

Endogenous uveitis is caused by micro-organisms or other agents from within the patient.

Classification of endogenous uveitis

The six main types of endogenous uveitis are:

1. Secondary to a systemic disease, such as: arthritis, e.g. ankylosing spondylitis; granuloma, e.g. sarcoidosis; chronic infection, e.g. tuberculosis.
2. Parasitic infestations, e.g. toxoplasmosis.
3. Viral infections, e.g. cytomegalovirus.
4. Fungal infections, e.g. candidiasis.
5. Idiopathic specific uveitis entities are a group of unrelated disorders which are not usually associated with any underlying systemic disease but which have special characteristics of their own to warrant a separate description, e.g. pars planitis.
6. Idiopathic non-specific uveitis entities which do not fall into any of the above categories make up about 25% of all cases of uveitis.

Pathological classification

Classified pathologically, uveitis is granulomatous or non-granulomatous. The main clinical differences between the two are summarized in *Table 6.1*. Clinically, this distinction is not always useful because some forms of granulomatous uveitis, e.g. sarcoidosis, may present with non-granulomatous features and, occasionally, non-granulomatous inflammation may have granulomatous characteristics.

Table 6.1 Main differences between granulomatous and non-granulomatous uveitis

Feature	*Granulomatous*	*Non-granulomatous*
Onset	Insidious	Acute
Course	Long	Short
Anterior segment		
Injection	+	+++
Pain	±	+++
Iris nodules	+++	–
Keratic precipitates	'Mutton fat'	Usually small
Fundus	Nodular lesions	Diffuse involvement

Clinical features

Anterior uveitis

Symptoms

The main symptoms of acute anterior uveitis are photophobia, pain, redness, decreased vision and lacrimation. In chronic anterior uveitis, however, the eye may be white and symptoms minimal, even in the presence of severe inflammation.

Signs

Injection

In acute anterior uveitis the circumcorneal 'ciliary' injection has a violaceous hue (*Figure 6.2*). The degree of injection should be graded from 0 to +4.

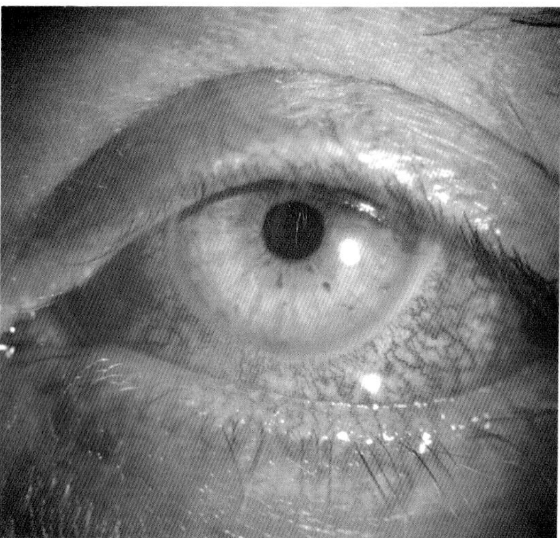

Figure 6.2 *Ciliary injection in acute anterior uveitis*

Keratic precipitates

The characteristics and distribution of keratic precipitates (KPs) may provide clues as to the possible aetiology of the uveitis. The following observations should be made and recorded.

Distribution

KPs most commonly form in the mid and inferior zones of the cornea. However, in Fuchs' uveitis syndrome, they are scattered throughout the endothelium.

Size

1. Endothelial dusting by many hundreds of small cells occurs in acute anterior uveitis, as well as during subacute exacerbations of chronic inflammation.
2. Small KPs are characteristic of herpes zoster and Fuchs' uveitis syndrome.
3. Medium KPs occur in most types of acute and chronic anterior uveitis (*Figure 6.3*).

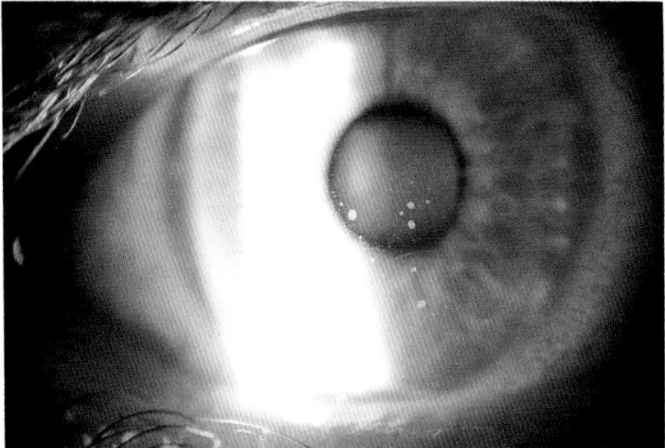

Figure 6.3 Small and medium-size keratic precipitates

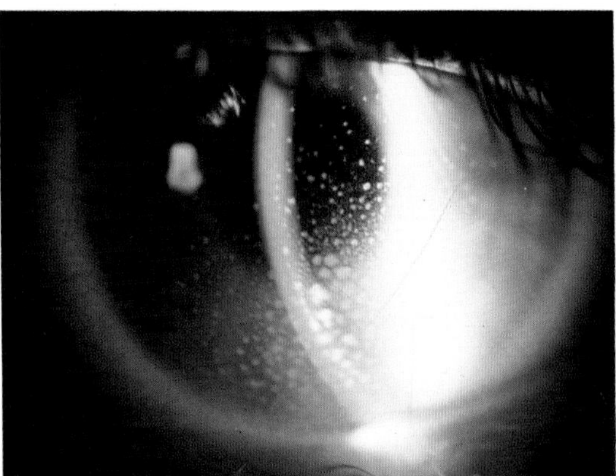

Figure 6.4 'Mutton fat' keratic precipitates

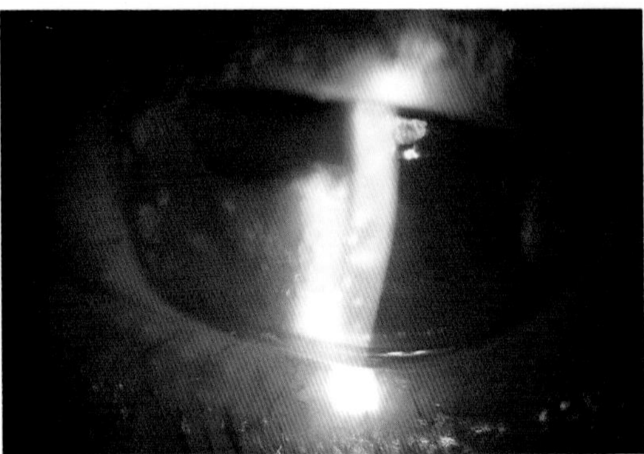

Figure 6.5 Old keratic precipitates

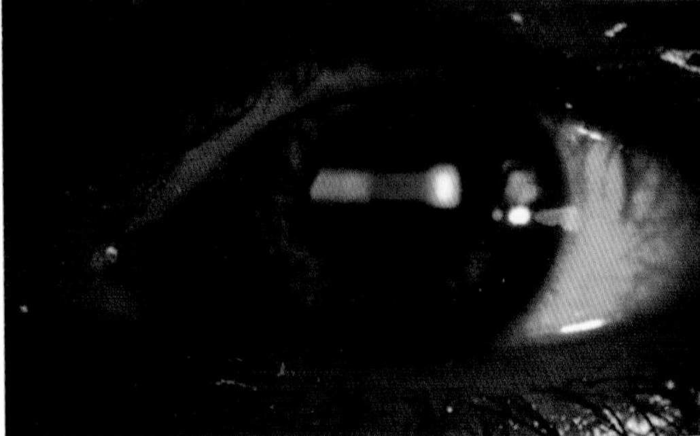

Figure 6.6 Aqueous cells (+4) and dense flare

4. Large KPs are usually of the 'mutton fat' variety and have a greasy or waxy appearance (*Figure 6.4*). They are composed of clusters of epithelioid cells and mononuclear macrophages and they typically occur in granulomatous uveitis.

Fresh or old?

Fresh KPs tend to be white and round. As they age, they shrink, fade, and become pigmented. Fading 'mutton fat' KPs usually take on a 'ground-glass' (hyalinized) appearance (*Figure 6.5*).

Aqueous cells (*Figure 6.6*)

The cells should be graded according to the number observed in the oblique slit beam. The light intensity and magnification of the slitlamp should be maximal and the beam 3-mm long and 1-mm wide. The cells should be counted and graded from 0 to +4 as shown in *Table 6.2*.

Table 6.2 Grading of aqueous cells

Cells per field	*Grade*
0	–
1–5	±
5–10	+
10–20	++
20–50	+++
Over 50	++++

Aqueous flare

The grading of flare is performed using the same setting on the slitlamp as for counting cells. The beam should be passed obliquely to the plane of the iris in order to evaluate the degree of obscuration of iris details. The flare is graded from 0 to +4 as shown in *Table 6.3*.

A flare is due to leakage of proteins into the aqueous humour through damaged blood vessels and is not necessarily a sign of active uveitis. For this reason, the presence of a flare in the absence of cells is *not* an indication for steroid therapy.

Table 6.3 Grading of aqueous flare

Description	*Grade*
Complete absence	0
Faint – just detectable	+
Moderate – iris details clear	++
Marked – iris details hazy	+++
Intense – fixed coagulated aqueous with considerable fibrin	++++

Iris nodules (*Figure 6.7*)

Koeppe nodules are situated at the pupillary border and are smaller than Busacca nodules which are less common and which are located on the surface of the iris away from the pupil.

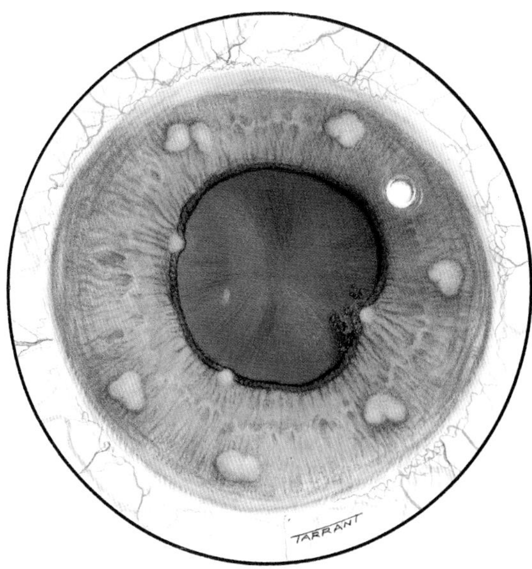

Figure 6.7 Koeppe and Busacca iris nodules in granulomatous anterior uveitis

Iris atrophy

This is an important feature of Fuchs' uveitis syndrome and it also occurs in uveitis due to herpes simplex and herpes zoster.

Rubeosis iridis

Rubeosis iridis (iris neovascularization) develops in some eyes with chronic anterior uveitis and in Fuchs' uveitis syndrome. In severe cases, a fibrovascular membrane covers the anterior lens surface and occludes the pupil (occlusio pupillae). In a few cases, neovascularization also develops in the chamber angle.

Posterior synechiae (*Figure 6.8*)

Posterior synechiae (adhesions between the anterior lens surface and the iris) form with ease during an attack of acute anterior uveitis because the pupil is small. They may also form in eyes with moderate to severe chronic anterior uveitis. Posterior synechiae extending for 360° (seclusio pupillae) prevent the passage of aqueous humour from the posterior to the anterior chamber giving rise to a forward bowing of the peripheral iris (iris bombé), which may lead to elevation of intraocular pressure due to secondary closure of the angle by the peripheral iris. In some eyes with chronic anterior uveitis, seclusion and occlusion of the pupil occur together.

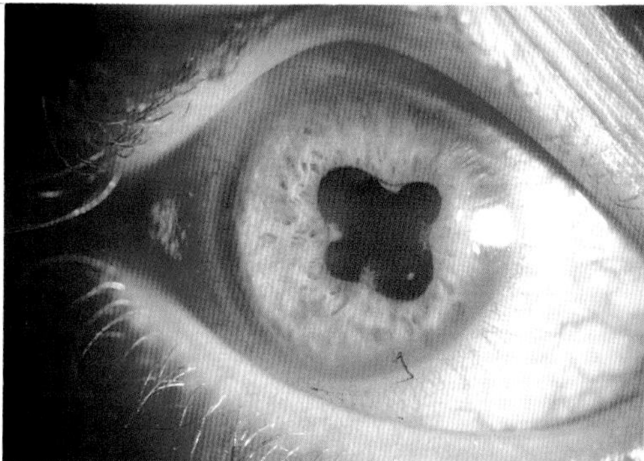

Figure 6.8 Posterior synechiae

Anterior vitreous

The cell density in the anterior vitreous should be compared with that in the aqueous. In iritis, aqueous cells far exceed the number of vitreous cells, whereas in iridocyclitis the cells are distributed equally between the two compartments.

Posterior segment

A careful examination should be performed of the macula for evidence of cystoid macular oedema which is an occasional complication of chronic anterior uveitis and a common complication of intermediate uveitis.

Intermediate uveitis

Symptoms

The presenting symptom is usually floaters, although occasionally the patient presents with impairment of central vision due to chronic cystoid macular oedema.

Signs

Intermediate uveitis is characterized by vitritis with few, if any, cells in the anterior chamber and the absence of a focal inflammatory lesion in the fundus.

Posterior uveitis

Symptoms

The two main symptoms of posterior segment inflammation are floaters and impaired vision. A patient with a peripheral inflammatory lesion will complain of seeing floaters and may have only minimal blurring of vision. On the other hand, active choroiditis involving the fovea or papillomacular bundle will primarily cause loss of central vision and the patient may not notice the presence of floaters.

Signs

Vitreous

Posterior segment inflammation causes vitreous opacities, vitreous flare, and frequently posterior vitreous detachment. The opacities should be classified according to size, shape, and position within the vitreous cavity.

Fine opacities are composed of individual inflammatory cells. In some cases the detached posterior hyaloid face is covered by inflammatory precipitates comparable to KPs.

Coarse opacities are usually the result of severe tissue destruction.

'Snowball opacities' are characteristic of pars planitis, although they may also occur in candidiasis and sarcoidosis.

Stringy opacities (*Figure 6.9*) are usually caused by alterations in the vitreous gel itself.

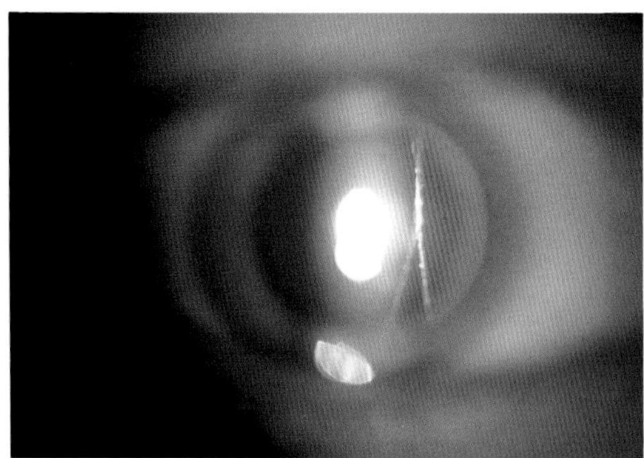

Figure 6.9 *Stringy vitreous opacities*

Grading of vitreous activity

Grading of vitreous activity is less satisfactory than grading of anterior chamber activity. It can be performed with either the direct or indirect ophthalmoscope.

With direct ophthalmoscope. The old grading system proposed by Kimura, Thygeson and Hogan (1959) is shown in *Table 6.4.*

Table 6.4 Grading of vitreous activity using direct ophthalmoscope

Description	*Grade*
No opacities	0
Few scattered fine and coarse opacities with a clear view of the fundus	+
Scattered fine and coarse opacities with fundus details somewhat obscured	++
Many opacities with marked blurring of fundus	+++
Dense opacities with no view of fundus	++++

With indirect ophthalmoscope. The disadvantage of the old grading system is that, in some eyes with active inflammation, vitreous cells and opacities may persist for many months despite the fact that the vitreous haze has resolved and visual acuity has returned to normal. For this reason, Nussenblatt and associates (1985) have proposed that the severity of *vitreous activity* is best assessed by grading the extent of vitreous haze. This is performed with the pupil maximally dilated with the indirect ophthalmoscope beam set at midpower and a +20 D lens. The clarities of three fundus landmarks are used as criteria: optic nerve head, retinal blood vessels, and normal striations and reflex of the retinal nerve fibres. The haze is then graded as shown in *Table 6.5.*

Table 6.5 Grading of vitreous activity with indirect ophthalmoscope

Description	*Grade*
Optic nerve head obscured	++++
Optic herve head visible but borders blurred	+++
Better visualization of retinal blood vessels	++
Better definition of optic nerve head and retinal blood vessels	+
Blurring of retinal nerve fibre striations	±
Nerve fibre striations well defined	0

Fundus

Choroiditis (*Figure 6.10*) is characterized by yellow or greyish patches with reasonably well-demarcated borders. Inactive lesions appear as white well-defined areas of chorioretinal atrophy with pigmented borders. The retinal blood vessels, which may be sheathed, pass over the lesions undisturbed.

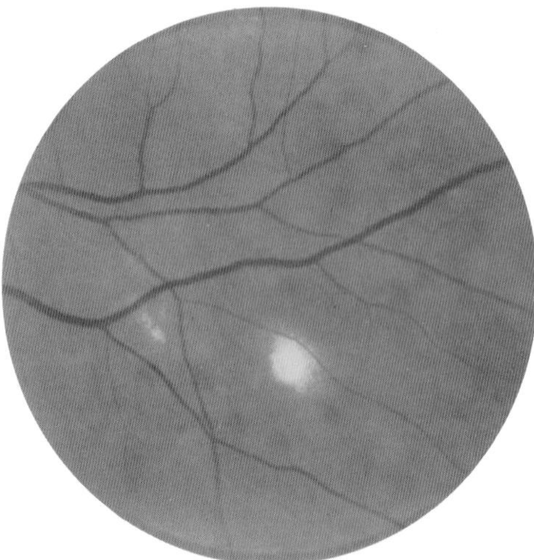

Figure 6.10 *Active focal choroiditis (courtesy of Mr A. Shun-Shin)*

Retinitis (*Figure 6.11*) gives the retina a white cloudy appearance. Because the outline of the inflammatory focus is indistinct, exact demarcation between healthy and inflamed retina may be difficult to discern.

Note. Posterior segment inflammation can be focal (*see Figure 6.10*), multifocal (*Figure 6.12*), geographical (*Figure 6.13*) and diffuse.

Vasculitis may involve the retinal veins (periphlebitis) or, less commonly, the arterioles (periarteritis). Active periphlebitis is characterized by a fluffy white haziness surrounding the blood column (*Figure 6.14*). Involvement is patchy, with irregular extensions outside the vessel wall. It represents a chronic inflammatory cell infiltrate within and surrounding the vessel wall, which may resolve without sequelae or it may be replaced by venous sclerosis.

Perivascular accumulation of granulomatous tissue in severe periphlebitis gives rise to 'candlewax drippings' or 'candlewax exudates'.

Neovascularization is relatively rare in eyes with posterior segment inflammation, although sarcoidosis may be associated with both peripheral as well as disc new vessels.

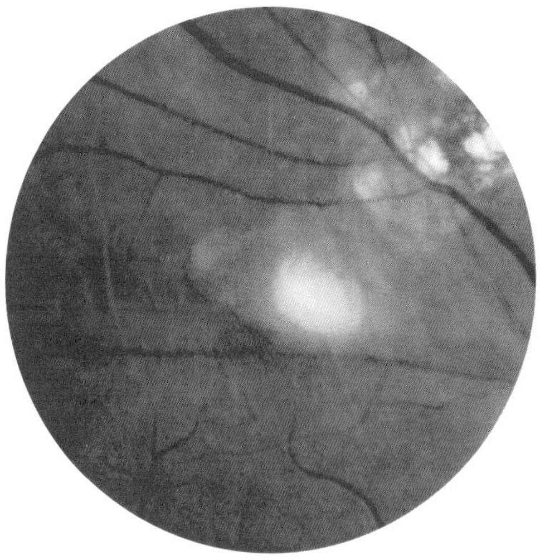

Figure 6.11 Active focal retinochoroiditis

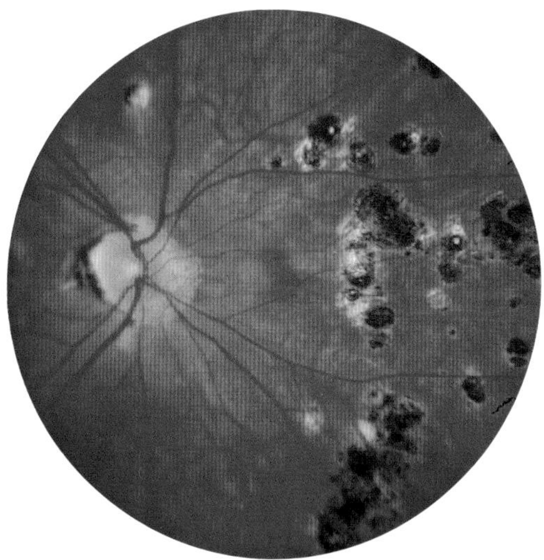

Figure 6.12 Old multifocal retinochoroiditis

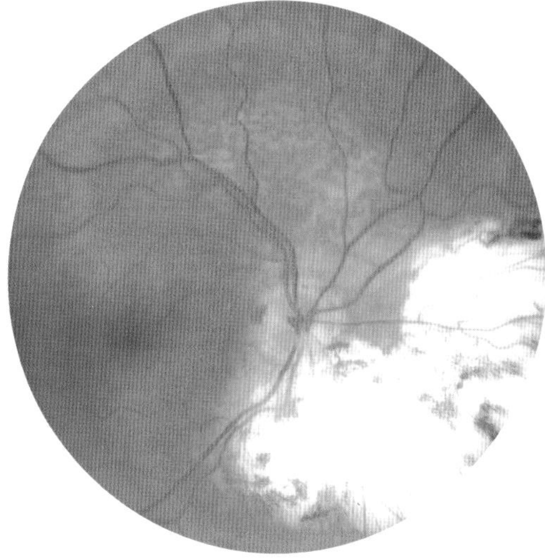

Figure 6.13 Old geographical retinochoroiditis

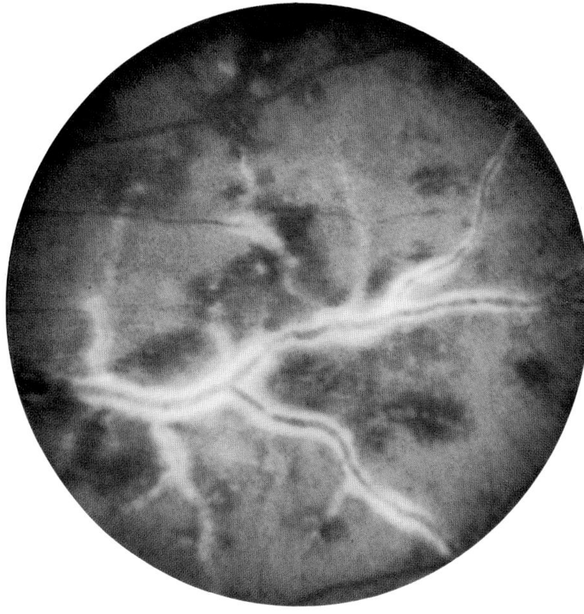

Figure 6.14 Severe periphlebitis

Because the new vessels are not usually associated with significant areas of capillary closure, they frequently regress once the inflammation is controlled although, on occasion, they may cause vitreous haemorrhage.

Retinal detachment. Exudative retinal detachment is the hallmark of Harada's disease. Rhegmatogenous and/or tractional retinal detachment is a common complication of acute retinal necrosis, and it occasionally occurs in eyes with severe toxoplasmosis and pars planitis.

Optic nerve head findings include papillitis (from contiguous or distant inflammatory foci), oedema (from hypotony), granuloma (sarcoidosis), and optic atrophy (secondary to retinal damage).

Differential diagnosis

It is important to remember that tumours may occasionally present with inflammatory signs which may be mistaken for endogenous uveitis (masquerade syndromes).

Retinoblastoma

In all young children with uveitis, it is extremely important to exclude the possibility of a retinoblastoma, which may mimic a posterior uveitis or cause a 'pseudohypopyon'.

Melanoma

A necrotizing malignant melanoma may also give rise to a 'pseudo-uveitis'.

Histiocytic lymphoma (reticulum cell sarcoma)

This very rare tumour should be considered in the differential diagnosis of chronic vitritis in patients between the ages of 40 and 60 years. The fundus shows yellow subretinal and choroidal infiltrates, frequently with multiple hyperpigmented spots.

Arthritis

Ankylosing spondylitis

Systemic features

Ankylosing spondylitis (AS) is a chronic inflammatory arthritis of unknown aetiology that predominantly affects the axial skeleton. The disease typically affects males between the ages of 20 and 40 years who are positive for HLA-B27 but negative for rheumatoid factor ('seronegative'). In females, AS has a more benign course than in males, and in children the disease frequently presents with a peripheral lower limb arthropathy without backache. Some patients with AS also have ulcerative colitis or Crohn's disease.

Diagnostic tests

X-rays

All young adult males with acute unilateral iridocyclitis should have X-rays of the sacroiliac joints irrespective of the presence or absence of low back symptoms. This is because, in early cases, the X-rays may be positive before the patient is symptomatic. The diagnosis of subclinical AS is important because appropriate therapy may prevent the development of more severe structural changes in the spine.

Tissue typing

Between 80 and 90% of patients with AS are positive for HLA-B27, as opposed to an incidence of about 8% in the general population. The incidence of HLA-B27 in patients with acute iridocyclitis is about 45% and, in those with both AS and acute iridocyclitis, the incidence rises to about 95%. The presence of HLA-B27 in a patient with early X-ray findings, therefore, merely confirms the diagnosis of AS. Patients with acute anterior uveitis, who are positive for HLA-B27 but radiologically normal, should be examined by a rheumatologist at 2-yearly intervals for evidence of sacroiliac involvement as there is a strong likelihood that they will eventually develop AS.

Ocular features

The typical ocular complication of AS is an acute, recurrent, non-granulomatous iridocyclitis. The active inflammation is invariably unilateral although both eyes are frequently involved at different times. The incidence of acute iridocyclitis in patients with AS is 30% and conversely about 30% of males with acute unilateral iridocyclitis will also have AS. However, there is no correlation between the severity and activity of eye and joint involvement and uveitis may either precede or follow the diagnosis of AS.

Signs

Initially the corneal endothelium shows 'dusting' and later small keratic precipitates may form. The aqueous contains many cells (usually between +3 and +4) as well as a flare. In severe cases, the anterior chamber contains a fibrinous exudate (*Figure 6.15*) which also coats the anterior lens surface and a hypopyon (*Figure 6.16*) may also be seen.

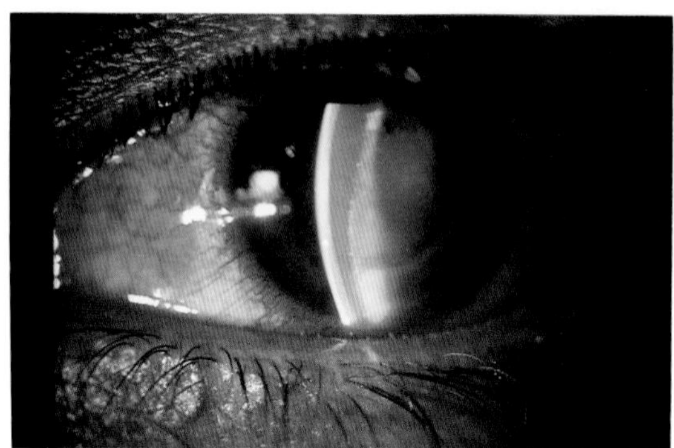

Figure 6.15 *Fibrinous exudate in anterior chamber*

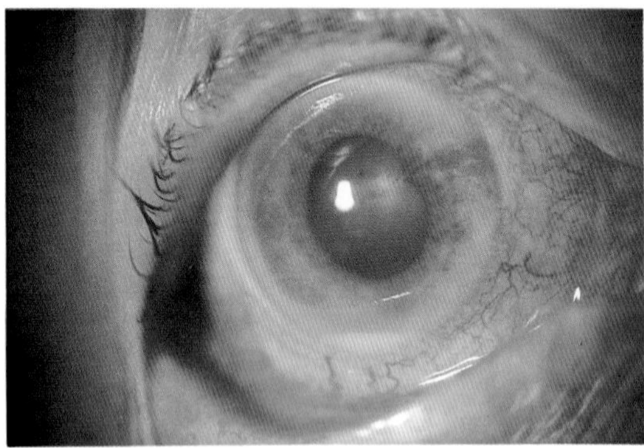

Figure 6.16 *Hypopyon*

Clinical course and complications

The attack of iridocyclitis seldom lasts longer than 6 weeks. The main complication is the formation of posterior synechiae which, if severe, may lead to secondary glaucoma from iris bombé. Although there is a high risk that the uveitis will recur in one or other eye, the long-term visual prognosis is good and vision-threatening complications such as secondary cataract and chronic cystoid macular oedema are rare. In a few patients with many recurrent attacks the inflammation eventually becomes chronic.

Management

The treatment of acute iridocyclitis is with topical or periocular steroids and mydriatics. Details of treatment are discussed later.

Reiter's syndrome

Systemic features

Reiter's syndrome consists of a triad of urethritis, conjunctivitis and 'seronegative' arthritis. This relatively uncommon disease which typically affects young men, 70% of whom are positive for HLA-B27, has three modes of presentation.

1. *Postvenereal.* The most common presentation is with a non-specific (i.e. non-gonococcal) urethritis, 2 weeks following sexual intercourse.
2. *Postdysenteric.* A less common presentation is following an attack of dysentery without a preliminary urethritis.
3. *Articular.* In some patients, acute arthritis is the first feature of the disease, with either urethritis or dysentery being insignificant. The inflammation typically affects the knees, ankles, and Achilles tendon. A periostitis may cause a calcaneal spur and some patients subsequently develop ankylosing spondylitis.

Other systemic features of Reiter's syndrome include keratoderma blennorrhagica of the palms or soles, circinate balanitis, nail dystrophy, painless mouth ulceration and plantar fasciitis.

Ocular features

Conjunctivitis

Although a mucopurulent conjunctivitis without follicles is common, it is not universal. It usually follows the urethritis by about 2 weeks, and it typically precedes the arthritis.

Keratitis

A punctate epithelial or subepithelial keratitis with anterior stromal infiltrates may accompany the conjunctival inflammation.

Iridocyclitis

An acute unilateral iridocyclitis occurs in about 20% of patients, either with the first attack of Reiter's syndrome or during a recurrence.

Psoriatic arthritis

Systemic features

Psoriatic arthritis is a 'seronegative', anodular, erosive, inflammatory arthritis occurring in about 5% of patients with psoriasis. The disease has no sexual preferential but is associated with an increased prevalence of HLA-B27 and HLA-B17. Typically, the arthritis is asymmetrical and involves the interphalangeal joints of the hands and feet. In some cases, the sacroiliac joints and the spine are also affected. Many patients show the typical pitting of psoriasis.

Ocular features

Conjunctivitis

About 20% of patients develop conjunctivitis.

Keratoconjunctivitis sicca

This is a relatively rare complication.

Keratitis

Some patients with anterior uveitis develop raised corneal infiltrates just inside the limbus.

Iridocyclitis

An acute unilateral iridocyclitis occurs less frequently in psoriatic arthritis than in either ankylosing spondylitis or Reiter's syndrome.

Juvenile chronic arthritis

Systemic features

Juvenile chronic arthritis (JCA) is a 'seronegative' idiopathic inflammatory arthritis developing in children under the age of 16 years. In the United States, the disease is frequently referred to as 'juvenile rheumatoid arthritis'. Based on the mode of onset of the disease and the extent of joint involvement during the first 3 months, three different subgroups of JCA are recognized.

Systemic onset JCA

Systemic onset JCA, which accounts for about 30% of cases, is characterized by a high remittent fever and at least one of the following features: transient maculopapular rash, generalized lymphadenopathy, hepatomegaly, splenomegaly, and pericarditis. Initially, arthralgia or arthritis may be absent or minimal and only a minority of patients subsequently develop a progressive polyarthritis.

The term 'Still's disease' is now usually reserved for patients in this subgroup, in which uveitis is extremely rare.

Polyarticular onset JCA

Polyarticular onset JCA accounts for about 20% of all cases. The disease affects five or more joints during the first 3 months. The most frequently involved joints are the knees followed by the wrists and ankles. In some patients, the arthritis persists for many years and causes crippling deformities. Uveitis is fairly rare in this subgroup.

Pauciarticular onset JCA

Pauciarticular onset JCA is the most frequent accounting for about 50% of all cases. In this subgroup, four or fewer joints are involved during the first 3 months. The most commonly affected joints are the knees, although occasionally the arthritis involves only a single finger or toe. Some patients in this subgroup remain pauciarticular while others subsequently develop a polyarthritis. About 20% of patients in this subgroup develop uveitis.

Diagnostic tests

Rheumatoid factor

All patients with uveitis and JCA are seronegative for rheumatoid factor. This confirms the fact that seropositive children with 'true' juvenile rheumatoid arthritis resemble their adult counterparts and are not at increased risk of uveitis.

Antinuclear antibodies

About 75% of children with JCA and uveitis are positive for antinuclear antibodies (ANA) as compared to an incidence of 30% in those without ocular involvement. It has been suggested that ANA formation precedes rather than follows the onset of uveitis and that a rising titre should arouse suspicion as to the increased risk of uveitis. However, there is no correlation between the level of ANA titre and the severity of either eye or joint disease.

Because the onset of intraocular inflammation is invariably *asymptomatic*, it is extremely important for children at risk to have regular *slitlamp biomicroscopy*. The frequency of examination is governed by the various risk factors just discussed which are summarized in *Table 6.6*.

Ocular features

The anterior uveitis in JCA is chronic, non-granulomatous and bilateral in 70% of cases. It is unusual for patients with initially unilateral uveitis to develop involvement of the second eye after more than 1 year. In those with bilateral uveitis, the severity of intraocular inflammation is usually symmetrical.

Table 6.6 Risk factors for JCA

Onset of JCA	*Risk of uveitis*	*Examination frequency*
Systemic	±	Annual
Polyarticular	+	9-monthly
Polyarticular + ANA	++	6-monthly
Pauciarticular	+++	4-monthly
Pauciarticular + ANA	++++	3-monthly

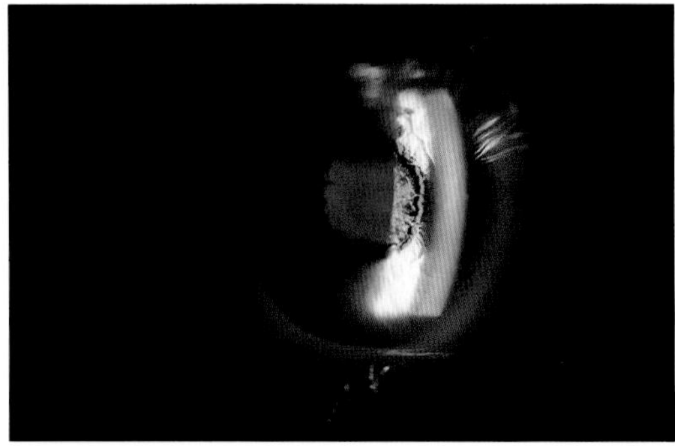

Figure 6.17 *Pupillary tags and pigment on anterior lens surface*

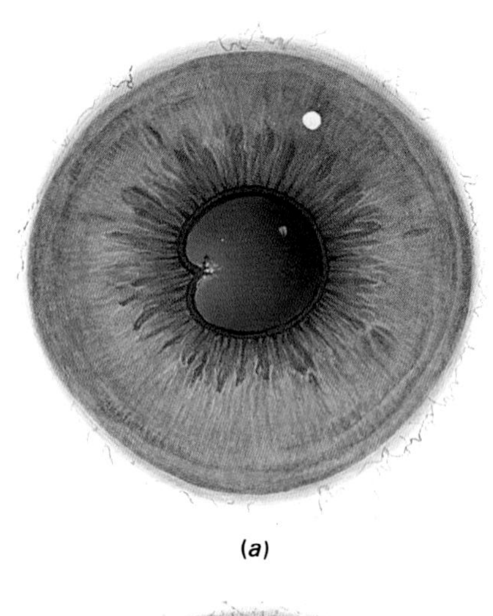

(*a*)

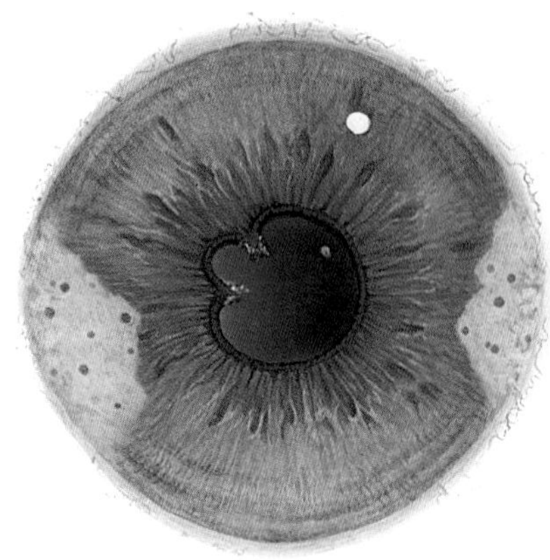

(*b*)

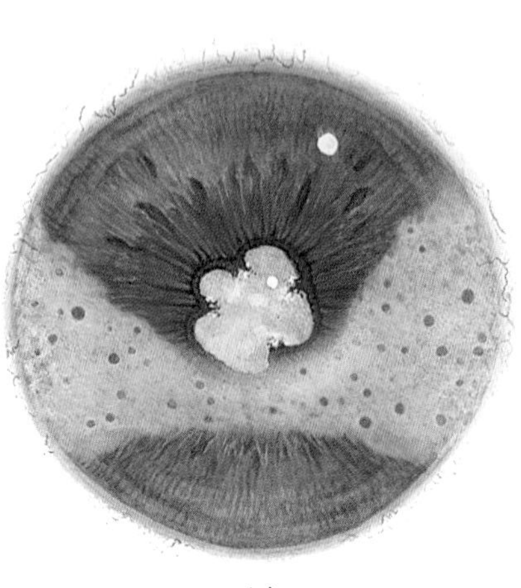

(*c*)

Figure 6.18 *Progression of complications of chronic iridocyclitis associated with juvenile chronic arthritis:* (a) *posterior synechiae;* (b) *increase in number of posterior synechiae and early band keratopathy;* (c) *extensive band keratopathy and mature complicated cataract*

Symptoms

As the onset of intraocular inflammation is invariably asymptomatic, the uveitis is frequently detected on routine slitlamp examination. Even during acute exacerbations with +4 cells in the aqueous humour, it is rare for patients to complain, although a few report an increase in vitreous floaters.

Signs

The eye is white, even in the presence of severe uveitis. The keratic precipitates are usually small to medium in size. During acute exacerbations, the entire corneal endothelium shows 'dusting' by many hundreds of cells, but hypopyon is very rare. Posterior synechiae are common in eyes with long-standing undetected uveitis. In some eyes the iris surface shows dilated blood vessels which may extend onto the lens. Although the intraocular inflammation is essentially non-granulomatous, some eyes show small Koeppe nodules. Pigment deposition on the anterior lens surface is common and some eyes also have pupillary tags (*Figure 6.17*).

Clinical course and complications

The severity of uveitis can be divided into four groups (*Figure 6.18*):

1. In about 10% of cases the intraocular inflammation is very mild, unassociated with keratic precipitates, with never more than +1 aqueous cells and persists for less than 12 months.
2. About 15% of patients have one attack of uveitis which lasts less than 4 months, with the severity of inflammation varying from +2 to +4 aqueous cells.
3. In 50% of cases, the uveitis is moderate to severe and persists for more than 4 months. The majority of acute exacerbations can be controlled by frequent instillation of topical steroids.
4. In 25% of cases, the intraocular inflammation is very severe, lasts for several years and responds poorly to treatment. In this subgroup, band keratopathy occurs in 40% of patients, complicated cataract in 30%, and secondary inflammatory glaucoma in 15%.

Management

Most patients can be controlled with topical steroids. Those that respond poorly to topical medication are also frequently resistant to systemic steroid therapy, although they may respond to periocular injections. The therapeutic value of cytotoxic agents such as chlorambucil is undetermined. Details of management of chronic anterior uveitis are discussed later.

Non-infectious systemic diseases

Sarcoidosis

Systemic features

The definition of sarcoidosis proposed by the Seventh International Conference on Sarcoidosis and other Granulomatous Disorders is as follows:

'Sarcoidosis is a multisystem granulomatous disorder of unknown aetiology, most commonly affecting young adults and presenting most frequently with bilateral hilar lymphadenopathy, pulmonary infiltration, skin, and eye lesions. The diagnosis is established most securely when clinicoradiographic findings are supported by histological evidence of widespread non-caseating epithelioid-cell granulomas in more than one organ or a positive Kveim–Slitzbach skin test. Immunological features are depression of delayed-type hypersensitivity suggesting impaired cell-mediated immunity and raised or abnormal immunoglobulins. There may also be hypercalciuria, with or without hypercalcaemia. The course and prognosis may correlate with the mode of onset: an acute onset with erythema nodosum (*Figure 6.19*) heralds a self-limiting course and spontaneous resolution, whereas an insidious onset may be followed by relentless, progressive fibrosis. Corticosteroids relieve symptoms and suppress inflammation and granuloma formation.'

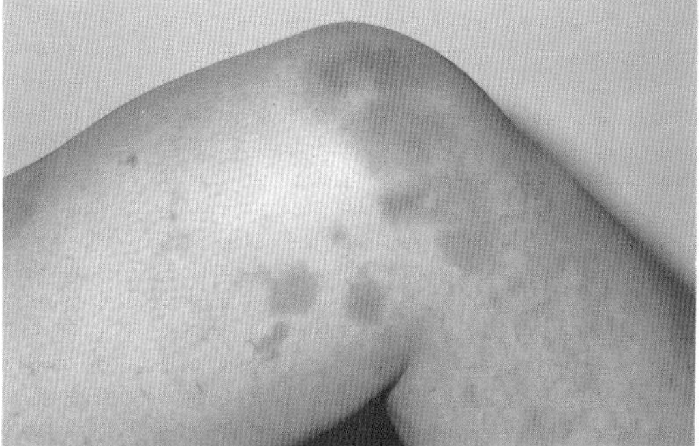

Figure 6.19 *Erythema nodosum*

Diagnostic tests

Although the diagnosis is usually easy, in some patients many of the features are missing and the following special investigations may be useful.

Chest X-ray

Over 90% of patients with ocular sarcoid will have an abnormal chest X-ray. The most common initial finding is bilateral hilar fullness (stage 1). This is followed by the appearance of reticulonodular infiltrates (stage 2). The hilar involvement then wanes and only pulmonary fibrosis remains (stage 3).

Biopsy

Lung biopsy by the tracheobronchial fibreoptic technique is now frequently carried out and is accurate in about 90% of patients in diagnosing sarcoidosis. Biopsy of lacrimal gland, conjunctiva, lymph nodes, tonsil and liver may also give histological confirmation of sarcoidosis.

Kveim–Slitzbach test

This is positive in 80% of patients with sarcoidosis. It relies on the fact that a saline suspension of sarcoid tissue (antigen) obtained from the spleen of a patient with active sarcoidosis, introduced intradermally, induces granuloma of sarcoid type when biopsied 4 weeks later.

Mantoux test

Although this is negative in a very high percentage of patients with sarcoidosis, it is now of limited value except in areas with a high incidence of positive tuberculin tests.

Angiontensin converting enzyme

Angiotensin converting enzyme (ACE) is produced by many cells in the body. In sarcoidosis the enzyme is thought to be synthesized by monocytes that have transformed from phagocytic into storage or secretory cells. Normal serum levels of ACE are 12–35 nmol/min per μl in men and 11–29 nmol/min per μl in women. Serum ACE is usually elevated in patients with active sarcoidosis and is normal in patients in remission.

Calcium

Calcium metabolism is abnormal in sarcoidosis and hypercalciuria is common (although hypercalcaemia is unusual).

Gallium-67 scan of head, neck and thorax

This frequently shows increased uptake in patients with active systemic sarcoidosis because the gallium is taken up by mitotically active liposomes of granulocytes.

Ocular features

The eye is involved in about 30% of patients with systemic sarcoidosis. Ocular involvement may occur in patients with few, if any, constitutional symptoms, as well as in those with inactive systemic disease. In acute sarcoidosis the ocular inflammation is usually unilateral and, as the disease becomes chronic, bilateral involvement usually develops.

Signs

External *(Figure 6.20)*

Sarcoidosis may involve the conjunctiva, the episclera and, rarely, the orbit and sclera. The skin of the eyelids may show violaceous sarcoid plaques (lupus pernio). Sarcoid granulomas of the lid margins may be mistaken for small chalazia. Granulomatous infiltration of the lacrimal gland, if severe, may be responsible for keratoconjunctivitis sicca.

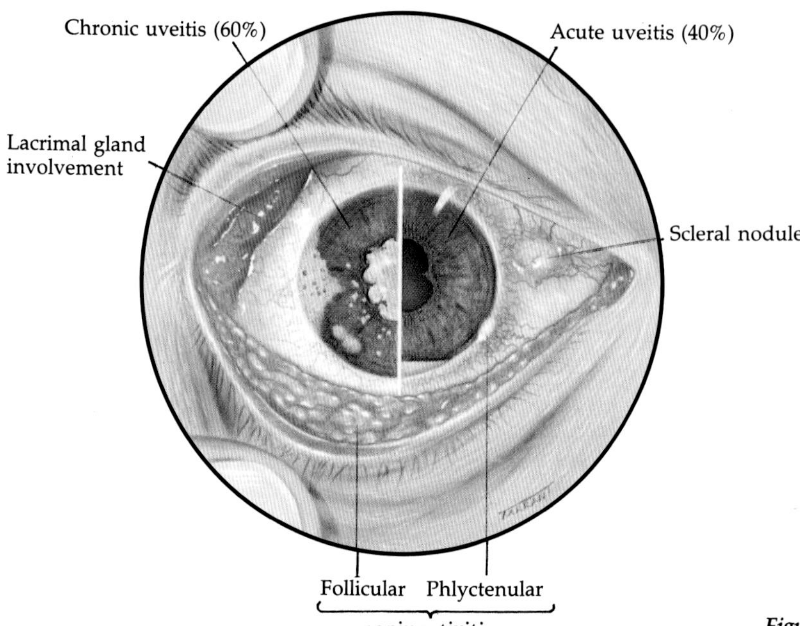

Figure 6.20 *Anterior segment complications of sarcoidosis*

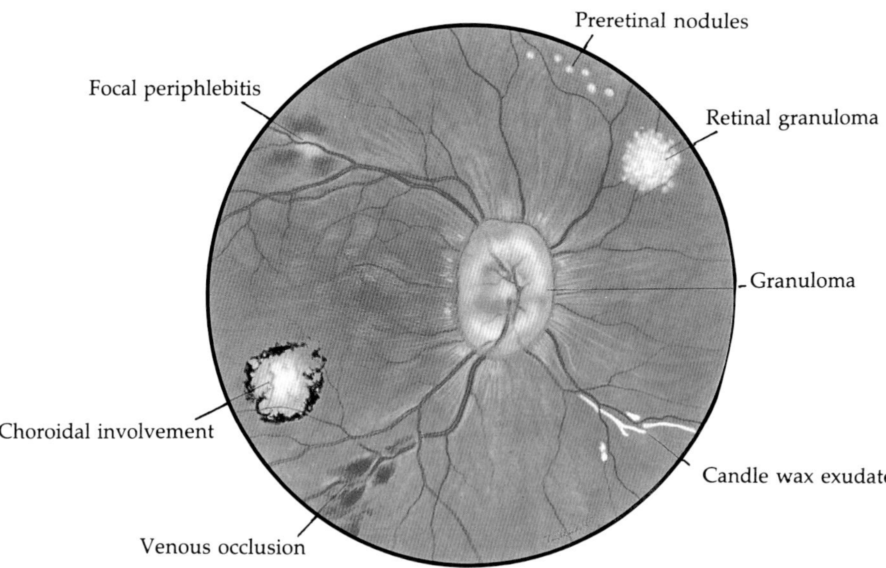

Figure 6.21 *Posterior segment complications of sarcoidosis*

Slitlamp

Iridocyclitis is by far the most common ocular complication; it may be acute or chronic.

Acute iridocyclitis, which is frequently unilateral, typically affects young patients with acute sarcoidosis.

Chronic granulomatous iridocyclitis, which is frequently bilateral, is more common than the acute form. It typically affects older patients with chronic lung fibrosis in whom the systemic disease may be inactive. The intraocular inflammation may be difficult to control and complications such as band keratopathy, complicated cataract and secondary glaucoma are frequent.

Vitreous

Diffuse vitritis is common, and more dense inferiorly. 'Snowball', opacities may also be present in a few patients.

Fundus (*Figure 6.21*)

The posterior segment is involved in about 25% of patients with ocular sarcoid and is usually associated with anterior uveitis. The posterior segment manifestations are caused by granulomatous penetration of the retinal and choroidal vessels with secondary damage involving: the blood vessels, the retina, the choroid, and the optic nerve.

Blood vessels

The most subtle and common sign of posterior segment sarcoidosis is a peripheral retinal periphlebitis involving only one or two segments of a retinal vein. Active periphlebitis is characterized by soft, white, perivenous infiltration (cutting) (*Figure 6.22*) associated with increased vascular permeability which may lead to peripheral globular retinal haemorrhages and intraretinal oedema. The acute lesions stain on fundus fluorescein angiography. Although acute periphlebitis may resolve spontaneously or with the use of systemic steroids, vascular sheathing, once established, usually persists. An advanced stage of periphlebitis caused by perivascular accumulation of granulomatous tissue (periphlebitic nodules) is known as 'candlewax drippings' (*Figure 6.23*). Two complications of periphlebitis are retinal branch vein occlusion and peripheral 'seafan' neovascularization (fronds).

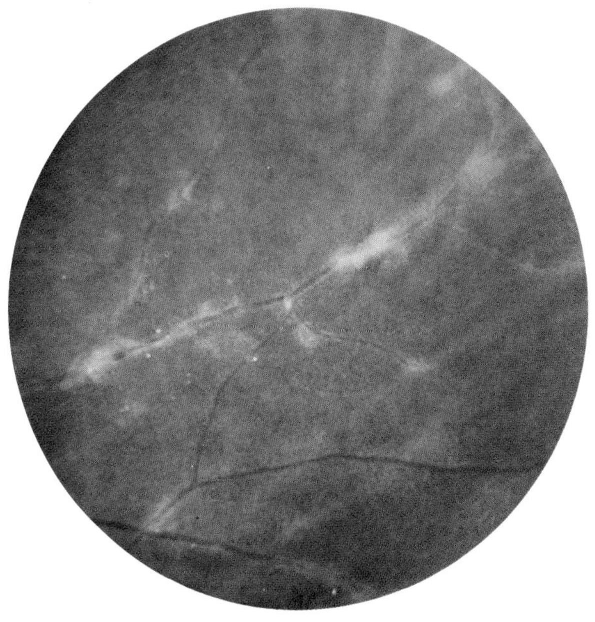

Figure 6.22 *Active peripheral periphlebitis in sarcoidosis*

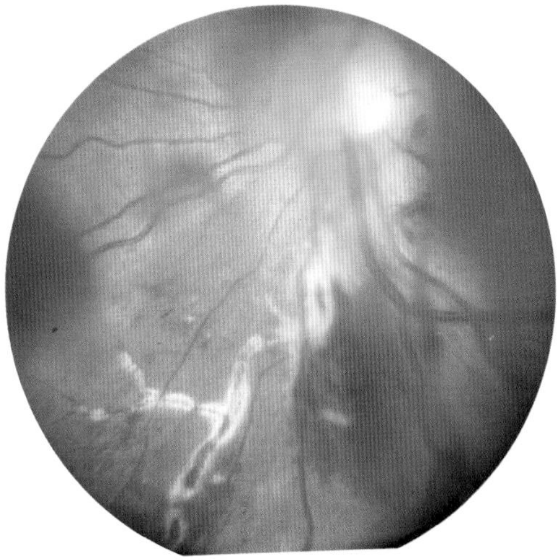

Figure 6.23 *Severe periphlebitis with 'candlewax drippings' and vitreous haemorrhage (courtesy of Mr J. Shilling)*

Retina

The 'spillover' of granulomatous tissue may result in retinal granulomas which may be associated with secondary neovascularization. In advanced cases, the sarcoid nodules may be located on the retinal surface and they may also extend into the vitreous. Preretinal nodules are typically discrete, grey-white, and located inferiorly and anterior to the equator (Landers' sign) (*Figure 6.24*). The most severe form of retinal sarcoid is called 'acute sarcoid retinopathy' which is characterized by a vitreous haze, candlewax drippings, retinal and preretinal granulomas, and retinal haemorrhages.

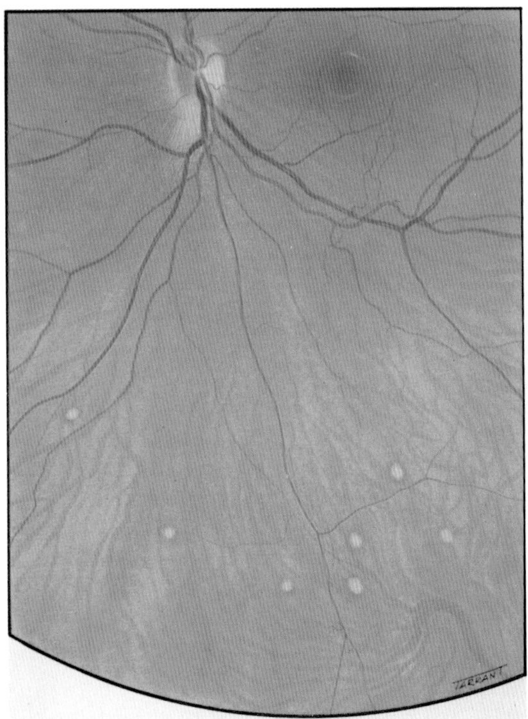

Figure 6.24 *Preretinal nodules in sarcoidosis (Landers' sign)*

Choroid

Choroidal sarcoidosis is relatively rare and is usually not associated with retinal or vitreous inflammation. The choroidal granulomas are typically bilateral, multiple, pale-yellow, elevated lesions at the posterior pole. They vary in size from small subpigment epithelial granulomas to large choroidal masses. Visual acuity may be reduced due to secondary elevation of the sensory retina at the fovea. Occasionally, the lesions may be associated with the formation of subretinal neovascular membranes.

Optic nerve

Sarcoidosis may give rise to the following lesions of the optic nerve:

1. Focal granulomas may involve the optic nerve but do not usually affect visual acuity.
2. Papilloedema is usually secondary to extensive involvement of the central nervous system and it may occur in the absence of other ocular lesions.
3. Neovascularization of the optic nerve head is an occasional complication of retinal branch vein occlusion secondary to severe periphlebitis or, rarely, it may be associated with an optic nerve head granuloma.

Management

Most ocular complications can be treated by topical and/or periocular steroids. Systemic steroids may be necessary in patients with severe posterior segment disease, particularly if the optic nerve is involved. Fundus neovascularization can be treated by laser photocoagulation provided the intraocular inflammation is adequately controlled.

Behçet's disease

Systemic features

Behçet's disease is an idiopathic multisystem disease which typically affects young men from the eastern Mediterranean region and Japan who are positive for HLA-B5. The basic lesion is an obliterative vasculitis probably caused by abnormal circulating immune complexes. The four 'major' features of Behçet's disease are the following:

1. Recurrent oral ulceration is a universal finding and, in the majority of patients, the presenting sign. The aphthous ulcers are painful and shallow with a central yellowish necrotic base. They tend to occur in crops and may involve the tongue, gums, lips and buccal mucosa.
2. Genital ulceration is present in about 90% of patients and is more obvious and troublesome in men than in women.
3. Skin lesions which include erythema nodosum, pustules, cutaneous hypersensitivity, and ulceration.
4. Uveitis.

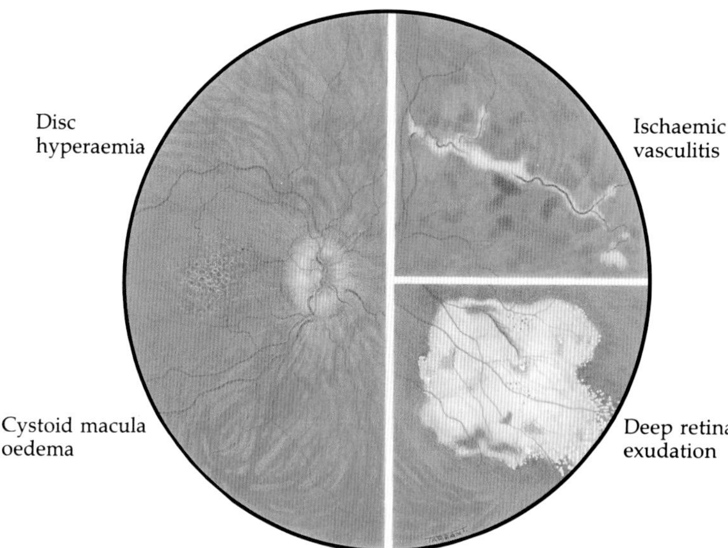

Figure 6.25 *Posterior segment complications of Behçet's disease*

Ocular features

About 70% of patients with Behçet's disease develop recurrent bilateral, non-granulomatous intraocular inflammation. In any individual patients, either anterior or posterior segment involvement can predominate.

Signs

External

Conjunctivitis, episcleritis, and keratitis occur in a few patients.

Slitlamp

Acute recurrent iridocyclitis which may be associated with a transient hypopyon is common.

Vitreous

Vitritis which may be severe and persistent is universal in eyes with uveitis.

Fundus

The posterior segment changes can be of three main types (*Figure 6.25*):

1. Diffuse vascular leakage through the fundus is the most common and persistent finding. It frequently gives rise to diffuse retinal oedema, cystoid macular oedema, and occasionally oedema or hyperaemia of the optic disc.
2. Retinal vasculitis predominantly involving the veins (periphlebitis) is also frequent. In severe cases it caused occlusion of major retinal veins which may subsequently lead to neovascularization.
3. Retinitis, in the form of white necrotic infiltrates of the inner retina which may be associated with intraretinal haemorrhages, may be seen during the active stages of the systemic disease. The infiltrates are usually transient and do not lead to secondary scarring. In some patients, however, acute massive retinal exudation involving the outer retinal layers with associated obliteration of the overlying blood vessels leads to areas of retinal necrosis and atrophy.

Clinical course and complications

The uveitis associated with Behçet's disease has a relatively poor visual prognosis. The acute iridocyclitis may become chronic and lead to phthisis bulbi. Posterior segment involvement may lead to severe attenuation of the retinal vasculature and blindness from secondary optic atrophy (*Figure 6.26*).

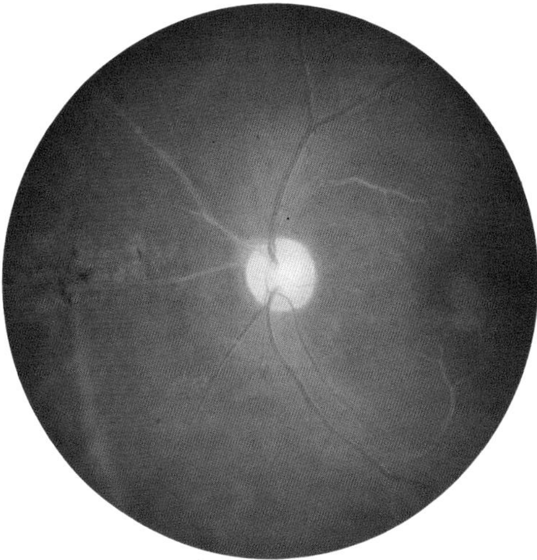

Figure 6.26 *Optic atrophy and vascular occlusion in Behçet's disease*

Management

Initially, the acute anterior uveitis usually responds well to topical steroid therapy. However, posterior segment involvement is frequently unresponsive to systemic steroid medication, although in some cases it is sensitive to chlorambucil.

Vogt–Koyanagi–Harada syndrome

Systemic features

The Vogt–Koyanagi–Harada (V-K-H) syndrome is an idiopathic, multisystem disorder which typically affects pigmented individuals. Japanese patients, in whom the disorder is relatively common, have an increased prevalence of HLA-B22. In order to establish the diagnosis of V-K-H, at least three of the following four groups of signs must be present:

1. *Cutaneous signs:*
   a. *Alopecia* (baldness) occurs in about 60% of patients and is usually confined to small areas.
   b. *Poliosis* (whitening of eyelashes) is also common and usually develops several weeks after the onset of the disease.
   c. *Vitiligo* (patches of skin depigmentation) usually follows the onset of visual symptoms by several weeks.
2. *Neurological signs:*
   a. *Neurological irrigation,* such as headache and stiffness develop simultaneously with ocular involvement.
   b. *Encephalopathy* is less frequent than meningeal involvement. It may be manifest as convulsions, cranial nerve palsies, and paresis.
   c. *Auditory symptoms* include tinnitus, vertigo, and deafness.
   d. *Cerebrospinal fluid lymphocytosis* is present during the acute phase of the disorder.
3. *Anterior uveitis.*
4. *Posterior uveitis.*

Ocular features

Symptoms

These depend on the site of initial involvement. Although both eyes are usually affected, one may become involved several days or weeks before the other.

Signs

Slitlamp

A granulomatous iridocyclitis is present.

Fundus

Posterior segment involvement usually starts with the appearance of a multifocal choroiditis (*Figure 6.27*) which may be associated with disc hyperaemic or oedema. Later, exudative retinal detachments develop which may be either extensive and bullous or relatively flat and confined to the posterior pole.

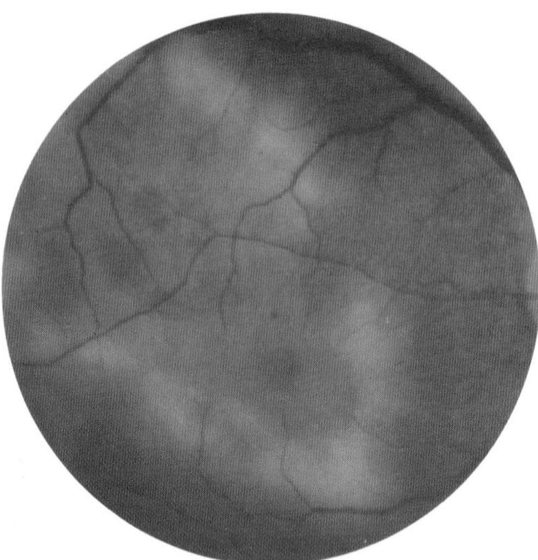

Figure 6.27 *Multifocal choroiditis in Vogt–Koyanagi–Harada syndrome (courtesy of Mr E. Glover)*

Clinical course and complications

Anterior uveitis

This has a chronic course and frequently leads to posterior synechiae, secondary glaucoma and cataract.

Posterior uveitis

The exudative retinal detachments gradually subside either spontaneously or with the help of systemic steroids leaving mottled scars corresponding to atrophy and proliferation of the retinal pigment epithelium. Visual acuity may remain good even with involvement of the macula.

Management

Anterior uveitis is treated vigorously with topical steroids and, if necessary, also with periocular and systemic therapy. The exudative retinal detachments may settle after only a few days of systemic steroid therapy.

Chronic systemic infections

Acquired syphilis

Syphilis is a chronic infection caused by a spirochaete called *Treponema pallidum*. The disease may be acquired or congenital.

Systemic features

Acquired syphilis is a venereal infection which can be divided into four stages.

Primary

This stage occurs between 10 days and 10 weeks following sexual contact. It is characterized by a painless indurated ulcer (chancre) usually located on the genitalia.

Secondary

The hallmark of secondary syphilis, which usually develops between 3 and 6 weeks after the chancre, is the appearance of a macular, papular, or mixed skin rash involving the palms and soles. Other features include malaise, fever generalized lymphadenopathy, condylomata lata, mucous patches and meningitis.

Latent

This follows resolution of secondary syphilis and can be detected only by serological tests.

Tertiary

About 15% of patients with untreated latent syphilis eventually develop tertiary syphilis, although many patients have tertiary syphilis without definite preceding manifestations of the primary and secondary stages. The four types of tertiary syphilis are: meningovascular, tabes dorsalis, general paralysis of the insane (GPI), and gummatous.

Diagnostic tests

FTA-ABS (fluorescent treponemal antibody absorption)

This is a specific test to detect antitreponemal antibodies. Once positive, the test will remain positive throughout the patient's life despite treatment. However, the test is not titratable and is read as: reactive, weakly reactive, or non-reactive.

VDRL (Veneral Disease Research Laboratory)

This is a non-specific reagin test which is useful for screening. It becomes positive shortly after the development of the primary chancre. The test is titratable, but it may become negative after many years in about 40% of patients. It also frequently becomes negative following adequate antisyphilitic therapy.

Ocular features

Syphilis is now a relatively rare cause of uveitis accounting for about 1% of cases. The disease must be suspected in any case of intraocular inflammation that is resistant to treatment with conventional therapy.

Signs

External

A primary chancre may, very occasionally, occur in the conjunctiva. The patient may also have loss of eyebrows and eyelashes (madarosis).

Slitlamp

An iridocyclitis occurs in about 4% of patients with secondary syphilis. The intraocular inflammation is usually acute and it may be granulomatous or non-granulomatous and, unless adequately treated, it becomes chronic. Both eyes are involved in about 50% of cases. In some patients, the iridocyclitis is first associated with the presence of roseolae (*Figure 6.28*) which consist of hyperaemic bright-red spots representing engorged pre-existing superficial vascular loops of the iris. The roseolae may then develop into more localized papules and subsequently into larger well-defined yellowish nodules. Gummas, which are characteristically located at the root of the iris, are extremely rare.

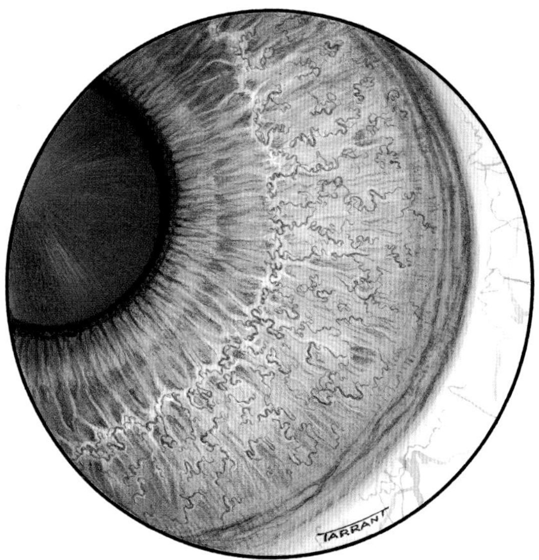

Figure 6.28 *Early roseolae in secondary syphilis*

Fundus

Syphilis can involve the choroid and retina.

Chorioretinitis, which is bilateral in about 50% of cases, is usually either multifocal or diffuse. The former is non-specific but the latter is characterized by a diffuse greyish-yellow exudation which may be most marked in the midretinal periphery and may surround the optic disc. A periarteritis and periphlebitis, similar to that seen in sarcoidosis, may also be present.

Neuroretinitis consists of primary involvement of the retina and optic nerve head and is independent of choroidal inflammation. It occurs usually during secondary syphilis and it may be associated with meningitis. The fundus shows a greyish clouding of the retina due to oedema, most marked at the posterior pole. The optic disc is elevated and its margins indistinct. The retinal veins may be engorged and peripapillary cotton-wool spots or flame-shaped haemorrhages may appear, as well as perimacular waxy exudates.

Clinical course and complications

Chorioretinitis

Unless adequately treated, the intraocular inflammation runs a protracted course. Its healed stage is occasionally characterized by extensive pigmentary changes with perivascular bone spicules similar to those seen in retinitis pigmentosa. These changes may be associated with night blindness and a ring scotoma.

Neuroretinitis

Unless treated with antisyphilitic drugs the disease progresses and the retinal vessels are replaced by white strands, the optic disc becomes atrophic, and areas of hyperpigmentation develop.

Management

Treatment of syphilitic uveitis is as follows: the patient should be hospitalized and a lumbar puncture performed to rule out neurosyphilis. The following antibiotics should be administered if the patient is not sensitive to penicillin:

1. Aqueous crystalline penicillin G, 2–4 $\times$ 10^6 units intravenously every 4 h for 10 days.
2. Aqueous penicillin G procaine, 2–4 $\times$ 10^6 units intramuscularly daily for 10 days.

Oral probenecid 500 mg every 6 h for 10 days should also be administered to elevate and prolong the plasma level of penicillin. Patients who are allergic to penicillin can be treated with oral erythromycin 500 mg four times a day for 15 days.

Tuberculosis

Systemic features

Tuberculosis (TB) is a chronic granulomatous infection caused by either bovine or human tubercle bacilli. The former causes TB by the drinking of milk from infected cattle and the latter is spread by 'droplet infection'. The two main forms of TB are primary and postprimary.

Primary TB

This occurs in subjects not previously exposed to the bacillus. It typically causes the 'primary complex' in the chest (Ghon focus + regional lymphadenopathy) which usually heals spontaneously and causes little if any systemic symptoms.

Postprimary TB

This is due to reinfection or, rarely, recrudescence of a primary lesion, usually in a patient with impaired immunity as from diabetes, systemic steroid therapy, or malnutrition. Clinical features of postprimary TB include fibrocaseous pulmonary lesions, and miliary TB from haematogenous spread to many parts of the body. Theoretically, uveal seeding by live bacilli may occur during the primary and miliary stages giving rise to either caseating nodules or small miliary tubercles.

Diagnostic tests

Examination of sputum

This is for acid-fast bacilli.

Chest X-ray

A chest X-ray compatible with TB is of significance in a patient with uveitis. However, a negative chest X-ray does not necessarily exclude the possibility of TB.

Tuberculin test

This may be useful in the diagnosis of extrathoracic TB. In the United Kingdom, less than 4% of English-born children have a positive test when tested at the age of 12 years. However, no importance can be attached to a positive result in a subject who has either received BCG or who has had TB in the past. A negative test usually excludes the possibility of TB whereas a positive test does not necessarily distinguish between previous exposure and active disease.

Isoniazid test

If TB uveitis is suspected, a therapeutic test is isoniazid 300 mg daily for 3 weeks has been recommended. If this causes a dramatic improvement in the ocular inflammation within 1 or 2 weeks then the diagnosis of TB is highly likely.

Ocular features

TB is now a rare cause of uveitis accounting for only about 1% of all cases. Despite this, it is important not to miss the diagnosis as it is one of the few cases of uveal inflammation which can be cured with specific medication. The possibility of TB is always presumptive and is based on indirect evidence, such as: intractable uveitis which is unresponsive to steroid therapy, negative findings for other causes of uveitis, positive systemic findings for TB and, occasionally, a positive response to the isoniazid test.

Signs

There is no specific finding in TB uveitis and the clinical picture is pleomorphic.

External

Virtually any ocular and periocular structure can be involved including the orbit, skin, conjunctiva and cornea.

Slitlamp

The most common finding is a chronic granulomatous iridocyclitis although occasionally the inflammation is non-granulomatous.

Fundus

TB primarily involves the choroid. The most frequent finding is a focal or multifocal choroiditis. Rarely, a large solitary choroidal granuloma, which may be mistaken for a choroidal tumour, may be present in one eye of a patient with chronic pulmonary TB.

Management

Treatment is with isoniazid 300 mg/day and 10 mg/day of pyridoxine hydrochloride (to prevent peripheral neuritis) combined with one other antituberculous drug such as rifampicin for 12 months. Ocular penetration of isoniazid is very good although some patients become intolerant.

Leprosy

Systemic features

Leprosy (Hansen's disease) has the highest incidence of ocular complications of any systemic disease. The pathogenic agent responsible for leprosy is *Mycobacterium leprae* which has an affinity for skin, peripheral nerves and the anterior segment of the eye. The two types are lepromatous and tuberculoid leprosy. Uveal involvement in tuberculoid disease is less common than in the lepromatous form.

Ocular features

Signs

External

The many lesions of the anterior segment include madarosis, keratitis (due to a combination of trichiasis, lagophthalmos, loss of corneal sensation, and secondary infection), conjunctivitis, scleritis, and episcleritis.

Slitlamp

The complications of anterior uveitis are the most common causes of blindness in leprosy. The uveitis can be of two types: acute and chronic iritis.

Acute iritis is thought to be caused by the deposition of immune complexes in the anterior uvea and it may be associated with systemic symptoms such as fever and swelling of skin lesions. Occasionally, the intraocular inflammation is precipitated by the initiation or withdrawal of anti-lepromatous systemic therapy.

Chronic iritis is due to direct invasion of the anterior uvea by bacilli. A relatively common finding is the presence at the pupillary margin of small glistening 'iris pearls' which resemble a necklace (*Figure 6.29a*). These lesions, which are composed of bacilli within histiocytes, are pathognomonic of lepromatous leprosy. The 'pearls' slowly enlarge and coalesce before becoming pedunculated and dropping into the anterior chamber (*Figure 6.29b*) from which they eventually disappear. Much less common than 'iris pearls' are nodular lepromata which are yellow, globular, polymorphic, single masses which, just like 'iris pearls', may be seen in uninflamed eyes. Eventually, the iris becomes atrophic and the associated formation of holes in the iris stroma may give rise to an appearance similar to essential iris atrophy.

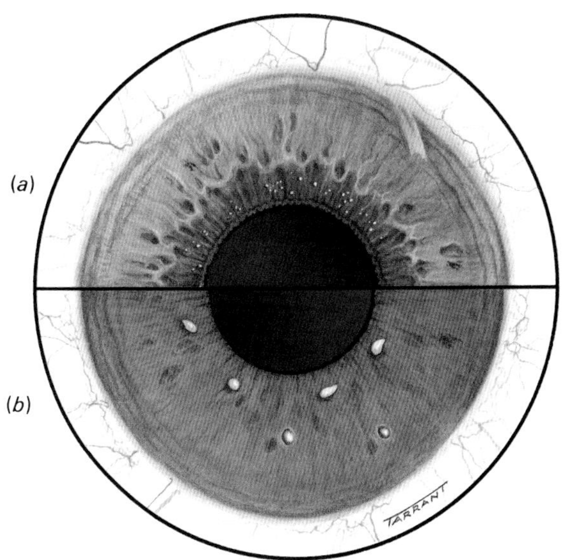

Figure 6.29 *Chronic lepromatous iridocyclitis.* (a) *Small 'iris pearls';* (b) *large 'iris pearls' some of which have dropped into the anterior chamber*

Management

Acute anterior uveitis is treated with topical mydriatics and steroids. By contrast the chronic form is more resistant to conventional therapy. It is thought that this is because it is not a true inflammation, but rather a form of neuroparalytic uveitis caused by early involvement of the iris nerves. Eyes with chronic uveitis usually tolerate surgery for secondary cataracts very well.

Parasitic infestations

Toxoplasmosis

Toxoplasmosis is an infestation by a ubiquitous, obligatory, intracellular protozoan parasite *Toxoplasma gondii*. The cat is the definitive host of the parasite and other animals, such as mice and livestock (cattle, sheep and pigs), as well as humans, are intermediate hosts.

Forms of *Toxoplasma gondii*

The three main forms of the parasite are:

1. The *oocyst* is the spore form which is excreted in cat faeces.
2. The *bradyzoite* is the inactive slowly metabolizing form which is encysted in tissues.
3. The *tachyzoite* (trophozoite) is the proliferating active form which is responsible for tissue destruction and inflammation. It has a particular affinity for neural tissue and causes acute retinitis in humans.

Modes of infestation of humans

Humans can become infested by toxoplasmosis in three main ways.

Ingestion of undercooked meat

It is thought that the most common mode of infestation is by the ingestion of raw meat such as steak tartare or undercooked hamburgers. In this way humans acquire toxoplasmosis by eating the flesh of an intermediate host which contains tissue cysts.

Ingestion of oocysts

This is probably a less common way of human infestation although it is the primary mode of infestation of animal intermediate hosts. Humans may accidentally contaminate their hands when disposing of cat litter trays and then transfer the oocysts onto food. Small children may also become infested by eating dirt (pica) containing oocysts. The oocyst may also be transferred to food by vectors such as flies.

Transplacental

If a pregnant woman develops acute toxoplasmosis, the parasites (tachyzoites) may pass through the placenta to infest the fetus.

Three stages of toxoplasmosis

In humans, toxoplasmosis can be divided into three stages:

1. *Acute.* When ingested by humans, the parasites penetrate the intestinal mucosa, gain access to the blood stream and become disseminated throughout the body. They then enter the cells of the reticuloendothelial system, the brain, the retina, the lungs and striated muscles where they rapidly multiply and cause the acute form of the disease (which is usually asymptomatic). At this stage, the host defence mechanism reacts to the parasite and specific antitoxoplasma antibodies are produced.
2. *Chronic (inactive).* When the acute proliferative phase of toxoplasmosis is curtailed, the parasites form intracellular cysts which contain slowly metabolizing inactive parasites (bradyzoites).
3. *Recurrent.* In some cases the patient's immune mechanism is suppressed, the cyst walls rupture, releasing active and proliferating parasites (tachyzoites) which invade and destroy healthy cells, causing recurrence of the disease.

Diagnostic tests

Dye test (Sabin–Feldman)

This test is based on the fact that live organisms exposed to normal serum take up methylene blue, whereas those exposed to serum containing antitoxoplasma antibodies fail to take up the dye.

Indirect fluorescent antibody test

This test utilizes killed organisms which are exposed to the patient's serum and antihuman globulin labelled with fluorescein and examined under the fluorescent microscope.

Haemagglutination test

In this test, lysed organisms are coated onto red blood cells which are then exposed to the patient's serum. Positive sera cause the red blood cells to agglutinate.

Enzyme-linked immunosorbent assay

In this test, the patient's antibodies bind to an excess of solid-phase antigen. This complex is then incubated with an enzyme-linked second antibody. Assessment of enzyme activity provides the measurement of specific antibody concentration. The test can also be used to detect antibodies in the aqueous humour and the vitreous.

Acute acquired systemic toxoplasmosis

Clinical features

The infestation may present in the following ways.

Subclinical

The vast majority of patients are completely asymptomatic when they acquire the infestation.

Febrile lymphadenitis

In some patients the disease causes a generalized lymphadenopathy, malaise, and headaches. This 'lymphadenopathic' form resembles glandular fever and persists for about 4 weeks.

'Influenza-like'

In a few patients, the acute infestation resembles influenza and is characterized by malaise, headache, inertia, fever, and muscle aching which lasts for about 10 days.

Meningoencephalitis

Very occasionally, acute toxoplasmosis gives rise to convulsions, unconsciousness, fever, and lymphadenopathy.

Exanthematous form

By far the rarest and most serious form of acute toxoplasmosis, which may be fatal, resembles a rickettsial infection and is characterized by fever, chills, a macular rash, and cough.

Congenital systemic toxoplasmosis

Clinical features

Toxoplasmosis is transmitted to the fetus through the placenta when a pregnant woman contracts the acute infestation (which is usually asymptomatic). If the mother is infested before pregnancy the fetus will not be affected. About 40% of infants born to recently infested mothers will acquire toxoplasmosis which may be inactive or active at the time of birth.

Active at birth

The severity of involvement of the fetus varies with the duration of gestation at the time of maternal infestation.

Death. If the infestation is acquired during early pregnancy the fetus may be stillborn.

Severe damage or miscarriage. If the infestation is acquired in midpregnancy, the fetus may be spontaneously aborted or it may have severe brain damage in the form of hydrocephalus or microcephalus.

Convulsions. If the infestation is acquired during late pregnancy, the fetus may suffer from generalized convulsions, paralysis, fever, visceral involvement and chorioretinitis. Skull X-rays may show intracranial calcification (*Figure 6.30*).

The 'three Cs' of congenital toxoplasmosis are convulsions, chorioretinitis, and calcification.

Inactive at birth

Just as in the acquired form, most cases of congenital systemic toxoplasmosis are subclinical. In these children, bilateral healed chorioretinal scars (*Figure 6.31*) may be discovered later in life either by chance on a routine fundus examination or when the child is found to have defective vision.

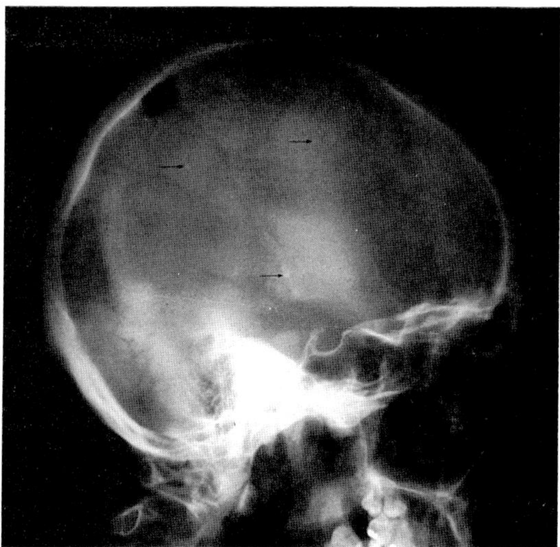

Figure 6.30 *Intracranial calcification in congenital toxopasmosis (courtesy of Dr I. Yentis)*

Recurrent toxoplasmic retinochoroiditis

Recurrence of old healed congenital ocular toxoplasmosis is responsible for between 50% and 75% of all cases of posterior uveitis in the United States and the United Kingdom. The recurrences usually take place between the ages of 10 and 35 years (average age is 25 years) when the cysts rupture and release hundreds of parasites (tachyzoites) into normal retinal cells.

The primary lesion is a retinitis and the inflammatory reaction seen in the choroid, iris, and retinal blood vessels is believed to be immune in origin and not actually due to direct infestation.

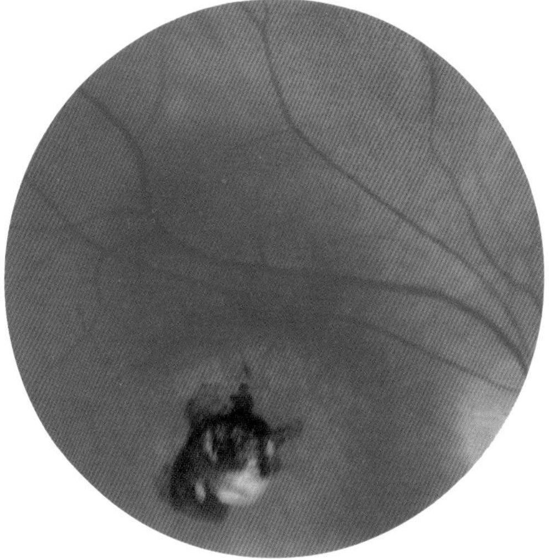

Figure 6.31 *Healed toxoplasma retinochoroiditis involving fovea*

Signs

Slitlamp

The anterior chamber may be quiet or it may occasionally show a non-granulomatous or granulomatous iridocyclitis.

Vitreous

The retinitis is usually accompanied by a severe vitritis which can frequently be traced back to the inflammatory focus. The posterior vitreous may become detached and the posterior hyaloid face covered by inflammatory precipitates comparable to keratic precipitates. In severe cases the vitritis may preclude visualization of the fundus with the direct ophthalmoscope.

Fundus

1. *Focal necrotizing retinitis*, adjacent to the edge of an old inactive pigmented scar ('satellite lesion'), is by far the most common finding. The lesion is most commonly solitary although multifocal retinitis may also occur and occasionally the lesion develops in an area of the retina that appears ophthalmoscopically normal. Although all parts of the fundus are at risk, the retinitis typically affects the post-equatorial fundus. Active retinitis is characterized by a white or yellow-white lesion with fluffy indistinct edges (*Figure 6.32*). It may vary in size from one-tenth to five disc diameters and is associated with an overlying vitreous haze and vitreous condensation.

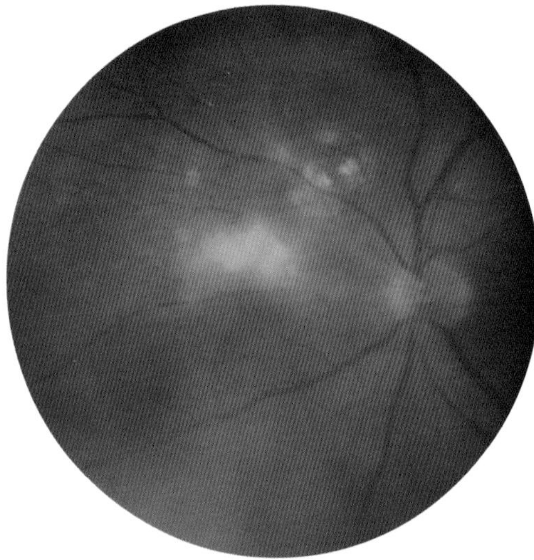

Figure 6.32 *Active toxoplasma retinochoroiditis*

2. *Deep retinitis* is much less common than the superficial retinitis just described. Here the inflammatory focus is located in the deeper retinal layers and appears yellow, has more distinct borders and is not associated with an overlying vitritis. In some cases the deep focus evolves into the more typical lesion within 1 or 2 weeks.
3. *Punctate outer retinal toxoplasmosis* is very rare. It is characterized by multifocal punctate outer retinal lesions with little or no vitreous involvement. The lesions are at the level of the deep retina and retinal pigment epithelium, and appear grey-white in colour. They resolve slowly and recur in a satellite fashion in adjacent areas.
4. *Massive granuloma* is another rare finding characterized by lesions that are greater than 6 disc diameters in size with sharply defined borders and amorphous centres. The granuloma may be difficult to visualize because of extensive involvement of the vitreous.
5. *Papillitis*—not infrequently the active retinitis is located in the juxtapapillary area (Jensen's choroiditis) and occasionally the optic nerve head itself is the primary site of involvement. The papillitis is characterized by a white inflammatory mass on the optic disc with an overlying vitreous haze. Visual acuity is usually relatively good unless the macula or the papillomacular bundle is also involved.

Clinical course and complications

The rate of healing is dependent on the virulence of the organism, the competence of the host's immune system, and the use of antimicrobial drugs. In uncompromised hosts the retinitis heals within 1–4 months and is replaced by a sharply demarcated atrophic scar surrounded by a hyperpigmented border. The vitreous haze gradually clears although vitreous condensation may remain. Resolution of anterior uveitis is a reliable sign of posterior segment healing. In a small percentage of cases, the intraocular inflammation persists for up to 2 years despite intensive antimicrobial and steroid therapy. Fulminating inflammation occurs most commonly when the retinitis is treated with steroids alone or in immunosuppressed patients. After the first attack, the rate of further recurrences is 2.7 per patient.

Eyes with toxoplasmosis may lose vision from various direct or indirect causes.

Direct

1. Involvement of the fovea.
2. Involvement of the papillomacular bundle.
3. Involvement of the optic nerve head (rare).

Indirect

1. Cystoid macular oedema from an extrafoveal lesion.
2. Macular pucker with wrinkling of the fovea may occur in some eyes in which the fovea is not directly involved.
3. Subretinal neovascularization leading to subretinal haemorrhage has been reported.
4. Retinal neovascularization, which may lead to secondary vitreous haemorrhage, is a very rare sequel to the inactive phase.
5. Tractional retinal detachment due to extensive vitreous fibrosis is also rare.
6. Rhegmatogenous retinal detachment due to breaks occurring during active retinitis.

Management

Indications

It is important to realize that not all active lesions need treatment because small peripheral foci may be self-limiting and relatively innocuous (*Figure 6.33*). There are three main indications for medical therapy of active toxoplasma retinitis:

1. A lesion involving or threatening the macula or the papillomacular bundle.
2. A lesion threatening or involving the optic nerve head.
3. A very severe vitritis that has caused severe visual impairment and which subsequently may be responsible for vitreous fibrosis and tractional retinal detachment.

Unless at least one of the criteria apply, treatment is unnecessary because the drugs currently available may have serious side-effects. The following drugs are used in the treatment of toxoplasma retinitis.

Steroids

1. Topical steroids are useful in the management of associated anterior uveitis but they have no effect on posterior segment inflammation.
2. Periocular steroid injections—anterior sub-Tenon's injection can be used to treat severe anterior uveitis and some authorities recommend the use of posterior sub-Tenon's injection in preference to systemic steroids for posterior segment inflammation.
3. Systemic therapy is recommended in eyes with vision-threatening lesions, particularly if associated with severe vitritis.

Antimicrobial drugs

The three drugs currently most widely used in the treatment of ocular toxoplasmosis are clindamycin, sulphonamides and pyrimethamine. Because of its toxicity, pyrimethamine is usually now considered as the third drug of choice in patients unresponsive to clindamycin and sulphonamides.

1. *Clindamycin* is given orally 300 mg four times a day for 3 weeks. However, if used alone it may cause a pseudomembranous colitis in some patients so that the patient should be advised to report any persistent cramps and diarrhoea immediately. Treatment of colitis is with oral vancomycin 500 mg every 6 hours for 10 days. The risk of colitis seems to be very much reduced when clindamycin is used together with sulphonamides, as the latter appears to inhibit clostridial overgrowth which is responsible for the colitis.
2. *Sulphonamides* either in the form of sulphadiazine or the mixed sulphonamide Sulphatriad (if available). A loading dose of 2 g is given orally followed by 1 g four times a day for 3–4 weeks. Rare side-effects of sulphonamides are renal stones and allergic reactions. The Stevens–Johnson syndrome is, very occasionally, triggered off by these drugs.

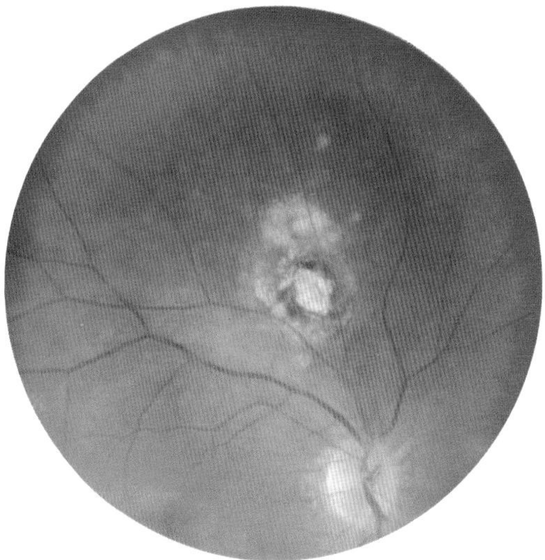

Figure 6.33 *Small 'satellite' active lesions not requiring treatment*

3. *Pyrimethamine* (Daraprim) is a folic acid antagonist which may cause thrombocytopenia and leucopenia. For this reason weekly blood counts should be performed and the drug used only in combination with folinic acid 10 mg/day orally (mixed with orange juice) as this counteracts the toxic side-effects of folic acid antagonists. The loading dose of pyrimethamine is 75–150 mg followed by 25 mg daily for 3–4 weeks. Only a 1-week course should be given if it is combined with clindamycin.

Toxocariasis

Toxocariasis is an infestation caused by a common intestinal roundworm of cats (*Toxocara cati*) and dogs (*Toxocara canis*). Human infestation is due to accidental ingestion of soil or food contaminated with ova which are shed in dog's faeces. Young children who eat dirt (pica) or are in close contact with puppies are at particular risk of acquiring the disease. Surveys have shown that the prevalence of infestation in puppies 2–6 months of age is greater than 80%. In the human intestine, the ova develop into larvae which penetrate the intestinal wall and travel to various organs such as the liver, lungs, skin, brain and eyes. When the larvae die they disintegrate and cause an inflammatory reaction followed by granulation. Clinically, human infestation can take one of two forms: visceral larva migrans and ocular toxocariasis.

Visceral larva migrans

Visceral larva migrans (VLM) is due to severe systemic infestation which usually occurs at about the age of 2 years. It is characterized by a low-grade fever, hepatosplenomegaly, pneumonitis which causes wheezing, and convulsions if the brain is involved. The patient's blood film shows a leucocytosis and a marked eosinophilia. The severity of VLM varies from patient to patient and those with very severe infestation may die.

Diagnostic tests

The ELISA (enzyme-linked immunosorbent assay) test is very useful in identifying patients with toxocariasis as it is highly sensitive and specific. Although, at present, a dilution of 1:8 is considered positive, recent evidence suggests that the presence of any antibody (even in undiluted serum) may be significant.

Ocular toxocariasis

The clinical syndrome of ocular toxocariasis differs markedly from VLM. The patients are otherwise healthy and they have a normal white cell count with absence of eosinophilia. A history of pica is less common, and the average age of patients with ocular involvement is considerably older (7.5 years) as compared with VLM (2 years). The three most common ocular lesions are: a chronic endophthalmitis-like picture, a peripheral granuloma, and a posterior pole granuloma. Other less common manifestations include: a pars planitis-like syndrome, anterior uveitis with or without hypopyon, optic papillitis, localized vitreous abscess and retinal tracks. Only the three most common lesions, all of which are unilateral, will be described in detail.

Chronic endophthalmitis

This usually presents between the ages of 2 and 9 years with leukocoria, strabismus, or a unilateral loss of vision.

Signs

A mild anterior uveitis is common but the cells and flare are rarely more than +2. Posterior synechiae may develop in severe cases. The vitreous shows inflammatory cells and debris. In some cases a peripheral granuloma is seen, while in others the peripheral retina and pars plana are covered by a dense greyish-white exudate similar to the 'snowbanking' seen in pars planitis (*see* later).

Clinical course and complications

The visual prognosis is very poor and some eyes eventually require enucleation. The main causes of visual impairment are:

1. *Retinal detachment.* The vitritis may result in the formation of vitreoretinal membranes which, on contraction, may cause either tractional or rhegmatogenous retinal detachments.
2. *Cyclitic membranes.* In severe cases, retrolental cyclitic membranes form and, by circumferential traction, pull the ciliary body away from the sclera causing ocular hypotony and, eventually, phthisis bulbi.
3. *Macular oedema* may be present in some eyes.
4. *Cataract.*

Posterior pole granuloma

This usually presents between the ages of 6 and 14 years with unilateral loss of vision.

Signs

The granuloma is round, solitary and located either at the macula (*Figure 6.34*) or between the macula and the optic disc. The lesion has a yellow-white colour, is slightly elevated above the retinal surface and is usually between one and two disc diameters in size. Retinal stress lines and distortion of the retinal vasculature are frequent associated findings and occasionally retinal blood vessels disappear into the umbilicated lesion. Occasionally, the granuloma is surrounded by hard yellow exudates.

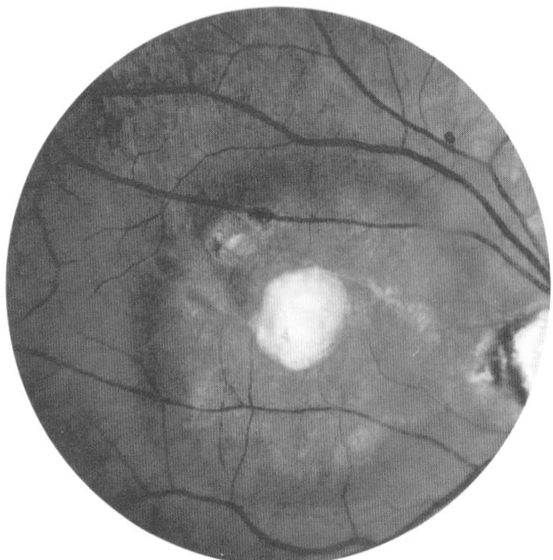

Figure 6.34 *Toxocaral granuloma at posterior pole (courtesy of Mr C. Migdal)*

Clinical course and complications

Once formed, the granuloma is usually stationary and the extent of visual loss is dependent on its location. Rare complications include serous retinal detachment and subretinal haemorrhage.

Peripheral granuloma

This usually presents between the ages of 6 and 40 years. In uncomplicated cases, visual acuity is normal and the lesion remains undetected throughout the patient's life. In other cases, vision becomes impaired either from distortion of the macula or retinal detachment.

Signs

The granuloma is white and hemispherical and is located at or anterior to the equator in any quadrant of the eye (*Figure 6.35*). The lesion is frequently associated with vitreous

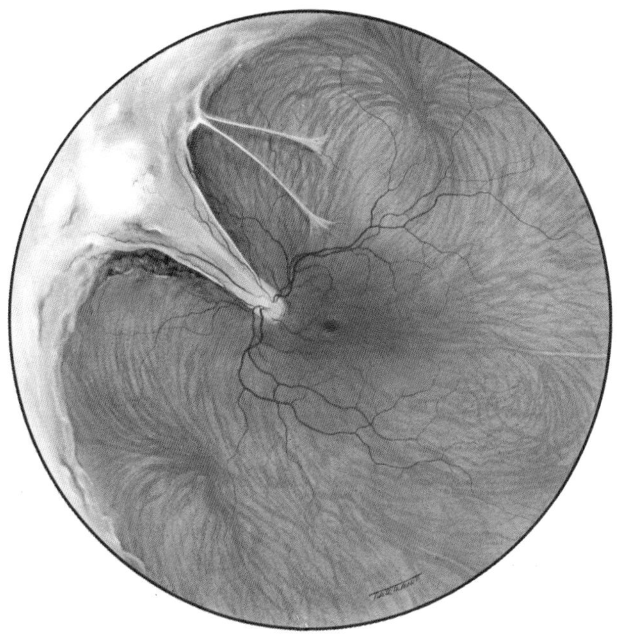

Figure 6.35 Peripheral toxocaral granuloma

bands which extend to the posterior fundus. In severe cases a fold of retina joins the granuloma to the optic nerve head.

Clinical course and complications

In the majority of cases the visual prognosis is excellent. In some eyes with severe involvement, vision may become impaired due to the following tractional phenomena.

Heterotopia of the macula. The traction bands connecting the granuloma with the optic nerve head may pull the blood vessels off the disc towards the lesion and also distort the macula. The 'dragging' of the macula may give rise to a pseudoexotropia.

Retinal detachment. Both tractional and rhegmatogenous retinal detachments may develop as a result of contraction of vitreoretinal membranes and bands.

Management

Nil. The majority of granulomas in quiet eyes require no specific therapy as the disease is 'burnt out'. Patients with dense vitreous membranes should, however, be observed in case they develop retinal detachment.

Medical. Antihelminthic drugs such as thiabendazole and diethylcarbamazine are of minimal value in treating toxocaral endophthalmitis and they may even result in increased inflammation due to death of the toxocara organism. The majority of cases of endophthalmitis will respond well to a course of systemic or periocular steroids.

Scleral buckling surgery. Eyes with rhegmatogenous retinal detachments may respond to conventional scleral buckling procedures.

Pars plana vitrectomy is indicated for the following reasons:

1. Endophthalmitis—eyes with chronic intraocular inflammation unresponsive to medical therapy may benefit from pars plana vitrectomy. Theoretically, the operation removes the larval antigen from the vitreous and makes the eye more quiet.
2. Retrolental cyclitic membrane—this can be excised with a vitreous cutter and the optical pathway restored. In addition, vitrectomy may prevent the subsequent development of phthisis bulbi.
3. Vitreoretinal traction—vitrectomy may relieve vitreoretinal traction involving the macula, as well as correcting tractional retinal detachment.

Prophylaxis

Puppies should be dewormed with piperazine.

Viral infections

Herpes zoster

Herpes zoster ophthalmicus (HZO) is an infection with the varicella-zoster virus of the first division of the trigeminal nerve. It accounts for between 10% and 25% of all dermatomal herpes zoster infections. The incidence of HZO increases with age and the infection is more common and usually more severe in immunosuppressed individuals and those with leukaemia and lymphoma. About 40% of patients with HZO develop an ipsilateral iridocyclitis usually within 2 weeks of the onset of the rash. Those with a vesicular eruption on the tip of the nose, from involvement of the external nasal branch of the nasociliary nerve (Hutchinson's sign), are at particular risk.

Signs

External

The typical rash of HZO is present and the eye is usually injected due to associated conjunctivitis or episcleritis.

Slitlamp

The iridocyclitis is non-granulomatous with small keratic precipitates. The anterior chamber reaction is usually fairly mild with a faint flare and a moderate number of cells, although very occasionally severe iris ischaemia causes hypopyon which may be tinged with blood. *Note:* various forms of keratitis may also be present (*see* Chapter 5).

Fundus

This is usually normal, although a very small minority of cases show a retinitis characterized by yellow retinal exudates, retinal haemorrhages and vascular sheathing.

Clinical course and complications

Unless treated vigorously with topical steroids, the anterior uveitis becomes chronic. The main complications of anterior uveitis are:

1. *Iris atrophy* (*Figure 6.36*). About 20% of cases develop distortion of the pupil followed a few days later by iris atrophy, characterized by sectorial loss of the iris pigment epithelium which can be seen on transillumination. Fluorescein angiography of the iris shows occluded blood vessels at the site of atrophy.

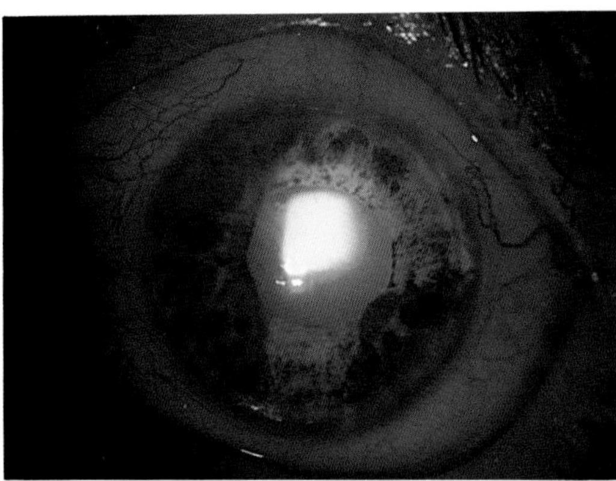

Figure 6.36 *Iris atrophy due to herpes zoster*

2. *Secondary glaucoma*. About 10% of eyes develop a rise in intraocular pressure which can sometimes be abrupt. The pressure elevation is caused by a combination of inflammation of the trabecular meshwork (trabeculitis) and trabecular obstruction by inflammatory debris.
3. *Secondary cataract*. This develops in a few patients with chronic anterior uveitis.
4. *Phthisis*. This is very rare and is caused by severe ischaemia of the ciliary body.

Management

In most cases treatment with topical steroids has to be continued for several months and then tapered very gradually. Systemic therapy is indicated in patients with posterior segment involvement.

Differential diagnosis

Although, in the majority of cases, the diagnosis is straightforward, it is important to remember that severe uveitis may occur in patients with only a slight rash anywhere on the forehead. In these cases, the initial diagnosis of HZO might have been missed and the patient may present several months later with a chronic unilateral iridocyclitis. In order not to miss the diagnosis, always think of the possibility of HZO as a cause of anterior uveitis and perform the following tests:

1. Test corneal sensation as this is frequently diminished following zoster keratitis.
2. Examine the cornea for evidence of nummular lesions which may persist for many months.
3. Transilluminate the iris for evidence of atrophy.
4. Examine the patient's scalp at the hairline for evidence of postherpetic scarring and pigmentation.

Herpes simplex

Controversy exists concerning the occurrence of herpes simplex uveitis in the absence of keratitis. Some authorities believe that this never occurs, while others are of the opinion that some cases of iridocyclitis are due to direct invasion of the anterior uvea by virus particles. In most eyes with herpes simplex keratitis and anterior uveitis, the latter is probably due to a hypersensitivity phenomenon, not associated with the presence of virus particles in the uvea. Herpes simplex anterior uveitis occurs in three different settings.

Associated with dendritic or geographical ulceration

Signs

An active fluorescein-staining corneal lesion is present (*see Figure 5.14*). The associated anterior uveitis is acute and follows the development of keratitis by 1 or 2 days. Secondary glaucoma may occur in severe cases and recurrent attacks may cause iris atrophy. The iris atrophy consists of small, sharply defined, areas with scalloped borders, in contrast to the larger segmental iris atrophy of herpes zoster.

Management

The keratitis is treated with topical antiviral agents (*see* Chapter 5). The pupil should be kept mobile to prevent posterior synechiae, but topical steroids should never be used in the presence of active epithelial keratitis.

Associated with disciform keratitis

Signs

A typical disciform keratitis consists of a central zone of epithelial oedema overlying an area of stromal thickening (*see Figure 5.15*). Some eyes also show folds in Descemet's membrane. The anterior uveitis is usually mild with +1 or +2 aqueous cells. The keratic precipitates are small or medium in size and they are characteristically located on the back of the disciform lesion. Occasionally, the intraocular pressure is elevated despite the presence of only mild uveitis.

Management

Treatment is with mydriatics and topical steroids (*see* Chapter 5).

Unassociated with keratitis

Signs

External

Nil apart from diminished corneal sensation in some patients. In these cases it seemed likely that the patient originally had a corneal lesion, but all traces of the infection had disappeared by the time the diagnosis of uveitis was made and the only possible clue to previous keratitis was diminished corneal sensation. It is also possible that the uveitis is unassociated with a previous attack of keratitis.

Slitlamp

A mild to moderate anterior uveitis is present.

Management

Treatment is with topical steroids and mydriatics. The patient should be examined at frequent intervals to ensure that he does not develop a dendritic ulcer.

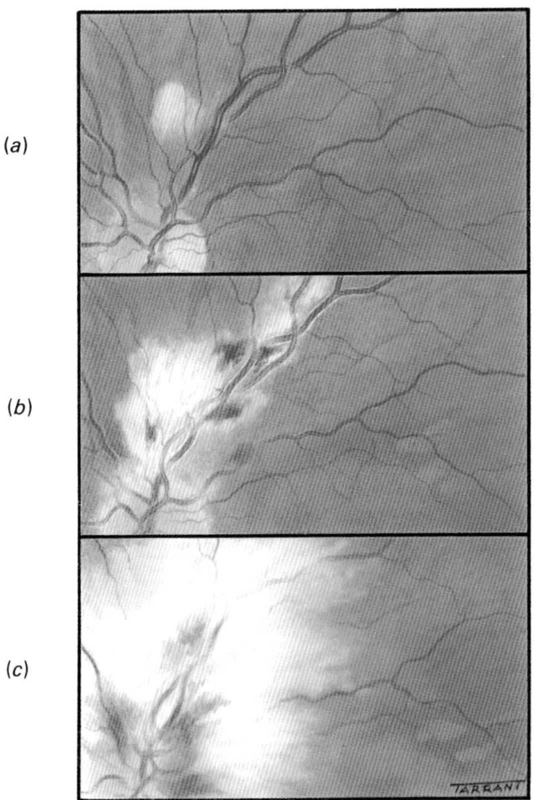

Figure 6.37 *Progression of CMV retinitis*

Acquired cytomegalovirus

Cytomegalovirus (CMV) retinitis is a rare chronic diffuse exudative infection of the retina caused by the CMV virus which occurs, with rare exceptions, in patients with an impaired immune system due to one of the following causes:

1. *AIDS—see* later.
2. *Cytotoxic chemotherapy*—for malignancies, such as leukaemia and lymphoma.
3. *Long-term immunosuppression*—following organ transplantation.

Signs

The earliest findings are white lesions (*Figure 6.37a*), similar to cotton-wool spots. These are followed by the appearance of geographical, yellow-white granular areas which represent areas of full-thickness retinal necrosis and oedema (*Figure 6.37b*) which starts either peripherally (*Figure 6.38*) or at the posterior pole. Later the lesions coalesce (*Figure 6.37c*) and are associated with retinal haemorrhages and vasculitis at their advancing border. The associated retinal nerve fibre haemorrhages may resemble retinal branch vein occlusions. The infective process spreads slowly and relentlessly along the course of the retinal blood vessels to involve the entire fundus (*Figure 6.39*) and leads to total retinal atrophy and, occasionally, also to involvement of the optic nerve. Some eyes develop exudative or rhegmatogenous retinal detachments.

Management

A recent study has shown that treatment with intravenous dihydroxypropoxymethyl guanine causes regression in some cases.

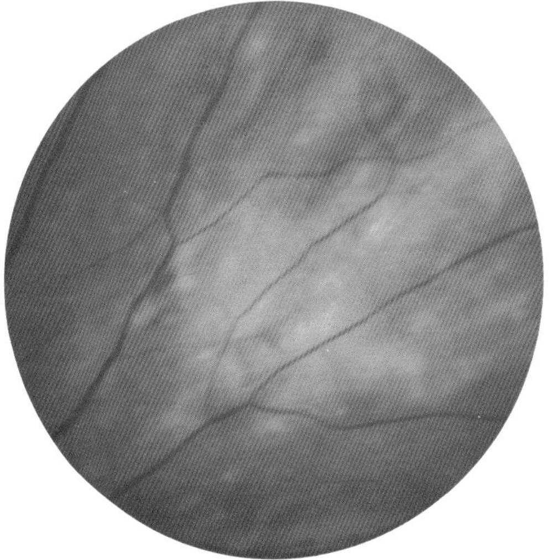

Figure 6.38 *Peripheral CMV retinitis (courtesy of Mr D. Spalton)*

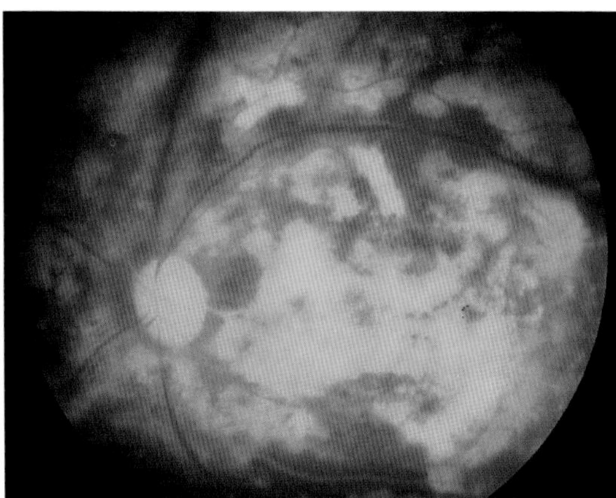

Figure 6.39 Extensive CMV retinitis (courtesy of Mr R. Marsh)

Acquired immune deficiency syndrome

Systemic features

The acquired immune deficiency syndrome (AIDS) is defined by the occurrence of Kaposi's sarcoma or opportunistic infections, or both, in previously healthy persons less than 60 years of age whose immunosuppression has no known cause. The syndrome most commonly affects homosexual men, but it may also affect haemophiliacs, and Haitian immigrants to the United States. Female sexual partners of men with AIDS and infants of women in known risk groups from AIDS are also at risk. The human immunodeficiency virus (HIV) is the causative pathogen of this invariably fatal disease. The opportunistic infections in AIDS include the following:

1. *Protozoa*
   Pneumocystis carinii pneumonia
   disseminated toxoplasmosis
2. *Viruses*
   disseminated CMV
   persistent invasive HSV
   herpes zoster
   Epstein–Barr virus
   adenovirus
3. *Fungi*
   systemic cryptococcosis
   oral and oesophageal candidiasis
4. *Bacteria*
   Mycobacterium avium-intracellulare.

Ocular features

Ocular complications occur in about 75% of AIDS patients.

Signs

External

Kaposi's sarcoma may involve the eyelids and conjunctiva. It appears as a bright-red mass, most frequently in the lower fornix. Skin tumours appear as elevated, non-tender purple nodules.

Severe herpes zoster ophthalmicus can sometimes be an early manifestation of the disease.

Slitlamp

The uveitis due to herpes zoster is usually severe and prolonged in AIDS patients.

Vitreous

A vitritis is present in eyes with CMV retinitis, candida endophthalmitis, and toxoplasmic retinitis.

Fundus

Cotton-wool spots identical to those seen in hypertension and diabetes are seen in about 50% of patients. They are usually transient and resolve over a period of 4–6 weeks. Some patients also develop scattered retinal nerve fibre haemorrhages, usually in the absence of cotton-wool spots. At present the cause of the cotton-wool spots and haemorrhages is unknown.

CMV retinitis (*Figures 6.37, 6.38, 6.39*) occurs in about 30% of homosexual AIDS patients and is the major cause of visual loss. Its appearance is a grave prognostic sign as most patients are dead within 6–8 weeks.

Management

A temporary regression of CMV retinitis has been reported in some patients following intravenous administration of dihydroxypropoxymethyl guanine. Kaposi's sarcoma is sensitive to radiotherapy.

Other viruses

Infectious mononucleosis

Glandular fever is occasionally associated with a mild bilateral transient anterior uveitis and rarely a chorioretinitis.

Influenza

Both influenza and parainfluenza viruses may cause a transient mild bilateral anterior uveitis which usually develops about 2 weeks after an attack of influenza.

Fungal infections

Presumed ocular histoplasmosis syndrome

Histoplasmosis is a fungal infection caused by *Histoplasma capsulatum*. The disease is acquired by inhalation and the organisms pass via the blood stream to the spleen, liver and, on occasion, to the choroid, setting up multiple foci of granulomatous inflammation. In the vast majority of patients, the fungaemia is innocuous and asymptomatic as the organisms disappear after a few weeks. A small minority of patients with severe disseminated systemic histoplasmosis develop an endophthalmitis.

Although the presumed ocular histoplasmosis syndrome (POHS) has never been reported in patients with active disseminated systemic histoplasmosis, the disease has an increased prevalence in areas where histoplasmosis is endemic, such as the Mississippi–Ohio–Missouri river valley. So far *Histoplasma capsulatum* has not been recovered from an eye with POHS.

Note. A syndrome identical to POHS has been reported in the United Kingdom where histoplasmosis does not occur.

Diagnostic tests

Histoplasma skin test

This is positive in about 90% of patients with POHS.

Complement fixation tests

These are of limited value because they usually become negative several years after the original infection.

X-rays

In some patients, plain X-rays will show old calcified granulomas in the lungs and spleen.

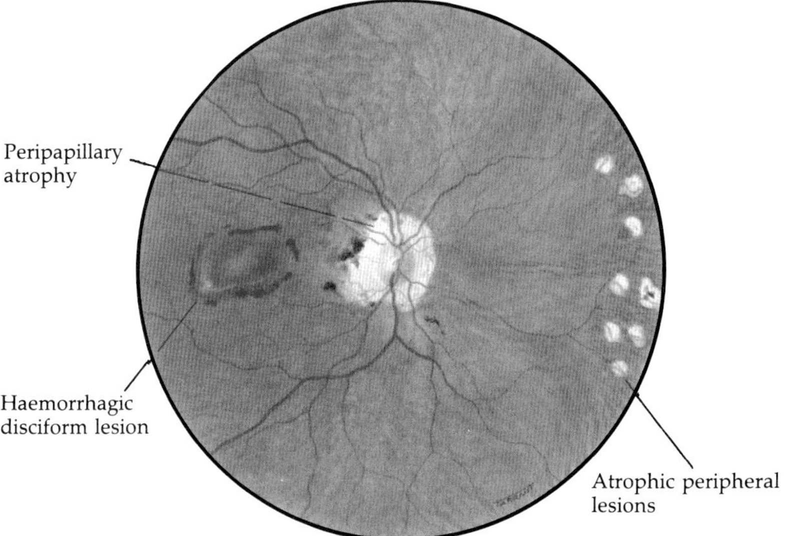

Figure 6.40 *Presumed ocular histoplasmosis syndrome*

Tissue typing

Patients with POHS, particularly if associated with maculopathy, have an increased prevalence of HLA-B7.

Fundus fluorescein angiography

This is extremely useful in detecting early subretinal neovascular membranes.

Clinical features

Symptoms

The POHS is asymptomatic unless it causes a maculopathy. The earliest symptom of macular involvement is metamorphopsia.

Signs

Four types of fundus lesion are observed (*Figure 6.40*):

1. *Atrophic spots* called 'histo spots' consist of roundish, slightly irregular, yellowish-white lesions measuring between 0.2 and 0.7 disc diameter in size. Small pigment clumps may be present within or at the margins of the scars although some spots are not associated with pigmentation (*Figure 6.41*). The lesions are scattered in the mid-retinal periphery and the posterior pole.
2. *Peripapillary atrophy* (*Figure 6.42*) is characterized, most frequently, by a diffuse circumferential choroidal atrophy extending up to 0.5 disc diameter beyond the border of the optic disc. Less commonly, the peripapillary lesions are irregular and punched out, resembling the peripheral spots. In some eyes both diffuse and focal lesions are seen.

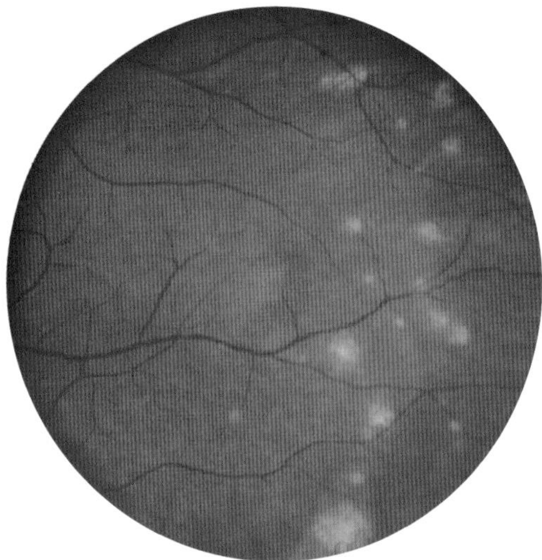

Figure 6.41 Peripheral 'histo spots' in presumed ocular histoplasmosis syndrome

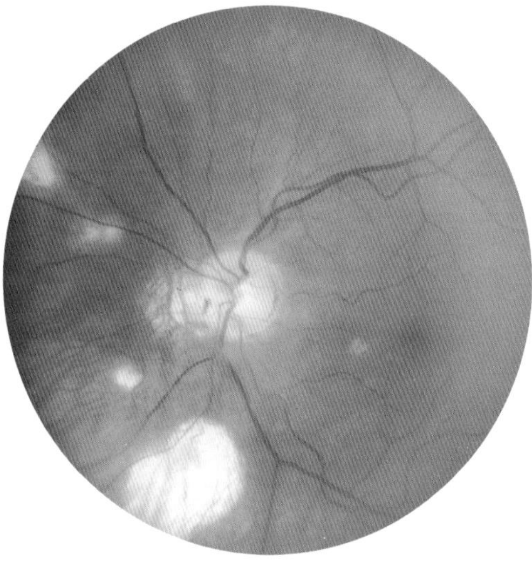

Figure 6.42 Peripapillary atrophy in presumed ocular histoplasmosis syndrome

3. *Linear streaks of chorioretinal atrophy* in the fundus periphery have recently been described.
4. *Subretinal choroidal neovascularization* is a late manifestation of POHS which usually develops between the ages of 20 and 45 years. In the majority of cases, the neovascular membranes are associated with an old macular 'histo spot', although occasionally they develop within a peripapillary lesion. Very rarely the membranes occur in the absence of a pre-existing scar and they have also been reported in association with peripheral 'histo spots'.

   Note that the vitreous is *never* involved.

Clinical course and complications

The clinical course of maculopathy is variable.

Serous detachment

The neovascular membrane may initially leak fluid and give rise to metamorphopsia, blurring of central vision and a positive relative scotoma. Careful slitlamp biomicroscopy with a fundus contact lens shows that the macula is elevated by serous fluid and an underlying focal yellow-white or grey lesion. In some eyes the subretinal fluid absorbs spontaneously and visual symptoms regress.

Haemorrhagic detachment

Frequently, a dark green-black ring develops on the surface of the yellow-white lesion and bleeding occurs into the subsensory retinal space causing a marked drop in visual acuity. In a few eyes, the subretinal haemorrhage resolves and visual acuity improves.

Disciform scar

In some eyes, the initial neovascular complex remains active for about 2 years giving rise to repeated haemorrhages. This finally causes a profound and permanent impairment of central vision due to the development of a fibrous disciform scar at the fovea.

Note. Patients with maculopathy in one eye and an asymptomatic atrophic macular scar in the other eye are likely to develop a disciform lesion in the second eye. They should therefore test themselves every day with an Amsler grid to detect early metamorphopsia.

Management

The mainstay of treatment of subretinal neovascular membranes in eyes with POHS is argon laser photocoagulation. Without treatment, 60% of eyes have a final visual acuity of less than 6/60. Most favourable results of photocoagulation are in eyes with neovascular complexes not closer than 0.25 disc diameter from the centre of the fovea and with intact capillary free zones. Pre-treatment fundus fluorescein angiography is vital in evaluating the extent and location of neovascular membranes.

Candidiasis

Candida albicans, a yeast-like fungus, is a frequent commensal of the human skin, mouth, gastrointestinal tract, and vagina. Candidiasis is an opportunistic infection in which the organism acquires pathogenic properties. Candidaemia, which may result in ocular involvement, occurs in three main groups of patients:

1. Drug addicts may acquire the disease through the use of non-sterile needles and syringes. Not infrequently, they have no obvious evidence of disseminated candidiasis and negative blood and urine cultures for *Candida*. In this group of patients the diagnosis may be missed unless the skin is carefully examined for evidence of injection site scars.

2. Patients with long-term indwelling catheters used for haemodialysis or intravenous nutrition following extensive bowel surgery are at increased risk.
3. 'Compromised host'—these are usually severely debilitated patients with decreased immunity either from an underlying systemic disease (AIDS, malignancies) and/or patients on long-term treatment with drugs such as antibiotics, steroids, and cytotoxic agents.

Signs

Slitlamp

Anterior uveitis is common and may be associated with a hypopyon.

Fundus

Although the initial foci involve the choroid, the organisms soon invade the retina and give rise to a multifocal retinitis manifest as small, round, white, slightly elevated lesions with indistinct borders (*Figure 6.43a*). As the lesions grow they may be associated with haemorrhages which, on occasion, have pale centres (Roth's spots). With appropriate antifungal therapy, the retinal lesions heal leaving behind a faint glial scar or a focal defect in the retinal pigment epithelium.

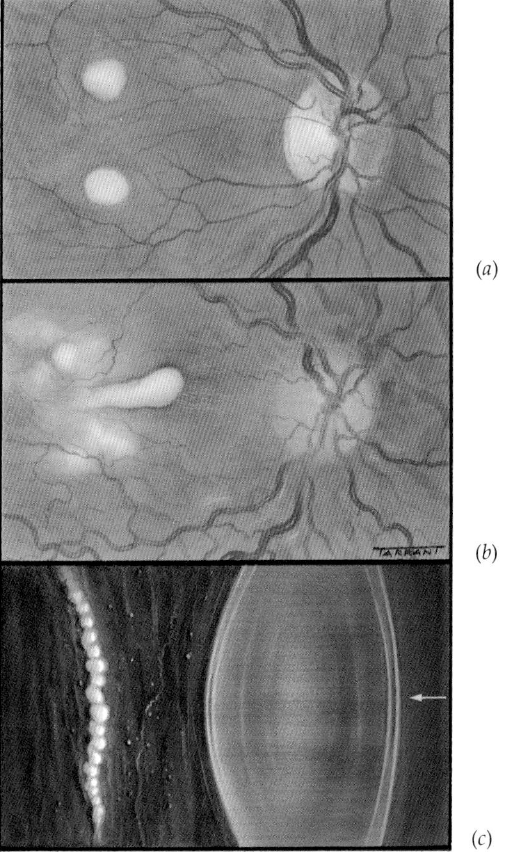

Figure 6.43 *Progression of ocular candidiasis:* (a) *multifocal retinitis;* (b) *extension into vitreous;* (c) *'string of pearls'*

Vitreous

Unless antifungal therapy is instituted, the small retinal lesions enlarge and extend into the vitreous gel giving rise to floating white 'puff-ball' or 'cotton-ball' colonies (*Figure 6.43b*). Several colonies joined together by opalescent strands are referred to as a 'string of pearls' (*Figure 6.43c*).

Clinical course and complications

Some mild cases of retinitis heal spontaneously. Advanced cases are characterized by a vitreoretinal abscess and severe retinal necrosis (*Figure 6.44*). Secondary vitreous organization may give rise to a tractional retinal detachment.

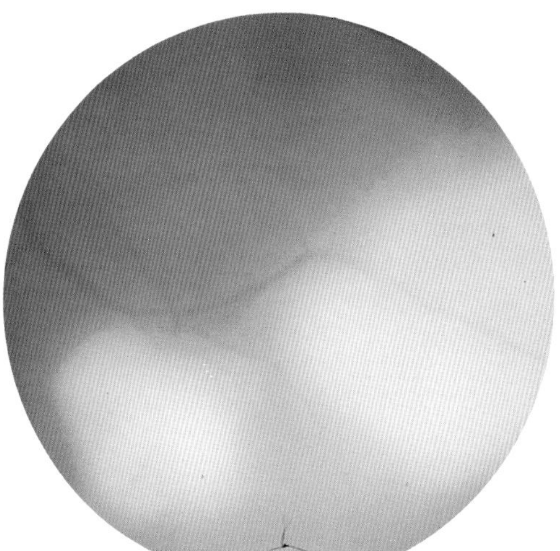

Figure 6.44 *Candida endophthalmitis (courtesy of Mr R. Marsh)*

Medical treatment

In the past, amphotericin B was the mainstay of therapy for ocular candidiasis. However, newer and less toxic drugs are now available which can be given orally. Initial treatment should be with a combination of 5-fluorocytosine (flucytosine) 150 mg/kg per day and ketoconazole 200 mg/kg per day for 3 weeks. Alternative therapy in resistant cases is intravenous amphotericin B in 5% dextrose given over a period of several days until a cumulative dose of 200 mg has been reached. The initial dose is 5 mg/day and after a few days this can be increased to 20 mg/day.

Pars plana vitrectomy

Cases with moderate to severe vitreous involvement (endophthalmitis) are best treated by pars plana vitrectomy and injection of 5 μg of amphotericin B into the central vitreous cavity. At the time of vitrectomy, smears and cultures should be taken to confirm the diagnosis and test the sensitivity of the organisms to antifungal agents.

Common idiopathic specific uveitis syndromes

Fuchs' uveitis syndrome

Fuchs' uveitis syndrome (FUS) or Fuchs' heterochromic cyclitis is a chronic, non-granulomatous anterior uveitis which has an insidious onset. It typically affects one eye of a middle-aged adult, although it can also occur during childhood and may very occasionally be bilateral. Although FUS accounts for about 2% of all cases of uveitis, it is probably misdiagnosed and overtreated more than any other uveitis entity. The heterochromia (difference in iris colour) may be absent in some patients or it may be difficult to detect, particularly in brown-eyed individuals, unless the patient is examined in daylight with undilated pupils.

Symptoms

The vast majority of patients are asymptomatic until the development of secondary cataract. A few patients complain of vitreous floaters and some notice a colour difference between the two eyes. Not infrequently the condition is detected by chance.

Signs
Slitlamp

Cornea. KPs are characteristic and possibly pathognomonic. They are small, round or stellate, grey-white in colour and are scattered throughout the corneal endothelium (*Figure 6.45*). They may come and go but they never become confluent or pigmented. Feathery fibrin filaments may be seen in between the KPs.

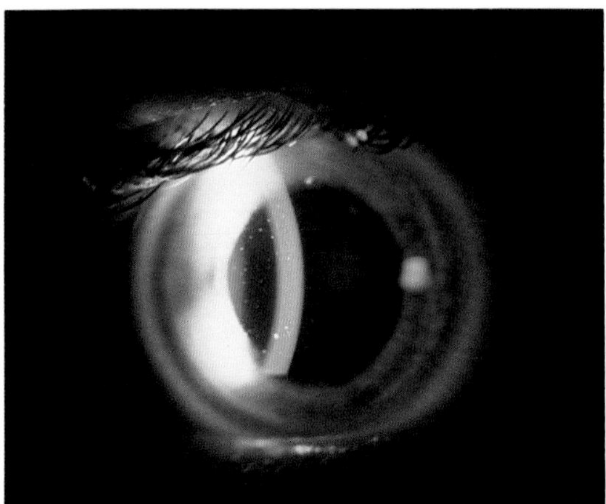

Figure 6.45 *Keratic precipitates in FUS*

Aqueous humour. A faint flare and cells (never more than +2) are usually present.

Iris:

1. Posterior synechiae are invariably *absent.*
2. Atrophy (*Figure 6.46*)—the typical findings are diffuse stromal atrophy which may be associated with patchy atrophy of the posterior pigment layer of the iris. In early cases the only abnormal finding is a loss of iris crypts. More advanced stromal atrophy makes the affected iris appear dull with loss of detail giving rise to a 'washed out' appearance, particularly in the pupillary zone. The patchy atrophy of the posterior pigment layer can be detected on iris transillumination (*Figure 6.47*) and gaps in pigmented pupillary frill make the border of the pupil appear moth-eaten. The normal radial iris blood vessels appear prominent due to lack of stromal support.
3. Heterochromia—most frequently the affected eye is hypochromic although this is an inconsistent feature. In some patients it may be hyperchromic, while in others heterochromia is absent. In a small proportion of cases the heterochromia is congenital. The factors determining the degree of heterochromia are the degree of atrophy of the stroma and posterior pigment layer, as well as the patient's natural iris colour. In some patients with predominantly stromal atrophy, the posterior pigmented layer shows through and becomes the dominant pigmentation so that the eye becomes hyperchromic. In general, a brown eye becomes less brown and blue eye assumes a more saturated blue colour.
4. Koeppe nodules are seen occasionally.

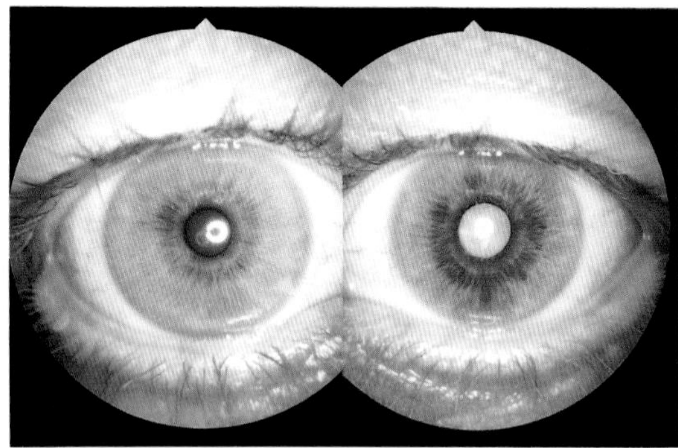

Figure 6.46 *Left eye: FUS with secondary cataract. Right eye: normal eye for comparison*

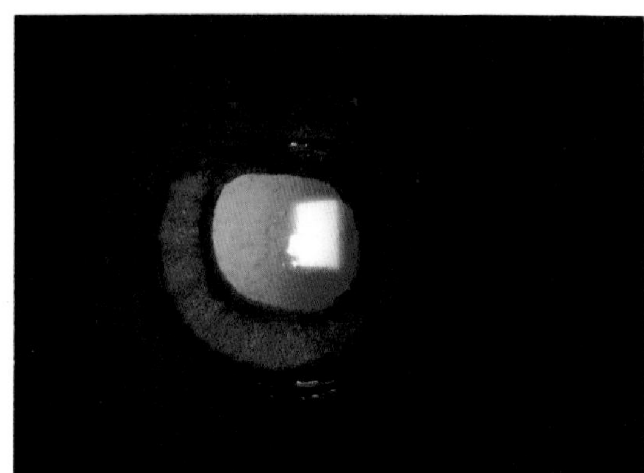

Figure 6.47 *Iris atrophy in FUS seen on iris transillumination*

5. Rubeosis is a fairly common finding manifest as fine irregular neovascularization on the iris surface. These vessels are more fragile than normal iris vessels, and they may bleed when the pressure in the anterior chamber is suddenly reduced, as with paracentesis.
6. Enlarged pupil—atrophy of the iris sphincter may make the pupil irregular and larger than its fellow.

Vitreous

A small number of cells and stringy opacites are common.

Gonioscopy

The angle may be normal or show the following abnormalities.

Neovascularization characterized by the presence of fine radial twig-like vessels in the chamber angle is common (*Figure 6.48*). These vessels are probably responsible for the filiform haemorrhages which develop with anterior chamber paracentesis 180° away from the puncture site (Amsler's sign).

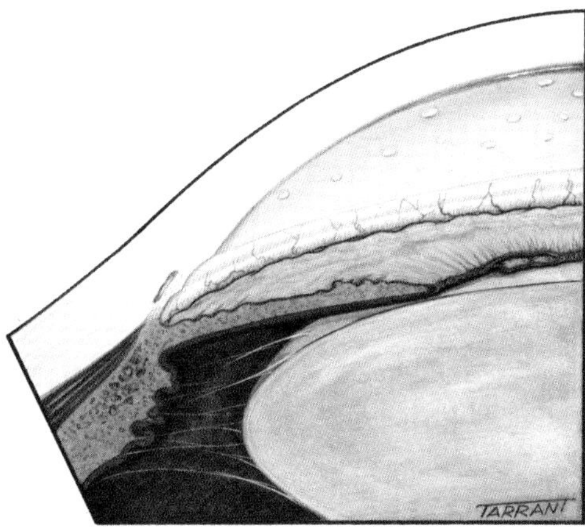

Figure 6.48 *Angle blood vessels in Fuchs' uveitis syndrome*

Membrane. An abnormal membrane which obscures the crisp angle details may be present in the angle.

Peripheral anterior synechiae. Small, non-confluent, irregular peripheral anterior synechiae are seen in some eyes.

Clinical course and complications

FUS runs a chronic course lasting many years. The two main complications are cataract and glaucoma both of which may be related to the inadvertent use of topical steroids in some patients.

Cataract

This is extremely common and does not differ from that associated with other types of anterior uveitis. The results of cataract surgery are usually good, although in some cases the operation is complicated by bleeding. Short-term results of posterior-chamber intraocular lens implantation have been encouraging.

Glaucoma

This is by far the most serious threat to the patient's vision and is frequent when the follow-up period is prolonged. Initially, the elevation of intraocular pressure is intermittent before becoming chronic. The glaucoma is usually of the open-angle type and is thought to be caused by trabecular sclerosis. As already mentioned, fine rubeosis and peripheral anterior synechiae do not necessarily correlate with the presence of raised intraocular pressure. The glaucoma usually becomes resistant to medical therapy and filtration surgery has only a moderate degree of success.

Management

In the vast majority of cases, treatment with topical steroids produces no objective improvement. Mydriatics are unnecessary as posterior synechiae do not develop. However, the patient should be examined at 4–6-monthly intervals in order to detect glaucoma.

Intermediate uveitis

Intermediate uveitis consists of three uveitis syndromes: pars planitis, chronic cyclitis, and senile vitritis. They are all characterized by cells in the vitreous, absent or minimal anterior uveitis, and the absence of a focal fundus lesion, although some eyes have a mild peripheral retinal periphlebitis.

Pars planitis

Pars planitis accounts for about 8% of all cases of uveitis. It is an insidious chronic idiopathic intraocular inflammation which typically affects a child or a young adult.

Although both eyes are affected in about 80% of cases, the severity of involvement is frequently asymmetrical.

Symptoms

The presenting symptom is usually floaters, although occasionally the patient presents with impairment of central vision due to macular oedema. In some cases the condition is diagnosed by chance.

Signs

Slitlamp

The anterior chamber may be quiet or it may show a slight flare, a few cells and several small keratic precipitates. Posterior synechiae, however, are absent.

Vitreous

In early cases cells are seen in the anterior vitreous. Later they assume a sheet-like configuration and small gelatinous exudates ('snowballs' or 'cotton-balls') appear (*Figure 6.49*). Posterior vitreous detachment is common.

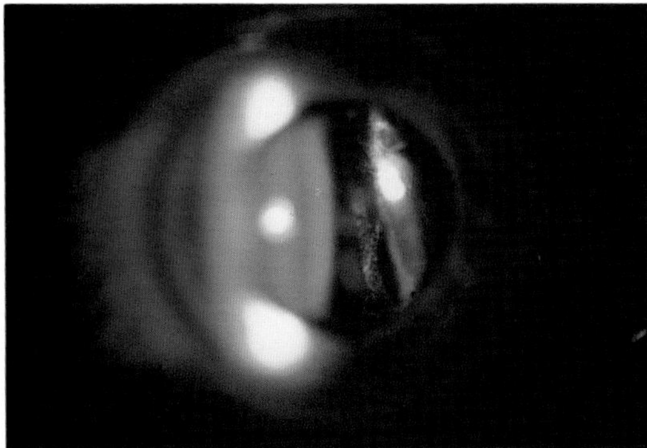

Figure 6.49 *'Snowball' vitreous opacities in pars planitis*

Pars plana and peripheral retina

A mild peripheral vasculitis with sheathing of the terminal venules is common. The hallmark of pars planitis is the presence of a grey-white plaque involving the inferior pars plana (*Figure 6.50*). The plaque which is referred to as 'snowbanking' can be seen only with indirect ophthalmoscopy and scleral indentation. In advanced cases, the plaque extends nasally and towards the temporal periphery as well as posteriorly to cover the peripheral retina.

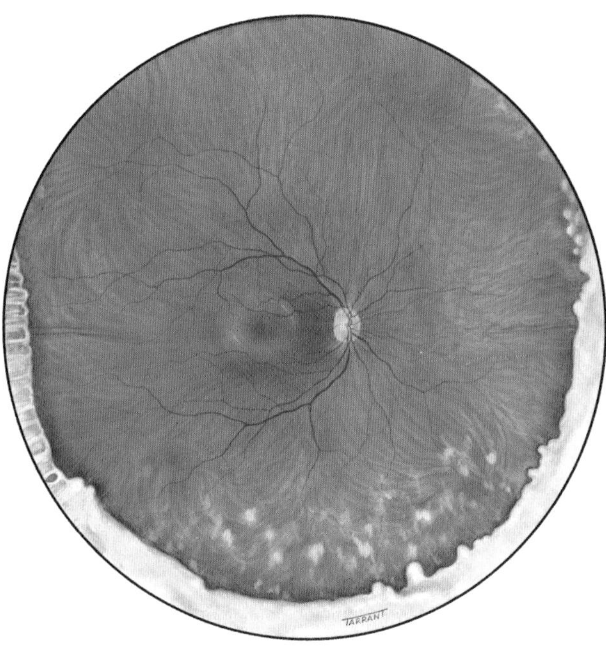

Figure 6.50 *Pars planitis*

Clinical course and complications

The clinical course is variable. A few patients have a single low-grade self-limiting episode lasting several months. The majority, however, have a chronic smouldering course lasing several years which may be associated with subacute exacerbations and incomplete remissions. Despite this, the visual prognosis in the majority of patients is relatively good. The three main vision threatening complications are: cystoid macular oedema, cataract and tractional retinal detachment.

Cystoid macular oedema

Clinically, early macular oedema appears as a loss of the foveal reflex with a wet appearance of the posterior pole associated with many glistening highlights reflected from the irregularly thickened retina. If the oedema becomes chronic, cystoid changes develop which may subsequently lead to a permanent impairment of visual acuity from lamellar hole formation (*see Figure 11.42*).

Cataract

As would be expected, secondary lens opacities tend to develop more frequently in eyes with severe and prolonged inflammation.

Tractional retinal detachment

In advanced cases, the pars plana exudate becomes vascularized from the ciliary body. The contraction of fibrovascular tissue may lead to tractional retinal detachment and vitreous haemorrhage, as well as 'dragging' of the vessels from the optic disc and heterotopia of the macula. Very rarely, a massive vascularized exudate proliferates onto the posterior lens capsule and forms a cyclitic membrane.

Management

It is important not to overtreat this condition. The main indication for treatment is a visual acuity of less than 6/9 due to chronic cystoid macular oedema. Most cases can be controlled and visual acuity improved by repeated posterior sub-Tenon steroid injections of methylprednisolone (Depomedrone). The necessity for repeated injections is governed by the patient's visual acuity and not the severity of vitritis. Systemic steroids can be used in the event of resistance to periocular injections. In severe steroid-resistant cases, cytotoxic agents may be of benefit.

Chronic cyclitis

Clinically, the only difference between pars planitis and chronic cyclitis is the absence of 'snowbanking' in the latter. It has been postulated that chronic cyclitis may be a forerunner or a milder form of pars planitis. Treatment is the same as for pars planitis.

Senile vitritis

This occurs in elderly patients who present with a vitritis, with absence of 'snowbanking'. In contrast to pars planitis, the cystoid macular oedema responds poorly to treatment.

Juvenile chronic iridocyclitis

Although juvenile chronic arthritis (JCA) is the most common systemic association of chronic iridocyclitis in children, the vast majority of patients with juvenile chronic iridocyclitis are otherwise healthy. However, as in the case of chronic iridocyclitis in patients with JCA, about 75% of patients with idiopathic juvenile chronic iridocyclitis are girls. Since the onset of intraocular inflammation is frequently insidious and asymptomatic, the majority of cases are not diagnosed until visual acuity is reduced from complicated cataract or the parents notice a white patch on the cornea due to band keratopathy (*Figure 6.51*). In a small number of cases the uveitis is detected by chance.

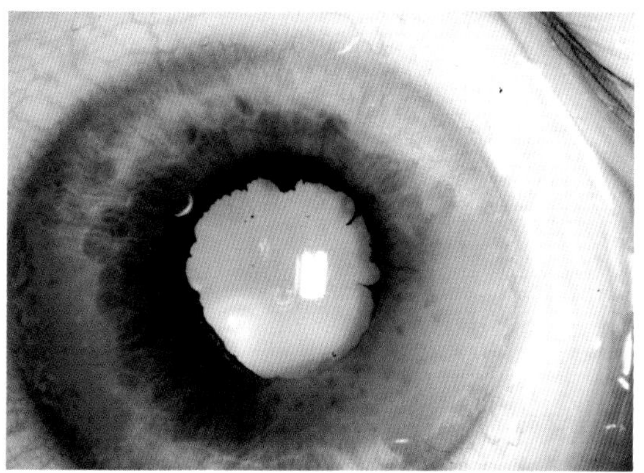

Figure 6.51 *Band keratopathy and cataract in idiopathic juvenile chronic iridocyclitis*

Acute anterior uveitis in young adults

Although ankylosing spondylitis is the most common systemic association of acute anterior uveitis, many patients have no underlying systemic disease, although about 45% are carriers of HLA-B27. The risk to HLA-B27 negative patients (particularly females) of subsequently developing ankylosing spondylitis is very small, although some HLA-B27 positive patients (particularly males) will subsequently develop the disease.

Rare idiopathic specific uveitis syndromes

Sympathetic uveitis

Sympathetic uveitis (ophthalmitis) is a very rare, *bilateral*, granulomatous panuveitis which occurs after accidental penetrating ocular trauma (usually associated with uveal prolapse) or, less frequently, following intraocular surgery. The traumatized eye is referred to as the 'exciting eye' and the fellow eye which also develops uveitis is called the 'sympathizing eye'. Sixty-five per cent of cases of sympathetic uveitis occur between 2 weeks and 3 months after injury and 90% of cases occur within the first year.

Symptoms

The prodromal symptoms in the 'sympathizing eye' are photophobia, and blurring of vision due to loss of accommodation.

Signs

External

The 'exciting' eye shows evidence of the initial insult and is frequently excessively red and irritable.

Slitlamp

Since the inflammation starts in the ciliary body, the earliest features in the 'sympathizing eye' are cells in the retrolental space. As the inflammation becomes more severe and chronic, both eyes show Koeppe nodules, mutton fat keratic precipitates and iris thickening. Unless treated early with mydriatics, posterior synechiae form very readily.

Fundus

Small, deep, yellow-white spots corresponding to Dalen–Fuchs' nodules are seen scattered throughout both fundi. Oedema of the optic nerve head and subretinal oedema are also frequent features.

Note. Very occasionally the inflammation starts in the posterior segment, but irrespective of the initial site the eventual outcome is a panuveitis.

Clinical course and complications

In a few cases, the uveitis has a relatively mild and self-limited course. In the majority, however, the intraocular inflammation persists for years and may lead to cataract, glaucoma, and eventual blindness from phthisis bulbi.

Management

In the vast majority of cases, enucleation (not evisceration) within 2 weeks of the injury will prevent sympathetic uveitis. It also seems likely that enucleation of the 'exciting' eye within 2 weeks of the onset of sympathetic uveitis favourably affects the eventual prognosis of the 'sympathizing' eye. The intraocular inflammation should be vigorously treated with topical, periocular and systemic steroids. Once the uveitis is controlled, steroid therapy can be gradually tapered but any acute exacerbations should be treated intensively. In severe steroid-resistant cases, cytotoxic agents, such as chlorambucil and cyclophosphamide, may be required.

Eales' disease

Eales' disease is an idiopathic peripheral periphlebitis which typically affects both eyes of a young male. The diagnosis should be made only after other causes of retinal periphlebitis have been excluded.

Symptoms

The presenting feature is usually a sudden blurring of vision due to vitreous haemorrhage.

Signs

Initially the small peripheral retinal venules show sheathing. The periphlebitis then extends more posteriorly and may be associated with peripheral retinal neovascularization.

Clinical course and complications

Advanced cases are characterized by massive proliferative retinopathy with extensive retinal and vitreous haemorrhage (*Figure 6.52*) and occasionally tractional retinal detachment. Some eyes also develop rubeosis iridis, neovascular glaucoma, and cataract.

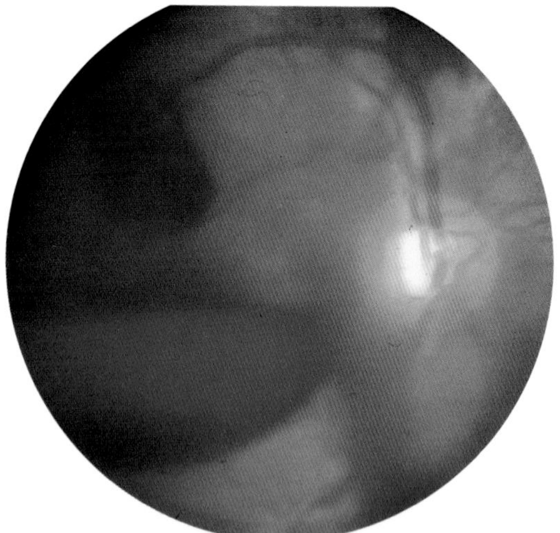

Figure 6.52 *Preretinal and vitreous haemorrhage in advanced Eales' disease (courtesy of Mr P. Rosen)*

Management

Treatment is unsatisfactory. In some cases, laser panretinal photocoagulation may be effective in eliminating areas of retinal ischaemia and thereby induce regression of neovascular tissue. Eyes with persistent vitreous haemorrhage or tractional retinal detachment may benefit from pars plana vitrectomy.

Acute posterior multifocal placoid pigment epitheliopathy

Acute posterior multifocal placoid pigment epitheliopathy (APMPPE) is a rare idiopathic disease which typically affects both eyes of a young adult. About 50% of patients have a prodromal influenza-like illness which may be associated with erythema nodosum. The retinal pigment epithelium has been implicated as the primary site of involvement, although it has also been suggested that the disease might represent a 'vasculopathy' of the choriocapillaris.

Symptoms

The initial symptom is a subacute unilateral impairment of central vision. Within a few days the fellow eye usually becomes similarly involved.

Signs

The typical lesions consist of deep, placoid, cream-coloured or grey-white areas involving the postequatorial retina and posterior pole (*Figure 6.53*). A few eyes also develop vascular sheathing and disc oedema as well as serous detachment of the sensory retina. Within a few days the fellow eye shows similar changes. On fundus fluorescein angiography, the acute lesions show early blockage of background choroidal fluorescence (*Figure 6.54, left*) with late staining (*Figure 6.54, right*).

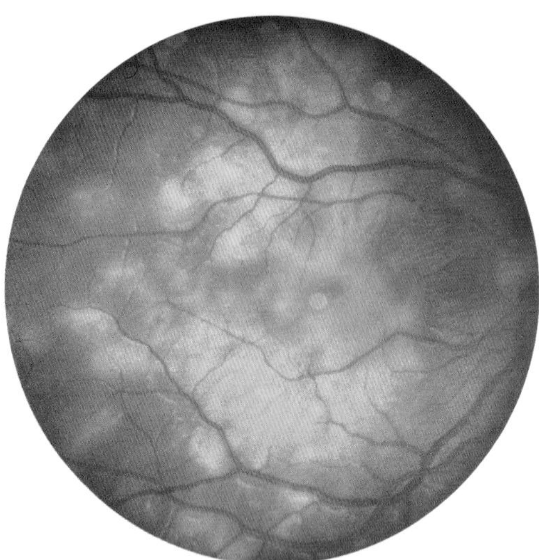

Figure 6.53 *APMPPE: active stage*

Clinical course and complications

In the vast majority of cases, the placoid lesions and vitritis resolve within a few weeks, and visual acuity returns to normal or near normal despite the presence of residual multifocal areas of depigmentation and clumping involving the retinal pigment epithelium (*Figure 6.55*). In a few cases visual acuity does not improve but recurrences do not occur.

Management

There is no effective treatment.

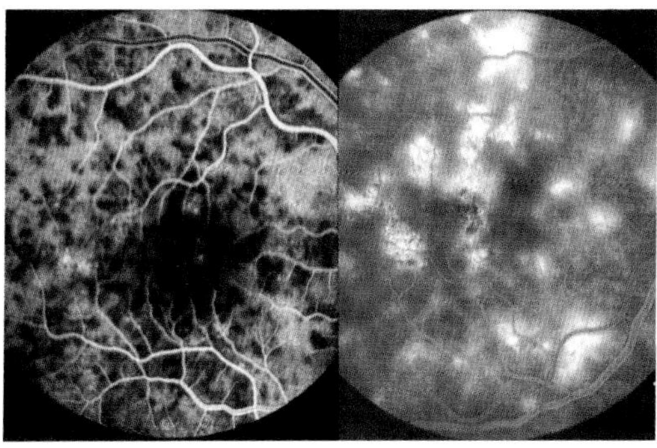

Figure 6.54 Fundus fluorescein angiogram in APMPPE. Left: early phase; right: late phase (courtesy of Professor A. C. Bird)

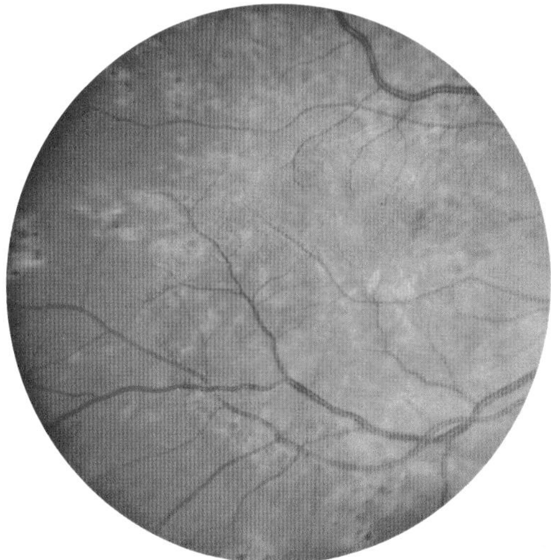

Figure 6.55 Changes in retinal pigment epithelium following resolution of APMPPE

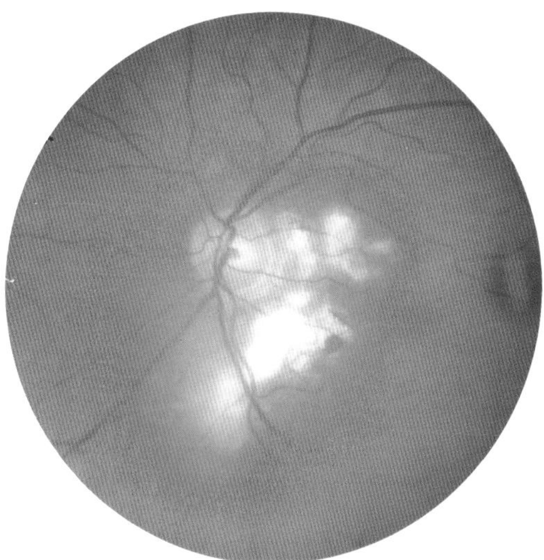

Figure 6.56 Active serpiginous choroidopathy

Serpiginous choroidopathy

Serpiginous (geographical) choroidopathy is a rare, idiopathic, recurrent disease of the retinal pigment epithelium and choriocapillaris which typically affects patients between the fourth and sixth decades of life. Involvement is bilateral although its extent is frequently asymmetrical.

Symptoms

The patient is asymptomatic unless the fovea is involved.

Signs

The chorioretinal lesions usually start around the optic disc (*Figure 6.56*) and spread outwards in all directions. The acute lesions consist of cream-coloured opacities with hazy borders at the level of the retinal pigment epithelium. They persist for a few weeks, eventually becoming lighter in colour and over the subsequent months they become inactive, leaving scalloped 'punched out' areas of retinal pigment epithelial and choroidal atrophy. Large choroidal blood vessels in the base of an area of atrophy frequently are the only visible remnants of the choroid. Fresh acute lesions then usually arise as extensions from old inactive scars.

Clinical course and complications

Successive attacks result in pseudopodal extension of the destructive process peripherally from the peripapillary area in an irregular, convoluted, snake-like manner. Involvement of the fovea causes a profound and permanent impairment of central vision (*Figure 6.57*). Eyes in which the fovea is bypassed are not always safe from future foveal involvement, as occasionally the lesions begin in an extrapapillary location and subsequently spread centrally towards the optic disc. Subretinal neovascularization occurs in some cases.

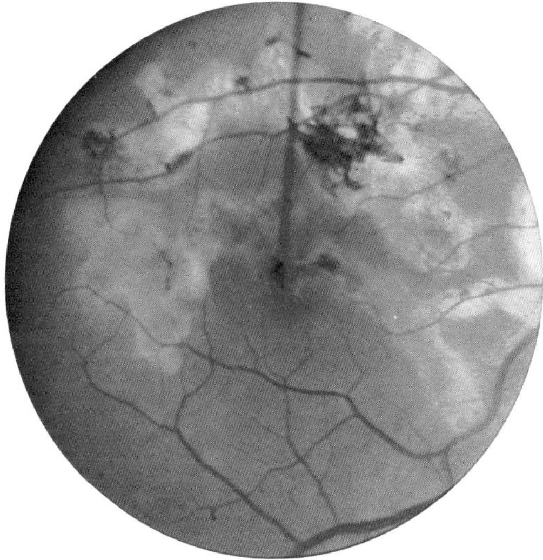

Figure 6.57 Involvement of fovea by serpiginous choroidopathy (courtesy of Professor A. C. Bird)

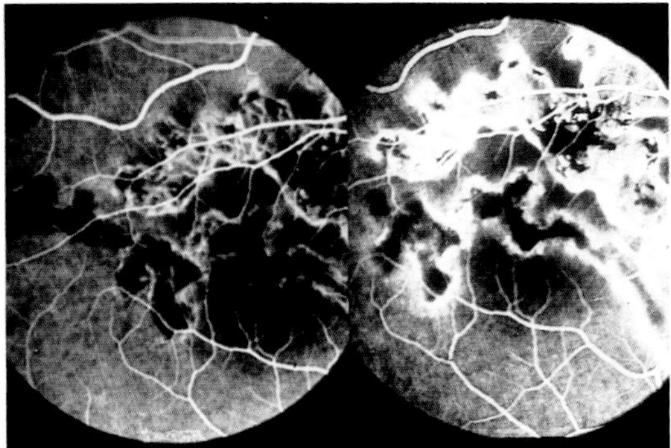

Figure 6.58 Fundus fluorescein angiogram in serpiginous choroidopathy. Left: early phase; right: late phase (courtesy of Professor A. C. Bird)

On fundus fluorescein angiography, the old inactive lesions show early hypofluorescence due to decreased background choroidal fluorescence from atrophy of the choriocapillaris (*Figure 6.58, left*). However, later there is hyperfluorescence at the margins of the atrophic areas due to diffusion of dye from the bordering normal choriocapillaris (*Figure 6.58, right*) and, in very late pictures, the atrophic areas themselves are diffusely hyperfluorescent as the dye stains the sclera and fibrous tissue.

Management

There is no effective treatment.

Birdshot retinochoroidopathy

Birdshot retinochoroidopathy (vitiliginous retinochoroiditis) is a very rare, idiopathic, bilateral, chronic, multifocal choroidopathy and vasculopathy. It typically affects healthy middle-aged individuals who are positive for HLA-A29 and is more common in women than in men.

Symptoms

The initial symptoms are either vitreous floaters or, less commonly, blurring of central vision due to macular oedema.

Signs

The postequatorial regions of both fundi show varying numbers of flat creamy-yellow spots due to focal hypopigmentation of the choroid and retinal pigment epithelium (*Figure 6.59*). The diameter of each lesion is between half to one disc and their borders are not sharply demarcated. The retinal vessels are undisturbed as they pass over the lesions and the larger choroidal vessels can be seen within each individual lesion. Although initially the spots do not involve the macula, later they may become more confluent and spread to the macula. After a few weeks or months, the individual spots evolve into more atrophic white depigmented lesions which are more circumscribed but which are not associated with secondary hyperpigmentation.

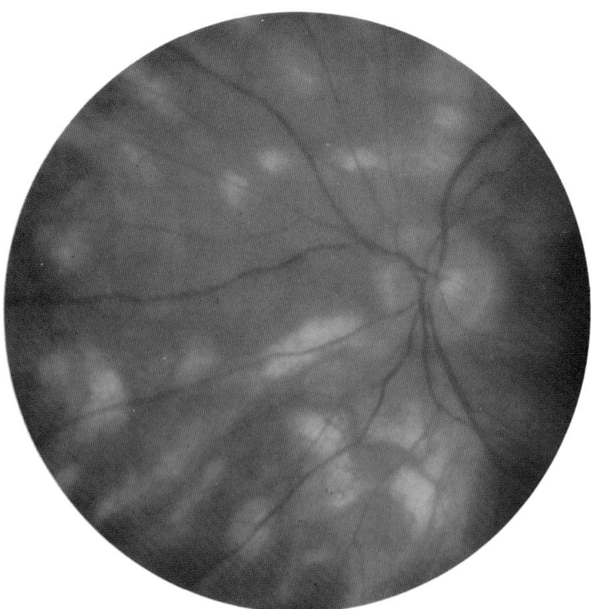

Figure 6.59 Birdshot retinochoroidopathy

Clinical course and complications

The disease runs a chronic course lasting several years with remissions and exacerbations with eventual stabilization and retention of useful vision in at least one eye. The main causes of visual impairment are: chronic cystoid macular oedema, geographical atrophy of macula, serous detachment of sensory retina, secondary cataract, optic atrophy and, occasionally, subretinal neovascularization.

Management

Topical, periocular and systemic steroids have been tried but have not been found to be beneficial.

Acute retinal necrosis

Acute retinal necrosis (ARN) is an extremely rare but devastating necrotizing retinitis. It affects otherwise healthy individuals of all ages and is bilateral in 30–50% of cases.

Symptoms

The initial symptoms are periorbital pain followed by blurring of vision.

Signs

The initial findings may involve either the posterior pole or the fundus periphery. The retinal arterioles appear sheathed and deep, multifocal, yellow-white patches begin to appear within the retina. The lesions, which may be associated with retinal haemorrhages, gradually become confluent and represent a full-thickness necrotizing retinitis. In cases that start in the periphery, the posterior fundus

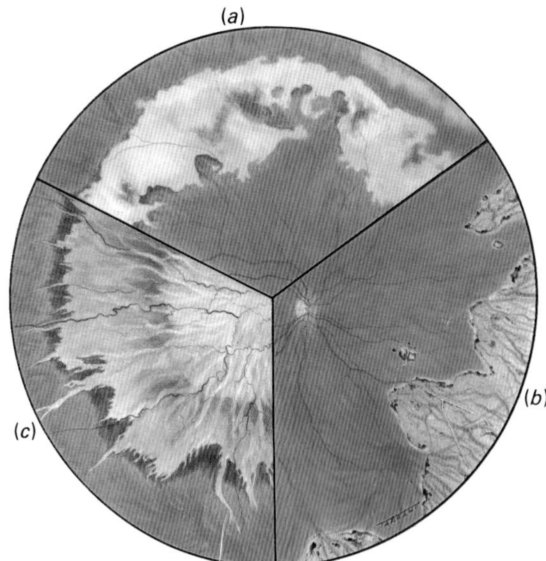

Figure 6.60 *Progression of acute retinal necrosis*

central to the vascular arcades is spared so that visual acuity may remain fairly good despite severe necrosis of the surrounding retina (*Figure 6.60a*).

Clinical course and complications

The acute retinitis resolves within 4–12 weeks leaving behind transparent and necrotic retina with atrophy of the retinal pigment epithelium (*Figure 6.60b*). About 70% of eyes develop retinal holes, usually at the margin of uninvolved and involved zones, which lead to rhegmatogenous retinal detachment (*Figure 6.60c*). In some eyes, secondary vitreous fibrosis gives rise to tractional retinal detachments. In both instances, the retinal detachment is extremely difficult to repair due to the development of gross proliferative vitreoretinopathy.

Management

Treatment with antibiotics, steroids, and cytotoxic agents has been tried, but found to be ineffective.

Glaucomatocyclitic crisis

Glaucomatocyclitic crisis (Posner–Schlossman syndrome) is characterized by recurrent attacks of secondary open-angle glaucoma with mild anterior uveitis. The disease typically affects young adults, 40% of whom are positive for HLA-Bw54. During an attack, the intraocular pressure is usually severely elevated (40–60 mmHg) for between a few hours to several days. The attacks are unilateral, although 50% of patients have bilateral involvement at different times.

Symptoms

Haloes around lights are frequent during an acute attack, although pain is rare.

Signs

Epithelial oedema may be present but the anterior chamber is not shallow. The aqueous contains a few cells but no flare. A few fine non-pigmented keratic precipitates are also present, but posterior synechiae do not develop.

Clinical course and complications

Although the intervals between attacks vary in length, with the passage of time they usually become longer and, in rare cases, a chronic rise in intraocular pressure develops. This may lead to cupping of the optic disc and loss of visual field. Some patients develop a mild heterochromia.

Management

During an attack, the intraocular pressure can be reduced medically and surgical intervention is rarely necessary. The beneficial effect of topical steroids is doubtful.

Management of uveitis

Aims of therapy

The three main aims of treating uveitis are:

1. To prevent vision threatening complications, such as glaucoma, cataract, chronic cystoid macular oedema, and retinal detachment.
2. To relieve the patient's discomfort.
3. To treat the underlying cause if possible.

The four main groups of drugs used in the treatment of uveitis are mydiatrics, steroids, cytotoxic agents, and cyclosporin. Patients with uveitis caused by infections should be treated with the appropriate antimicrobial or antiviral agent.

Mydriatics

In *Table 6.7* are shown the properties of the main topical mydriatics used in the management of uveitis.

Indications

Mydriatics are used for three reasons.

1. *To give comfort.* The discomfort caused by severe acute anterior uveitis is due to spasm of the ciliary muscle and the sphincter of the pupil. This can be relieved by using atropine which is the most powerful cycloplegic available. It is usually unnecessary to use atropine for more

Table 6.7 Topical mydriatics used in uveitis

Drug	*Mydriasis*		*Cycloplegia*	
	Maximal effect (min)	*Full recovery (days)*	*Maximal effect (h)*	*Full recovery (days)*
Atropine 1%	40	10+	6	14
Hyoscine (0.25% and 0.5%) (scopolamine)	30	7	1	7
Homatropine (1%–5%)	60	3	1	3
Cyclopentolate (0.5–2%) (Mydrilate, (Cyclogyl)	60	1	1	1
Tropicamide (0.5% and 1%) (Mydriacyl)	40	0.25	0.5	0.25
Phenylephrine 10% (Neosynephrine)	20	0.25	Nil	–

The values given are for the strongest concentrations.

than 1 or 2 weeks. Once the inflammation is showing signs of subsiding it can be substituted by a short-acting mydriatic, such as tropicamide or cyclopentolate.

2. *To prevent posterior synechiae.* This is best achieved by using a short-acting mydriatic which keeps the pupil mobile. In mild cases of chronic anterior uveitis the mydriatic can be instilled once a day at bedtime to prevent difficulties with accommodation during the day. In eyes with chronic anterior uveitis, the pupil should not be kept constantly dilated as posterior synechiae can still form in the dilated position. In young children, constant atropinization of one eye may induce amblyopia.
3. *To break down synechiae.* The formation of posterior synechiae is undesirable as it interferes with the normal action of the pupil, it may cause pupil block glaucoma due to seclusio pupillae, and also it promotes the development of complicated cataract. Once significant synechiae have formed, intensive topical mydriatic therapy with atropine, phenylephrine, and cocaine is seldom effective in breaking them down, although an anterior sub-Tenon's injection of Mydricaine (adrenaline, atropine and procaine) may be effective if the synechiae are new and unassociated with fibrosis.

Steroids

Steroids are still the mainstay in the management of most cases of uveitis. They can be administered topically in the form of drops or ointment, by periocular injection, or systemically.

Topical administration

Preparations

In *Table 6.8* are shown the main topical steroid preparations (available in the United Kingdom) in decreasing order of anti-inflammatory power.

Severe forms of anterior uveitis can be treated with the powerful steroids, such as dexamethasone, betamethasone, and prednisolone, while the weaker preparations such as fluorometholone and clobetasone are reserved for relatively mild uveitis in patients who are steroid reactors. This is because the latter two drugs have a lesser propensity to elevate intraocular pressure in susceptible individuals than the more powerful preparations.

A solution penetrates the cornea better than a suspension or ointment. Ointment can, however, be instilled at bedtime.

Indications

Topical steroids can only be used in the treatment of anterior uveitis because they cannot reach a therapeutic level in tissues that are behind the lens.

Frequency of instillation

The frequency of instillation of drops depends on the severity of inflammation and can vary from one drop every 5 minutes to one drop every other day. In general, one should start with a high rate of instillation and then decrease as the inflammation lessens, rather than start with a low rate and work up. This principle applies to both topical and systemic administration of steroids. The management of acute anterior uveitis is relatively straightforward and treatment can usually be tapered after a few days and then discontinued after 5–6 weeks. The treatment of chronic anterior uveitis is very much more difficult because steroid therapy may have to be given for many months and even years. In these cases, acute exacerbations with +4 aqueous cells are treated with hourly instillation for 2–3 days and then the drops are tapered to four times a day. If the inflammation is under good control with no

Table 6.8 Topical steroids used in uveitis

Generic name	*Drops*	*Ointment*
Dexamethasone 0.1% (Maxidex)	+	
Betamethasone sodium phosphate 0.1% (Betnesol)	+	+
Prednisolone sodium phosphate 0.5% (Predsol)	+	
Fluorometholone 0.1% (FML)	+	
Clobetasone butyrate 0.1% (Eumovate)	+	

more than +1 aqueous cells, then the rate of instillation can be further reduced gradually over the next few months and then stopped. Following cessation of drops, the patient should be re-examined within a few days to ensure that the uveitis has not recurred.

Complications

The following complications may occur from topical steroid administration.

Glaucoma

The application of a potent steroid four times a day for 6 weeks will cause a marked elevation of intraocular pressure (to over 31 mmHg) in about 5% of the general population. A further 35% show a moderate rise (between 22 and 30 mmHg) and the remaining 60% show virtually no change. The stronger steroids, such as dexamethasone, betamethasone, and prednisolone, are probably equipotent in their ability to raise intraocular presure but weaker steroids, such as fluorometholone and clobetasone, have a low propensity for elevating intraocular pressure.

Cataract

Posterior subcapsular cataract can be promoted by both systemic and, less frequently, topical steroid administration. The risk increases with the amount and duration of therapy.

Corneal complications

These are as follows:

1. Reduction of immunological protection against secondary infection with bacteria and fungi.
2. Enhancement of recrudescences and multiplication of HSV.
3. Corneal melting may be enhanced due to the inhibition of collagen synthesis.

Systemic absorption

Systemic side-effects may be induced following prolonged administration, particularly in children.

Mydriasis and ptosis

These are transient and reversible and may be caused by the preservative and not the steroid.

Periocular injections

Preparations

In *Table 6.9* are shown the four main steroids available for periocular injection.

Table 6.9 Main steroids used for periocular injections

Short-acting (1 day)	*Long-acting (several weeks)*
Betamethasone 4 mg/ml	Methylprednisolone acetate 40 mg/ml
Dexamethasone 4 mg/ml	Triamcinolone acetonide 40 mg/ml

Advantages over drops

1. They are able to reach a therapeutic concentration behind the lens.
2. Drugs that are only water soluble and incapable of penetrating the cornea when given topically can enter the eye by penetrating the sclera when given by periocular injection.
3. A long-lasting effect can be achieved if a depot preparation such as methylprednisolone (Depomedrone) is used.

Indications

1. Severe acute anterior uveitis, especially in patients with ankylosing spondylitis with a marked fibrinous exudate in the anterior chamber or hypopyon.
2. As an adjunct to topical or systemic therapy in resistant cases of chronic anterior uveitis.
3. Intermediate uveitis.
4. Poor patient compliance.
5. At the time of surgery in eyes with uveitis.

Techniques of administration

Periocular injections can be subconjunctival, anterior sub-Tenon, posterior sub-Tenon, and retrobulbar. Subconjunctival injections are given mainly for the treatment of corneal inflammations and retrobulbar injections are now seldom used. For these reasons, only the two types of sub-Tenon's injections will be described.

Preparation of patient

It is extremely important to have the conjunctiva very well anaesthetized prior to attempting a periocular injection. If this is done correctly, the injection can be given with minimal discomfort to the patient. The conjunctiva is anaesthetized as follows:

1. Instil a topical anaesthetic such as amethocaine or cocaine at 1-min intervals for 10 min.
2. Place a small cotton pledget impregnated with cocaine into the conjunctival sac at the site of injection and leave it there for 5 min.

Anterior sub-Tenon injection technique

1. Draw up 1 ml of steroid into a 2-ml syringe and replace the drawing up needle with a number 25 gauge 3/8 inch (10 mm) disposable needle.
2. Ask the patient to look away from the site of injection.
3. With toothed (St Martin's) forceps grasp conjunctiva and Tenon's.

4. With the bevel away from the eye, pass the needle through conjunctiva and Tenon's at the point where they are grasped.
5. Slowly inject 0.5 ml of steroid.

Note. Anterior sub-Tenon's injections are used mainly in the treatment of severe or resistant anterior uveitis.

Posterior sub-Tenon injection technique

1. Draw up 1.5 ml of steroid into a 2-ml syringe (*Figure 6.61, left*) and replace the drawing up needle with a number 25 gauge 5/8 inch (16 mm) disposable needle (*Figure 6.61, right*).

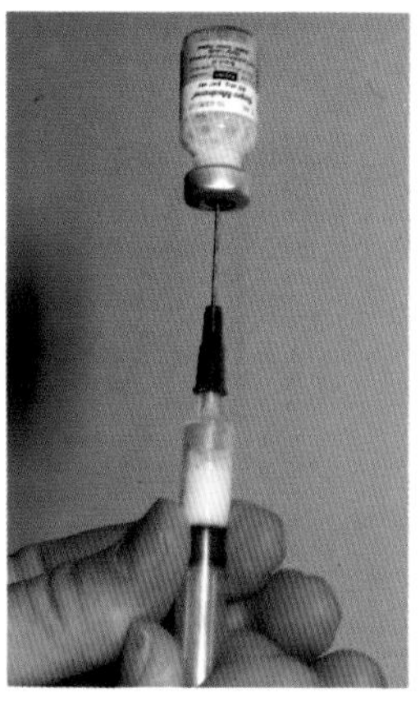

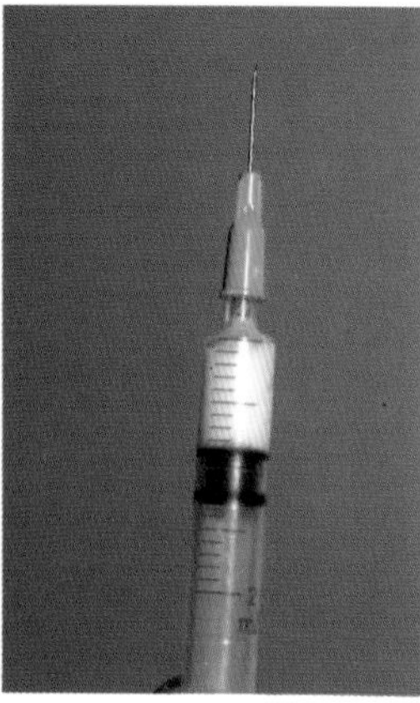

Figure 6.61 *Left: drawing up of methylprednisolone (Depomedrone); right: 25-gauge, 5/8 inch needle for posterior sub-Tenon injection*

2. Ask the patient to look away from the site of injection which is usually in the upper or lower temporal quadrant.
3. Evert the eyelid and penetrate the bulbar conjunctiva with the tip of the needle (bevel towards the globe) slightly on the global side of the fornix (*Figure 6.62*).
4. Slowly insert the needle posteriorly keeping it as close to the globe as possible. In order not to penetrate the globe accidentally with the top of the needle make wide side-to-side motions as you are inserting the needle and watch the limbus—movement of the limbus means that you have engaged the sclera!

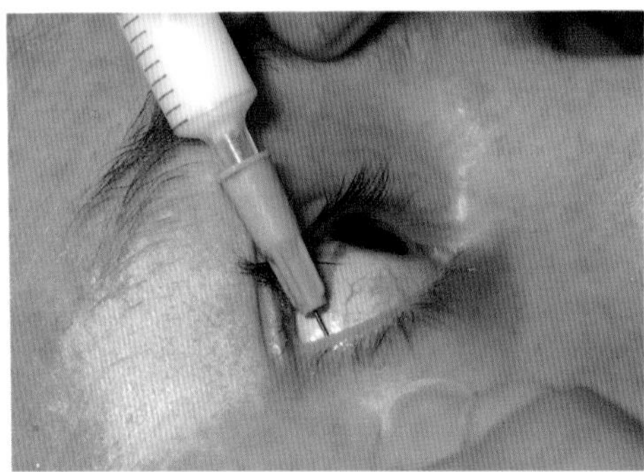

Figure 6.62 *Posterior sub-Tenon injection*

5. When the needle cannot be inserted any further withdrawn the plunger slightly and if no blood has entered the syringe inject 1 ml of steroid. If the needle is too far away from the globe, adequate trans-scleral absorption of the steroid will not occur. The posterior sub-Tenon injection is indicated for intermediate uveitis and as an alternative to systemic therapy of posterior uveitis.

Systemic therapy

Preparations

The main oral preparation for systemic use is prednisolone 5 mg. Enteric coated (2.5 mg) tablets can be used in patients with a history of gastric ulceration. Injections of adrenocorticotrophic hormone (ACTH) can be used in the few patients who are intolerant to oral therapy.

Indications

The main indications for systemic therapy are:

1. Intractable anterior uveitis which has failed to respond to both topical therapy and anterior sub-Tenon injections.
2. Intractable intermediate uveitis which has failed to respond to posterior sub-Tenon injections.
3. Posterior uveitis which has failed to respond to posterior sub-Tenon injections.

Rules in the use of systemic steroids

1. Start with a large dose and then reduce.
2. The initial dose of prednisolone is 1–1.5 mg/kg body weight.
3. The total dose should be taken before eating breakfast.
4. Switch to an every-other-breakfast regimen once the inflammation is brought under control and then taper gradually over several weeks.
5. If steroids are given for less than 2 weeks there is no need to reduce the dose gradually.

Side-effects

Short steroid therapy

1. Peptic ulceration.
2. Mental changes.
3. Aseptic necrosis of the head of the femur.
4. Hyperosmolar hyperglycaemic non-ketotic coma (very rare).

Long steroid therapy

1. Osteoporosis.
2. Cushingoid state.
3. Electrolyte imbalance.
4. Reactivation of infections, such as TB.
5. Cataract.
6. Increase in severity of pre-existing disease, such as diabetes.

7. Limitation of growth in children.
8. Myopathy.

When not to use steroids

1. In inactive disease with a chronic flare but no cells.
2. In mild anterior uveitis with not more than a +1 cell.
3. In intermediate uveitis with normal vision.
4. In Fuchs' uveitis syndrome.
5. When antimicrobial therapy is more appropriate, e.g. candidiasis.

Cytotoxic agents

Cytotoxic agents are drugs which were initially used for the treatment of certain malignant diseases. The three main groups that have been used in the treatment of uveitis are shown in *Table 6.10.*

Table 6.10 Main groups of cytotoxic agents used in uveitis

Group	*Drugs*
Antifoliates	Methotrexate
Antipurines	6-Mercaptopurine Azathioprine
Alkylating agents	Chlorambucil Cyclophosphamide

Since all of these drugs are potentially toxic, their administration should be supervised by a physician. Complications of cytotoxic drugs include: bone marrow depression, gastrointestinal ulceration, stomatitis, liver damage, sterility, alopecia, neoplasia, haemorrhagic cystitis, genetic damage, and nausea and vomiting. Methotrexate and 6-mercaptopurine are now seldom used because of their relatively serious side-effects and poor results in the treatment of uveitis.

Indications

The two main general indications for the use of cytotoxic agents are:

1. Potentially binding (usually bilateral) reversible intraocular inflammation which has failed to respond to *adequate* steroid therapy.
2. Intolerable side-effects from systemic steroid therapy.

Specific types of uveitis that have been treated with cytotoxic agents include the following:

1. *Behçet's disease.* Due to the poor visual prognosis, posterior uveitis associated with Behçet's disease is considered by many to be an absolute indication for cytotoxic agents. The most commonly used drug is chlorambucil. In about 50% of patients, the intraocular inflammation is stabilized, and in 25% it is improved. The remainder continue to deteriorate.
2. *Sympathetic uveitis.* This is probably only a relative indication for cytotoxic drugs, since the majority of cases can be controlled by adequate steroid therapy. Both chlorambucil and cyclophosphamide have been found to be beneficial in steroid-resistant cases.
3. *Intermediate uveitis.* This is a very rare condition as most cases can be controlled by periocular steroid injections. In severe intractable cases azathioprine, chlorambucil, and cyclophosphamide may be beneficial.
4. *Juvenile chronic arthritis.* The results of treatment of intractable uveitis with chlorambucil have been equivocal.

Cyclosporin

Cyclosporin is a powerful anti-T-cell immunosuppressive agent. Preliminary uncontrolled studies have shown that it is a promising agent in the treatment of steroid and/or cytotoxic resistant cases of Behçet's uveitis, intermediate uveitis, sympathetic uveitis, and sarcoid uveitis. Unfortunately, an unacceptably high rate of renal toxicity makes it an unacceptable drug for routine use.

Further reading

Introduction

Hogan, M.J., Kimura, S.J. and Thygeson, P. (1959) Signs and symptoms of uveitis. 1. Anterior uveitis. *American Journal of Ophthalmology*, **47**, 155–170

Kimura, S.J., Thygeson, P. and Hogan, M.J. (1959) Signs and symptoms of uveitis. 2. Classification of posterior manifestations of uveitis. *American Journal of Ophthalmology*, **47**, 171–176

Nussenblatt, R.B., Palestine, A.G., Chan, C-C. *et al.* (1985) Standardization of vitreal inflammatory activity in intermediate and posterior uveitis. *Ophthalmology*, **92**, 467–471

Arthritis

Ankylosing spondylitis

Beckinsale, A.B., Davies, J., Gibson, J.M. *et al.* (1984) Acute anterior uveitis, ankylosing spondylitis, back pain, and HLA-B27. *British Journal of Ophthalmology*, **68**, 741–745

Beckinsale, A.B., Guss, R.B. and Rosenthal, A.R. (1982) Acute anterior uveitis associated with HLA-B27 positive tissue type. A comparative study of two populations. *Transactions of the Ophthalmological Society of the United Kingdom*, **102**, 168–170

Brewerton, D.A. (1985) The genetics of acute anterior uveitis. *Transactions of the Ophthalmological Society of the United Kingdom*, **104**, 248–249

Brewerton, D.A., Caffrey, M., Hart, F.D. *et al.* (1973a) Ankylosing spondylitis and HLA-B27. *Lancet*, **i**, 904–907

Brewerton, D.A., Caffrey, M., Nicholls, A. *et al.* (1973b) Acute anterior uveitis and HLA-B27. *Lancet*, **ii**, 994–996

Kimura, S.J., Hogan, M.J., O'Connor, G.R. *et al.* (1967) Uveitis and joint disease. *Archives of Ophthalmology*, **77**, 309–316

Ohno, S., Kimura, S.J., O'Connor, G.R. *et al.* (1977) HLA antigens and uveitis. *British Journal of Ophthalmology*, **61**, 62–64

Reiter's disease

Purcell, J.J. Jr, Baldassare, A.R. and Tsai, C.C. (1980) Reiter's syndrome. *Perspectives in Ophthalmology*, **4**, 17–22

Juvenile chronic arthritis

Kanski, J.J. (1977) Anterior uveitis in juvenile rheumatoid arthritis. *Archives of Ophthalmology*, **95**, 1794–1797

Kanski, J.J. (1981) Care of children with anterior uveitis. *Transactions of the Ophthalmological Society of the United Kingdom*, **101**, 387–390

Kanski, J.J. and Shun-Shin, G.A. (1984) Systemic uveitis syndromes in childhood: An analysis of 360 cases. *Ophthalmology*, **91**, 1247–1251

Key, S.N. and Kimura, S.J. (1975) Iridocyclitis associated with juvenile rheumatoid arthritis. *American Journal of Ophthalmology*, **80**, 425–429

Perkins, E.S. (1966) Patterns of uveitis in children. *British Journal of Ophthalmology*, **50**, 169–185

Schaller, J.G., Johnson, G.D., Holborow, E.J. *et al.* (1974) The association of antinuclear antibodies with the chronic iridocyclitis in juvenile rheumatoid arthritis (Still's disease). *Arthritis and Rheumatism*, **17**, 409–416

Smiley, W.K. (1974) The eye in juvenile rheumatoid arthritis. *Transactions of the Ophthalmological Society of the United Kingdom*, **94**, 817–829

Non-infectious systemic diseases

Sarcoidosis

Asdourian, G.K., Goldberg, M.F. and Busse, B.J. (1975) Peripheral retinal neovascularization in sarcoidosis. *Archives of Ophthalmology*, **93**, 787–790

Campo, R.V. and Aaberg, T.M. (1984) Choroidal granuloma in sarcoidosis. *Ophthalmology*, **97**, 419–427

Doxanas, M.T., Kelly, J.S. and Prout, T.E. (1980) Sarcoidosis of the optic nerve head. *American Journal of Ophthalmology*, **90**, 347–351

James, G.D., Neville, E. and Langley, D.S. (1976) Ocular sarcoidosis. *Transactions of the Ophthalmological Society of the United Kingdom*, **96**, 133–139

Marcus, D.F., Bovino, J.A. and Burton, T.C. (1982) Sarcoid granuloma of the choroid. *Ophthalmology*, **89**, 1326–1330

Nicholson, C.W., Eagle, R.C. Jr, Yanoff, M. *et al.* (1980) Conjunctival biopsy as an aid in the evaluation of the patient with suspected sarcoidosis. *Ophthalmology*, **87**, 287–291

Obenauf, C.D., Shaw, H.E., Sydnor, C.F. *et al.* (1978) Sarcoidosis and its ocular manifestations. *American Journal of Ophthalmology*, **86**, 648–655

Perkins, E.S. (1981) (Editorial) Ocular sarcoidosis. *Archives of Ophthalmology*, **99**, 1193

Sanders, M.D. and Shilling, J.S. (1976) Retinal, choroidal and optic disc involvement in sarcoidosis. *Transactions of the Ophthalmological Society of the United Kingdom*, **96**, 140–144

Weinreb, R.N. (1984) Diagnosing sarcoidosis by transconjunctival biopsy of the lacrimal gland. *American Journal of Ophthalmology*, **97**, 573–576

Weinreb, R.N., Barth, R. and Kimura, S.J. (1980) Limited gallium scans and angiotensin converting enzyme in granulomatous uveitis. *Ophthalmology*, **87**, 202–206

Weinreb, R.N. and Kimura, S.J. (1980) Uveitis associated with sarcoidosis and angiotensin converting enzyme. *American Journal of Ophthalmology*, **89**, 180–185

Behçet's disease

Collum, L.M.T., Mullaney, J. and Bowell, R. (1981) Current concepts of Behçet's disease. *Transactions of the Ophthalmological Society of the United Kingdom*, **101**, 422–428

Colvard, D.M., Robertson, D.M. and O'Duffy, J.D. (1977) The ocular manifestations of Behçet's disease. *Archives of Ophthalmology*, **95**, 1813–1817

James, G.D. and Spiteri, M.A. (1982) Behçet's disease. *Ophthalmology*, **89**, 1279–1284

O'Duffy, J.D., Robertson, D.M. and Goldstein, N.P. (1984) Chlorambucil in the treatment of uveitis and meningoencephalitis of Behçet's disease. *American Journal of Medicine*, **76**, 75–78

Ohno, S. (1981) Immunological aspects of Behçet's and Vogt–Koyanagi–Harada disease. *Transactions of the Opthalmological Society of the United Kingdom*, **101**, 335–341

Page, N.G.R., Thomson, A. and James, D.G. (1982) Behçet's disease. *Transactions of the Ophthalmological Society of the United Kingdom*, **102**, 174–177

Palimeris, G., Koliopoulos, J., Theodossiadis, G. *et al.* (1980) Adamantiadis–Behçet's syndrome. Clinical and immunological observations. *Transactions of the Ophthalmological Society of the United Kingdom*, **100**, 527–530

Vogt–Koyanagi–Harada syndrome

Carlson, M.R. and Kerman, B.M. (1977) Hemorrhagic macular detachment in the Vogt–Koyanagi–Harada syndrome. *American Journal of Ophthalmology*, **84**, 632–635

Ohno, S., Char, D.H., Kimura, S.J. *et al.* (1977) Vogt–Koyanagi–Harada syndrome. *American Journal of Ophthalmology*, **83**, 735–740

Snyder, D.A. and Tessler, H. (1980) Vogt–Koyanagi–Harada syndrome. *American Journal of Ophthalmology*, **90**, 69–73

Chronic systemic infections

Syphilis

Arruga, J., Valentines, J., Mauri, F. *et al.* (1985) Neuroretinitis in acquired syphilis. *Ophthalmology*, **92**, 262–270

Belin, M.W., Baltch, A.L. and Hay, P.B. (1981) Secondary syphilitic uveitis. *American Journal of Ophthalmology*, **92**, 210–214

Folk, J.C., Weingeist, T.A., Corbett, J.J. *et al.* (1983) Syphilitic neuroretinitis. *American Journal of Ophthalmology*, **95**, 480–486

Ross, W.H. and Sutton, H.F.S. (1980) Acquired syphilitic uveitis. *Archives of Ophthalmology*, **98**, 496–498

Schlaegel, T.F. Jr and Kao, S.F. (1982) A review (1970–1980) of 28 presumptive cases of syphilitic uveitis. *American Journal of Ophthalmology*, **93**, 412–414

Schwartz, L.K. and O'Connor, G.R. (1980) Secondary syphilis with iris papules. *American Journal of Ophthalmology*, **90**, 380–384

Zwink, F.B. and Dunlop, E.M.C. (1976) Clinically silent anterior uveitis in secondary syphilis. *Transactions of the Ophthalmological Society of the United Kingdom*, **96**, 148–150

Tuberculosis

Abrams, J. and Schlaegel, T.F. Jr (1982) The role of the Isoniazid therapeutic test in tuberculous uveitis. *American Journal of Ophthalmology*, **94**, 511–515

Jabbour, N.M., Faris, B. and Trempe, C.L. (1985) A case of tuberculosis presenting with choroidal tuberculoma. *Ophthalmology*, **92**, 834–837

Schlaegel, T.F. Jr (1981) Bacterial and protozoal uveitis. *Transactions of the Ophthalmological Society of the United Kingdom*, **101**, 312–316

Leprosy

Ffytche, T.J. (1981) Iritis in leprosy. *Transactions of the Ophthalmological Society of the United Kingdom*, **101**, 325–327

Ffytche, T.J. (1981) Role of iris changes as a cause of blindness in leprosy. *British Journal of Ophthalmology*, **65**, 231–239

Ffytche, T.J. (1981) Cataract surgery in the management of the late complications of lepromatous leprosy in South Korea. *British Journal of Ophthalmology*, **65**, 243–248

Spaide, R., Nattis, R., Lipka, A. *et al.* (1985) Ocular findings in leprosy in the United States. *American Journal of Ophthalmology*, **100**, 411–416

Parasitic infestations

Toxoplasmosis

Doft, B.H. and Gass, J.D.M. (1985) Punctate outer retinal toxoplasmosis. *Archives of Ophthalmology*, **103**, 1335–1336

Dutton, G.N. and Hay, J. (1983) Toxoplasmic retinochoroiditis—current concepts in pathogenesis. *Transactions of the Ophthalmological Society of the United Kingdom*, **103**, 503–507

Fitzgerald, C.R. (1980) Pars plana vitrectomy for vitreous opacities secondary to presumed toxoplasmosis. *Archives of Ophthalmology*, **98**, 321–323

Folk, J.C. and Lobes, L.A. (1984) Presumed toxoplasmic papillitis. *Ophthalmology*, **91**, 64–67

Michelson, J.B., Shields, J.A., Federman, J.L. *et al.* (1978) Retinitis secondary to acquired systemic toxoplasmosis with isolation of the parasite. *American Journal of Ophthalmology*, **86**, 548–552

Nozik, R.A. (1977) Results of treatment of ocular toxoplasmosis with injectable corticosteroids. *Ophthalmology*, **83**, 811–818

Saari, M., Vourre, I., Niminen, H. *et al.* (1976) Acquired toxoplasmic chorioretinitis. *Archives of Ophthalmology*, **94**, 1485–1490

Stern, G.A. and Romano, P.E. (1978) Congenital toxoplasmosis. Possible occurrence in siblings. *Archives of Ophthalmology*, **96**, 615–618

Tabbara, K.F. and O'Connor, G.R. (1980) Treatment of ocular toxoplasmosis with clindamycin and sulfadiazine. *Ophthalmology*, **87**, 129–134

Toxocariasis

Belmont, J.B., Irvine, A., Benson, W. *et al.* (1982) Virectomy in ocular toxocariasis. *Archives of Ophthalmology*, **100**, 1912–1915

Biglan, A.W., Glickman, L.T. and Lobes, L.A. Jr (1979) Serum and vitreous toxocara antibody in nematode endophthalmitis. *American Journal of Ophthalmology*, **88**, 898–901

Hagler, W.S., Pollard, Z.F. and Jarrett, W.M. (1981) Results of surgery for *Toxocara canis*. *Ophthalmology*, **88**, 1081–1086

Luxemberg, M.N. (1979) An experimental approach to the study of intraocular *Toxocara canis*. *Transactions of the American Ophthalmological Society*, **77**, 542–602

Pollard, Z.F., Jarrett, W.H., Hagler, W.S. *et al.* (1979) ELISA for diagnosis of ocular toxocariasis. *Ophthalmology*, **86**, 743–749

Schantz, P.M. and Glickman, L.T. (1978) Toxocaral visceral larva migrans. *New England Journal of Medicine*, **298**, 436–439

Viral infections

Herpes zoster

Cobo, L.M., Foulks, G.N., Liesegang, T. *et al.* (1985) Oral acyclovir in the therapy of acute herpes zoster ophthalmicus. *Ophthalmology*, **92**, 1574–1582

Coles, E.L., Meisler, D.M., Calabrese, L.H. *et al.* (1984) Herpes zoster ophthalmicus and acquired immune deficiency syndrome. *Archives of Ophthalmology*, **102**, 1027–1029

Hedges, T.R. and Albert, D.M. (1982) The progression of the ocular abnormalities of herpes zoster: Histopathologic observations of nine cases. *Ophthalmology*, **89**, 165–176

Liesegang, T.J. (1985) Corneal complications from herpes zoster ophthalmicus. *Ophthalmology*, **92**, 316–324

Lightman, S., Marsh, R.J. and Powell, D. (1981) Herpes zoster ophthalmicus: a medical review. *British Journal of Ophthalmology*, **65**, 539–541

McGill, J., Chapman, C. and Mahakashingham, M. (1983) Acyclovir therapy in herpes zoster infection—a practical guide. *Transactions of the Ophthalmological Society of the United Kingdom*, **103**, 111–114

Marsh, R.J. (1976) Current management of herpes zoster ophthalmicus. *Archives of Ophthalmology*, **96**, 334–337

Womack, L.W. and Liesegang, T.J. (1983) Complications of herpes zoster ophthalmicus. *Archives of Ophthalmology*, **101**, 42–45

Cytomegalovirus infection

Berger, B.B., Weinberg, R.S. and Tessler, H. (1979) Bilateral cytomegalovirus panuveitis after high dose corticosteroid therapy. *American Journal of Ophthalmology*, **88**, 1020–1025

Meredith, T.A., Aaberg, T.M. and Reeser, F.H. (1979) Rhegmatogenous retinal detachment complicating cytomegalovirus retinitis. *American Journal of Ophthalmology*, **87**, 793–796

Palestine, A.G., Stevens, G., Lane, H.C. *et al.* (1986) Treatment of cytomegalovirus retinitis with dihydroxypropoxymethyl guanine. *American Journal of Ophthalmology*, **101**, 95–101

Acquired immune deficiency

Freeman, W.R., Lerner, C.W., Mines, J.A. *et al.* (1984) A prospective study of the ophthalmic findings in the acquired immune deficiency syndrome. *American Journal of Ophthalmology*, **97**, 133–142

Holland, G.N., Pepose, J.S., Petitt, T.H. *et al.* (1983) Acquired immune deficiency syndrome. Ocular manifestations. *Ophthalmology*, **90**, 859–873

Khadem, M., Kalish, S.B., Goldsmith, J. *et al.* (1984) Ophthalmic findings in acquired immune deficiency syndrome (AIDS). *Archives of Ophthalmology*, **102**, 201–206

Newman, N.M., Mandel, M.R., Gullett, J. *et al.* (1983) Clinical and histologic findings in opportunistic ocular infections. Part of a new syndrome of acquired immunodeficiency. *Archives of Ophthalmology*, **101**, 396–401

Palestine, A.G., Rodriguez, M.M., Macher, A.M. *et al.* (1984) Ophthalmic involvement in acquired immune deficiency syndrome. *Ophthalmology*, **91**, 1092–1099

Rosenberg, P.R., Uliss, A.E., Friedland, G.H. *et al.* (1983) Acquired immunodeficiency syndrome. Ophthalmic manifestations in ambulatory patients. *Ophthalmology*, **90**, 874–878

Fungal infections

Histoplasmosis

Archer, D.B., Maguire, C.J.F. and Newell, F.W. (1975) Multifocal choroiditis. *Transactions of the Ophthalmological Society of the United Kingdom*, **95**, 184–191

Dreyer, R.F. and Gass, J.D.M. (1984) Multifocal choroiditis and panuveitis. *Archives of Ophthalmology*, **102**, 1776–1784

Ganley, J.P. (1984) Epidemiology of presumed ocular histoplasmosis. *Archives of Ophthalmology*, **102**, 1754–1756

Kahill, M.K. (1982) Histopathology of presumed ocular histoplasmosis. *American Journal of Ophthalmology*, **94**, 369–376

Lewis, M.L., Vannewkirk, M.R. and Gass, J.D.M. (1980) Follow-up study of presumed ocular histoplasmosis syndrome. *Ophthalmology*, **87**, 390–398

Macher, A., Rodrigues, M.M., Kaplan, W. *et al.* (1985) Disseminated bilateral choroiditis due to *Histoplasma capsulatum* in a patient with acquired immune deficiency syndrome. *Ophthalmology*, **92**, 1159–1164

Roth, A.M. (1977) *Histoplasma capsulatum* in the presumed ocular histoplasmosis syndrome. *American Journal of Ophthalmology*, **84**, 293–298

Schlaegel, T.F. Jr (1977) The prognosis in the presumed ocular histoplasmosis syndrome. *Perspectives in Ophthalmology*, **1**, 140–145

Smith, R.E. (1981) Studies in the presumed ocular histoplasmosis syndrome. *Transactions of the Ophthalmological Society of the United Kingdom*, **101**, 328–334

Watzke, R.C. and Claussen, R.W. (1981) The long-term course of multifocal choroiditis (presumed ocular histoplasmosis). *American Journal of Ophthalmology*, **91**, 750–760

Candidiasis

Aguilar, G.L., Blumenkranz, M.S., Egbert, P.R. *et al.* (1979) Candida endophthalmitis after intravenous drug abuse. *Archives of Ophthalmology*, **97**, 96–102

Brownstein, S., Mahoney-Kinsner, J. and Harris, R. (1983) Ocular candida with pale centre haemorrhages. *Archives of Ophthalmology*, **101**, 1745–1748

McDonnell, P.J., McDonnell, J.M., Brown, R.H. *et al.* (1985) Ocular involvement in patients with fungal infections. *Ophthalmology*, **92**, 706–709

Parke, D.W. III, Jones, D.B. and Gentry, L.O. (1982) Endogenous endophthalmitis among patients with candidemia. *Ophthalmology*, **89**, 789–796

Salmon, J.F., Partridge, B.M. and Spalton, D.J. (1983) Candida endophthalmitis in a heroin addict. *British Journal of Ophthalmology*, **67**, 306–309

Servant, J.B., Dutton, G.N., Ong-Toneg, L. *et al.* (1985) Candida endophthalmitis in Glaswegian heroin addicts: Reports of an epidemic. *Transactions of the Ophthalmological Society of the United Kingdom*, **104**, 297–308

Common idiopathic specific uveitis syndromes

Intermediate uveitis

Chester, G.H., Blach, R.K. and Cleary, P.E. (1976) Inflammation in the region of the vitreous base. *Transactions of the Ophthalmological Society of the United Kingdom*, **96**, 151–154

Fleder, K.S. and Brockhurst, R.J. (1982) Neovascular fundus abnormalities in peripheral uveitis. *Archives of Ophthalmology*, **100**, 750–754

Green, W.R., Kincaid, M.C., Michels, R.D. *et al.* (1981) Pars planitis. *Transactions of the Ophthalmological Society of the United Kingdom*, **101**, 361–367

Pederson, J.E., Kenyon, K.R., Green, W.R. *et al.* (1978) Pathology of pars planitis. *American Journal of Ophthalmology*, **86**, 762–774

Smith, R.E., Godfrey, W.A. and Kimura, S.J. (1976) Complications of chronic cyclitis. *American Journal of Ophthalmology*, **82**, 277–282

Tessler, H.H. (1985) What is intermediate uveitis? In *Year Book of Ophthalmology*, edited by J.T. Ernest, pp. 155–157. Chicago: Year Book Medical Publications

Fuchs' uveitis syndrome

Arffa, R.C. and Schlaegel, T.F. Jr (1984) Chorioretinal scars in Fuchs' heterochromic iridocyclitis. *Archives of Ophthalmology*, **102**, 1153–1155

Berger, B.B., Tressler, H.H. and Kattow, M.H. (1980) Anterior segment ischaemia in Fuchs' heterochromic cyclitis. *Archives of Ophthalmology*, **98**, 499–501

Kimura, S.J. (1978) Fuchs' syndrome of heterochromic cyclitis in brown-eyed patients. *Transactions of the American Ophthalmological Society*, **76**, 76–86

Liesegang, T.J. (1982) Clinical features and prognosis in Fuchs' uveitis syndrome. *Archives of Ophthalmology*, **100**, 1622–1626

O'Connor, G.R. (1985) Doyne Lecture: Heterochromic cyclitis. *Transactions of the Ophthalmological Society of the United Kingdom*, **104**, 219–231

Rare idiopathic specific uveitis syndromes

Sympathetic uveitis

Lubin, J.R., Albert, D.M. and Weinstein, M. (1980) Sixty-five years of sympathetic ophthalmia: a clinicopathologic review of 105 cases (1913–1978). *Ophthalmology*, **87**, 109–121

Mackley, T.A. and Azar, A. (1978) Sympathetic ophthalmia: a long-term follow-up. *Archives of Ophthalmology*, **96**, 257–262

Marak, G.E. (1979) Recent advances in sympathetic ophthalmia. *Survey of Ophthalmology*, **24**, 141–156

Rao, N.A., Robin, J., Dartman, S. *et al.* (1983) The role of penetrating wound in the development of sympathetic ophthalmia—experimental observations. *Archives of Ophthalmology*, **101**, 102–104

Rao, N.A. and Wong, V.G. (1981) Aetiology of sympathetic ophthalmitis. *Transactions of the Ophthalmological Society of the United Kingdom*, **101**, 357–360

Acute posterior multifocal placoid pigment epitheliopathy

Damato, B.E., Nanjiani, M. and Foulds, W.S. (1983) Acute posterior multifocal placoid pigment epitheliopathy. A follow-up study. *Transactions of the Ophthalmological Society of the United Kingdom*, **103**, 517–522

Holt, W.S., Regan, C.D.J. and Trempe, C. (1976) Acute posterior multifocal placoid pigment epitheliopathy. *American Journal of Ophthalmology*, **81**, 403–412

Lewis, R.A. and Martonyi, C.L. (1975) Acute posterior multifocal placoid pigment epitheliopathy. A recurrence. *Archives of Ophthalmology*, **93**, 235–238

Murray, S.B. (1979) Acute posterior multifocal placoid pigment epitheliopathy. Not so benign? *Transactions of the Ophthalmological Society of the United Kingdom*, **99**, 497–500

Serpiginous choroidopathy

Chisholm, I.H., Gass, J.D.M. and Hutton, W.L. (1976) The late stage of serpiginous (geographic) choroiditis. *American Journal of Ophthalmology*, **82**, 343–351

Hamilton, A.M. and Bird, A.C. (1974) Geographical choroidopathy. *British Journal of Ophthalmology*, **58**, 784–797

Laatikainen, L. and Erkkila, H. (1974) Serpiginous choroiditis. *British Journal of Ophthalmology*, **58**, 777–783

Birdshot retinochoroidopathy

Freust, D.J., Tressler, H.H., Fishman, G.A. *et al.* (1984) Birdshot retinochoroidopathy. *Archives of Ophthalmology*, **102**, 214–219

Gass, J.D.M. (1981) Vitiliginous chorioretinitis. *Archives of Ophthalmology*, **99**, 1778–1787

Kaplan, H.J. and Aaberg, T.M. (1980) Birdshot retinochoroidopathy. *American Journal of Ophthalmology*, **90**, 773–782

Nussenblatt, R.B., Mittal, K.K., Ryan, S. *et al.* (1982) Birdshot choroidopathy associated with HLA-A29 antigen and immune responsiveness to retinal S-antigen. *American Journal of Ophthalmology*, **94**, 147–158

Ryan, S.J. and Maumenee, A.E. (1980) Birdshot retinochoroidopathy. *American Journal of Ophthalmology*, **89**, 31–45

Acute retinal necrosis

Culbertson, W.W., Clarkson, J.G., Blumenkranz, M.S. *et al.* (1983) (Editorial) Acute retinal necrosis. *American Journal of Ophthalmology*, **96**, 683–685

Fisher, J.P., Lewis, M.L., Blumenkranz, M. *et al.* (1982) The acute retinal necrosis syndrome. Part 1. Clinical manifestations. *Ophthalmology*, **89**, 1309–1316

Gorman, B.D., Nadel, A.J. and Coles, R.S. (1982) Acute retinal necrosis. *Ophthalmology*, **89**, 809–814

Price, F.W. Jr and Schlaegel, T.F. Jr (1980) Bilateral acute retinal necrosis. *American Journal of Ophthalmology*, **89**, 419–424

Saari, K.M., Boke, W., Manthey, K.F. *et al.* (1982) Bilateral acute retinal necrosis. *American Journal of Ophthalmology*, **93**, 403–411

Young, N.J.A. and Bird, A.C. (1978) Bilateral acute retinal necrosis. *British Journal of Ophthalmology*, **62**, 581–590

Glaucomatocyclitic crisis

Hirose, S., Ohno, S. and Matsuda, H. (1985) HLA-Bw54 and glaucomatocyclitic crisis. *Archives of Ophthalmology*, **103**, 1837–1839

Raitta, C. and Vannas, A. (1977) Glaucomatocyclitic crisis. *Archives of Ophthalmology*, **95**, 608–612

Management of uveitis

Dinning, W.J. (1981) Treatment of uveitis. *Transactions of the Ophthalmological Society of the United Kingdom*, **101**, 391–393

Dinning, W.J. (1983) Therapy—selected topics. In *Uveitis, Pathophysiology and Therapy*, edited by E. Kraus-Mackiw and G.R. O'Connor, pp. 198–220. New York: Thième-Stratton Inc.

Graham, E.M., Sanders, M.D., James, D.G. *et al.* (1985) Cyclosporin A in the treatment of posterior uveitis. *British Journal of Ophthalmology*, **104**, 146–151

Nussenblatt, R.B., Palestine, A.G. and Chan, C.C. (1983) Cyclosporin A in the treatment of intraocular inflammatory disease resistant to systemic corticosteroid and cytotoxic agents. *American Journal of Ophthalmology*, **96**, 275–282

Palmer, R.G., Kanski, J.J. and Ansell, B.M. (1985) Chlorambucil in the treatment of intractable uveitis associated with juvenile chronic arthritis. *Journal of Rheumatology*, **12**, 967–970

7

Glaucoma

Introduction

Aqueous humour dynamics

Classification

Pathogenesis of damage

Methods of examination

Slitlamp biomicroscopy

Tonometry

Tonography

Gonioscopy

Perimetry

Primary open-angle glaucoma

Introduction

Clinical features

Corticosteroid responsiveness

Ocular associations

Systemic associations

Differential diagnosis

Antiglaucoma drugs

Management

Primary angle-closure glaucoma

Introduction

Latent

Intermittent (subacute) PACG

Acute

Chronic

Absolute

Plateau iris syndrome

Laser iridotomy

Secondary glaucomas

Inflammatory

Neovascular

Pigment dispersion syndrome

Pseudoexfoliation syndrome

Phacolytic

Phacomorphic

Glaucoma and ectopia lentis

Traumatic

Ghost cell

Glaucoma and intraocular tumours

Iridocorneal endothelial syndromes

Iridoschisis

Glaucoma due to raised episcleral venous pressure

Congenital glaucomas

Primary

Rubella syndrome

Aniridia

Mesodermal dysgenesis

Peters' anomaly

Congenital ectropion uveae

Phacomatoses

Introduction

Glaucoma is a name given to a group of diseases in which the intraocular pressure (IOP) is sufficiently elevated to damage vision.

Aqueous humour dynamics

The principal factors determining the level of IOP are the rate of aqueous humour production and the resistance encountered in the outflow channels.

Production of aqueous occurs in the secretory ciliary epithelium by two mechanisms:

1. *Secretion* is the result of an active metabolic process and is independent of the level of IOP.
2. *Ultrafiltration*, the rate of which is influenced by the level of blood pressure in the ciliary capillaries, the plasma oncotic pressure, and the level of IOP.

Outflow of aqueous is by two routes:

1. *Trabecular meshwork.* Approximately 80% of total outflow of aqueous is through the trabecular meshwork into Schlemm's canal, and then into the venous circulation by way of the aqueous veins.
2. *Uveoscleral pathways* account for the remaining 20% of aqueous outflow. Here the aqueous flows through the ciliary body into the suprachoroidal space, to be drained by the venous circulation in the ciliary body, choroid, and sclera.

Classification

The many types of glaucoma are classified, primarily, as being of the *open-angle* or *angle-closure* type, according to the manner in which aqueous outflow is impaired. In open-angle glaucoma, the elevation in IOP is caused by increased resistance in the drainage channels, whereas in angle-closure glaucoma the obstruction to aqueous outflow is caused by closure of the chamber angle by the peripheral iris.

Further classification describes the disorder as *primary* or *secondary* depending on the absence or presence of associated factors contributing to the IOP rise.

In some cases the age of the patient at the onset of glaucoma is also taken into consideration, and the condition is then described as *congenital, infantile, juvenile,* or *adult* accordingly.

Pathogenesis of damage

Observations of visual field changes and axoplasmic flow point to the optic nerve head, rather than any other point along the nerve axon, as being the primary site of damage. The progression of visual field loss can be explained most easily by a lesion involving the optic nerve head. Studies of axoplasmic flow show vulnerability of nerve axons to elevated IOP as they pass through the optic disc. Currently there are two hypotheses concerning the mechanism of damage.

1. *The indirect ischaemic theory* postulates that raised IOP causes death of nerve fibres by interfering with the microcirculation to the optic nerve head. Therefore, according to this theory, it is the difference between the IOP and the intracapillary pressure (perfusion pressure) that determines whether or not damage will result.
2. *The direct mechanical theory* suggests that elevated IOP directly damages the retinal nerve fibres.

Both factors may be operative in some patients.

Methods of examination

Slitlamp biomicroscopy

Much can be learned from a careful initial examination of the anterior segment in glaucoma suspects. Some of the possible findings are summarized in *Figure 7.1*.

Tonometry

A measurement of IOP using a tonometer is an essential part of the evaluation of all glaucoma suspects. Tonometry may be by indentation or applanation.

Indentation

This is based on the principle that a plunger will indent a soft eye more than a hard eye. The Schiötz tonometer (*Figure 7.2*) is constructed in such a way that, when placed on the eye, the plunger together with a preset weight indents the cornea. The amount of indentation is measured on a scale and then the reading is converted into millimetres of mercury (mmHg) by the use of special tables.

The main advantage of the Schiötz tonometer is that it is cheap, easy to use, convenient to carry, and it does not require a slitlamp for measurements to be made.

Its main disadvantage becomes apparent when it is used in eyes with abnormal scleral rigidity. Increased elasticity of the outer coats of the eye (low scleral rigidity) may occur in high myopia, dysthyroid exophthalmos, and in eyes treated with miotics as well as in those that have been subjected to surgery. In these cases, the Schiötz tonometer may register a falsely low level of IOP when compared with

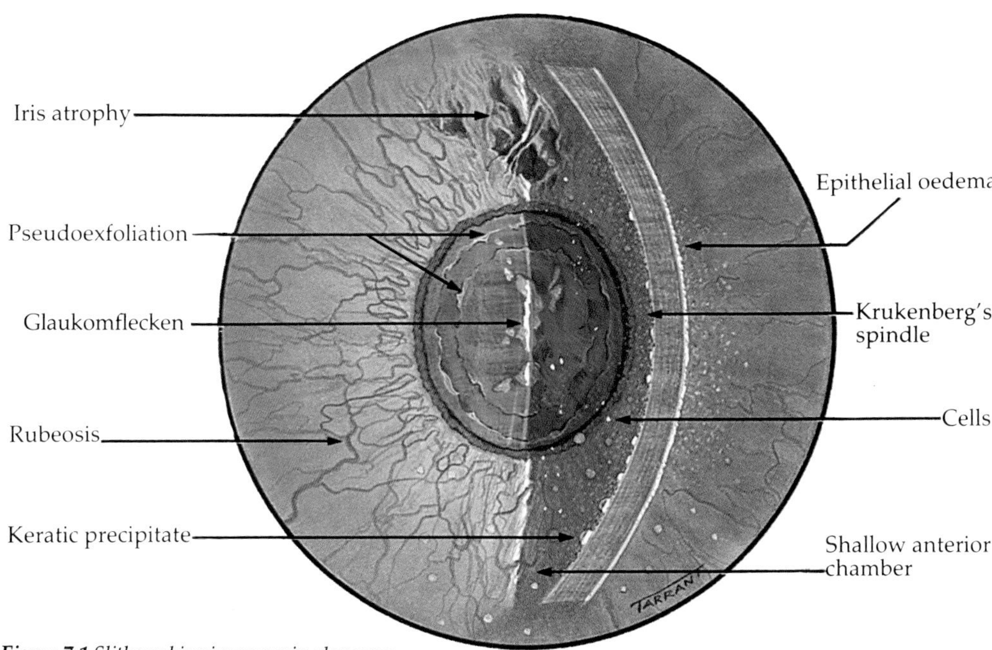

Figure 7.1 *Slitlamp biomicroscopy in glaucoma*

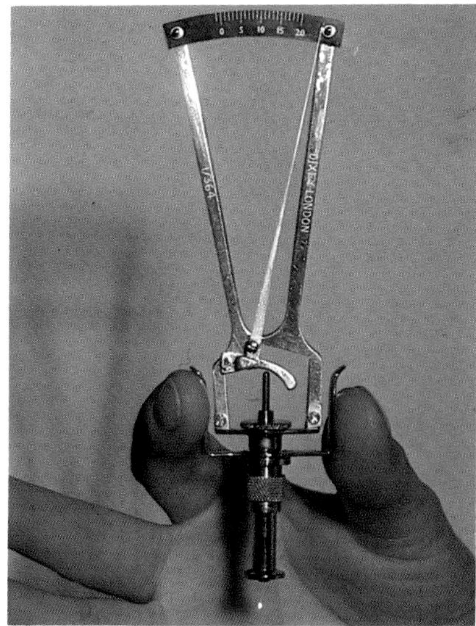

Figure 7.2 *Schiötz tonometer*

an applanation tonometer (Schiötz–applanation disparity). If the eye has an abnormally high scleral rigidity, a falsely high level of IOP may be obtained. Abnormalities of scleral rigidity can be detected with the Schiötz tonometer by using two different weights. If the two measurements are identical then scleral rigidity is normal. If there is a discrepancy, then abnormal scleral rigidity is present and an alternative method of measurement should be used.

Applanation

This is based on the Imbert–Fick law which states that for an ideal, dry, thin-walled sphere the pressure inside the sphere (P) equals the force necessary to flatten its surface (F) divided by the area of flattening (A).

$$P = F/A$$

However, the human eye is not an ideal sphere and the cornea resists flattening. In addition, capillary attraction of the tear meniscus tends to pull the tonometer towards the cornea. When measurements of IOP are made with the Goldmann tonometer, these two forces cancel each other out when the flattened area has a diameter of about 3 mm. The flattening of such a small segment of the cornea causes only minimal displacement of fluid in the eye and, therefore, the pressure reading is unaffected by variations in scleral rigidity. Six applanation tonometers are in current use.

The Goldmann (*Figure 7.3*)

This is a variable force applanation tonometer consisting of a double prism that has a diameter of 3.06 mm. In order to take a reading, the tear film is stained with fluorescein and a cobalt blue filter is used. When the prism touches the apex of the cornea two yellow semicircles will be seen. These represent the fluorescein-stained tear film touching the upper and lower outer halves of the prism. When the cornea has been perfectly flattened, the inner edges of the two semicircles will just touch. The IOP is then determined by reading the number on the dial and multiplying by 10. In order to obtain an accurate measurement, it is essential for the two semicircles to be correctly centred on the cornea and to be of the right thickness (*Figure 7.4*). Too much fluorescein will make the semicircles appear thick with a small radius, whereas insufficient fluorescein will make the radius large and the semicircles too thin. At present, the Goldmann tonometer is the most widely used and gives the most accurate readings.

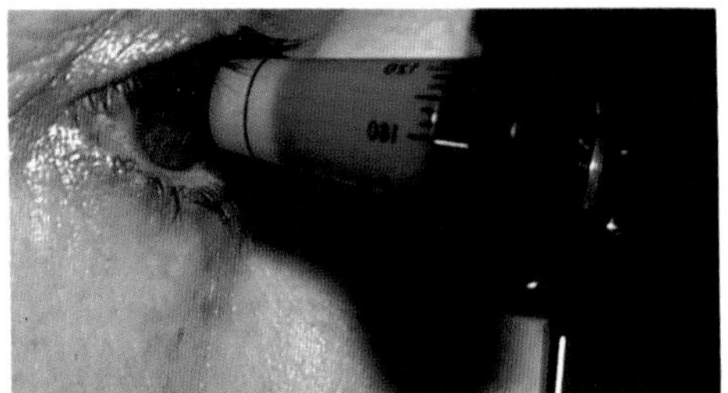

Figure 7.3 Goldmann tonometer

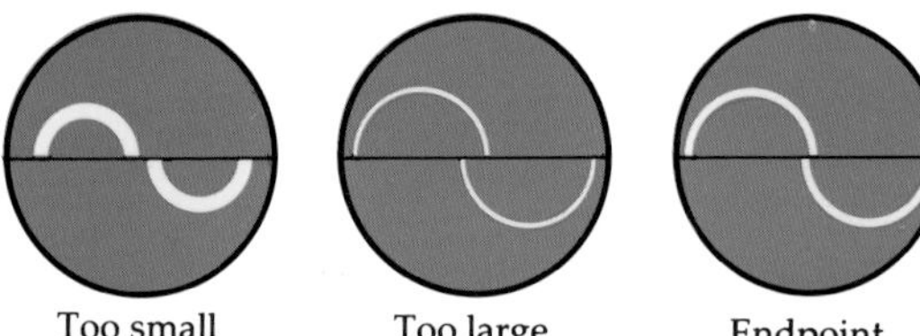

Figure 7.4 Applanation tonometry

The Perkins

This is a hand-held tonometer, which uses a Goldmann prism adapted to a small light source, and is spring counterbalanced. Its main advantage is that it does not require a slitlamp and it can be used with the patient in the supine position (*Figure 7.5*). It is therefore extremely useful in measuring the IOP in bed-bound or anaesthetized patients.

The pneumatonometer (*Figure 7.6*)

This is a sophisticated device which measures the IOP by indenting the cornea by a graded flow of gas against a flexible diaphragm. Its main advantages are its ease of application and the production of a permanent record.

The 'air-puff' tonometer (*Figure 7.7*)

This tonometer (not to be confused with the pneumatonometer) uses the Goldmann principle but, instead of using a prism, the central part of the cornea is flattened by a jet of air. Light is then reflected from the flattened corneal surface to a photoreceptor which is activated to turn the air off. The time required to sufficiently flatten the anterior cornea relates directly to the level of IOP. Its main advantages are that a local anaesthetic is not required and there is no danger of spreading infection from one patient to another.

The Mackay–Marg

This is a portable electronic tonometer which has an action that can be considered as lying between the indentation and applanation principles. It measures the force required to flatten a small area of the cornea against a 1.5 mm plunger protruding 5 µm beyond the surface footplate. A non-optical method of recording IOP is used. Although this instrument gives slightly higher readings than the Goldmann, it can be used on scarred or irregular corneas.

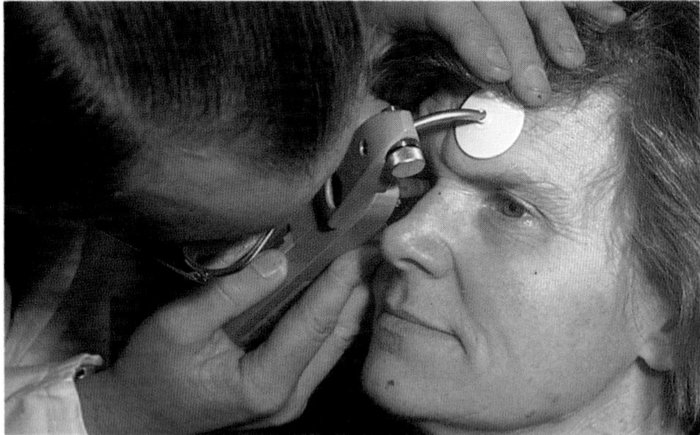

Figure 7.5 Perkins hand-held applanation tonometer

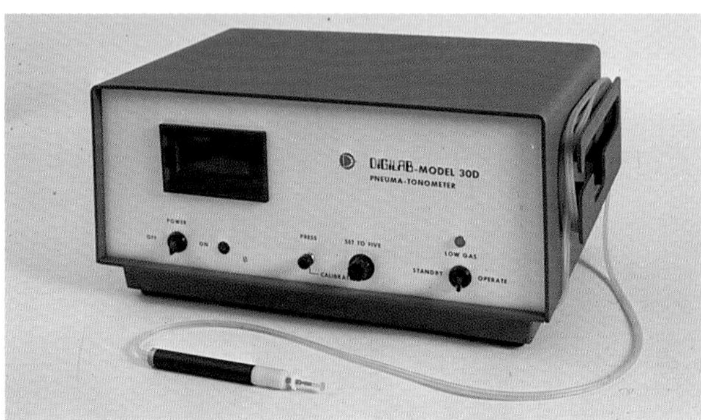

Figure 7.6 Pneumatonometer (courtesy of Keeler Ltd)

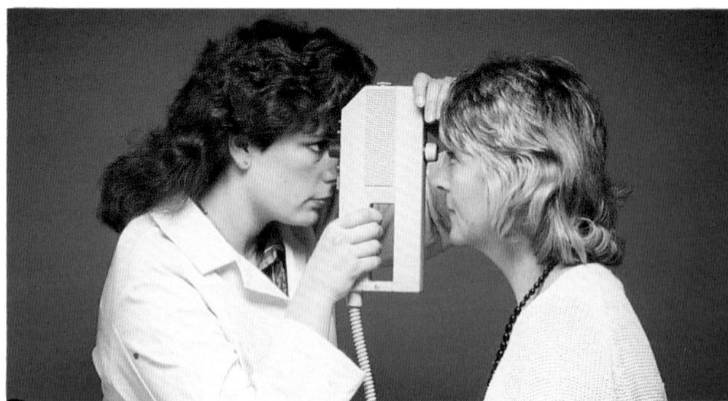

Figure 7.7 Non-contact Pulsair tonometer (courtesy of Keeler Ltd)

The microelectronic Tono-Pen

This works by a principle similar to the Mackay–Marg tonometer. It employs a microscopic strain-gauge transducer that applanates the cornea, converting intraocular pressure into electrical waves. A single-chip computer in the instrument analyses the waveforms obtained from several corneal touches, and displays this along with an estimate of the reading's reliability on a digital readout. The Tono-Pen correlates favourably with the Goldmann. The area of applanation surface is small allowing increased accuracy in measuring IOP after keratoplasty, radial keratotomy, and irregular astigmatism.

Tonography

This is a special form of tonometry based on the principle that, when a Schiötz tonometer indents the eye, the displaced aqueous causes an increase in IOP. If the tonometer is then kept on the eye, its weight will 'massage' additional aqueous out of the eye causing the IOP to fall.

The facility of outflow (denoted by *C*) is a measure of the ability of aqueous to leave the eye in a given period of time. It is expressed in microlitres per minute per millimeter of mercury. It is detected by placing an electronic Schiøtz tonometer on the eye for 4 minutes while recording the pressure change on a galvanometer. *C* is determined by comparing the initial and final pressure readings and then using a special nomogram.

Although in the past tonography helped to elucidate some of the pathophysiological mechanisms in glaucoma, its clinical value in managing individual patients is severely limited by difficulties of interpretation. Although, in general, *C* values of over 0.20 are considered normal and those below 0.11 pathological, both healthy and glaucomatous eyes exhibit values between these limits.

Gonioscopy

The purpose of gonioscopy is to identify abnormal angle structures and to estimate the width of the chamber angle. It is a difficult technique that can only be mastered by many hours of practice on both normal and abnormal eyes.

Optical principles

The angle cannot be visualized directly through an intact cornea because light emitted from angle structures undergoes total internal reflection (*Figure 7.8*). A goniolens eliminates total internal reflection by replacing the cornea–air interface by a new lens–air interface that has a refractive index greater than that of cornea and tears.

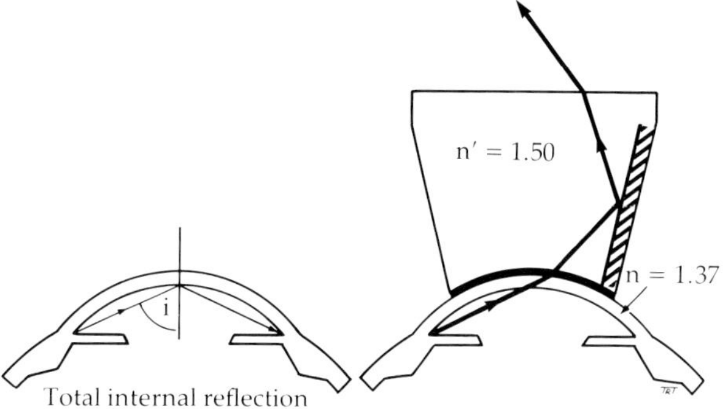

Figure 7.8 *Optical principles of gonioscopy: n = refractive index*

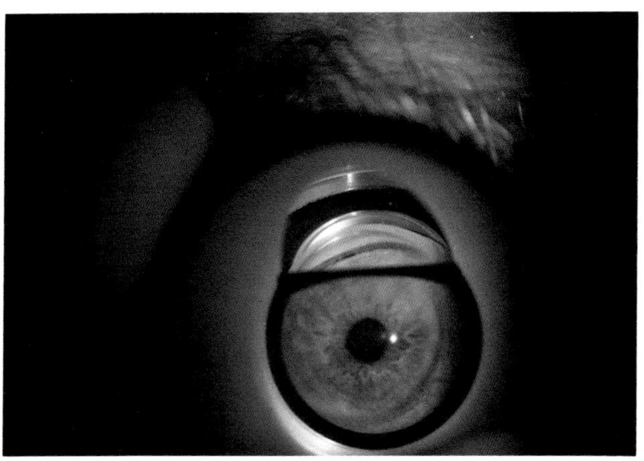

Figure 7.9 *Indirect gonioscopy showing angle hyperpigmentation in pigmentary glaucoma*

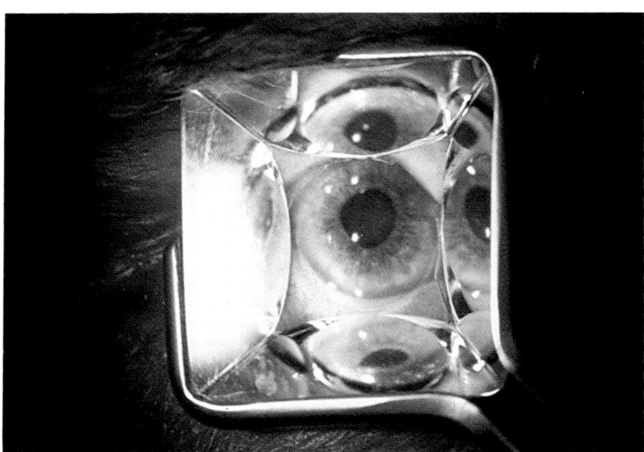

Figure 7.10 *Indirect gonioscopy using a Zeiss goniolens*

Goniolenses

Indirect

Indirect goniolenses provide a mirror image of the opposite angle and can only be used at a slitlamp.

The Goldmann goniolens (*Figure 7.9*) has a curvature that is steeper than that of the cornea. For this reason, a viscous coupling fluid is necessary to bridge the gap between the cornea and the goniolens during gonioscopy. Because the goniolens usually has only one mirror, it has to be rotated 360° in order to inspect the entire angle.

The Zeiss (*Figure 7.10*) goniolens does not require a coupling fluid because its curvature is flatter than that of the cornea. It is held in place by a handle and its four mirrors enable the entire extent of the angle to be visualized simultaneously. When using the Zeiss goniolens, an estimation of the angle width has to be interpreted with caution as an undue posterior pressure on the cornea will distort angle structures, making a narrow angle appear artificially wide.

Direct

Direct goniolenses provide a direct view of the angle and are usually used with the patient in the supine position. They may be used for diagnostic purposes or during the operation of goniotomy.

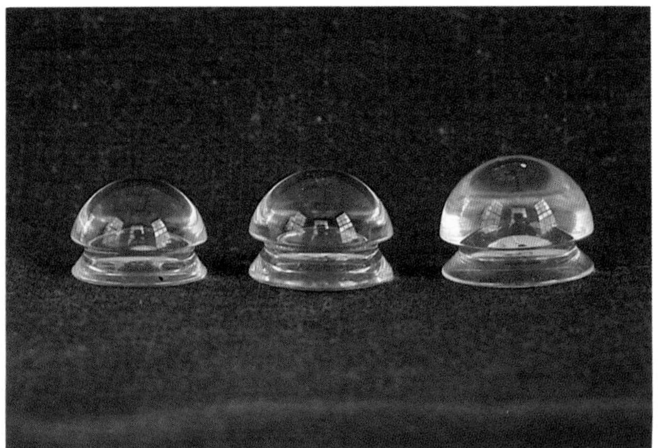

Figure 7.11 Koeppe goniolenses

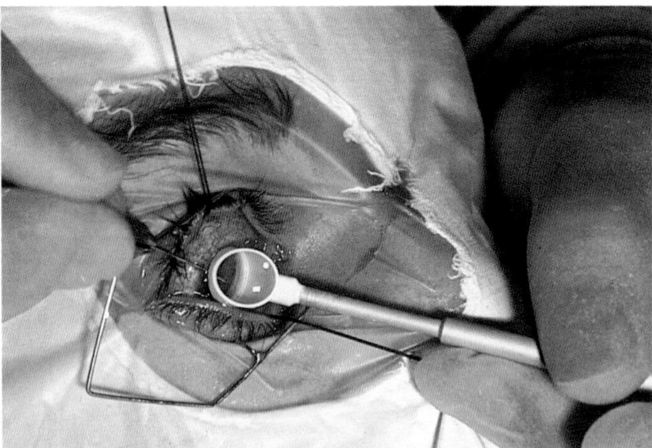

Figure 7.12 Direct gonioscopy using a Swan–Jacob goniolens

The Koeppe (*Figure 7.11*) is the most popular of the direct diagnostic goniolenses. It has a dome shape and comes in several sizes. It is particularly useful for simultaneous comparison of the two angles. When the lens is used in conjunction with a hand-held microscope, it offers great flexibility, allowing detailed inspection of the various subtleties of angle structures both by direct and retroillumination.

The *Swan–Jacob* (*Figure 7.12*), the *Barkan*, the *Medical Workshop prismatic* and the *Thorpe* (*Figure 7.13*) are all surgical goniolenses that can also be used for diagnostic purposes.

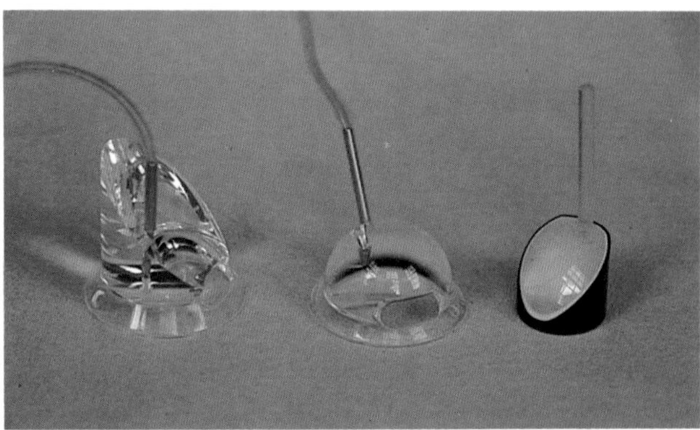

Figure 7.13 Direct surgical goniolenses. *Left:* Medical Workshop; *middle:* Barkan; *right:* Thorpe

Identification of angle structures (*Figure 7.14*)

Schwalbe's line

This is the most anterior structure, appearing as an opaque line. Anatomically it represents the peripheral termination of Descemet's membrane and the anterior limit of the trabeculum. In some eyes it is inconspicuous and can only be located by noting the termination of the corneal wedge. Using a narrow slit beam, two linear reflections can be seen, one from the external surface of the cornea and its junction with the sclera, the other from the internal surface of the cornea. The two reflections meet at Schwalbe's line which is also the anterior limit of the trabeculum. In certain eyes, Schwalbe's line is very prominent and displaced anteriorly. This is referred to as 'posterior embryotoxon'.

The trabeculum

The trabeculum (trabecular meshwork) stretches from Schwalbe's line to the scleral spur, the innermost portion being the uveal meshwork, and the outermost fibres the corneoscleral portion. The part immediately adjacent to Schwalbe's line has a whitish colour and is thought to be non-functional, while the remaining functional part of the trabeculum has a greyish-blue translucent appearance.

Trabecular pigmentation is very rare in the normal eye prior to puberty. In normal senile eyes it varies in degree, being most marked inferiorly. Four pathological causes of

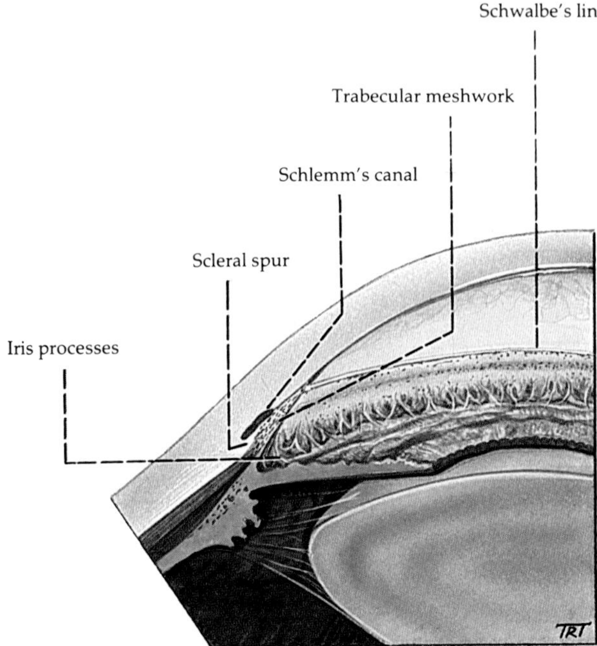

Figure 7.14 Angle structures

increased pigmentation are trauma, acute glaucoma, uveitis, and pseudoexfoliation. In these cases, the pigment is most marked inferiorly and usually lies on the surface of the trabeculum, reaching anteriorly towards Schwalbe's line. In contrast, the pigment in eyes with the pigment dispersion syndrome lies within the trabecular tissue itself and involves 360° of the angle.

Schlemm's canal

This can occasionally be identified in eyes without trabecular pigment as a slightly darker line in the lower trabeculum. Blood in Schlemm's canal can sometimes be seen if the goniolens compresses the episcleral veins so that the episcleral venous pressure exceeds the IOP. Pathological causes of raised episcleral venous pressure include carotid–cavernous fistula, superior vena caval obstruction, and the Sturge–Weber syndrome. All of these, as well as ocular hypotony, may be associated with blood in Schlemm's canal.

The scleral spur

This is the most anterior projection of the sclera and the site of attachment of the longitudinal muscle of the ciliary body. Gonioscopically, it is situated just posterior to the trabeculum and appears as a narrow whitish band.

The ciliary body

This stands out just behind the scleral spur as a dull-brown or slate-grey band. Its width depends on the position of iris insertion.

The angle recess

This represents the dipping of the iris as it inserts into the ciliary body.

Iris processes

These stretch from the iris to be inserted at the level of the scleral spur. They are most prominent during childhood and with increasing age they tend to wither and lose their continuity. They should not be confused with peripheral anterior synechiae which are broader and represent adhesions between the iris and chamber angle structures.

Blood vessels

These can often be observed in normal eyes as they run in a radial pattern at the base of the iris and angle recess. Abnormal vessels, which run randomly in various directions, occur in neovascular glaucoma, anterior uveitis, and Fuchs' uveitis syndrome.

Shaffer grading system

An estimation of the angle width is achieved by observing the amount of separation between two imaginary tangent lines constructed to the inner surface of the trabeculum and the anterior iris surface, respectively. The Shaffer grading system was conceived to provide a convenient method of comparing the widths of different chamber angles. The system assigns a numerical grade (0–4) to each angle with associated anatomical description, the angle width in degrees, and implied clinical interpretation (*Figure 7.15*).

Grade 4 (35–45°)

This is the widest angle characteristic of high myopia and aphakia. The ciliary body can be visualized with ease. This angle is judged incapable of closure.

Grade 3 (20–35°)

This is also an open angle in which at least the scleral spur can be identified. This angle is also judged incapable of closure.

Grade 2 (20°)

This is a moderately narrow angle in which only the trabeculum can be seen. Angle closure is possible but unlikely.

Grade 1 (10°)

This is a very narrow angle in which only Schwalbe's line, and perhaps also the top of the trabeculum, can be visualized. Closure is not inevitable, although the risk is high. A slit angle is one in which there is no obvious iridocorneal contact but no angle structures can be identified. This type of angle has the greatest danger of imminent closure.

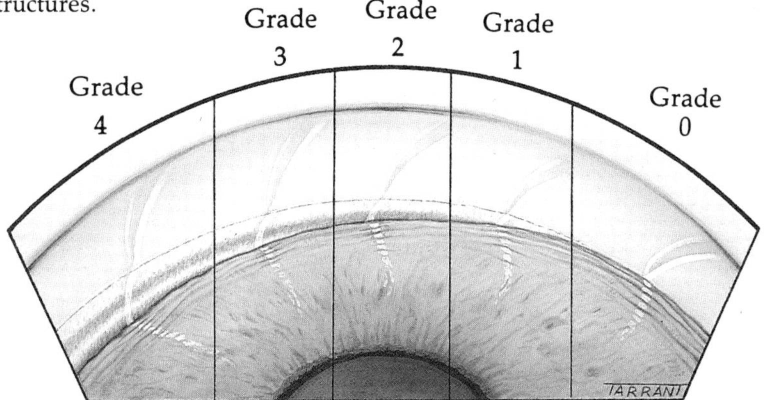

Figure 7.15 *Shaffer grading of angle*

Grade 0 (0°)

This is a closed angle from iridocorneal contact, recognized by the non-appearance of the apex of the corneal wedge. In this situation, indentation gonioscopy with the Zeiss goniolens is necessary to differentiate between 'appositional' and 'synechial' angle closure.

Spaeth grading system

Although the Shaffer grading is extremely useful, the configuration of the angle recess is frequently more complex and varied to permit valid description by a single characteristic. At least three different aspects of the configuration of the angle should be identified: the angular approach, the curvature of the peripheral iris and the point of insertion of the iris. Because these characteristics vary independently, each must be described separately.

The angular approach (*Figure 7.16a*)

This is a function of the depth of the anterior chamber. The point of reference is a line tangential to the inner surface of the trabeculum, and the angle width is estimated by constructing a tangent to the anterior iris surface approximately one-third of the distance from the most peripheral portion of the iris.

The curvature of the peripheral iris (*Figure 7.16b*)

This can be graded as follows:

R = *regular*, in which the iris appears to course regularly from its root without significant anterior or posterior bowing. In most normal eyes there is little curvature.
S = *steep*, in which the iris rises from its root with a sudden, steep, convex curve. Eyes with marked anterior iris convexity are at increased risk of developing angle-closure glaucoma.
Q = *queer*, in which there is marked posterior concavity of the peripheral iris as might occur in a high myope or with lens subluxation.

Iris insertion (*Figure 7.16c*)

This can be in five different locations indicated by the letters A to E.

A = *above Schwalbe's line*. The angle is totally occluded by contact between the peripheral iris and the cornea above Schwalbe's line.
B = *behind Schwalbe's line*. The peripheral iris is in contact with the trabeculum behind Schwalbe's line.
C = *scleral spur*. The iris root is at the level of the scleral spur.
D = *deep*. This signifies a deep angle recess in which the anterior ciliary body is visible.

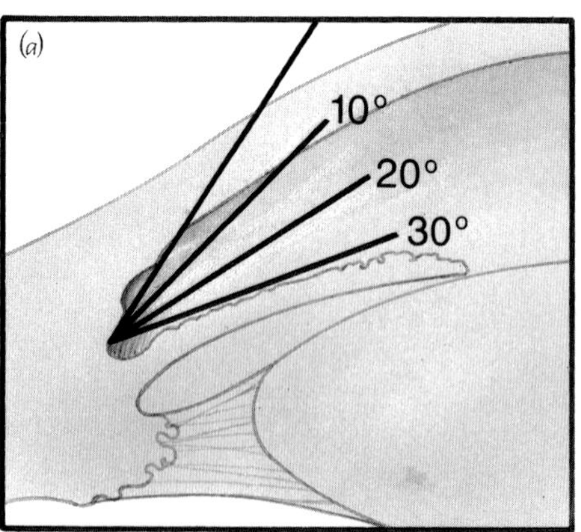

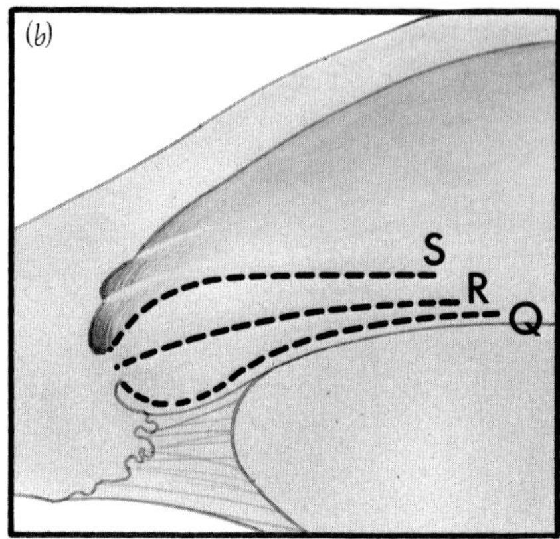

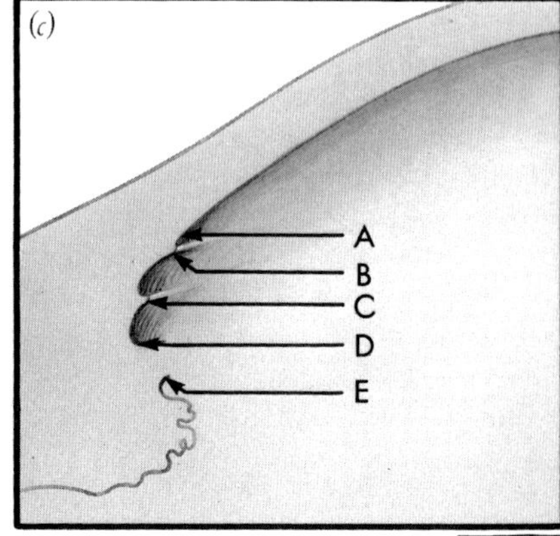

Figure 7.16 *Spaeth grading of angle*

E = extremely deep. This signifies an extremely deep angle recess which allows an unusually large part of the ciliary body to be visualized. It should be emphasized that only C, D, and E are normal configurations, and A and B are pathological.

Perimetry

Perimetry is important in both diagnosis and management of glaucoma. Its first role is to detect visual field changes at the earliest possible stage. This requires knowledge of the type of defects characteristic of early glaucoma. The second role of perimetry is a quantitative assessment of the defects regarding their size, shape, and density.

Definitions

Visual field

It is convenient to imagine the visual field (*Figure 7.17*) as an island of vision surrounded by a sea of darkness. The outer aspect of the island extends approximately 60° nasally, 90° temporally, 50° superiorly, and 70° inferiorly. It should be remembered that the visual field is not a flat plane but a three-dimensional structure. The visual acuity is most acute at the very top of the island and then it declines progressively towards the periphery (the nasal slope being steeper than the temporal).

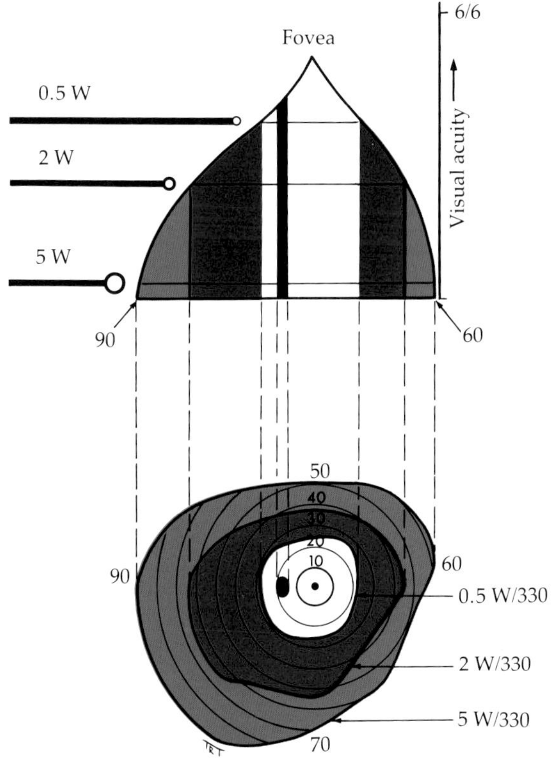

Figure 7.17 *Visual field and isopters*

Isopters

As the size of a target is decreased, the area within which it can be perceived becomes smaller, so that a series of ever-diminishing circles called isopters is formed. Isopters therefore resemble the contour lines on a map which enclose an area above a certain height, and so an isopter encloses an area within which a target of a given size is visible. An erosion of the coastline of the island of vision will cause an indentation of all isopters in the affected area.

Scotoma

An absolute scotoma is an area of the visual field where there is a total loss of vision. A relative scotoma is caused by partial visual damage so that some targets can be seen and others cannot. Frequently, a scotoma (*Figure 7.18*) will have sloping edges so that an absolute scotoma may be surrounded by a relative scotoma.

The smallest test object indicates the actual area of damage, whereas the largest test object will reveal the severity of damage.

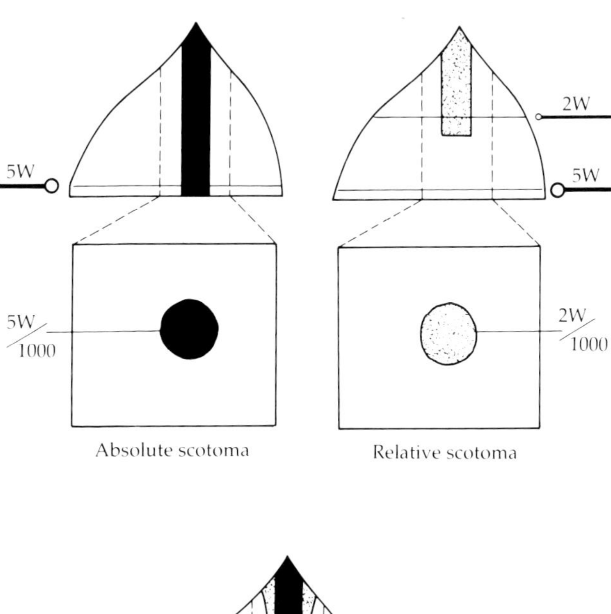

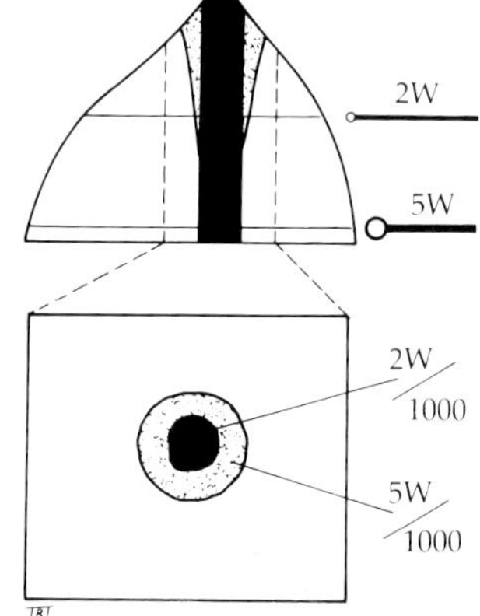

Figure 7.18 *Upper left: absolute scotoma; upper right: relative scotoma; lower: absolute scotoma surrounded by a relative scotoma*

Visible threshold

The visible threshold is defined as the threshold at which a stimulus is perceived 50% of the time when presented statically. This is found by increasing the intensity of the stimulus by 0.1 log unit steps.

Kinetic perimetry

This involves moving a stimulus of known luminance from the periphery towards the centre to establish isopters. The main types of kinetic perimetry are: confrontation, Lister, tangent screen and Goldmann.

Static perimetry

Here a stimulus is presented in a predetermined position for a preset duration. Automated perimeters test a grid of points in the visual field with fixed stimuli of varying luminance.

Perimetric methods

Many techniques are available for examining visual fields. In essence, most methods depend on the patient's subjective response to a visual stimulus.

Confrontation tests

These tests are useful for the detection of hemianopias and altitudinal defects but not subtle field defects due to early glaucoma. They are discussed in Chapter 15.

Lister perimeter

Although the Lister perimeter is seldom more useful than confrontation in the detection of a peripheral field defect, it is of considerable value in documenting the natural course of a peripheral defect. The perimeter consists of a semicircular frame that can be rotated about a central axis. The target is brought in from various directions and the patient indicates when he first sees the target by tapping a coin. The Aimark perimeter is similar.

Tangent screen

This test evaluates the central 30° of the visual field. The patient is seated 1 or 2 metres from a black screen and is instructed to report when he first sees the target and then when it disappears.

Goldmann perimeter

This is a hemispherical dome that has a rest for the patient's chin (*Figure 7.19*). The instrument has controls in the rear to change the test object size, colour, or brightness. A special photometric device keeps the contrast between the target and background luminosity at a constant ratio. A telescope with an incorporated fixation target is used to observe the patient's fixation at all times. The main advantage of this instrument over the tangent screen is that the test conditions and the intensity of the target are always the same, whenever the patient is tested. This permits greater reproducibility and standardization of the results.

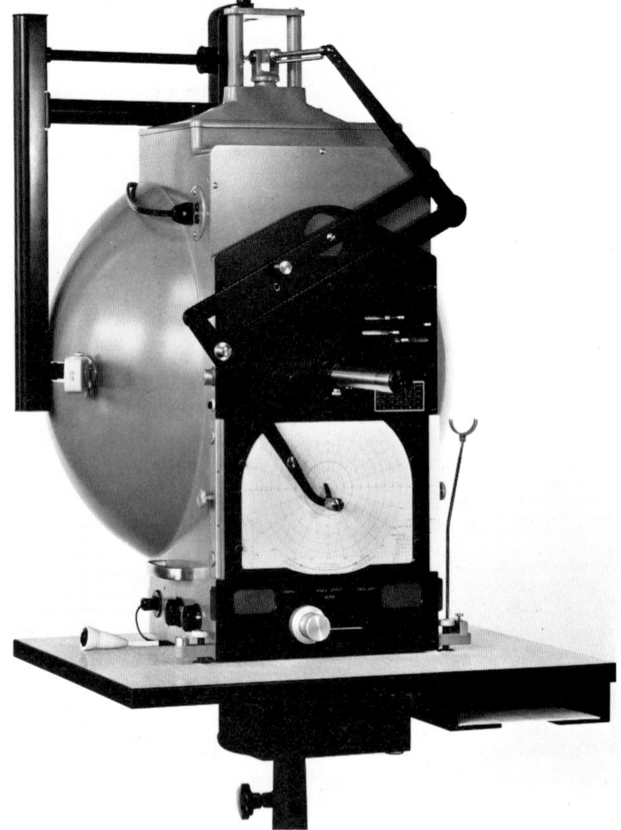

Figure 7.19 *Goldmann perimeter*

Automated perimeters

Automated perimeters test visual fields by a static method. Suprathreshold static perimetry consists of presenting targets at luminance levels above normal threshold values for various strategic locations in the visual field. Targets

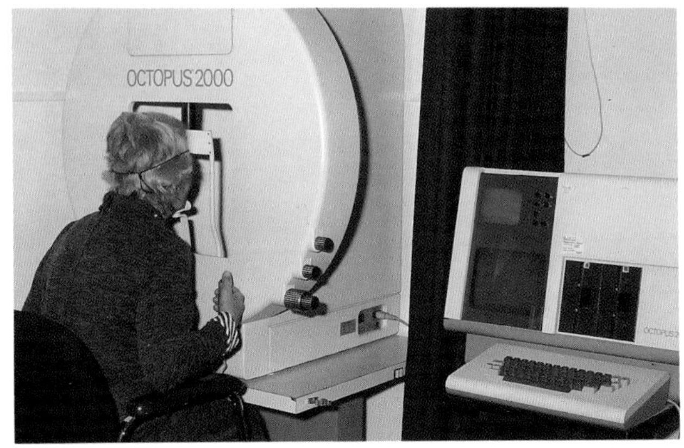

Figure 7.20 *Octopus perimeter*

that are detected indicate normal visual function, whereas missed targets reflect areas of visual field sensitivity loss. Most of the automated perimeters compare favourably with the Goldmann perimeter in their ability to detect visual field defects.

One of the most sophisticated of the automated perimeters is the *Octopus* (*Figure 7.20*). This consists of a hemispherical bowl and a projection system capable of placing stimuli anywhere in the visual field. Fixation is monitored on a console which also houses the computer. The computer performs the perimetry and records the results in both geographical and numerical forms. The Octopus can also represent visual fields in terms of 'normal areas', 'absolute defects', and 'relative defects'.

Other automated perimeters in current use are the *Fieldmaster*, the *Humphrey*, and the *Dicon*.

Primary open-angle glaucoma

Introduction

Primary open-angle glaucoma (POAG) which is also referred to as chronic simple glaucoma is characterized by the following:

1. An IOP of over 21 mmHg.
2. An open angle.
3. Glaucomatous cupping and visual field loss.

It is a chronic, slowly progressive, usually bilateral disease with an insidious onset. It is the most prevalent of all glaucomas affecting approximately 1 in 200 of the general population over the age of 40 years and is responsible for about 20% of all cases of blindness in the United Kingdom and United States, affecting both sexes equally.

Inheritance

POAG is frequently inherited, probably in a multifactorial manner. The responsible gene is thought to show a lack of penetrance and variation in expressivity in some families. Because about 10% of first-degree relatives of POAG sufferers eventually develop the disease, periodic examination of those at risk is important. The risk is higher if a sibling has the disease.

Pathogenesis

In POAG, the rise in IOP is caused by increased resistance of the drainage channels. Most authorities believe that the main site of resistance to aqueous outflow, in both normal and glaucomatous eyes, probably lies in the dense juxtacanalicular trabecular meshwork, or the endothelium lining the inner wall of Schlemm's canal. There is evidence to suggest that in POAG the drainage system of Schlemm's canal may also be at fault.

Anatomy of retinal nerve fibres

The retinal nerve fibres are arranged in a precise pattern that forms the basis for the optic disc and visual field changes in POAG (*Figure 7.21*). The *macular* fibres follow a straight course to the optic nerve head forming a spindle-shaped area (papillomacular bundle). The *nasal* fibres also follow a relatively straight course to the optic nerve head. Fibres arising from the retina *temporal* to the macula have to follow an arcuate path around the papillomacular bundle in order to reach the optic nerve head. They do not cross the horizontal raphe that extends from the fovea to the temporal retinal periphery and forms the boundary between the superior and inferior halves of the retina. The arcuate fibres reaching the superotemporal and inferotemporal aspects of the optic nerve head are particularly susceptible to damage. This might be explained by regional differences in the fine structure of the lamina cribrosa. The superior and inferior parts of the lamina at the level of the sclera appear to contain larger pores and thinner connective tissue supports for the passage of nerve fibre bundles than the nasal and temporal aspects, making these parts of the optic nerve head most vulnerable.

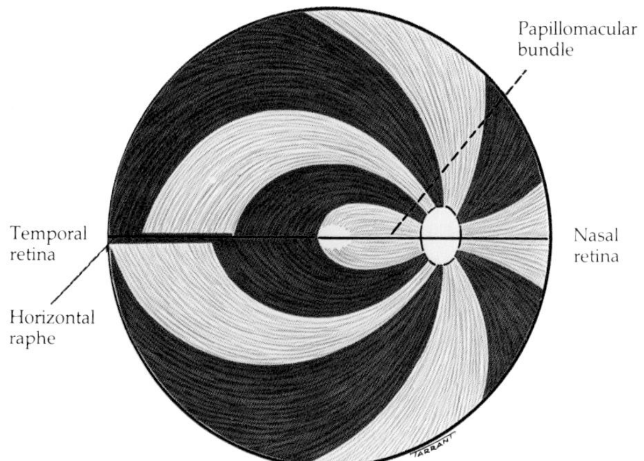

Figure 7.21 *Anatomy of retinal nerve fibres*

Clinical features

Symptoms

Because of its insidious onset, POAG is usually asymptomatic until it has caused a significant loss of visual field.

Optic disc changes

In most patients, POAG is suspected by finding an abnormal optic disc on routine examination. Documentation of arrest or progression of cupping, combined with perimetry, plays a vital part in assessing the efficacy of treatment

Normal disc

The optic nerve head can be thought of as a channel through which retinal nerve fibres leave the globe. The optic cup therefore represents the volume of the channel not occupied by neural disc tissue. The actual dimensions of the cup seem to be related to the diameter of the disc. A small disc will therefore have a small cup as the nerve fibres have to be bunched up to leave the eye (*Figure 7.22, left*). The cup will be bigger in a larger disc as there will be less crowding of nerve fibres (*Figure 7.22, right*). However, for all normal eyes, the actual area of pink disc tissue is constant, irrespective of the overall size of the disc.

A large cup is therefore due to a mismatch between the size of the channel and the number of traversing nerve fibres.

A physiologically large cup occurs when the channel is larger than necessary to accommodate all existing fibres, whereas in pathological cupping it is caused by a decrease in the number of nerve fibres.

Cup–disc ratio

In all eyes the diameter of the cup can be expressed as a fraction of the diameter of the disc both in the vertical and horizontal meridian. This 'cup–disc ratio' is genetically determined. Most normal eyes have a horizontal cup–disc ratio of 0.3 or less. However, half of those with early POAG have a ratio greater than 0.3; therefore a ratio greater than 0.3 should be regarded with suspicion although it may not necessarily be pathological. A difference in ratio between the eyes greater than 0.1 is seen in 8% of the normals. Because 70% of patients with early POAG demonstrate unequal ratios, any difference should be regarded with suspicion until the possibility of glaucoma has been excluded.

It is important to bear in mind that glaucomatous expansion of the optic cup will be superimposed upon the amount of physiological cupping present prior to the onset of glaucoma. For example, if an eye with a small cup develops glaucoma the cup will increase, but in its early stages its dimensions may still be smaller than that of a large physiological cup. An estimation of cup size alone is therefore of limited value in the diagnosis of early glaucoma, unless it is found to be increasing. Nevertheless, glaucomatous cups are usually larger than physiological cups, although a large cup is not necessarily pathological.

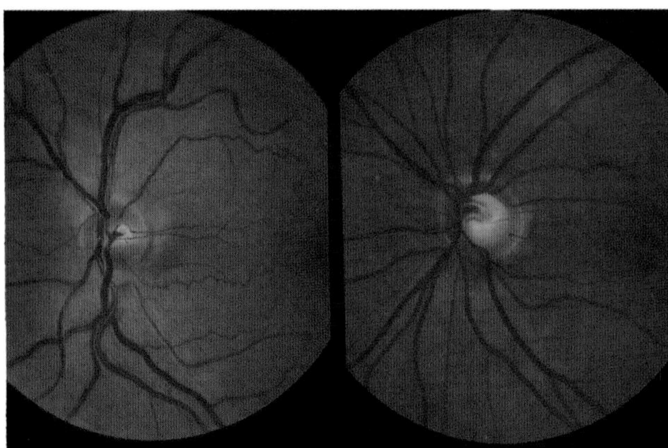

Figure 7.22 *Normal optic discs. Left: small cup; right: large cup*

Pallor and cupping

When evaluating a suspicious disc it is important not to confuse pallor with cupping. Pallor is defined as the maximal area of colour contrast, or the area of the optic disc lacking small blood vessels. Cupping, on the other hand, is best evaluated by observing the bending of small blood vessels as they cross the optic disc. In some eyes the area of cupping and pallor correspond (*Figure 7.23, left*), whereas in others the area of cupping is greater than the area of pallor (*Figure 7.23, right*). In normal eyes the area of cupping increases slightly with age but the area of pallor remains essentially unaltered. In glaucomatous eyes both cupping and pallor increase.

Signs of early damage

In some eyes, subtle signs of glaucomatous retinal nerve fibre damage can be detected prior to the development of pathological cupping and detectable loss of visual field.

The normal retinal nerve fibres appear as fine parallel striations that cross over the larger blood vessels and enter the disc (*Figure 7.24, top left*). Visualization of these striations can be enhanced by:

1. Use of monochromatic 'red-free' light.
2. An ophthalmoscope with a bright light.
3. A well dilated pupil.
4. Clear media.
5. A darkly pigmented retinal pigment epithelium and choroid.

In eyes with early glaucomatous damage some of the striations will be replaced by slit-like defects or grooves which are best detected one disc diameter above and below the disc (*Figure 7.24, top right*). In some cases the appearance of a flame-shaped disc haemorrhage is a sign of imminent damage.

Progression of cupping

The spectrum of disc damage in glaucoma ranges from highly localized tissue loss with notching of the neuroretinal rim to diffuse concentric enlargement of the optic cup.

In the detection of early cupping, particular attention should be paid to neural tissue loss, especially in the vertical sectors of the optic disc. It is more convenient to think in terms of vertical expansion or elongation of the cup into areas of the optic nerve head where tissue has been destroyed, leading to a vertically oval cup. In *Figure 7.25a*, the cup has expanded inferotemporally but has not yet

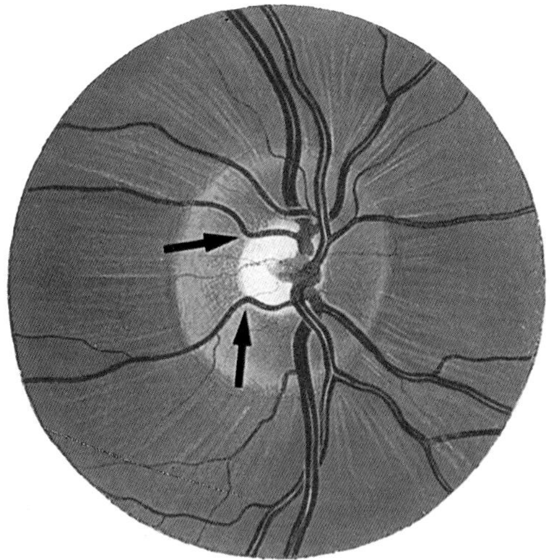

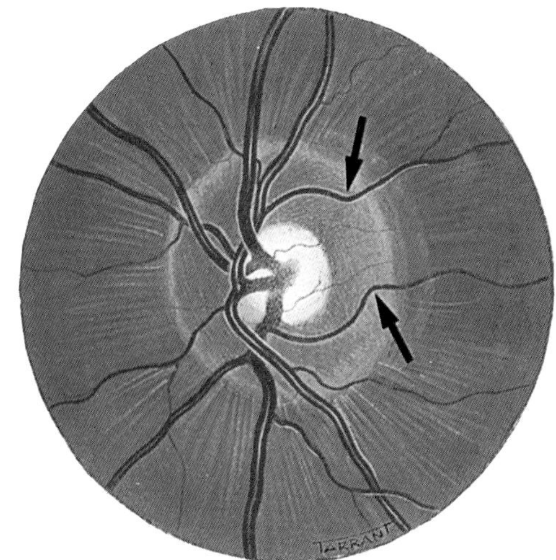

Figure 7.23 *Pallor and cupping of optic discs: arrows delineate area of cupping*

reached the disc margin. A splinter-shaped haemorrhage on the disc margin is also seen. In *Figure 7.25b*, the cup has extended both superiorly and inferiorly to a moderate degree. The double angulation of the blood vessels as they dive sharply backwards and then turn along the steep wall of the excavation before angling again onto the floor of the cup is a common, but not necessarily a pathognomonic, finding in glaucoma, and is sometimes referred to as the 'bayonetting sign'.

Ophthalmoscopy using red-free light will reveal wedge-shaped defects in the inferior peripapillary region and baring of the large retinal blood vessels (*Figure 7.24, bottom left*).

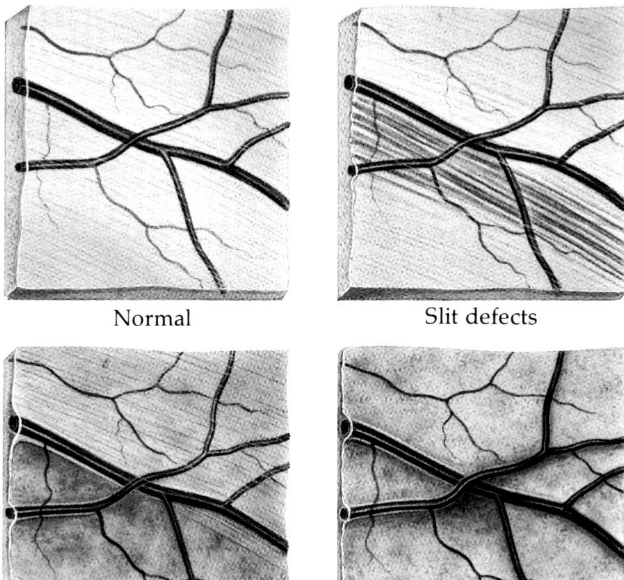

Figure 7.24 *Progression of nerve fibre damage in glaucoma*

The localized loss of tissue just described is the easiest to recognize and is the most characteristic finding in glaucoma. However, the axon loss can also occur diffusely across the entire cross-section of the optic nerve. When this happens, the excavation simply enlarges concentrically without associated localized notching of the neuroretinal rim. A concentrically enlarged cup may be difficult to distinguish from a large physiological cup whose cup–disc ratio is still within normal limits. Sometimes the enlarging cup may leave behind, or 'bare', a characteristic curved (circumlinear) blood vessel that marks the previous boundary of the physiological cup. The best way to detect concentric enlargement of the cup is to compare it with a previous record of the disc.

Figure 7.25c shows advanced cupping with total loss of superior and inferior disc tissue. The area of pallor, representing the floor of the cup, is vertically oval. The openings of the lamina cribrosa are visible up to the margin of the disc. This 'lamellar dot sign', just like the 'bayonetting sign', indicates that in these meridia all neural disc tissue has been destroyed. The progressive loss of nasal disc tissue causes a nasal displacement of the central blood vessels. This finding, especially occurring asymmetrically, may occasionally serve as a clue to the presence of glaucoma. As the damage progresses, the temporal margin of the disc atrophies and then the nasal rim also disappears. Eventually, all neural disc tissue is destroyed and the optic nerve head appears white and deeply excavated (*Figure 7.25d*).

Ophthalmoscopy using red-free light will show total atrophy of the retinal nerve fibre layer and complete baring of the large retinal blood vessels (*Figure 7.24, bottom right*). The atrophic area will appear darker and mottled because of enhanced visualization of the retinal pigment epithelium and choroid.

A stereoscopic evaluation of the optic nerve head using a slitlamp and a Hruby lens, or a +90 D lens may be necessary to detect glaucomatous changes in a highly

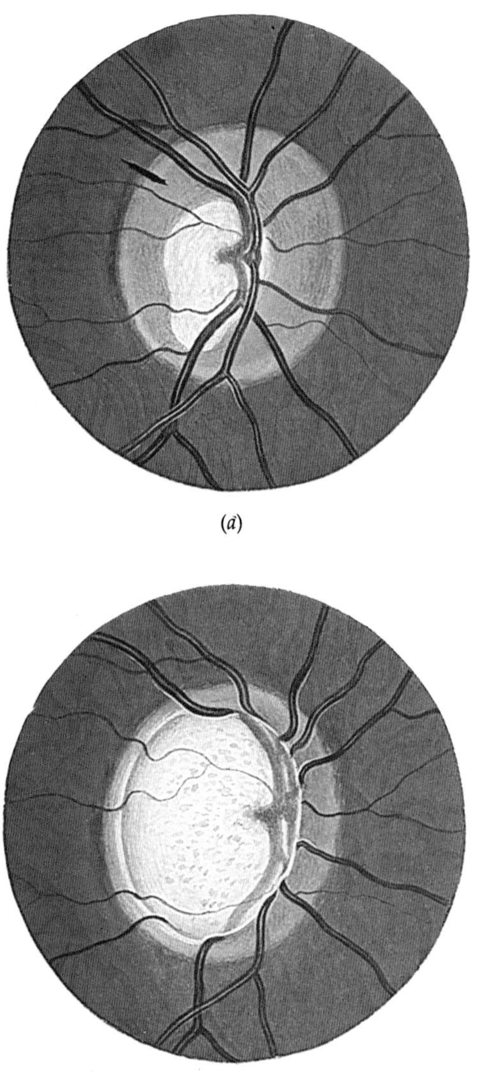

(a)

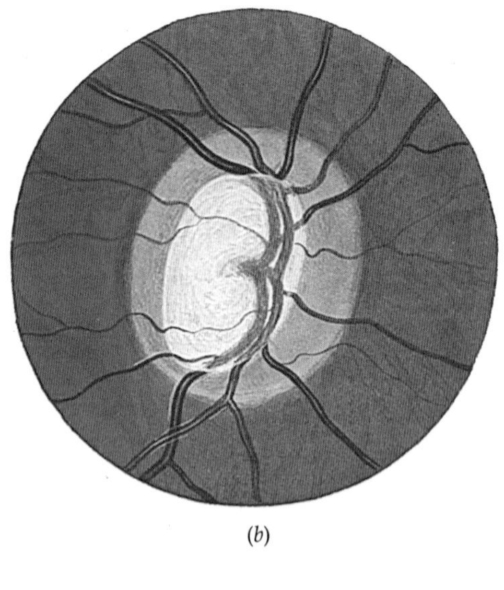

(b)

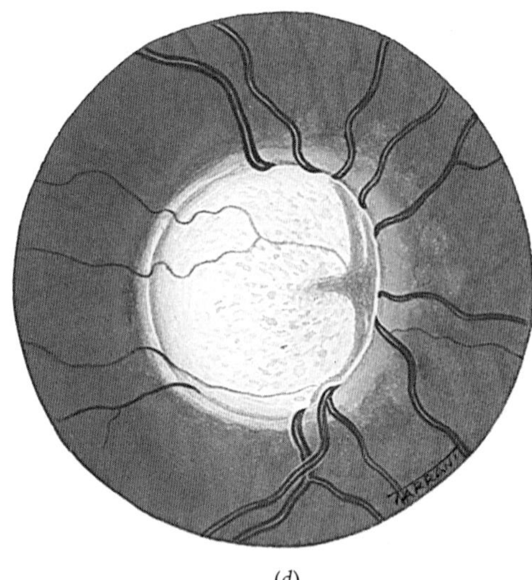

(c)

(d)

Figure 7.25 *Progression of glaucomatous cupping*

myopic eye. The findings should be carefully drawn in the notes with a record of the cup–disc ratio. This will provide a useful basis for subsequent comparison and ensures that a careful examination has been performed. Ideally, stereophotographs of suspicious cases should also be taken.

Visual field defects

The earliest *clinically significant* field defect is a scotoma that develops between 10 and 20° of fixation in areas constituting downward or, more commonly, upward extensions from the blind spot (Bjerrum area) (*Figure 7.26, left*). Initially, the defects do not connect with the blind spot but, with the passage of time, they tend to elongate circumferentially along the distribution of arcuate nerve fibres (Seidel scotoma). Isolated paracentral nasal scotomas may also be found in early glaucoma (*Figure 7.26, right*). Although these defects are frequently absolute when first detected, they may occasionally disappear after normalization of IOP.

Baring of the blind spot may occur in association with nerve fibre bundle defects but it is too non-specific a sign to be of diagnostic importance by itself. A nasal (Roenne) step is frequently associated with other defects but rarely may be present by itself. For this reason, the detection of a nasal step (or a temporal wedge, which is equally significant; *Figure 7.27*) should lead to a thorough search for paracentral scotomas. In uncontrolled glaucoma, the scotomas in the Bjerrum area coalesce to form an arcuate-shaped defect that arches from the blind spot around the macula reaching to within 5° of fixation nasally (*Figure 7.28, left*).

Damage to adjacent nerve fibres causes a peripheral breakthrough (*Figure 7.28, right*), and a ring or a double arcuate scotoma develops when defects arising in opposite halves of the visual field join together (*Figure 7.29, left*). In these cases, the asymmetrical involvement of independent nerve fibres causes the nasal step to be retained. The visual field loss gradually spreads to the periphery and also centrally so that eventually only a small island of central vision and an accompanying temporal island are left (*Figure 7.29, right*). The temporal island is usually extinguished before the central island, although occasionally this sequence is reversed.

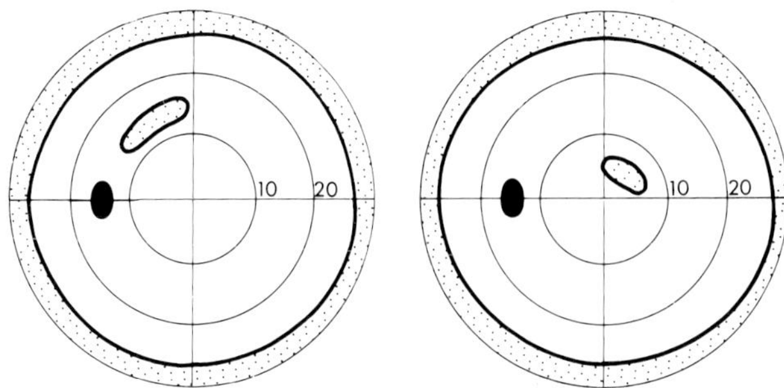

Figure 7.26 *Early glaucomatous visual field defects*

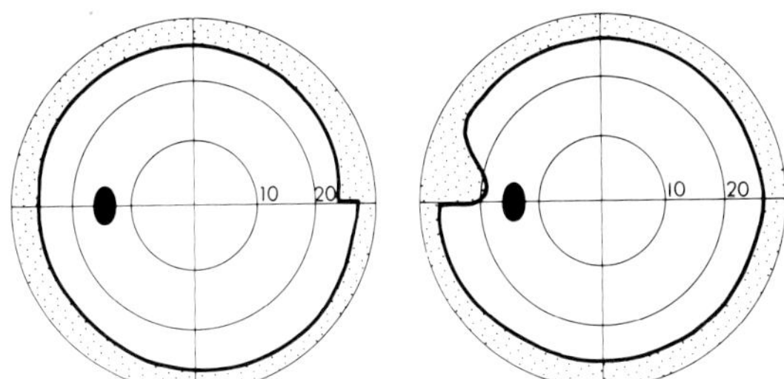

Figure 7.27 *Left: nasal step; right: temporal wedge*

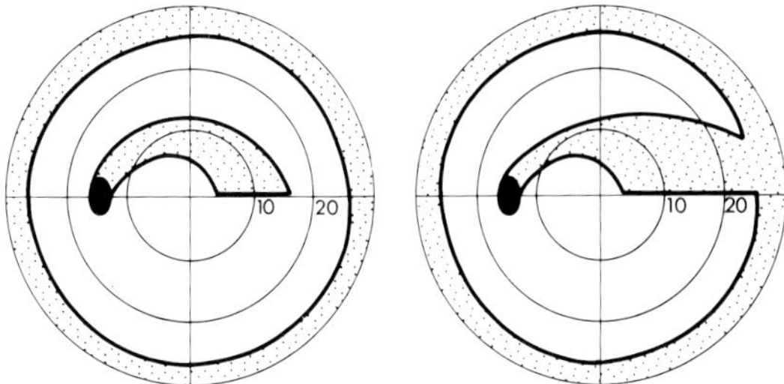

Figure 7.28 *Left: arcuate Bjerrum scotoma; right: arcuate scotoma with peripheral breakthrough*

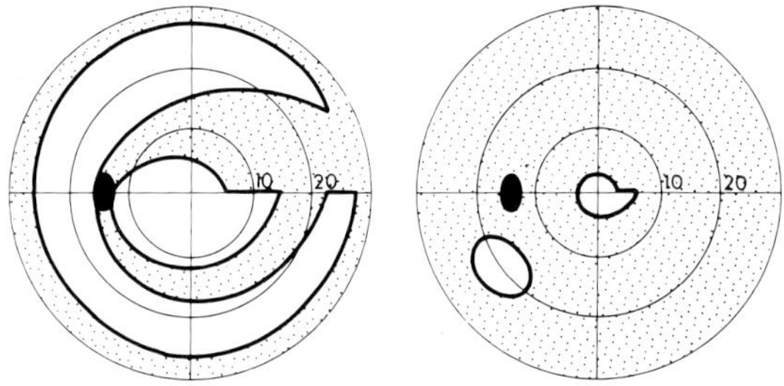

Double arcuate scotoma Temporal–central island

Figure 7.29 *Advanced glaucomatous visual field defects*

Tonometry

Patients with POAG frequently show a wider swing in IOP than normals. For this reason the finding of a single pressure reading of 21 mmHg or less does not exclude the diagnosis. In order to detect such fluctuations, it may be necessary to measure the IOP at different times of the day or, better still, at periodic intervals around the clock (phasing). A large discrepancy in the level of IOP between the two eyes should be viewed with suspicion on the assumption that, irrespective of the absolute pressure value, the eye with the higher reading is probably diseased.

Tonography

This test was initially advocated as a method of circumventing the diagnostic problems in patients with large diurnal pressure variations. Unfortunately, it has proven to be of very little value in the detection of early POAG.

Gonioscopy

Although the angle must be open for a diagnosis of POAG to be made, there are no pathognomonic findings.

Corticosteroid responsiveness

It has been shown that the application of betamethasone drops four times a day for 6 weeks causes a marked elevation of IOP (to over 31 mmHg) in about 5% of the general population. A further 35% show a moderate rise (between 22 mmHg and 30 mmHg), and the remaining 60% show virtually no change. About 90% of patients with established POAG are high corticosteroid reactors, and the remaining 10% are moderate reactors. Approximately 30% of siblings of patients with established POAG are high corticosteroid reactors and 50% are moderate reactors. The incidence of high corticosteroid responsiveness in the offspring of sufferers from POAG is 25%, and of moderate responsiveness is 70%.

It has been postulated that the response of IOP to topical corticosteroid administration is determined genetically and the genes that determine corticosteroid responsiveness and POAG are closely related. Both high myopes and diabetics have a higher incidence of corticosteroid responsiveness and also of POAG than the general population.

For the foregoing reasons, topical corticosteroids should be used with caution in patients with POAG, in their first-degree relatives, and in high myopes and diabetics. Systemic corticosteroids are much less likely to cause elevation of IOP than topical preparations. No matter whether the patient is a high or intermediate corticosteroid responder, dexamethasone, betamethasone, and prednisolone are probably equipotent in their ability to raise IOP. Fluorometholone raises the IOP half as much as betamethasone, and medrysone only one-eighth as much. Clobetasone also has a low propensity for elevating IOP.

Ocular associations

High myopia

Although the diagnosis of POAG may occasionally be difficult in highly myopic eyes, there is no doubt that high myopes have an increased prevalence of POAG.

Retinal vein occlusion

Raised IOP makes the eye susceptible to retinal vein occlusion.

Retinal detachment

POAG occurs more frequently in patients with rhegmatogenous retinal detachment than in normals. However, should an eye with established POAG suddenly develop a dramatic drop in IOP, then a retinal detachment should be suspected.

Fuchs' endothelial dystrophy

Approximately 15% of patients with Fuchs' dystrophy have POAG.

Retinitis pigmentosa

The incidence of POAG in patients with retinitis pigmentosa is 3%.

Systemic associations

Diabetes mellitus

Diabetic patients have a higher prevalence of POAG than non-diabetics. Conversely, about 10% of POAG patients have either frank diabetes or abnormal glucose tolerance test results.

Phenylthiocarbamide (PTC) tasting

Seventy per cent of POAG patients are PTC non-tasters, whereas the proportion of non-tasting normal subjects is 20%.

Thyroid function

The incidence of PTC non-tasters is increased in individuals with a low protein-bound iodine. POAG patients also have a higher incidence of low levels of protein-bound iodine.

Differential diagnosis

'Low-tension glaucoma'

This is similar to POAG except that the IOP is 21 mmHg or less on initial screening. Most patients with these findings fall into one of the following categories.

True low-tension glaucoma is thought to be caused by a low vascular perfusion pressure which makes the optic nerve susceptible to damage, even from a normal IOP. Treatment of these patients is usually frustrating and unsatisfactory. In order to prevent progressive visual field loss, the IOP should be maintained at less than 12 mmHg.

Non-progressive low-tension glaucoma is frequently associated with a past history of sudden and profound systemic hypotension, usually due to acute blood loss or myocardial infarction. In these patients, even without therapy, the visual field changes are usually non-progressive.

Pseudo-low-tension glaucoma is true POAG with wide diurnal variations in IOP. It is best diagnosed by phasing.

Mimicking conditions include disorders that cause nerve fibre bundle defects such as congenital disc anomalies (hyaline bodies and tilted disc), and colobomatous optic discs that may be mistaken for glaucomatous cupping. Certain acquired compressive or ischaemic optic nerve or chiasmal lesions may, on cursory examination, be misinterpreted as being glaucomatous (*see* Chapter 15).

Ocular hypertension

This is similar to POAG except that there is no cupping or field loss. Long-term studies have shown that only a minority of eyes with elevated IOP will eventually develop glaucomatous damage. It appears that most cases of ocular hypertension merely represent the upper end of the IOP distribution curve and are not cases of early POAG.

Unfortunately, at present there is no infallible way of predicting which ocular hypertensives will subsequently develop POAG. For this reason some authorities prefer to use the term 'glaucoma suspect' to describe these patients in order to emphasize the need for long-term follow-up.

Intermittent angle-closure glaucoma

This can be mistaken for POAG if the patient is examined when the IOP is only mildly elevated and the angle moderately open.

Antiglaucoma drugs

The main drugs used in the treatment of glaucoma are: beta-adrenergic blocking agents, adrenaline, miotics, guanethidine and carbonic anhydrase inhibitors.

Pharmacology

Adrenergic neurones secrete noradrenaline at neuromuscular nerve endings. Adrenergic receptors are of three types (*Figure 7.30*):

1. *Alpha* receptors are situated in arterioles, the dilator muscle of the iris and in Müller's muscle. Alpha stimulation therefore causes an increase in blood pressure, mydriasis and lid retraction. An increase in the facility of aqueous outflow also occurs as a result of alpha stimulation.

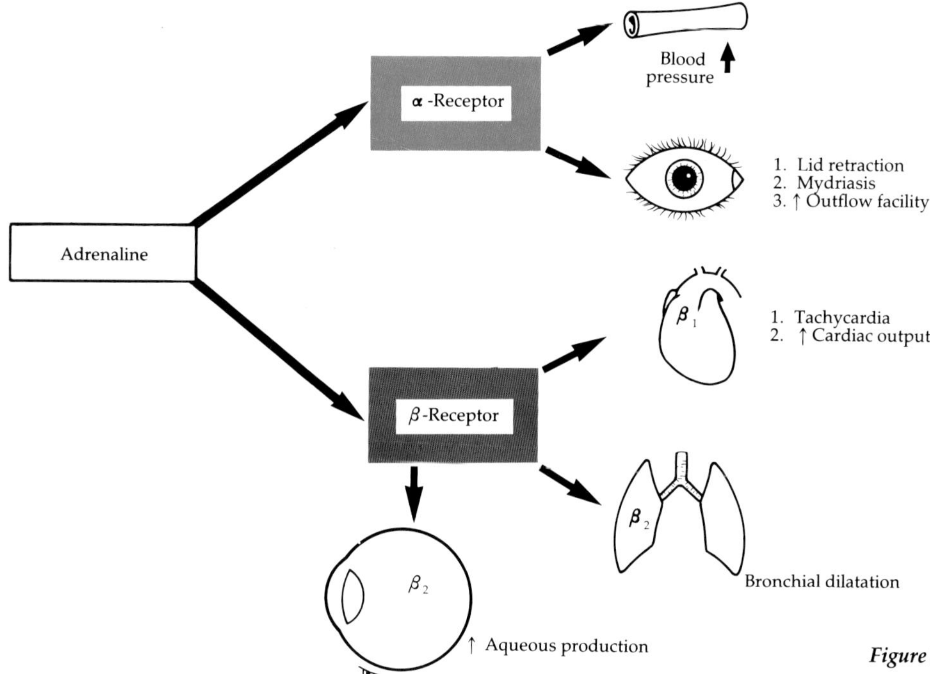

Figure 7.30 *Pharmacology of adrenergic neurones*

2. *Beta-1* receptors are present in heart muscle and cause tachycardia and increased cardiac output when stimulated.
3. *Beta-2* receptors are located in the bronchial musculature and when stimulated cause bronchial dilatation. Recent studies have shown that, contrary to previous teaching, beta-2 stimulation causes a slight increase and not a decrease in aqueous humour secretion.

Beta blockers are agents that compete with catecholamines for beta-adrenergic receptor sites.

Cholinergic neurones secrete acetylcholine at neuromuscular nerve endings. The acetylcholine then acts on receptors until its effect is terminated by the enzyme cholinesterase. Cholinergic neurones are of two types (*Figure 7.31*):

1. *Nicotinic* receptors are present in striated muscle such as the levator, the orbicularis, and the extraocular muscles.
2. *Muscarinic* receptors are situated in parasympathetically innervated structures such as the iris and the ciliary body.

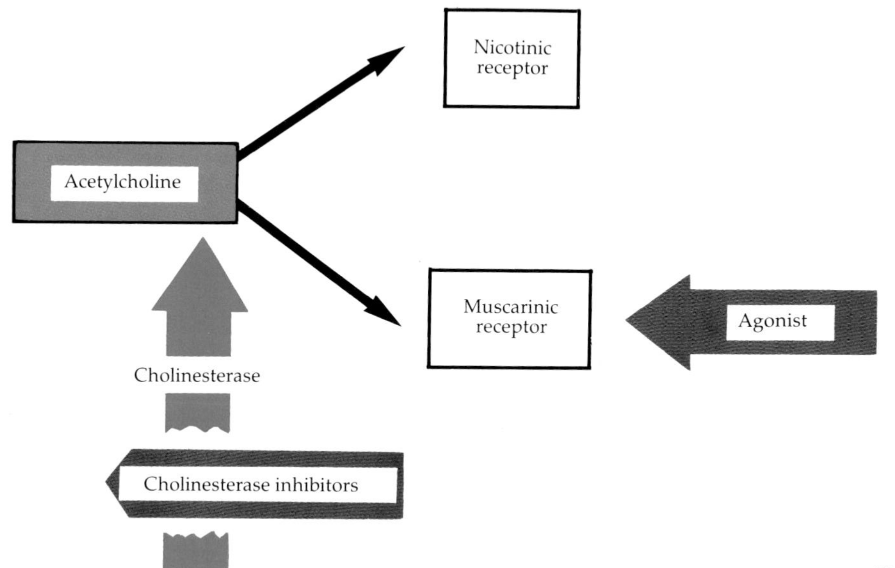

Figure 7.31 *Pharmacology of cholinergic neurones*

Parasympathomimetic drugs imitate or potentiate the action of acetylcholine. They are of two types: agonists and cholinesterase inhibitors.

The agonists exert their effects by directly stimulating receptors. Pilocarpine is a muscarinic agonist. (Nicotinic agonists play no part in the treatment of glaucoma.)

The cholinesterase inhibitors exert their effects indirectly by destroying cholinesterase, thus causing an accumulation of naturally produced acetylcholine. Although they enhance both nicotinic and muscarinic effects, in the treatment of glaucoma they are used solely for their muscarinic properties. The four cholinesterase inhibitors that have been used in the treatment of glaucoma are physostigmine (eserine), ecothiopate (Phospholine Iodide), demecarium bromide (Tosmilen, Humorsol), and isoflurophate (dyflos).

The effects of miotics on aqueous humour dynamics are still incompletely understood. It has been postulated that they lower IOP by causing a contraction in the longitudinal muscle of the ciliary body. When contracted, this muscle exerts a pull on the scleral spur and produces changes in the trabecular meshwork or in Schlemm's canal, causing an increase in aqueous outflow.

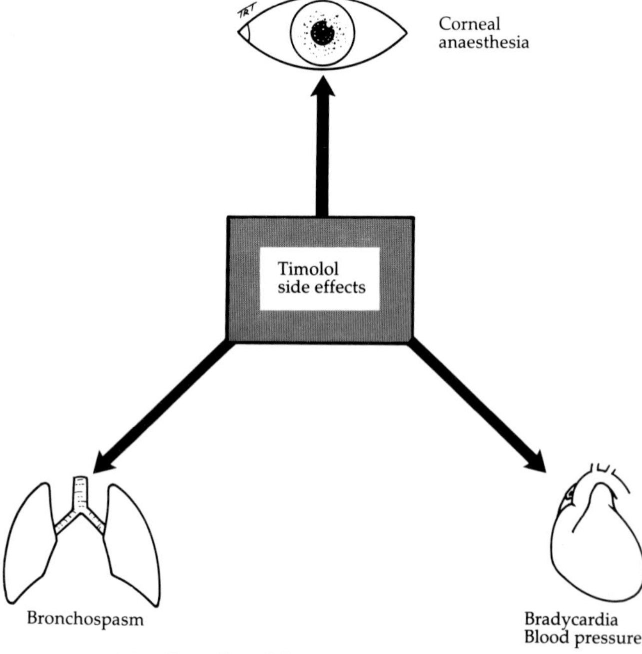

Figure 7.32 Side-effects of timolol

Beta-adrenergic blocking agents

The four beta blockers currently used in the management of glaucoma are: timolol, betaxolol, carteolol, and metipranolol.

Timolol (0.25%, 0.5%)

Timolol (Timoptol, Timoptic) is a non-selective beta-adrenergic blocking agent which lowers intraocular pressure by reducing aqueous secretion. The maximal pressure-lowering effect is reached within 1–2 hours and lasts for up to 24 hours. The drug like all topical beta-blockers is administered twice a day.

Although timolol may initially cause a dramatic lowering of IOP, in some patients this effect partially wanes during the ensuing days, an effect referred to as 'short-term' escape. Although in the majority of cases the drug continues to be effective after many months of therapy, a tendency for a slow rise in IOP has been noted in some patients. It is uncertain whether this phenomenon, which is termed 'long-term drift', is due to loss of efficacy of the drug, or worsening of the glaucoma, or both.

Side-effects (*Figure 7.32*)

Local side-effects include superficial punctate keratopathy and rarely corneal anaesthesia.

Systemic side-effects include bradycardia as a result of its beta-1 adrenergic blocking action. This effect may reduce cardiac contractility and cause systemic hypotension. Timolol should, therefore, not be used in patients with a slow pulse or heart block. The beta-2 adrenergic blocking action of timolol may cause bronchospasm. This may be particularly dangerous in asthmatics and patients with chronic obstructive airways disease. Other side-effects include fatigue, disorientation, confusion, and depression.

The incidence and severity of systemic side-effects can be reduced by performing punctal occlusion for 1 minute after instillation of the drops.

Betaxolol (0.5%)

Betaxolol (Betoptic) is a cardioselective beta-1 adrenergic blocking agent which is nearly as effective as timolol in lowering intraocular pressure and has the advantage of having little effect on the cardiopulmonary system. It is therefore safer to use than timolol in patients with pulmonary disease.

Other non-selective beta-adrenergic blocking agents in current use include:

1. Carteolol (Teoptic) 1% and 2%.
2. Metipranolol (Glauline) 0.1%, 0.3% and 0.6%.
3. Levobunolol (Betagan) 0.5%.

Adrenaline (epinephrine) (0.5%, 1%, 2%)

Adrenaline is an alpha and beta agonist. It lowers IOP by increasing aqueous outflow through its alpha agonist action. Its pressure-lowering effect is reached within 1–2 hours and lasts for 12–24 hours after twice daily administration.

Side-effects (*Figure 7.33*)

Local side-effects include stinging, headache, allergic blepharoconjunctivitis, conjunctival hyperaemia (2 hours

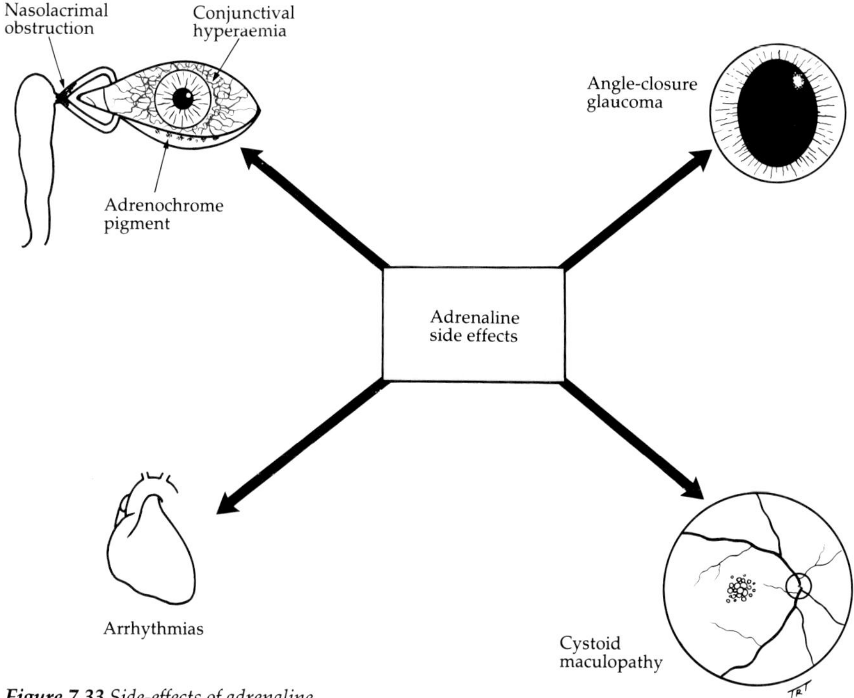

Figure 7.33 *Side-effects of adrenaline*

after instillation), nasolacrimal obstruction, and adrenochrome deposits in the conjunctiva (with long-term use).

Angle-closure glaucoma may be precipitated in eyes with narrow chamber angles due to its mydriatic effect (alpha agonist action). The mydriatic effects of adrenaline are enhanced by timolol.

Cystoid maculopathy may occur in aphakic eyes, especially if the 2% concentration is used. Careful monitoring of visual acuity, and possibly also fluorescein angiography, are necessary if adrenaline therapy is deemed essential in the treatment of glaucoma in an aphakic eye. Fortunately, the maculopathy is usually reversible on cessation of administration.

Systemic side-effects include premature cardiac contractions and occasionally other arrhythmias (due to its beta-1 agonist action).

Advantages

Adrenaline need only be administered twice a day. It does not cause miosis or spasm of accommodation. It is useful in the treatment of certain secondary glaucomas. It has an additive effect to pilocarpine, carbonic anhydrase inhibitors, and also probably to timolol.

Disadvantages

About 30% of patients with POAG are unresponsive to adrenaline medication. The drug does not appear to be as effective in lowering IOP as either timolol or pilocarpine. The relatively high incidence of side-effects necessitates its discontinuation in a significant number of patients.

Dipivalyl adrenaline (0.1%)

Dipivalyl adrenaline (Propine) is a prodrug which is converted into adrenaline after absorption into the eye. Its main advantage over adrenaline is that it penetrates the cornea 17 times better, and the hypotensive effect of 0.1% dipivalyl adrenaline is comparable to 1% adrenaline. This low concentration causes fewer side-effects such as conjunctival hyperaemia and headache.

Guanethidine

Guanethidine has a potentiating effect on adrenaline in the treatment of glaucoma. The combination of the two is called Ganda. The concentration of guanethidine in Ganda is either 1% or 3%; this is combined with either 0.2% or 0.5% adrenaline.

Miotics

Pilocarpine (1%, 2%, 3%, 4%)

In the treatment of POAG, pilocarpine is administered four times a day. Its pressure-lowering action begins within 20 minutes, reaches its peak in about 1.5 hours, and lasts for 4 hours. Concentrations above 4% do not appear to be more effective in lowering IOP although they may have a slightly more prolonged effect. Ocuserts are a controlled-release system for delivery of pilocarpine at a constant rate for 7 days. This improves diurnal pressure variations and increases patient compliance. The Pilo-20 system is equivalent to a 1% solution of pilocarpine and the Pilo-40 system is equivalent to the 2–4% concentration.

Carbachol (3%)

Carbachol used three times a day is a very useful alternative to pilocarpine in resistant or intolerant cases. It begins to act within 40 minutes and its duration of action is between 8 and 12 hours.

Long-acting miotics

Ecothiopate (0.06–0.25%), *demecarium bromide* (0.125–0.25%) and *isoflurophate* (0.01–0.1%) need be instilled only once or twice daily as their duration of action is 24 hours.

Side-effects of miotics

Local side-effects of miosis include diminished night vision, permanent miosis with prolonged use, reduced visual acuity in the presence of axial lens opacities, a generalized constriction of the visual field, and an apparent increase in size of visual field defects. Spasm of accommodation may induce myopia and cause considerable difficulties in young patients. As the degree of spasm is variable, it cannot always be overcome by the provision of spectacles. Frontal headache is a frequent symptom at the start of therapy, but it usually regresses after a few weeks. If severe it can be relieved by salicylates.

Angle-closure glaucoma may be precipitated in eyes with narrow angles due to aggravation of pupillary block.

Retinal detachment is a very rare complication that should be suspected if a glaucomatous eye suddenly develops a dramatic drop in IOP or in vision. Ideally, the peripheral retina should be examined and any predisposing lesions treated prophylactically before the commencement of miotic therapy.

Lens opacities may occur as a result of the use of long-acting cholinesterase inhibitors. For this reason, these drugs are usually reserved for the treatment of glaucoma in aphakic eyes.

Iris cysts may form along the pupillary border with the use of long-acting cholinesterase inhibitors. This complication can be avoided by the simultaneous administration of phenylephrine 2.5% or adrenaline 1%.

Systemic side-effects due to parasympathetic stimulation include bradycardia, increased sweating, diarrhoea, salivation, and anxiety. Ecothiopate may block other cholinesterases in the body and cause 'Scoline apnoea' following general anaesthesia in which the patient is unable to resume spontaneous respiration.

Advantages

Miotics are cheap and very effective pressure-lowering drugs.

Disadvantages

Miotics are contraindicated in the management of secondary glaucoma due to anterior uveitis as they increase the permeability of the blood–aqueous barrier, allowing the transfer of protein, fibrin, and cells into the aqueous. They may also promote the formation of synechiae in eyes with active uveitis. Other disadvantages are the disabling side-effects of miosis and the need to administer pilocarpine four times a day.

Carbonic anhydrase inhibitors

The four carbonic anhydrase inhibitors (CAIs) used in the treatment of glaucoma are:

Acetazolamide	(Diamox)	250 mg
Dichlorphenamide	(Daranide)	50 mg
Methazolamide	(Neptazane)	50 mg
Ethoxzolamide	(Cardrase)	125 mg

The CAIs are among the most potent of all antiglaucoma agents, reducing IOP by between 40 and 60% by their action on the secretory ciliary epithelium. Although acetazolamide is the only one that can be administered by injection as well as orally, there is, as yet, no clear evidence to suggest superiority of one over the others. The pressure-lowering effect is apparent within 1 hour, reaching a peak at 4 hours, and wearing off in about 6–12 hours. A long-acting preparation of acetazolamide 500 mg (Diamox Sustets) has an effect lasting for up to 24 hours.

Unfortunately, the usefulness of the CAIs in long-term therapy of POAG is often limited by their side-effects. Compliance is also poor with only about two-thirds of patients taking their medication regularly.

Side-effects (*Figure 7.34*)

Because *paraesthesiae* are a universal side-effect, compliance should be questioned if the patient denies this symptom.

The *'malaise symptom complex'* includes malaise, fatigue, depression, loss of weight, and decreased libido. This

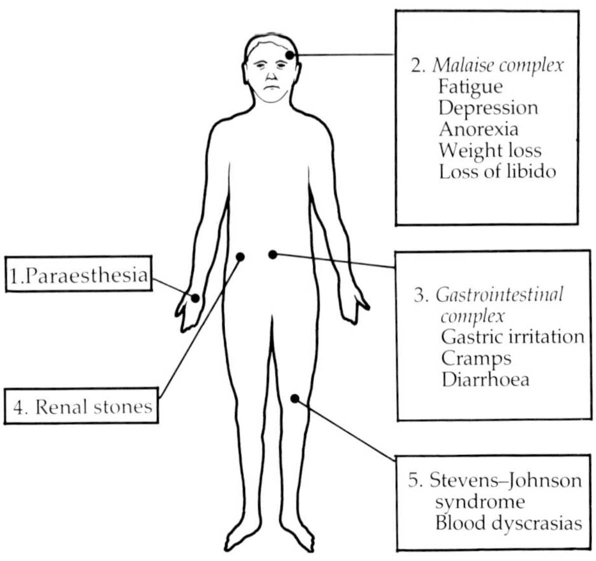

Figure 7.34 *Side-effects of carbonic acid anhydrase inhibitors*

syndrome is associated with excessive levels of the drug in the serum and with systemic metabolic acidosis. Fifty per cent of patients can be helped by supplemental 2-week courses of sodium acetate.

The *'gastrointestinal symptom complex'*, consisting of gastric irritation, abdominal cramps, diarrhoea and nausea, can occur independently of the malaise syndrome and does not appear to be related to changes in blood chemistry.

Renal stone formation is another rare complication that is related to decreased urinary citrate excretion without a corresponding fall in serum calcium.

Because the CAIs belong to the sulphonamide family of drugs, they may cause the Stevens–Johnson syndrome and blood dyscrasias. Other side-effects include transient myopia and altered taste of carbonated beverages.

Management

Indications for treatment

Established POAG

There is universal agreement that all eyes with POAG must be treated in order to prevent further damage.

POAG in one eye and ocular hypertension in the other

Because the risk of damage in the eye with ocular hypertension is significant (probably in the order of 65% in 5 years), most would advocate treatment even in the absence of visual field loss.

Ocular hypertension

If neither eye is glaucomatous but merely shows elevated IOP, the decision whether or not to treat is more difficult and controversial. In this situation other risk factors have to be taken into consideration.

Level of IOP

The risk of damage seems to be higher for eyes with very high pressures (over 30 mmHg) than for those with pressures in the 20s, although there is no 'magic number' which makes treatment mandatory. Fortunately, the actual number of patients with very high pressures but no field loss is small. In general, most ophthalmologists would treat ocular hypertensives with pressures over 30 mmHg.

Rising pressure

Eyes with ocular hypertension that show a steady and progressive rise in IOP over many months will probably eventually develop POAG. In these cases very careful monitoring of the optic discs and visual fields is necessary and, if there is any evidence of impending damage such as haemorrhage on the disc or an enlarging cup, treatment should be started even in the absence of demonstrable field loss.

Family history

In the presence of a family history of POAG, the risk of damage is increased eight-fold as it seems likely that the patient has inherited some of the factors that make the optic nerve head more vulnerable to damage. Most authorities would therefore advocate treatment of ocular hypertensives who have first-degree relatives with POAG.

Diabetes mellitus

It has been suggested that the optic nerve head in a diabetic patient is more vulnerable to damage by elevated IOP than in a healthy subject. This may be related to vascular compromise in diabetes.

Age of patient

The optic nerve heads of elderly patients appear to be less resistant to elevated IOP than in young people. In addition, about 10% of ocular hypertensives over the age of 65 years will develop retinal vein occlusion.

Only eye

Most would probably advocate treatment of ocular hypertension in a patient who has only one seeing eye.

Baseline evaluation

The key to effective treatment is careful and regular follow-up. It is important to perform a good baseline examination with which future progress can be compared.

The initial examination includes the following:

1. Visual acuity.
2. Slitlamp examination of the anterior segment with particular reference to lens opacities and secondary glaucomas masquerading as POAG.
3. Applanation tonometry.
4. Evaluation of the optic discs, ideally with photographs.
5. Gonioscopy.
6. Perimetry.

Treatment of POAG may be medical, by argon laser trabeculoplasty, or by filtration surgery.

Principles of medical therapy

The initial therapy of POAG is medical. The chosen drug should be used in its lowest concentration, as infrequently as possible, in order to achieve the desired effect. If possible, the drug with the fewest potential side-effects should be chosen.

In most cases the initial medical therapy is with a beta-blocker (e.g. timolol 0.25%, betaxolol 0.5%). If this is ineffective, the strength of the beta-blocker can be increased and/or Propine added. Pilocarpine is usually reserved for patients who are uncontrolled on a combination of a beta-blocker and Propine. Because of the risk of side-effects, carbonic anhydrase inhibitors should be considered only as short-term treatment.

Follow-up evaluation

After the initiation of therapy the patient is seen at 2- or 4-weekly intervals until the IOP is controlled and then at 3–4-monthly intervals. Unfortunately, the actual safe level of IOP is still unknown, although in most cases further damage is unlikely if the IOP has been reduced to the lower 'teens'. However, an optic nerve head showing minimal damage can tolerate a higher IOP than one with gross cupping and advanced visual field loss. Only stability of the visual fields and appearance of the optic disc are proof that the IOP is indeed at a safe level.

Gonioscopy

Because the anterior chamber gradually shallows with age, gonioscopy should be performed routinely once a year. Miotics may precipitate angle closure in eyes with shallow anterior chambers. For this reason, gonioscopy should be performed on all patients soon after the initiation of miotic therapy or whenever the IOP rises for an inexplicable reason.

Perimetry

If control of IOP is good and the appearance of the optic discs stable, twice yearly perimetry is sufficient. Because pupillary constriction reduces retinal sensitivity and may mimic progressive visual field loss, particularly in older patients with lens opacities, it is necessary to perform perimetry immediately before and soon after the initiation of miotic therapy in order to obtain a baseline. Alternatively, the pupil should be dilated with phenylephrine 2.5% at each subsequent visual field examination. Because of possible short-term fluctuations in the visual fields, it is usually necessary to assess a series of fields before diagnosing definitive field loss.

Argon laser trabeculoplasty

The advent of argon laser trabeculoplasty (ALT) has dramatically changed the treatment of patients with uncontrolled open-angle glaucoma. Theoretically, ALT causes a shrinkage of the collagen on the inner surface of the trabecular ring and contracts it inwards, thereby opening the intertrabecular spaces and increasing aqueous outflow.

Indications

ALT should be considered in cases of open-angle glaucoma that are uncontrolled despite maximal tolerated medical therapy. In order to perform ALT, the trabecular meshwork must be easily visible through a clear cornea and at least 180° of the angle has to be open.

Technique

1. The cornea is anaesthetized.
2. The laser is set at a spot size of 50 μm, a duration of 0.1 s, and power setting of between 500 and 750 mW.
3. A Goldmann triple-mirror goniolens with anti-reflection coating is inserted and the patient is instructed to look at the fixation light with the other eye.
4. Using the small semicircular mirror, the angle structures are identified. If the angle is relatively narrow, a few laser burns (200 μm, 0.1 s, 200 mW) can be applied to the peripheral iris close to the angle structures. This will cause the iris to retract and enhance visualization of the trabeculum.
5. The aiming beam is then precisely focused and burns applied to the junction of the non-pigmented with the pigmented trabeculum. The ideal reaction is the appearance of either a small bubble or blanching at the point of impact (*Figure 7.35a,b*). If this does not occur the power of the laser should be increased by 200-mW steps. In heavily pigmented angles, a power setting of as little as 400 mW may suffice, whereas some non-pigmented angles may require as much as 2000 mW. In general, most eyes require 100 burns for 360° to obtain the necessary fall of IOP. This can be done either during one session or in two separate sessions spaced 4–6 weeks apart.

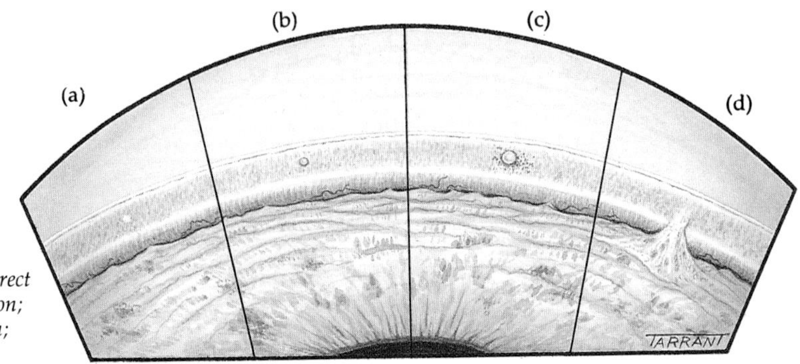

Figure 7.35 *Laser trabeculoplasty.* (a) *Transient blanching–correct reaction;* (b) *transient formation of small bubble – correct reaction;* (c) *large bubble with heavy pigment fall-out – excessive reaction;* (d) *peripheral anterior synechiae – burn applied too posteriorly*

Postoperative management

1. Following ALT the patient should be observed for at least 3 hours so that any excessive elevation of IOP can be detected and treated. This is particularly important in patients with advanced visual field loss. If after 3 hours, the IOP is not elevated the patient is sent home and instructed to use steroid drops four times a day for 1 week. Glaucoma medication should be continued as before.
2. The patient is re-examined 2 days later to evaluate the extent of laser-induced anterior uveitis and to record the level of IOP. Although occasionally there is an immediate drop of IOP, more frequently this takes between 4 and 6 weeks.
3. The patient is re-examined in 6 weeks. If the IOP is satisfactory, glaucoma medication may be gradually reduced although total withdrawal is rarely achieved. If the IOP is still uncontrolled, despite 360° treatment, then filtration surgery should be considered as repeating ALT is unlikely to be successful.

Complications

1. Transient, acute elevation of IOP occurs in about 25% of patients. Significant elevation of IOP is treated with pilocarpine 4% drops and Diamox (acetazolamide) 250 mg, both four times a day. Occasionally, hyperosmotic agents such as oral glycerol are required if the IOP is excessively high. Post-ALT elevation of IOP appears to be more common when the entire angle is treated in one session. In eyes with advanced field loss, it is therefore safer to initially treat only one-half of the angle.
2. Permanent increase in IOP occurs in about 3% of cases.
3. Iritis which is mild and usually innocuous is fairly common.
4. Peripheral anterior synechiae may occur from burns applied too posteriorly (*Figure 7.35d*).
5. Small haemorrhages may develop if the blood vessels on peripheral iris or ciliary body are inadvertently treated. The bleeding is usually innocuous and can usually be stopped by applying pressure on the globe with the goniolens.

Results

About 75% of eyes with POAG have an average drop of IOP of between 8 mmHg and 10 mmHg. The results of ALT are also excellent in cases of glaucoma capsulare, pigmentary glaucoma, and aphakic or pseudophakic eyes which have POAG prior to lens extraction. However, the results in eyes that develop glaucoma after cataract extraction are less good with a success rate of about 50%. The least favourable results are in secondary and congenital glaucomas.

Filtration surgery

Indications

In general, filtration surgery should be considered in cases of uncontrolled glaucoma, despite ALT and maximally tolerated medical therapy. However, some cases of very high IOP in association with advanced cupping and field loss, should have filtration surgery without first trying ALT.

Preoperative preparation

Any pre-existing inflammation should be controlled in order to reduce the amount of postoperative iritis which may cause scarring of the filtration bleb. If possible, strong miotics should be stopped 2 weeks prior to surgery as they may cause congestion and leakage of protein from the iris and contribute to subsequent scarring of the bleb. The IOP should be reduced as much as possible before the eye is entered in order to reduce the risk of expulsive choroidal haemorrhage.

Choice of operation

The aim of glaucoma filtration surgery is to create a fistula which will act as a new channel for aqueous outflow. The two most popular filtration operations are Scheie's thermosclerostomy and trabeculectomy. In the former the fistula passes through the entire thickness of the sclera, whereas in the latter the fistula is 'guarded' by a superficial scleral flap. Although trabeculectomy is associated with fewer complications, the drop of IOP may not always be as great as with Scheie's procedure.

Operative techniques

Trabeculectomy

1. A conjunctival incision is made about 10 mm posterior to the limbus and a conjunctival flap dissected anteriorly.
2. An area, based at the limbus and measuring about 4 mm by 4 mm is outlined on the sclera with wet-field cautery.
3. Incisions are made along the cautery marks through about half to two-thirds of scleral thickness (*Figure 7.36a*).
4. The superficial flap is dissected and extended anteriorly as far as clear cornea.
5. A deep rectangular block of sclera (1.5 mm × 3 mm) is excised anterior to the sclera spur (*Figure 7.36b*).
6. A peripheral iridectomy is performed.
7. The superficial scleral flap is repositioned and sutured (*Figure 7.36c*).
8. The conjunctiva is sutured.

To some extent the amount of drainage can be controlled by varying the thickness of the scleral flap and by the tightness of suturing.

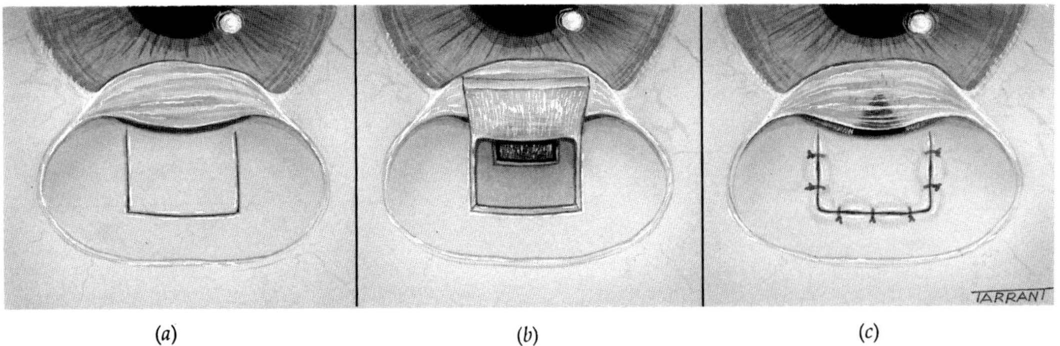

(a) (b) (c)

Figure 7.36 Trabeculectomy

Scheie's thermosclerostomy

1. A limbal-based conjunctival flap is dissected as for a trabeculectomy.
2. A partial thickness groove, about 4 mm long, is made at the limbus in the middle of the grey line.
3. The posterior lip of the groove is cauterized.
4. The incision is extended into the anterior chamber.
5. A peripheral iridectomy is performed.
6. The conjunctiva is sutured.

Postoperative management

Topical cycloplegics and corticosteroids should be administered until all inflammation has subsided. Because a good flow of aqueous through the new filtration site is necessary to maintain drainage postoperatively, drugs that inhibit aqueous secretion should be discontinued on the day of surgery.

Postoperative complications

These can be divided into early and late. The former occur within a few days of surgery and the latter within weeks, months or years.

The main early complications are:

1. Changes in refraction.
2. Hyphaema.
3. Shallow anterior chamber.
4. Endophthalmitis.
5. Total loss of visual field.

The main late complications are:

1. Endophthalmitis.
2. Cataract.

Early complications

Changes in refraction. A transient forward movement of the lens may induce a change in refraction and cause blurred vision. The condition resolves spontaneously within a few days and requires no specific treatment.

Hyphaema. Mild transient hyphaemas are fairly common and usually innocuous.

Shallow anterior chamber. A shallow or flat anterior chamber is a fairly common postoperative complication. If the eye is soft and no drainage bleb is present, then the cause of the flat anterior chamber is probably a 'button-hole' in the bleb. In this situation, a Seidel test using fluorescein should be performed to identify the site of leakage and the bleb repaired or a soft contact lens applied until the leak has healed. However, a flat anterior chamber in a soft eye with a good bleb is probably due to excessive filtration. In most instances, the chamber will reform spontaneously within a few days or with the aid of a pressure dressing.

If the anterior chamber is flat in a hard eye, the diagnosis is probably ciliary block (malignant) glaucoma. This very rare complication is presumably due to the blockage of aqueous flow at the secreting portion of the ciliary body, so that aqueous is forced backwards into the vitreous. Initial therapy is directed towards dilating the ciliary ring in order to increase the distance between the ciliary processes and the equator of the lens, thereby tightening the zonule and pulling the lens posteriorly into its normal position. In about 50% of cases this can be achieved by using atropine 2% and phenylephrine 10%. Intravenous mannitol is also very useful in shrinking the vitreous gel and allowing the lens to move posteriorly. If these measures are ineffective, aspiration of trapped aqueous through a pars plana incision should be performed in order to allow the lens to move posteriorly and break the blockage to aqueous flow.

Endophthalmitis. Intraocular infection following glaucoma filtration surgery is less common than following cataract extraction. Its management is discussed in Chapter 8.

Total loss of visual field. This extremely rare but devastating complication may occur in eyes with severe preoperative visual field loss.

Later complications

Endophthalmitis (*Figure 7.37*). Late intraocular infection appears to be directly related to the type of bleb formed rather than to the actual surgical procedure. The thin-walled cystic bleb with a positive Siedel test is particularly vulnerable as it drains transconjunctivally and is, therefore, most likely to provide a pathway for the entrance of bacteria into the eye. All patients with this type of bleb

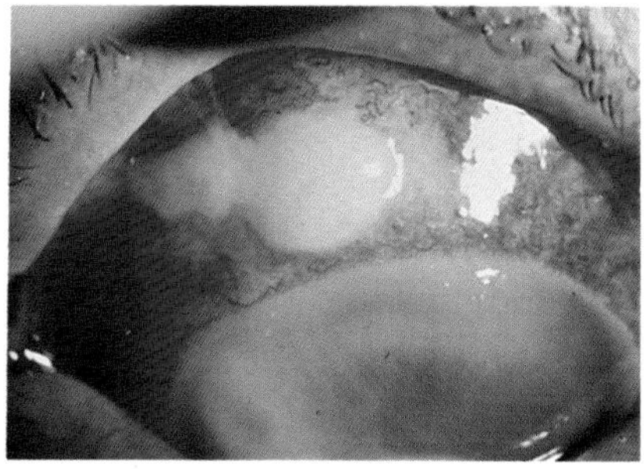

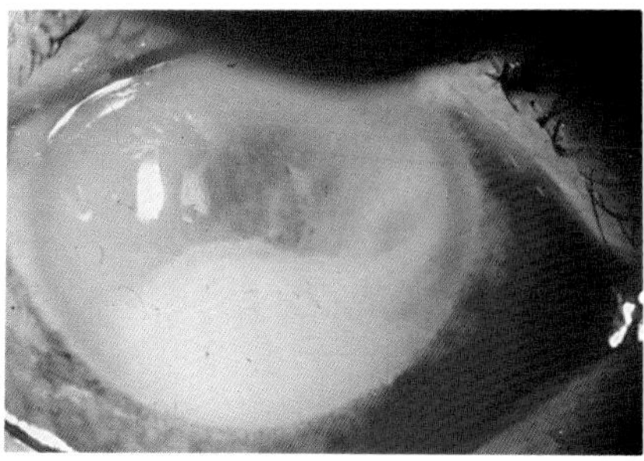

***Figure* 7.37** *Late endophthalmitis following filtration surgery*

should be warned of the possibility of late infection and told to report immediately should the eye become red or sticky, or the vision blurred. The fitting of contact lenses and unnecessary gonioscopy should also be avoided in eyes with filtering blebs as this may traumatize the bleb and increase the risk of infection.

Cataract. Glaucoma filtration surgery predisposes an eye to the subsequent development of lens opacities.

Results

In general, the success rate of filtration surgery in POAG is in the region of 80–90%. The results are, however, less good in black patients, young patients, and in aphakes.

Primary angle-closure glaucoma

Introduction

Primary angle-closure glaucoma (PACG) is a condition in which obstruction to aqueous outflow is brought about solely by closure of the angle by the peripheral iris. It occurs in anatomically predisposed eyes, and is frequently bilateral. The disease affects approximately 1 in 1000 individuals over the age of 40 years, affecting females more commonly than males by a ratio of four to one.

Inheritance

Like POAG it has a genetic basis, and it seems likely that it is the anatomical predisposition to the disease that is inherited.

Predisposing factors

Predisposing factors can be anatomical and physiological.

Anatomical

Eyes with PACG are characterized by a relatively anterior location of the iris–lens diaphragm, a shallow anterior chamber, and a narrow entrance to the chamber angle. The proximity of the peripheral iris to the cornea enables angle closure to occur more easily than in a normal eye. Three interrelated factors are responsible for these characteristics: lens size, corneal diameter, and axial length of the globe.

Lens size. The lens is the only ocular structure that continues to increase in size throughout life. Axial growth of the lens brings its anterior surface closer to the cornea. Equatorial growth tends to slacken the suspensory ligament, allowing the iris–lens diaphragm to move anteriorly. Both of these factors cause a very gradual and slowly progressive shallowing of the anterior chamber and a decrease in anterior chamber volume. Eyes with PACG have shallower anterior chambers than normal eyes (1.8 mm as opposed to 2.8 mm), and women have shallower anterior chambers than men.

Corneal diameter. The depth of the anterior chamber and width of the chamber angle are related to the corneal diameter. Eyes with PACG have a corneal diameter 0.25 mm less than normal eyes.

Axial length of globe. In normal eyes, lens thickness, relative position of the lens, and corneal diameter vary in relation to the axial length of the globe. A short eye, which is also frequently hypermetropic, has a small corneal diameter and a thick and relatively anteriorly located lens.

Physiological

The immediate physiological precipitating factors of PACG in predisposed eyes are not fully understood. At present two theories exist.

The dilator muscle theory postulates that contraction of the dilator muscle exerts a posterior vector. This increases the amount of apposition between the iris and the anteriorly located lens and enhances the degree of physiological pupillary block (*Figure 7.38a*). The simultaneous dilatation of the pupil renders the peripheral iris more flaccid. The relative pupillary block causes the pressure in the posterior chamber to increase and the peripheral iris to bow anteriorly (iris bombé) (*Figure 7.38b*). Eventually the angle becomes obstructed by the peripheral iris and the IOP rises (*Figure 7.38c*).

The sphincter muscle theory postulates that the sphincter of the pupil is the prime culprit in precipitating angle closure. The pupillary blocking force of the sphincter is greatest when the diameter of the pupil is about 4 mm.

The role played by emotional factors in precipitating angle closure is ill understood.

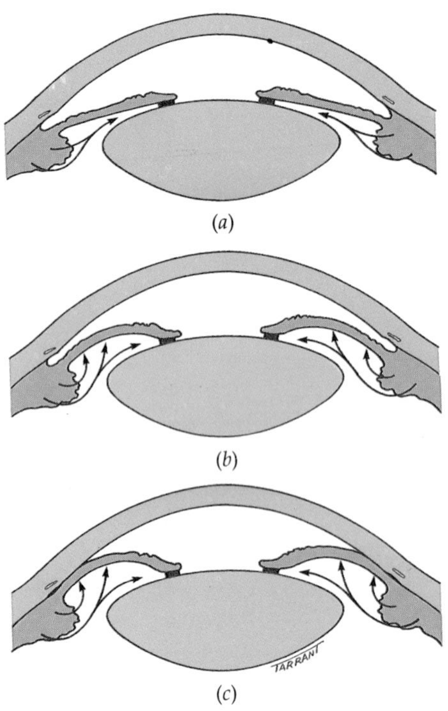

Figure 7.38 Mechanism of angle-closure glaucoma. (a) *Relative pupil block;* (b) *iris bombé;* (c) *iridotrabecular contact*

Classification

PACG can be divided into five overlapping phases. However, the disease does not necessarily progress from one stage to the next in an orderly manner.

Latent
Intermittent (subacute)
Acute
  congestive phase
  postcongestive phase
    postsurgical
    spontaneous reopening of angle
    hypotony due to reduced aqueous secretion
Chronic
Absolute

Latent

Diagnosis

The asymptomatic latent phase of PACG is characterized by a shallow anterior chamber, a convex-shaped iris–lens diaphragm, close proximity of the peripheral iris to the cornea (*Figure 7.39*), and a normal IOP. Gonioscopy shows a narrow angle capable of closure (grade 1 to 2).

Management

If the latent phase is present in the fellow eye of a patient who has already suffered an acute or subacute attack of PACG in the other eye, then peripheral iridectomy or laser iridotomy should be performed. This is because, without such treatment, the risk of an acute attack during the next 5 years is about 50%. However, if a narrow angle is found on routine gonioscopy in an eye with a suspiciously shallow anterior chamber, the clinician must decide whether or not the angle is capable of closure. In this situation provocative testing may be useful.

Physiological provocative tests

Before the test is commenced the IOP is measured and recorded.

1. *Dark room test.* The patient is left in a dark room (awake) for 1 hour.
2. *Prone test.* The patient lies in the prone position for 1 hour.
3. *Prone-dark room test.* The patient lies prone in a dark room for 1 hour. At present this appears to be the most popular and most physiological test.

After 1 hour, the IOP is measured and gonioscopy performed. A positive result is an increase in IOP of 8 mmHg or more, in the presence of a closed angle.

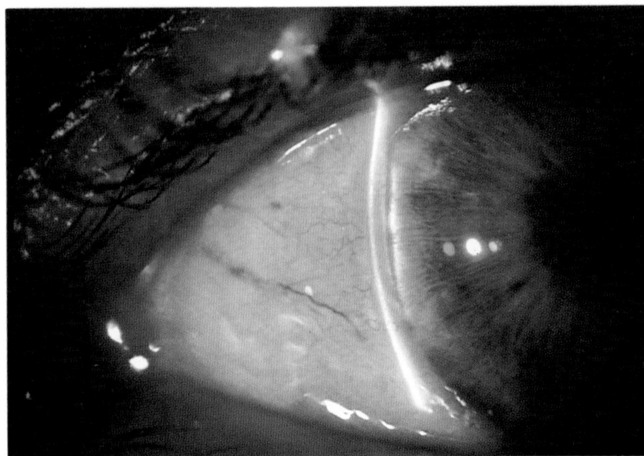

Figure 7.39 Close proximity of peripheral iris to cornea

Pharmacological (mydriatic) provocative tests

Before the test is commenced the IOP is measured and recorded. A mydriatic is then instilled into one eye. The most commonly used mydriatics are eucatropine 5% or hydroxyamphetamine (Paredrine) 5%. Mapstone has described a provocative test using phenylephrine 10% combined with pilocarpine 2%. When the pupil is dilated to 5 mm the IOP is measured every 10 minutes for 1 hour. A positive result is the same as in the physiological tests.

The main criticism of mydriatic provocative tests is that they are unphysiological no matter which mydriatic is used. They may also precipitate a severe attack of PACG. Because mydriatics are capable of causing an elevation of IOP in the presence of an open angle, gonioscopical evidence of angle closure is mandatory if the result is to be interpreted as positive.

If provocative testing is negative, this does not necessarily mean that the angle is incapable of closure in the years to come. The patient should therefore be warned of possible symptoms of angle closure and followed up periodically. A positive result means that the angle is capable of spontaneous closure but it does not mean that closure is imminent or inevitable. In this situation the possible complications of iridectomy or laser iridotomy have to be weighed against the risk of PACG.

Possible subsequent course

An eye with latent PACG may remain healthy with a normal pressure. Some eyes will develop intermittent attacks of angle closure while others will develop an acute attack. In some cases chronic angle closure develops without passing through a subacute or acute stage.

Intermittent (subacute)

Diagnosis

Intermittent attacks of PACG occur in eyes in which the angle is narrow in one part but not in another. A rapid partial closure and reopening of the angle occurs and the level of elevation of IOP is proportional to the extent of angle closure. The IOP is usually less than 45 mmHg during the attack. The attacks may be precipitated by physiological mydriasis (watching television in a dark room), or by a physiological shallowing of the anterior chamber when the patient assumes a prone or semiprone position (as when sewing or reading).

The symptoms of intermittent PACG are transient impairment of vision associated with haloes around lights due to corneal oedema (the blue end of the spectrum being near the light source). There is usually no associated congestion although the patient may complain of eye ache or frontal headache. The attacks are recurrent and are usually broken after 1–2 hours by physiological miosis (exposure to bright light or sleep).

The signs during a subacute attack are a dilated pupil and mild corneal epithelial oedema. In between attacks the eye looks perfectly normal although the angle is narrow.

Management

During attack

Because the iris sphincter is usually still functional when the IOP is below 45 mmHg, intensive miotic therapy (pilocarpine 2% every 5 minutes) is usually effective in pulling this iris away from the angle and aborting the attack. The fellow eye should be treated prophylactically with pilocarpine 1% four times a day, and then bilateral peripheral iridectomy or laser iridotomy should be performed.

Between attacks

If the patient is seen when the IOP is normal and the history is not typical, provocative tests may be helpful in deciding the correct management.

Possible subsequent course

Some eyes with intermittent attacks will develop an acute attack while others will pass straight into the chronic angle-closure phase.

Acute

Acute PACG can be divided into congestive and postcongestive phases.

Congestive phase

Diagnosis

The congestive phase of PACG is due to a sudden total angle closure which causes a severe elevation of IOP.

Symptoms

The symptoms include rapidly progressive impairment of vision, periocular pain, and congestion of the eye. In severe cases, nausea and vomiting may occur. Only 50% of patients with acute PACG give a history of typical previous intermittent attacks.

Signs

The signs include injection of the limbal and conjunctival vessels giving rise to the typical 'ciliary flush'. The severe elevation of IOP (usually between 50 mmHg and 100 mmHg) causes corneal oedema with epithelial vesicles. The anterior chamber is shallow and iridocorneal contact can be observed by directing a narrow slit beam onto the limbus at an angle of about 60° (*Figure 7.40*). After the cornea clears, the anterior chamber is found to contain a flare and cells, but no keratic precipitates. The iris vessels are congested and the pupil is vertically oval and fixed in the semidilated position (*Figure 7.41*). It is unreactive to both light and accommodation. If the angle can be visualized, it will be found to be completely closed by

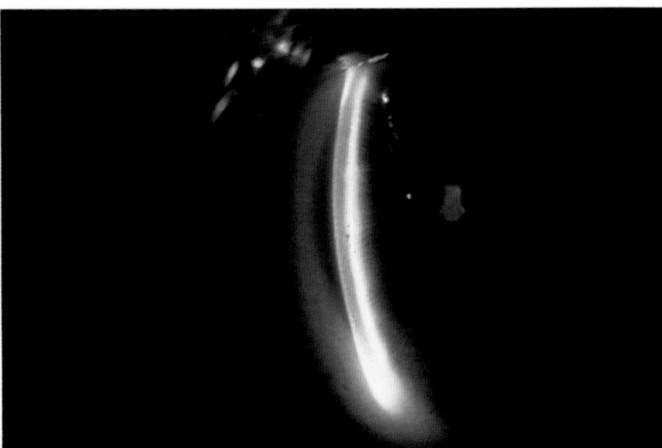

Figure 7.40 Iridocorneal contact in acute primary angle-closure glaucoma

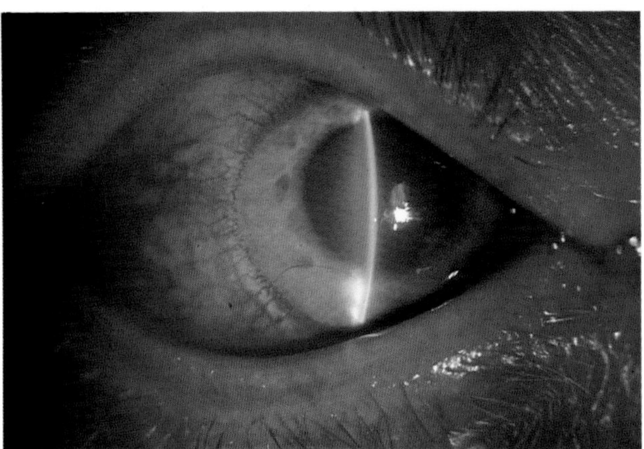

Figure 7.41 Acute primary angle-closure glaucoma

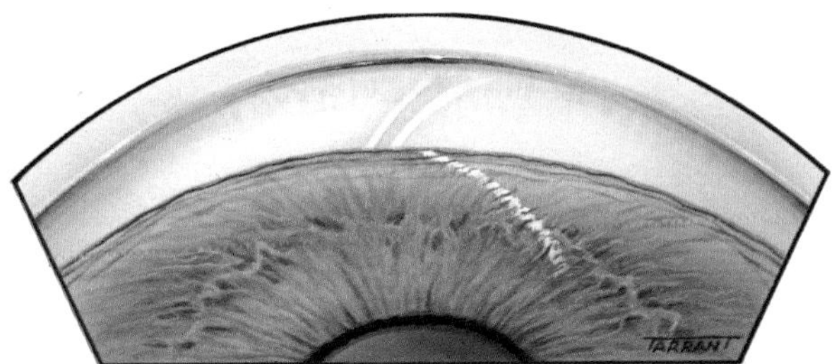

Figure 7.42 Total angle closure – apex of corneal wedge cannot be visualized

iridocorneal contact (grade 0) and the apex of the corneal wedge cannot be seen (*Figure 7.42*). The fellow eye usually has a shallow anterior chamber and a narrow angle. The optic nerve head is oedematous and hyperaemic.

Three conditions that may be mistaken for acute PACG are neovascular glaucoma, glaucomatocyclitic crisis, and phacolytic glaucoma.

Management

Although the management of acute PACG is essentially surgical, the initial treatment is medical.

Medical therapy

When the IOP exceeds 50 mmHg, the iris sphincter is usually paralysed due to ischaemia. For this reason intensive miotic therapy (pilocarpine 4% every 5 minutes) is seldom effective in pulling the peripheral iris away from the angle and the IOP has to be lowered by drugs that reduce aqueous secretion, such as timolol 0.5% and acetazolamide. A loading dose of acetazolamide 500 mg should be given intravenously, followed by 250 mg four times a day orally. Analgesics and antiemetics may be needed to make the patient more comfortable.

It is also mandatory to treat the unaffected eye prophylactically with pilocarpine 1% drops four times a day.

Corneal indentation

In the absence of significant 'synechial' closure of the angle, simple repeated indentations, each lasing about 30 seconds, of the central part of the cornea using a squint hook (*Figure 7.43*) or a cotton-tipped applicator may be effective in forcing aqueous into the peripheral part of the anterior chamber and thus artificially opening the angle. If the angle is kept open for a few minutes by this manoeuvre, aqueous will exit from the eye and the IOP will drop. Hopefully, iris ischaemia will also be relieved and the sphincter will respond to pilocarpine. If corneal indentation combined with intravenous injection of acetazolamide fails to decrease IOP, then treatment with hyperosmotic agents may be necessary.

Hyperosmotic agents

Because of their speed of action and effectiveness, hyperosmotic agents are of great value during the acute crisis of PACG. The four most commonly used agents are glycerol, isosorbide, mannitol, and urea. They all act by drawing water out of the eye and in this way reduce the IOP. The two principles of hyperosmotic therapy are:

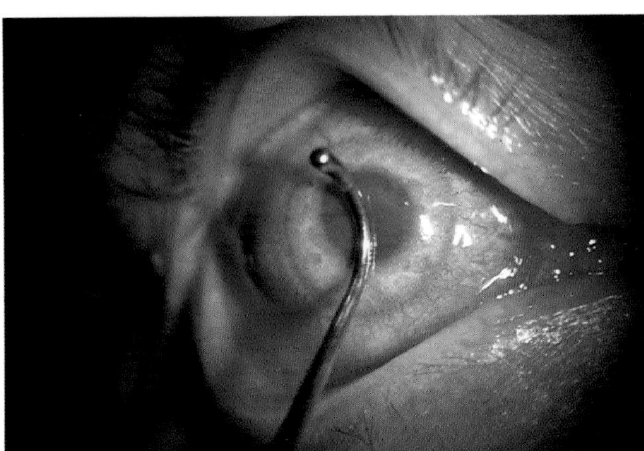

Figure 7.43 Corneal indentation by squint hook in treatment of primary angle-closure glaucoma

1. The osmotic pressure is dependent on the number of particles in solution and not the actual size of the particles. For this reason, the smaller the molecular weight, the greater will be its effectiveness per gram in osmotic therapy.
2. The osmotic agent must be unable to penetrate the blood–aqueous barrier. If penetration does occur, an equilibrium will be set up and any further effectiveness lost.

Oral hyperosmotic agents exert their maximal effect within 1 hour and this lasts for about 3 hours. The dose is 1–2 g/kg body weight (50% solution).

1. *Glycerol* is a clear syrupy liquid with a sweet sickening taste. It is given as a solution in water or pure lemon juice. It is not a strong diuretic but it may occasionally induce nausea and vomiting. Although it is metabolized to glucose in the body, it can be given to diabetic patients provided they are well controlled.
2. *Isosorbide* has a minty flavour but does not cause nausea. It has a diuretic action and may occasionally cause diarrhoea. Because it is metabolically inert, it can be administered to diabetic patients without insulin cover.

Intravenous hyperosmotic agents exert their maximal effect within 30 minutes and this lasts for about 4–6 hours.

1. *Mannitol.* The dose is 1–2 g/kg body weight of a 20% solution in water. This should be given over 30–40 minutes and the speed of administration should not exceed 60 drops per minute. Mannitol is a fairly large molecule which stays extracellular and does not penetrate the blood–aqueous barrier. Because it causes a marked diuresis, it is advisable to use a Foley catheter in elderly men in order to prevent urinary obstruction. Because a large volume is required, mannitol may cause problems due to cardiovascular overload and pulmonary oedema.
2. *Urea.* The dose is 1–2 g/kg body weight as a 30% solution in 10% invert sugar. Urea has a lower molecular weight than mannitol so that some of it enters the eye. It causes less of a diuresis than mannitol but should not be used in patients with impaired renal function. Sloughing of the skin and subcutaneous tissues may occur if it extravasates outside the vein wall. In general it is less popular than mannitol in the treatment of acute PACG.

Side-effects common to all hyperosmotic agents include headache, backache, nausea, vertigo, and mental confusion. They must be used with great caution in patients with cardiac, renal, or hepatic disease. In elderly patients the minimal dose required to produce the necessary effect should be used.

Once the IOP has been reduced medically three options are open for further management:

1. Continued medical therapy with pilocarpine 2% is only indicated in the case of a very elderly patient in poor general health, unable to stand a surgical peripheral iridectomy and where a laser is not available to perform an iridotomy.
2. Surgical peripheral iridectomy or laser iridotomy.
3. Filtration surgery.

Surgery

If at all possible, PACG should be treated by peripheral iridectomy (*Figure 7.44*) or laser iridotomy, as this is safer than a filtration procedure. However, simple iridectomy will only be successful in preventing a subsequent rise in IOP if not more than 50% of the angle is closed by permanent anterior synechiae. If more than half of the angle is permanently closed, a filtration operation is indicated. Some of the factors that should be taken into consideration when deciding on the correct procedure are as follows.

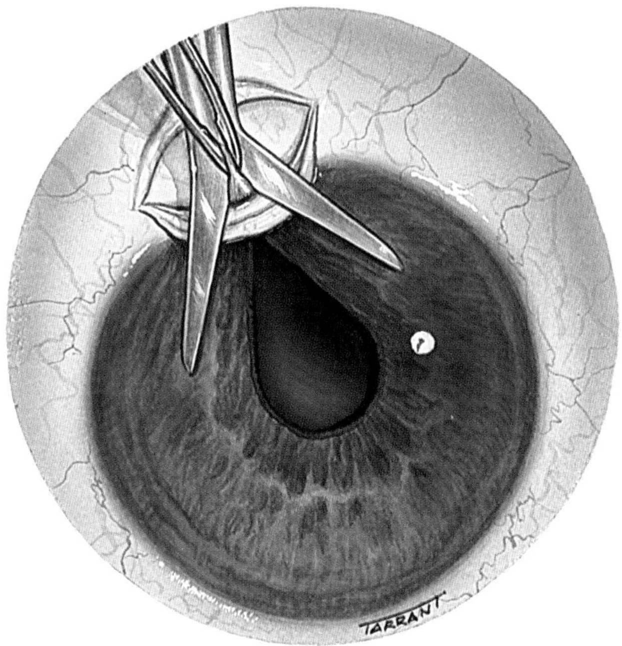

Figure 7.44 *Peripheral iridectomy*

Symptoms. The history is not a reliable guide.

Response to medication. If the IOP is adequately controlled by miotics alone this indicates that a sufficient portion of the angle is open for iridectomy to suffice.

Cupping and field loss usually means that filtration surgery is required.

Tonography. If this shows a normal or near-normal facility of outflow, this indicates that enough of the trabeculum is functioning for iridectomy to suffice.

Standard gonioscopy. If over half the angle is open then iridectomy should suffice.

Indentation gonioscopy (*Figure 7.45*). If, on standard gonioscopy, over half of the angle is seen to be closed, then indentation gonioscopy using the Zeiss four-mirror goniolens is necessary in deciding what percentage of the angle is closed by mere apposition between the peripheral

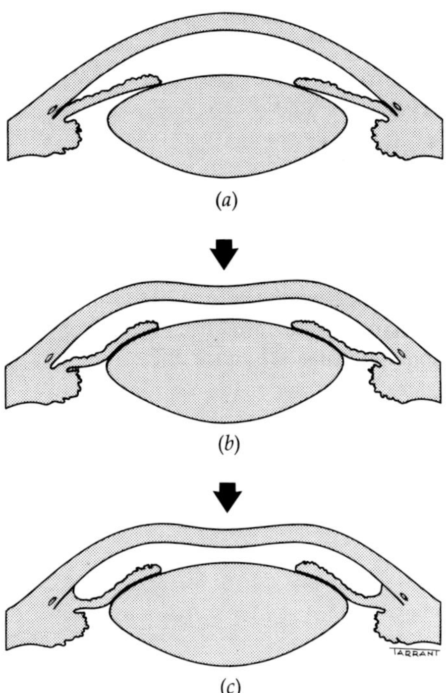

Figure 7.45 *Principles of indentation gonioscopy.* (a) *Appositional closure of angle;* (b) *indentation gonioscopy forces aqueous into peripheral part of anterior chamber and forces peripheral iris away from angle structures;* (c) *angle wide open*

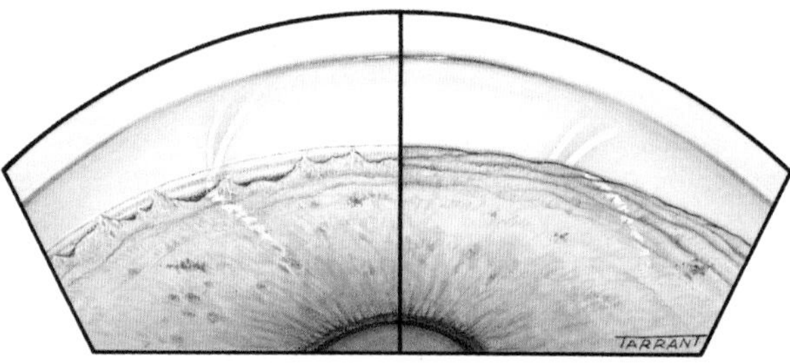

Figure 7.46 *Indentation gonioscopy. Right: appearance of angle before indentation gonioscopy showing complete angle closure; left: appearance during indentation gonioscopy showing reopening of portion of angle. Some permanent peripheral anterior synechiae remain*

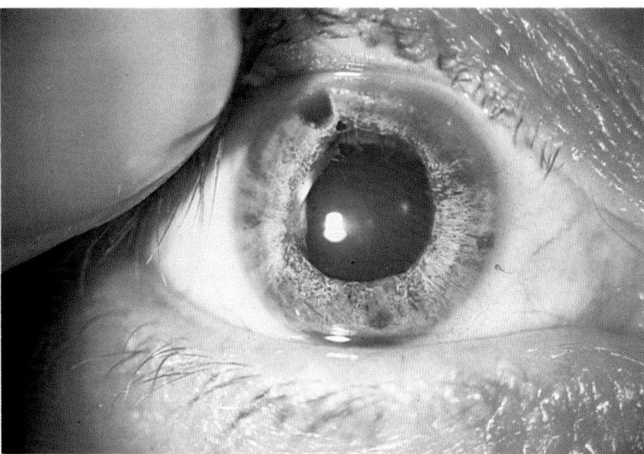

Figure 7.47 *Iris atrophy following acute primary angle-closure glaucoma*

iris and cornea and how much is permanently closed by anterior synechiae. When the small surface of the Zeiss lens is pressed against the cornea, aqueous will be forced into the peripheral part of the anterior chamber, driving the iris base posteriorly. If the angle is closed by mere apposition, then this manoeuvre will open the angle (*Figure 7.46*). If synechial closure is present, this procedure will not tear the adhesions away from the trabeculum and the angle will remain closed. If it is found that less than 50% of the angle is closed by synechiae, then a peripheral iridectomy should suffice.

Postcongestive phase

The postcongestive phase of acute PACG may occur in three different situations:

1. *Postsurgical* in which the IOP has been normalized by successful surgery or laser iridotomy. In some eyes treated by iridectomy alone, the IOP may still be somewhat elevated despite the fact that 50% or more of the angle is open. This is usually due to associated trabecular damage and requires additional medical therapy with either timolol or pilocarpine, or both.
2. *Spontaneous reopening of angle* may occur in some eyes. Management is the same as for intermittent PACG.
3. *Hypotony due to reduced aqueous secretion* may occur in some eyes despite the presence of a completely closed angle. This is caused by a temporary decrease in aqueous secretion by the ischaemic ciliary epithelium. When the secretory epithelium recovers its function, a chronic elevation of IOP may develop, leading to cupping and field loss as in POAG.

Diagnosis

The IOP may be normal, subnormal, or elevated. A rapid reduction of IOP may give rise to folds in Descemet's membrane. Ischaemic damage during the acute congestive phase may result in areas of stromal iris atrophy (*Figure 7.47*) and a slight flare with a few cells in the aqueous. Permanent paralysis of the sphincter associated with posterior synechiae may keep the pupil fixed and semi-dilated and the iris may show a spiral-like configuration. The angle may be open or show varying degrees of closure. If open, trabecular hyperpigmentation may be present, and a straight line of pigment may be seen at the site of previous iridocorneal contact anterior to Schwalbe's line. The lens may show small, grey-white, anterior subcapsular or capsular opacities (glaukomflecken) in the pupillary zone, which are diagnostic of a previous congestive attack (*Figure 7.48*). Fine pigment derived from the iris pigment epithelium may cover the corneal endothelium and the iris. If the eye is very soft, the optic disc may be congested and choroidal folds may be present at the posterior role. In other cases the disc may be white and atrophic due to infarction.

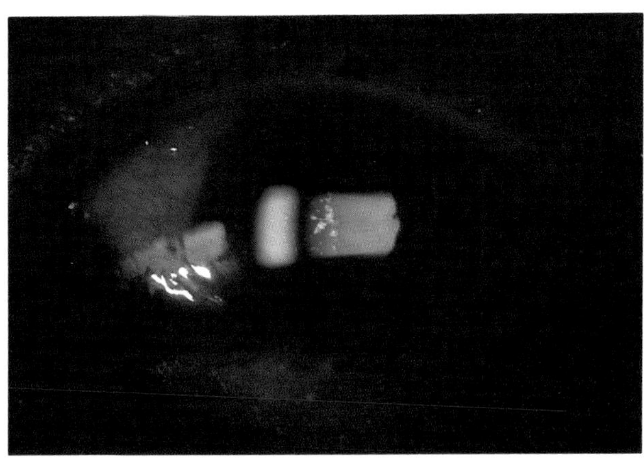

Figure 7.48 Glaukomflecken

Chronic

Diagnosis

This is also sometimes referred to as 'creeping angle closure' because the angle becomes slowly and progressively closed. The closure usually starts superiorly and spreads inferiorly. The symptoms are the same as in POAG. The IOP is usually only mildly elevated and there is a variable amount of angle closure. Permanent synechiae do not usually develop until late. Cupping of the optic disc and visual field loss is identical to that seen in POAG.

Management

Initial treatment is with laser iridotomy. If this is unsuccessful, a trabeculectomy should be performed.

Note. Some authorities include under the heading of 'chronic PACG' cases that show a moderate chronic elevation of IOP with cupping and field loss that have passed through the intermittent or congestive phase.

Absolute

This is the end-stage of acute congestive PACG in which the eye is completely blind. Treatment is symptomatic to relieve pain.

Plateau iris syndrome

This is a rare cause of acute glaucoma which occurs in an eye in which the iris is inserted anteriorly on the ciliary body. This makes the iris plane flat as it runs directly towards Schwalbe's line. When the pupil dilates, the iris becomes bunched up so that its peripheral part occludes the trabeculum. This condition should be suspected in an eye with acute glaucoma in which the axial anterior chamber depth appears to be normal. Treatment is with miotics and not peripheral iridectomy.

Laser iridotomy

Indications

In general, argon or yttrium–aluminium–garnet (YAG) laser iridotomy has replaced surgical iridectomy in the treatment of most forms of pupil-block glaucoma.

Contraindications

Corneal clouding poses a major obstacle as it impairs precise focusing and diminishes the power of the laser. In cases of acute PACG with corneal oedema, it is necessary to first clear the cornea with glycerin before attempting laser iridotomy. A flat anterior chamber is also a contraindication because of the risk of endothelial burns.

Technique of argon laser iridotomy

The pupil should be constricted with pilocarpine drops instilled 1 hour prior to treatment.

1. The cornea is anaesthetized.
2. The laser is set at a spot size of 50 μm, a duration of 0.2 s, and a power setting of 500 mW.
3. An Abraham iridotomy lens is inserted. This special contact lens provides extra magnification and concentrates the energy delivered to the iris. It also acts as a heat sink and minimizes the risk of corneal burns.
4. The aiming beam is precisely focused, preferably on an iris crypt, located in the upper nasal quadrant about two-thirds of the distance from the pupil to the limbus.
5. Repeated superimposed burns are applied. The sign of an adequate reaction is the appearance of a small hole in the stroma with release of pigment, often associated with the formation of a small bubble. If the response is inadequate, the power is increased by 200-mW steps. When the pigment epithelium is penetrated a mushroom-like cloud of pigment frequently emerges from the iridotomy site. The opening is then enlarged and deepened until the lens can be visualized. Although helpful, transillumination can be deceptive as it may be positive with an incomplete iridotomy.

The technique described above may have to be modified if the iris is either very dark brown or extremely light blue. Laser burns of 0.2 s to a thick brown iris may cause contraction of the stroma and produce a black char which is impossible to penetrate. This can be remedied by decreasing the duration of the burn to 0.02 s and increasing the power. In a very light-blue iris, the laser may burn through the pigment epithelium but fail to penetrate the stroma, since it contains little pigment to absorb the energy. In this case a few applications of 300 mW of long duration (0.5 s) will usually produce a stromal burn.

Technique of YAG laser iridotomy

The technique is essentially the same as for argon iridotomy except that a different contact lens is used and the iridotomy is placed more peripherally. The usual setting is 4–5 mJ with 3 pulses per shot.

YAG versus argon

The main advantages of YAG over argon are:

1. Iris colour is immaterial.
2. Fewer shots are required to penetrate the iris (average of 7 with YAG and 70 with argon).
3. Less laser-induced iritis.
4. Less failure of patency.
5. Patients prefer YAG.

The one slight disadvantage of YAG is a higher incidence of bleeding. However, this is usually transient and innocuous.

Postoperative management of argon and YAG iridotomy

1. Gonioscopy is performed to assess the state of the angle.
2. The patient is observed for 1 hour so that excessive elevation of IOP can be detected and treated.
3. Steroid drops are administered four times a day for 1 week to control laser-induced iritis.
4. Miotics are continued until it is certain the iridotomy is patent.

Complications

1. Transient, acute elevation of IOP within 1 hour of treatment is not uncommon.
2. Iritis is common but usually mild and transient.
3. Pupillary distortion is transient and innocuous.
4. Non-progressive lens opacities occasionally develop at the site of treatment.
5. Corneal burns may occur if a contact lens is not used or if the iridotomy is performed in an eye with a shallow anterior chamber.
6. Slight innocuous bleeding is common with YAG but rare with argon.
7. Macular burns are extremely rare. In order to minimize this risk, the iridotomy should be placed in the upper nasal quadrant and the beam directed peripherally.

Secondary glaucomas

Inflammatory

Secondary inflammatory glaucoma frequently presents the clinician with a considerable diagnostic and therapeutic challenge. Although in some cases the elevation of intraocular pressure (IOP) is transient and innocuous, frequently it is persistent and severely damaging. In fact, secondary glaucoma is now the most common cause of blindness in eyes with chronic anterior uveitis, particularly in children.

Diagnostic problems

Failure to monitor intraocular pressure

The clinician may be so preoccupied with suppressing the intraocular inflammation, that he may fail to suspect the presence of raised IOP. He may also have the mistaken belief that a young and healthy optic disc can withstand prolonged periods of raised IOP and remain unscathed.

High swings in intraocular pressure

The diurnal fluctuation of IOP, normally exaggerated in eyes with primary open-angle glaucoma, is even more dramatic in eyes with a compromised outflow facility due to chronic anterior uveitis. It is therefore important to monitor patients with borderline pressures over a 24-hour period (phasing).

Ciliary shutdown

Acute iridocyclitis or an acute exacerbation of chronic iridocyclitis is frequently associated with a temporary decrease in aqueous secretion due to inflammation of the secretory ciliary epithelium (ciliary shutdown). The finding of a normal or subnormal IOP may therefore lull the clinician into a false sense of security, so that he may overlook the fact that a return of ciliary body function, due to a decrease in uveitis activity, may be associated with a rise in IOP in an eye with a permanently compromised outflow facility. It is therefore important to perform gonioscopy on all eyes with chronic anterior uveitis and to continue to monitor the IOP and the appearance of the optic discs as the inflammation is resolving.

Mechanism

In some cases it may be difficult to determine the actual mechanism of the pressure rise and, in some cases, more than one mechanism may be responsible. In steroid responders, the IOP may become elevated as the inflammation is being brought under control.

Classification

Secondary glaucoma due to anterior uveitis can be divided into four main types. As already mentioned more than one mechanism may play a part in the same eye.

Angle closure due to pupil block
Angle closure without pupil block
Open angle
Specific hypertensive uveitis syndromes

Angle closure from pupil block

Mechanism

Secondary angle closure is caused by 360° iridolenticular adhesions (seclusio pupillae). Since the pupil block obstructs the passage of aqueous humour from the posterior to the anterior chamber, the increased pressure in the posterior chamber causes an anterior bowing of the peripheral iris (iris bombé). Severe iris bombé is associated with shallowing of the anterior chamber and apposition of the peripheral iris to the trabeculum and peripheral cornea. If the eye has active inflammation, the iridocorneal contact soon becomes permanent with the development of peripheral anterior synechiae (PAS).

Very occasionally, pupil block develops in an aphakic eye due to adhesion between the iris sphincter and an organized anterior vitreous face or an intact posterior capsule. This is one of the reasons for avoiding extracapsular cataract extraction in eyes with chronic anterior uveitis and performing an anterior vitrectomy following intracapsular cataract surgery.

Diagnosis

Secondary angle-closure glaucoma due to seclusio pupillae is now relatively rare. In fact, most eyes with seclusio pupillae have a normal or a subnormal IOP due to concomitant chronic ciliary shutdown or detachment of the ciliary body by a contracting cyclitic membrane.

Slitlamp biomicroscopy shows 360° posterior synechiae, iris bombé, and a shallow anterior chamber (*Figure 7.49*). Gonioscopy shows apposition of the peripheral iris to the trabeculum and, in advanced cases, also to the peripheral cornea. Indentation gonioscopy with a Zeiss four-mirror goniolens may be useful in assessing the extent of angle closure by reversible (appositional) contact and how much is closed by permanent PAS.

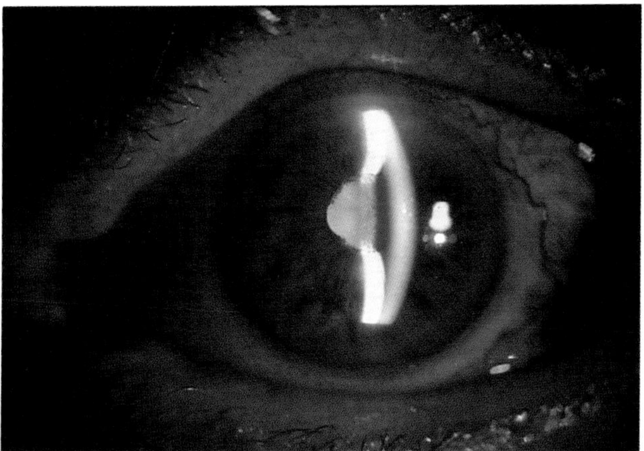

Figure 7.49 *Seclusio pupillae and iris bombé in chronic iridocyclitis*

Medical management

Prevention of seclusio pupillae

In the majority of cases, seclusio pupillae can be prevented by adequate therapy. In eyes with acute anterior uveitis, atropine should be used to prevent posterior synechiae, whereas in eyes with chronic anterior uveitis, a short-acting mydriatic such as tropicamide 1% or cyclopentolate 1%, instilled once or twice a day, is effective in preventing formation of posterior synechiae by keeping the pupil mobile. Once significant posterior synechiae have formed, topical mydriatics (atropine, phenylephrine, cocaine) are seldom effective in breaking them down although an anterior sub-Tenon injection of Mydricaine (a mixture of atropine, adrenaline, and procaine) may be effective if the synechiae are relatively new and unassociated with fibrosis.

Prevention of peripheral anterior synechiae

In an eye with active anterior uveitis, PAS will form quickly once the peripheral iris is apposed to the trabeculum. In the presence of appositional angle closure, it is therefore extremely important to reduce the 'stickiness' of the peripheral iris as quickly as possible with intensive topical steroids and an anterior sub-Tenon injection of methylprednisolone acetate (Depomedrone).

Lowering of intraocular pressure

Although some eyes with healthy optic discs are able to tolerate a moderately high IOP for several weeks, it is important to reduce the IOP as soon as possible, particularly if surgery is being contemplated. In relatively mild cases, topical therapy with timolol, adrenaline and propine may be effective, although when the pressure is very high carbonic anhydrase inhibitors (acetazolamide, dichlorphenamide) are usually also required. However, it is important to point out that hyperosmotic agents (mannitol, glycerol), whose action is dependent on an intact blood–aqueous barrier, may be less effective in lowering IOP than in eyes with primary angle-closure glaucoma.

Surgical management

Laser iridotomy

If medical therapy is ineffective, the communication between the posterior and anterior chambers should be re-established without delay by performing an iridotomy or iridectomy. However, this will be successful only if less than 75% of the angle is permanently closed with PAS. In eyes with relatively thick irides, a YAG laser may be more effective than an argon laser in penetrating the iris stroma. In eyes with shallow anterior chambers, great care should be taken not to damage the corneal endothelium. Although laser iridotomy is safer than surgical iridectomy in eyes with intraocular inflammation, it has the disadvantage that the opening in the iris is smaller (particularly with the YAG laser) and more prone to subsequent closure in eyes with persistent inflammation. For this reason, it is recommended that several iridotomies are performed and the patient is examined at frequent intervals to ensure that the openings remain patent.

Surgical iridectomy

This should be considered only if laser iridotomy is unsuccessful or if a laser is unavailable. Preoperatively, every effort should be made to reduce the amount of intraocular inflammation as much as possible and to lower the IOP medically. An incision should be made in clear cornea and care should be taken to avoid a rapid decompression of the globe. In order to lessen the possibility of postoperative closure, a sector (broad) rather than a peripheral iridectomy should be performed. The anterior chamber should be reconstituted with great care, because a shallow anterior chamber will predispose to PAS formation and negate the effects of the operation.

Angle closure without pupil block

Mechanism

In phakic eyes

In eyes with chronic iridocyclitis, the deposition and subsequent contraction of inflammatory debris may pull the peripheral iris over the trabeculum and cause a gradual and progressive closure of the angle by PAS. Eyes with pre-existing narrow angles are more at risk from angle closure than those with open angles. Eyes with granulomatous inflammation may also be more prone to this type of angle closure than those with non-granulomatous uveitis.

In aphakic eyes

Secondary glaucoma is a relatively common complication following surgery for complicated cataracts. It has been postulated that this may be due in part to failure to reconstitute the anterior chamber immediately after the completion of surgery. Air should be avoided as it may predispose to PAS formation and the anterior chamber should be reconstituted with either saline or balanced salt solution. In addition, inadequate postoperative suppression of surgically induced inflammation may promote the formation of PAS.

Diagnosis

Secondary angle closure unassociated with pupil block is a common cause of raised IOP in eyes with chronic iridocyclitis. As the angle becomes progressively compromised, the rise in IOP is usually gradual. Even severe elevations of IOP of 50 mmHg or more may be asymptomatic or the patient may merely report an occasional mild headache. Because of this relative lack of symptoms and a slitlamp examination which merely shows a deep anterior chamber, it is extremely important to constantly monitor the IOP, examine the angle gonioscopically, and evaluate the optic discs for evidence of glaucomatous damage. In very young and uncooperative children, tonometry and gonioscopy may be extremely difficult or impossible, and the first suspicion of glaucoma is the finding of a grossly cupped optic disc. As already mentioned, exacerbations of intraocular inflammation in eyes with chronic iridocyclitis are frequently associated with a lowering of IOP. Even glaucomatous eyes with a moderate elevation in IOP of 30–35 mmHg may become hypotonous during acute exacerbations. It is therefore extremely important to pay particular attention to the IOP as the uveitis is being brought under control.

Management

The problems encountered in the management of inflammatory glaucoma due to angle closure by extensive PAS are surpassed only by that of treatment of neovascular glaucoma. In fact, some eyes with inflammatory glaucoma develop a fibrovascular membrane in the angle, similar to that seen in neovascular glaucoma. The following options should be considered.

Non-intervention

In eyes with relatively mild iridocyclitis, it may be prudent not to treat the inflammation too vigorously for fear of upsetting the delicate balance between diminished aqueous outflow and decreased inflow as a result of relative ciliary body shutdown.

Medical

Topical therapy with timolol, adrenaline and Propine may be effective in mild cases, although moderate to severe cases require the addition of carbonic anhydrase inhibitors to bring the IOP down to a safe level.

Filtration surgery

This may be successful in some adult eyes, but the results are inferior to those in primary open-angle glaucoma. The results of filtration surgery are particularly disappointing in children. Two of the possible reasons are:

1. A low scleral rigidity in children predisposes to complications such as vitreous loss, scleral collapse, and scleral ectasia.
2. The increased thickness and more rapid healing of Tenon's capsule predisposes to obstruction of the sclerotomy site.

Trabeculodialysis

This procedure is performed with an irrigating goniotomy needle (*Figure 7.50*). The tip of the needle is passed across the anterior chamber into the inferior angle and PAS are retracted by depressing the base of the iris. An incision is then made just posterior to Schwalbe's line and the trabeculum is retracted (*Figure 7.51*). If possible, the incision should be extended for about 90°. It has been

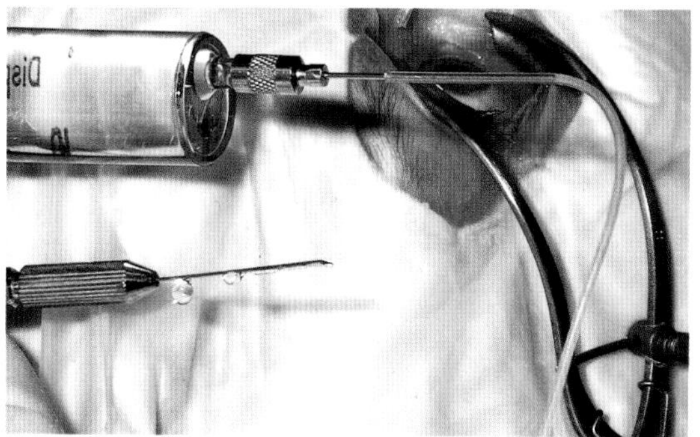

Figure 7.50 *Irrigating goniotomy needle used for trabeculodialysis*

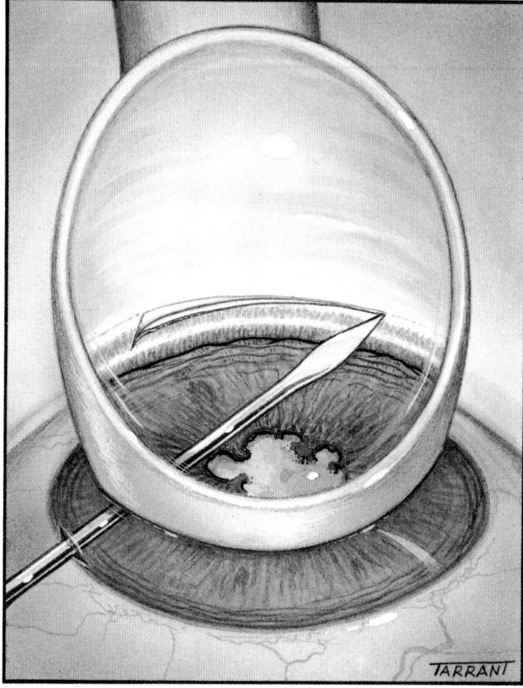

Figure 7.51 *Trabeculodialysis*

postulated that the mechanism by which trabeculodialysis lowers IOP is by providing a direct communication between the anterior chamber and Schlemm's canal. The main advantages of this procedure are:

1. It is relatively easy to perform.
2. It is free from serious complications.
3. It can be combined with lensectomy.

Trabeculodialysis is successful in lowering IOP in about 60% of eyes with severe inflammatory glaucoma although many patients still need medical therapy. Interestingly, the presence of aphakia and the extent of preoperative angle closure have no bearing on the surgical outcome.

Goniosynechialysis

This relatively new procedure involves first deepening of the anterior chamber with sodium hyaluronate (Healonid) followed by separation of the PAS under direct visualization with a special curved irrigating cyclodialysis spatula. This operation may be successful provided the angle has not been closed for longer than one year.

Valve implants

In some eyes, valve implants that drain aqueous from the anterior chamber to the subconjunctival space (Molteno, White, Schocket, Krupin–Denver) may be successful in lowering IOP (*Figure 7.52*).

Cyclocryotherapy

This procedure (*Figure 7.53*) consists of destruction of the secretory ciliary epithelium. A special glaucoma probe or a retinal cryoprobe is used with the applications placed 3 mm from the limbus with freezing at −80°C for 1 minute. Initially, 180° of the globe should be treated with six applications. When re-treatment is required the same area should be frozen and, only if this is ineffective, should the remaining 180° of the globe be treated in a similar fashion. The main disadvantages of this procedure are the risk of inducing phthisis bulbi and that, in many cases, the IOP drop is only temporary.

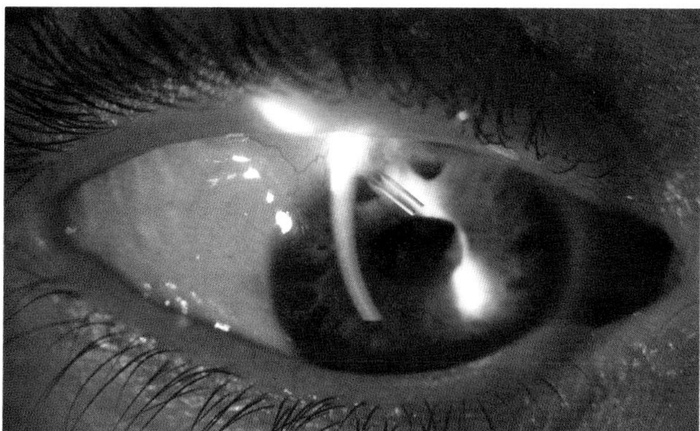

Figure 7.52 *Valve implant* in situ *showing end of drainage tube in anterior chamber*

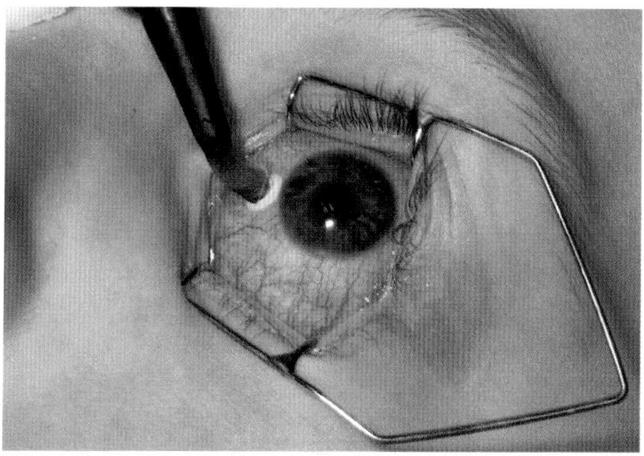

Figure 7.53 *Cyclocryotherapy*

Open-angle glaucoma

Mechanism

In acute iridocyclitis

As already mentioned during the acute phase of anterior uveitis, the IOP is usually normal or subnormal due to a concomitant ciliary shutdown. Occasionally, however, a secondary open-angle glaucoma develops due to obstruction of aqueous outflow, most commonly just as the acute inflammation is subsiding and ciliary body function is returning to normal. This effect, which is transient and fairly innocuous, may be steroid induced or caused by a combination of the following mechanisms.

Trabecular obstruction. Inflammatory cells and debris may clog the intertrabecular pores and the trabecular obstruction may be associated with increased aqueous viscosity due to leakage of proteins from the inflamed iris blood vessels. Eventually the cells and debris are phagocytosed by the trabecular endothelial cells and, provided the uveitis does not recur, the trabeculum regains its full facility of outflow and the IOP returns to normal.

Acute trabeculitis. A reduction in outflow facility may be caused by inflammation and oedema of the trabeculum itself, with a secondary reduction in the diameter of the trabecular pores. It is thought that acute trabeculitis is the probable cause of raised IOP in eyes with uveitis due to herpes zoster and herpes simplex.

Prostaglandins. These may be associated with raised IOP although the exact mechanisms are still uncertain.

In chronic iridocyclitis

It has been postulated that the main mechanism for reduced outflow facility in eyes with open angles and chronic anterior uveitis is trabecular scarring and/or sclerosis as a result of chronic trabeculitis. The exact incidence and importance of this mechanism is, however, difficult to determine with accuracy as most eyes also have PAS.

Diagnosis

Due to the variable appearance of the chamber angle on gonioscopy, a definitive diagnosis of elevated IOP as a result of reduced facility of outflow is very difficult. In theory, the angle should be open and, in some eyes, a gelatinous exudate resembling 'mashed potatoes' may be seen on the trabeculum.

Management

In acute iridocyclitis, the IOP usually returns to normal once the inflammation has subsided. In steroid-responders, it may be necessary to discontinue strong steroid (dexamethasone, betamethasone) and use a weaker steroid such as fluorometholone which has a lower propensity for elevating IOP. In chronic iridocyclitis the treatment is similar to that of secondary angle-closure glaucoma by PAS.

Specific hypertensive uveitis syndromes

Fuchs' uveitis syndrome

See Chapter 6.

Glaucomatocyclitic crisis (Posner–Schlossman syndrome)

See Chapter 6.

Neovascular

Neovascular glaucoma occurs as a complication of rubeosis iridis (new vessels on the iris surface). By far the two most frequent causes of rubeosis are retinal ischaemia associated with central retinal vein occlusion and diabetes mellitus.

Clinical features and management

It is convenient to divide the progression of rubeosis iridis into three stages.

Stage 1

The neovascularization starts as dilated capillary tufts at the pupillary margin and then extends radially towards the angle, sometimes joining a dilated vessel at the collarette. It is important to realize that, at this stage, the IOP is usually normal and the condition may regress either spontaneously or with treatment.

Panretinal photocoagulation may be successful in causing regression. If the rubeosis is present in a postvitrectomy diabetic eye with a persistent retinal detachment, reattachment of the retina will frequently induce regression and prevent neovascular glaucoma.

Stage 2

The new vessels then continue to grow across the iris surface and join the circumferential ciliary body artery (*Figure 7.54, left*). New vessels arising from the circumferential ciliary body artery then proliferate across the face of the ciliary body, cross the scleral spur, and invade the trabeculum where they arborize. At this stage contraction of fibrovascular tissue within the angle leads to the formation of PAS and the IOP starts to rise.

Stage 3

As the fibrovascular tissue continues to contract the whole angle becomes closed by PAS in a zipper-like fashion (*Figure 7.54, right*). The iris becomes pulled up over the whole of the trabecular meshwork and hides all angle structures posterior to Schwalbe's line. The pupil shows distortion and ectropion (*Figure 7.55*). The IOP becomes markedly elevated and the globe becomes painful and congested.

At this stage the main aim of treatment is to relieve pain and congestion as there is usually very little hope of preserving sight. Several modalities can be tried.

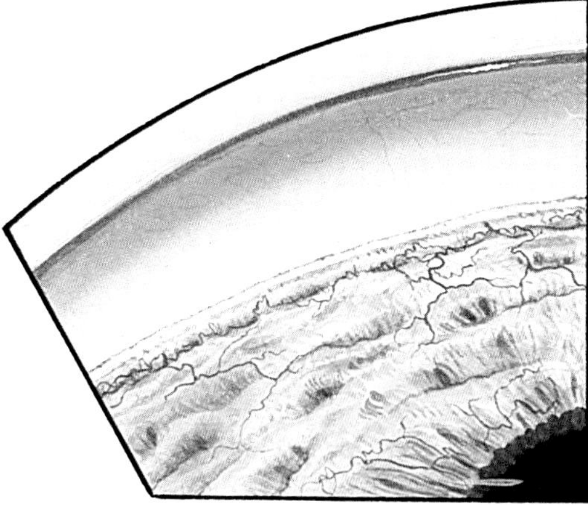
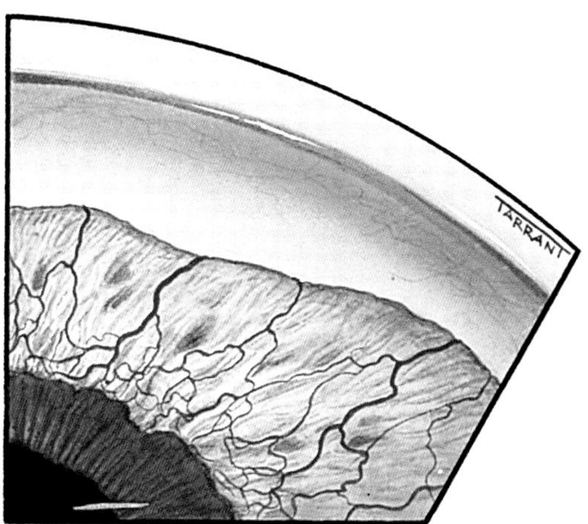

Figure 7.54 *Neovascular glaucoma. Left: early; right: late with peripheral anterior synechiae*

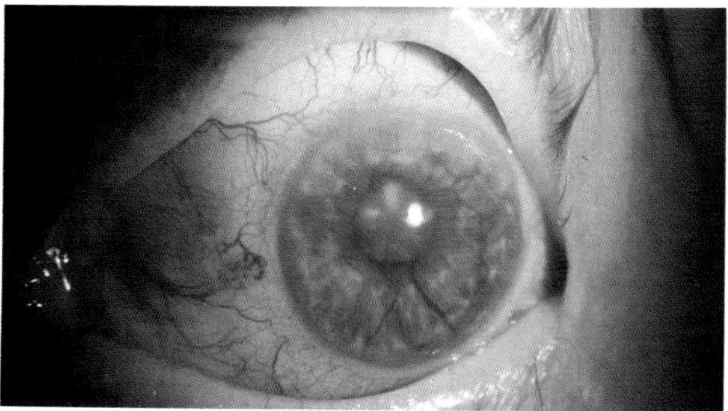

Figure 7.55 *Advanced neovascular glaucoma*

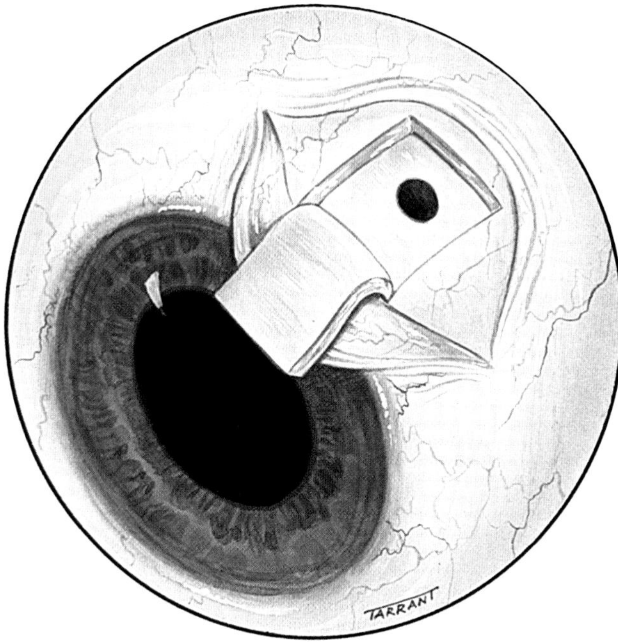

Figure 7.56 *Pars plana filtration*

Medical treatment with atropine and topical corticosteroids may decrease the amount of pain, congestion, and inflammation by reducing the amount of leakage from the rubeotic vessels. Antiglaucoma therapy with timolol, adrenaline, and carbonic anhydrase is usually of limited benefit. Miotic therapy is absolutely contraindicated as this only increases inflammation and discomfort.

Routine filtration surgery usually gives disappointing results due to obstruction of the drainage site by the prolonged postoperative inflammation or continued fibrovascular proliferation.

Modified trabeculectomy with bipolar cautery to the sclerostomy site, the iris vessels, and to the exposed ciliary processes (a potential source of future neovascularization) may occasionally be successful in lowering IOP and, provided the condition is not too advanced, in preserving some vision.

Valve implants may be successful in some cases.

Pars plana filtration can only be performed in an aphakic eye that has undergone a pars plana vitrectomy. The operation is similar to a conventional trabeculectomy, but the scleral flap is fashioned over the pars plana (*Figure 7.56*). A piece of deep scleral tissue and a ciliary body are excised together with any residual vitreous. The risk of haemorrhage is small as the engorged vessels in the anterior segment remain undisturbed. This procedure is usually performed for neovascular glaucoma following pars plana vitrectomy in a diabetic eye.

Cyclocryotherapy. Prior to the advent of modified trabeculectomy and valve implants, cyclocryotherapy was a popular method of treating neovascular glaucoma. However, it does nothing to open the angle or provide an alternative route for the drainage of aqueous humour. It may actually intensify the amount of ocular ischaemia and lead to anterior segment necrosis and late phthisis bulbi.

Retrobulbar alcohol injection is very useful in relieving pain but it may cause a permanent ptosis and does nothing to relieve congestion.

Enucleation may have to be performed if all else fails.

Pigment dispersion syndrome

This rare condition, characterized by dispersion of pigment throughout the anterior segment, typically affects young moderately myopic white males. It is thought that the pigment shedding is caused by mechanical contact between the posterior surface of the iris and anterior surface of zonular fibrils as a result of excessive posterior bowing of the midperipheral portion of the iris.

Clinical features

Cornea

Pigment deposition on the corneal endothelium typically assumes a vertical spindle shape (Krukenberg spindle) (*Figure 7.57, upper left*), the size and density of which is usually proportional to the extent of associated iris atrophy. In some cases the pigment is distributed more diffusely.

Anterior chamber

This is frequently excessively deep particularly in the midperiphery where the iris tends to bow posteriorly.

Iris

The anterior surface is coated by fine pigment granules. The loss of pigment epithelium from the midperiphery gives rise to striking slit-like transillumination defects (*Figure 7.57, upper right*). A few advanced cases with severe iris atrophy may even show a mild heterochromia iridis.

Angle

This is wide open and hyperpigmented throughout due to pigment deposition on and within the trabeculum (*Figure 7.57, lower*).

Lens

Pigment deposition occurs on both lens surfaces and on the zonules.

Retina

Very occasionally, the extreme retinal periphery shows pigment deposition.

Glaucoma

About 10% of patients with the pigment dispersion syndrome eventually develop raised IOP; the condition is then termed 'pigmentary glaucoma'. It is therefore extremely important to check the IOP of all patients with signs suggestive of pigment dispersion. The elevation of IOP appears to be caused by pigmentary obstruction and damage to the trabeculum. Patients with asymmetrical pigmentary glaucoma have more severe glaucoma in the eye with greater pigment dispersion. The natural history of pigmentary glaucoma is still incompletely defined. Many patients have progressive optic nerve damage and visual field loss, although a few show a decrease in the extent of pigment dispersion with age with stabilization or even spontaneous resolution of glaucoma.

Management

Medical treatment is the same as that of POAG although advanced cases may be more difficult to control. The results of treatment by argon laser trabeculoplasty are good.

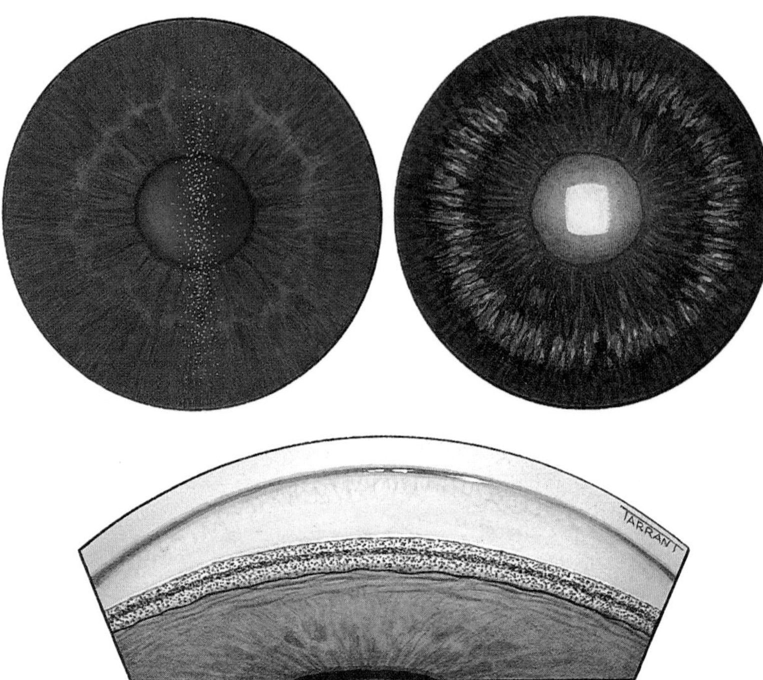

Figure 7.57 *Main features of pigment dispersion syndrome. Upper left: Krukenberg spindle; upper right: iris atrophy; bottom: hyperpigmentation of angle*

Pseudoexfoliation syndrome

This condition is due to the secretion of a grey-white, flake-like, basement membrane material akin to amyloid. It typically affects elderly patients and is particularly common in Scandinavians. Both eyes are affected in about 45% of cases.

Clinical features (*Figure 7.58*)

Glaucoma

About 60% of affected eyes develop open-angle glaucoma and 20% of fellow unaffected eyes also develop elevated IOP. The combination of glaucoma and pseudoexfoliation is referred to as 'glaucoma capsulare'.

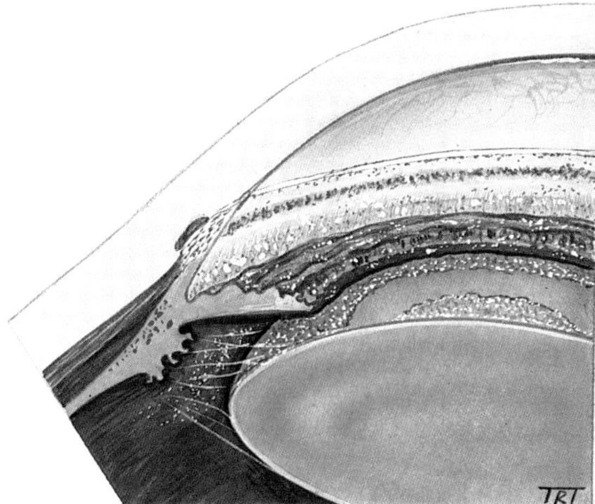

Figure 7.58 *Pseudoexfoliation syndrome*

Lens

The material becomes deposited on the anterior lens capsule (*Figure 7.59*). The constant rubbing action of the pupil then scrapes the material off the midzone of the lens, giving rise to a central disc, a peripheral band, and a clear zone in between.

Iris

The flake-like substance becomes deposited at the pupillary margin. In addition, the sphincter may show atrophic changes due to its constant rubbing action.

Angle

The material that has been rubbed off the anterior lens capsule by the iris then floats in the aqueous and comes to rest in the trabecular meshwork, becoming trapped within the pores. On gonioscopy these deposits look like dandruff. The trabecular meshwork is also hyperpigmented and in some eyes a wavy line of pigment extends anterior to Schwalbe's line (Sampaolesi's line).

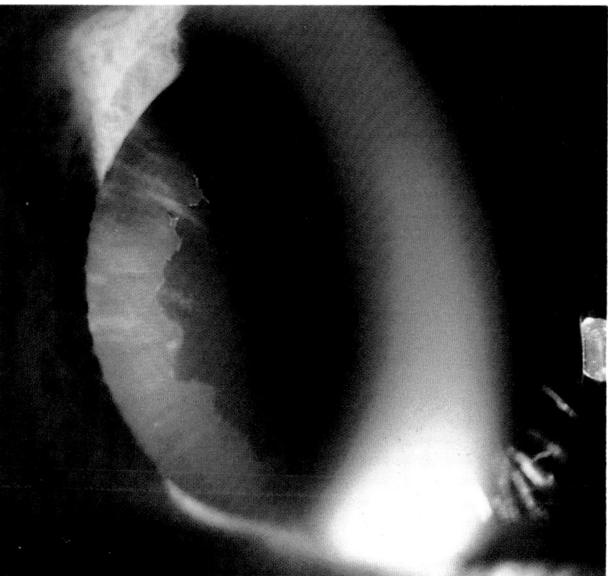

Figure 7.59 *Pseudoexfoliation of anterior lens capsule*

Other structures such as the *zonule, ciliary processes,* and adjacent *conjunctival vessels* may also show white flake-like deposits.

Management

Treatment is similar to POAG although the IOP may be more difficult to control medically. The response to argon laser trabeculoplasty is usually good. Lens extraction is of no benefit.

Phacolytic

Clinical features

This typically occurs in eyes with mature or hypermature cataracts. Leakage of denatured lens proteins through an intact capsule stimulates a macrophagic reaction so that the macrophages ingest the protein (*Figure 7.60*). Usually keratic precipitates are absent. The pressure rise is due to obstruction of the trabecular pores by the macrophages, or the protein itself, or both. The pressure rise may be acute with pain and congestion.

Management

The IOP should be reduced medically and then the lens should be extracted without delay.

Phacomorphic

This is a secondary angle-closure glaucoma that occurs when a swollen intumescent cataract blocks the pupil.

Lens extraction is the only possible treatment after the acute pressure rise has been controlled medically.

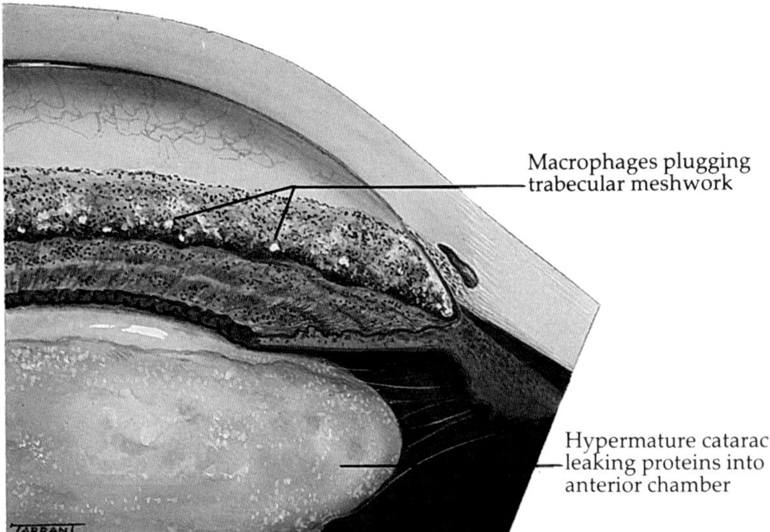

Figure 7.60 Phacolytic glaucoma

Glaucoma and ectopia lentis

There are basically five ways in which an eye with a displaced lens can develop a pressure rise (*Figure 7.61*).

Dislocation into the anterior chamber

This causes a sudden and sharp elevation of IOP. It is an acute emergency because the lens may cause permanent damage to the corneal endothelium.

An attempt can be made to replace the lens by dilating the pupil. If the lens is soft it can be removed through a small limbal incision with a vitreous cutter.

Anterior dislocation

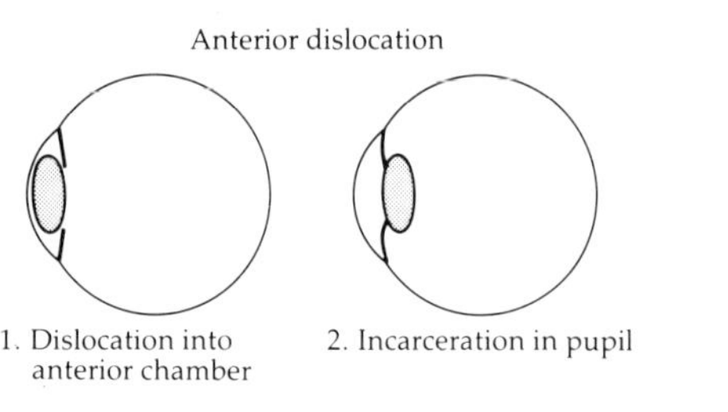

Posterior dislocation

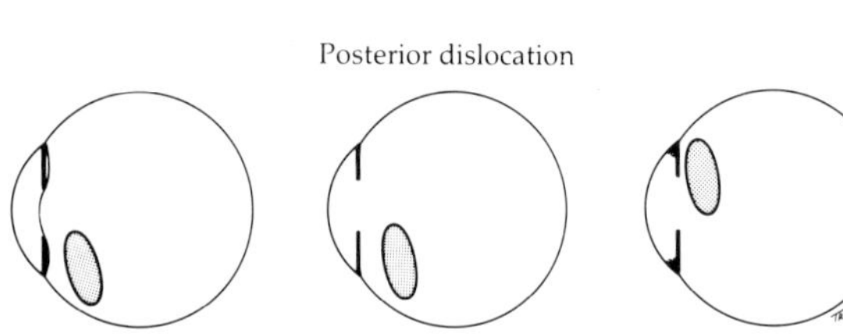

Figure 7.61 Mechanisms of secondary glaucoma in eyes with displaced lenses

Incarceration in the pupil

This usually occurs when the lens is small and spherical in shape (microspherophakia) and only part of the zonule has been disrupted so that the remaining part of the zonule acts as a hinge.

In this situation miotics are contraindicated as they make the pupil block worse. Treatment is with mydriatics or peripheral iridectomy. The pupil in the fellow eye has to be miosed in order to prevent a similar occurrence.

Pupil block by vitreous

In posterior dislocation vitreous may block the pupil.

Treatment is by mydriatics, peripheral iridectomy, or anterior vitrectomy.

Phacolytic glaucoma

This is due to leakage of lens protein.

If possible the cataractous lens should be extracted. However, if it is hard and dislocated posteriorly, this may be very difficult and hazardous.

Angle anomaly

The pressure rise may be caused by an associated angle anomaly and unconnected with the displaced lens.

Traumatic

Trauma may cause early glaucoma due to bleeding into the anterior chamber or late glaucoma associated with angle recession (*Figure 7.62*).

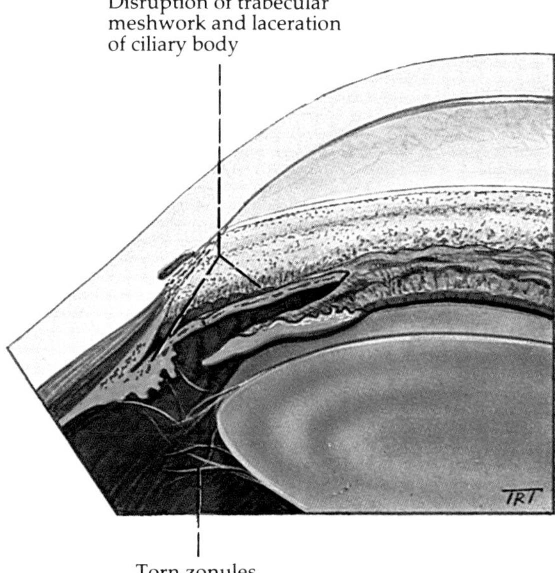

Figure 7.62 *Angle recession*

Hyphaemia

Blood in the anterior chamber may cause elevation of IOP from blockage of the trabecular meshwork with red blood cells. Secondary glaucoma almost invariably accompanies a total hyphaema (*Figure 7.63*). The blood clot may also occlude the pupil and an angle-closure component may be superimposed.

Angle recession

This is usually due to a blunt ocular injury that causes a laceration of the anterior face of the ciliary body. It is thought that the pressure rise is caused by trabecular damage and not by the angle recession itself. However, the larger the area of recessed angle the higher the incidence of glaucoma. It is important to be aware of the fact that the glaucoma may not develop until many years following the initial injury. For this reason all patients with recessed angles should be examined periodically for late glaucoma.

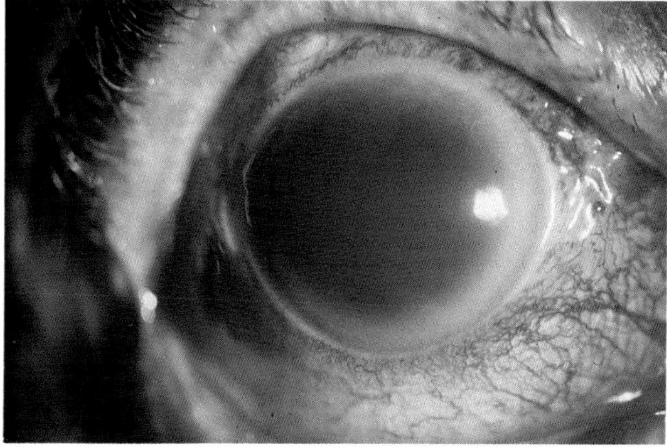

Figure 7.63 *Total hyphaema*

Ghost cell glaucoma

Aetiology

In this recently described condition, the obstruction to aqueous outflow is due to degenerate and less pliable red blood cells rather than to macrophages and debris. It appears that after 2 weeks in the vitreous, red blood cells degenerate into ghost cells when haemoglobin leaks out of them. They then pass through a defect in the anterior vitreous face into the anterior chamber. Because their normal pliability is lost, they become entrapped within the pores of the trabeculum and obstruct aqueous outflow. In aphakic eyes ghost cell glaucoma may occur in three situations.

1. The most common form occurs when a cataract extraction is complicated by a large vitreous haemorrhage and hyphaema. The red blood cells in the anterior chamber clear, but those in the vitreous persist and are turned into ghost cells. Weeks or months later the ghost cells pass into the anterior chamber and cause glaucoma.
2. Ghost cells pass into the anterior chamber following removal of the lens in eyes that have suffered a vitreous haemorrhage prior to cataract extraction.
3. Ghost cell glaucoma is also caused by late vitreous haemorrhage in an eye that is already aphakic.

Clinical features

Ghost cell glaucoma can be recognized by the presence of reddish-brown or khaki cells in the anterior chamber. These findings can sometimes be confused with uveitis and endophthalmitis, leading to excessive use of steroids and antibiotics.

Management

If medical treatment fails to control the glaucoma, irrigation of the anterior chamber should be performed and the ghost cells washed out.

Glaucoma and intraocular tumours

There are four main mechanisms by which intraocular tumours can cause glaucoma:

1. *Trabecular blockage* by tumour cells may either be caused by direct extension through the ciliary body, or by the carriage of tumour cells in the aqueous.
2. *Melanomalytic glaucoma* is caused by the ingestion of tumour cells by macrophages and blockages of trabecular pores similar to phacolytic glaucoma.
3. *Angle-closure glaucoma* may be caused by a forward displacement of the iris–lens diaphragm by an iris or ciliary body tumour.
4. *Neovascular glaucoma* may occur in eyes harbouring a melanoma or retinoblastoma. It is important to exclude the possibility of a tumour by performing ultrasonography in eyes with opaque media and glaucoma.

Iridocorneal endothelial syndromes

The iris naevus (Cogan–Reese) syndrome, Chandler's syndrome and progressive essential iris atrophy represent a continuum of clinical manifestations of a single disease process involving the proliferation of corneal endothelium and characteristic iris abnormalities. Some have suggested the term 'proliferative endotheliopathy' to describe this very rare condition.

Clinical features

The iridocorneal endothelial (ICE) syndromes typically affect one eye of young to middle-aged women. Glaucoma is secondary to endothelial overgrowth in the anterior chamber and formation of PAS. The synechiae develop in a previously open anterior chamber angle and extend up to Schwalbe's line. Corneal endothelial abnormalities, iris nodules, and varying degrees of iris atrophy have been described in all three syndromes. In their purest forms, the three syndromes are easily distinguished from each other. However, there is frequently considerable overlap and a clear differentiation is difficult. Differentiation depends primarily on the changes in the iris.

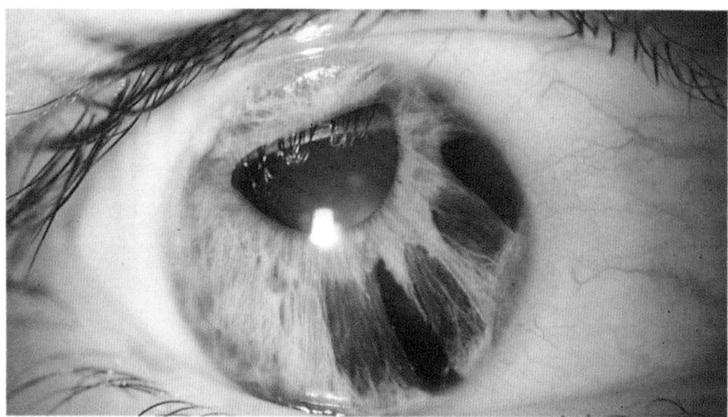

Figure 7.64 *Essential iris atrophy*

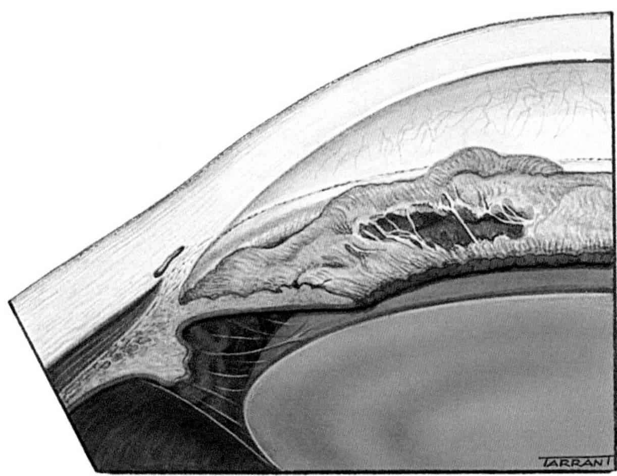

Figure 7.65 *The angle in essential iris atrophy*

Essential iris atrophy (*Figure 7.64*) is characterized by a displacement of the pupil towards an area of PAS. There is mild to moderate ectropion uveae, stromal atrophy, and full-thickness iris hole formation opposite the side of synechiae (*Figure 7.65*). Between areas of atrophy the iris stroma appears normal.

Iris naevus (Cogan–Reese) syndrome is characterized by a diffuse naevus involving the anterior iris. Iris nodules may or may not be present. The normal pattern of the iris surface appears smudged and matted.

Chandler's syndrome falls between the other two entities.

Management

Surgery for glaucoma may be necessary as more PAS form and medical treatment becomes ineffective. Unfortunately it is difficult and hazardous because defects in the iris may expose the zonule and anterior vitreous. The value of prophylactic broad iridectomy to prevent PAS formation is doubtful.

Iridoschisis

This is a rare bilateral senile cleavage of the iris stroma in which the atrophic anterior stroma splits into fibres containing blood vessels (*Figure 7.66*). About 50% of eyes with this condition develop angle-closure glaucoma. It is unclear whether the iris changes are responsible, or whether iridoschisis occurs more frequently in eyes predisposed to angle closure.

Glaucoma due to raised episcleral venous pressure

This occurs in carotid–cavernous fistula (*see* Chapter 15), superior vena caval obstruction, and the Sturge–Weber syndrome (*see* later).

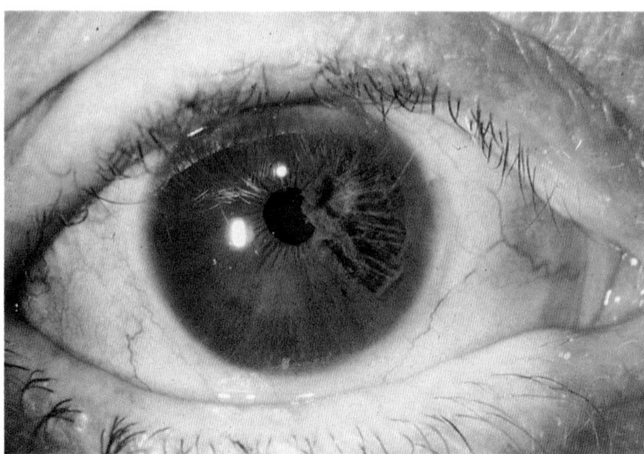

Figure 7.66 *Iridoschisis (courtesy of Mr R. Marsh)*

Congenital glaucomas

The congenital glaucomas are a diverse group of usually inherited disorders in which an ocular anomaly present at birth is responsible for the pressure rise. Because glaucoma may not occur until several years after birth, some prefer to use the term 'developmental' glaucoma to describe these disorders.

Primary

Although it is the most common of the congenital glaucomas it is still an extremely rare disease affecting only 1 in 10 000 births.

The disease is inherited as an autosomal recessive trait with incomplete penetrance. About 65% of patients are boys.

Pathogenesis

Despite extensive investigation, the pathogenesis of primary congenital glaucoma remains an enigma. At present two theories predominate.

1. *Barkan and Worst* postulate the presence of a continuous cellular membrane that obstructs aqueous outflow. The drainage angle itself, although immature, is considered to be functional once the membrane has been incised.
2. *Allen and Maumenee* state that an abnormal cleavage of the chamber angle is responsible. The subsequent failure of the iris and ciliary body to separate from the trabecular meshwork results in an anterior insertion of the longitudinal muscle of the ciliary body with decrease in facility of outflow.

Considerable discrepancies exist between the clinical appearance of the drainage angle and histological findings.

Clinical features

In about 40% of cases, the IOP is elevated during intrauterine life and the child is born with ocular enlargement (true congenital glaucoma). In about 50% of cases the disease becomes manifest some time after birth but prior to the patient's first birthday (infantile glaucoma). The clinical features depend on the age of onset and the severity of the pressure rise. Both eyes are affected in 75% of cases although the severity of involvement is frequently asymmetrical.

Buphthalmos

If the IOP becomes elevated prior to the age of 3 years, the cornea and also the sclera will enlarge. The enlarged eye due to glaucoma is referred to as buphthalmos (*Figure 7.67*). As the cornea continues to enlarge, mainly at the corneoscleral junction, the anterior chamber deepens. In severe cases the lens may become subluxated from stretching of the zonule. Unfortunately, buphthalmos is usually not reported by the parents unless it is unilateral or very advanced.

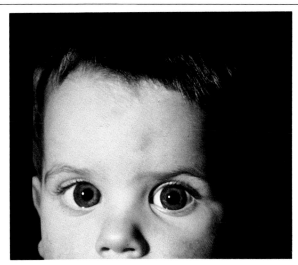

Figure 7.67 *Buphthalmos*

Cornea

Oedema. The elevated IOP gives rise to epithelial oedema which is frequently the first sign noticed by the parents as it gives the cornea a hazy appearance.

Breaks on Descemet's membrane may occur as a result of corneal enlargement and allow a sudden influx of aqueous into the stroma. The stromal oedema may lead to permanent corneal scarring.

Haab's striae appear as curvilinear lines on the corneal endothelium (*Figure 7.68*). They represent healed breaks of Descemet's membrane.

Cupping

In infants, cupping of the optic disc occurs early but it may regress when the IOP is normalized. Recent studies have shown that, in contrast to adult eyes, the scleral canal in infants apparently enlarges with high IOPs as part of the general enlargement of the globe. Thus, the cup–disc ratio increase in children could occur from neural loss, scleral canal enlargement, or both. The glaucomatous disc in infants may show round central cupping or it may be vertically oval as in adults.

Lacrimation

This is a very important feature of infantile glaucoma after the age of 3 months. It is occasionally misdiagnosed as being due to failure of canalization of the nasolacrimal duct.

Photophobia

This is another feature that tends not to become manifest until after several months of life.

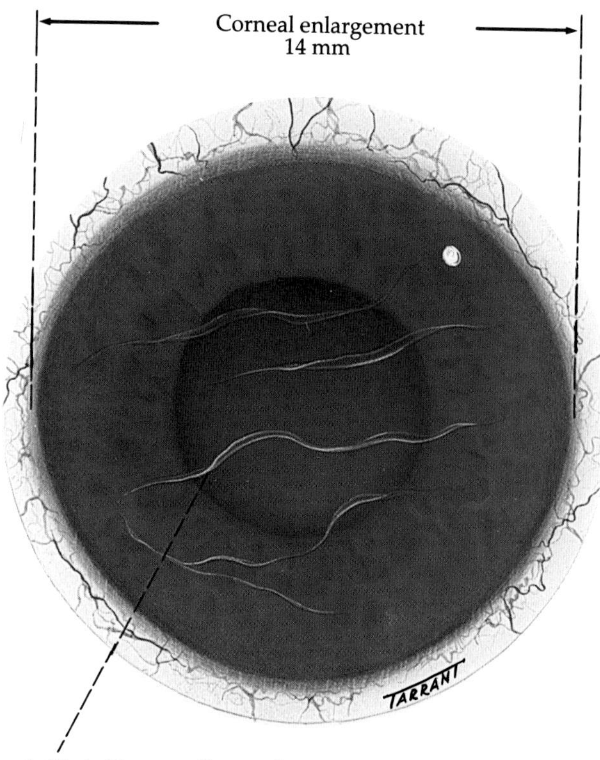

Figure 7.68 *Haab's striae*

Differential diagnosis

Corneal clouding present at birth may be due to trauma, intrauterine infections, or the mucopolysaccharidoses. Large corneas may represent megalocornea. Lacrimation may be due to failure of canalization of the nasolacrimal duct. Important causes of secondary glaucoma include persistent hyperplastic primary vitreous, retinoblastoma, retinopathy of prematurity, xanthogranuloma, and trauma.

Evaluation

The initial examination should be performed under anaesthesia using ketamine. Intraocular pressure measurement can be done using the Schiötz tonometer or one of the hand-held tonometers such as the Perkins.

Corneal diameter measurement

In infants the mean horizontal corneal diameter is 10.00 mm, and in adults it is 11.8 mm. Most of the increase in corneal diameter occurs within the first year of life. Corneal diameters greater than 12 mm are therefore suspect if present before the age of 1 year and 13 mm or more is suspect at any age; diameters of 14 mm are typical of advanced cases.

Gonioscopy

The Koeppe goniolens is excellent for a simultaneous comparison of the two angles. If this is unavailable one of the surgical goniolenses can be used.

The gonioscopical findings in normal neonate eyes are somewhat different from those in adult eyes. In the past this has led to confusion between normal and pathological findings. In normal neonate eyes, angle recess is small or absent, the peripheral iris and radial blood vessels 'lift' slightly at the junction of the trabeculum, producing a scalloped border, and the trabecular sheets are more translucent than in adults.

Some of the gonioscopical findings in congenital glaucoma include (*Figure 7.69*):

1. Barkan's membrane extending from Schwalbe's line over the angle.
2. Thickening of trabecular sheets.
3. Hypoplasia of peripheral iris stroma making the iris blood vessels appear unprotected and the pigment layer of the iris visible.
4. High insertion of iris at or above the level of the scleral spur.

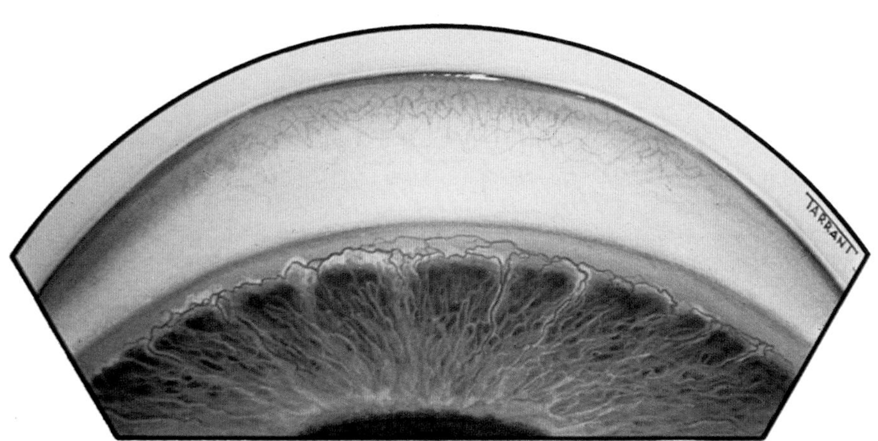

Figure 7.69
Angle anomalies in primary congenital glaucoma

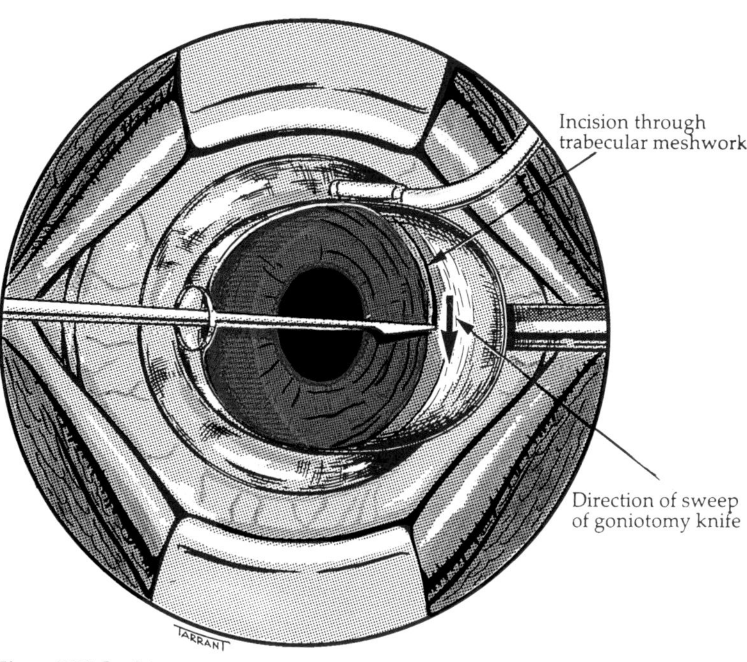

Figure 7.70 *Goniotomy*

Management

Treatment of congenital glaucoma is essentially surgical.

Goniotomy

This is the procedure of choice. In this operation an arcuate incision is made, using a special knife, halfway between the root of the iris and Schwalbe's line (*Figure 7.70*). Although the operation may have to be repeated it is successful in 85% of cases.

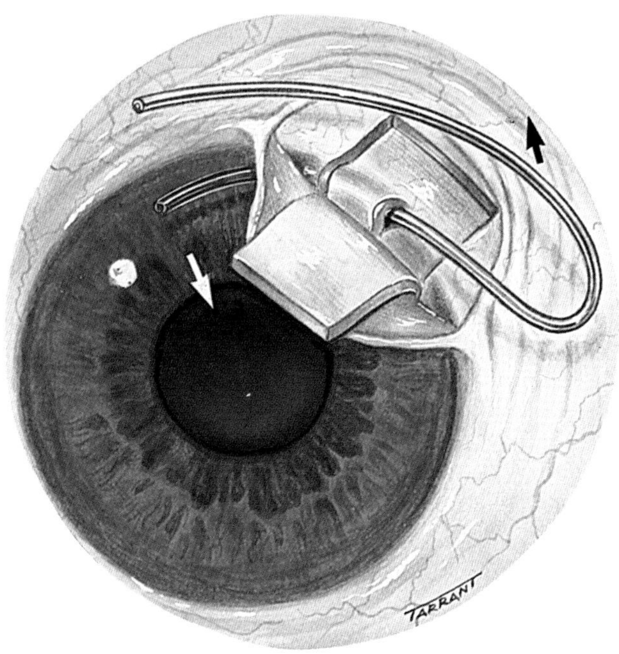

Figure 7.71 *Trabeculotomy*

Trabeculotomy

This may be necessary in complicated cases, either when corneal clouding prevents visualization of the angle or in the rare cases where goniotomy has failed. In this operation a fine metal probe is passed into Schlemm's canal (*Figure 7.71*). It is then swept into the anterior chamber, thus exposing Schlemm's canal directly to aqueous humour. Following surgery, it is extremely important to detect and treat refractive errors and amblyopia. As in all glaucomas, long-term follow-up is essential. A progressive enlargement of the corneal diameter is as important a sign of uncontrolled congenital glaucoma, as progressive loss of visual field is in adult glaucoma.

Note. Occasionally the angle anomalies of congenital glaucoma may not cause a rise in IOP until the teens or even early adult life. In these cases the clinical manifestations simulate primary adult open-angle glaucoma and the correct diagnosis can only be made by careful gonioscopy.

Rubella syndrome

Glaucoma occurs in about 10% of cases. The diagnosis may be missed as the eye may not be significantly enlarged due to pre-existing microphthalmos and the corneal haze may be mistaken for rubella keratitis. As a consequence of this the prognosis is poor. The angle anomaly is similar to that of primary congenital glaucoma although fine dust-like black specks may be seen on the trabecular meshwork and peripheral iris. Occasionally, glaucoma does not develop until later in life.

The systemic and other ocular complications of the rubella syndrome are discussed in Chapter 8.

Aniridia

This is a very rare bilateral disorder the main features of which are congenital absence of the iris and foveal hypoplasia. Most patients have very poor vision and nystagmus. About one-third of cases are sporadic and two-thirds are inherited as an autosomal dominant trait. Of the sporadic cases, two-thirds represent a fresh autosomal dominant mutation. Deletion of a portion of the short arm of chromosome 11 is present in some cases.

Systemic associations

Wilms' tumour (malignant kidney tumour) develops in about 20% of sporadic aniridia cases, usually before the age of 2 years. Other systemic associations include mental retardation, and abnormalities of the genitourinary system and digits.

Ocular features

1. *Aniridia.* This varies from almost total absence (*Figure 7.72*) to mild hypoplasia. However, even in marked cases some iris remnants can be seen on gonioscopy.

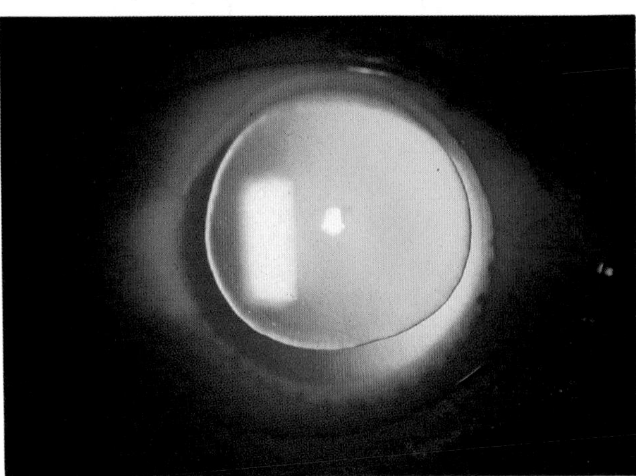

Figure 7.72 *Aniridia*

2. *Glaucoma* develops during late childhood or early adolescence in about 50% of cases. The rise in IOP is thought to be caused by trabecular obstruction by the stump of residual iris tissue (*Figure 7.73*). Control of IOP is extremely difficult, although trabeculectomy or cyclocryotherapy is successful in some cases.
3. *Other ocular defects* include foveal hypoplasia, optic nerve hypoplasia, corneal pannus, epibulbar dermoids, cataract, and lens subluxation. The vast majority of patients have very poor vision and nystagmus.

Mesodermal dysgenesis

This consists of four overlapping disorders some of which are associated with glaucoma.

Posterior embryotoxon

This is a prominent Schwalbe's line. It is found in about 10% of normal eyes and is a universal finding in mesodermal dysgenesis.

Axenfeld's anomaly

This is characterized by strands of peripheral iris tissue attached to a prominent Schwalbe's line. Glaucoma is an uncommon association (*Figure 7.74*).

Rieger's anomaly

This very rare dominantly inherited disorder is characterized by the following features which are usually bilateral but not invariably symmetrical:

1. *Posterior embryotoxon.*
2. *Angle anomalies* which in mild cases are similar to those seen in Axenfeld's anomaly. In advanced cases, broad leaves of stroma adhere to the cornea anterior to Schwalbe's line (*Figure 7.75*). Synechiae extending anterior to Schwalbe's line are associated with pupillary distortion and peripheral corneal opacification.

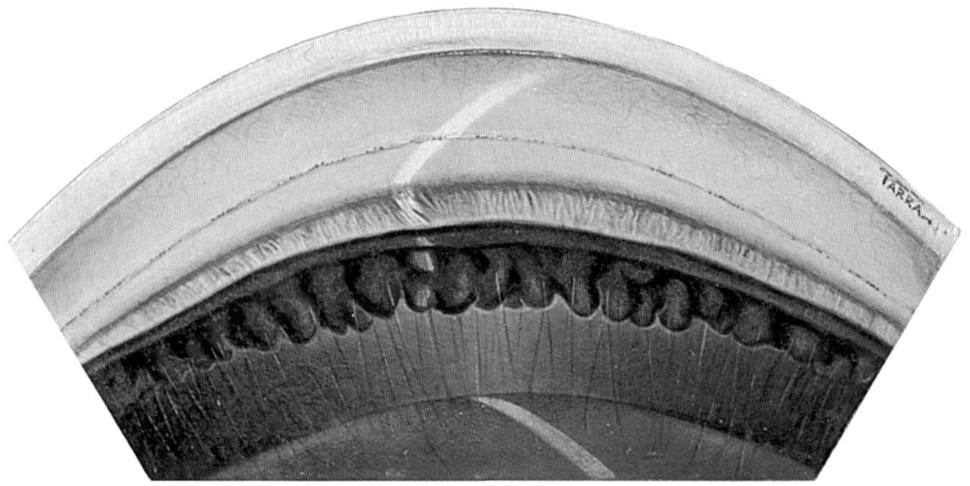

Figure 7.73 *Aniridia*

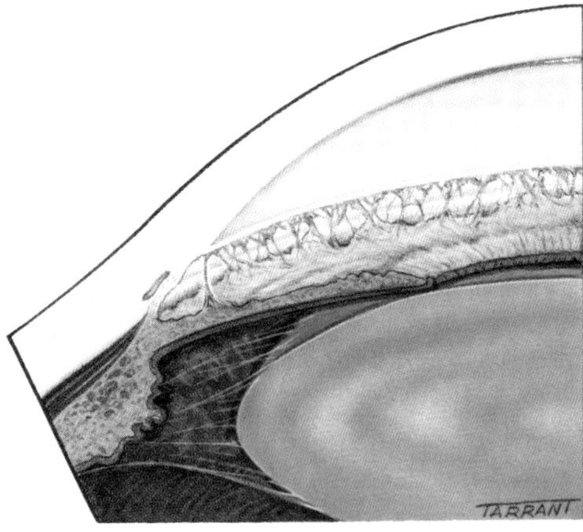

Figure 7.74 Angle in Axenfeld's syndrome

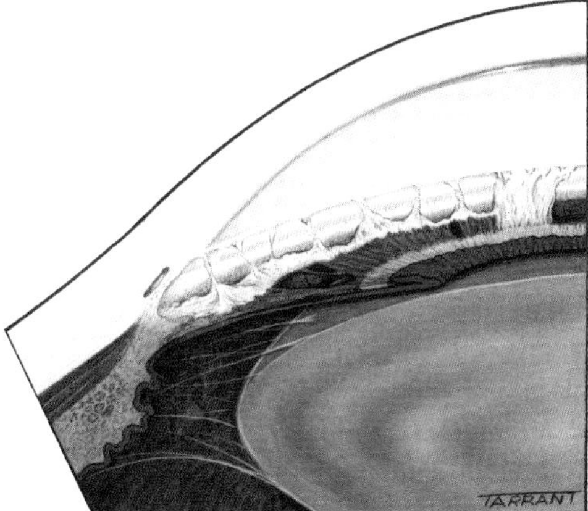

Figure 7.75 Angle in Reiger's anomaly

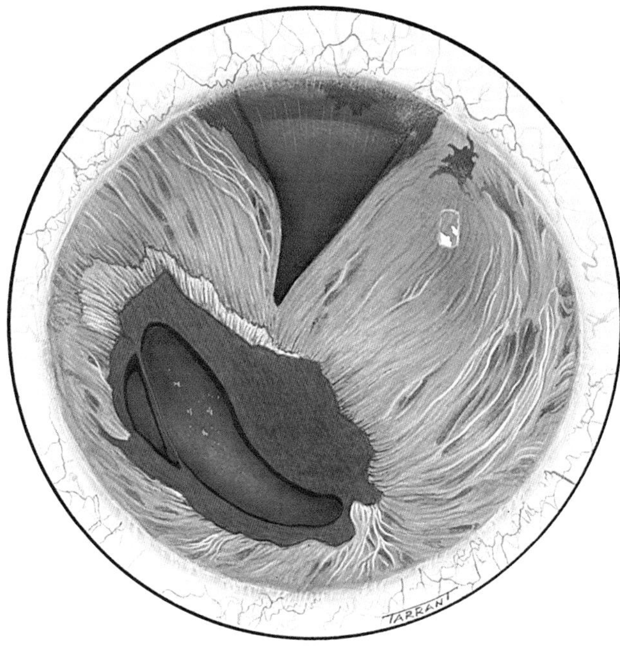

Figure 7.76 Iris anomalies in Reiger's anomaly

3. *Stromal hypoplasia* of the iris which, if severe, may be associated with full-thickness holes (pseudopolycoria) (*Figure 7.76*).
4. *Pupillary anomalies* such as displacement (corectopia), and ectropion uveae.
5. *Glaucoma* is present in about 50% of cases and is usually detected in childhood. The pressure rise is due either to an associated developmental anomaly of the trabeculum and Schlemm's canal or to synechial angle closure.

Rieger's syndrome

This consists of Reiger's anomaly in association with the following:

1. *Dental anomalies* consisting of a decrease in the number of teeth (hypodontia) and a decrease in size of existing teeth (microdontia) (*Figure 7.77*).
2. *Facial anomalies* which include hypoplasia of the maxilla causing a relative flattening of the face, a broad flat nasal bridge, and hypertelorism.

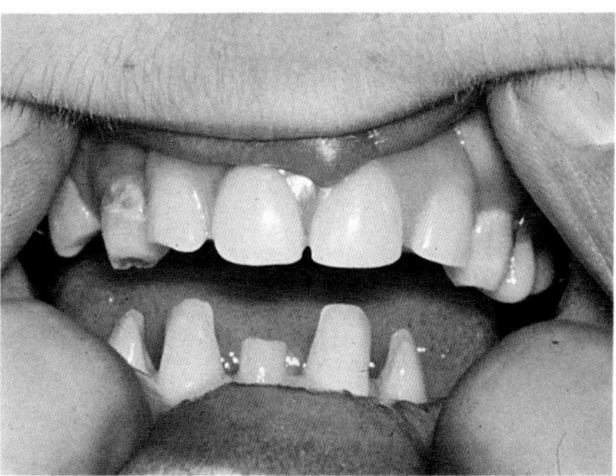
Figure 7.77 Dental anomalies in Reiger's syndrome

Peters' anomaly

This extremely rare congenital anomaly of the anterior segment is inherited as an autosomal recessive trait. It can be manifest in one of three ways:

1. A corneal opacity with a posterior central stromal defect and attenuation or absence of Descemet's membrane.
2. A posterior central corneal opacity with iris adhesions to its margins (*Figure 7.78*).
3. A posterior central corneal defect with lens apposition, or keratolenticular strands with or without iris adhesions.

Glaucoma due to angle malformation occurs in about 50% of cases.

Other occasional features include cornea plana, sclerocornea, microphthalmos, and iridolenticular and vitreoretinal defects.

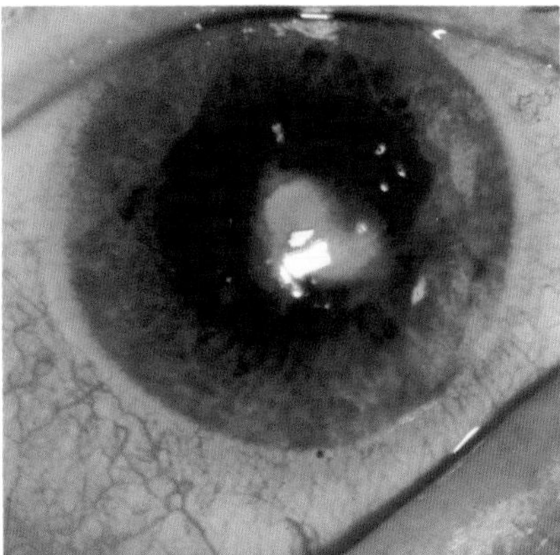

Figure 7.78 Peter's anomaly (courtesy of Mr A. Fielder)

Congenital ectropion uveae

Congenital ectropion uveae (hyperplasia of the iris pigment border) is a rare, non-progressive unilateral anomaly characterized by the presence of iris pigment on the anterior surface of the iris stroma (*Figure 7.79*). The size of the lesion and extent to which the pupillary circumference is involved is variable. The pupil is usually round and reactive to light. The condition may be a solitary finding or it may be associated with neurofibromatosis and other congenital ocular malformations. A significant percentage of eyes with congenital ectropion uveae have an associated angle anomaly which causes glaucoma most commonly between early childhood and the onset of puberty. It is therefore extremely important for patients with congenital ectropion uveae to be carefully followed for the development of elevated IOP.

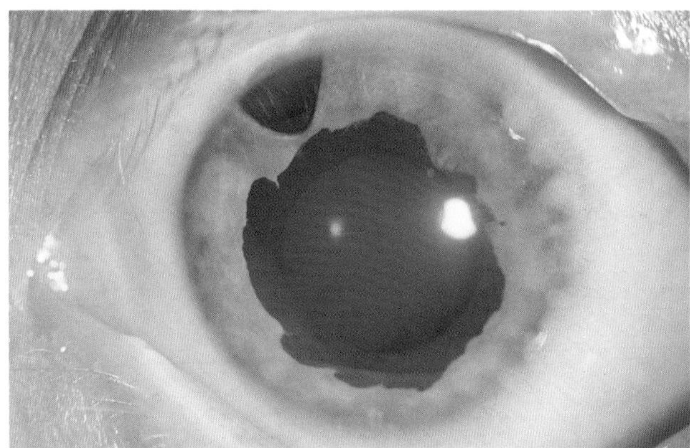

Figure 7.79 Congenital ectropion uveae

Phacomatoses

Sturge–Weber syndrome

The Sturge–Weber syndrome (encephalotrigeminal angiomatosis) is the only phacomatosis without a hereditary tendency.

Systemic features

Cutaneous angioma (*naevus flammeus; Figure 7.80*)

This is present at birth and roughly involves the area of distribution of the first and second divisions of the trigeminal nerve. It may be associated with hypertrophy of the involved area of the face. Occasionally the lesion extends across the midline and may even involve the upper trunk and upper extremities.

Meningeal angioma

A frequent finding is an ipsilateral angioma of the meninges and brain which most commonly involves the parieto-occipital region. The brain lesion is usually accompanied by jacksonian-type epilepsy which may lead to hemiparesis and hemianopia. Atrophy of the neighbouring cerebral cortex may lead to varying degrees of mental deficiency. The intracranial lesion frequently calcifies and presents a characteristic appearance on plain skull X-ray.

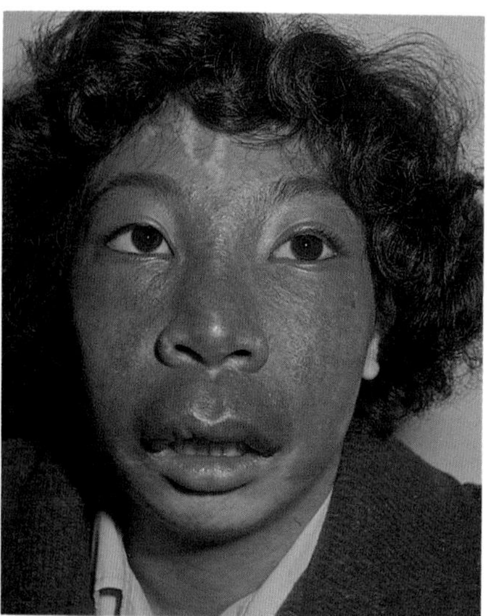

Figure 7.80 Sturge–Weber syndrome showing bilateral naevus flammeus

Ocular features

Glaucoma

About 30% of patients with the Sturge–Weber syndrome develop glaucoma. The glaucomatous eye invariably corresponds to the side of the facial angioma (which is bilateral in 10% of cases), particularly when the upper eyelid is involved. In 60% of patients, the intraocular pressure elevation develops within the first 2 years of life and gives rise to buphthalmos. Most of these patients have an angle anomaly. The remaining 40% do not develop glaucoma till late childhood or early adulthood. In these patients the chamber angle has a more normal appearance. Some authorities believe that, in some of these late-onset cases, the elevation of intraocular pressure is secondary to raised episcleral venous pressure due to an arteriovenous communication caused by an associated episcleral haemangioma.

Choroidal angioma

A diffuse choroidal haemangioma is present in about 40% of patients with the Sturge–Weber syndrome (*see* Chapter 13).

Neurofibromatosis

Neurofibromatosis (von Recklinghausen's disease) is inherited as an autosomal dominant trait with irregular penetrance and variable expressivity. The stigmata of this not uncommon condition may be present at birth or may appear later.

Systemic features

Central nervous system

The disease is characterized by multiple tumours which may involve the brain, spinal cord and meninges, as well as cranial, peripheral, and sympathetic nerves. A few patients develop phaeochromocytomas.

Bone defects

These are present at birth and most commonly involve the greater wing of the sphenoid giving rise to pulsating proptosis. Occasionally vertebral and longbone defects are also seen.

Skin lesions

These may be of three types:

1. *Café-au-lait spots* are hyperpigmented patches with ill-defined serrated edges which typically involve the trunk and axilla, although they may be seen on other parts of the body (*Figure 7.81*). In some cases, these lesions may be the only manifestations of the disease. Similar skin patches are seen in some patients with tuberous sclerosis.
2. *Fibroma molluscum* is a pedunculated, flabby, pigmented nodule which is frequently widely distributed over the body.
3. *Plexiform neurofibromas* consist of enlarged peripheral nerves. On palpation they may resemble a bag of worms. Involvement of the upper eyelid by one of these lesions may cause ptosis and a characteristic S-shaped deformity (*see Figure 1.27*). Facial hemiatrophy may be seen in some patients (*Figure 7.82*).

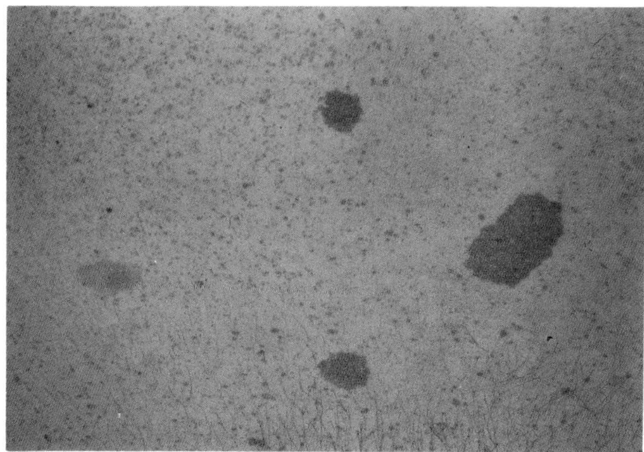

Figure 7.81 *Café-au-lait patches in neurofibromatosis*

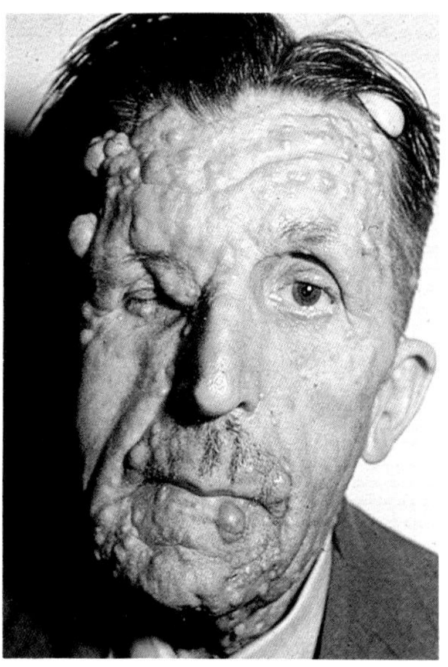

Figure 7.82 *Right facial hemiatrophy in severe neurofibromatosis*

Ocular features

Glaucoma

Glaucoma is less common in neurofibromatosis than in the Sturge–Weber syndrome. When present it is associated in 50% of cases with an ipsilateral plexiform neurofibroma of the upper eyelid and facial hemiatrophy. Four theories have been postulated to explain the mechanism of glaucoma in patients with neurofibromatosis:

1. Obstruction to outflow of aqueous by neurofibromatous tissue in the angle.
2. A developmental angle anomaly.
3. Angle closure by a ciliary body tumour.
4. Angle closure by PAS secondary to fibrovascular membrane formation in the angle.

Iris nodules

These nodules are very common. They are dome shaped and are located superficially or in the stroma. They vary in number and seem to increase in number with age. The lesions are melanocytic naevi and do not consist of neurofibromatous tissue. Some patients may have ectropion uveae.

Fundus lesions

These are rare. Choroidal naevi and patches of hypopigmentation of the choroid and retinal pigment epithelium may be seen in a few patients. Astrocytic hamartomas identical to those seen in patients with tuberous sclerosis have also been described in a few cases.

Proptosis

This may be caused by an optic nerve glioma, an orbital tumour (neurilemmoma, plexiform neuroma, or meningioma), or a spheno-orbital-encephalocele due to a bony defect in the sphenoid bone.

Further reading

Primary-open angle glaucoma

Abedin, S., Simmons, R.J. and Grant, W.M. (1982) Progressive low-tension glaucoma. *Ophthalmology,* **89,** 1–6

Airaksinen, P.J. and Nieminen, H. (1985) Retinal nerve fibre layer photography in glaucoma. *Ophthalmology,* **92,** 877–879

Anderson, G.R. (1983) What happens to the optic disc and retina in glaucoma? *Ophthalmology,* **90,** 766–770

Akingbehin, A.O. (1983) Comparative study of the intraocular pressure effects of fluorometholone 0.1% versus dexamethasone 0.1%. *British Journal of Ophthalmology,* **67,** 661–663

Caspel, E.F. and Engstrom, P.F. (1981) The normal, cup–disc ratio. *American Journal of Ophthalmology,* **91,** 588–597

Drance, S.M., Keltner, J.L. and Johnson, C.A. (1983) Automated perimetry. *Clinical Modules for Ophthalmologists,* Vol. 1, Module 11

Fellman, R.L., Spaeth, G.L. and Starita, R.J. (1984) Gonioscopy: key to successful management of glaucoma. *Clinical Modules for Ophthalmologists,* Vol. 2, Module 7

Grant, W.M. and Burke, B. (1982) Why do some people go blind from glaucoma? *Ophthalmology,* **89,** 991–998

Hart, W.M. and Becker, B. (1982) The onset and evolution of glaucomatous visual field defects. *Ophthalmology,* **89,** 268–279

Henkind, P. (1983) Technology: its role in our concept of glaucoma. The 35th Mark J. Schoenberg Lecture. *Ophthalmology,* **90,** 753–757

Hitchings, R. (1977) Disc field correlation in glaucoma. *Perspectives in Ophthalmology,* **1,** 167–172

Hodapp, E.A. and Anderson, D.R. (1986) Treatment of early glaucoma. *Clinical Modules for Ophthalmologists,* Vol. 4, Module 4

Hoskins, H.D., Hetherington, J., Minckler, D.S. *et al.* (1983) Complications of laser trabeculoplasty. *Ophthalmology,* **90,** 796–799

Hoskins, H.D. and Migliazzo, C.V. (1986) Filtering surgery for glaucoma. *Clinical Modules for Ophthalmologists,* Vol. 4, Module 9

Katz, L.J., Cantor, L.B. and Spaeth, G.L. (1985) Complications of surgery in glaucoma. *Ophthalmology,* **92,** 959–963

Keltner, J.L., Johnson, C.A. and Lewis, R.A. (1985) Quantitative office perimetry. *Ophthalmology,* **92,** 862–872

Lieberman, M.F., Hoskins, H.D. and Hetherington, J. (1983) Laser trabeculoplasty and the glaucomas. *Ophthalmology,* **90,** 790–795

Maumenee, A.E. (1983) Causes of optic nerve damage in glaucoma. Robert N. Shaffer Lecture. *Ophthalmology,* **90,** 741–752

Migdal, C. and Hitchings, R.A. (1984) Primary therapy for chronic simple glaucoma. The role of argon laser trabeculoplasty. *Transactions of the Ophthalmological Society of the United Kingdom,* **104,** 62–66

Migdal, C. and Hitchings, R.A. (1986) Control of chronic simple glaucoma with primary medical, surgical and laser treatment. *Transactions of the Ophthalmological Society of the United Kingdom,* **105,** 653–656

Mikenberg, F.S. and Drance, S.M. (1984) The mode of progression of visual field defects in glaucoma. *American Journal of Ophthalmology,* **98,** 443–445

Morrison, E. and Archer, D.B. (1984) Effect of fluorometholone (FML) on the intraocular pressure of corticosteroid responders. *British Journal of Ophthalmology,* **68,** 581–584

Rosenthal, A.R. and Perkins, E.S. (1985) Family studies in glaucoma. *British Journal of Ophthalmology,* **69,** 664–667

Schwartz, L.W., Spaeth, G.L., Traverso, C. *et al.* (1983) Variation of techniques on the results of argon laser trabeculoplasty. *Ophthalmology,* **90,** 781–784

Watson, P.G. and Grierson, I. (1981) The place of trabeculectomy in the treatment of glaucoma. *Ophthalmology,* **88,** 175–196

Wilson, R., Walker, A.M., Dueker, D.K. *et al.* (1982) Risk factors for rate of progression of glaucomatous visual field loss. *Archives of Ophthalmology,* **100,** 737–741

Wise, J.B. (1981) Long-term control of adult open-angle glaucoma by argon laser treatment. *Ophthalmology,* **88,** 197–202

Primary angle-closure glaucoma

Anderson, D.R. (1979) Corneal indentation to relieve acute angle-closure glaucoma. *American Journal of Ophthalmology,* **88,** 1091–1093

Campbell, D.G. (1980) Angle-closure glaucoma, an update. *Perspectives in Ophthalmology,* **4,** 123–127

Gieser, D.K. and Wilensky, J.T. (1984) Laser iridectomy in the management of chronic angle-closure glaucoma. *American Journal of Ophthalmology,* **98,** 446–450

Klapper, R.M. (1984) Q-switched neodymium: YAG laser iridotomy. *Ophthalmology,* **91,** 1017–1021

Mapstone, R. (1981) The fellow eye. *British Journal of Ophthalmology,* **65,** 410–413

Moser, M.R., Schwartz, L.W., Spaeth, G.L. *et al.* (1986) Laser iridotomy. *Ophthalmology,* **93,** 20–24

Quigley, H.A. (1981) Long-term follow-up of laser iridotomy. *Ophthalmology,* **88,** 218–224

Robin, A.L. and Pollack, I.P. (1984) A comparison of neodymium: YAG and argon laser iridotomies. *Ophthalmology,* **91,** 1011–1016

Inflammatory glaucomas

Campbell, D.G. and Vela, A. (1984) Modern goniosynechialysis for the treatment of synechial angle-closure glaucoma. *Ophthalmology,* **91,** 1052–1060

Caprioli, J., Strang, S.L. and Spaeth, G.L. (1985) Cyclocryotherapy in the treatment of advanced glaucoma. *Ophthalmology,* **92,** 947–954

Herschler, J. and Davis, E.B. (1980) Modified goniotomy for inflammatory glaucoma; histologic evidence for the mechanism of pressure reduction. *Archives of Ophthalmology,* **98,** 684–687

Hoskins, H.D. Jr, Hetherington, J. Jr and Shaffer, R.N. (1977) Surgical management of inflammatory glaucoma. *Perspectives in Ophthalmology,* **1,** 173–181

Kanski, J.J. and McAllister, J.A. (1985) Trabeculodialysis for inflammatory glaucoma in children and young adults. *Ophthalmology,* **92,** 927–929

Ritch, R. (1981) Pathophysiology of glaucoma in uveitis. *Transactions of the Ophthalmological Society of the United Kingdom,* **101,** 321–324

Sarkies, N.J.C. and Hitchings, R.A. (1985) Silicone tube and gutter in advanced glaucoma. *Transactions of the Ophthalmological Society of the United Kingdom*, **104**, 133–136

Schocket, S.S., Nirankari, V.S., Lakhanpal, V. *et al.* (1985) Anterior chamber tube shunt to an encircling band in the treatment of neovascular glaucoma and other refractory glaucomas. *Ophthalmology*, **92**, 553–562

Neovascular glaucoma

Brown, G.C., Magargal, L.E., Schachat, A. *et al.* (1983) Neovascular glaucoma. *Ophthalmology*, **91**, 315–320

Flanagan, D.W. and Blach, R.K. (1983) Place of panretinal photocoagulation and trabeculectomy in the management of neovascular glaucoma. *British Journal of Ophthalmology*, **67**, 526–528

Herschler, J. and Agness, D.A. (1979) A modified filtering operation for neovascular glaucoma. *Archives of Ophthalmology*, **97**, 2339–2341

Krupin, T., Kaufman, P., Mandell, A. *et al.* (1980) Filtering valve implant surgery for eyes with neovascular glaucoma. *American Journal of Ophthalmology*, **89**, 338–343

Krupin, T., Mitchell, K.B. and Becker, B. (1978) Cyclocryotherapy in neovascular glaucoma. *American Journal of Ophthalmology*, **86**, 24–26

Magargal, L.E., Brown, G.C., Augsburger, J.J. *et al.* (1981) Neovascular glaucoma following central retinal vein occlusion. *Ophthalmology*, **88**, 1095–1101

Molteno, A.C.B., Van Rooyen, M.M.B. and Bartholomew, R.S. (1977) Implants for draining neovascular glaucoma. *British Journal of Ophthalmology*, **61**, 120–125

Shields, M.B. (1985) Trends in the therapy of secondary glaucomas. *Clinical Modules for Ophthalmologists*, Vol. 3, Module 4

Sinclair, S.H., Aaberg, T.M. and Meredith, T.A. (1982) A pars plana filtering procedure combined with lensectomy and vitrectomy for neovascular glaucoma. *American Journal of Ophthalmology*, **93**, 185–191

Tasman, W., Magargal, L.E. and Augsburger, J.J. (1980) Effects of argon laser photocoagulation on rubeosis and angle neovascularization. *Ophthalmology*, **87**, 400–402

Teich, S.A. and Walsh, J.B. (1981) A grading system for iris neovascularization. *Ophthalmology*, **88**, 1102–1106

Wand, M. (1985) Diagnosis and treatment of neovascular glaucoma. *Clinical Modules for Ophthalmologists*, Vol. 3, Module 8

Pigment dispersion syndrome

Campbell, D.G. (1979) Pigment dispersion and glaucoma. A new theory. *Archives of Ophthalmology*, **97**, 1667–1672

Davidson, J.A., Brubaker, R.F. and Ilstrup, D.M. (1983) Dimensions of the anterior chamber in pigment dispersion syndrome. *Archives of Ophthalmology*, **101**, 81–83

Lunde, M.W. (1983) Argon laser trabeculoplasty in pigment dispersion syndrome with glaucoma. *American Journal of Ophthalmology*, **96**, 721–725

Richter, C.U., Richardson, T.M. and Grant, W.M. (1986) Pigmentary dispersion syndrome and pigmentary glaucoma. *Archives of Ophthalmology*, **104**, 211–215

Speakman, J.S. (1981) Pigmentary dispersion. *British Journal of Ophthalmology*, **65**, 249–251

Sugar, S. (1983) Pigmentary glaucoma and glaucoma associated with exfoliation–pseudoexfoliation syndrome: Update. Robert N. Shaffer Lecture. *Ophthalmology*, **91**, 307–310

Iridocorneal endothelial syndrome

Eagle, R.C., Font, R.L., Yanoff, M. *et al.* (1979) Proliferative epitheliopathy with iris abnormalities. *Archives of Ophthalmology*, **97**, 2104–2119

Frangoulis, M.A., Sherrard, E.S., Kerr-Muir, M.G. *et al.* (1985) Clinical features of the irido-corneal endothelial syndrome. *Transactions of the Ophthalmological Society of the United Kingdom*, **104**, 775–781

Kupfer, C., Kaiser-Kupfer, M.I., Datiles, M. *et al.* (1983) The contralateral eye in the iridocorneal endothelial (ICE) syndrome. *Ophthalmology*, **90**, 1343–1350

Shields, M.B., Campbell, D.G. and Simmons, R.J. (1978) The essential iris atrophies. *American Journal of Ophthalmology*, **85**, 749–759

Congenital glaucomas

Anderson, D.R. (1983) Trabeculectomy compared with goniotomy for glaucoma in children. *Ophthalmology*, **90**, 805–806

Brownstein, S. and Little, J.M. (1983) Ocular neurofibromatosis. *Ophthalmology*, **90**, 1595–1599

Chisholm, I.A. and Chudney, A.E. (1983) Autosomal dominant iridocorneal dysgenesis with associated somatic anomalies: four-generation family with Rieger's syndrome. *British Journal of Ophthalmology*, **67**, 529–534

Cibis, G.W., Tripathi, R.C. and Tripathi, B.J. (1984) Glaucoma in the Sturge–Weber syndrome. *Ophthalmology*, **91**, 1061–1071

Dowling, J.L., Albert, D.M., Nelson, L.B. *et al.* (1985) Primary glaucoma associated with iridotrabecular dysgenesis and ectropion uveae. *Ophthalmology*, **92**, 912–921

Gregor, Z. and Hitchings, R.A. (1980) Rieger's anomaly: a 42-year follow up. *British Journal of Ophthalmology*, **64**, 56–58

Hoskins, H.D., Shaffer, R.N. and Hetherington, J. (1984) Anatomical classification of the developmental glaucomas. *Archives of Ophthalmology*, **102**, 1331–1336

Kivlin, J.D., Fineman, R.M., Crandall, A.S. *et al.* (1986) Peters' anomaly as a consequence of genetic and nongenetic syndromes. *Archives of Ophthalmology*, **104**, 61–64

Morgan, K.S., Black, B., Ellis, F.D. *et al.* (1981) Treatment of congenital glaucoma. *American Journal of Ophthalmology*, **92**, 799–803

Morin, J.D. and Bryars, J.H. (1980) Causes of loss of vision in congenital glaucoma. *Archives of Ophthalmology*, **98**, 1575–1576

Phelps, C.D. (1978) The pathogenesis of glaucoma in the Sturge–Weber syndrome. *Ophthalmology*, **85**, 276–286

Quigley, H.A. (1982) Childhood glaucoma. *Ophthalmology*, **89**, 219–226

Ritch, R., Forbes, M., Hetherington, J. *et al.* (1984) Congenital ectropion uveae with glaucoma. *Ophthalmology*, **91**, 326–331

Waring, G.O., Rodrigues, M.M. and Laibson, P.R. (1975) Anterior chamber cleavage syndromes. A stepladder classification. *Survey of Ophthalmology*, **20**, 3–10

8

The Lens

Classification of cataract

Aetiological

Morphological

According to maturity

According to age of onset

Management of infantile cataract

Evaluation

Indications for surgery

Surgical techniques

Correction of aphakia

Management of cataract in adults

Indications for extraction

Intracapsular vs extracapsular extraction

Intraocular lenses

Technique of ICCE and implantation of an anterior chamber IOL

Technique of ECCE and implantation of a posterior chamber IOL

Phacoemulsification

Vitreous loss

Early postoperative complications of cataract surgery

Late postoperative complications of cataract surgery

Ectopia lentis

Inherited

Acquired

Surgical techniques

Abnormalities of lens shape

Classification of cataract

Aetiological (*Table 8.1*)

Senile

Senile cataracts are of three types (*Figure 8.1*).

Subcapsular

These cataracts may be anterior or posterior. The anterior variety lies directly under the lens capsule and is associated with fibrous metaplasia of the anterior epithelium of the lens. The posterior type lies just in front of the posterior capsule and is associated with posterior migration of the epithelial cells of the lens. Patients with posterior subcapsular opacities are particularly troubled by headlights of oncoming cars and by bright sunlight. Their vision for near is also frequently diminished more than their distance vision.

Table 8.1 Aetiological classification of cataract

Senile	
Traumatic	Penetrating Concussion Infrared irradiation Electric shock Ionizing irradiation
Metabolic	Diabetes Hypoglycaemia Galactosaemia Galactokinase deficiency Mannosidosis (alpha-mannosidase) Fabry's disease (alpha-galactosidase A) Lowe's syndrome (amino acids) Wilson's disease (alpha-2-globulin ceruloplasmin) Hypocalcaemia
Toxic	Corticosteroids Chlorpromazine Miotics Busulphan Gold Amiodarone
Secondary (complicated)	Anterior uveitis Hereditary retinal and vitreoretinal disorders High myopia Glaukomflecken
Maternal infection	Rubella Toxoplasmosis Cytomegalic inclusion disease
Maternal drug ingestion	Thalidomide Corticosteroids
Three important causes of presenile cataract	Dystrophia myotonica Atopic dermatitis GPUT and GK enzyme deficiency
Syndromes associated with cataract	Down's Werner's Rothmund's Lowe's
Hereditary	

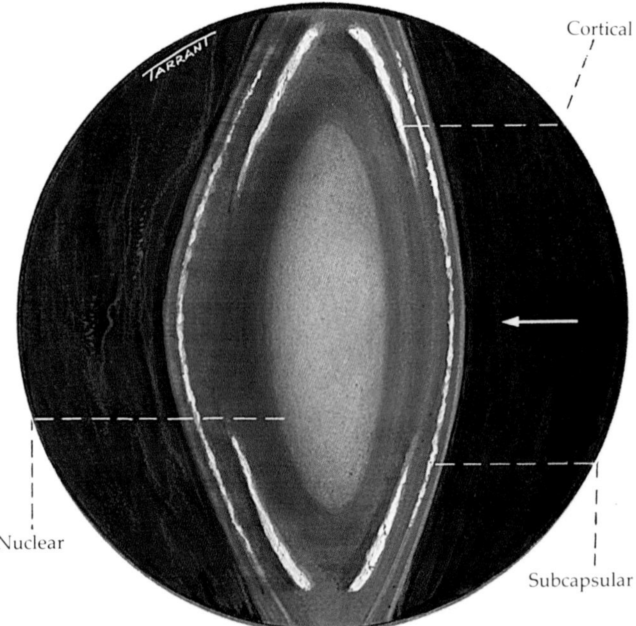

Figure 8.1 *Senile cataract*

Nuclear

This cataract is an exaggeration of the normal ageing change involving the lens nucleus. It is frequently associated with myopia due to an increase in the refractive index of the lens nucleus and also with increased spherical aberration. Some elderly patients with nuclear cataracts may be able to read again without spectacles, due to induced myopia ('second sight of the aged').

Cortical

This cataract is one in which the opacification involves the anterior, posterior, or equatorial cortex. The opacities frequently assume a radial spoke-like or shield-like configuration, and eventually the entire cortex becomes opacified.

Traumatic

Trauma is the most common cause of unilateral cataract in young individuals. Lens opacities may be due to various types of injury.

Penetrating injuries with direct injury to the lens may cause lens opacities.

Concussion injuries may lead to the development of Vossius' ring, due to an 'imprinting' of iris pigment onto the anterior lens capsule.

Glass-blowers' cataract is caused by infrared energy and is characterized by 'scrolls' of peeled anterior lens capsule (exfoliation).

Electric shock is a rare cause of cataract.

Ionizing irradiation to ocular tumours, such as retinoblastoma, may cause lens opacities.

Metabolic

Diabetes

Diabetes is associated with two types of cataract:

1. *Senile* cataract which appears earlier and may progress more rapidly in a diabetic patient than in a non-diabetic.
2. *True diabetic* cataract which is due to osmotic overhydration of the lens and appears as bilateral white punctate or snowflake posterior or anterior opacities (*Figure 8.2*). In certain cases the cataract may mature in a few days. Diabetic cataracts have been seen as early as 1 year of age.

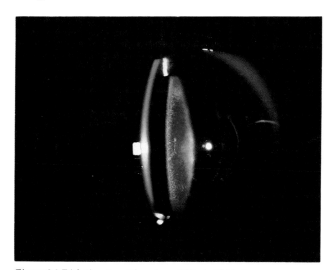

Figure 8.2 *Diabetic cataract (courtesy of Mr A. Fielder)*

Galactosaemia

Cataract is associated with two kinds of recessively inherited galactosaemic enzyme deficiencies.

Classic galactosaemia

This is the result of severe impairment of galactose utilization due to the absence of galactose-1-phosphate uridyltransferase (GPUT).

Systemic features which become manifest during infancy include vomiting, diarrhoea, renal disease, hepatosplenomegaly, cirrhosis, anaemia, deafness, nutritional failure, and mental retardation. The disease is fatal unless galactose in the form of milk and milk products is removed from the diet.

Ocular features. A large percentage of infants with galactosaemia develop bilateral 'oil droplet' central lens opacities (reminiscent of a drop of oil floating in water) within the first few days or weeks of life. The exclusion of galactose (in milk products) from the diet will prevent the development of cataract. The lens changes may be reversible if recognized early, before their progression to maturity, which often occurs within a few months.

Galactokinase deficiency

This is a related disorder due to deficiency of galactokinase (GK), which is the first enzyme in the metabolic pathway of galactose utilization. However, in contrast to classic galactosaemia, affected children are healthy, although they are at increased risk of developing cataracts in the first few years of life. It is also now thought that some presenile cataracts are due to mild GK deficiency.

It should be noted that galactose is only indirectly cataractogenic through its reduction to dulcitol within the lens. Dulcitol accumulation within the metabolizing lens cells leads to an increase in intralenticular osmotic pressure with disruption of the lens fibres and opacification.

Mannosidosis

This disorder is due to a deficiency of the enzyme α-mannosidase leading to the accumulation in the tissues of mannose-rich oligosaccharide.

Systemic features may resemble the mucopolysaccharidoses with a mild to severe (Hurler-like) facial coarseness, mental retardation, short stature, skeletal changes, and hepatosplenomegaly.

Ocular features consist of 'spoke-like' or 'wheel-like' posterior capsular opacities. The absence of corneal changes may aid in clinical differentiation from Hurler's disease.

Fabry's disease

This disorder is due to a deficiency in the enzyme α-galactosidase A.

Systemic features include angiokeratomas (purple telangiectatic skin lesions), cardiovascular and renal impairment, and episodes of excruciating pain involving the fingers and toes.

Ocular features include cornea verticillata (*see Figure 5.51*; which resembles chloroquine and amiodarone toxicity), and spoke-like lens opacities (in 25% of cases) similar to those seen in mannosidosis. The ocular lesions do not impair vision but are unique and diagnostic.

Lowe's (oculocerebrorenal) syndrome

This disorder is a rare inborn error of amino acid metabolism which predominantly affects boys.

Systemic features include mental retardation, renal dwarfism, osteomalacia, muscular hypotonia, and frontal prominence.

Ocular features. Lowe's syndrome is one of the few conditions in which congenital glaucoma (in 50% of cases) is associated with congenital cataract (in 100% of cases). The lens is small, thin, and disc-like (microphakia). The lens opacities may be capsular, lamellar, nuclear, or total. Mothers of affected children may also show multiple punctate lens opacities.

Wilson's disease (hepatolenticular degeneration)

This disorder is due to a deficiency of the alpha-2 globulin, ceruloplasmin, which leads to inadequate copper binding and a widespread deposition of copper in the tissues. Treatment is with D-penicillamine.

Systemic features. Five main types of presentation are described:

1. During childhood with jaundice and hepatosplenomegaly.
2. During infancy with a flapping tremor of the wrists and shoulder and normal liver function.
3. Juvenile cerebral degeneration with spasticity, dysarthria, and dysphagia.
4. Cirrhosis as the initial presentation without CNS signs.
5. Mental changes and emotional instability without neurological signs.

Ocular features include the classic Kayser–Fleischer ring which is present in nearly all cases. It is located at the peripheral part of Descemet's membrane and appears as a zone of granules that change colour under different types of illumination. The copper appears to be deposited preferentially in the vertical meridian of the cornea. The green 'sunflower cataract' is a much less common manifestation. Lenticular copper is deposited in both anterior and posterior parts of the lens. Like the corneal changes, it may disappear with treatment and seldom results in visual impairment.

Hypocalcaemic syndromes

Both hypoparathyroidism and pseudohypoparathyroidism may be associated with multicoloured crystals, or small, discrete, white flecks. In contrast to true diabetic cataracts, those associated with tetany seldom progress to maturity.

Toxic

Corticosteroids (*Figure 8.3*)

The association between posterior subcapsular cataract formation with prolonged corticosteroid therapy, whether systemic or topical, is beyond dispute. However, the exact relationship between the total dose, weekly dose, and duration of administration of systemic corticosteroids and cataract formation is still unclear. Earlier studies showed that cataract developed only in patients receiving moderate or high maintenance doses for longer than 1 year. Patients receiving less than 10 mg/day of prednisone equivalent or those treated for less than 1 year were considered immune. While it is generally believed that children are more susceptible than adults to the cataractogenic effects of systemic corticosteroids, the role of individual (genetic) susceptibility has been stressed recently by some authors, who have found that lens changes may develop after short-term therapy and are not invariably present following prolonged administration of corticosteroids.

On the basis of these findings, it has been suggested that the concept of a 'safe' dose should be abandoned. Patients in whom lens changes develop should have their therapy reduced to a minimum consistent with the control of the disease and should if possible be considered for alternate-day therapy, because lens changes occur less frequently in patients receiving intermittent therapy. Regression of early opacities may occur when the drug is stopped or reduced although progression may occur despite withdrawal.

Chlorpromazine

This may cause the deposition of fine yellowish-brown granules under the anterior lens capsule. The deposits are initially situated within the pupillary area but are rarely

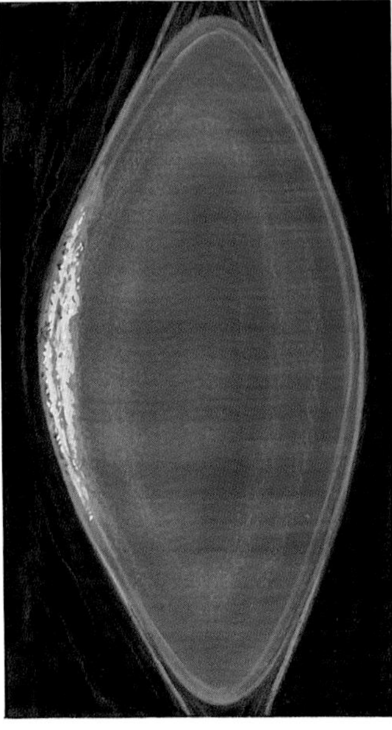

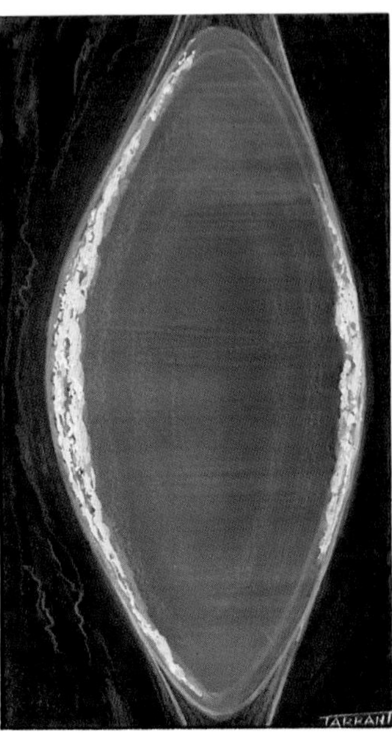

Figure 8.3 *Progression of steroid-induced cataract*

sufficiently dense to interfere with vision. If the drug is used in high doses, it may also cause retinal damage.

Miotics

The long-term use of miotics, particularly the long-acting cholinesterase inhibitors such as ecothiopate (Phospholine Iodide), isoflurophate (dyflos), and demecarium bromide (Tosmilen, Humorsol) may cause the formation of tiny anterior subcapsular vacuoles and occasionally more advanced opacities. Cessation of medication may stop, retard, or occasionally reverse their progression.

Busulphan (Myleran)

This which is a drug used in the treatment of chronic myeloid leukaemia, and may very occasionally cause lens opacities.

Amiodarone

This is a drug used to treat a variety of cardiac arrhythmias. Visually inconsequential anterior subcapsular lens opacities occur in about 50% of patients using moderate to high doses. Cornea deposits may also occur (*see* Chapter 5).

Gold

This is occasionally used to treat patients with rheumatoid arthritis. About 50% of patients who have received treatment for 3 years or longer develop innocuous anterior capsular lens deposits.

Secondary (complicated)

This is a cataract that occurs as a result of some other primary ocular disease.

Anterior uveitis

This is the most common cause of secondary cataract. The earliest finding is a polychromatic lustre at the posterior pole of the lens (*Figure 8.4*). If the uveitis is controlled, the progression of cataract may be arrested. If the inflammation cannot be controlled, anterior and posterior subcapsular opacities develop and the lens may become completely opaque. The lens opacification seems to progress more rapidly in the presence of posterior synechiae. Occasionally, the anterior lens surface becomes covered by a fibrovascular membrane derived from the iris and the pupil may become completely occluded (occlusio pupillae). The membrane may also render the pupil completely immobile so that 360° posterior synechiae develop (seclusio pupillae). Frequently seclusion and occlusion of the pupil occur together, both resulting from the same fibrovascular membrane.

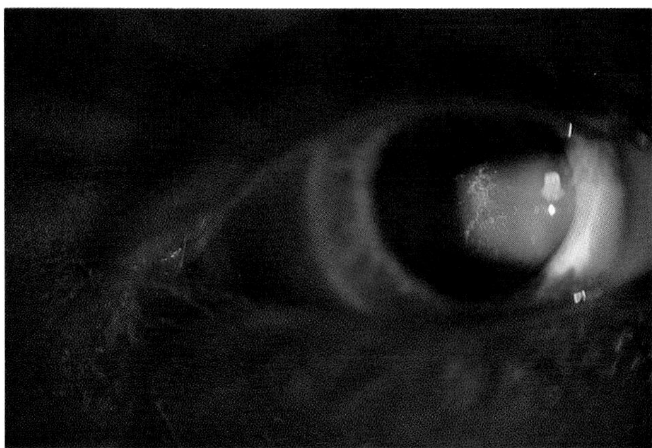

Figure 8.4 *Early posterior cataract secondary to chronic anterior uveitis*

Hereditary retinal

Hereditary retinal (retinitis pigmentosa, Leber's congenital amaurosis, gyrate atrophy) and *vitreoretinal* disorders (Wagner's and Stickler's syndromes) may be associated with posterior subcapsular lens opacities (*see* Chapter 12). The removal of the cataracts may occasionally be indicated and vision improved even in the presence of severe retinal changes.

High myopia

This is frequently associated with secondary posterior lens opacities as well as early development of nuclear sclerosis.

Glaukomflecken

These are small, grey-white, anterior subcapsular or capsular opacities in the pupillary zone that are diagnostic of a previous attack of congestive angle-closure glaucoma (*see* Chapter 7).

Maternal infections

Rubella

Serological studies have shown that about 15% of all women of child-bearing age are susceptible to rubella. Transmission of the virus appears to require close contact and probably occurs through the respiratory route since the virus is shed consistently from oropharyngeal secretions. Immunity following natural infection is long-lasting.

Fetal infection is probably the direct result of maternal viraemia (which may be clinical or subclinical) with seeding of the virus in the placenta. The risk to the fetus is closely related to the stage of gestation at the time of maternal infection. Fetal infection is about 50% during the first 8 weeks, 33% between week 9 and 12, and about 10% between week 13 and 24. Each of the various organs that may be affected has its own period of sensitivity to the infection, after which no gross malformations are produced.

Systemic defects

1. *Spontaneous abortions* and stillbirths are common.
2. *Congenital heart lesions* (patent ductus arteriosus, and pulmonary artery malformations) are present in 70% of cases.

3. *Deafness* is probably the most common manifestation and is usually the only one that occurs alone.
4. *Other manifestations* of congenital rubella include microcephaly, intrauterine growth retardation, mental retardation, hypotonia, hepatosplenomegaly, thrombocytopenic purpura, and pneumonitis.

Ocular defects

These occur in 30–60% of cases.

1. *Cataracts* are present in about 50% of cases. After the gestational age of about 6 weeks, the virus is incapable of traversing the lens capsule so that the lens is immune. Although the lens opacities (which may be unilateral or bilateral) are usually present at birth, they may occasionally develop several weeks or even months later. The opacity can involve the nucleus and have a dense pearly appearance or it may present as a more diffuse opacity involving most of the lens. The virus has been shown to be capable of persisting within the lens for up to 3 years postnatally.
2. *Microphthalmos* is present in about 15% of cases and is often associated with cataract.
3. *Retinopathy* is a common ocular manifestation and probably represents viral involvement of the cells of the retinal pigment epithelium. The retina has a 'salt-and-pepper' appearance, consisting of discrete, patchy, black pigmentation interspersed with similar patches of depigmentation, most frequently involving the macula but occasionally extending into the retinal periphery. Vision is usually unaffected although recent reports have described choroidal neovascularization in a few cases.
4. *Glaucoma* is found in about 10% of cases and usually presents during the neonatal period. It may or may not be associated with cataract.
5. *Other defects* include a corneal haze (which may be transient), strabismus, nystagmus, optic atrophy, and extreme refractive errors.

Other causes of cataract due to maternal infections include *toxoplasmosis* and *cytomegalic inclusion disease.*

Maternal drug ingestion

Congenital cataracts have also been reported in the children of mothers who have taken certain drugs during pregnancy (thalidomide, corticosteroids).

Important causes of presenile cataract

Dystrophia myotonica

This is an uncommon genetically determined disorder which can affect many parts of the body.

Systemic features include excessive contractility and difficulty in relaxation of skeletal muscle, hypogonadism, prefrontal baldness, expressionless face, ptosis (*Figure 8.5*), and cardiac anomalies.

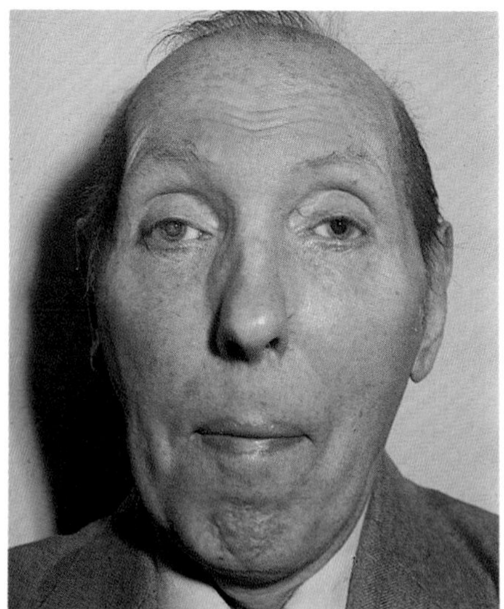

Figure 8.5 *Dystrophia myotonica*

Ocular features include lens opacities which consist of a cortical carpet of polychromatic dust with or without a posterior subcapsular stellate (christmas-tree) figure, abnormal pupillary reactions (light–near dissociation), and pigmentary changes involving the macula or peripheral retina.

Atopic dermatitis

Cutaneous features are discussed in Chapter 1. *Ocular features* include bilateral posterior or occasionally anterior stellate opacities, which develop during the third decade of life and frequently spread to involve the entire lens, chronic keratoconjunctivitis and keratoconus.

Syndromes associated with cataract

Down's syndrome (mongolism)

Down's syndrome is a relatively common condition with a wide variety of clinical findings. Trisomy-21 is by far the most common cytogenetic type, followed by a translocation form and mosaicism, respectively.

Systemic features include mental retardation, stunted growth, mongoloid facies and congenital heart defect.

Ocular features Lens opacities, severe enough to cause a decrease of visual acuity, occur in about 15% of patients. Other ocular manifestations include: narrowed and slanted palpebral fissures, blepharitis, strabismus, nystagmus, light-coloured and spotted irides (Brushfield spots), keratoconus, and myopia.

Werner's syndrome

Systemic features include premature senility, diabetes, hypogonadism, and arrested growth. *Ocular features* consist of bilateral cataracts which develop between the ages of 20 and 40 years.

Rothmund's syndrome

This is a rare hereditary disease predominantly affecting females.

Systemic features include skin changes (atrophy, pigmentation, and telangiectasis) beginning in early infancy, saddle-shaped nose, bony defects, disturbance of hair growth, and hypogonadism.

Ocular features consist of bilateral cataracts which develop during the second to fourth decades of life.

Hereditary

About one-third of all congenital cataracts are hereditary and unassociated with any of the metabolic or systemic disorders already described. The mode of inheritance is usually dominant. The morphology of the opacity as well as the need for surgery is usually similar in parent and offspring.

Morphological

Six main morphological cataract types are recognized.

Capsular

1. *Congenital* capsular thickening may be associated with both anterior and posterior polar opacities as well as with pyramidal cataracts in which the opacity projects into the anterior chamber.
2. *Acquired* capsular opacities occur in pseudoexfoliation syndrome, gold toxicity, glass-blowers' cataract, and Vossius' ring.

Subcapsular

These may be posterior or (more rarely) anterior.

1. *Posterior* subcapsular opacities are typical of *secondary (complicated) cataracts* but may also be found in association with dystrophia myotonica, drugs (corticosteroids), irradiation, and senile (cupuliform) cataract.
2. *Anterior* subcapsular opacities occur in glaukomflecken, Wilson's disease, miotic therapy and chlorpromazine and amiodarone administration.

Nuclear

1. *Congenital* nuclear opacities (*Figure 8.6*) occur in rubella, galactosaemia, and cataracta centralis pulverulenta in which the entire embryonic nucleus is opaque.
2. *Senile* nuclear sclerosis.

Cortical

1. *Congenital* cortical opacities are very common and do not usually interfere with vision. They may be white or have a deep-blue hue. A subtype of a congenital cortical opacity is a coronary cataract which surrounds the lens nucleus like a crown. It is sometimes classified as a supranuclear cataract.
2. *Senile* cortical (cuneiform) cataracts start as vacuoles and clefts between the lens fibres. Opacification of the clefts leads to the formation of the typical radial spoke-like pattern which is best appreciated against the red reflex.

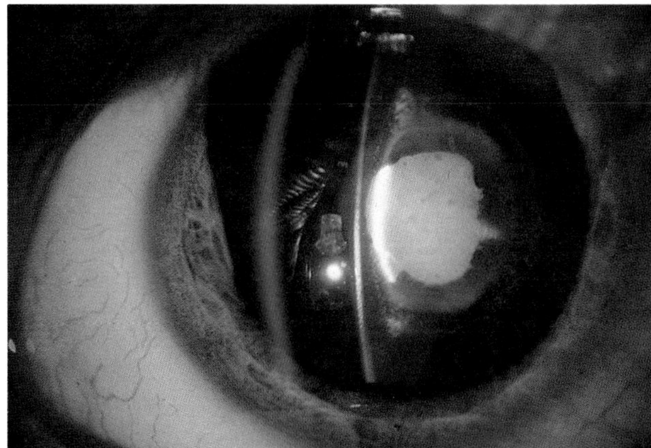

Figure 8.6 *Congenital cataract*

Lamellar

This type of opacity, which is invariably congenital, involves one lamella of the fetal or nuclear zones. Radial spoke-like opacities (riders) frequently surround the cataract (*Figure 8.7*).

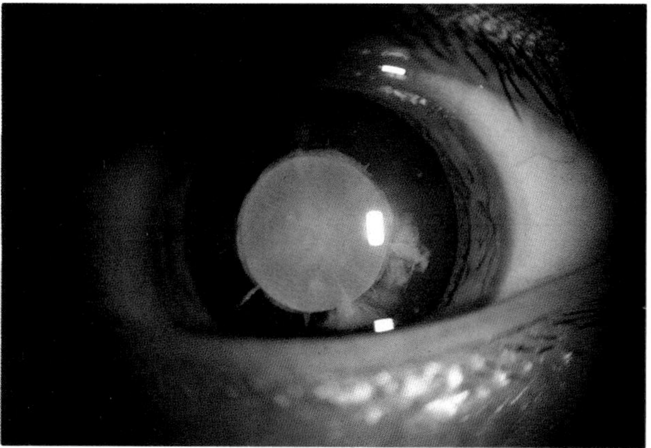

Figure 8.7 *Congenital cataract with riders*

Sutural

These are very common, congenital, Y-shaped opacities within the lens nucleus. They are of no clinical significance.

According to maturity

1. *Immature* cataract is one in which scattered opacities are separated by clear zones.

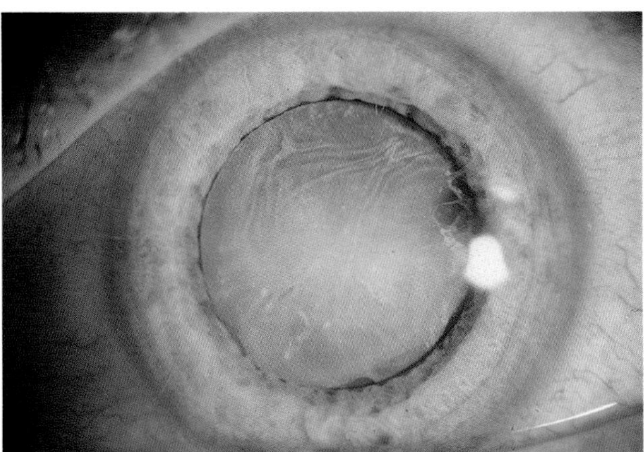

Figure 8.8 *Hypermature cataract with wrinkled anterior lens capsule*

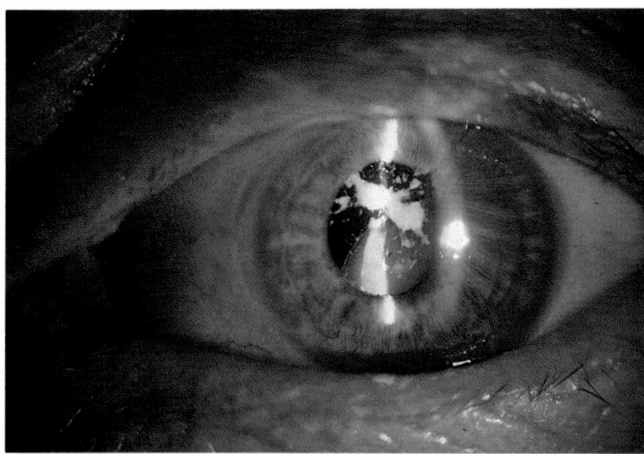

Figure 8.9 *Morgagnian cataract*

2. *Mature* cataract is one in which the cortex is totally opaque.
3. *Intumescent* cataract is one in which the lens has become swollen by imbibed water. It can be mature or immature.
4. *Hypermature* cataract is a mature cataract which has become smaller and has a wrinkled capsule due to leakage of water out of the lens (*Figure 8.8*).
5. *Morgagnian cataract* is a hypermature cataract in which the total liquefaction of the cortex has allowed the nucleus to sink inferiorly (*Figure 8.9*).

According to age of onset

This classification is into congenital, infantile, juvenile, presenile, and senile.

Management of infantile cataract

The recent advent of extended-wear contact lenses and newer surgical techniques have improved the results of treatment of infantile cataract.

Evaluation

In the evaluation of infants with cataract three aspects should be considered: the eyes, the patient, and the parents.

The eyes

Unilateral versus bilateral

In the general prognosis for visual improvement of dense unilateral cataract is much less favourable than for bilateral cataracts. This is based on the works of Hubel and Wiesel, and Van Noorden which show that unilateral visual deprivation in very young animals leads to permanent structural changes in the geniculocortical visual pathways which produce severe and irreversible amblyopia.

Density

Density of the opacity is assessed using both the direct and indirect ophthalmoscope. A very dense opacity will preclude any detailed view with either. A less dense opacity will allow the fundus to be seen with the indirect, but not with the direct, ophthalmoscope. In the presence of an insignificant opacity, the fundus can be seen with both instruments.

Morphology

The morphology of the opacity can give important clues as to the possible aetiology. This is best assessed by slitlamp biomicroscopy.

Associated pathology

This may involve the anterior segment (corneal clouding, microphthalmos, glaucoma, persistent hyperplastic primary vitreous) or the posterior segment (chorioretinitis, Leber's amaurosis, rubella retinopathy, foveal hypoplasia). Occasionally, examination under anaesthesia may be required and repeated examinations may be necessary to document the possible progression of cataract or associated disease.

Visual function

This can be determined by various methods. Clinical tests include the presence or absence of central fixation, nystagmus, or strabismus. The presence of nystagmus and strabismus would indicate severe visual impairment.

Special tests include *Catford Drum, visually evoked response,* and *preferential looking*.

Preferential looking is based on the observation that infants are more interested in looking at patterned than otherwise equivalent stimuli. The test apparatus consists of a large grey screen with right and left apertures through which targets with stripes of varying widths are presented, either in the right or left aperture (*Figure 8.10*). Each striped

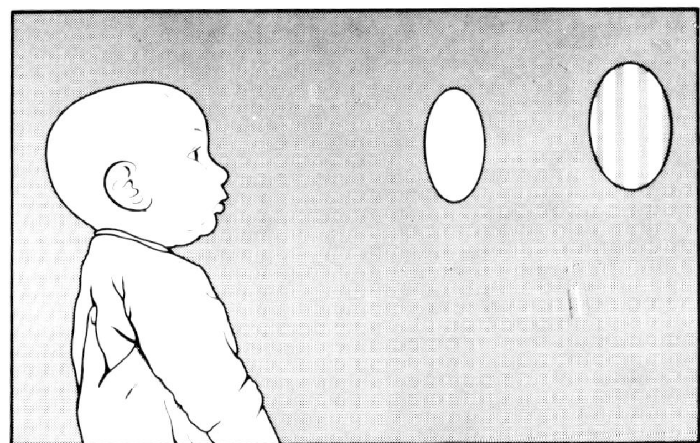

Figure 8.10 *Preferential looking*

pattern is paired with a homogeneous grey card. By turning a wheel the striped and grey cards can be interchanged and the stripe width can be varied. It is assumed that an infant will look at stripes that are wide enough for him to see. Each series of stripes is then compared with an equivalent Snellen type value. Visual acuity measurements by this method have shown that at birth normal visual acuity is about 3/60 and this improves to about 6/12 by the age of 1 year.

The patient

The overall evaluation of the patient should be performed by a paediatrician with special reference to associated systemic disease (rubella, and metabolic or biochemical defects), as well as mental retardation which is present in a significant number of cases.

Rubella

1. Serological tests for specific IgM rubella antibody.
2. Virus cultures from the nasopharynx, urine, lens, or other tissues may be taken to confirm the diagnosis.
3. Platelet count for thrombocytopenia if bruising is present.
4. Maternal rubella titres are now seldom necessary.

Galactosaemia

1. Urinalysis for the presence of a reducing substance.
2. Red blood cell GPUT and GK activity for confirmation.

Hypoglycaemia

Blood glucose determination.

Lowe's syndrome

Urine chromatography for amino acids.

Hypocalcaemic syndromes

1. Serum calcium and phosphorus.
2. Skull X-rays for presence of calcification of basal ganglia in idiopathic (autoimmune) hypoparathyroidism.

The parents

The assessment of the parents should include two factors:

1. *Search for the cause of cataract* including hereditary cataract and maternal intrauterine infections or ingestion of drugs during pregnancy.
2. *Motivation* of the parents and their understanding and willingness to participate in the frequently demanding and complicated postoperative care of their child.

Indications for surgery

1. *Bilateral advanced cataracts* through which the fundus details cannot be visualized with the indirect ophthalmoscope require surgery within a few weeks of birth.
2. *Bilateral immature cataracts* in which the fundus details can be visualized with both the direct and indirect ophthalmoscopes do not require surgery. In cases in which the fundus details can be seen with the indirect but not with the direct ophthalmoscope, surgery can be postponed if the patient appears to have good near vision. If near vision is poor then surgery should be considered.
3. *Unilateral cataracts.* It is important to realize that, in an infant, unilateral uncorrected aphakia is as good a stimulus for amblyopia as is the presence of a dense cataract. Surgery for visual improvement is usually contraindicated unless it can be performed within the first few weeks (and preferably the first few days) of life and then only if parental motivation is extremely good.

Surgical techniques

The techniques available for the treatment of infantile cataracts are simple aspiration and lensectomy.

Simple aspiration

Simple aspiration, using either separate infusion and aspiration cannulae or a single aspiration–infusion cannula, has proved to be a safe and effective procedure for the treatment of certain soft cataracts. However, in infants the posterior capsule invariably becomes opacified and requires subsequent surgery.

Lensectomy

This operation in which the whole lens including both anterior and posterior capsules is removed with a vitreous cutter has now largely replaced simple aspiration. Lensectomy can be performed either through a limbal incision or through the pars plana (or pars plicata).

1. A small peritomy is made and extended posteriorly to make a T-shaped incision (*Figure 8.11a*). The conjunctiva and Tenon's capsule are reflected down to the sclera.
2. With cautery a mark is made on the sclera 3.5 mm behind the limbus (*Figure 8.11b*).
3. With a Ziegler's knife (or equivalent), a stab incision is made in the sclera 3.5 mm from the limbus. If a fully functioning probe (i.e. one with an infusion sleeve) is not being used, a second incision is made and the infusion cannula secured.
4. The knife is introduced into the equator of the lens and the anterior capsule is punctured and sliced (*Figure 8.11c*). The lens is then stirred up to facilitate its subsequent excision with the cutter. As the knife is withdrawn from the eye the sclerotomy is enlarged slightly. If the knife does not enter the lens nucleus with ease or if it pushes the lens to the opposite side, this means that the nucleus is too hard to be aspirated into the cutting port. In this situation, the lensectomy should be aborted and one of the following two options considered: either the sclerotomy is sutured and the procedure converted to a large incision extracapsular extraction or the lens nucleus is softened with an ultrasonic fragmentor and then the lensectomy continued as follows.
5. The infusion system is turned on and the tip of the cutter introduced into the lens. If the pupil is very small and will not dilate it is enlarged with the cutter (*Figure 8.11d*)
6. The lens is gradually excised whilse working within the capsular bag (*Figure 8.12a*). Relatively soft lens material can be aspirated without activating the cutting mechanism, although harder pieces require both aspiration and cutting. Initially the aspiration pressure should be about 100 mmHg and then, if necessary, it can be increased to 200 mmHg. In order to visualize and excise peripheral lens matter from under the iris, the sclera is indented and the globe is simultaneously rotated towards the indentation. When peripheral lens matter is being excised from under the iris, the port of the cutter should be pointing sideways. Pointing the port anteriorly may aspirate the iris, and pointing it posteriorly may cause premature damage to the posterior capsule and result in dislocation of lens particles into the vitreous cavity.
7. The cutting port is turned posteriorly and the posterior capsule is excised (*Figure 8.12b*).
8. The anterior vitreous is excised (*Figure 8.12c*).
9. The anterior capsule is excised (*Figure 8.12d*). If the anterior capsule is covered by a dense rubbery fibrous plaque which cannot be excised with the cutter, it should first be cut free from the surrounding tissue with microscissors and then removed with microforceps. Hard calcified plaques of lens matter that resist excision with the cutter can also be removed with microforceps.
10. The infusion system is turned off and a small amount of fluid aspirated through the cutter in order to lower the intraocular pressure. This will prevent herniation of intraocular contents through the sclerotomy when the cutter is withdrawn.
11. The sclerotomy is closed with 6-0 Vicryl. Care is taken to ensure that the anterior chamber is adequately reconstructed because active uveitis in an eye with a shallow anterior chamber promotes the development of peripheral anterior synechiae and secondary angle-closure glaucoma.

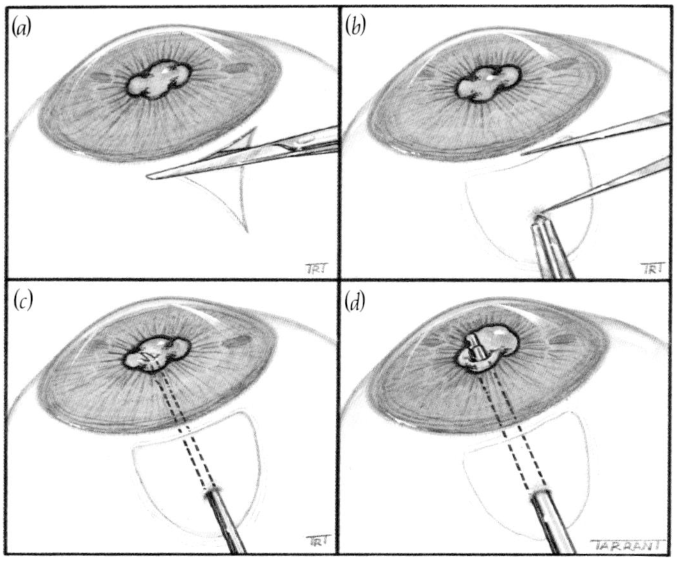

(a) (b) (c) (d)

Figure 8.11 *Lensectomy* (see *text*)

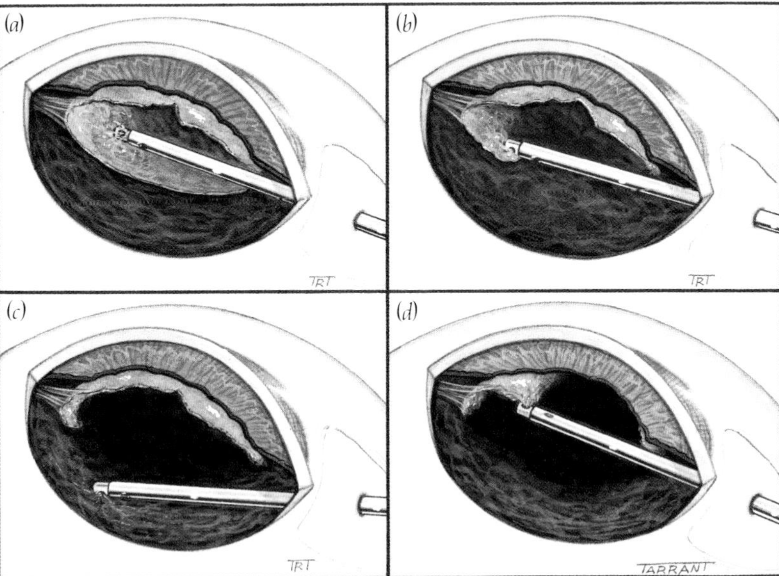

Figure 8.12 *Lensectomy* (see *text)*

12. The conjunctiva is sutured with 6-0 Vicryl and an anterior sub-Tenon's injection of methylprednisolone (Depomedrone) and gentamicin is given.

Complications

Figure 8.13a. Accidental excision of iris tissue can be avoided by pointing the aspiration away from the iris and by avoiding excessive suction.

Figure 8.13b. Posterior dislocation of lens material can be avoided by taking great care not to damage the posterior capsule prematurely and also by not trying to remove hard lenses.

Figure 8.13c. Retinal dialysis formation can be avoided by keeping well away from the vitreous base at all times.

Correction of aphakia

At present, the two ways of correcting infantile aphakia is with either contact lenses or epikeratophakia (*see* Chapter 5). If necessary, the contact lenses can be substituted for spectacles at the age of about 2 years.

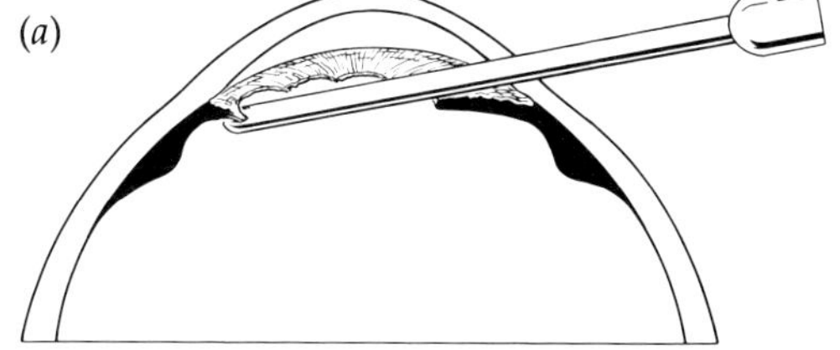

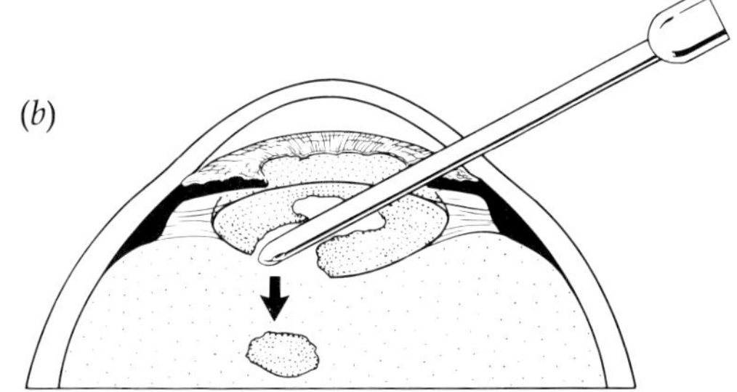

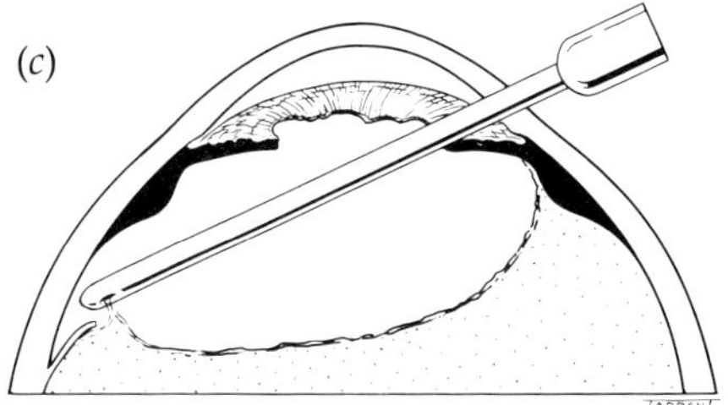

Figure 8.13 *Complications of lensectomy* (see *text)*

Management of cataract in adults

Indications for extraction

Cataract extraction is indicated for one of three reasons: visual improvement, medical, or cosmetic. It is extremely important for the patient to have a clear understanding for which of these reasons cataract extraction is being performed.

Visual improvement

This is by far the most common indication and varies from person to person. For example, a librarian with a posterior subcapsular cataract may need surgery, if when reading in bright light his near vision falls to less than N6 even though his distance vision is still 6/12, enabling him to drive. A farmer with dense nuclear cataract reducing his vision to 6/36 may need surgery although he can still read N5. On the other hand, an elderly lady with the same level of vision may be quite content provided she can still see television.

In patients with bilateral dense cataracts, surgery is usually performed first on the eye with the worse vision. Opinions differ as to when surgery should be performed on the second eye. Some surgeons operate on the second eye within a few days of the first. The main advantages are one period of hospitalization, convalescence, and rehabilitation. However, others feel that the second eye should be operated only after the first is fully rehabilitated.

Medical

Occasionally the presence of a cataract is adversely affecting the health of the eye. This may be due to several causes:

1. Phacolytic glaucoma.
2. Phacoanaphylactic endophthalmitis.
3. Angle-closure glaucoma caused by an intumescent lens.
4. Retinal disease such as diabetic retinopathy or retinal detachment, treatment of which is being hampered by the presence of lens opacities.

Cosmetic

Cataract extraction is indicated for cosmetic reasons in order to obtain a black pupil.

Intracapsular vs extracapsular cataract extraction

Intracapsular extraction

In intracapsular cataract extraction (ICCE), the entire lens is removed with a cryoprobe.

The disadvantages of ICCE as compared with extracapsular cataract extraction are:

1. Posterior chamber intraocular lens (IOL) implantation is impossible because the posterior capsule is absent.
2. ICCE cannot be performed with safety on patients under the age of 35 years in whom the congenital adhesion between the anterior hyaloid face and the posterior capsule (capsulohyaloidal ligament) is still intact. If ICCE is attempted in young individuals, the risk of vitreous loss is unacceptably high. Although the enzyme α-chymotrypsin (Zonulysin) will dissolve the zonules of a young person; it has no effect on the capsulohyaloidal ligament. Extracapsular extraction is therefore the technique of choice in young patients.
3. The incidence of vitreous-related anterior segment problems (e.g. pupil block, vitreous touch syndrome, vitreous wick syndrome) is higher. In uncomplicated extracapsular extraction, the barrier between the anterior and posterior segments remains intact so that vitreous cannot herniate into the anterior chamber.
4. The incidence of postoperative retinal break formation and aphakic retinal detachment is higher.
5. The incidence of postoperative cystoid macular oedema is higher.

Extracapsular extraction

Extracapsular cataract extraction (ECCE) involves excision of a portion of the anterior capsule followed by expression of the nucleus and cortical clean-up. The posterior capsule is left intact.

The disadvantages of ECCE as compared with ICCE are:

1. ECCE is more difficult to master and is more reliant on instrumentation. Consequently, the incidence of operative complications such as rupture of the posterior capsule, vitreous loss, and endothelial damage is significant when the operation is performed by a novice.
2. Postoperative opacification of the posterior capsule occurs in a significant number of cases.
3. ECCE is contraindicated in eyes with active chronic anterior uveitis. This is because the intact posterior capsule may act as a 'scaffold' along which inflammatory membranes can grow during the postoperative period. This is undesirable as it not only impairs vision but contraction of the membranes may detach the ciliary body and precipitate phthisis bulbi.
4. ECCE cannot be performed if the zonules are not intact.

Intraocular lenses

Patient selection

Age

Most surgeons do not perform implantation in children as they feel that, in the present state of knowledge, there is no guarantee that the material from which the lenses are made will remain inert over a span of several decades.

Proliferative diabetic retinopathy

This is a relative contraindication because, in the presence of an IOL, particularly if associated with a pupil that is difficult to dilate, treatment of retinopathy by photocoagulation may be difficult.

Anterior uveitis

The presence of Fuchs' uveitis syndrome is a relative contraindication to implantation. Eyes with other types of active chronic anterior uveitis should not be implanted because an IOL may cause exacerbation of the intraocular inflammation and also act as a 'scaffold' for secondary membrane formation.

High myopia

This is usually a contraindication because the aphakic spectacle correction is weak and free from the aberrations associated with high-power plus lenses.

Main designs of intraocular lenses

The two main designs of IOLs in current use are anterior chamber and posterior chamber. Each IOL consists of two parts: an optical portion and haptics which give the lens stability.

Materials and methods of manufacture

The optics are manufactured from polymethylmethacrylate (PMMA) and the haptics from either PMMA or polypropylene (Prolene). In some IOLs both the optic and haptics are made from PMMA. The manufacturing methods of IOLs are lathe cut, injection moulded, compression moulded, and spin cast. Because PMMA transmits ultraviolet light, a possible source of retinal damage, the optics of some IOLs absorb ultraviolet light.

Anterior chamber intraocular lenses

These lie in front of the iris and have flexible or semiflexible angle-supported haptics. Anterior chamber IOL implantation is possible with both ICCE and ECCE. They are, therefore, very useful as a standby if the posterior capsule is accidentally ruptured during ECCE making posterior chamber implantation impossible. Anterior chamber IOLs are also used for secondary implantation in eyes that had previously undergone ICCE.

Posterior chamber intraocular lenses

These lie behind the iris and have flexible haptics which are inserted either into the capsular bag or into the ciliary sulcus (a groove between the root of the iris and the ciliary body). In some posterior chamber IOLs, the optic and haptic lie in the same plane, while in others the haptics are angled slightly anteriorly enabling easier insertion into the ciliary sulcus and allowing for a greater separation between the pupil and the optic. The optics of some IOLs have a 'laser ridge' which separates the posterior surface of the optic from the posterior capsule so that the IOL is not damaged during YAG laser capsulotomy.

Optimal postoperative refraction

This will differ according to whether the patient requires a monocular or binocular correction.

Monocular correction

If the fellow eye has poor visual acuity due to a dense cataract or amblyopia, the best postoperative refraction is about −1 D as this will enable the patient to carry out most ordinary tasks without spectacles and he can wear bifocals when finer visual acuity is required. Some of the most dissatisfied patients are low myopes who have been turned into hypermetropes after IOL implantation.

Binocular correction

When prescribing spectacles it is important that the difference in power between the two lenses is not greater than 3 D. This is because although the patient will have excellent visual acuity in both eyes when he looks straight ahead, he will develop double vision on looking up or down due to induced vertical prism differences between the two eyes. If a patient has good visual acuity in the unoperated eye, the postoperative refraction in the operated eye ideally should be within 1 or 2 D of the prescription in the unoperated eye. For example, if a patient has +4 D in the unoperated eye, a postoperative refraction of −1 D would produce a 5-D difference between the two lenses resulting in double vision.

Calculation of intraocular lens power

The suitable power of the IOL is calculated by using a special formula which incorporates keratometry readings and the length of the globe as determined by A-scan ultrasonography. Because an anterior chamber IOL has to be slightly weaker than a posterior chamber IOL to achieve the same postoperative refraction, the 'K' constant used in the formula is different according to which type of IOL is to be implanted.

Technique of ICCE and implantation of an anterior chamber IOL

1. A superior rectus (bridle) suture is inserted in order to stabilize the eye and to keep it rotated slightly downwards (*Figure 8.14a*).

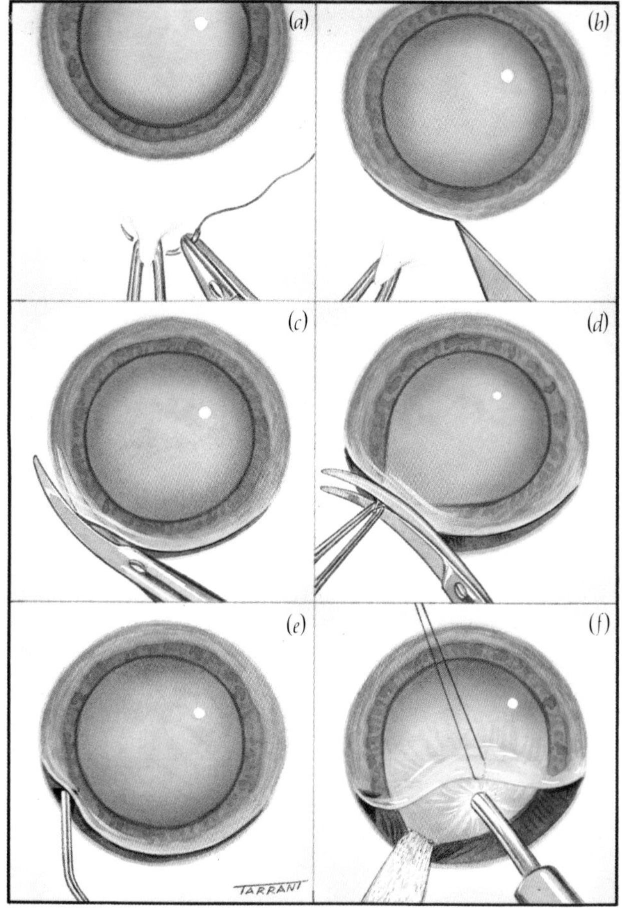

Figure 8.14 Intracapsular cataract extraction

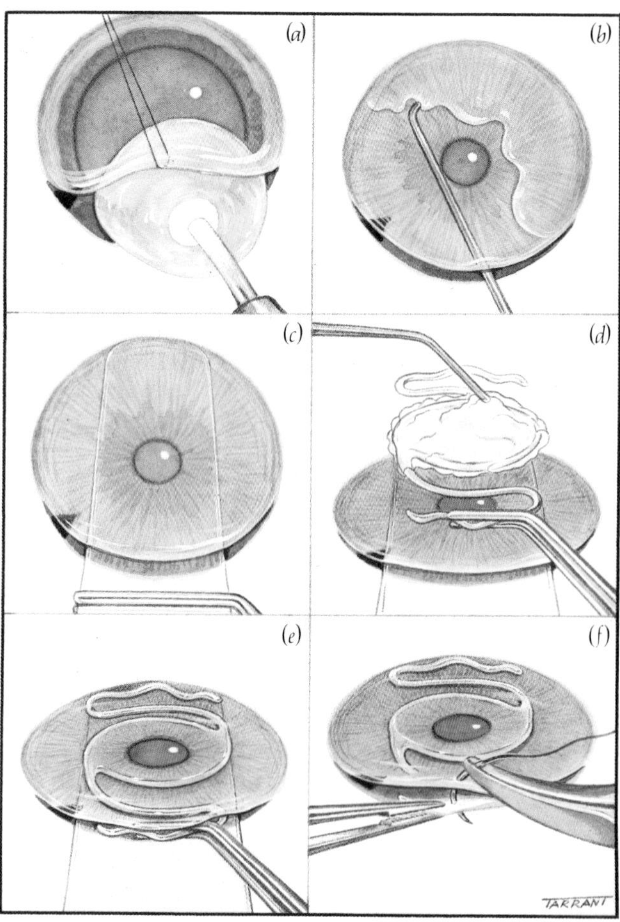

Figure 8.15 Implantation of anterior chamber lens

2. A vertical groove is made through about two-thirds depth of peripheral clear cornea from 2.30 to 9.30 o'clock (*Figure 8.14b*). An incision of inadequate size predisposes to rupture of the anterior capsule during lens delivery.
3. The anterior chamber is entered with the knife at the distal end of the groove and the full-thickness incision enlarged to about 5 mm.
4. The full-thickness incision is completed with scissors (*Figure 8.14c*).
5. A peripheral iridectomy is performed to prevent postoperative pupil block (*Figure 8.14d*).
6. The zonules are dissolved by injecting α-chymotrypsin (Zonulysin) through the iridectomy into the posterior chamber (*Figure 8.14e*). Failure to use Zonulysin in a relatively young person with strong zonules may result in rupture of the anterior capsule during lens delivery.
7. The bridle suture is released and lid speculum is checked to ensure that it is not pressing on the globe as excessive external pressure during lens delivery increases the risk of vitreous loss.
8. The surface of the lens is dried with a triangular cellulose swab. Inadequate drying may cause the iceball to expand too quickly and freeze to the iris.
9. The iris is retracted with a dry swab and the tip of the warm cryoprobe is applied to the superior pre-equatorial part of the lens (*Figure 8.14f*). Inadequate retraction of the iris with a wet swab may also result in freezing of the iceball to the iris. In this event, freezing should be immediately terminated and the cause corrected.
10. Freezing is activated and the lens is extracted by initially elevating it straight up and then gently sliding it from side to side (*Figure 8.15a*). A premature attempt at lens delivery in the presence of an inadequate cryoadhesion may result in a rupture of the anterior capsule. In this event, the nucleus should be expressed and residual cortex aspirated as in a planned extra-capsular extraction (*see* later). Any residual large capsular tags are trimmed with scissors and removed with forceps.
11. The pupil is constricted by injecting Miochol (acetylcholine 1%) into the anterior chamber. This tightens the iris and reduces the risk of iris tuck during insertion of the IOL. A small pupil is also helpful in preventing vitreous entering the anterior chamber.
12. Healonid (sodium hyaluronate 1%) is injected in order to prevent possible collapse of the anterior chamber

and damage to the corneal endothelium during insertion of the IOL (*Figure 8.15b*).

13. A lens glide is slid into the inferior angle (optional) in order to prevent iris tuck at 6 o'clock (*Figure 8.15c*).
14. The IOL of predetermined power is grasped by the superior haptic and the surface of the optic is covered with Healonid in order to protect the corneal endothelium during implantation (*Figure 8.15d*).
15. The inferior haptic is introduced through the lips of the incision and the IOL is slid along the glide into the inferior angle (*Figure 8.15e*).
16. The glide is withdrawn and the superior haptic is gently pushed downwards into the superior angle.
17. Any iris tuck at 12 o'clock can be corrected by gently pushing the optic towards 6 o'clock.
18. The Healonid is washed out because if left *in situ* it may cause postoperative elevation of intraocular pressure.
19. The incision is closed (*Figure 8.15f*).
20. An anterior sub-Tenon's injection of Betnesol (betamethasone) and gentamicin is given.

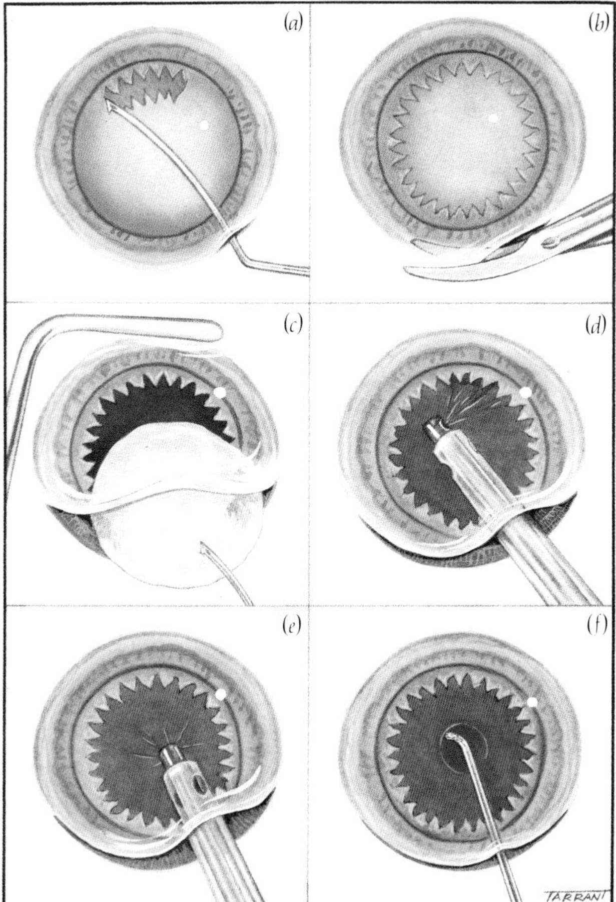

Figure 8.16 *Extracapsular extraction*

Technique of ECCE and implantation of a posterior chamber IOL

1. A superior rectus (bridle) suture is inserted.
2. A vertical groove is made through about two-thirds of peripheral clear cornea from 2 o'clock to 10 o'clock.
3. The anterior chamber is entered with the knife near the distal end of the groove.
4. The cystitome (infusion on) is introduced into the anterior chamber and advanced towards the edge of the dilated pupil at 6 o'clock.
5. Multiple small radial cuts are made in the anterior capsule for 360° (*Figures 8.16a*).
6. The full-thickness incision is completed with scissors (*Figure 8.16b*).
7. The anterior capsule is removed with forceps.
8. With the tip of the cystitome, posterior pressure is exerted first on the sclera at 12 o'clock and then with a squint hook at 6 o'clock. The nucleus is expressed by alternating pressure from above and below (*Figure 8.16c*). If the nucleus fails to present the incision is enlarged.
9. The tip of the infusion–aspiration (I–A) cannula, with the infusion turned on and the aspiration port pointing up, is introduced into the anterior chamber and passed under the iris at 6 o'clock.
10. Strands of cortex are engaged into the port by activating the suction mechanism (*Figure 8.16d*). The cortex is then dragged centrally and aspirated under direct visualization. This manoeuvre is repeated sequentially until all cortex has been removed. Inadequate cortical clean-up is usually due to the inability to remove lens material from under the iris at 12 o'clock as a result of pupillary constriction. When performing cortical clean-up, it is important not to accidentally aspirate the posterior capsule as this may cause it to rupture and make implantation of a posterior chamber IOL impossible. A sign of imminent rupture is the appearance of fine sharp lines radiating from the aspiration port (*Figure 8.16e*). If the posterior capsule is ruptured after most of the cortex has been removed and there is no vitreous loss, it is safe to implant a 'back-up' anterior chamber IOL. If, however, a significant amount of cortex is still present it should be excised with a vitreous cutter together with the ruptured posterior capsule. The management of vitreous loss is discussed later.
11. The posterior capsule is polished with special sand-blasted cannula (*Figure 8.16f*) (Kratz scratcher) to remove any small residual subcapsular plaques. Great care should be taken not to rupture the capsule during this manoeuvre.
12. Healonid is injected into the capsular bag to facilitate subsequent insertion of the IOL (*Figure 8.17a*).
13. The IOL is grasped by the optic and its anterior surface coated with Healonid (*Figure 8.17b*).
14. The inferior haptic is inserted through the lips of the incision and then passed under the iris at 6 o'clock (*Figure 8.17c*).

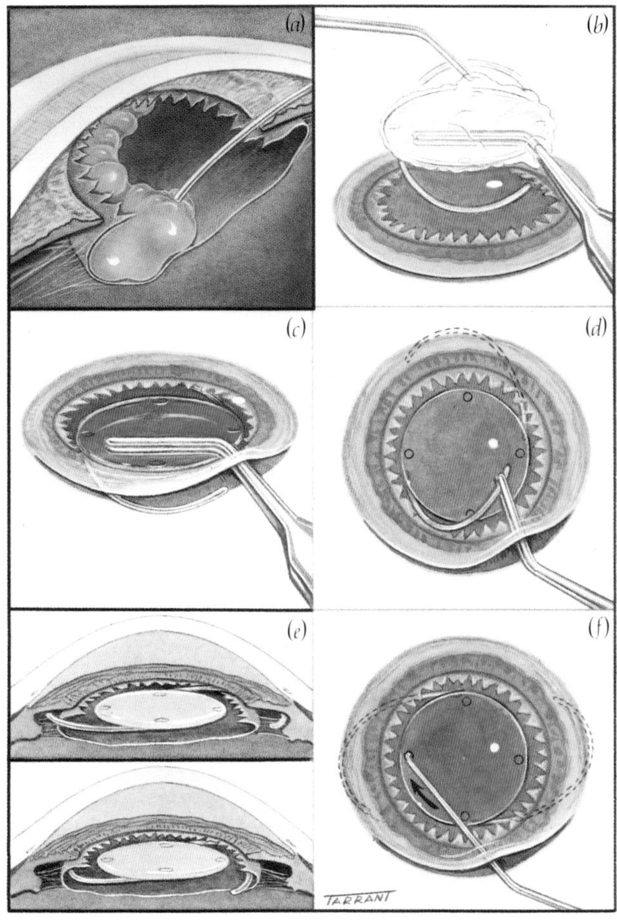

Figure 8.17 Implantation of posterior chamber lens

15. The tip of the superior haptic is grasped with forceps and advanced into the anterior chamber. As the superior pole of the haptic is clearing the edge of the pupil (*Figure 8.17d*), the arm is pronated to ensure that when the haptic is released it will spring open under the iris and not out of the incision. Preferably both haptics should be placed into the capsular bag (*Figure 8.17e, bottom*) and not into the ciliary sulcus (*Figure 8.17e, top*).
16. The IOL is dialled into the horizontal position by engaging the guide holes with a special hook (*Figure 8.17f*). This prevents iris tuck and confirms the integrity of the zonules.
17. The IOL is gently pushed from side to side to check for correct centring.
18. The pupil is constricted by injecting Miochol into the anterior chamber to ensure that the optic is behind the iris.
19. The incision is closed.
20. An anterior sub-Tenon's injection of Betnesol and gentamicin is given.

Phacoemulsification

The Kelman unit basically consists of a hollow 1-mm titanium needle which is activated by an ultrasonic mechanism to vibrate at 40 000 times a second in its longitudinal axis. This mechanical vibration transforms the lens matter into an emulsion which can be aspirated from within the capsular bag and replaced by infusion fluid. The nucleus can be emulsified in the posterior chamber or it can be first dislocated into the anterior chamber, emulsified, and then aspirated.

Advantages of the Kelman Cavitron unit (KPE) include a small incision (much smaller than in simple extracapsular extraction), more rapid wound healing, short convalescence, and early stabilization of refractive error with less astigmatism.

Disadvantages of KPE are a higher incidence of complications by beginners due to the fact that the technique is difficult, lens material is more likely to become mixed with vitreous, the iris may become damaged, it cannot be used in eyes with grade +3 and +4 nuclear sclerosis, and the equipment is expensive.

Vitreous loss

Vitreous loss may occur both during ICCE and following accidental rupture of the posterior capsule during planned ECCE. It is potentially a serious complication because it is associated with an increased incidence of the following postoperative problems:

Updrawn pupil
Iris prolapse
Vitreous touch syndrome
Vitreous wick syndrome
Uveitis
Retinal detachment
Chronic cystoid macular oedema

The clinical features and management of these complications will be discussed later.

Prevention

Preoperative

Because with ICCE, vitreous loss tends to occur in both eyes, it may be safer to perform a planned ECCE in the second eye if vitreous loss occurred during an ICCE in the first. However, irrespective of the technique of extraction, the risk of vitreous loss can be further reduced by shrinking the vitreous by the preoperative intravenous administration of mannitol 20%. The dose is 1–2 g/kg body weight, given over about 40 minutes and not exceeding 60 drops per minute. Because the maximal effect is reached within about 30 minutes and lasts between 4–6 hours, the infusion should be started about one and a half hours prior to surgery.

Intraoperative

The risk of vitreous loss can be reduced by checking that neither the lid speculum nor the bridle suture is exerting pressure on the globe prior to lens extraction. If the operation is being performed under general anaesthesia, the anaesthetist should make sure that the patient is not performing the Valsalva manoeuvre as this tends to increase vitreous pressure.

Management

The aim of management is to clear the incision and anterior chamber of formed vitreous. This can be achieved by one of two methods.

Sponge vitrectomy

In this procedure vitreous is excised by the use of small triangular sponges and scissors. The tip of the sponge is applied to the vitreous, the sponge is then retracted slightly and the vitreous which has become adherent to the sponge is excised with scissors. This may have to be repeated many times until the desired effect has been achieved.

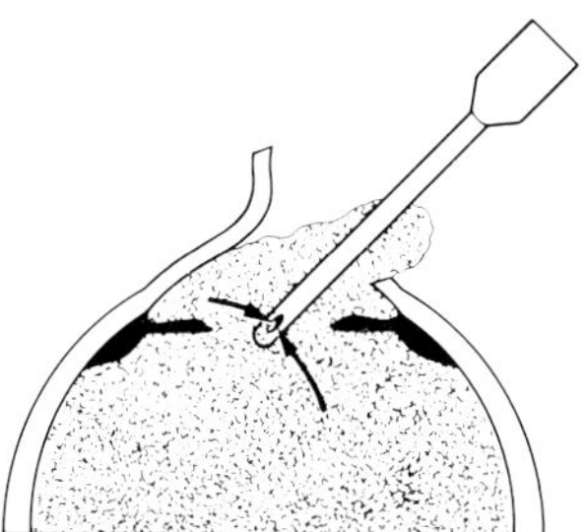
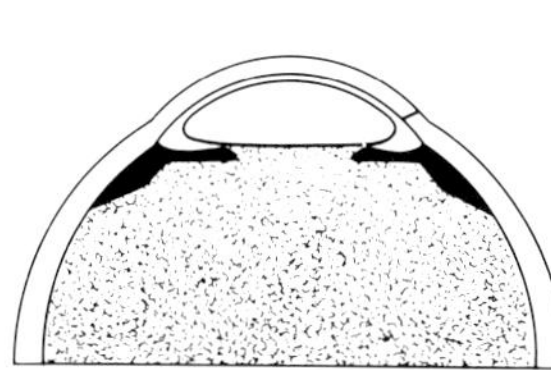

Figure 8.18 *Management of vitreous loss*

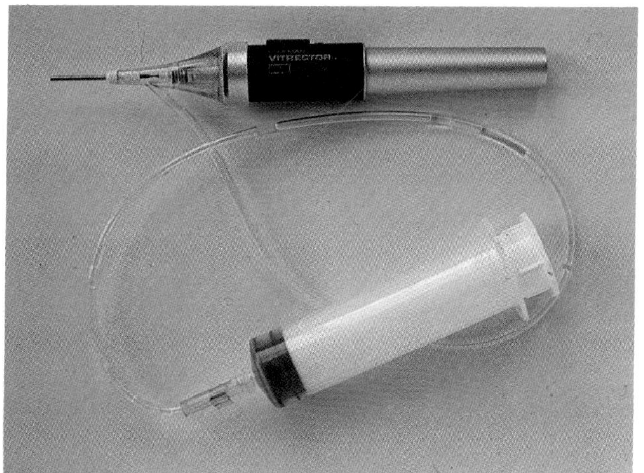

Figure 8.19 *Kaufman vitrector*

Automated vitrectomy

In this procedure the vitreous is excised from the anterior chamber (*Figure 8.18*) with the Kaufman vitrector (*Figure 8.19*).

Early postoperative complications of cataract surgery

These occur within a few days of cataract surgery. The main early complications are:

Iris prolapse
Hyphaema
Striate keratopathy
Wound leak
Pupil block
Bacterial endophthalmitis

Iris prolapse

This, now relatively uncommon, complication is usually caused by inadequate suturing of the incision. It is more frequent following inappropriate management of vitreous loss. Complications of untreated iris prolapse include: defective healing of the incision, excessive astigmatism, chronic anterior uveitis, epithelial ingrowth, cystoid macular oedema, and endophthalmitis.

Treatment

The prolapsed iris tissue is excised and the incision resutured.

Hyphaema

This fairly common, but usually innocuous, complication is caused by bleeding from small blood vessels crossing the incision. It most frequently occurs between the second and seventh postoperative day and may be precipitated by minor ocular trauma.

Treatment

Small hyphaemas require no specific treatment. Large hyphaemas which have caused a secondary elevation of intraocular pressure should be evacuated in order to prevent bloodstaining of the cornea.

Striate keratopathy

Corneal oedema with folds in Descemet's membrane may occur as a result of damage to the corneal endothelium by instruments, IOLs, or excessive bending. The risk of damage to the corneal endothelium during insertion of an IOL can be reduced by using Healonid.

Treatment

Most cases are innocuous and self-limiting and clear within a few days. The rare severe and persistent cases may require penetrating keratoplasty.

Wound leak

This relatively rare complication is most frequently due to inadequate closure of the incision. The site of leakage can be identified by performing the Seidel test. In this test, the incision is examined with a blue light following the instillation of fluorescein into the lower fornix. The fluorescein will become diluted by escaping aqueous at the leakage site.

Treatment

Although small leaks may seal spontaneously with the aid of padding or a bandage contact lens, large leaks require resuturing of the incision.

Pupil block

This may occur following ICCE with or without an anterior chamber IOL, but not after an uncomplicated ECCE. It is caused by blockage of the pupil and the peripheral iridectomy by formed vitreous. The aqueous humour entrapped in the posterior chamber leads to iris bombé and shallowing of the anterior chamber (*Figure 8.20*). If left untreated, the eventual outcome is secondary angle-closure glaucoma due to the formation of peripheral anterior synechiae.

Treatment:

1. *Medical treatment.* Carbonic anhydrase inhibitors should be administered if the intraocular pressure is elevated and an attempt made to break the pupil block by dilating the pupil.
2. *Laser ididotomy* (argon or YAG) should be performed if medical treatment is unsuccessful. The technique is described in Chapter 7.
3. *Surgical iridectomy* is an alternative to laser iridotomy if a laser is unavailable.

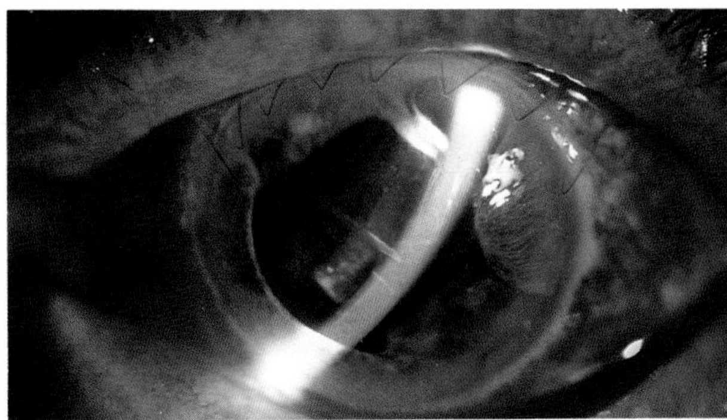

***Figure 8.20** Pupil block in eye with an anterior chamber lens*

Bacterial endophthalmitis

This is a devastating, but fortunately now a very rare, complication of cataract surgery.

Aetiology

In order of frequency the most common causative organisms are *Staphylococcus epidermidis. Staph. aureus, Pseudomonas* sp. and *Proteus* sp. The main sources of infection are contaminated solutions and instruments, the patient's own bacterial flora, and occasionally air-borne bacteria.

Prevention

1. Treatment prior to surgery of pre-existing infections such as staphylococcus blepharitis, conjunctivitis, and dacryocystitis.
2. Preoperative prophylactic antibiotics (gentamicin every 10 minutes for 1 hour prior to surgery) to decrease the patient's own bacterial conjunctival flora.
3. Postoperative prophylactic anterior sub-Tenon's injection of antibiotics (gentamicin 20 mg).
4. Meticulous attention to aseptic surgical technique.

Clinical features

Most cases become evident within the first 24–48 hours with pain, visual loss, oedema of the eyelids, chemosis, corneal haze, a fibrinous exudate or hypopyon in the anterior chamber, vitritis, and an absent or diminished red reflex. Occasionally the above features are delayed in onset and less severe. This is likely to occur when the offending organism is relatively avirulent (e.g. *Staphylococcus epidermidis*) or when prophylactic antibiotics and steroids have been administered postoperatively.

Successful treatment depends on identification and elimination of the offending organisms with antibiotics (and possibly vitrectomy), and control of host inflammatory response with steroids.

Identification of organisms

1. With the patient in the operating theatre a small bevelled partial thickness incision is made in peripheral clear cornea.
2. With a 25-gauge needle attached to a tuberculin syringe, 0.2 ml of aqueous is aspirated and samples are inoculated onto the following culture media: blood agar, chocolate agar, liquid thioglycolate, and Sabouraud's agar.
3. Several drops are placed onto slides for Gram and Giemsa staining.
4. The incision is slightly enlarged and, with a 22-gauge needle attached to a tuberculin syringe, about 0.3 ml is aspirated from the midvitreous cavity. In an eye with an IOL, vitreous samples can be obtained through a sclerotomy 3.5 mm posterior to the limbus. Inoculation

is the same as for aqueous samples. Vitreous cultures give a better yield than aqueous cultures.

Antibiotic therapy

Until culture results are available (usually 48 hours), antibiotics that cover both Gram-positive and Gram-negative organisms should be administered. In order to obtain the highest possible intraocular concentration, every possible route should be utilized.

Intravitreal

After the culture specimens have been obtained, the following antibiotics should be injected slowly into the midvitreous cavity using a 25-gauge needle.

1. Gentamicin 0.1 mg in 0.1 ml which is prepared as follows: 0.1 ml (4 mg) is withdrawn from a fresh vial containing gentamicin sulphate for injection (40 mg/ml); this is added to 3.9 ml of sterile (not bacteriostatic) saline; 0.1 ml of this solution is injected into the vitreous.
2. Cephazolin 2.25 mg in 0.1 ml which is prepared as follows: the powder in a 500 mg vial is reconstituted using 2 ml of sterile (not bacteriostatic) saline; 1 ml of the solution is withdrawn and diluted with 9 ml of sterile saline; 0.1 ml of the solution is injected into the vitreous.

Periocular injections

An anterior sub-Tenon's injection is given containing gentamicin 40 mg and cephazolin 125 mg. The technique of injection is described in Chapter 6. The injections are repeated daily for 5–7 days according to the response to therapy.

Systemic

1. Oral—sodium fusidate 500 mg three times a day.
2. Intravenous—cephazolin 1 g four times a day.

Topical

Fortified gentamicin and cephazolin drops every 30 minutes.

Corticosteroid therapy

The simultaneous administration of steroids will not interfere with the control of the infection, provided the organisms are sensitive to the antibiotics.

Periocular injections

Betamethasone 4 mg or dexamethasone 4 mg (1 ml) daily for 5–7 days according to response to therapy.

Systemic

Oral prednisolone 20 mg four times a day for 10–14 days. In relatively early and mild cases systemic steroids can be omitted.

Topical

Dexamethasone 0.1% drops every 30 minutes.

Subsequent therapy

This is governed by the culture results.

1. *Resistant bacteria*—modify antibiotic therapy accordingly.
2. Negative—prognosis is excellent. Antibiotics can be gradually discontinued.
3. *Staphylococcus epidermidis*—prognosis is relatively good. The present therapeutic regimen should be continued for 7–10 days and then gradually discontinued.
4. *Virulent bacteria*—if the infection is responding well to present therapy no change in treatment is necessary.
5. *Virulent bacteria*—if the infection is not responding despite appropriate antibiotic therapy, the prognosis is very poor. In this case, a pars plana vitrectomy should be performed and further antibiotics together with dexamethasone 0.4 mg injected into the vitreous.

Late postoperative complications of cataract surgery

These occur within weeks, months or years. The main late complications are:

Cystoid macular oedema
Opacification of the posterior capsule
Retinal detachment
Epithelial ingrowth
Filtering bleb
Vitreous touch syndrome
Vitreous wick syndrome
'UGH' syndrome
'Sunset' syndrome

Cystoid macular oedema (Irvine–Gass syndrome)

Aetiology

The exact cause of cystoid macular oedema (CMO) following cataract extraction is still unknown, although inflammation, vitreous traction, and generalized vascular incompetence have been postulated as predisposing factors. Prostaglandins have been implicated as direct mediators of the noxious stimulus. Recent studies have shown that the prophylactic treatment with topical indomethacin, a non-steroidal anti-inflammatory agent, reduces the incidence of CMO.

Risk factors

1. *ICCE vs ECCE.* The incidence of CMO is highest with ICCE and lowest with ECCE and an intact posterior capsule.
2. *IOL.* Regardless of the surgical technique, the presence of an IOL does not appear to significantly affect the

incidence of CMO. However, about 30% of eyes develop CMO following secondary IOL implantation.
3. *Capsulotomy.* When a primary capsulotomy is performed at the time of ECCE, the incidence of postoperative CMO is increased four-fold and is virtually the same as with ICCE. However, if capsulotomy is delayed for 6 months or more, the risk of CMO is significantly reduced.
4. *Vitreous loss* at the time of cataract extraction is associated with an increased incidence of CMO, irrespective of the surgical technique.
5. *Systemic vascular disease,* such as hypertension or diabetes, is thought to increase the risk of CMO.
6. *Fellow eye.* Patients with CMO in one eye are at increased risk of developing it in the second eye, even after uncomplicated cataract extraction.
7. *Ultraviolet light.* It has been suggested but unproven that ultraviolet light may play an adverse role.

Clinical features

It is important to differentiate 'angiographic' from 'clinical' CMO.

Angiographic CMO

This develops soon after cataract extraction and probably represents a physiological response to surgical trauma. Its incidence is about 60% following uncomplicated ICCE and about 20% after uncomplicated ECCE. Fluorescein angiography shows the typical 'flower-petal' pattern due to leakage of eye from the perifoveal capillaries (*see Figure 11.21*). In the vast majority of cases, the condition is mild, asymptomatic, transient, and innocuous.

Clinical CMO

This is much less common and more severe than the 'angiographic' type:

1. *Symptoms.* The patient typically presents between 2 and 4 months following surgery with diminished visual acuity which is occasionally associated with mild ocular irritation and photophobia. Rarely CMO first develops many months and even years following catarat extraction.
2. *Slitlamp examination* of the anterior segment may be either normal or it may show the following: ciliary flush, mild anterior uveitis and vitritis, ruptured anterior vitreous face with adhesion of formed vitreous to the inside of the incision, and pupillary distortion. The clinical course is less favourable in eyes with abnormal than with normal anterior segments.
3. *Ophthalmoscopical features*—these are described in Chapter 11.

Treatment

1. *Conservative.* Most cases resolve spontaneously within 6 months and require no specific treatment. CMO of less than 6 months' duration does not usually lead to lamellar hole formation.
2. *Corticosteroids.* In some persistent cases corticosteroids may be beneficial although their effects are frequently transient. The initial treatment is with topical steroids every 2 hours for 3 weeks. If there is no improvement, a posterior sub-Tenon's injection of a long-acting steroid such as methylprednisolone (Depomedrone) or triamcinolone (Kenalog) should be given. The technique of posterior sub-Tenon's injection is described in Chapter 6.
3. *Neodymium YAG laser.* If steroid therapy is unsuccessful in an eye with vitreous adhesions to the cataract incision, an attempt should be made to disrupt the adhesions with a YAG laser.
4. *Anterior vitrectomy.* If both medical and YAG treatment fail, then the vitreous should be removed from the anterior segment with a vitreous cutter.
5. *Removal of the IOL* should be considered if it appears to be contributing to or aggravating intraocular inflammation. This applies particularly to iris-supported and anterior chamber IOLs.

Opacification of the posterior capsule

This is the most frequent late complication of uncomplicated ECCE. Three types are recognized:

1. *Elschnig's pearls*—due to the proliferation of lens epithelium onto the posterior capsule at the site of apposition between the remnants of the anterior capsule with the posterior capsule. This, the most frequently seen type of opacification, is related to the patient's age. It is extremely common in children and occurs in about 50% of adults after 3–5 years.
2. *Primary*—due to a residual subcapsular plaque.
3. *Capsular fibrosis* (*Figure 8.21*).

Indications for treatment

1. Diminished visual acuity.
2. Impaired visualization of the fundus for diagnostic or therapeutic purposes.
3. Monocular diplopia or severe glare due to wrinkling of the posterior capsule.

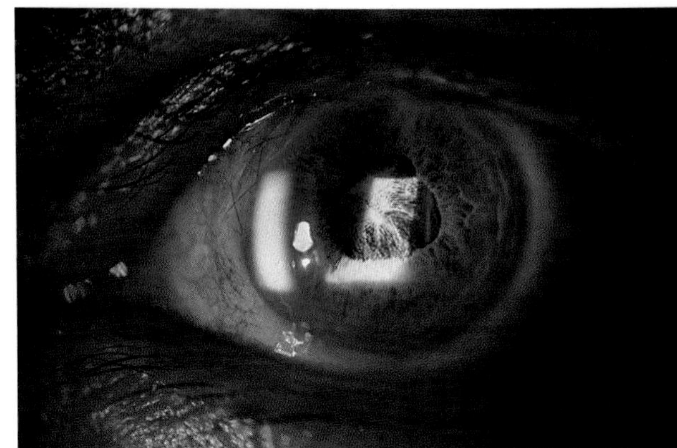

Figure 8.21 *Thickened posterior capsule following extracapsular extraction*

Neodymium-YAG laser capsulotomy

This is by far the most convenient method because it is relatively safe, painless, and can be performed as an out-patient procedure. The key to safe and successful laser capsulotomy is accurate focusing and using the minimal amount of energy required to puncture the capsule. With a Q-switched laser, the power setting is between 1 and 2.5 mJ/pulse and, with a mode-locked laser, between 3 and 5 mJ/pulse.

Technique

1. The cornea is anaesthetized.
2. A special high-plus power anterior segment laser contact lens is inserted. The lens enlarges the 'cone angle' of the beam at the focus and, because the diameter of the focus is smaller, facilitates laser puncture of the capsule.
3. To avoid induced astigmatism, the aiming beam is adjusted so that it forms an angle of no more than 30° with the visual axis.
4. When performing YAG laser capsulotomy it is important not to damage the IOL. In an eye with an anterior chamber IOL, the risk is small because the IOL is not in contact with the posterior capsule. However, in the presence of a posterior chamber IOL, laser capsulotomy may be more difficult because, in the absence of a 'laser ridge', the posterior capsule and the IOL may be in apposition. If the laser is focused directly on the posterior capsule the IOL may be damaged and, if focused too far posteriorly, the capsule will not be punctured. In the absence of an automatic defocusing control, the safest method is initially to focus the laser beam just behind the posterior surface of the capsule and then to bring the focus gradually more anteriorly until the capsule is punctured.
5. The capsulotomy is performed by applying a series of punctures in a cruciate pattern (either '×' or '+'), with the first puncture aimed at the visual axis (*Figure 8.22*). An opening of 3 mm is usually sufficient to improve visual acuity, but larger openings are necessary for adequate retinal examination or retinal photocoagulation.

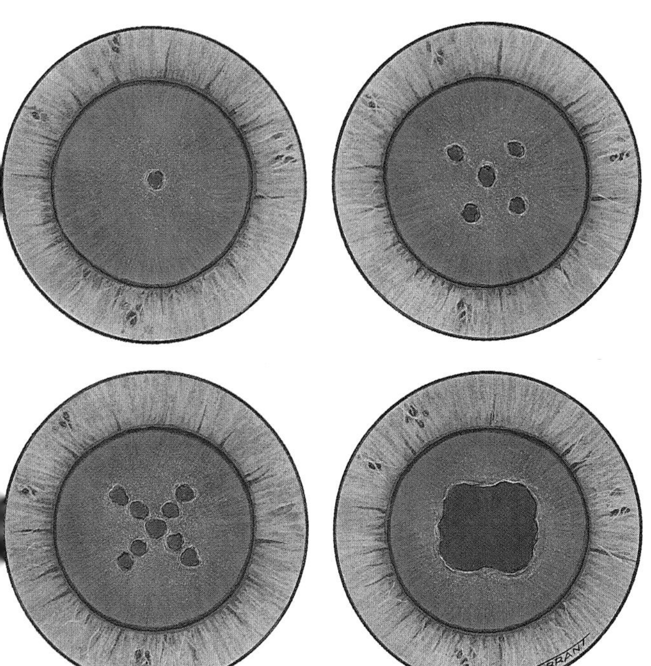

Figure 8.22 *Technique of YAG laser capsulotomy*

Postoperative management

1. Following YAG laser capsulotomy, the patient should be observed for at least 3 hours so that any excessive elevation of intraocular pressure (IOP) can be detected and treated. This is particularly important in patients who also have glaucoma.
2. Cycloplegics and mydriatics are unnecessary as patient discomfort and anterior segment inflammation are usually minimal.

Complications

1. *Elevation of IOP* develops within 3 hours of capsulotomy in about 50% of cases. The rise in IOP is probably caused by 'clogging' of the trabeculum by debris. In otherwise normal eyes, a mild elevation of IOP is of no consequence as it usually resolves within 1 week. However, in eyes with pre-existing glaucoma, the incidence of IOL elevation is higher and its duration longer than in otherwise normal eyes. Some glaucomatous eyes may therefore require additional glaucoma therapy for several weeks or months following laser capsulotomy.
2. *Rupture of the anterior hyaloid face* with herniation of vitreous into the anterior chamber is relatively common and usually innocuous. Very occasionally, however, it may cause secondary pupil block glaucoma in an eye without a peripheral iridectomy.
3. *Damage to the IOL* may occur if the laser is poorly focused. Although undesirable, the presence of a few laser marks on the IOL does not alter visual function or change the ocular tolerance of the IOL.
4. *Cystoid macular oedema* is an occasional complication. Its incidence appears to be less when capsulotomy is delayed for 6 months or longer following cataract extraction.
5. *Retinal detachment* is rare. Its incidence appears tobe less when capsulotomy is delayed for 1 year or longer following cataract extraction.

Surgical capsulotomy

Indications

1. When a YAG laser is unavailable.
2. Corneal opacity which prevents adequate focusing of the laser.
3. Uncooperative patient.
4. An opaque lens capsule associated with significant residual cortical remnants.

Retinal detachment

Mechanism

It has been postulated that cataract surgery induces a loss of hyaluronic acid from within the vitreous gel, which in turn causes synchysis and posterior vitreous detachment which may result in retinal tear formation.

Risk factors

Extracapsular vs intracapsular

Preservation of the posterior capsule following uneventful ECCE reduces the risk of subsequent RD as compared with uneventful ICCE. However, the risk is increased if capsulotomy is performed within the first year following extraction.

Vitrous loss

Particularly if it is inappropriately managed, vitreous loss is associated with about 7% risk of RD.

Myopia

Myopia greater than −6 D is associated with a 7% risk of RD following uncomplicated ICCE. If vitreous is lost, the risk is increased to 15%.

Predisposing lesions

Eyes with lattice degeneration or breaks in flat retina have an increased risk of RD following cataract extraction. If possible, these lesions should be treated prophylactically prior to cataract surgery, or as soon as possible following surgery.

Epithelial ingrowth

This extremely rare but devastating complication is caused by invasion of the anterior segment by epithelial cells derived from the conjunctiva through a defect in the incision. The frequent eventual outcome is intractable glaucoma due to trabecular obstruction. Epithelial ingrowth is characterized by persistent postoperative anterior uveitis and the appearance of a translucent membrane with a scalloped border in the superior part of the posterior corneal surface (*Figure 8.23*). Later the membrane grows across the iris and anterior vitreous, and distorts the pupil.

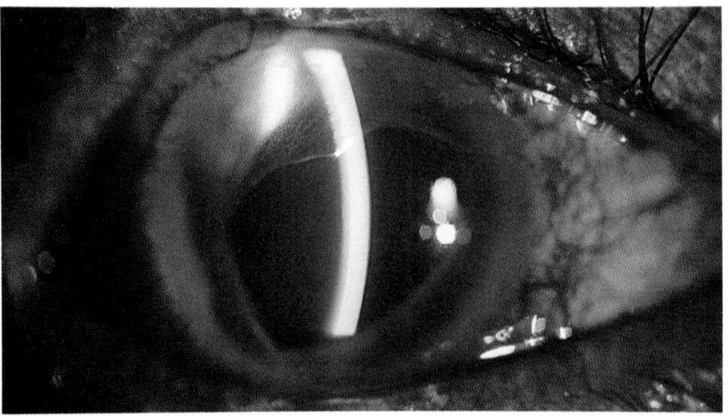

Figure 8.23 Epithelial ingrowth

Treatment

The epithelial cells on the corneal endothelium and ciliary body are destroyed by cryotherapy and the membrane on the iris and anterior vitreous is excised with a vitreous cutter.

Filtering bleb

This relatively rare complication is caused by defective healing of the incision with leakage of aqueous under the conjunctiva.

Treatment

Surgical intervention is indicated in eyes with chronic irritation and hypotony. The bleb should also be repaired, even if asymptomatic, in patients wishing to wear a contact lens because of the increased risk of endophthalmitis.

The two techniques of repairing a bleb are:

1. Freezing of the bleb with a retinal cryoprobe once for 60 seconds and twice for 30 seconds.
2. Surgical excision of the bleb and suturing of the fistula.

Vitreous touch syndrome

This rare complication, which occurs several weeks or months following ICCE, is caused by vitreo-endothelial contact. The endothelial cells in contact with formed vitreous decompensate and the cornea becomes oedematous. Fortunately, not all eyes with vitreocorneal touch develop endothelial decompensation.

Treatment

If the corneal oedema is progressive, treatment is excision of all vitreous in the anterior chamber with a vitreous cutter.

Vitreous wick syndrome

In this rare complication, a bead of formed vitreous prolapses through a small dehiscence in the incision. The condition usually occurs between the second and fourth weeks and is characterized by the onset of ocular irritation and the presence of a plug of vitreous in the incision. If a strand of vitreous connects the externalized vitreous with the iris, gentle traction on the plug with a cotton bud will cause the pupil to peak. Continued exposure of the externalized vitreous to bacterial contamination may lead to endophthalmitis.

Treatment

All vitreous is excised from the anterior chamber with a vitreous cutter and the fistula is sutured.

'UGH' syndrome

This is a triad of uveitis, glaucoma, and hyphaema. Although now relatively rare, it appears to be more common in eyes with anterior chamber IOLs than with other designs.

Treatment

Mild cases in which the optic of the IOL is covered by inflammatory and pigment cells can usually be controlled with topical steroids. In severe and persistent cases, the offending IOL may need to be removed.

'Sunset' syndrome

This very rare complication (*Figure 8.24*) occurs months or years after implantation of a posterior chamber IOL. It is characterized by dislocation of the IOL into the vitreous, probably as a result of zonular rupture during implantation. It appears to be more frequent when the optic has been dialled into position.

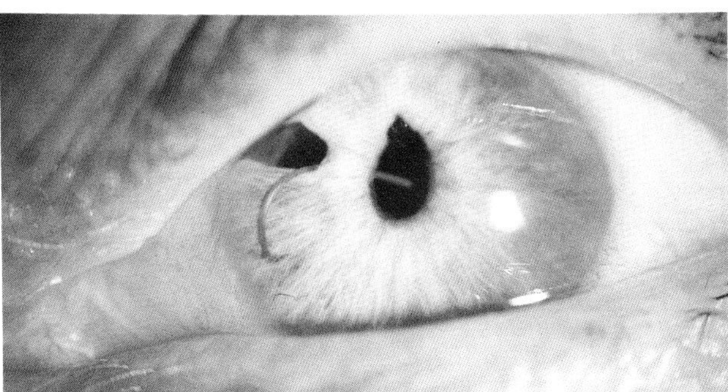

Figure 8.24 *'Sunset' syndrome*

Treatment

If the lens is completely dislocated and not causing any problems, it is best left alone. Partially dislocated IOLs located in the anterior vitreous can be removed and, if necessary, replaced by an anterior chamber IOL.

Ectopia lentis

Inherited

Marfan's syndrome

Systemic features

This is a dominantly inherited disorder characterized by a widespread abnormality of connective tissue. However, in about 15% of cases, no other family member shows any of the stigmas of the disorder.

In its classic form, Marfan's syndrome is characterized by the following:

1. *Cardiac anomalies* such as aneurysms of the ascending aorta and aortic regurgitation.
2. *Skeletal anomalies* in which the patient's limbs are inappropriately long compared with the trunk (*Figure 8.25*). Long spider-like fingers (arachnodactyly), pectus deformities, mild joint laxity, and high arched palate are also frequently seen.
3. *Muscular underdevelopment*, leading to a high incidence of hernias.

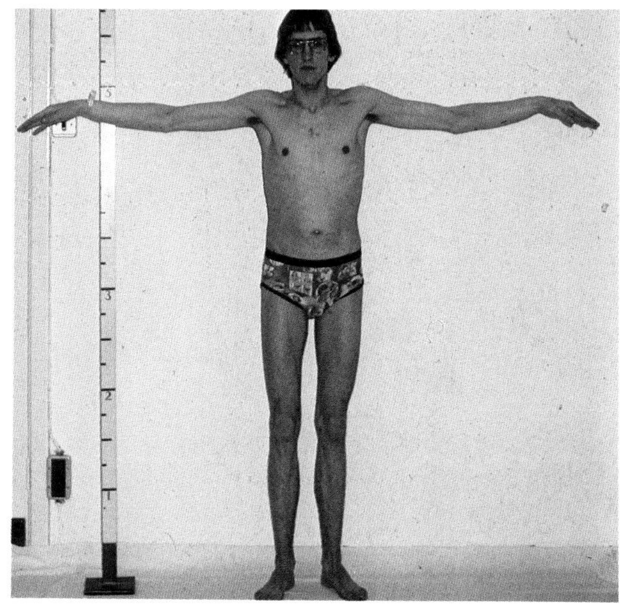

Figure 8.25 *Marfan's syndrome*

Ocular features

1. *Lens subluxation* which is bilateral, symmetrical, non-progressive and upward is present in 80% of cases (*Figure 8.26*). Because the zonule is frequently intact, the ability to accommodate is retained. In some cases the lens may also be small and spherical (microspherophakia; *Figure 8.27*).

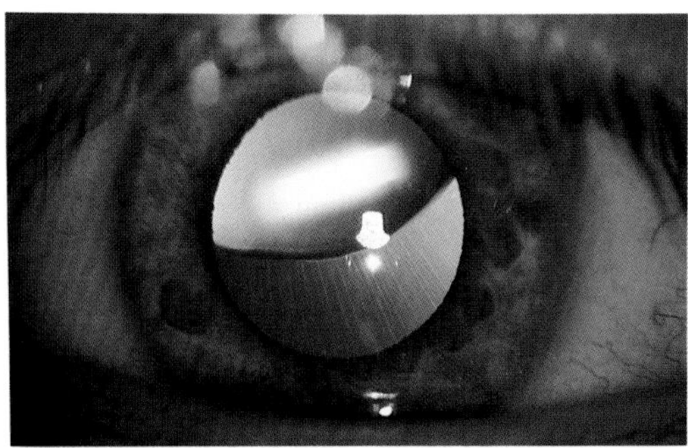

Figure 8.26 *Upward lens subluxation in Marfan's syndrome*

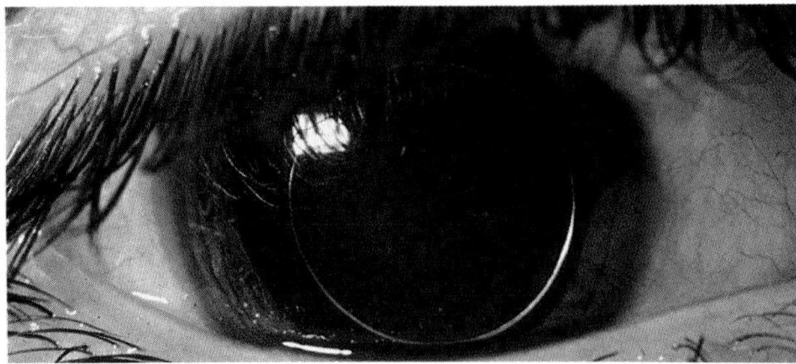

Figure 8.27 *Microspherophakia*

2. *Angle anomaly* is present in 75% of eyes, and is characterized by dense iris processes and thickened trabecular sheets.
3. *Glaucoma* may be the result of the angle anomaly or it may be associated with lens subluxation. (The mechanisms of glaucoma with lens subluxation are discussed in Chapter 7.)
4. *Hypoplasia of dilator muscle* makes the pupil very difficult to dilate.
5. The *cornea* may be flattened.
6. *Axial myopia* is a very frequent finding.
7. *Retinal detachment* due to a very high incidence of predisposing peripheral retinal degenerations such as lattice is common, and is the most serious ocular complication of Marfan's syndrome.

Weill–Marchesani syndrome

Systemic features

This is a rare, recessively inherited disorder characterized by short stature, short stubby fingers, and mental retardation.

Ocular features

1. *Microspherophakia* is the dominant ocular feature. Inferior dislocation may occur during the 'teens' or early 20s.
2. *Angle anomaly* from mesodermal dysgenesis may be associated with this syndrome.
3. *Glaucoma* is usually caused by an incarceration of the lens in the pupil. Treatment is by mydriasis or iridectomy. The fellow eye should be kept on miotics to prevent a similar occurrence.

Homocystinuria

Systemic features

This is an inborn error of metabolism due to a deficiency in the enzyme cystathione synthetase. This gives rise to abnormally high levels of homocystine in the plasma and urine. On cursory examination, the condition can be confused with Marfan's syndrome. However, unlike Marfan's syndrome, it is inherited in a recessive manner, arachnodactyly is less frequent, skeletal anomalies consist of osteoporosis with fractures, and mental retardation is frequent. Vascular complications are due to an increase in platelet stickiness giving rise to thrombosis of intermediate-sized arteries and veins, particularly following general anaesthesia. The hair of patients with homocystinuria is frequently fine and fair, and a malar flush is a common finding.

Ocular features

1. *Lens subluxation* is typically downwards. Accommodation is lost due to disintegration of the zonule.
2. *Glaucoma* may occur as a result of pupil block due to lens incarceration in the pupil, or by a total dislocation into the anterior chamber.

Hyperlysinaemia

This is a very rare inborn error of metabolism due to a deficiency in the enzyme lysine dehydrogenase. It is characterized by motor, mental, and growth retardation. In these patients microspherophakia is the main ocular feature.

Familial ectopia lentis

This is unassociated with systemic defects. In these patients the pupil may also be ectopic (*Figure 8.28*).

Aniridia

This is occasionally associated with ectopia lentis.

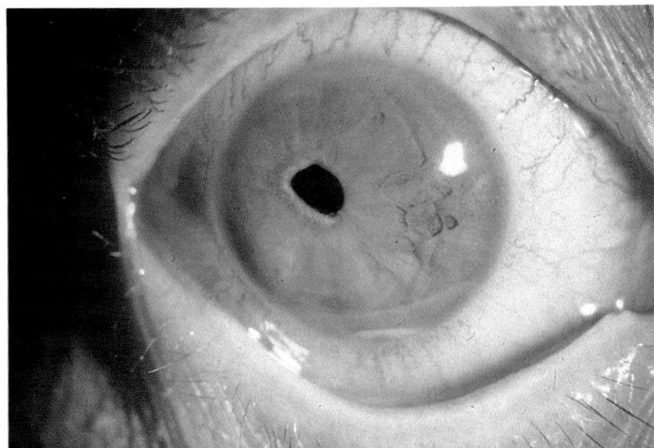

Figure 8.28 *Dislocated lens in eye with an ectopic pupil and lens-induced uveitis*

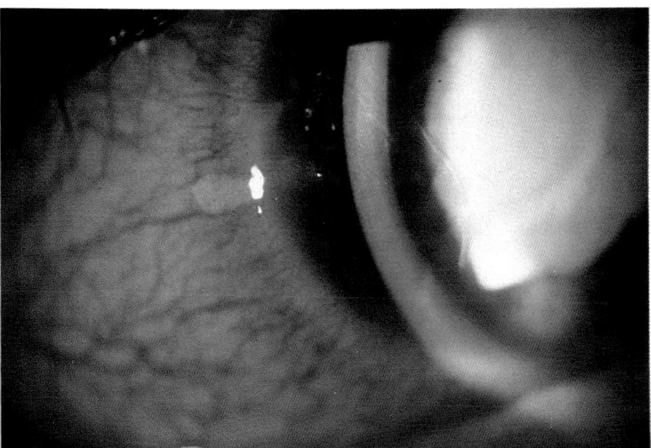

Figure 8.29 *Dislocated lens in buphthalmos – note Haab's striae*

Acquired

1. Trauma (common).
2. Large eye (high myopia, buphthalmos; *Figure 8.29*).
3. Anterior uveal tumours.
4. Chronic cyclitis (rare).
5. Hypermature cataract.
6. Syphilis.

Indications for removal of an ectopic lens are secondary glaucoma, uniocular diplopia, and lens-induced uveitis.

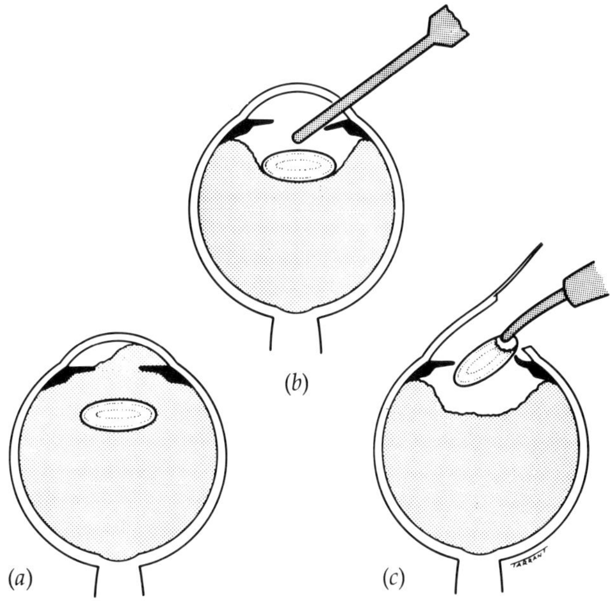

Figure 8.31 *Removal of hard dislocated lens*

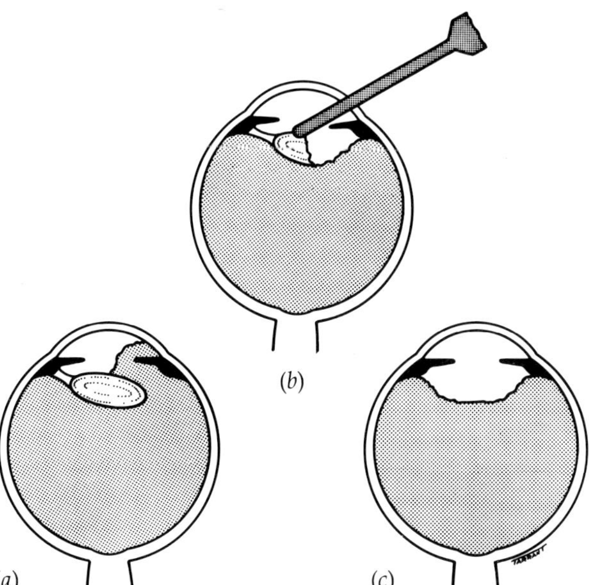

Figure 8.30 *Lensectomy for soft subluxated lens*

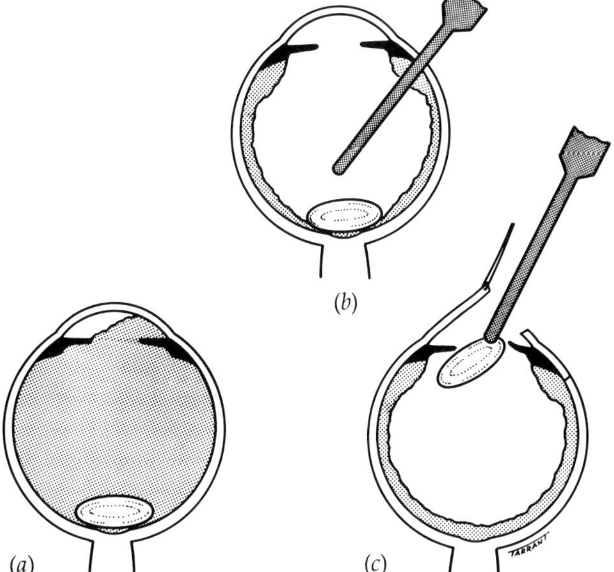

Figure 8.32 *Removal of hard posteriorly dislocated lens*

Surgical techniques

The technique depends on the hardness of the lens as well as its location within the vitreous cavity. Soft lenses can be removed easily with the vitreous cutter, irrespective of their location within the vitreous cavity (*Figure 8.30*). If the lens is lying on the retina, the open cutting port is positioned adjacent to the lens and then gentle suction is applied. The probe together with the lens is slowly retracted into the midvitreous cavity and then stronger suction is used to mould and remove the lens by aspiration and cutting.

If a hard lens is dislocated posteriorly an open-sky approach is more appropriate. If the lens is situated in the anterior vitreous and can be seen through the pupil without the aid of a contact lens, a preliminary half-thickness corneal section is prepared but the anterior chamber is not entered. A small stab incision is then made at the limbus and an anterior vitrectomy is performed so that all vitreous lying anterior to the lens is excised. The corneal section is then completed and the lens removed with a cryoprobe (*Figure 8.31*). If the lens is located in the posterior vitreous or has settled on the retina, the preliminary steps are similar but a total vitrectomy is performed. The eye is then opened and the saline filling the vitreous cavity removed. The lens is then extracted under direct visualization using either an insulated vitreous cryoprobe or the aspiration facility of the vitreous cutter (*Figure 8.32*).

Abnormalities of lens shape

Coloboma

This is usually located inferiorly and if large it may be associated with similar defects involving the iris and choroid. Giant retinal tears may occur in these eyes.

Anterior lenticonus

This is an anterior axial projection of the central 3–4 mm of the lens (*Figure 8.33*). It occurs in some patients with Alport's syndrome which is clinically characterized by the familial occurrence of progressive, haematuric nephritis and sensorineural deafness. Other ocular features of Alport's syndrome include lens opacities and retinal flecks in the macula and retinal midperiphery.

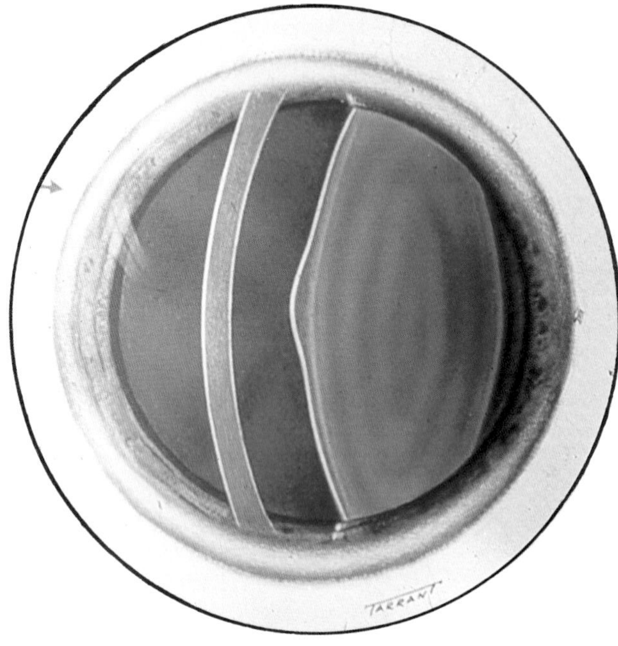

Figure 8.33 *Anterior lenticonus in Alport's syndrome (courtesy of Dr M. d'A. Crawfurd)*

Posterior lenticonus

This is a very rare condition which occurs in infancy or early childhood. It is characterized by a circumscribed round or oval bulge of the posterior 2–7 mm axial zone of the lens. With age, the posterior bulge increases progressively and the lens cortex of the cone may become opaque and obscure the lenticonus. Although the more common unilateral cases are usually sporadic bilateral cases may be familial.

Lentiglobus

This is a more generalized hemispherical deformity of the lens.

Microphakia

This is a lens with a smaller than normal diameter. It may be an isolated finding or it may occur in patients with Lowe's syndrome in which it is not only small but also disc-like. Any condition that causes an early arrest in the development of the eye will result in microphakia.

Microspherophakia

This is a lens that is not only small but spherical in shape. The main causes include familial microspherophakia which is unassociated with systemic defects, as well as Weill–Marchesani syndrome, Marfan's syndrome, and hyperlysinaemia.

Further reading

Cataract

Ederer, F., Hiller, R. and Taylor, H.R. (1981) Senile lens changes and diabetes in two population studies. *American Journal of Ophthalmology*, **91,** 381–395

Elman, M.J., Miller, M.T. and Matalon, R. (1986) Galactokinase activity in patients with idiopathic cataracts. *Ophthalmology*, **93,** 210–215

Eshagian, J., Rafferty, N.S. and Goossens, W. (1981) Human cataracta complicata. *Ophthalmology*, **88,** 155–163

Fisher, R.F. (1981) The lens in uveitis. *Transactions of the Ophthalmological Society of the United Kingdom*, **101,** 317–320

Flach, A.J., Dolan, B.J., Sudduth, B. *et al.* (1983) Amiodarone-induced lens opacities. *Archives of Ophthalmology*, **101,** 1554–1556

Maumenee, I.H. (1979) Classification of hereditary cataracts in children by linkage analysis. *Ophthalmology*, **86,** 1554–1559

McCormick, S.A., DiBartolomeo, A.G., Raju, V.K. *et al.* (1985) Ocular chrysiasis. *Ophthalmology*, **92,** 1432–1435

Shapiro, M.B. and France, T.D. (1985) The ocular features of Down's syndrome. *American Journal of Ophthalmology*, **99,** 659–663

Skalka, H.W. and Prachal, J.T. (1980) Presenile cataract formation and decreased activity of galactosemic enzymes. *Archives of Ophthalmology*, **98,** 269–273

Skalka, H.W. and Prachal, J.T. (1980) Effect of corticosteroids on cataract formation. *Archives of Ophthalmology*, **98,** 1773–1777

Urban, R.C. and Cotlier, E. (1986) Corticosteroid-induced cataracts. *Survey of Ophthalmology*, **31,** 102–110

Winder, A.F. (1981) Laboratory screening in the assessment of human cataracts. *Transactions of the Ophthalmological Society of the United Kingdom*, **101,** 127–130

Management of infantile cataract

Beller, R., Hoyt, C.S., Marg, E. *et al.* (1981) Good visual function after neonatal surgery for congenital monocular cataracts. *American Journal of Ophthalmology*, **91,** 559–565

Davies, P.D. and Tarbuck, D.T.M. (1977) Management of cataracts in infancy and childhood. *Transactions of the Ophthalmological Society of the United Kingdom*, **97,** 148–149

Gelbart, S.S., Hoyt, C.S., Jastrebski, G. *et al.* (1982) Bilateral congenital cataract. *American Journal of Ophthalmology*, **93,** 615–621

Hoyt, C.S. (1983) Management of congenital cataracts. *Clinical Modules for Ophthalmologists*, Vol. 1, Module 6

Jacobson, S.G., Mohindra, I. and Held, R. (1982) Visual acuity in infants with ocular disease. *American Journal of Ophthalmology*, **93,** 198–209

Kanski, J.J. and Crick, M.D.P. (1977) Lensectomy. *Transactions of the Ophthalmological Society of the United Kingdom*, **97,** 52–57

Price, R.L., Conforto, J.R., Yeh, H. *et al.* (1978) Medical and surgical management of children with cataract. *Perspectives in Ophthalmology*, **2,** 49–54

Stark, W.J., Taylor, H.R., Michels, R.G. *et al.* (1979) Management of congenital cataracts. *Ophthalmology*, **86,** 1571–1578

Willshaw, H.E. (1985) Traditional clinical methods of visual assessment in childhood. *Transactions of the Ophthalmological Society of the United Kingdom*, **104,** 641–645

Management of cataract in adults

Cheng, H., Law, A.B., McPherson, K. *et al.* (1981) Longitudinal study of intraocular lenses after intracapsular extraction. *Transactions of the Ophthalmological Society of the United Kingdom*, **101,** 79–83

Fastenburg, D.M., Schwartz, P.L. and Lin, H.Z. (1984) Retinal detachment following neodymium : YAG laser capsulotomy. *American Journal of Ophthalmology*, **97,** 288–291

Galin, M.A., Tuberville, A.W., Obstbaum, S.A. *et al.* (1981) Why do some implants fail? *Transactions of the Ophthalmological Society of the United Kingdom*, **101,** 84–86

Gaasterland, D.E. (1984) Clinical applications of neodymium : YAG lasers. *Clinical Modules for Ophthalmologists*, Vol. 2, Module 8

Green, W.R. and McDonnell, P.J. (1985) Opacification of the posterior capsule. *Transactions of the Ophthalmological Society of the United Kingdom*, **104,** 727–739

Hiles, D.A. and Biglan, A.W. (1981) Intraocular lens implantation in children: Indications, contraindications, complications and results. *Perspectives in Ophthalmology*, **5,** 39–46

Jaffe, N.S. (1985) Current and future concepts of the design of intraocular lenses. *Transactions of the Ophthalmological Society of the United Kingdom*, **104,** 703–714

Kanski, J.J. and Ramsay, J.H. (1980) Vitrectomy techniques in the management of complications in cataract surgery. *Transactions of the Ophthalmological Society of the United Kingdom*, **100,** 216–218

Kaufman, H.E. (1980) The corrections of aphakia. *American Journal of Ophthalmology*, **89,** 1–10

Moses, L. (1984) Complications of rigid anterior chamber implants. *Ophthalmology*, **91,** 819–825

Percival, S.P.B., Anand, V. and Das, S.K. (1983) Prevalance of aphakic retinal detachments. *British Journal of Ophthalmology*, **67,** 43–45

Polack, F.M. (1980) Management of anterior segment complications of intraocular lenses. *Ophthalmology*, **87,** 881–886

Roper-Hall, M.J. (1985) Sophistication in intraocular lens surgery. Rayner Lecture 1984. *Transactions of the Ophthalmological Society of the United Kingdom*, **104,** 500–506

Terry, A.C., Stark, W.J., Maumenee, A.E. *et al.* (1983) Neodymiumn : YAG laser for posterior capsulotomy. *American Journal of Ophthalmology*, **96,** 716–720

Van Buskirk, E.M. and Weleber, R.G. (1986) Intraocular lenses in glaucoma. *Clinical Modules for Ophthalmologists*, Vol. 4, Module 7

Yannuzzi, L.A. (1985) Cystoid macular oedema following cataract surgery. *Clinical Modules for Ophthalmologists*, Vol. 3, Module 10

Abnormalities of lens shape

Govan, J.A.A. (1983) Ocular manifestations of Alport's syndrome: a hereditary disorder of basement membrane? *British Journal of Ophthalmology*, **67,** 493–503

Khalil, M. and Saheb, N. (1984) Posterior lenticonus. *Ophthalmology*, **91,** 1429–1430

Pollard, Z.F. (1983) Familial bilateral posterior lenticonus. *Archives of Ophthalmology*, **101,** 1238–1240

9

Retinal Detachment

Introduction

Definitions

Classification

Applied anatomy

Examination techniques

Indirect ophthalmoscopy

Scleral indentation

Fundus drawing

Slitlamp biomicrosopy with fundus contact lens

How to find the primary retinal break

Pathogenesis

Rhegmatogenous retinal detachment

Tractional retinal detachment

Exudative retinal detachment

Clinical features

Rhegmatogenous retinal detachment

Tractional retinal detachment

Exudative retinal detachment

Differential diagnosis

Acquired retinoschisis

Choroidal detachment

Miscellaneous conditions

Prophylaxis

Retinal breaks

Predisposing peripheral retinal degenerations

Treatment modalities

Benign degenerations

Surgical principles

Scleral buckling

Drainage of subretinal fluid

Intravitreal injections

Pars plana vitrectomy

Surgical techniques

Local buckling

Encirclement

Clinical examples

Causes of failure

Early

Late

Postoperative complications

Early

Late

Introduction

Definitions

Retinal break

A full-thickness defect in the sensory retina.

Retinal detachment

A separation of the sensory retina from the retinal pigment epithelium (RPE) by subretinal fluid (SRF).

Posterior vitreous detachment

A separation of the cortical vitreous from the internal limiting membrane (ILM) of the sensory retina posterior to the vitreous base.

Retinoschisis

A splitting of the sensory retina into two layers.

Choroidal detachment

An effusion of fluid into the suprachoroidal space.

Vitreoretinal traction

A force exerted on the retina by structures originating in the vitreous. In centripetal traction the pull is towards the vitreous, and in tangential traction the force is parallel to the surface of the retina.

Syneresis

A contraction of gel which separates its liquid from solid components.

Synchysis

A liquefaction of gel.

Classification

All retinal detachments (RDs) are divided into two main types—rhegmatogenous and non-rhegmatogenous; the Greek word *rhegma* means a break in continuity. The two forms of non-rhegmatogenous RDs (sometimes also referred to as secondary) are tractional and exudative.

Rhegmatogenous

SRF derived from synchytic vitreous gains access to the subretinal space through a retinal break. Rhegmatogenous RDs may be spontaneous or traumatic.

Tractional

The sensory retina is pulled away from the RPE by contracting vitreoretinal membranes; the source of SRF is unknown. Two important causes of tractional RD are the proliferative retinopathies and penetrating ocular trauma.

Exudative

SRF derived from the choroid gains access to the subretinal space through damaged RPE. Important causes are choroidal tumours and inflammation.

Applied anatomy (*Figure 9.1*)

Ora serrata

The ora serrata is the junction between the retina and ciliary body. The nasal ora is characterized by tooth-like extensions of retina onto the pars plana (dentate processes) which are separated by oral bays. In the temporal ora the dentate processes are blunt or absent. Clinically insignificant congenital lesions are small glistening 'oral pearls'.

Visualization

In the phakic eye, the ora cannot be visualized without scleral indentation. In the aphakic eye, visualization is possible without indentation, provided the pupil is large.

Surgical anatomy

Externally the ora corresponds to the insertions of the rectus muscles. In the emmetropic eye this is located 7 mm behind the limbus temporally and 6 mm nasally.

Retinochoroidal adhesion

At the ora, the sensory retina is fused with the RPE and choroid. This adhesion, which is weaker nasally than temporally, acts as a barrier to the spread of SRF into the pars plana. However, there is no equivalent adhesion between the choroid and sclera, so choroidal detachments invariably progress anteriorly to involve the ciliary body.

Congenital anomalies

These may occasionally have clinical significance.

Cystic retinal tufts are white, ovoid, inward projections of sensory retina located just posterior to the vitreous base. An abnormally strong adhesion of cortical vitreous to a cystic retinal tuft may result in retinal tear formation during acute posterior vitreous detachment (PVD).

Meridional folds are small folds of sensory retina in line with a dentate process. Rarely, a retinal break at the base of a fold may cause RD.

Enclosed oral bays are small islands of pars plana surrounded by retina, and should not be mistaken for peripheral retinal holes.

Pars plana

The ciliary body is located 1 mm from the limbus and extends posteriorly for about 6 mm. The first 2 mm consists of the pars plicata and the remaining 4 mm consists of the flattened pars plana. Clinically insignificant congenital

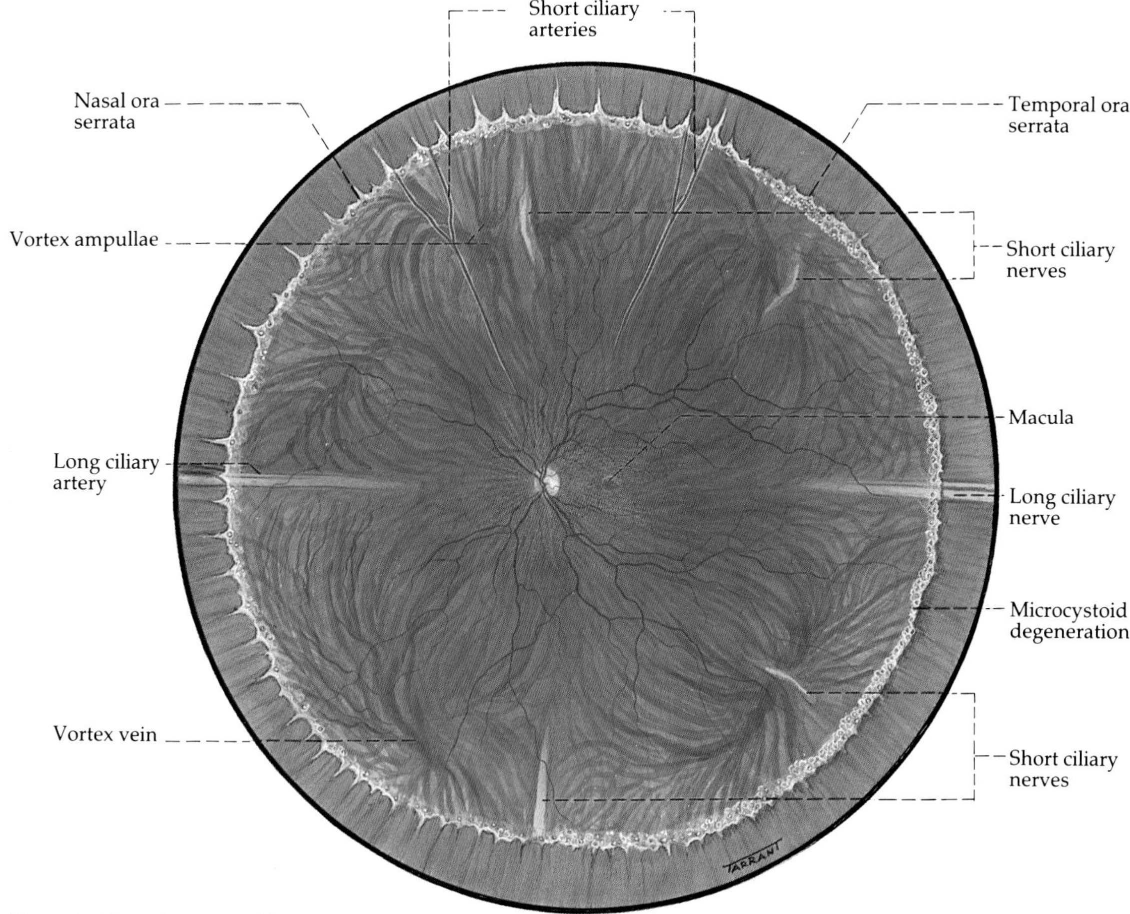

Figure 9.1 *Normal anatomical landmarks of fundus*

anomalies are transparent cysts located between the non-pigmented and the pigmented ciliary epithelium (pars plana cysts).

Surgical anatomy

In order not to endanger the lens or retina, the ideal location for surgical incisions is the mid-pars plana, which is located between 4 and 5 mm from the limbus.

Vitreous base

The vitreous base (*Figure 9.2*) is a 3–4 mm wide zone that straddles the ora serrata.

Surgical anatomy

The collagen fibres of the vitreous are exceptionally dense and strongly adherent to the posterior pars plana and perioral retina. An incision through the mid-part of the pars plana (4–5 mm from the limbus) will usually be located anterior to the vitreous base. If blunt-ended instruments are introduced into the eye through the vitreous base, they may exert traction and give rise to a peripheral retinal tear. Because of the strong adhesion of the cortical vitreous at the vitreous base, following an acute PVD the posterior hyaloid surface remains attached to the posterior border of the vitreous face and so any pre-existing perioral retinal holes within the vitreous base do not lead to RD. Severe blunt ocular trauma may cause an avulsion of the vitreous base with tearing of the non-pigmented epithelium of the pars plana along its anterior border and of the retina along its posterior border.

Congenital anomalies

Posterior tongue-like extensions and isolated islands of dense cortical vitreous associated with abnormally strong vitreoretinal adhesions may be the sites of retinal tears in eyes with acute PVD.

Aphakic RDs

These are frequently caused by small U-shaped tears located near the posterior border of the vitreous base.

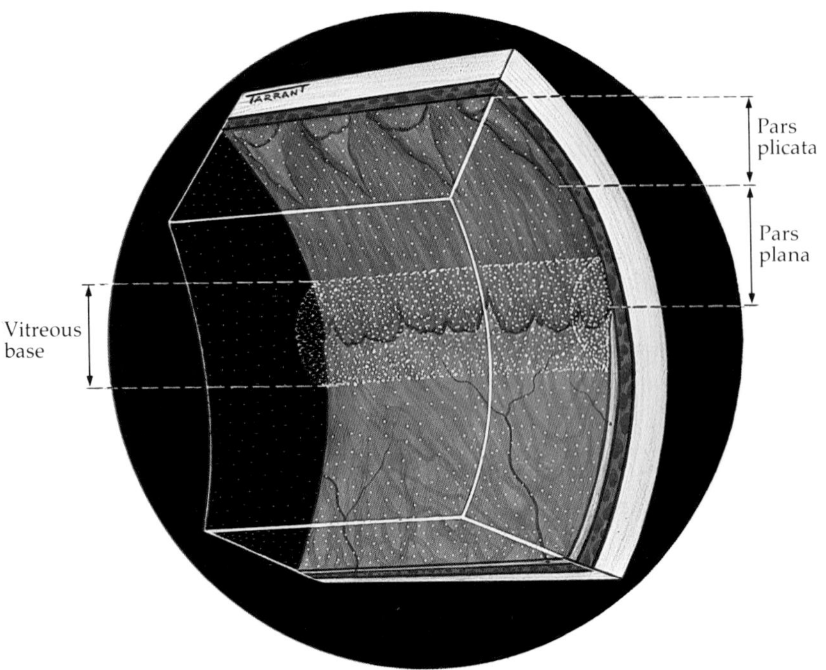

Figure 9.2 Anatomy of vitreous

Vitreoretinal adhesions

Normal

In the healthy eye the peripheral cortical vitreous is loosely attached to the ILM of the sensory retina. Stronger attachments occur at the following sites:

1. *Vitreous base*—very strong.
2. *Optic disc margin*—fairly strong.
3. *Around fovea*—fairly weak.
4. *Peripheral blood vessels*—usually weak.

Abnormal

Occasionally the following abnormally strong vitreoretinal adhesions are associated with retinal tear formation in eyes with acute PVD (*see* later).

1. Posterior border of lattice degeneration.
2. Congenital cystic retinal tufts.
3. Retinal pigment clumps.
4. Peripheral blood vessels.
5. Vitreous base anomalies—such as posterior tongue-like extensions and isolated islands.
6. Areas of 'white with pressure' and 'white without pressure'.

Long posterior ciliary arteries

Fundus landmarks

The arteries accompanied by nerves are recognized as yellow lines that start behind the equator and run anteriorly in the 3 and 9 o'clock meridians. They divide the fundus into upper and lower zones.

Surgical anatomy

The arteries run in the suprachoroidal space in line with the horizontal recti. Care should be taken not to damage them when draining SRF or performing intravitreal injections. Because the arteries supply the anterior uvea, obstruction to blood flow by a tight encircling band may result in anterior segment ischaemia.

Vortex veins

Fundus landmarks

The vortex ampullae are located just posterior to the equator in the 1, 5, 7, and 11 o'clock meridia.

Surgical anatomy

Externally the vortex veins emerge from their scleral canals at variable distances from the equator. Not infrequently, more than four vortex veins are present, and great care should be taken not to damage the veins when inserting a squint hook under the rectus muscles. The inferior vortex veins are at particular risk because they are usually located more anteriorly than the superior veins. Because the venous drainage of the anterior uvea is mainly via the vortex system, occlusion of the veins by a posteriorly placed tight encircling strap will cause congestion of the anterior segment. The vortex veins limit posterior extension of a choroidal detachment as they pass through the suprachoroidal space into their scleral canals.

Examination techniques

Indirect ophthalmoscopy

Indirect ophthalmoscopy is essential in all eyes with RD. Unfortunately, the technique is not easy and can be mastered only by many hours of practice. Because RD is a bilateral disease it is essential to examine both eyes.

Advantages over direct ophthalmoscopy

Low magnification. In direct ophthalmoscopy, the amount of magnification of the fundus is dependent on the refractive error of the patient's eye. In an emmetropic eye the magnification is 15 and this enables only a small area (about 10° in diameter) to be visualized at one time. In the highly myopic eye, the amount of magnification is even greater and the area visualized correspondingly smaller. When using indirect ophthalmoscopy, the magnification is independent of the patient's refractive error and is determined by the power of the condensing lens. For example, a +20 D lens magnifies ×3.5 and the field of view is about 40°, while a +30 D lens magnifies ×2 and the field of view is about 60°, irrespective of the patient's refractive error. The main advantages of low magnification are:

1. A larger area of the fundus can be visualized simultaneously and the likelihood of overlooking important lesions is reduced.
2. Most optical distortions are eliminated and highly myopic eyes (which are particularly susceptible to RD) can be examined more easily.
3. The topography of large fundus lesions can be more readily appreciated.

Stereoscopic view and depth of focus enable elevated and solid lesions to be interpreted with greater accuracy.

Stronger illumination and superior resolution enhance visualization of the fundus through hazy media.

Peripheral retina can be seen more easily. This is very important because most breaks and predisposing lesions are located at or anterior to the equator.

Long working distance. This is particularly helpful when drawing the fundus and examining young uncooperative patients.

During surgery a lightweight indirect ophthalmoscope with a teaching mirror is extremely useful. The long working distance is also very helpful.

Scleral indentation can be used.

Preparation of patient

Pupils. Make sure that both pupils are well dilated and will not constrict when exposed to the bright light of the indirect opthalmoscope. Topical tropicamide 1% combined with phenylephrine 10% is usually adequate.

Position. Ideally, the patient should be in the supine position, with one pillow , on a bed or couch (*Figure 9.3*) and not sitting upright in a chair.

Darken examination room.

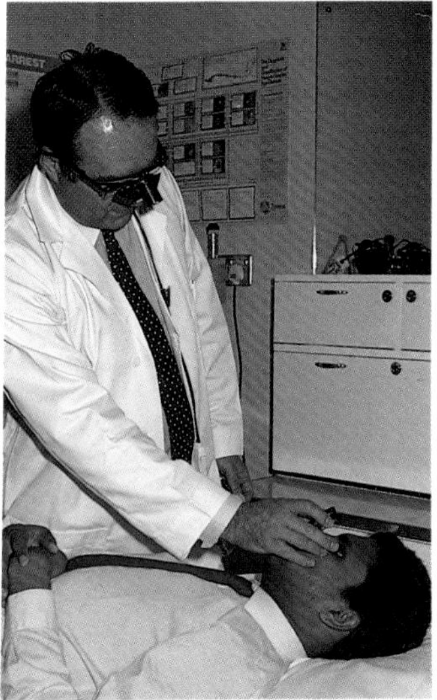

Figure 9.3 *Indirect ophthalmoscopy – correct position*

Condensing lenses

1. *+20 D* is used for routine examination.
2. *+30 D* is sometimes preferred by beginners as it causes less magnification. It is also very useful for detecting highly elevated lesions and for visualizing the fundus in eyes with small pupils.

Technique

1. *Check the indirect ophthalmoscope* for correct interpupillary distance and align the beam so that it is located in the centre of the viewing frame.
2. *Instruct the patient* to keep both eyes open at all times.
3. *Take the lens into one hand* and, if necessary, gently separate the patient's eyelids with the fingers.
4. *Find the red reflex* but do not turn the power of the light beam to maximum.
5. *First examine the vitreous* and resist the temptation to immediately visualize the retina. Hold the flat surface of the lens facing the patient.
6. *Focus on the posterior pole* but avoid the tendency to move towards the patient if you are having difficulty in seeing the fundus.
7. *Be prepared to move around the patient.* For example, stand opposite the clock hour position to be examined, so that when examining the 3 o'clock meridian in the right eye, you are on the patient's right-hand side and when viewing the 9 o'clock meridian you are on his left-hand side.
8. *Ask the patient* to move his eyes and head into optimal positions for examination. For example, when examining the extreme retinal periphery, ask the patient to look away from you.

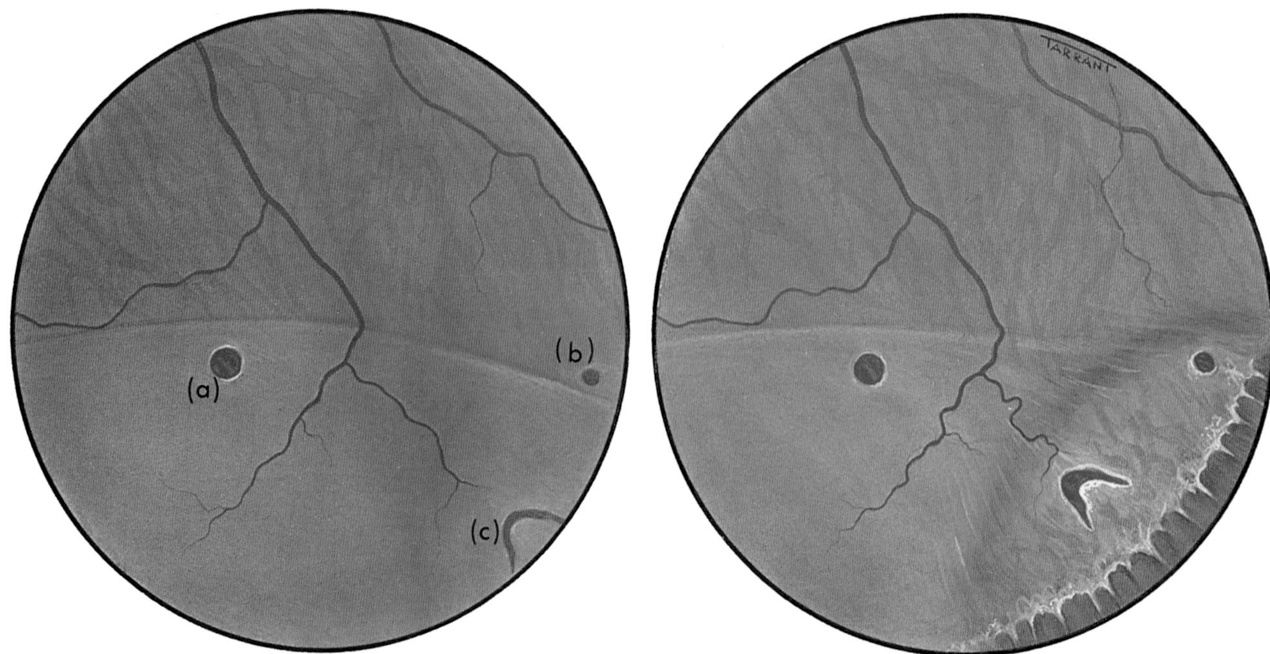

Figure 9.4 *Advantages of scleral indentation. Left: without indentation; right: with indentation*

Scleral indendation

Purpose

The purpose of scleral indentation is to enhance visualization of the peripheral retina anterior to the equator and to perform a kinetic evaluation of the retina. For example, *Figure 9.4, left,* shows a retinal hole (*a*) near the equator which can be seen without scleral indentation because the underlying choroid provides good contrast and the hole appears red. However, a small round hole (*b*) near the ora serrata or a small U-shaped tear (*c*) near the posterior border of the vitreous base may be overlooked without scleral indentation. *Figure 9.4, right,* shows that with scleral indentation the small hole (*b*) is seen more easily because the contrast between the choroid and sensory retina is enhanced. Indentation also brings the peripheral fundus into view and enables the flap of the small U-shaped tear (*c*) to be seen in profile.

Technique

1. To view the ora serrata at 12 o'clock, first ask the patient to look down and then apply the scleral indenter to the outside of the upper eyelid at the margin of the tarsal plate.
2. With the indenter in place, ask the patient to look up; at the same time advance the indenter into the anterior orbit parallel with the globe.
3. Align your eyes with the condensing lens and indenter (*Figure 9.5*) and then exert gentle pressure and observe the mound created by the indentation in the fundus. At all times keep the indenter tangential to the globe because you will cause pain if you indent perpendicularly.
4. Move the indenter to an adjacent part of the fundus, making sure that your eyes, the condensing lens, the fundus image and the indenter are all in a straight line.
5. The entire fundus can usually be examined while indenting through the eyelids. Occasionally, in patients with very tight eyelids, indentation directly over the conjunctiva may be necessary in the 3 and 9 o'clock positions. If this is done gently, a topical anaesthetic may not be required.

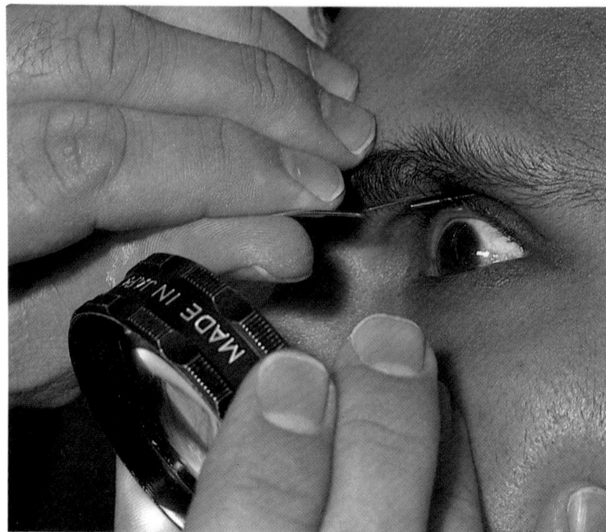

Figure 9.5 *Scleral indentation*

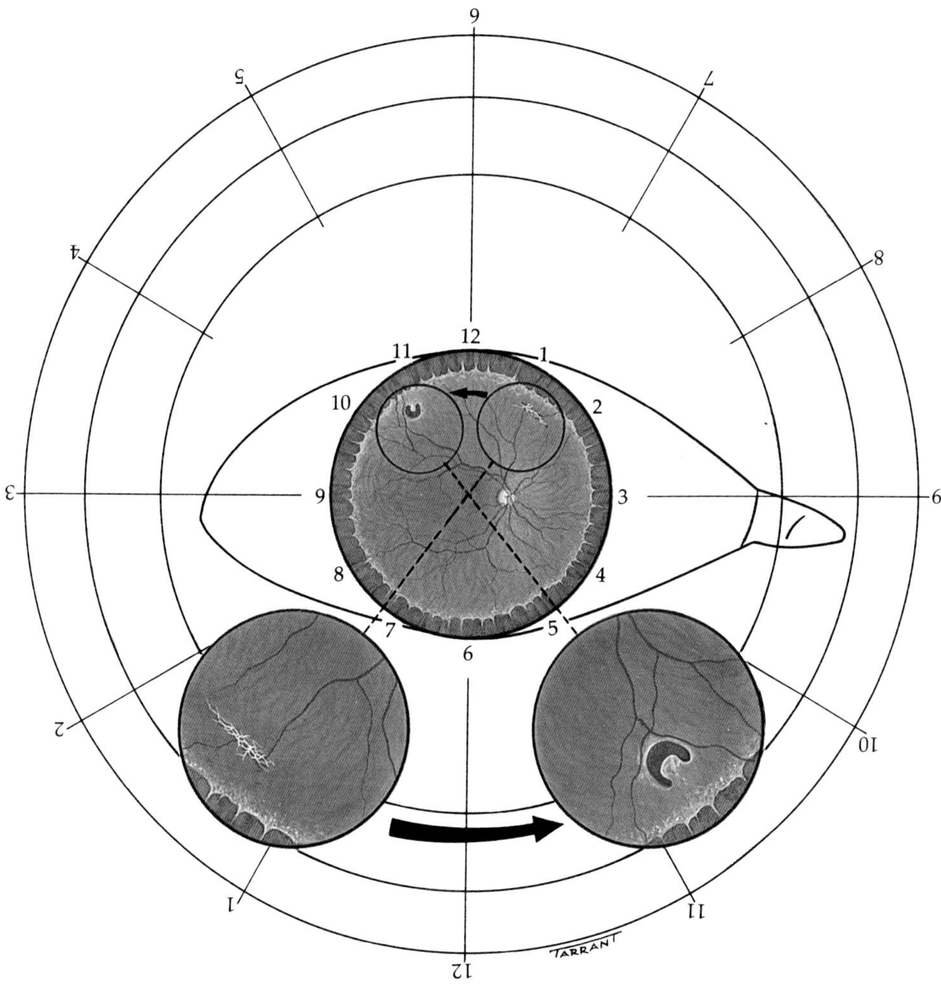

Figure 9.6 Drawing retinal lesions

Fundus drawing

Technique

The image seen with the indirect ophthalmoscope is vertically inverted and laterally reversed. This phenomenon can be used to good advantage when drawing the fundus if the top of the chart is placed towards the patient's feet (upside down). In this way the inverted position of the chart in relation to the patient's eye corresponds to the image of the fundus obtained by the observer. For example, a U-shaped tear at 11 o'clock in the patient's right eye will correspond to the 11 o'clock position on the chart (*Figure 9.6*). The same applies to the area of lattice degeneration between 1 and 2 o'clock.

Colour code (*Figure 9.7*)

Have available coloured pencils (red, blue, yellow, black, green).

1. *Record the boundaries of the RD* by starting at the optic nerve and then extending peripherally.

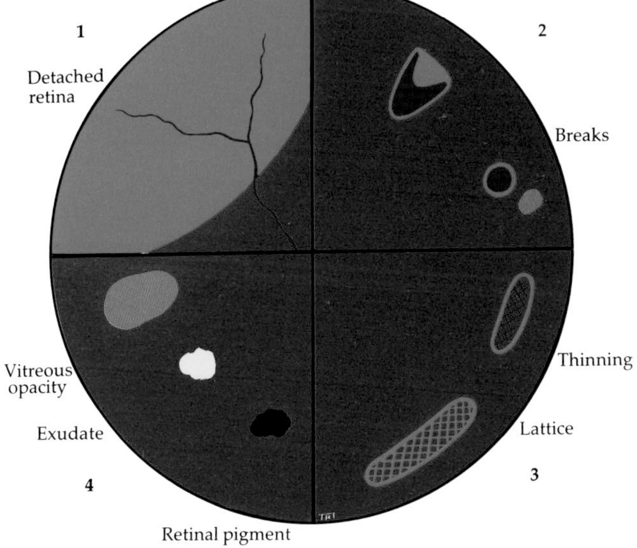

Figure 9.7 Colour code for retinal drawing

2. *Draw detached retina* in *blue*, and *flat retina* in *red*.
3. *Indicate the course of retinal veins* with a *blue* pencil.
4. *Examine the peripheral retina with scleral indentation:*
   a. Draw retinal breaks in *red* with *blue* outlines; the flap of a retinal tear is also drawn in *blue*.
   b. Thin retina is indicated by *red* hatchings outlined in *blue*.
   c. Lattice degeneration is shown as *blue* hatchings outlined in *blue*.
   d. Retinal pigment is shown in *black*, and retinal exudates *yellow*.
   e. Vitreous opacities such as blood and opercula are shown in *green*.

Slitlamp biomicroscopy with fundus contact lens

Purpose

This examination is performed after the fundus has been drawn. The particular advantages are as follows:

1. *Detection of breaks*. The magnification of the slitlamp is useful in detecting small peripheral retinal breaks, especially in eyes with choroidal atrophy in which the colour contrast between the choroid and sensory retina is reduced. It is also useful in deciding whether or not an area of very thin retina (as in lattice degeneration) contains small retinal holes.
2. *Evaluation of vitreous cavity* with respect to the presence of transvitreal membranes, vitreous opacities and PVD.
3. *Evaluating lesions at posterior pole* with high magnification is extremely useful.

Fundus contact lenses

Goldmann triple-mirror contact lens (*Figure 9.8, left*)

Make sure you are familiar with the function of each part of the lens.

The central part provides a 30° view of the posterior pole.

The equatorial mirror (largest and oblong in shape) enables visualization from 30° to the equator.

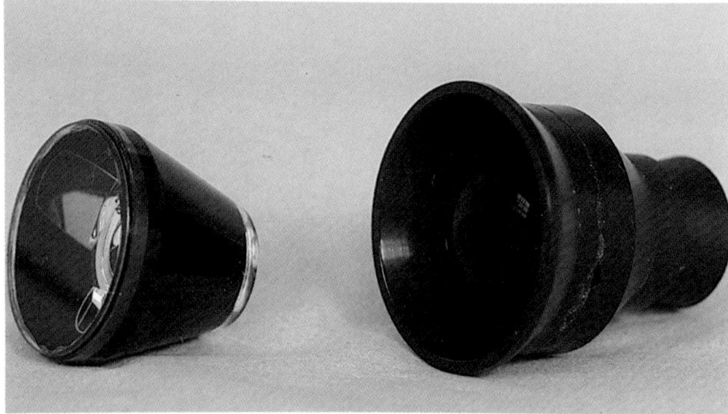

Figure 9.8 *Fundus contact lenses: Left: Goldmann triple-mirror; right: Rodenstock panfunduscope*

The peripheral mirror (intermediate in size and square shaped) enables visualization between the equator and the ora serrata.

The gonioscopic mirror (smallest and dome shaped) may be used for visualizing the extreme retinal periphery and pars plana.

Rodenstock panfunduscope (*see Figure 9.8, right*)

This lens is easier to use by the beginner because it provides a single wide-angled view of the fundus without employing mirrors. The image is vertically inverted and laterally reversed as in indirect ophthalmoscopy.

Insertion of contact lens

1. Insert coupling fluid into the cup of the contact lens but do not overfill—it should be no more than half full.
2. Hold the lens in your dominant hand.
3. With his head firmly in place, ask the patient to look up but not to move his head away.
4. Insert the inferior rim of the lens into the lower fornix and then press it quickly against the cornea so that the coupling fluid has no time to escape.
5. Ask the patient to look straight ahead.
6. If viewing the patient's left eye hold the contact lens in your right hand, and vice versa.

Technique

Image in mirror

Remember that the image viewed in the Goldmann triple-mirror is vertically inverted (upside down) but not reversed laterally. This means that in order to view the 12 o'clock position in the fundus, you shoud place the mirror at 6 o'clock and fundus lesions located to the right of 12 o'clock will also appear in the mirror on the right-hand side. This is unlike the image viewed with the panfunduscope and the indirect ophthalmoscope, which is not only vertically inverted but also *laterally reversed*.

Tilt of illumination column

Always tilt except when viewing the 12 o'clock position in the fundus (i.e. with the mirror at 6 o'clock).

Position of illumination column (*Figure 9.9*)

1. *Horizontal meridians*: when viewing the 3 and 9 o'clock positions in the fundus keep the column central.
2. *Vertical meridians*: when viewing the 6 and 12 o'clock positions the column can be right or left of centre.
3. *Oblique meridians*: when viewing the 1.30 and 7.30 o'clock positions keep the column right of centre, and vice versa when viewing the 10.30 and 4.30 o'clock positions.

Axis of beam

When viewing different positions of the peripheral retina rotate the axis of the beam so that it is always at right angles to the mirror.

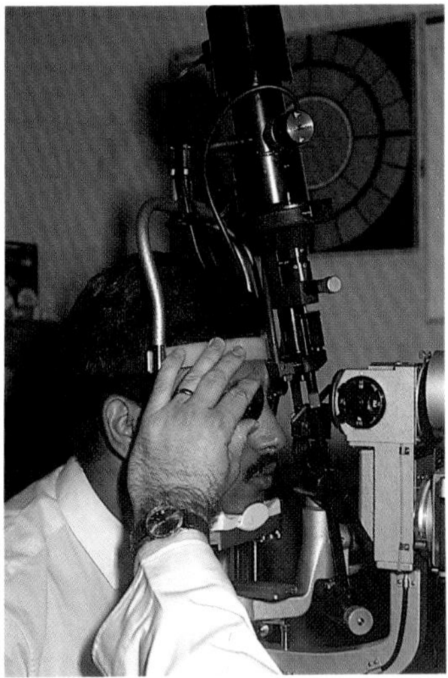

Figure 9.9 Illumination column tilted and right of centre

Rotation of lens

To visualize the entire fundus rotate the lens for 360° using first the equatorial mirror and then the peripheral mirror.

Tilting of lens

In order to obtain a more peripheral view of the retina tilt the lens to the opposite side and ask the patient to move his eyes to the same side, e.g. to obtain a more peripheral view of 12 o'clock (with mirror at 6 o'clock) tilt the lens down and ask the patient to look up.

Central lens

Examine the vitreous cavity with both a horizontal and a vertical slitbeam and then examine the posterior pole.

Interpretation of findings

Normal vitreous

The healthy gel in a young individual appears homogeneous with the same density throughout. Swift ocular movements produce undulating folds in the gel and a few small opacities may be seen.

Synchysis

The central vitreous cavity contains optically empty spaces (lacunae). The condensed lining of a large cavity may be mistaken for a detached posterior hyaloid surface (pseudo-PVD).

PVD

The detached posterior hyaloid surface can be traced to its insertion into the vitreous base above. *An annular opacity (Weiss ring)* representing a ring of glial tissue detached from the margin of the optic disc is virtually pathognomonic of PVD.

Cells

Pigment cells ('tobacco dust') in the anterior vitreous in a patient complaining of sudden photopsia and floaters are strongly suggestive of a retinal tear. A careful examination of the peripheral retina (particularly superiorly) is mandatory. *Numerous small opacities* within the anteriorly displaced gel or in the retrohyaloid space are strongly suggestive of blood.

How to find the primary retinal break

Quadrantic distribution

About 60% of all retinal breaks are located in the upper temporal quadrant, 15% in the upper nasal quadrant, 15% in the lower temporal quadrant, and 10% in the lower nasal quadrant. The upper temporal quadrant is by far the most common site for retinal breaks and should be examined in great detail if a retinal break cannot be detected initially.

Multiple breaks

About 50% of eyes with RD have more than one break. In the vast majority of eyes the breaks are located within 90° of each other.

Configuration of SRF

SRF usually spreads in a gravitational fashion, and its shape is governed by anatomical limits (ora serrata and optic nerve) and the location of the primary retinal break. If

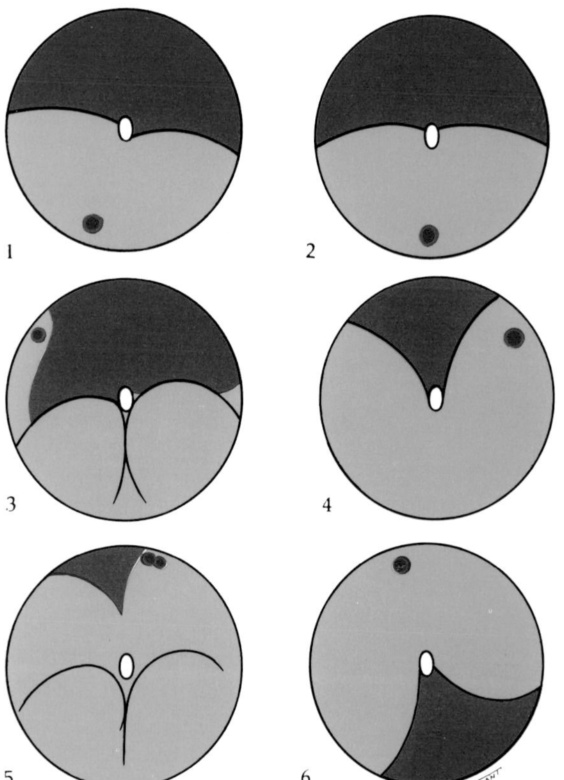

Figure 9.10 Shape of retinal detachment in relation to position of primary retinal break (right eye)

the primary break is located superiorly, the SRF first spreads inferiorly on the same side as the break and then spreads superiorly on the opposite side of the fundus. The likely location of the primary retinal break can therefore be predicted by studying the shape of the RD. Several examples are shown in *Figure 9.10*.

1. A shallow inferior RD in which the SRF is slightly higher on the temporal side points to a primary break on that side.
2. A primary break located at 6 o'clock will cause an inferior RD with equal fluid levels.
3. In a bullous inferior RD the primary break usually lies above the horizontal meridian, especially in aphakic eyes.
4. If the primary break is located in the upper nasal quadrant the SRF will revolve around the optic disc and then rise on the temporal side until it is level with the primary break.
5. A subtotal RD with a superior wedge of attached retina points to a primary break located in the periphery nearest its highest border.
6. When the SRF crosses the vertical midline above, the primary break is near to 12 o'clock, the lower edge of the RD corresponding to the side of the break.

History

Although the quadrantic location of photopsia is of no value in predicting the location of the primary break, the quadrant in which the shadow first appears may be of considerable value. For example, if the shadow started in the upper nasal quadrant the primary break is probably located in the lower temporal quadrant.

Pathogenesis

Rhegmatogenous retinal detachment

Rhegmatogenous RD affects about 1:10 000 of the population each year and is bilateral in about 10% of cases. The retinal breaks responsible for RD are caused by an interplay between vitreoretinal traction and an underlying weakness in the peripheral retina (predisposing degeneration). The relatively high prevalence of retinal breaks (about 5%) in the general population suggests that there are still unknown factors associated with RD.

Vitreoretinal traction

Mechanism of acute PVD

Synchysis senilis is an age-related liquefaction of the vitreous gel caused by alterations of its micromolecular structure (*Figure 9.11, upper left*). Some eyes with synchysis senilis develop a hole in the thinned posterior vitreous cortex which overlies the fovea. The synchytic fluid from within the centre of the vitreous cavity passes through this defect into the newly formed retrohyaloid space. This process forcibly detaches the posterior vitreous surface from the ILM of the sensory retina as far as the posterior border of the vitreous base (*Figure 9.11, upper right*). The remaining solid vitreous gel collapses inferiorly and the retrohyaloid space is occupied entirely by synchytic fluid. This process is called acute rhegmatogenous PVD with collapse (it will be referred to as acute PVD from now on).

Complications of acute PVD

Following PVD, the sensory retina is no longer protected by the stable vitreous cortex and can be directly affected by dynamic vitreoretinal tractional forces. The vision-threatening complications of acute PVD are dependent on the strength and extent of pre-existing vitreoretinal adhesions.

Nil

In the majority of eyes vitreoretinal attachments are weak and the vitreous cortex detaches completely from the ILM of the sensory retina without sequelae.

Retinal tear

About 10% of eyes develop retinal tears due to the transmission of traction at sites of abnormally strong vitreoretinal adhesions (*Figure 9.11, lower left*). Although tears usually develop at the time of PVD, very occasionally they may be delayed by several weeks or even months. Tears due to acute PVD are usually symptomatic (photopsia and floaters), U-shaped, located in the upper fundus and frequently associated with vitreous haemorrhage due to rupture of a peripheral retinal blood vessel. After the tear has formed, the retrohyaloid synchytic fluid has direct access to the subretinal space. Unless the tear is treated prophylactically by photocoagulation or cryotherapy the risk of RD is high.

Avulsion of blood vessels

Very occasionally, PVD may cause avulsion of a peripheral retinal blood vessel and vitreous haemorrhage in the absence of a retinal tear (*Figure 9.11, lower right*).

Predisposing peripheral retinal degenerations

About 60% of all breaks develop in areas of the peripheral retina that show specific changes. These lesions may be associated with a spontaneous breakdown of pathologically

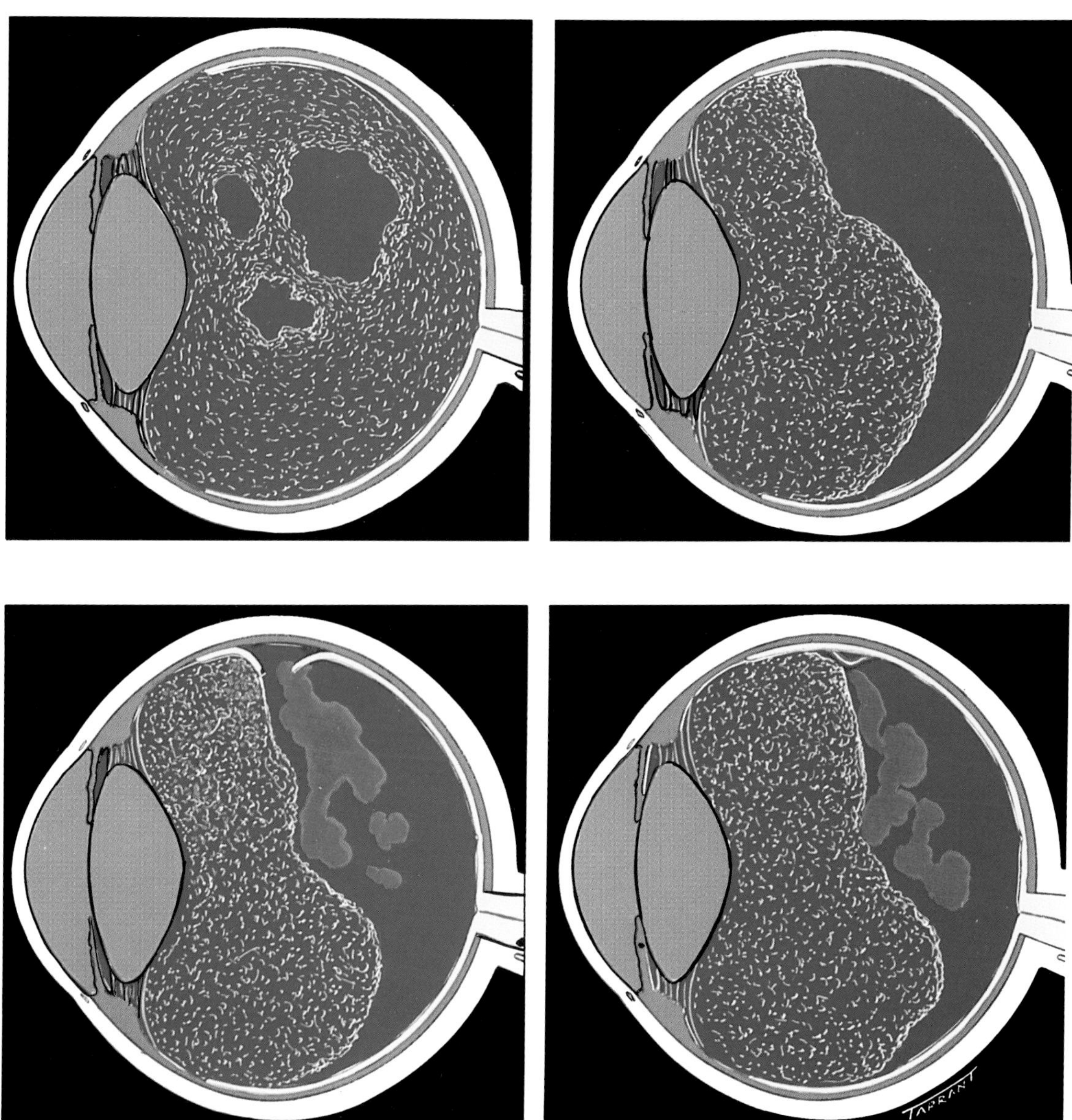

***Figure 9.11** Upper left: synchysis; upper right: uncomplicated PVD; lower left: retinal tear and vitreous haemorrhage due to PVD; lower right: avulsed blood vessel and vitreous haemorrhage due to PVD*

thin retinal tissue to cause a retinal hole, or they may predispose to retinal tear formation in eyes with acute PVD. Retinal holes are round or oval in shape. They are usually smaller than tears and are less likely to cause RD.

Lattice (palisade) degeneration

Lattice degeneration is present in about 8% of the general population. It probably develops early in life, with a peak incidence during the second and third decades. It is therefore not an age-related disease. Although the condition may be familial it shows no sexual preference. It is found more commonly in myopes over −3 D. Lattice is the most important degeneration directly related to RD. It is present in about 40% of eyes with RD and is an important cause of RD in young myopes. Lattice-like lesions are frequently found in patients with Marfan's syndrome, Ehlers–Danlos syndrome and Wagner's disease, all of which are associated with an increased incidence of RD.

Clinical features (*Figure 9.12a–d*)

Typical lattice consists of sharply demarcated, circumferentially orientated, spindle-shaped areas of retinal thinning, most frequently located between the equator and the posterior border of the vitreous base. The islands of lattice may form two, three or even four circumferentially orientated rows. Occasionally they are radially, usually

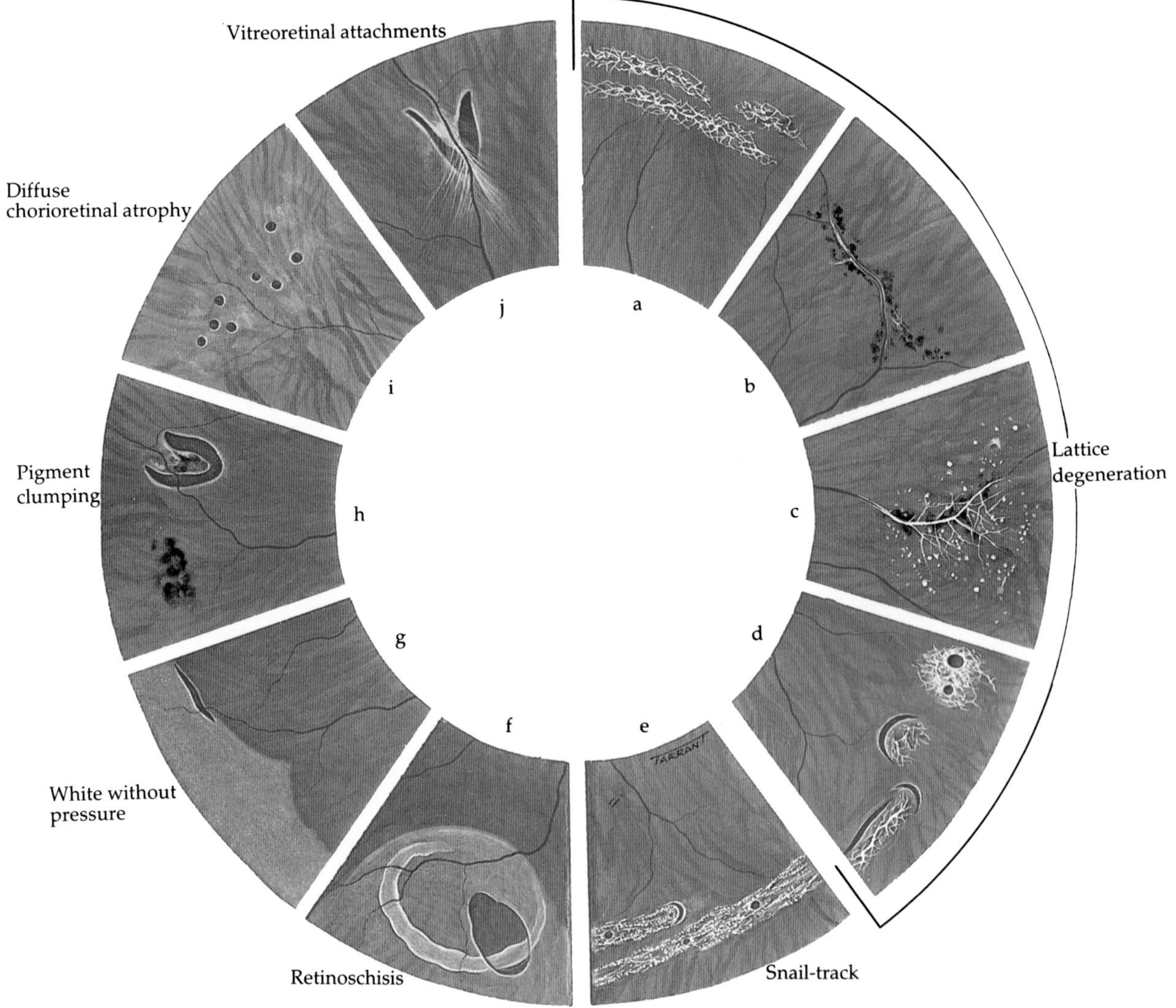

Figure 9.12 *Predisposing peripheral retinal degenerations*

paravascularly, orientated and extend posterior to the equator (*see Figure 9.14, upper left*). Lattice is usually bilateral and is more frequently present in the temporal than nasal half of the fundus and is more common superiorly than inferiorly. Associated features present within lattice lesions include 'snowflakes', hyperplasia of the RPE and 'white with pressure'. A very characteristic feature of advanced lesions is an arborizing network of white lines often continuous with peripheral blood vessels. The vitreous overlying an area of lattice is synchytic but the vitreous attachments around the margin of a lesion are exaggerated (*Figure 9.13*).

Complications

1. *Nil.* In the vast majority of cases there are no complications, even if holes are present.
2. *Retinal holes.* Small round holes frequently found within islands of lattice (*Figure 9.14, lower right*) may occasionally be responsible for RD, particularly in young myopes. In these patients the RD may not be preceded by symptoms of acute PVD (photopsia and floaters) and the SRF usually spreads slowly.
3. *Retinal tears.* Usually located at the posterior edge of an island of lattice (*Figure 9.14, lower left*), retinal tears may develop in eyes with acute PVD due to vitreoretinal traction at the site of an exaggerated vitreous attachment. Occasionally a small island of lattice is present on the flap of a retinal tear (*Figure 9.14, upper right*). RDs due to lattice tears typically occur in myopes over the age of 50 years. The SRF progresses more rapidly than in RDs caused by small round lattice holes.

Snailtrack degeneration

This lesion is probably an early form or variant of lattice degeneration.

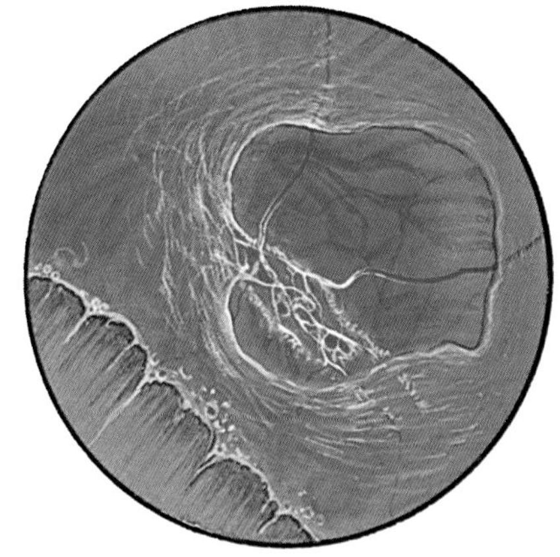

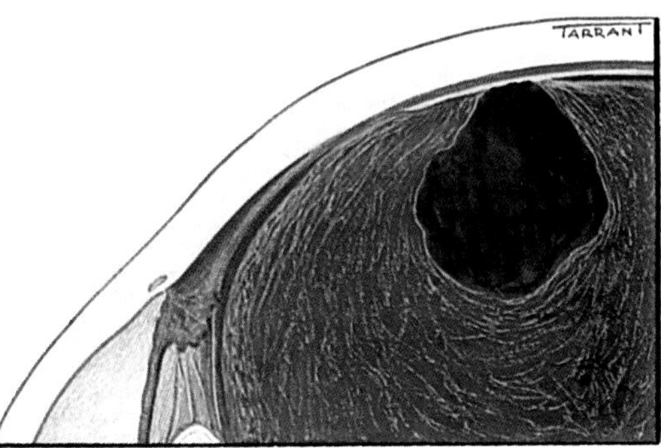

Figure 9.13 *Vitreous changes in lattice degeneration*

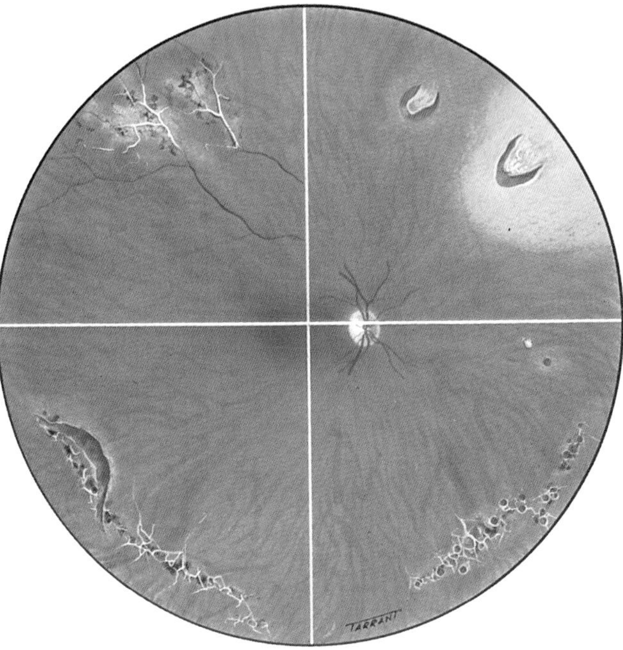

Figure 9.14 *Upper left: radial lattice degeneration; upper right: lattice degeneration on flap of a U-shaped tear; lower right: small round holes in lattice degeneration; lower left: tear along posterior border of lattice degeneration*

Clinical features (*Figure 9.15*)

Snailtrack degeneration consists of sharply demarcated bands of tightly packed 'snowflakes' which give the peripheral retina a white frost-like appearance. White lines are absent and the incidence of small round holes within the lesions (*Figure 9.12e*) is less than in true lattice. The lesions are associated with the phenomenon of 'white with pressure'.

Complications

These are the same as with lattice degeneration.

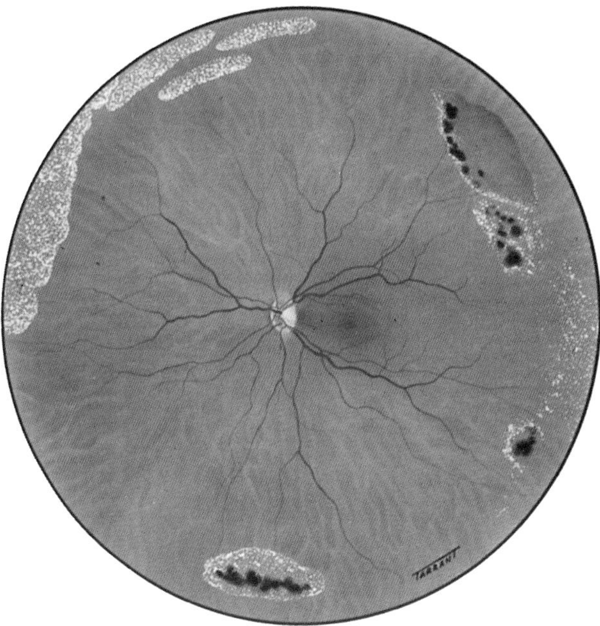

Figure 9.15 *Snailtrack degeneration*

Acquired retinoschisis

Retinoschisis is a splitting of the sensory retina into two layers—an outer (choroidal layer) and an inner (vitreous layer). In typical retinoschisis the split occurs at the outer plexiform layer, and in the less common reticular form the split is at the level of the nerve fibre layer. The condition is present in about 5% of the population over the age of 20 years and is particularly prevalent in hypermetropes (70% of patients are hypermetropic).

Clinical features (*Figure 9.16*)

In its early stages retinoschisis involves the extreme inferotemporal periphery of both fundi, appearing as an exaggeration of microcystoid degeneration with a smooth elevation of the retina. The lesion may progress circumferentially until it has involved the entire fundus periphery. The typical form usually remains anterior to the equator, although the reticular type may spread beyond the equator and may, rarely, threaten the fovea. In some cases the inner

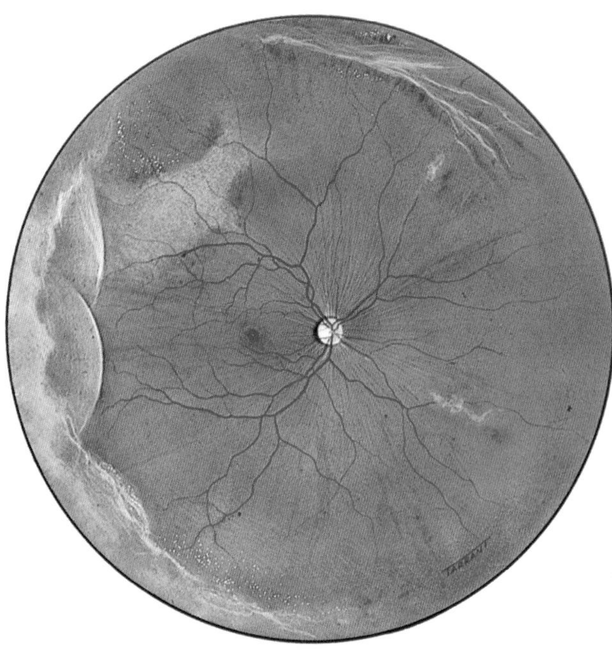

Figure 9.16 *Acquired retinoschisis involving temporal periphery*

layer has 'snowflakes' on its surface and blood vessels which are sheathed or have a 'silver-wire' appearance (*Figure 9.17*). The outer layer has a beaten-metal appearance and shows the phenomenon of 'white with pressure'. The schisis cavity may be bridged by rows of torn grey-white tissue.

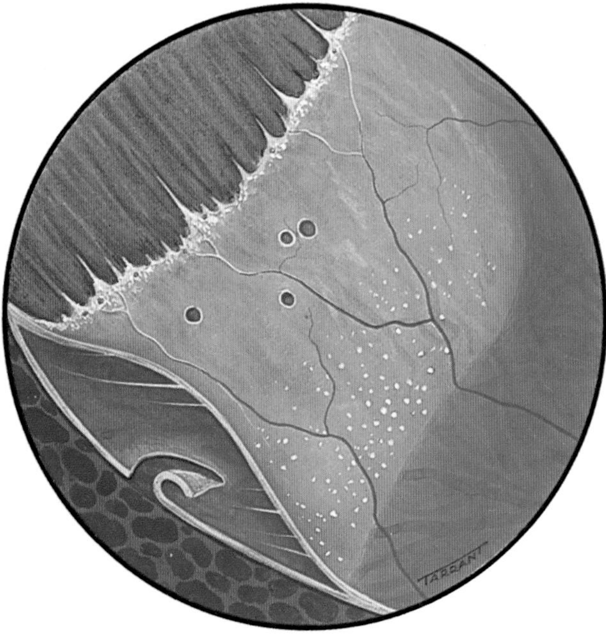

Figure 9.17 *Acquired retinoschisis*

Complications

1. *Nil.* In the vast majority of cases the condition is innocuous and asymptomatic.
2. *Breaks.* These may occur in the reticular type. Inner layer breaks are small and round, while the less common outer layer breaks are usually larger, have rolled edges and are located behind the equator (*Figure 9.12f* and *see Figure 9.25f*). Eyes with only inner layer breaks do not develop RD as there is no communication with the subretinal space.
3. *RD.* This is a very rare complication of acquired retinoschisis. Very occasionally, eyes with breaks in both layers develop extensive RD, especially in the presence of PVD. Eyes with only outer layer breaks do not as a rule develop RD because the fluid within the schisis cavity is viscous and does not pass through the break into the subretinal space. Rarely, however, the schisis fluid loses its viscosity and passes through the break into the subretinal space, giving rise to a localized non-progressive RD.

'White with pressure' and 'white without pressure'

Clinical features

The phenomenon of 'white with pressure' is a translucent grey appearance of the retina, induced by indenting the sclera. Each area has a fixed configuration which does not change when the scleral depressor is moved to an adjacent area. In particularly marked cases, the retina has the same appearance even without scleral indentation—this is termed 'white without pressure' (*Figure 9.12g*).

'White with pressure' is frequently seen in normal eyes which do not develop retinal breaks. It is also frequently observed along the posterior border of islands of lattice degeneration, snailtrack degeneration and the outer layer of acquired retinoschisis. On cursory examination a normal area of retina surrounded by 'white without pressure' may be mistaken for a retinal break (*Figure 9.18, left*).

Complications

Giant tears. These occasionally develop along the posterior border of an area of 'white without pressure' (*Figure 9.18, right*). For this reason, if 'white without pressure' is found in the fellow eye of a patient with a spontaneous giant retinal tear, prophylactic cryotherapy should be performed (*see Figure 9.28*).

Pigment clumps

Clinical features (*Figure 9.12h*)

These are small, localized, irregular patches of pigmentation often associated with vitreoretinal traction tufts which sometimes raise the retinal surface.

Complications

Occasionally an equatorial pigment clump is found on the flap of a U-shaped tear.

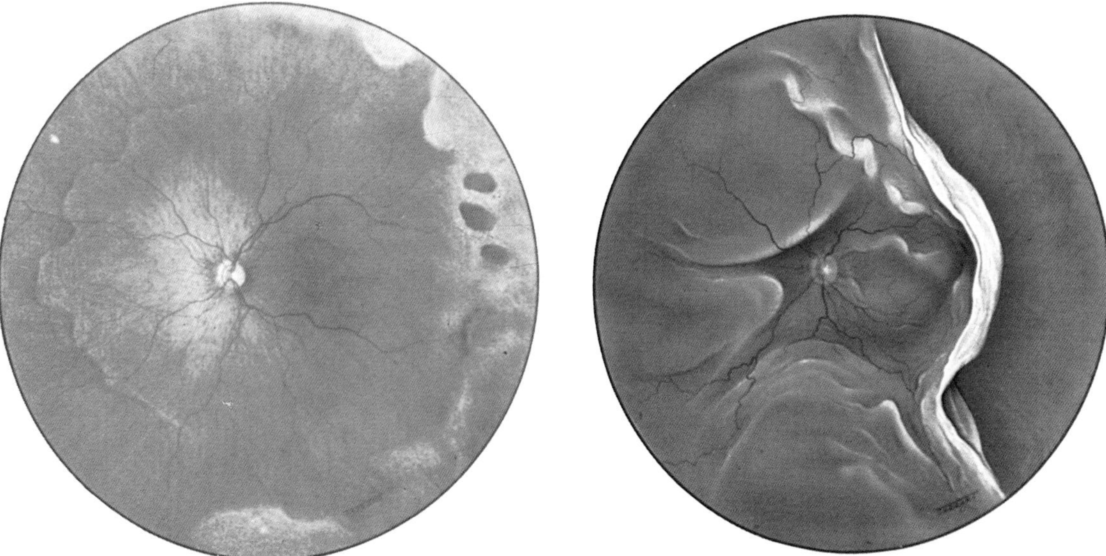

Figure 9.18 Left: 'white without pressure' with pseudoholes in upper temporal quadrant; right: giant retinal tear

Diffuse chorioretinal atrophy

Clinical features (*Figure 9.12i*)

This consists of a diffuse choroidal depigmentation and thinning of the overlying retina in the equatorial area of highly myopic eyes.

Complications

Retinal holes developing in the atrophic retina may lead to RD.

Paravascular vitreoretinal attachments

Clinical features

These cannot be detected ophthalmoscopically.

Complications

Strong attachments may lead to the formation of retinal tears in eyes with acute PVD (*Figure 9.12j*).

Significance of myopia

Although myopes make up 10% of the general population, over 40% of all RDs occur in myopic eyes. The following interrelated factors predispose a myopic eye to RD:

1. *Lattice degeneration*—more common in myopes over −3 D.
2. *Diffuse chorioretinal atrophy*—may give rise to small round holes in highly myopic eyes.
3. *Vitreous*—syneresis, synchysis and PVD are more common.
4. *Cataract surgery*—7% of eyes over −6 D develop RD following uncomplicated intracapsular cataract extraction. If vitreous loss occurs, the incidence of RD is about 15%.

Significance of trauma

Trauma is responsible for about 10% of all cases of RD. It is the most common cause of RD in children, particularly boys.

Blunt trauma

Severe blunt ocular trauma causes a compression of the anteroposterior diameter of the globe and a simultaneous expansion at the equatorial plane. The relatively inelastic vitreous gel causes traction along the posterior aspect of the vitreous base with tearing of the retina (dialysis). In some cases the vitreous base is avulsed and a tear in the non-pigmented epithelium of the pars plana develops in addition to a retinal dialysis. Traumatic dialyses may occur in any quadrant but are said to be more frequent in the upper nasal quadrant. Other less common postcontusive breaks are macular holes and equatorial holes. Although traumatic dialyses develop at the time of injury, the RD usually does not develop until several months later. Progression is frequently slow, probably because the vitreous gel is healthy in a young individual.

Penetrating trauma

RD develops in about 20% of eyes following posterior segment trauma. The RD may be rhegmatogenous, due to retinal tears caused by foreign bodies, or tractional.

Tractional retinal detachment

Diabetic

See Chapter 10.

Traumatic

Traumatic tractional RD is the result of vitreous incarceration in the wound and the presence of blood within the vitreous gel which acts as a stimulus to fibroplastic proliferation. The contraction of epiretinal membranes leads to a shortening and a rolling effect on the peripheral retina in the region of the vitreous base. Vitreous scaffold traction is due to the contraction of cellular proliferation which extends from the wound to the peripheral retina.

Exudative retinal detachment

Exudative RDs are much less common than either rhegmatogenous or tractional RDs. They are caused by subretinal disorders which damage the RPE and thereby allow the passage of fluid derived from the choroid into the subretinal space. A more correct description would therefore be 'transudative'.

Aetiology

1. *Choroidal tumours.* Melanomas, haemangiomas and metastases are the most common tumours to cause exudative RD. It is important always to consider that an RD is caused by an intraocular tumour until proved otherwise.
2. *Inflammation* due to Harada's disease and posterior scleritis.
3. *Following RD surgery.* Postoperative exudative RD should not be mistaken for a recurrence of a rhegmatogenous RD.
4. *Following panretinal photocoagulation* of proliferative retinopathies.

Management

Treatment depends on the cause. Some exudative RDs resolve spontaneously (postoperative), while others are treated with systemic corticosteroids (Harada's disease and posterior scleritis).

Clinical features

Rhegmatogenous retinal detachment

Symptoms

The classic premonitory symptoms reported in about 60% of patients with RD are flashing lights and vitreous floaters caused by acute PVD with collapse. After a variable period of time, the patient notices a relative peripheral visual field defect which may progress to involve central vision.

Photopsia

Photopsia is a subject sensation perceived as a flash of light. In eyes with acute PVD, it is probably caused by traction at sites of vitreoretinal adhesion. The cessation of photopsia is due either to separation of the adhesion or to the complete tearing away of a piece of retina (operculum) around the site of adhesion. In eyes with PVD, the photopsia may be induced by eye movements and tends to be more noticeable in dim illumination. It tends to be projected into the patient's temporal peripheral visual field and, unlike floaters, it has no lateralizing value. Photopsia due to vitreoretinal traction should be differentiated from that due to migraine.

Floaters

A floater is a moving vitreous opacity which is perceived when it casts a shadow onto the retina. Vitreous opacities in eyes with acute PVD are of three types: large ring, cobweb and small spots.

Large ring

A solitary ring-shaped opacity represents the detached annular attachment to the margin of the optic disc (Weiss ring).

Cobwebs

These are caused by condensation of collagen fibres within the collapsed vitreous cortex.

Small spots

A sudden shower of minute red-coloured or dark spots is an ominous symptom as it usually indicates vitreous haemorrhage due to tearing of a peripheral retinal blood vessel.

Visual field defect

A visual field defect is due to the spread of SRF posterior to the equator. It is perceived by the patient as a 'black curtain'. The defect is usually progressive, although in some cases it may not be present on waking in the morning (due to spontaneous absorption of SRF), only to reappear later on during the day. A lower field defect is usually appreciated more quickly by the patient than an upper field defect.

Loss of central vision

Loss of central vision may be due either to involvement of the fovea by SRF or, less frequently, to obstruction of the visual axis by a large upper bulbous RD in an eye in which the fovea is still uninvolved.

Signs of fresh retinal detachment

Anterior segment

Pupil

A relative afferent pupillary conduction defect (Marcus Gunn pupil) is present in eyes with extensive RDs irrespective of the type.

Intraocular pressure

This is usually lower by about 5 mmHg as compared with the normal fellow eye.

Anterior chamber

A mild anterior uveitis is a very common finding. Occasionally, the inflammation may be severe enough to cause posterior synechiae. In these cases the underlying RD may be overlooked and the poor visual acuity incorrectly ascribed to secondary cystoid macular oedema.

Posterior segment

Retinal breaks

These appear as discontinuities in the retinal surface. Due to the colour contrast between the sensory retina and underlying choroid they are usually red. However, in eyes with hypopigmented choroid (as in high myopia), the colour contrast is decreased and small breaks may be overlooked unless slitlamp examination with a fundus contact lens is performed.

Configuration

This is convex. The detached retina has a slightly opaque and corrugated appearance (due to intraretinal oedema) with loss of the underlying choroidal pattern (*Figure 9.19*). The retinal blood vessels appear darker than in flat retina, so the colour contrast between venules and arterioles is less apparent. The SRF extends up to the ora serrata except in the very rare cases due to a macular hole in which the SRF is initially confined to the posterior pole.

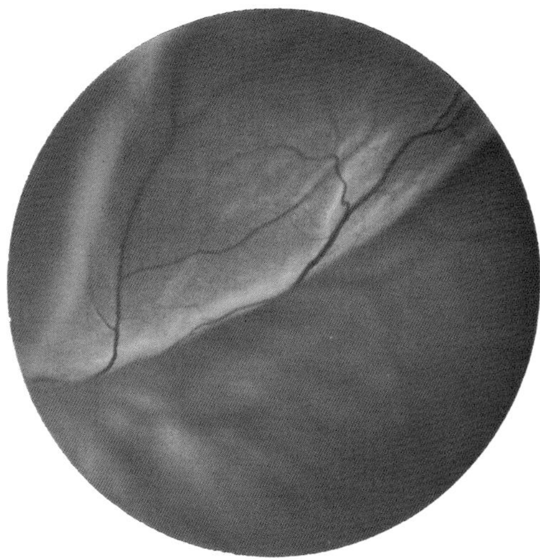

Figure 9.19 *Fresh superior RD*

Mobility

The detached retina undulates freely with eye movements except in cases of severe proliferative vitreoretinopathy (*see* later).

Shifting fluid

This is absent (*see* later).

Macular pseudohole

Due to the thinness of the retina at the fovea, a pseudohole is frequently seen in eyes with detachments involving the posterior pole. This should not be mistaken for a true macular hole which may give rise to RD in highly myopic eyes or following blunt ocular trauma.

Vitreous

1. *PVD* is a universal finding.
2. *'Tobacco dust'* in the anterior vitreous is present in all cases. If it is absent, suspect a simulating lesion such as retinoschisis.
3. *Transvitreal membranes* are present in advanced proliferative vitreoretinopathy (*see* later).
4. *Blood* may be present within the vitreous gel or in the retrohyaloid space.

Signs of long-standing retinal detachment (*see Figure 9.40a*)

Retinal thinning

This must not be confused with retinoschisis.

Secondary intraretinal cysts

These take about 1 year to develop, and disappear following retinal reattachment.

Subretinal demarcation lines

These 'high-water marks' are initially pigmented and then tend to lose their pigment. They develop at the junction of flat and detached retina and take about 3 months to develop. They are convex with respect to the ora serrata and, although they represent sites of increased adhesion, SRF not infrequently spreads beyond a demarcation line.

Subretinal fibrosis (*Figure 9.20*)

Multiple opaque strands are present on the outer retinal surface.

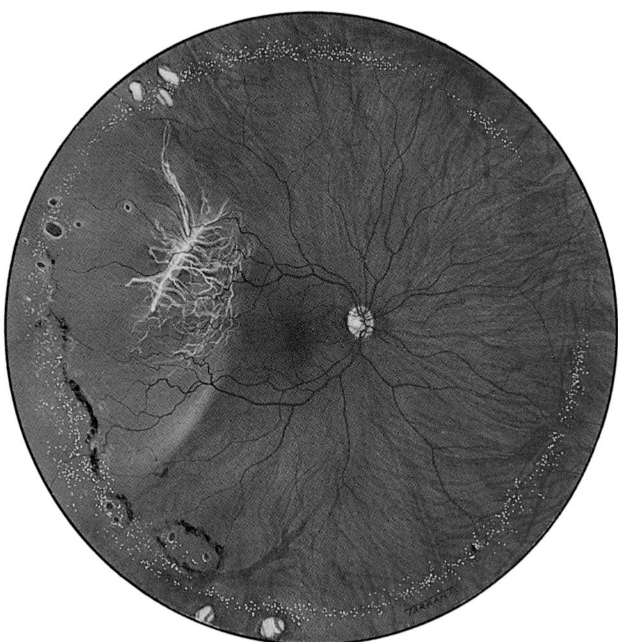

Figure 9.20 Temporal rhegmatogenous RD with subretinal fibrosis; also note multiple small round holes in both flat and detached retina, patches of pavingstone degeneration at 7 and 11 o'clock, and circumferential 'snowflakes'

Proliferative vitreoretinopathy

Pathogenesis

Proliferative vitreoretinopathy (PVR) is caused by the proliferation of membranes on the inner retinal surface (epiretinal membranes), on the posterior surface of the detached hyaloid and occasionally also on the outer retinal surface (subretinal membranes). These membranes are thought to be caused by the proliferation and metaplasia of cells derived from the RPE and retinal glia. Mild PVR is found in about 5% of eyes with RD. In some eyes, contraction of the fibrous component of epiretinal and, sometimes, subretinal membranes causes tangential traction with varying degrees of distortion of affected retina. Severe postoperative contraction of these membranes associated with contraction of transvitreal membranes is now the most common cause of failure in RD surgery.

Clinical features

PVR is divided into four stages but progression from one stage to the next is not inevitable.

Grade A (minimal)

This grade has diffuse vitreous haze and 'tobacco dust' consisting of pigmented macrophages. Although these findings occur in most eyes with RD, they are particularly severe in eyes with early PVR.

Grade B (moderate)

This grade comprises rolled edges of retinal breaks and/or wrinkling of the inner retinal surface with tortuosity of blood vessels. The epiretinal membranes responsible for these findings cannot be identified clinically.

Grade C (marked)

This grade has full-thickness retinal folds which may be radial, circular or star-shaped, affecting one quadrant of detached retina (grade C-1), two quadrants (grade C-2) (*see Figure 9.41, left*) or three quadrants (grade C-3). The affected area of retina appears rigid and shows little or no mobility during eye movements or movements induced by scleral indentation. The membranes responsible for these changes have a high collagen content and can usually be detected ophthalmoscopically. In all categories of grade C PVR, the RD may be partial or total.

Grade D (massive) (*Figure 9.21*)

This grade is characterized by full-thickness retinal folds involving all four quadrants of totally detached retina. Bridging traction caused by the contraction of transvitreal membranes which stretch from one part of the retina to another (usually at the equator) induce a funnel-like configuration to the postequatorial retina. In grade D-1 the funnel is open, in grade D-2 it is open but narrow and in grade D-3 it is closed so even the optic disc cannot be visualized.

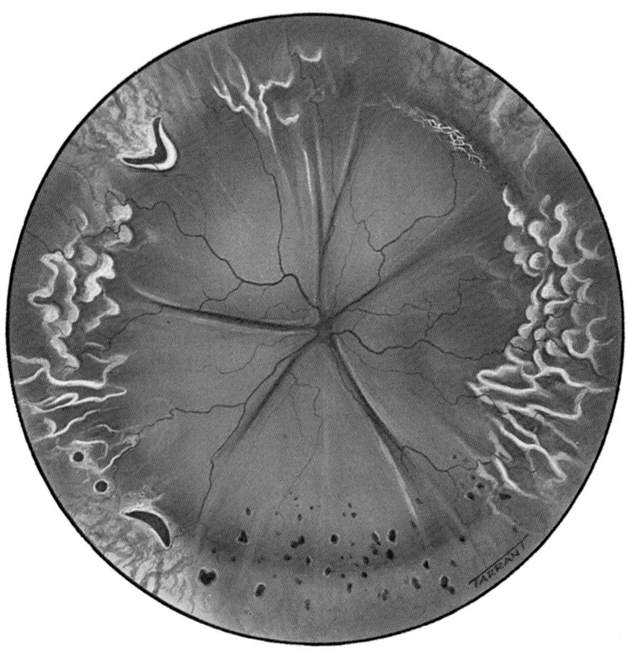

Figure 9.21 PVR grade D

Subsequent course of untreated RD

Unless they are successfully treated surgically, the vast majority of RDs become total and eventually give rise to secondary cataract, chronic uveitis, hypotony and, eventually, phthisis bulbi. A minority of RDs remain stationary for many years or indefinitely due to the formation of demarcation lines. Very rarely, a small RD may reattach spontaneously, particularly if the patient is subjected to prolonged bed rest.

Tractional retinal detachment

Symptoms

Photopsia and floaters usually are absent because vitreoretinal traction develops slowly and is not associated with acute PVD. *Visual field defect* progresses slowly and may become stationary for months and even years.

Signs

1. *Breaks* are absent unless a secondary rhegmatogenous component develops.
2. *Configuration* is concave. The SRF is less than in a rhegmatogenous RD and seldom extends to the ora serrata. The highest elevation of the retina occurs at sites of vitreoretinal traction (*see Figure 10.23*).
3. *Mobility* is severely reduced.
4. *Secondary intraretinal cysts* are absent despite the fact that the RD may be of long standing.
5. *Subretinal demarcation lines* are absent.

Exudative retinal detachment

Symptoms

Photopsia is absent as there is no vitreoretinal traction and *floaters* occasionally are present due to associated vitritis. *Visual field defect* may develop suddenly and progress rapidly. In some cases of Harada's disease both eyes are involved simultaneously.

Signs

1. *Breaks* are absent.
2. *Configuration* is convex. The detached retina is smooth and not corrugated as in a rhegmatogenous RD. Occasionally the SRF is so deep that the RD can be seen with the slitlamp without the aid of a contact lens, and it may even touch the back of the lens.
3. *Shifting fluid* is the hallmark of exudative RD. The SRF responds to the force of gravity and detaches the area of retina under which it accumulates. For example, in the upright position the SRF collects under the inferior retina but, on assuming the supine position, the inferior retina flattens and the SRF shifts posteriorly and detaches the macula and superior retina. In eyes with exudative RDs due to posterior scleritis the SRF may be turbid.
4. *Other features.* The cause of the RD, such as a choroidal tumour, may be apparent when the fundus is examined, or the patient may have an associated systemic disease responsible for the RD (rheumatoid arthritis, Harada's disease, toxaemia etc.).

Differential diagnosis

Acquired retinoschisis

Symptoms

Photopsia and floaters are usually absent because there is no vitreoretinal traction. *Visual field defect* is seldom present because spread posterior to the equator is very rare. If it does occur the field defect is absolute.

Signs

1. *Breaks* may be present in one or both layers in eyes with reticular retinoschisis.
2. *Configuration* is convex, but the retina is not opaque and corrugated as in rhegmatogenous RD (*Figure 9.22*). However, the smooth and thin inner leaf of the schisis cavity may be mistaken for an atrophic long-standing rhegmatogenous RD on cursory examination. The schisis cavity starts at the ora serrata (just like a rhegmatogenous RD) but seldom spreads posterior to the equator. The most common site is the inferotemporal quadrant, with frequent symmetrical involvement in both eyes. Findings associated with retinoschisis are 'snowflakes' and sheathed vessels on the inner leaf, 'white with pressure' and a beaten metal appearance of the outer leaf, and rows of torn grey–white tissue bridging the schisis cavity (*see Figure 9.17*).
3. *Mobility* is severely restricted.
4. *Subretinal demarcation lines* are absent.

Choroidal detachment

Symptoms

Photopsia and floaters are absent because there is no vitreoretinal traction. *Visual field defect* present if the detachment spreads posterior to the equator is rare.

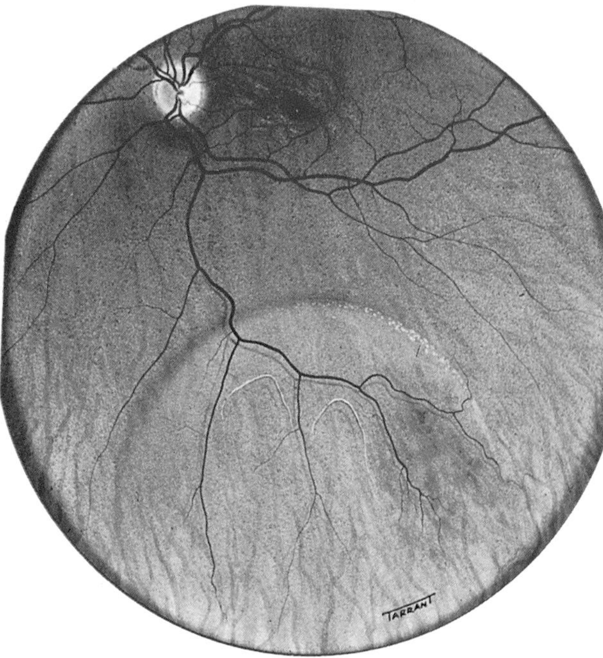

Figure 9.22 Inferior acquired retinoschisis with outer layer breaks and 'snowflakes'

Signs

Anterior segment

Intraocular pressure is usually very low as a result of hyposection of aqueous humour due to a concomitant detachment of the ciliary body. *Anterior chamber* is usually of normal depth but may be shallow in eyes with extensive choroidal detachments.

Posterior segment

1. *Configuration* is convex. The elevations are smooth and bullous and have a brown colour. Temporal and nasal bullae tend to be most prominent (*Figure 9.23*). Because the detachments are only limited anteriorly by the scleral spur, the peripheral retina and ora serrata can be seen with ease without scleral indentation. The elevations do not extend to the posterior pole because they are limited by the firm adhesion between the suprachoroidal lamellae where the vortex veins enter their scleral canals.
2. *Mobility* is severely reduced.

Miscellaneous conditions

On cursory examination without the aid of indirect opthalmoscopy, the following lesions may be mistaken for RD:

1. *'Solid' detachments*—due to choroidal tumours (*Figure 9.24*) or scleral masses which elevate the RPE and sensory retina.
2. *Vitreous haemorrhage*—compacted in the midvitreous cavity to form an ochre membrane.
3. *Retinal artery occlusion*—the retinal oedema caused by an acute central retinal artery occlusion may be mistaken for a shallow RD.

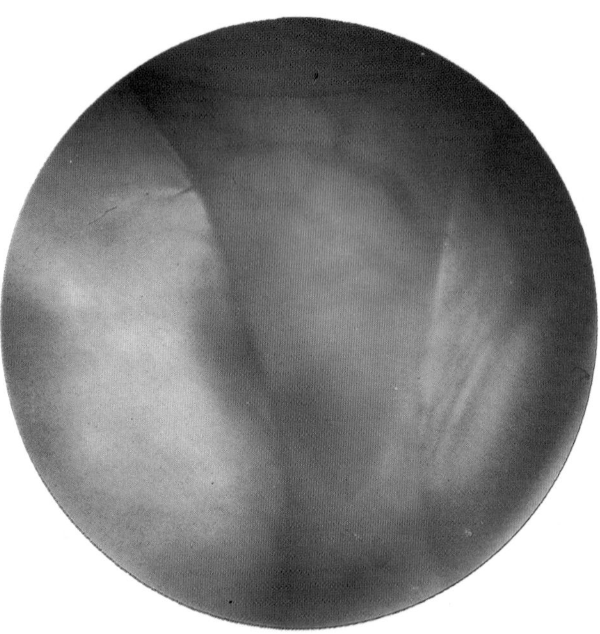

Figure 9.23 Large choroidal detachment

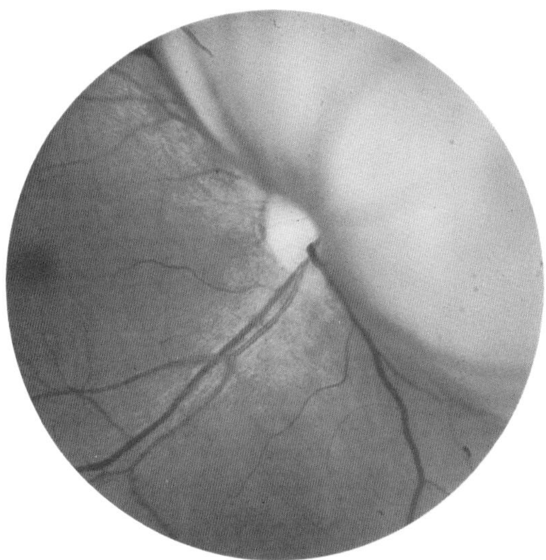

Figure 9.24 'Solid' RD due to a choroidal tumour

Prophylaxis

Retinal breaks

Although, given the right circumstances, most retinal breaks are capable of causing RD, there is no doubt that some are more dangerous than others. Important criteria to be considered in the selection of patients for prophylactic treatment can be divided into three main groups.

Characteristics of break

Type

A tear is more dangerous than a hole.

Size

A large break is more dangerous than a small break.

Symptoms

Tears associated with symptoms of acute PVD are more dangerous than those detected on routine examination.

Location

Superior breaks are more dangerous than inferior breaks because, due to gravity, SRF is likely to spread more quickly. Upper temporal tears are particularly dangerous because the macula is likely to be involved early in the event of RD. Equatorial breaks are more dangerous than those located near the ora serrata.

'Subclinical RD'

This refers to a break surrounded by a small amount of SRF. Because the SRF is usually located anterior to the equator it does not give rise to a peripheral visual field defect. Frequently 'subclinical RDs' become 'clinical' within a short period of time.

Pigment

Pigmentation around a retinal break indicates that it has been present for a long time and the danger of progression to clinical RD is fairly small.

Other ocular considerations

Aphakia

A retinal break in an aphakic eye is more dangerous than an identical lesion in a phakic eye. Even a relatively innocuous small peripheral round hole may give rise to RD following cataract extraction, particularly if it is associated with vitreous loss.

Myopia

Because myopic patients are more prone to RD, a retinal break in a myopic eye should be taken more seriously than an identical lesion in a non-myopic eye.

Only eye

Retinal breaks should be taken very seriously, particularly if the fellow eye has lost vision from RD.

Patient

Family history

Any break or predisposing degeneration should be taken seriously if the patient gives a family history of RD.

Reliability

It may be necessary to treat a relatively innocuous break prophylactically if the patient cannot be relied upon to report new symptoms indicative of acute PVD or RD.

Systemic disease

RDs in patients with Marfan's syndrome, Stickler's syndrome and Ehlers–Danlos syndrome usually have a poor prognosis, so any break or predisposing degeneration should be treated prophylactically.

Clinical examples

The following clinical examples illustrate the various risk factors just discussed (*Figure 9.25*).

Large equatorial U-shaped tear associated with 'subclinical RD' and located in upper temporal quadrant (*Figure 9.25a*)

Prophylaxis

This should be carried out without delay because the risk of progression to a clinical RD is very high. Because the tear is located in the upper temporal quadrant, early macular involvement by SRF is likely.

Technique

Cryotherapy combined with an explant has the greatest chance of success. Argon laser photocoagulation alone is less likely to be successful because the break is surrounded by SRF.

Large U-shaped tear in upper temporal quadrant in eye with symptomatic acute PVD (*Figure 9.25b*)

Prophylaxis

This should be carried out without delay because the risk of progression to clinical RD is high. Although the tear is not associated with a 'subclinical RD', it is still dangerous because it is large, located in the upper temporal quadrant and symptomatic. Fresh tears such as this in patients with symptoms of acute PVD frequently progress to clinical RD within a few days or weeks unless treated prophylactically.

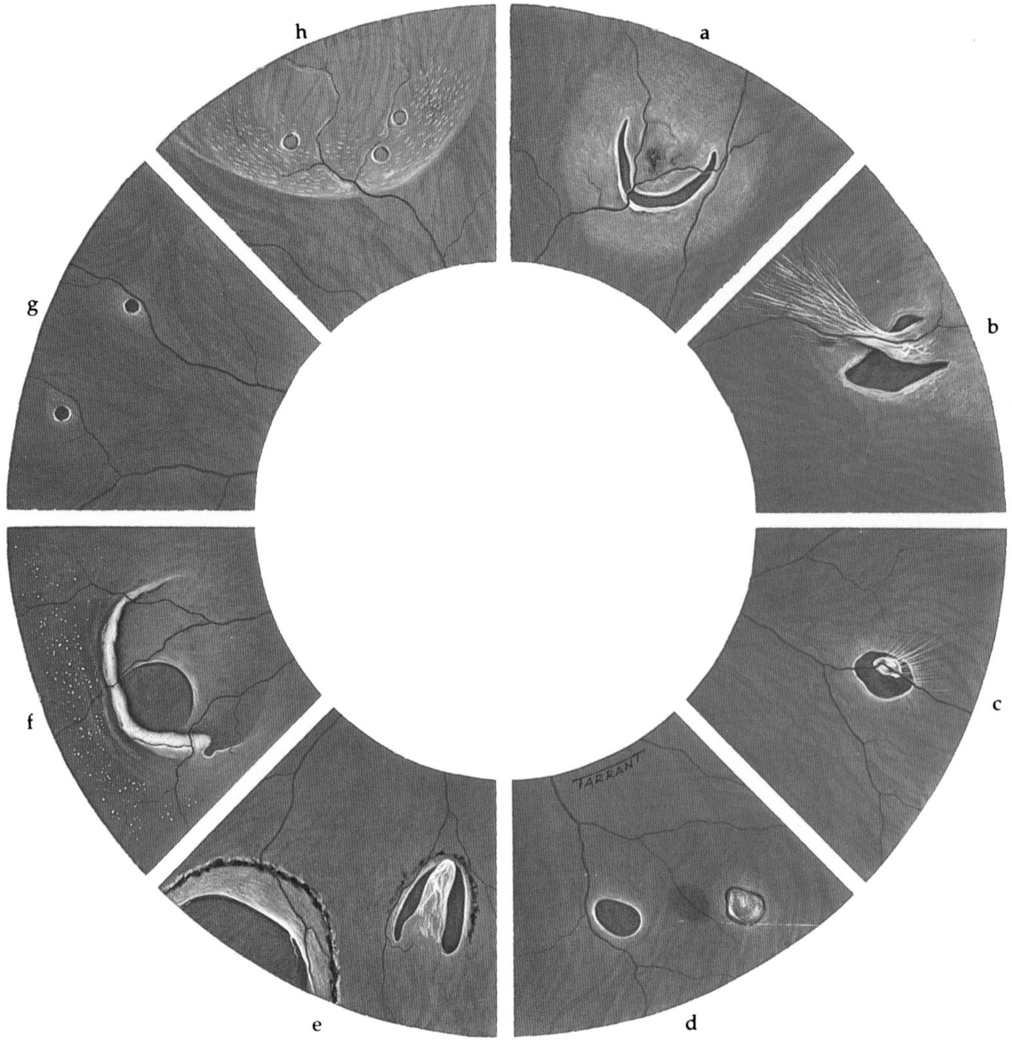

Figure 9.25 *Retinal breaks*

Technique

Cryotherapy should be combined with a radial explant because vitreoretinal traction is still present on the flap of the tear. Argon laser photocoagulation alone is less likely to be effective although it has more chance of success than the previous example (*Figure 9.25a*).

Operculated tear bridged by patent blood vessel (*Figure 9.25c*)

Prophylaxis

This should be carried out because persistent vitreoretinal traction on the operculum may cause an RD. In addition, persistent traction on the bridging blood vessel may cause recurrent vitreous haemorrhage.

Technique

Although many eyes with breaks associated with avulsed or bridging blood vessels have been successfully treated by argon laser photocoagulation alone, the possibility of an explant to release traction on the operculum and blood vessel should be considered.

Operculated tear in lower temporal quadrant of aphakic eye discovered on routine examination (*Figure 9.25d*)

Prophylaxis

Since vitreoretinal traction is released an operculated tear that has not led fairly quickly to RD can be considered safer than a similar tear with persistent traction (as in *Figure 9.25c*). However, because any break in an aphakic eye is much more dangerous than in a phakic eye, prophylactic treatment should be advised.

Technique

Because the operculum is floating freely on the detached posterior vitreous surface an explant is unnecessary and the break can be treated either with laser photocoagulation or with cryotherapy depending on its location in relation to the equator. Relatively posterior lesions are easier to treat by photocoagulation whereas anterior lesions are easier to approach by transconjunctival cryotherapy. Both methods of treatment can be carried out under local anaesthesia as outpatient procedures.

Inferior U-shaped tear and dialysis surrounded by pigment found on routine examination (*Figure 9.25e*)

Prophylaxis

Because these breaks have been present for a long time the risk of RD is small. However, the presence of pigmentation around a large U-shaped tear is not always a guaranteee against progression, particularly when associated with other risk factors such as aphakia, myopia or RD in the fellow eye.

Technique

Cryotherapy or laser photocoagulation can be carried out (if necessary).

Acquired retinoschisis with breaks in both layers (*Figure 9.25f*)

Prophylaxis

This is probably unnecessary unless the fellow eye has suffered RD due to acquired retinoschisis. Although this lesion represents a full-thickness defect in the sensory retina, the fluid within the schisis cavity is usually viscid and rarely passes into the subretinal space.

Technique

Cryotherapy can be performed around the outer layer break (if necessary). This can be combined with a barrier of laser photocoagulation just outside the schisis in order to prevent macular involvement in lesions extending posterior to the equator.

Two small round asymptomatic holes near ora serrata (*Figure 9.25g*)

Prophylaxis is unnecessary as the risk of RD is extremely small because the holes are probably located within the vitreous base. About 5% of the general population have similar lesions.

Small inner layer holes in acquired retinoschisis (*Figure 9.25h*)

Prophylaxis is unnecessary as there is no communication between the vitreous cavity and the subretinal space.

Predisposing peripheral retinal degenerations

Lattice and snailtrack

In the absence of associated retinal breaks neither of these degenerations is treated prophylactically unless it is associated with one or more of the following risk factors:

1. RD in fellow eye—most frequent indication.
2. Aphakia—an already aphakic eye or one about to become aphakic.
3. High myopia—particularly if associated with extensive lattice degeneration.
4. Strong family history of RD.
5. Marfan's syndrome, Stickler's syndrome or Ehlers–Danlos syndrome.

'White without pressure'

This is not treated prophylactically unless the fellow eye has suffered a spontaneous giant retinal tear.

Treatment modalities

Cryotherapy vs photocoagulation

Most lesions can be adequately treated with either cryotherapy or laser photocoagulation. In the majority of cases the treatment modality is based on the surgeon's preference and experience as well as on the availability of instrumentation. The other considerations are:

1. *Location of lesion:*
   a. Equatorial lesions can be treated by either photocoagulation or cryotherapy.
   b. Postequatorial lesions can only be treated by photocoagulation unless the conjunctiva is incised.
   c. Peripheral lesions near the ora serrata can only be treated adequately by cryotherapy. It is particularly important to treat the base of a U-shaped tear.
2. *Clarity of media*—eyes with hazy media are much easier to treat by cryotherapy.
3. *Pupil size*—eyes with small pupils are easier to treat by cryotherapy.

Laser photocoagulation technique

1. Select a spot size of 200 μm and set the duration to 0.1 to 0.2 second.
2. Insert the triple-mirror contact lens.
3. Surround the lesion with two rows of confluent burns of moderate intensity (*Figure 9.26*). When treating islands of lattice degeneration do not apply burns to the lesion itself as this may induce or enlarge a retinal break.

Serious complications from peripheral retinal photocoagulation are rare. When they do occur, they are usually associated with excessively heavy treatment to large areas of the retina and may involve both anterior and posterior segments (*see* Chapter 10).

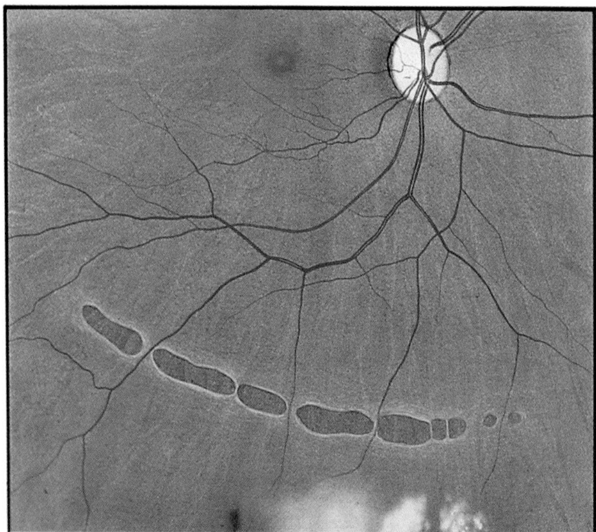

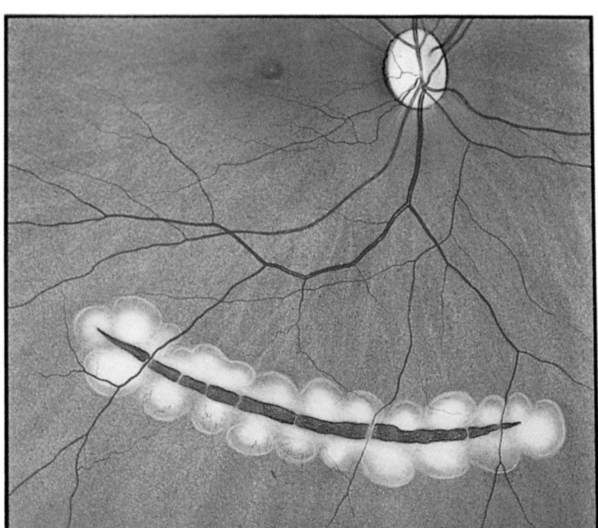

Figure 9.26 *Row of retinal holes. Top: before treatment; bottom: after prophylactic photocoagulation*

Cryotherapy technique

1. Anaesthetize the eye with topical cocaine. Some surgeons also inject lignocaine (Xylocaine) subconjunctivally in the same quadrant as the lesion to be treated.
2. Insert a Barraquer speculum.
3. Check the cryoprobe for correct freezing and defrosting and also make sure that the rubber sleeve is not covering the tip.
4. While viewing with the indirect ophthalmoscope, gently indent the sclera with the tip of the probe.
5. Surround the lesion with a single row of cryoapplications, terminating freezing as soon as the retina whitens.
6. Do not remove the cryoprobe until it has defrosted completely because premature removal may 'crack' the choroid and give rise to a choroidal haemorrhage.

Benign degenerations

It is extremely important for the clinician to be able to recognize benign peripheral retinal degenerations (*Figure 9.27*) in order to avoid unnecessary prophylactic treatment.

Microcrystoid (peripheral cystoid) degeneration (*Figure 9.27a*)

This consists of tiny, often red-coloured vesicles with indistinct boundaries on greyish-white background which make the retina appear thickened and less transparent. The condition always commences adjacent to the ora serrata and extends posteriorly and circumferentially with a smooth undulating posterior border. It is present in every adult eye, increasing in severity with age, and is not in itself causally related to RD, but may give rise to acquired retinoschisis.

Snowflakes (*Figure 9.27b*)

These are minute, glistening, yellow-white dots which are frequently found scattered diffusely in the fundus periphery. Occasionally, more circumscribed areas of snowflakes may be seen near the equator. Foci composed solely of snowflakes are most unlikely to lead to the formation of retinal breaks and require no treatment. These lesions are, however, of considerable clinical importance as they are frequently associated with other vitreoretinal degenerations, such as lattice or snailtrack degeneration, and acquired retinoschisis.

Pavingstone degeneration (*Figure 9.27c*)

This consists of discrete yellow-white areas of chorioretinal thinning, and is present to some extent in 25% of normal eyes.

Honeycomb (reticular) degeneration (*Figure 9.27d*)

This is a senile change characterized by a fine network of perivascular hyperpigmentation.

Drusen (*Figure 9.27e*)

These are small clusters of pale lesions which frequently have a pigmented border. They are similar to drusen at the posterior pole.

Oral pigmentary degeneration (*Figure 9.27f*)

This is a senile change consisting of a hyperpigmented band running adjacent to the ora serrata.

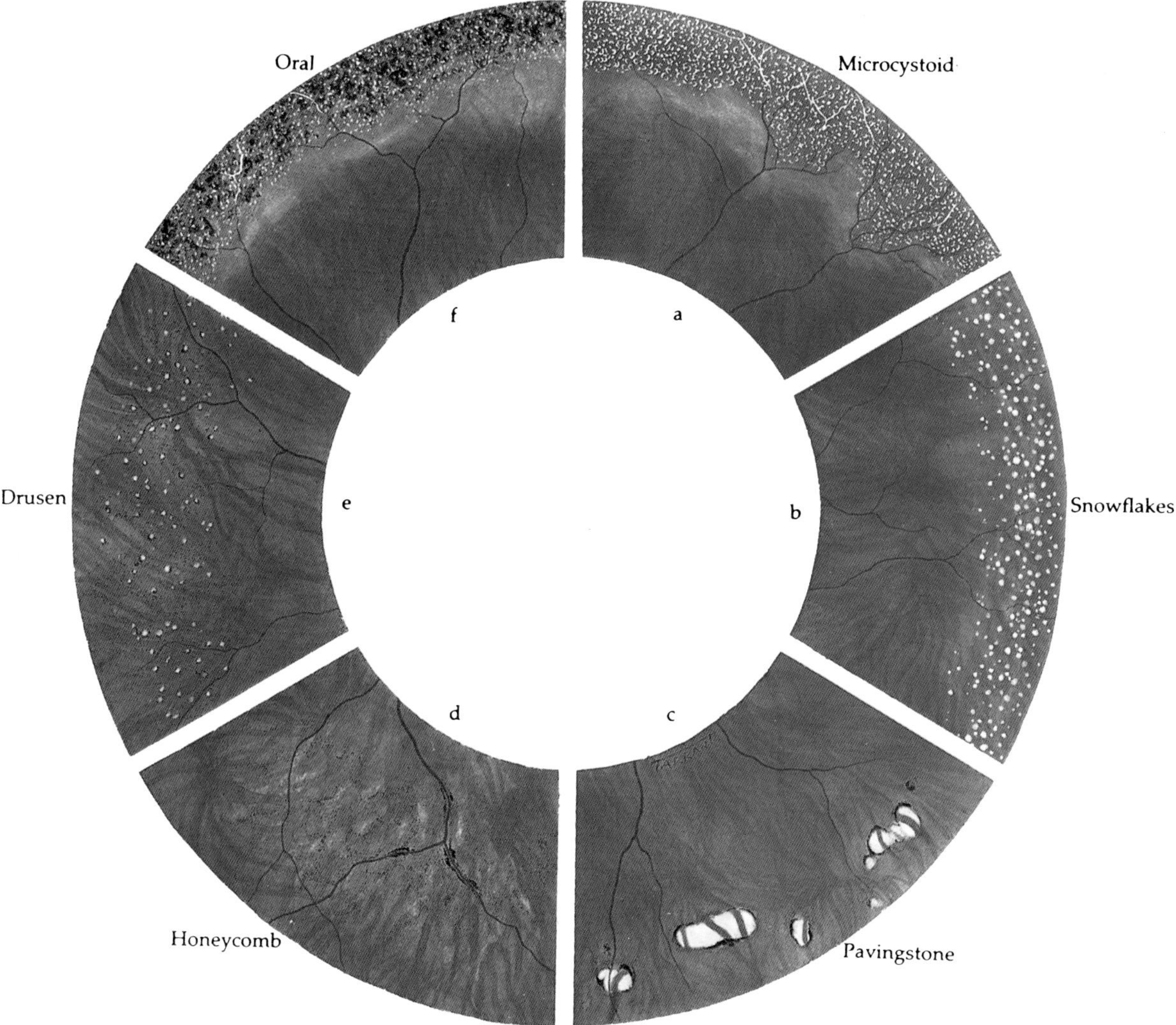

Figure 9.27 *Benign peripheral retinal degenerations*

Surgical principles

Scleral buckling

Definitions

1. *Scleral buckling.* A surgical procedure to create an inward indentation of the sclera ('buckle').
2. *Explant.* Material sutured directly onto the sclera to create a buckle.
3. *Implant.* Material placed within the sclera to create a buckle (now abandoned by most surgeons).

Purpose

1. To close retinal breaks by apposing the RPE to the sensory retina.
2. To release vitreoretinal traction.

Configuration of explants

1. *Radial.* This is placed at right angles to the limbus.
2. *Segmental circumferential.* This is placed circumferentially with the limbus to create a segmental buckle.
3. *Encircling circumferential.* This is placed around the entire circumference of the globe to create a 360° buckle.

Explant material

All explants are made of soft or hard silicone.

Soft silicone (Silastic) sponges. Round sponges have a diameter of 3 mm, 4 mm and 5 mm, and oval sponges are 5.5 × 7.5 mm. Sponges can be used for both radial and circumferential buckling.

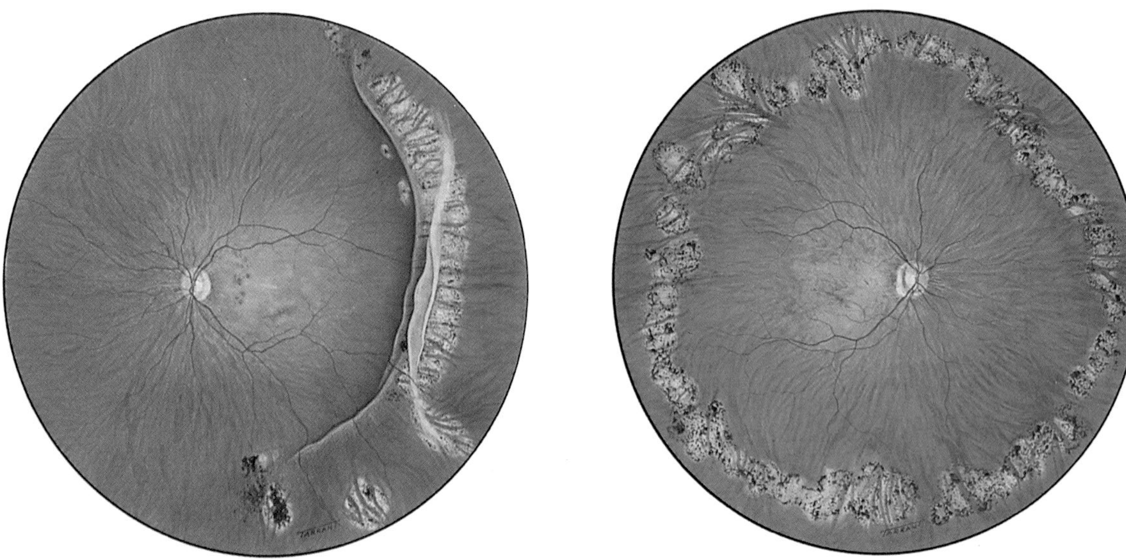

Figure 9.28 *Left: giant retinal tear treated by a wide circumferential buckle; right: fellow eye following 360° prophylactic cryotherapy*

Hard silicone straps. These are used for 360° buckling.

Hard silicone tyres. This is of various dimensions and is used to supplement an encircling buckle.

Indications

Radial buckling

1. *Large U-shaped tears*—particularly when 'fishmouthing' is anticipated (*see* later).
2. *Posterior breaks*—because sutures are easier to insert.

Segmental circumferential buckling

1. *Multiple breaks*—located in one or two quadrants and/or at varying distances from the ora serrata.
2. *Anterior breaks.*
3. *Wide breaks*—such as dialyses and giant tears (*Figure 9.28, left*).

Encircling buckles

1. *Breaks* involving three or more quadrants.
2. *Lattice degeneration* involving three or more quadrants.
3. *Extensive RD without detectable breaks* particularly in eyes with hazy media, intraocular lens implants or aphakia. A broad buckle is used in an attempt to seal breaks anterior to the equator.
4. *PVR grade C* to create a permanent 360° buckle by reducing the diameter of the globe at the equator.
5. *Failed local procedures* in which the reason for failure is not apparent.
6. *Inexperienced surgeon* who is unfamiliar with the accurate localization of breaks.

Drainage of subretinal fluid

Indications

Difficulty in localization

Localization of relatively posterior retinal breaks may be extremely difficult in eyes with highly elevated bullous RDs unless the retina is first partially flattened by draining the SRF.

Immobile retina

Non-drainage is successful only if the detached retina is sufficiently mobile to move back against the buckle during the postoperative period. If it is rendered relatively immobile by PVR, a high buckle is required to seal the break. This can be achieved only if the eye is first softened by draining the SRF.

Long-standing RD

Eyes with long-standing RDs tend to have viscous SRF which takes a long time (many months) to absorb. Drainage is therefore essential even if the break can be closed without drainage.

Inferior tears

RDs associated with inferior equatorial tears are better drained because, when the patient assumes the upright position postoperatively, any residual SRF will gravitate inferiorly and may reopen the tear. Most dialyses, however, can be closed without drainage.

Fear of complication from raised intraocular pressure

With the non-drainage procedure the scleral sutures have to be tightened over the sponge in order to achieve the desired buckling effect. This causes a significant elevation of intraocular pressure for several hours. As the pressure gradient is reduced, the sponge expands inwards and closes the retinal tear. After the tear is closed, any residual SRF usually absorbs within 24–48 hours. The temporary elevation of intraocular pressure is usually harmless although in the following situations it may have detrimental effects:

1. In eyes with advanced glaucomatous field loss it may cause a complete loss of all vision.
2. In eyes with thin sclera the sutures may cut out as they are being tightened over the sponge.
3. In eyes that have had recent cataract extraction the incision may rupture. If possible, wait at least 6 weeks before contemplating detachment surgery.

Advantages

Although non-drainage of SRF avoids most of the complications, which will be described later, it is important to point out that drainage provides immediate contact between the sensory retina and RPE with flattening of the fovea. If this contact is delayed for more than 5 days, a satisfactory adhesion will not develop around the retinal break because the 'stickiness' of the RPE will have worn off. This may result in non-attachment of the retina or, in some cases, reopening of the break during the postoperative period.

Intravitreal injections

Air

Indications

1. *Hypotony.* The most frequent indication is to reconstitute the globe and prevent excessive hypotony following drainage of SRF.
2. *'Fishmouthing'* of a large retinal tear may result in failure to reattach the retina unless the tear can be closed internally by the air bubble (tamponade).
3. *Radial retinal folds* can be flattened.
4. *Giant retinal tears.* The posterior flap can be unrolled (*see Figure 9.30*).
5. *Posterior breaks* especially if they are large, may need air for tamponade.
6. *Macular hole* giving rise to an RD can be tamponaded.

Duration

Air starts to absorb immediately and usually by the fifth postoperative day it will have completely absorbed. A mixture of 70% air and 30% sulphur hexafluoride (SF_6) lasts twice as long as air alone. This is because the SF_6 component of the bubble takes up nitrogen and expands as the air is absorbing.

Balanced salt solution

Indications

1. *Hypotony.* Balanced salt solution (BSS) does not impair visualization of the fundus, as may occur from small air bubbles. It is therefore particularly useful when SRF has been drained early in the procedure in order to facilitate accurate localization of breaks in eyes with bullous RDs.
2. *Radial folds.* BSS will flatten radial folds but it must not be used in eyes with 'fishmouthing' tears because it will pass through the tear into the subretinal space and increase the RD.

Silicone oil

This substance is used only in eyes with very complicated RDs.

Indications

1. *Grade D PVR.* Silicone oil is a highly viscous substance which will push an immobile retina against the RPE.
2. *Giant tears.* In eyes with RD caused by giant tears, postoperative redetachment due to PVR is extremely common. The use of silicone oil as a primary procedure (frequently combined with vitrectomy) has greatly improved long-term results.

Duration

Unless removed, silicone oil remains permanently in the eye.

Pars plana vitrectomy

Definition

Pars plana vitrectomy is an intraocular microsurgical procedure during which vitreous opacities and membranes are excised with cutting instruments introduced through a pars plana incision (*see* Chapter 10). Frequently vitrectomy is combined with the following intraocular manipulations:

1. Segmentation of epiretinal and occasionally also subretinal membranes.
2. Internal drainage of SRF.
3. Internal gas/fluid exchange.

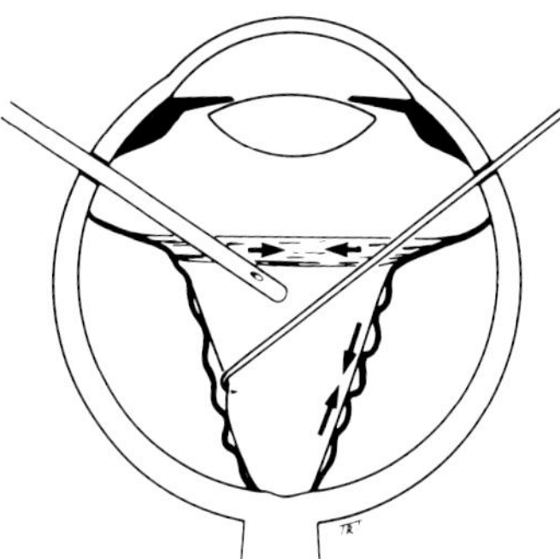

Figure 9.29 *Pars plana vitrectomy for PVR grade D; epiretinal membranes are separated from the retina*

4. Internal silicone oil/fluid exchange.
5. Intraocular bipolar diathermy.
6. Endophotocoagulation.

Indications

1. *Tractional RD.* Because diabetic tractional RDs frequently remain stationary for many months, vitrectomy is carried out only in the event of macular involvement (*see* Chapter 10).
2. *PVR grade D* (*Figure 9.29*) to mobilize the detached retina by segmenting epiretinal membranes and transvitreal bands.
3. *Giant tears* (*Figure 9.30*) to mobilize the posterior flap of a giant tear which extends for 180° or more.

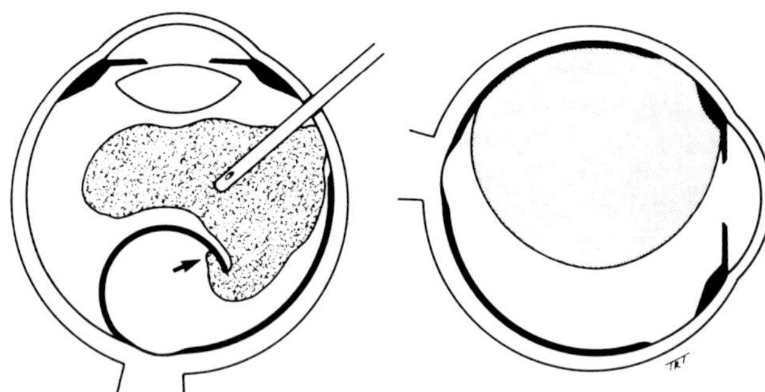

Figure 9.30 *Pars plana vitrectomy (left) and intravitreal air injection (right) for RD due to a giant tear*

Surgical techniques

Local buckling

1. The conjunctiva and Tenon's capsule are incised near the limbus (peritomy) (*Figure 9.31*).
2. With a cellulose sponge the episcleral tissue is cleared from the sclera.
3. A squint hook is inserted under a rectus muscle and a reverse mounted needle with a 4-0 silk suture is passed under the tendon (*Figure 9.32*).
4. The retinal break is localized by inserting a 5-0 Dacron suture into the sclera at the site calculated to correspond to the break.
5. The cut end of the suture is grasped close to the knot with curved mosquito forceps.
6. While viewing with the indirect ophthalmoscope, the sclera is indented with the forceps. If the indentation does not coincide with the break, the procedure is repeated until the break is accurately localized.
7. The retinal break together with any predisposing lesions in detached and flat retina are treated by cryotherapy (*Figure 9.33*).
8. The appropriate-sized sponge is selected.
9. Mattress-type sutures, which will straddle the sponge, are inserted (*Figure 9.34*).
10. The sponge is fed through the sutures and the sutures are tightened with a temporary bow (*Figure 9.35*).
11. The position of the buckle in relation to the break is checked.
12. If necessary, SRF is drained as follows:
    a. A 3 mm sclerotomy down to choroid is performed.
    b. A 5-0 Dacron suture is passed across the lips of the sclerotomy.
    c. Low-intensity diathermy is applied to the choroid.
    d. The choroid is gently perforated with a 25-gauge needle.
13. The fundus is inspected for correct positioning of the buckle.

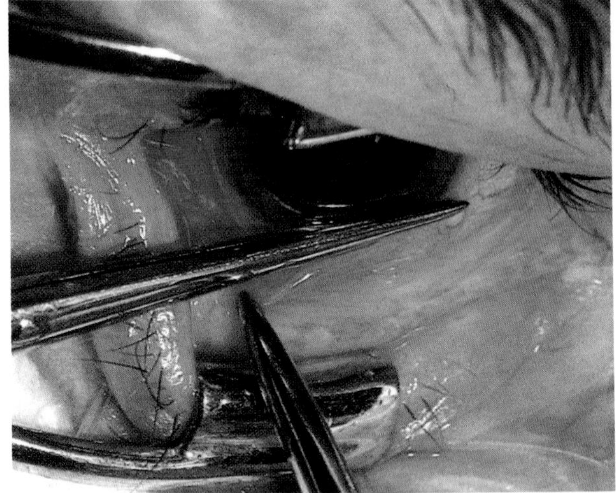

Figure 9.31 *Circumferential incision at limbus*

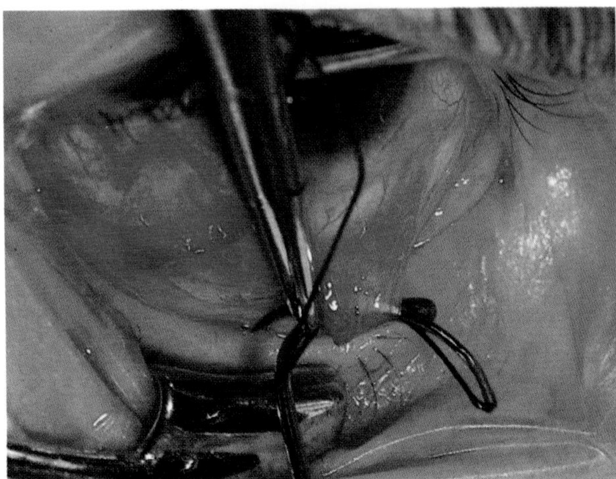

Figure 9.32 *Insertion of bridle suture*

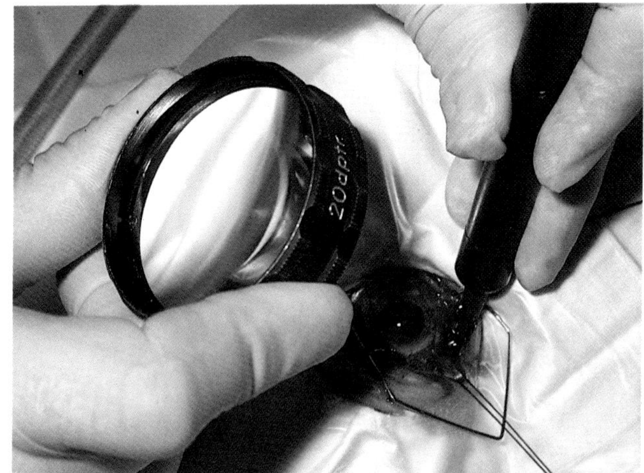

Figure 9.33 *Cryotherapy*

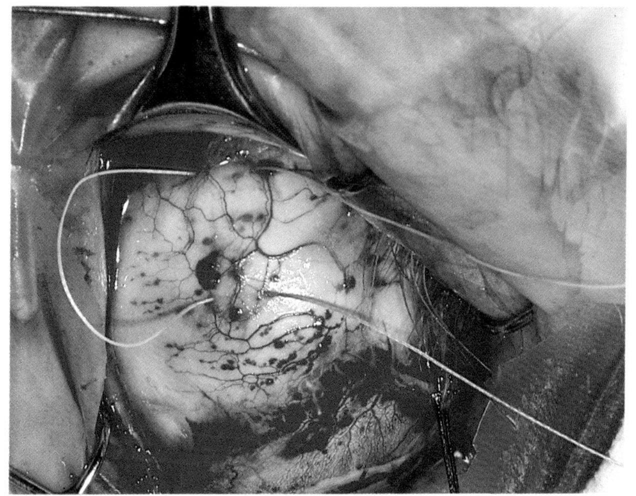

Figure 9.34 *Insertion of mattress suture*

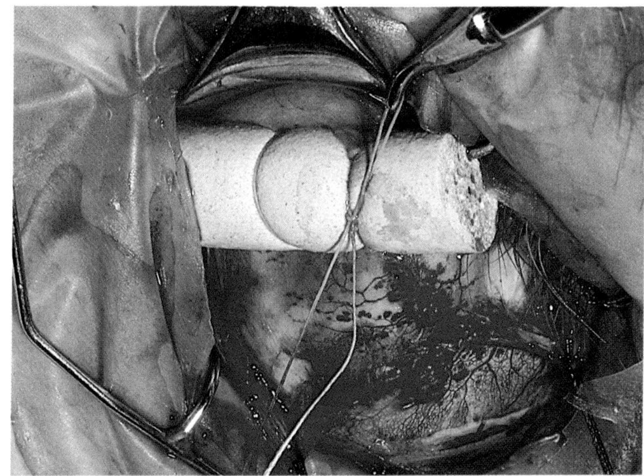

Figure 9.35 *Temporary bow*

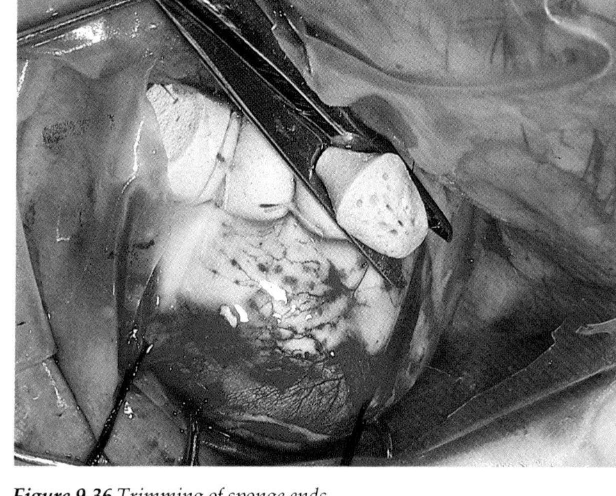

Figure 9.36 *Trimming of sponge ends*

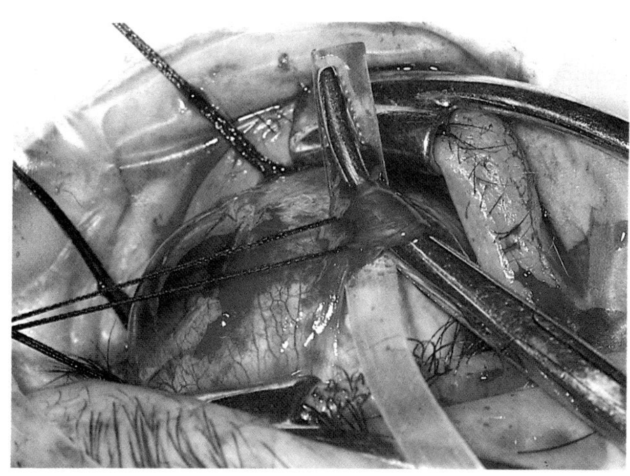

Figure 9.37 *Insertion of strap under superior rectus muscle*

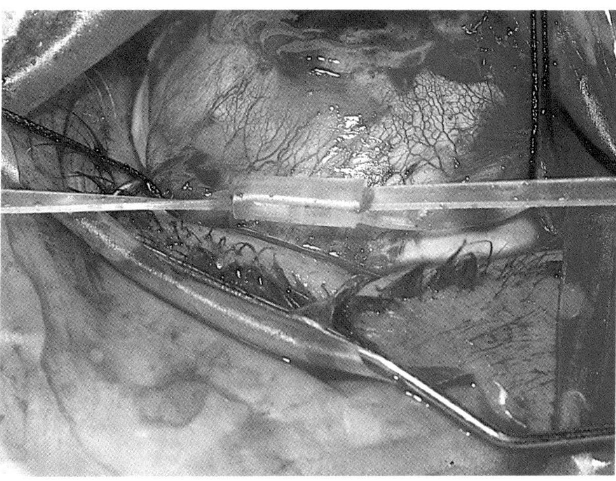

Figure 9.38 *Strap being tightened*

14. The temporary bow is converted into a permanent bow.
15. The edges of the sponge are trimmed (*Figure 9.36*).
16. The conjunctiva is sutured.

Encirclement

The initial steps are essentially the same as for local buckling except that the peritomy extends for 360° and all four recti are exposed.

1. The end of the strap (usually a no. 40) is grasped with curved mosquito forceps and is fed under the four recti (*Figure 9.37*).
2. The two ends of the strap are secured with a Watzke sleeve.
3. The strap is tightened by pulling its two ends until it fits snugly around the ora serrata (*Figure 9.38*).
4. The strap is slid posteriorly (about 4 mm) and secured in each quadrant with a short holding suture.
5. Retinal breaks are treated with cryotherapy and, if necessary, SRF is drained.
6. The strap is tightened.
7. The conjunctiva is sutured.

Clinical examples

The following clinical examples will emphasize the most important aspects of management just discussed.

Management of fresh RD (*Figure 9.39*)

Clinical features

There is a localized right upper temporal RD due to a U-shaped tear (*Figure 9.39a*).

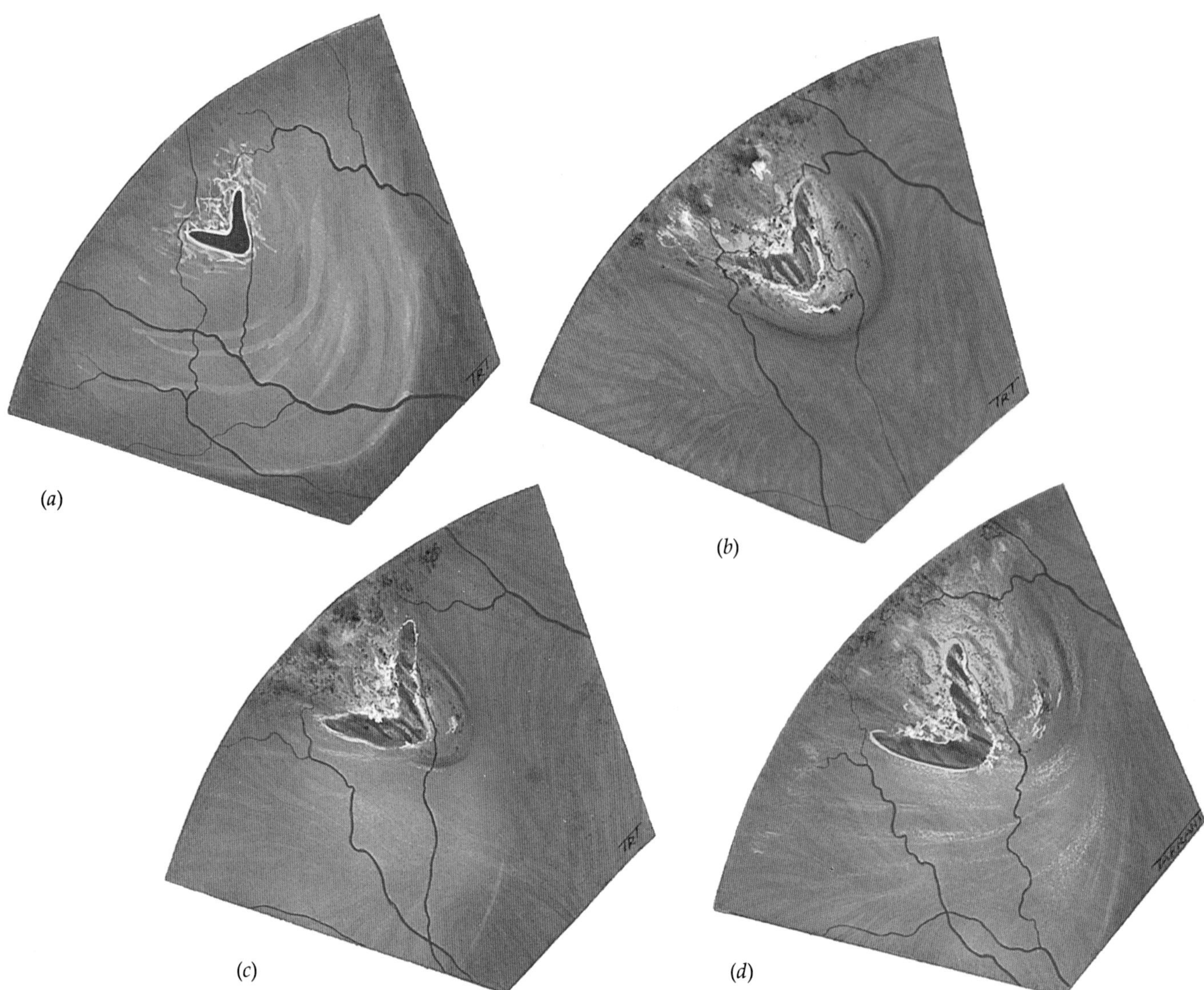

Figure 9.39 (a,b) *Management of fresh upper temporal RD;* (c,d) *cause of failure*

Preoperative considerations

1. *Prognosis for central vision.* This is good because the macula is uninvolved.
2. *Indications for bed rest.* The patient should be admitted immediately, rested flat in bed and operated on as soon as possible because the macula is in great danger as the break is located in the upper temporal quadrant.

Surgical technique

1. *Peritomy* from 8.30 to 12.30 o'clock to expose the lateral and superior recti.
2. *Buckling.* Most U-shaped tears can be sealed with a 5-mm sponge explant (*Figure 9.39b*). *Figure 9.39c* shows an undersized buckle. The sutures should be about 8 mm apart to obtain adequate height to the buckle. The buckle should be placed radially to prevent the possibility of 'fishmouthing'. Accurate positioning of the explant is vital in this case. *Figure 9.39d* shows a malpositioned buckle.
3. *Drainage of SRF.* This is unnecessary because the retina is freely mobile, the break can be apposed to the RPE without difficulty, the RD is fresh and the SRF watery.

Management of long-standing RD (*Figure 9.40*)

Clinical features (*Figure 9.40*)

There is an extensive right RD with macular involvement associated with a U-shaped tear in the upper temporal quadrant and two small round holes in the lower temporal quadrant. A partially pigmented demarcation line is present at the junction of detached and flat retina. A secondary intraretinal cyst is present inferiorly.

Preoperative considerations

1. *Prognosis for central vision.* This is very poor because the fovea has been detached for at least 12 months.
2. *Indications for bed rest.* There is none because the macula has been detached for several months and the RD is not bullous. Surgery can be performed at the patient's and surgeon's convenience.

Surgical technique

1. *Peritomy* from 5.30 to 12.30 o'clock to expose the superior, lateral and inferior recti.

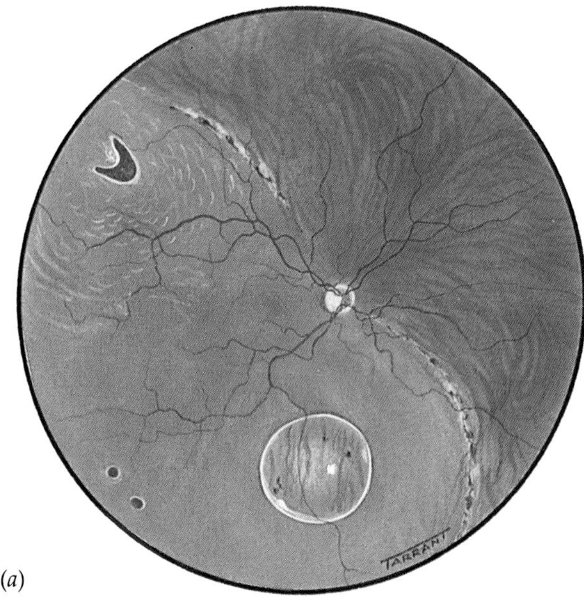

(*a*)

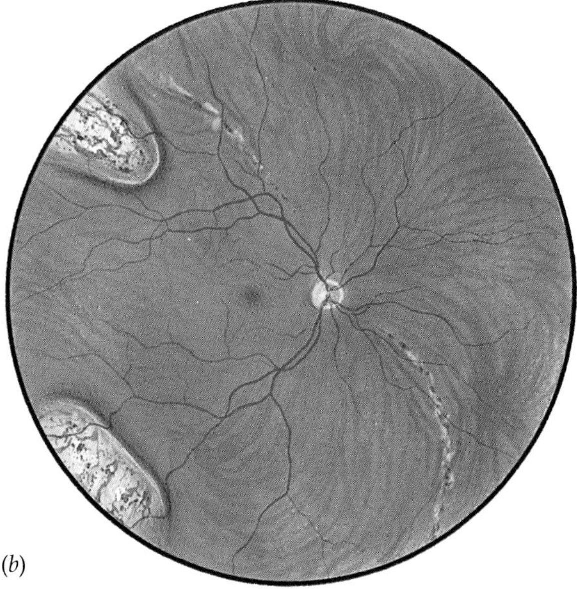

(*b*)

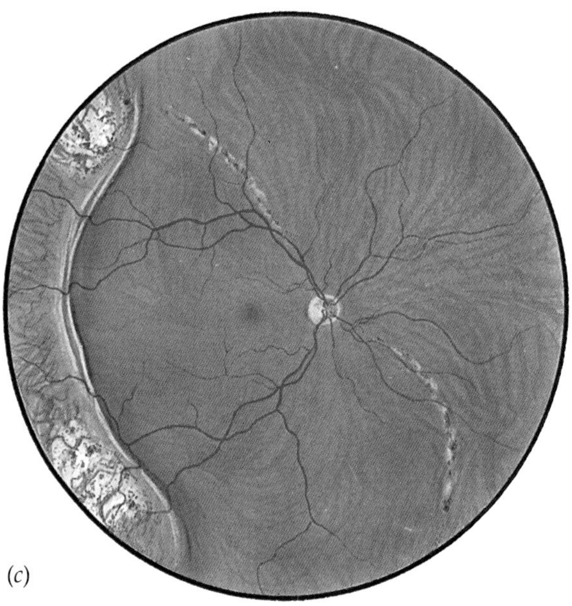

(*c*)

Figure 9.40 *Management of long-standing RD*

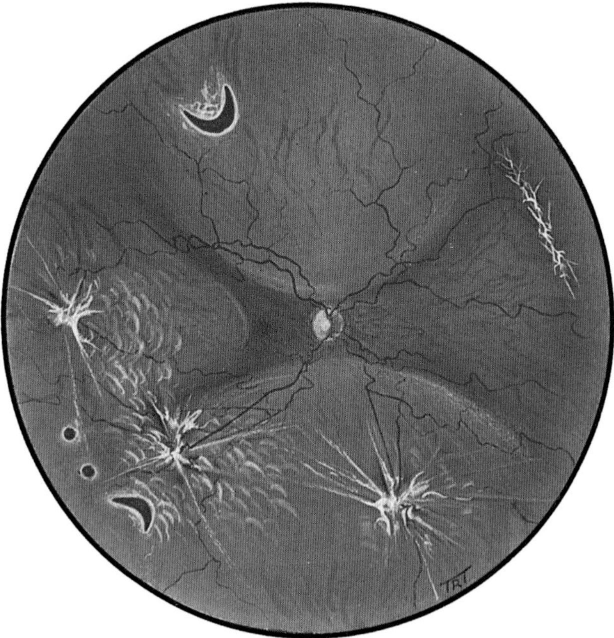

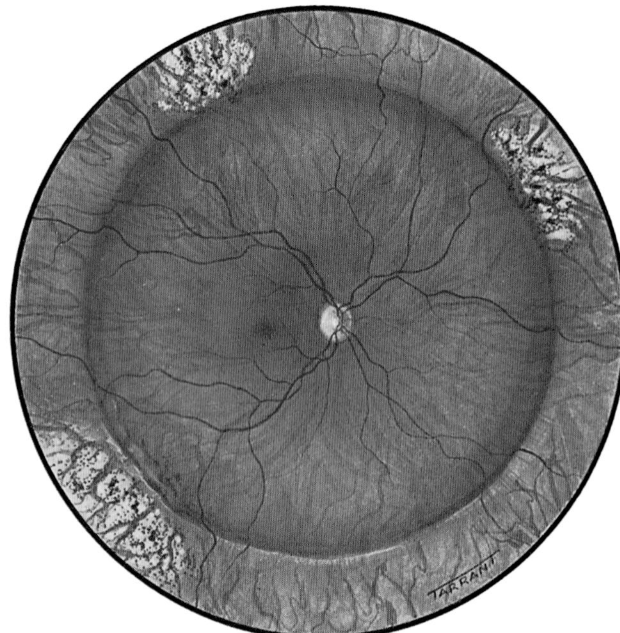

Figure 9.41 *Management of RD complicated by PVR grade C-2*

2. *Buckling*. The U-shaped tear can be sealed with a 5-mm-wide radial sponge explant and the two holes can be sealed with a 4-mm-wide circumferential sponge explant (*Figure 9.40b*). Alternatively, all breaks can be sealed with a long 4-mm-wide circumferential sponge explant extending from 7 to 10.30 o'clock (*Figure 9.40c*).
3. *Drainage of SRF*. This is necessary because in an RD of long standing the SRF is viscous and will take a long time to absorb unless it is drained.

Management of RD complicated by PVR (*Figure 9.41*)

Clinical features (*Figure 9.41, left*)

There is a total right RD, with breaks and lattice degeneration in three separate quadrants. Star-shaped retinal folds present in two quadrants of detached retina are indicative of grade C-2 PVR.

Preoperative considerations

1. *Prognosis for central vision*. This is poor because the macula is involved and the presence of PVR reduces the prognosis for reattachment.
2. *Indications for bed rest*. There is none because the macula is involved and the SRF will not absorb because the retina is not freely mobile.

Surgical technique

1. *Peritomy*. 360°, to expose all four recti.
2. *Buckling*. 360° (*Figure 9.41, right*) because retinal breaks and lattice degeneration involve three quadrants of the detached retina. A permanent buckle is desirable because PVR grade C also is present.
3. *Drainage of SRF*. This is necessary to close the breaks because the retina is not freely mobile.

Causes of failure

Early

By far the most common cause for failure to reattach the retina is an open retinal break. The causes can be preoperative or operative.

Preoperative

It should be emphasized that about 50% of all RDs are associated with more than one break. In the vast majority of these the breaks are located within 90° of each other. Do not be satisfied, if you have found only one break, until you have made a thorough search for the presence of other breaks and have satisfied yourself that the configuration of the SRF corresponds to the position of the primary break. In eyes with hazy media or intraocular lens implants, visualization of the peripheral retina may be very difficult and retinal breaks impossible to detect. As a last resort, consider the possibility of a true macular hole if no peripheral break is evident.

Operative

Buckle failure

This may be due to:

1. Inadequate size (*see Figure 9.39c*)—replace.
2. Incorrect position (*see Figure 9.39d*)—reposition.
3. Inadequate height—drainage of SRF may be necessary.

'Fishmouthing'

This may or may not be associated with a communicating radial retinal fold. In some cases the tear can be closed by applying heavy photocoagulation (xenon or argon) to the retina around the tear in order to induce swelling. If this is unsuccessful, reoperation is necessary to reposition the sponge and also probably to inject air into the vitreous cavity.

Missed iatrogenic break

Reoperation is necessary to seal the break.

Late

This is defined as initial reattachment of the retina and subsequent redetachment after the patient has been sent home (late failure)

Proliferative vitreoretinopathy

The postoperative development of PVR is now the most common cause of late failure, accounting for about 25% of all cases. The incidence of PVR is 8% after the first operation, 12% after the second and 18% after the third.

Clinical features

1. *Onset* is typically between the fourth and sixth postoperative weeks.
2. *Symptoms*. After an initial period of visual improvement following successful retinal reattachment the patient reports a sudden and progressive loss of vision, which may develop within a few hours.
3. *Signs*. Ophthalmoscopy usually reveals PVR grade D (*see Figure 9.21*).

Reopening of retinal break

A retinal break may reopen due to inadequate chorioretinal reaction or to late buckle failure.

Inadequate chorioretinal reaction

Small round holes do not usually leak postoperatively, even if they have not been adequately treated by cryotherapy, provided they are located on the buckle. U-shaped tears of moderate to large dimensions may leak postoperatively even though they are initially closed by the buckle, unless they are well surrounded by cryotherapy. This is because persistent traction on the flap of the tear may pull the sensory retina away from the RPE and allow SRF to reaccumulate.

Late buckle failure

This can be due to:

1. Slipping of an encircling element anteriorly or posteriorly.
2. Spontaneous extrusion of the sponge explant.
3. Removal of the sponge explant because of infection or exposure.

New break

Occasionally, new retinal breaks develop in areas of the retina subjected to persistent vitreoretinal traction following local buckling. This is less likely to occur following encircling procedures which give a permanent buckle.

Postoperative complications

These can be divided into early and late. Early complications occur within a few days of surgery and late complications occur within weeks, months or years.

Early

Acute orbital cellulitis

Cause

This rare complication is due to the insertion of a contaminated sponge.

Prevention

Preoperative soaking of the sponge in a bath containing an antibiotic (gentamicin). *Postoperative* subconjunctival injection of gentamicin 20 mg.

Clinical features

1. *Onset*—first few days.
2. *Symptom*—pain.
3. *Signs*—variable eyelid swelling and tenderness, chemosis and mucopurulent discharge.

Treatment

Mild infection may respond to systemic antibiotics such as oral sodium fusidate (Fucidin) 500 mg three times a day or intramuscular methicillin 1 g four times a day. *Severe infection* requires removal of the sponge. This should be delayed for at least 5 days in order to reduce the risk of retinal redetachment.

Choroidal detachment

Cause

This fairly common but usually innocuous complication is due to transudation of choroidal fluid into the potential space between the sclera and uvea (suprachoroidal space).

Predisposing factors

Prolonged severe ocular hypotony

This is invariably associated with drainage of a large volume of SRF. It causes a temporary insufficiency of the choroidal vasculature, resulting in a transudation.

Damage to vortex veins

Such damage, particularly by large posteriorly placed buckles, may occasionally be a contributory factor.

Clinical features

1. *Onset*—during the first 3 days.
2. *Symptoms*—usually are absent.
3. *Signs—see Figure 9.23.*

Treatment

Because the vast majority of choroidal detachments are innocuous and resolve spontaneously within 2 weeks, no specific treatment is usually required.

Vitritis

Cause

Vitritis is a result of excessive cryotherapy due to:

1. Failure to detect the end-point correctly in eyes with bullous RDs, resulting in excessively long applications.
2. Treatment or accidental retreatment of large areas of the retina.

Clinical features

1. *Onset*—usually after the fourth day (later than infection).
2. *Symptoms*—slight pain and hazy vision.

Signs

Vitreous—hazy with the haze initially most intense adjacent to the implant and it then spreads throughout the entire vitreous cavity.

Retina:

1. *Early findings*—at sites of excessive freezing the retina will be oedematous, and occasionally a self-limiting exudative RD may also be present.
2. *Late findings*—severe atrophy of the RPE and choroid. Excessive cryotherapy may also cause dispersion of pigment derived from the RPE into the subretinal space. Following retinal reattachment, multiple subretinal polymorphic black spots may be present. The pigment may also cause a pseudodemarcation line along the border of previously detached and flat retina.

Treatment

Topical and periocular steroids are usually effective. *Systemic steroids* – prednisolone 40 mg daily in divided doses may be necessary in severe cases to speed up resolution.

Bacterial endophthalmitis

This devastating complication is much less common after RD surgery than following cataract extraction.

Causes

1. Entry of bacteria through the sclerotomy site following drainage of SRF.
2. Introduction of bacteria into the eye during intravitreal injection.
3. Entry of bacteria through necrotic sclera—very rare.

Prevention

1. Avoid drainage of the SRF, if possible.
2. Avoid intravitreal injections, if possible.
3. Inject gentamicin 20 mg subconjunctivally at the completion of surgery.

Clinical features

1. *Onset*—usually within 24–48 hours of surgery.
2. *Symptoms*—pain and severe progressive loss of vision.
3. *Signs*—oedema of the eyelids, chemosis, corneal haze, fibrinous exudate in the anterior chamber, hypopyon and vitritis with loss of the red reflex. The appearance of a creamy-white exudate over the buckle is suggestive of intraocular spread of an extraocular infection through a necrotic sclera.

Treatment

This is discussed in Chapter 8.

Late

Exposure of explant

The explant (usually Silastic sponge) may become exposed several weeks or months postoperatively (*Figure 9.42*).

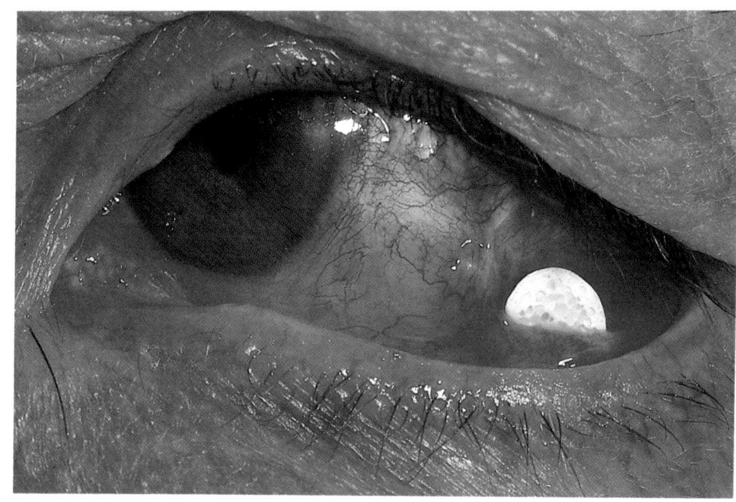

Figure 9.42 *Exposed sponge explant*

Causes

1. *Inadequate coverage* of the sponge with Tenon's capsule and conjunctiva during closure.
2. *Inadequate suturing* of the sponge to the sclera.
3. *Failure to trim the ends of the sponge* so a sharp edge erodes through the conjunctiva.
4. *Large sponge placed too anteriorly.*

Clinical features

1. *Onset*—no specific time.
2. *Symptoms.* The patient may report something white in the eye or that the explant has dropped out.
3. *Signs.* Exposed sponge is evident and chronic conjunctivitis may or may not be present.

Management

1. *Spontaneous complete extrusion.* No specific therapy is required. A short course of topical antibiotics should be administered until the conjunctiva has healed.
2. *Partial extrusion.* Small, loosely attached sponges can be pulled out with forceps following the instillation of a topical anaesthetic.
3. *Large sponges still tightly attached to the sclera.* These may require to be removed under a general anaesthetic.

Infection of explant

Although rare, this is more common than acute early infection.

Causes

1. *Contamination* of the explant at the time of surgery.
2. *Fistula.*

Clinical features

1. *Onset*—at any time.
2. *Symptoms*—pain and tenderness.
3. *Signs.* Erythema over the explant, subconjunctival haemorrhages, local granuloma, chronic conjunctivitis or a fistula may be seen.

Management

The explant is removed, although an associated encircling band may be left *in situ.*

Maculopathy

Following successful surgery the macula may appear clinically normal or specific changes may be seen which may or may not be associated with impaired visual acuity.

Clinical features

1. *Cellophane maculopathy* is characterized by an abnormal reflex at the macula which is not associated with distortion of the surrounding blood vessels. This finding is compatible with normal visual acuity.
2. *Macular pucker* is characterized by an opaque membrane and distortion of blood vessels (*see Figure 11.46*). It is probably a more advanced stage of cellophane maculopathy caused by the proliferation and subsequent contraction of an epiretinal membrane. This complication appears not to be related to the type, extent or duration of RD, nor to the type of surgical procedure, and it may even occur following prophylactic photocoagulation (or, less commonly, cryotherapy). Most eyes with macular pucker have a visual acuity of 6/36 or less.
3. *Pigmentation* due to pigment fallout as a result of excessive cryotherapy is thought not to be responsible for poor visual acuity.

4. *Cystoid macular degeneration* unassociated with leakage of fluorescein from the perifoveal capillaries typically occurs in eyes with long-standing involvement of the macula by SRF. Visual acuity is usually very poor, and when the cystoid changes resolve they are replaced by degenerative lesions involving the RPE without any improvement in visual function.
5. *Atrophic maculopathy* is usually caused by the gravitation of blood in the subretinal space due to intraoperative choroidal haemorrhage.

Extraocular muscle imbalance

Transient diplopia is fairly common during the immediate postoperative period and is a good prognostic sign indicating macular reattachment. Persistent diplopia may be due to one of the following:

1. *Insertion of a large sponge* under one of the rectus muscles—in most cases the diplopia resolves spontaneously after a few weeks and requires no specific therapy apart from reassurance or the temporary use of prisms. Very rarely the sponge has to be removed.
2. *Disinsertion of a rectus muscle* (usually superior or inferior rectus) in order to place a buckle under the muscle. This is now a rare cause of diplopia as muscle disinsertion is usually unnecessary. In persistent cases, strabismus surgery may be required.
3. *Rupture of the muscle belly* due to excessive traction on the sutures. This may cause a complete palsy unless the cut ends can be approximated. Treatment may be very difficult and requires muscle operations on both eyes.
4. *Excessive conjunctival scarring*, usually associated with repeated operations, may cause mechanical restriction of eye movements.
5. *Decompensation of a large heterophoria* due to poor postoperative visual acuity in the operated eye. Strabismus surgery may be required if the decompensation is persistent.

Ptosis

Postoperative stretching of an already attenuated levator aponeurosis by lid oedema may cause a mild aponeurotic ptosis, especially in elderly patients. This is due to the failure of transmission of force from a functioning levator to the upper eyelid.

Management

As the ptosis is usually mild, a Fasanella–Servat procedure is usually sufficient to correct a persistent defect (*see* Chapter 1).

Cataract

Causes

1. Anterior segment necrosis.
2. Injury to the lens during intravitreal injection.
3. Progression of pre-existing lens opacities.
4. Silicone oil.
5. Intraocular gas (SF_6).
6. Persistent RD.

Further reading

Introduction

Foos, R.Y. (1974) Vitreous base, retinal tufts, and retinal tears. In *Retina Congress*, edited by C.D.J. Regan, pp. 259–280. New York: Appleton-Century-Crofts

Grignolo, A., Schepens, C.L. and Health, P. (1957) Cysts of the pars plana ciliaris. Ophthalmoscopic appearance and pathological description. *Archives of Ophthalmology*, **58**, 530–543

Lonn, L.I. and Smith, T.R. (1967) Ora serrata pearls. *Archives of Ophthalmology*, **77**, 809–813

Spencer, L.M., Foos, R.Y. and Straatsma, B.R. (1970) Enclosed bays of the ora serrata. *Archives of Ophthalmology*, **83**, 420–425

Spencer, L.M., Foos, R.Y. and Straatsma, B.R. (1970) Meridional folds, meridional complexes and associated abnormalities of the peripheral retina. *American Journal of Ophthalmology*, **70**, 697–714

Straatsma, B.R., Landers, M.B. and Kreiger, A.E. (1968) The ora serrata in the adult human eye. *Archives of Ophthalmology*, **80**, 3–20

Pathogenesis

Ashrafzadeh, M.T., Schepens, C.L., Elzeneiny, I.H. *et al.* (1973) Aphakic and phakic retinal detachment. *Archives of Ophthalmology*, **89**, 476–483

Benson, W.E., Grand, M.G. and Okun, E. (1975) Aphakic retinal detachment. *Archives of Ophthalmology*, **93**, 245–247

Campbell, C.J. and Rittler, M.C. (1972) Cataract extraction in the retinal detachment prone patient. *American Journal of Ophthalmology*, **73**, 17–21

Eagling, E.M. (1974) Ocular damage due to blunt trauma. *British Journal of Ophthalmology*, **58**, 126–140

Foulds, W.S. (1975) Aetiology of retinal detachment. *Transactions of the Ophthalmological Society of the United Kingdom*, **95**, 118–128

Gregor, Z. and Ryan, S.J. (1982) Combined posterior contusion and penetrating injury in the pig eye. II. Histological features. *British Journal of Ophthalmology*, **66**, 799–804

Jaffe, N.A. (1968) Complications of acute posterior vitreous detachment. *Archives of Ophthalmology*, **79**, 568–571

Jaffe, N.S., Clayman, H.M. and Jaffe, M.S. (1984) Retinal detachment in myopic eyes after intracapsular and extracapsular cataract extraction. *American Journal of Ophthalmology*, **97**, 48–52

Kanski, J.J. (1975) Complications of acute posterior vitreous detachment. *American Journal of Ophthalmology*, **80**, 44–46

Osterlin, S. (1977) Preludes to retinal detachment in the aphakic eye. *Modern Problems in Ophthalmology*, **18**, 464–467

Percival, S.P.B., Anand, V. and Das, S.K. (1983) Prevalence of aphakic retinal detachments. *British Journal of Ophthalmology*, **67**, 43–45

Ruben, M. and Rajpurohit, P. (1976) Distribution of myopia in aphakic retinal detachment. *British Journal of Ophthalmology*, **60**, 517–521

Schepens, C.L. and Marden, S. (1966) Data on the natural history of retinal detachment. *American Journal of Ophthalmology*, **61**, 213–226

Tasman, W.S. (1968) Posterior vitreous detachment and peripheral retinal breaks. *Transactions of the American Academy of Ophthalmology and Otolaryngology*, **72**, 217–224

Clinical features

Benson, W.E., Nantawan, P. and Morse, P.H. (1977) Characteristics and prognosis of retinal detachments with demarcation lines. *American Journal of Ophthalmology*, **84**, 641–644

Boldrey, E.E. (1983) Risk of retinal tears in patients with vitreous floaters. *American Journal of Ophthalmology*, **96,** 783–787
Hagler, W.S. and North, A.W. (1967) Intraretinal macrocysts and retinal detachment. *Transactions of the American Academy of Ophthalmology and Otolaryngology*, **71,** 442–454
Hamilton, A.M. and Taylor, W. (1972) Significance of pigment granules in the vitreous. *British Journal of Ophthalmology*, **56,** 700–702
Kanter, P.J. and Goldberg, M.F. (1974) Bilateral uveitis with exudative retinal detachment. *Archives of Ophthalmology*, **91,** 13–19
Machemer, R. (1978) Pathogenesis and classification of massive periretinal proliferation. *British Journal of Ophthalmology*, **62,** 737–747
Machemer, R., Van Horn, D. and Aaberg, T.M. (1978) Pigment epithelial proliferation in human retinal detachment with massive periretinal proliferation. *American Journal of Ophthalmology*, **85,** 181–191
Morse, P.H. (1974) Fixed retinal star folds in retinal detachment. *American Journal of Ophthalmology*, **78,** 930–934
Retina Society Terminology Committee (1983) The classification of retinal detachment with proliferative vitreoretinopathy. *Ophthalmology*, **90,** 121–125

Prophylaxis of rehgmatogenous retinal detachment

Aaberg, T.M. and Stevens, T.R. (1972) Snail track degeneration of the retina. *American Journal of Ophthalmology*, **73,** 370–376
Byer, N.E. (1974) Changes in and progression of lattice degeneration of the retina. *Transactions of the American Academy of Ophthalmology and Otolaryngology*, **78,** 114–125
Byer, N.E. (1976) The natural history of senile retinoschisis. *Transactions of the American Academy of Ophthalmology and Otolaryngology*, **81,** 458–471
Byer, N.E. (1982) The natural history of asymptomatic retinal breaks. *Opthalmology*, **89,** 1033–1039
Chignell, A.H. and Shilling, J.S. (1973) Prophylaxis of retinal detachment. *British Journal of Ophthalmology*, **57,** 291–298
Davis, M.D. (1974) Natural history of retinal breaks without detachment. *Archives of Ophthalmology*, **92,** 183–194
Govan, J.A.A. (1981) Prophylactic circumferential cryopexy: a retrospective study of 106 eyes. *British Journal of Ophthalmology*, **65,** 364–370
Hagler, W.S. and Waldorff, H.S. (1973) Retinal detachment in relation to senile retinoschisis. *Transactions of the American Academy of Ophthalmology and Otolaryngology*, **77,** 99–113
Kanski, J.J. (1975) Anterior segment complications of retinal photocoagulation. *American Journal of Ophthalmology*, **79,** 424–427
Kanski, J.J. (1978) Prophylaxis of retinal detachment. *Perspectives in Ophthalmology*, **2,** 263–273
Kanski, J.J. and Daniel, R. (1975) Prophylaxis of retinal detachment. *American Journal of Ophthalmology*, **79,** 197–205
Lemesurier, R. and Chignell, A.H. (1981) Prophylaxis of aphakic retinal detachment. *Transactions of the Ophthalmological Society of the United Kingdom*, **101,** 212–213
Morse, P.H. (1974) Lattice degeneration of the retina and retinal detachment. *American Journal of Ophthalmology*, **78,** 930–934
Morse, P.H. and Eagle, R.C. (1975) Pigmentation and retinal breaks. *American Journal of Ophthalmology*, **79,** 190–193
Robertson, D.M. and Norton, E.W.D. (1973) Long term follow up of treated retinal breaks. *American Journal of Ophthalmology*, **75,** 395–404
Robertson, D.M. and Priluck, I.A. (1979) 360° prophylactic cryotherapy. *Archives of Ophthalmology*, **97,** 2130–2134

Surgical principles

Chignell, A.H. (1974) Retinal detachment surgery without drainage of subretinal fluid. *American Journal of Ophthalmology*, **77,** 1–5
Chignell, A.H. and Markham, R.H.C. (1978) Buckling procedures and drainage of subretinal fluid. *Transactions of the Ophthalmological Society of the United Kingdom*, **97,** 474–477
Chignell, A.H. and Markham, R.H.C. (1981) Retinal detachment surgery without cryotherapy. *British Journal of Ophthalmology*, **65,** 371–373
Crick, M.D.P. and Chignell, A.H. (1977) Treatment of rhegmatogenous retinal detachment without apparent holes. *Transactions of the Ophthalmological Society of the United Kingdom*, **97,** 272–275
Grey, R.H.B. and Leaver, P.K. (1979) Silicone oil in the treatment of massive preretinal retraction. 1. Results in 105 eyes. *British Journal of Ophthalmology*, **63,** 355–360
Griffith, R.D., Ryan, E.A. and Hilton, G.F. (1976) Primary retinal detachments without apparent breaks. *American Journal of Ophthalmology*, **81,** 420–427
Grizzard, W.S. and Hilton, G.F. (1982) Scleral buckling for retinal detachments complicated by periretinal proliferation. *Archives of Ophthalmology*, **100,** 419–422
Kanski, J.J. (1975) Giant retinal tears. *American Journal of Ophthalmology*, **79,** 846–852
Lean, J.S. and Chignell, A.H. (1981) Limitations of conventional treatment of fibrotic retinal detachment. *Transactions of the Ophthalmological Society of the United Kingdom*, **101,** 186–188
Leaver, P.K., Cooling, R.J., Feretis, E.B. *et al.* (1984) Virectomy and fluid/silicone-oil exchange for giant retinal tears: results at six months. *British Journal of Ophthalmology*, **68,** 432–438
Lincoff, H.A. and Kreissig, I. (1975) Advantages of radial buckles. *American Journal of Ophthalmology*, **79,** 955–957
Lincoff, H.A., Kreissig, I. and Parver, L. (1976) Limits of constriction in the treatment of retinal detachment. *Archives of Ophthalmology*, **94,** 1473–1477
McLean, E.B. and Norton, E.W.D. (1974) Use of intraocular air and sulfur hexafluoride gas in repair of selected retinal detachments. *Modern Problems in Ophthalmology*, **12,** 428–435
Michels, R.G. (1979) Vitrectomy techniques in retinal reattachment surgery. *Ophthalmology*, **86,** 556–586
Morse, P.H. (1977) Encirclement versus 360° buckling and prognostic factors in retinal separation surgery. *Transactions of the Ophthalmological Society of the United Kingdom*, **97,** 36–38
Pruett, R.C. (1977) The fishmouthing phenomenon. *Archives of Ophthalmology*, **95,** 1777–1787
Scott J.D. (1977) A rationale for use of liquid silicone. *Transactions of the Ophthalmological Society of the United Kingdom*, **97,** 235–237

Surgical techniques

Aaberg, T.M. and Wiznia, R.A. (1976) The use of solid soft silicone rubber exoplants in retinal detachment surgery. *Ophthalmic Surgery*, **7,** 96–105
Birchall, C.H. (1979) The fishmouth phenomenon in retinal detachment: old concepts revisited. *British Journal of Ophthalmology*, **63,** 507–510
Brown, P. and Chignell, A.H. (1982) Accidental drainage of subretinal fluid. *British Journal of Ophthalmology*, **66,** 625–626
Chawla, H.B. (1982) A review of techniques employed in 1100 cases of retinal detachment. *British Journal of Ophthalmology*, **66,** 636–642
Chignell, A.H. (1977) Retinal mobility in retinal detachment surgery. *British Journal of Ophthalmology*, **61,** 446–449
King, L.M. and Schepens, C.L. (1974) Limbal peritomy in retinal detachment surgery. *Archives of Ophthalmology*, **91,** 295–298
Morse, P.H. and Burch, J. (1978) Essentials of scleral buckling surgery. *Perspectives in Ophthalmology*, **2,** 245–250
Scott, J.D. and Stern, W.H. (1979) Radial buckling in posterior retinal tears. *American Journal of Ophthalmology*, **88,** 941–942

Causes of failure and complications

Abraham, R.K. and Shea, M. (1969) Significance of pigment dispersion following cryoretinopexy. Scotoma and atrophy. *Modern Problems in Ophthalmology*, **8,** 455–461

Chignell, A.H., Revie, I.H.S. and Clemett, R.S. (1971) Complications of retinal cryotherapy. *Transactions of the Ophthalmological Society of the United Kingdom*, **91,** 635–651

Cleary, P.E. AND Leaver, P.K. (1978) Macular abnormalities in the reattached retina. *British Journal of Ophthalmology*, **62,** 595–603

Hagler, W.S. and Ataraliya, V. (1971) Macular pucker after retinal detachment surgery. *British Journal of Ophthalmology*, **55,** 441–457

Hahn, Y.S., Lincoff, A., Lincoff, H. *et al.* (1979) Infection after sponge implantation for scleral buckling. *American Journal of Ophthalmology*, **87,** 180–185

Hilton, G.F. (1974) Subretinal pigment migration: effects of cryosurgical retinal reattachment. *Archives of Ophthalmology*, **91,** 445–450

Hilton, G.F. and Wallyn, R.H. (1979) The removal of scleral buckles. *Archives of Ophthalmology*, **96,** 2061–2063

Kanski, J.J., Elkington, A.R. and Davies, M.S. (1973) Diplopia after retinal detachment surgery. *American Journal of Ophthalmology*, **76,** 38–40

Lobes, L.A. Jr and Burton, T.C. (1978) The incidence of macular pucker after retinal detachment surgery. *American Journal of Ophthalmology*, **85,** 72–77

Schwartz, P.L. and Pruett, R.C. (1977) Factors influencing retinal detachment after removal of buckling elements. *Archives of Ophthalmology*, **95,** 804–808

Sewell, J., Knobloch, W.H. and Eifrig, D.E. (1974) Extraocular muscle imbalance after surgical treatment for retinal detachment. *American Journal of Ophthalmology*, **78,** 321–323

Ulrich, R.A. and Burton, T.C. (1974) Infection following scleral buckling procedures. *Archives of Ophthalmology*, **92,** 213–215

10

Retinal Vascular Disorders

Principles of retinal photocoagulation

Wavelengths of light
Ocular pigments
Laser
Xenon
Indications
Complications

Diabetic retinopathy

Introduction
Classification
Background
Maculopathy
Preproliferative
Proliferative
Advanced diabetic eye disease
Pars plana vitrectomy

Retinal vein occlusion

Introduction
Branch vein occlusion
Central vein occlusion

Retinal artery occlusion

Aetiology
Clinical features
Emergency treatment
Cardiovascular investigations
Treatment of carotid disease

Hypertensive retinopathy

Introduction
Hypertensive features
Arteriosclerotic features

Sickle-cell retinopathy

Introduction
Ocular features

Retinopathy of prematurity

Active
Cicatricial (regressed)

Retinal telangiectasias

Introduction
Idiopathic juxtafoveolar retinal telangiectasia
Leber's miliary aneurysms
Coats' disease

Principles of retinal photocoagulation

Photocoagulation is essentially a destructive form of therapy dependent on the absorption of light energy by ocular pigments (melanin, haemoglobin, and xanthophyll) and its conversion into heat energy. The purpose of treatment is to produce a therapeutic burn to a preselected area of the eye while causing minimal damage to surrounding tissues.

Wavelength of light

At present the three main photocoagulators in use are:

1. *Xenon arc* emits white light from 350 to 1600 nm. This is absorbed well by the melanin in the retinal pigment epithelium (RPE) but poorly by haemoglobin and xanthophyll.
2. *Argon laser* emits coherent blue-green light of about 488–515 nm. This is absorbed by all three ocular pigments.
3. *Krypton laser* emits red light at about 647 nm. This is absorbed well by melanin but poorly or not at all by haemoglobin and xanthophyll. The main effect of krypton is on the choroid, RPE and outer retinal layers.

Ocular pigments

1. *Melanin* is present in the cells of the RPE and choroid. The light absorbed by melanin in the RPE is the main source of heat energy in all three types of photocoagulation. Highly pigmented fundi absorb light energy better than pale fundi.
2. *Haemoglobin* best absorbs argon laser energy and is only a significant source of heat when most of the energy is concentrated on a blood vessel.
3. *Xanthophyll* is a yellow pigment present in the inner retinal layers of the macula. It becomes a heat source only when blue argon laser wavelength photocoagulation is applied close to the fovea. This makes treatment inside the foveal avascular zone dangerous. The main advantage of krypton over argon is that it is not absorbed by xanthophyll pigment so that lesions inside the foveal avascular zone and in the papillomacular bundle may be amenable to treatment with less morbidity.

Laser

LASER = Light Amplification by Stimulated Emission of Radiation.

1. *Delivery system* is through a slitlamp. This stereoscopic viewing system and magnification enables more accurate focusing on small targets than when using xenon photocoagulation.
2. *Burn.* The spot size varies from 50 µm to 1000 µm (1 mm). The exposure time can be varied from 0.01 to 5 seconds, and the power setting from 0 to 3 W (0–3000 mW). It must be remembered that the smaller the spot size the greater the energy. Therefore, when changing to a smaller spot size during photocoagulation, the power level must be turned down, and vice versa. This is the reverse to the xenon arc.
3. *Advantages.* Elevated blood vessels can be treated by argon because the light is absorbed by haemoglobin. The small spot size enables lesions close to the fovea to be photocoagulated. This applies particularly to krypton which is not well absorbed by xanthophyll pigment. Because krypton is not absorbed by haemoglobin, it may be possible to treat the retina through vitreous haemorrhage with krypton but not with argon. In addition, krypton is more effectively transmitted through nuclear sclerosis than argon because it is not absorbed by the xanthophyll pigment in the lens.
4. *Disadvantages.* Treatment of large areas of the retina is more time consuming than with xenon, although the 'rapid fire' capability shortens photocoagulation time considerably when performing panretinal photocoagulation (PRP).

Xenon

1. *Delivery system* is through a direct ophthalmoscope and requires a retrobulbar anaesthetic.
2. *Burn.* The three variables are the spot size, duration, and power level. When using the xenon arc, the smaller the spot size, the greater the energy required to produce a given burn, and vice versa. This means that a 1.5° spot has only one-sixteenth the energy of a 6° spot. When the spot size is decreased it is therefore necessary to increase the energy level. The four spot sizes are 1.5°, 3°, 4.5°, and 6°. The 1.5° burn corresponds to 450 µm and the 6° burn to 1800 µm. In practice a retinal burn cannot be produced with the xenon arc using less than 1.5° and a duration shorter than 0.2 second. In photocoagulation with the xenon arc, the power level is determined only after the spot size and duration (usually 0.5 second) have been decided.
3. *Advantages.* The large xenon burn is advantageous when extensive areas of the retina have to be ablated as this can be performed quickly. It is also the treatment of choice when severe tissue destruction is required in the treatment of certain fundus tumours.
4. *Disadvantages.* Although xenon is not significantly absorbed by xanthophyll pigment, it cannot be used close to the fovea because the spot size is too large. The need for a retrobulbar injection is another disadvantage.

Indications

The three main indications for fundus photocoagulation are:

1. *To create adhesions.* This applies mainly to the treatment of predisposing vitreoretinal degenerations and retinal breaks.
2. *To close blood vessels.* This can be done indirectly by panretinal photocoagulation (PRP) in order to reduce or eliminate 'vasoformative substance' in eyes with proliferative retinopathies or by direct destruction of abnormal leaking or bleeding vessels.
3. *To cause tissue necrosis.* This applies mainly in the treatment of certain fundus tumours and in flattening serous elevations of the neurosensory retina or RPE.

In practice the three most frequent indications for fundus photocoagulation are:

1. *Retinal and disc neovascularization* secondary to diabetes or retinal vein occlusion (*see* later).
2. *Retinal breaks and other predisposing lesions (see* Chapter 9).
3. *Subretinal neovascular membranes (see* Chapter 11).

Complications

Posterior segment

1. *Foveal burn* is the most disastrous complication. It usually occurs when treating the temporal retinal periphery with the equatorial mirror. In order to avoid this complication, it is essential to make constant reference to the fovea.
2. *Occlusion of a major vein or artery* is a very rare complication. If the vein is still closed after completion of treatment, the area of the retina drained by the vein should be ablated. Closure of an artery will result in infarction.
3. *Retinal haemorrhage* can usually be stopped by pressing on the contact lens and thereby elevating the intraocular pressure.
4. *Choroidal haemorrhage* may be caused by small high energy laser burns due to rupture of Bruch's membrane. This may later lead to the formation of choroidal subretinal neovascular membranes.
5. *Macular oedema* is fairly common following extensive PRP. Fortunately it usually resolves spontaneously within a few weeks.
6. *Macular pucker* is a more serious complication as it invariably causes a permanent impairment of central vision. It is more common following xenon than argon photocoagulation.
7. *Contraction of fibrous tissue.* Special care should be taken when treating neovascularization associated with large areas of fibrous tissue, because the energy generated may induce contraction of fibrous tissue and subsequent tractional retinal detachment. However, the presence of a localized tractional retinal detachment does not preclude photocoagulation provided argon burns are not applied within 2 disc diameters (3 mm) of the edge of the detachment.
8. *Effects on visual function* include night blindness, altered colour and light brightness appreciation, constriction of visual fields, retinal nerve fibre bundle defects, and a decrease of visual acuity. These effects are more common following xenon than argon treatment.

Anterior segment

1. *Corneal complications* include burns, erosions, superficial punctate keratopathy, striate keratitis and, very occasionally, bullous keratopathy.
2. *Iris complications* are usually caused by inadvertent burns to the iris due to either faulty technique or small pupils. They include iritis, iris atrophy, and damage to the sphincter. The absorption of heat by the posterior pigmented epithelium of the iris may increase the temperature of the aqueous humour and be indirectly responsible for damage to the corneal endothelium.
3. *Lens complications* are rare. Here again increased temperature at the anterior lens surface from energy absorbed by the posterior pigmented iris epithelium is thought to be one of the mechanisms for the development of lens opacities. It also seems likely that ageing lens changes result in decreased transmission and increased absorption of light energy of the argon laser. This, combined with high-power, long duration exposures and difficulty in focusing due to poor visualization, may be sufficient to elevate the temperature of the anterior lens surface to a level capable of causing lens damage. Photocoagulation with the krypton laser may be safer in patients with lens opacities as penetration of xanthophyll pigment in the lens is easier.
4. *Shallowing of the anterior chamber* may occur following PRP within 48 hours of treatment. This is invariably associated with an annular ciliochoroidal detachment, although the exact relationship between these two events is unclear. The shallowing of the anterior chamber is associated with a variable myopia, and occasionally anterior displacement of the iris–lens diaphragm may lead to angle-closure glaucoma. Treatment is with acetazolamide until spontaneous resolution occurs, usually within 10 days.

Diabetic retinopathy

Introduction

Diabetes occurs either because of lack of insulin or due to the presence of factors that oppose the action of insulin. The end result is an increase in blood glucose concentration (hyperglycaemia). Nearly all diabetics have 'primary' diabetes which may be of two types:

1. *Insulin-dependent (type 1) diabetes* is due to damage to the beta-cells of the pancreatic islets of Langerhans. It is not directly inherited, although individuals may inherit a predisposition associated with certain HLA types. The peak incidence is 10–20 years although elderly patients can also be insulin dependent.
2. *Non-insulin-dependent (type 2) diabetes* has no known cause, although in many cases there is a strong genetic component, unrelated to the HLA system. It is most prevalent after middle age and occurs most frequently between the ages of 50 and 70 years, although there is a certain amount of overlap between the two types of diabetes.

In the United Kingdom 1–2% of the population have diabetes—about half are known to have the condition and the rest can be estimated by population studies.

Important facts

1. The risk of blindness is about 25 times greater in diabetics than in non-diabetics.
2. Diabetic retinopathy (DR) is the commonest cause of legal blindness in individuals between the ages of 20 and 65 years.
3. The incidence of DR is related more to the duration of diabetes than to any other factor. In patients diagnosed as diabetic prior to the age of 30 years, 50% will have DR after 10 years, and 90% will have DR after 30 years.

Pathogenesis

DR is essentially a microangiopathy affecting the retinal precapillary arterioles, the capillaries, and the venules. However, larger vessels may also become involved. The retinopathy has features of both microvascular occlusion and leakage. Despite long and extensive research, the pathogenesis of DR is still a matter for much speculation.

Microvascular occlusion

Aetiology

Some of the postulated interrelated factors responsible for or associated with microvascular occlusion (*Figure 10.1*) include:

1. Thickening of the capillary basement membrane—this is a well-documented histopathological change in diabetics.
2. Capillary endothelial cell damage and proliferation.
3. Changes in red blood cells leading to defective oxygen transport.
4. Increased stickiness and aggregation of platelets.

Consequences (*Figure 10.2*)

The most important consequence of retinal capillary non-perfusion is retinal ischaemia which, in turn, causes retinal hypoxia. Initially, the non-perfused area is located in the midretinal periphery. The two main effects of retinal hypoxia are the formation of arteriovenous shunts (communications) and neovascularization.

1. *Arteriovenous shunts* are due to a significant amount of capillary occlusion ('drop-out'). They run a straight course from venule to arteriole. Because it is unclear whether or not these lesions represent actual intraretinal new vessels, they are often referred to as 'intraretinal microvascular abnormalities' (IRMA).
2. *Neovascularization* is thought to be due to a 'vasoformative substance' elaborated by hypoxic retinal tissue in an attempt to revascularize hypoxic areas of the retina. For reasons that are not yet clear, this substance is not only capable of promoting neovascularization on the retina and optic nerve head (proliferative DR), but also on the iris (rubeosis iridis).

Microvascular leakage

Aetiology

The cellular elements of retinal capillaries are of two types: endothelial cells and pericytes (mural cells). The tight junctions of the endothelial cells constitute the inner blood–retinal barrier as they prevent the passage of large molecules across the vessel wall. The pericytes, which are wrapped around the capillaries, are thought to be responsible for the structural integrity of the vessel wall itself. In normal healthy individuals, there is one pericyte to each endothelial cell. In diabetic patients, there is a reduction in the number of pericytes which is thought to be responsible for distension of the capillary wall and disruption of the blood–retinal barrier leading to leakage of plasma constituents into the retina. Microaneurysms are saccular pouches which may form as a result of local capillary distension. They may either leak or become thrombosed.

Recent studies using quantitative fluorophotometry have documented a breakdown in the blood–retinal barrier prior to the appearance of angiographically or ophthalmoscopically demonstrable lesions. It has also been suggested that the blood–retinal barrier at the level of the retinal pigment epithelium may be altered in diabetes.

Consequences

The two consequences of increased vascular permeability are haemorrhage and retinal oedema (*Figure 10.3*). The latter may be diffuse or localized.

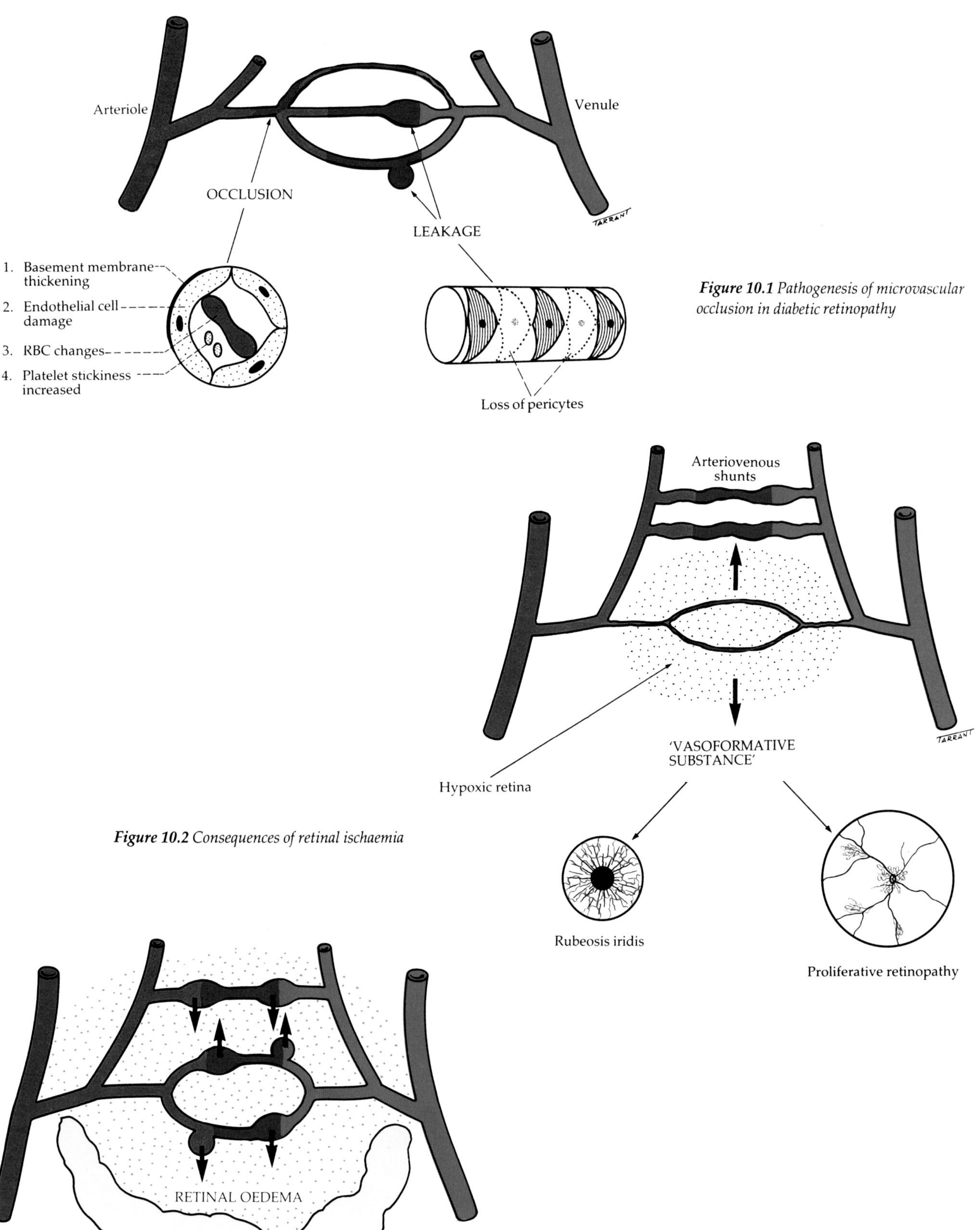

Figure 10.1 *Pathogenesis of microvascular occlusion in diabetic retinopathy*

Figure 10.2 *Consequences of retinal ischaemia*

Figure 10.3 *Consequences of retinal vascular leakage*

1. *Diffuse retinal oedema* is due to extensive capillary dilatation and leakage.
2. *Localized retinal oedema* is due to focal leakage from microaneurysms. Chronic localized retinal oedema leads to the deposition of hard exudates at the junction of healthy and oedematous retina. The exudates, which are composed of lipoprotein and lipid-laden macrophages, typically form in a circinate pattern. In some eyes they absorb spontaneously over a period of months or years, either into the healthy surrounding capillaries or by phagocytosis of their lipid content. In other cases, more chronic extravasation leads to enlargement of the exudates and the deposition of cholesterol.

Classification

Background
Maculopathy
  focal
  diffuse
  ischaemic
Preproliferative
Proliferative
Advanced diabetic eye disease
  persistent vitreous haemorrhage
  retinal detachment
  opaque membrane formation
  neovascular glaucoma

Background

Clinical features (*Figure 10.4*)

Microaneurysms

These are located in the inner nuclear layer of the retina and are the first clinically detectable lesions of DR, appearing as small round dots, usually located temporal to the macula. They vary in size from 20 to 200 µm in diameter and, when coated with blood, they may be indistinguishable from dot haemorrhages.

Haemorrhages

The clinical appearance of haemorrhages (*Figure 10.5*) depends on their location within the retina. 'Dot' and 'blot' haemorrhages originate from the venous end of the capillaries and are therefore located within the compact middle layers of the retina. Flame-shaped haemorrhages, which originate from the more superficial precapillary arterioles, follow the course of the retinal nerve fibre layer.

Hard exudates

These are located between the inner plexiform and inner nuclear layers of the retina. They vary in size, have a yellow waxy appearance with relatively distinct margins, and are frequently distributed in a circinate pattern peripheral to areas of chronic focal leakage (*Figure 10.6*). The centres of rings of hard exudates usually contain microaneurysms.

Retinal oedema

This is due to increased permeability of the retinal capillaries and is characterized by retinal thickening. Macular oedema is the most common cause of visual impairment in patients with background DR. Initially, the oedema is located between the outer plexiform and inner nuclear layers. Later it may involve the inner plexiform and nerve fibre layers, until eventually the entire thickness of the retina may become oedematous. Clinically, retinal oedema is best detected by slitlamp biomicroscopy combined with a Hruby lens, a fundus contact lens, or a +90 D (Volk) lens. On examination, the thickened oedematous retina obscures visualization of the underlying retinal pigment epithelium and choroid. With further accumulation of fluid, the macula assumes a cystoid appearance. The Diabetic Retinopathy Study defined 'clinically significant' macular oedema as follows:

1. Retinal oedema within 500 µm of the fovea.
2. Hard exudates within 500 µm of the fovea, if associated with adjacent retinal oedema.
3. Retinal oedema 1 disc area (1500 µm) or larger, any part of which is within 1 disc diameter of the fovea.

Management

Although there is no medical cure for DR, certain measures may be helpful.

1. *Good metabolic control.* There is increasing evidence to suggest that good initial control of diabetes retards, but does not prevent, the development of DR. It may also have a beneficial effect in established cases, particularly in type 1 patients receiving divided insulin injections.
2. *Hypertension.* Strict control of systemic hypertension is important in all diabetic patients in order to prevent detrimental effects to the retinal circulation.
3. *Anaemia* should also be treated as its presence may worsen DR.
4. *Aspirin and dipyridamole (Persantin)* decrease platelet stickiness and may have beneficial effects.

At present most ophthalmologists do not treat patients with simple background DR and normal visual acuity but merely perform an annual examination. In some cases, however, treatment may be instituted at an early stage if there is good evidence that central vision is threatened by the progression of oedema or hard exudates towards the fovea.

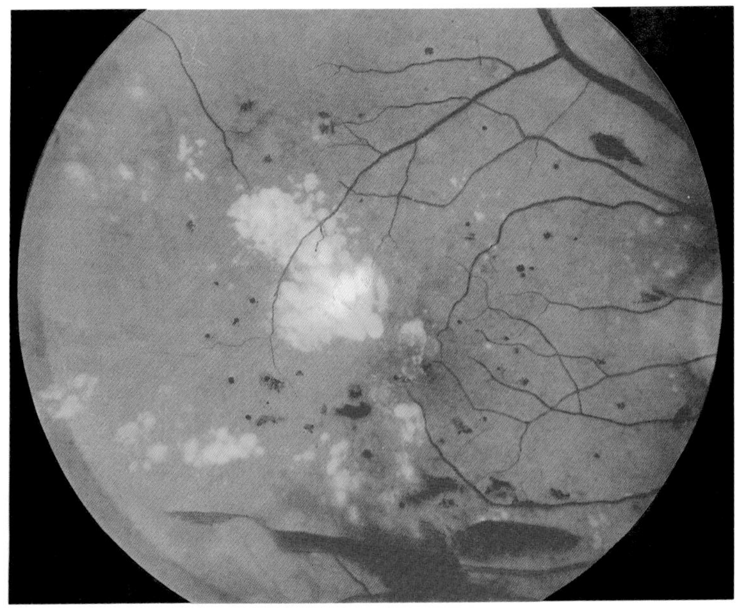

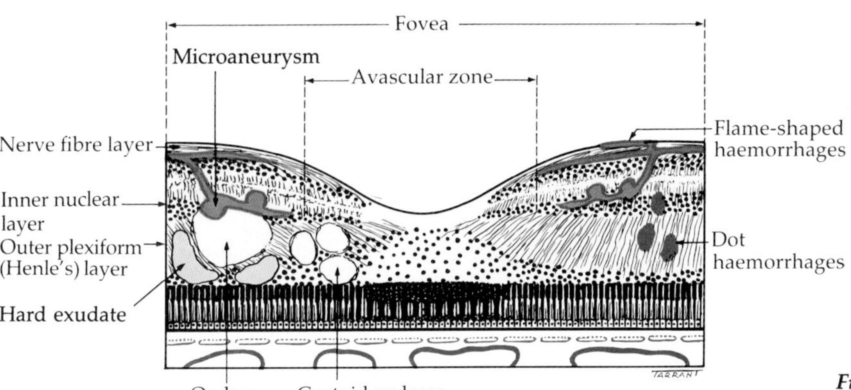

Figure 10.4 *Background diabetic retinopathy*

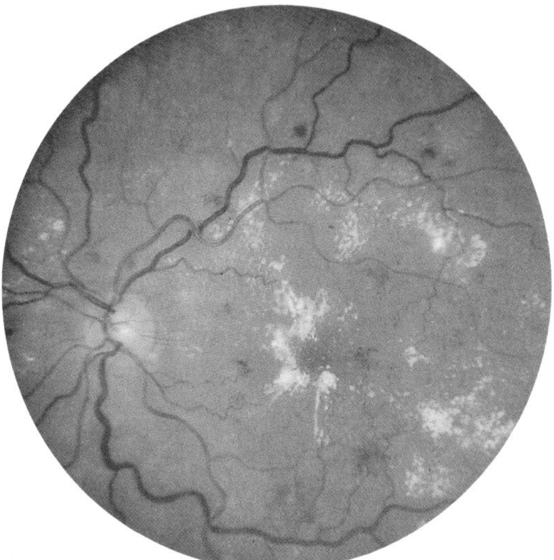

Figure 10.5 *Moderate background diabetic retinopathy showing microaneurysms, dot and blot haemorrhages and hard exudates*

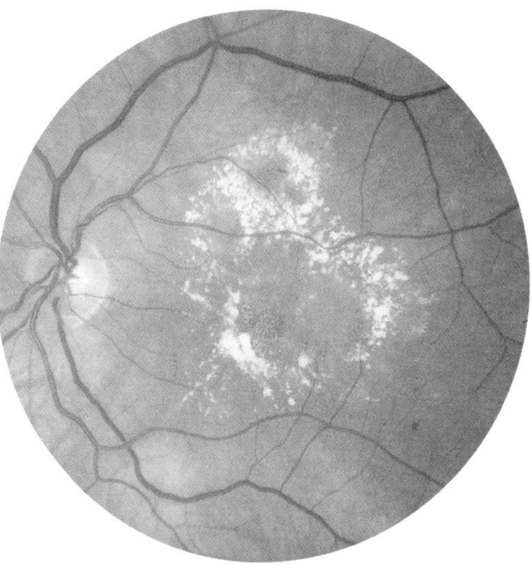

Figure 10.6 *Background diabetic retinopathy with hard exudates arranged in circinate rings*

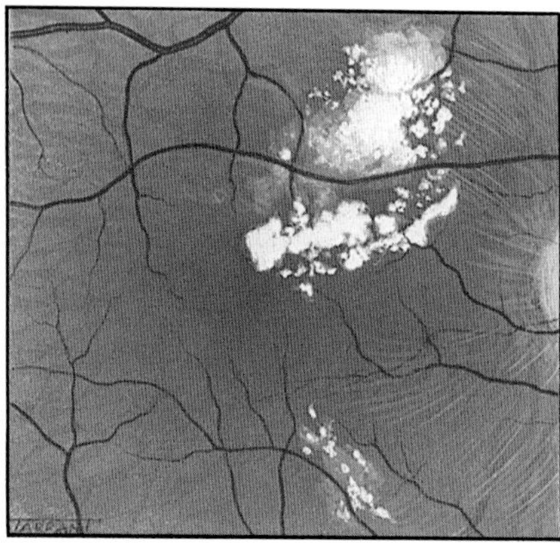

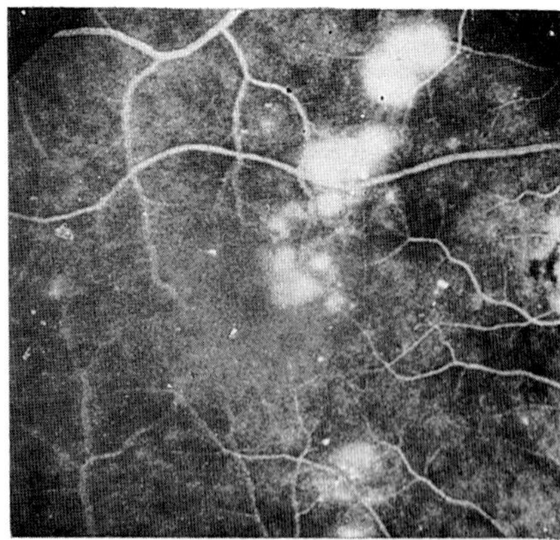

Figure 10.7 Focal diabetic maculopathy (courtesy of Mr R. Whitelocke and Editor of Transactions of the Ophthalmological Society of the UK)

Maculopathy

Maculopathy is the commonest cause of visual impairment in patients with DR, and is more frequent in type 2 diabetes. The three main types are focal, diffuse, and ischaemic.

Focal

Clinical features

This is caused by focal leakage from microaneurysms and dilated capillary segments. It is characterized by the presence of background DR associated with mild macular oedema and surrounding hard exudates (*Figure 10.7, left*). Visual impairment is caused by the 'spill-over' of oedema and/or exudates into the fovea. Usually there is a delay before the foveola itself becomes involved and visual acuity severely impaired.

Fluorescein angiography

This demonstrates focal areas of leakage, but adequate macular capillary perfusion (*Figure 10.7, right*). In the majority of cases, however, pre-treatment angiography is unnecessary because the site of primary leakage is usually evident clinically.

Treatment

Technique

The pupil is dilated with a combination of tropicamide 1% and phenylephrine 10%. Focal argon laser burns are then applied to individual microvascular malformations and centres of hard exudate rings (*Figure 10.8*). The spot size is between 50 and 200 μm with a duration of 0.1 second or less, with sufficient power to obtain definite whitening around the microaneurysm or leakage site. For all microaneurysms greater than 40 μm in diameter, an attempt should be made to either whiten or darken the microaneurysm itself.

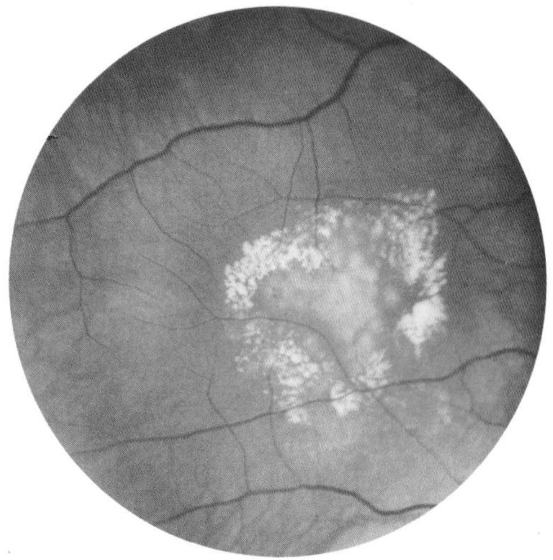

Figure 10.8 Laser burns applied to centre of ring of hard exudates

Results

In general, the results of treatment of focal diabetic maculopathy are reasonably good with resolution of retinal oedema and exudates with either stabilization or improvement of visual acuity in a significant proportion of cases. Patients who are treated early while they still have reasonably good visual acuity do much better than those treated late.

Diffuse

Clinical features

This is caused by leakage from diffusely dilated capillaries throughout the posterior pole. It is characterized by generalized retinal thickening in association with microaneurysms and haemorrhages but with relatively few, if any, hard exudates. In long-standing severe cases, microcystic spaces (cystoid macular oedema) (*Figure 10.9, left*) develop at the fovea which may subsequently result in a permanent impairment of visual acuity due to the formation of a lamellar hole.

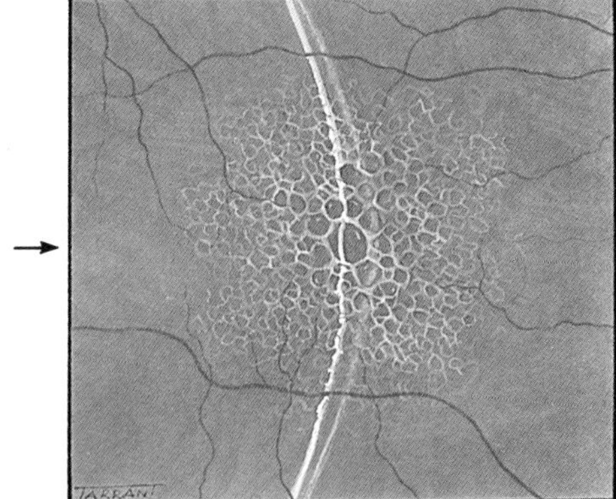

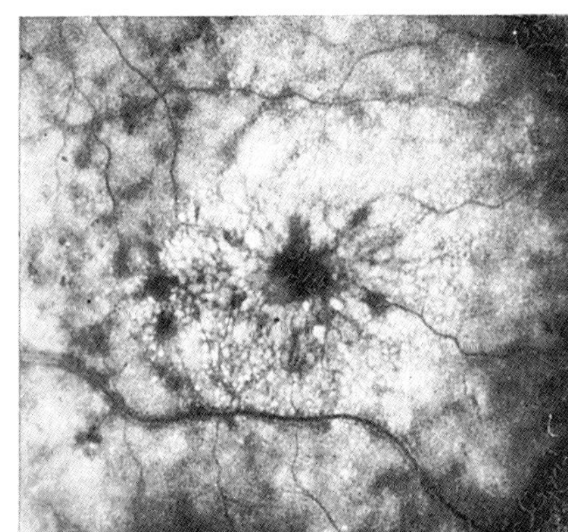

Figure 10.9 *Diffuse diabetic maculopathy (courtesy of Mr R. Whitelocke and Editor of* Transactions of the Ophthalmological Society of the UK)

Fluorescein angiography

This shows diffuse leakage at the posterior pole (*Figure 10.10a*). The presence of cystoid macular oedema is characterized by the typical 'flower-petal' pattern of leakage (*Figure 10.9, right*).

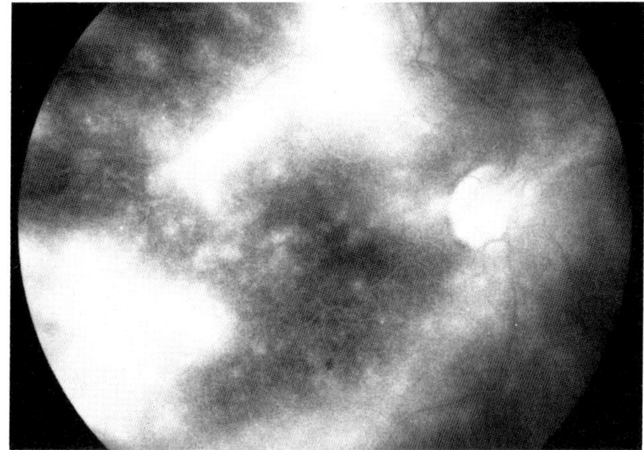

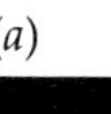

(*a*)

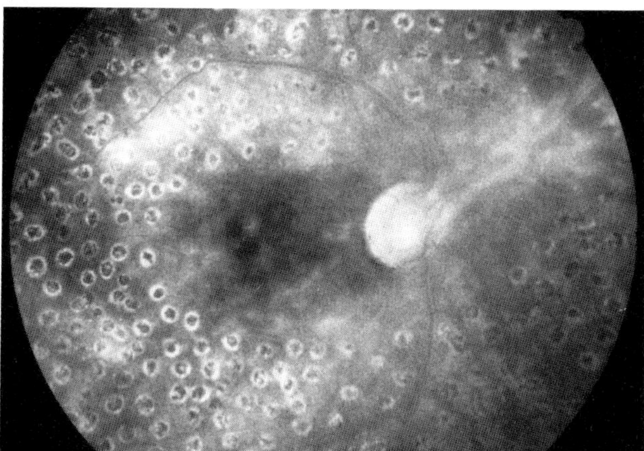

(*b*)

Figure 10.10 (a) *Fluorescein angiogram showing diffuse maculopathy;* (b) *fluorescein angiogram of same eye following grid laser photocoagulation showing resolution*

Treatment

Technique

This is with a grid pattern of between 150 and 200 low intensity burns applied to the macula but avoiding the fovea (*Figure 10.10b*). The spot size is between 50 and 200 μm with a duration of between 0.05 and 0.10 second. A space one burn wide is left between each lesion. The burns may be placed in the papillomacular bundle but not closer than 500 μm from the foveola. The exact indications for this type of treatment have still to be established by further trials. Occasionally, strict control of diabetes, associated hypertension, or renal failure may result in resolution of oedema and some improvement of visual acuity.

Results

These are much less favourable than for focal maculopathy.

Ischaemic

Clinical features

The ophthalmoscopical findings in ischaemic maculopathy may be similar to those seen in diffuse maculopathy (microaneurysms, haemorrhages, relatively few hard exudates, and macular oedema varying from mild to cystoid). Fluorescein angiography is therefore necessary in making the differentiation (*Figure 10.11*). In ischaemic maculopathy, fluorescein angiography will reveal areas of capillary non-perfusion in the macular and paramacular regions, whereas in diffuse maculopathy the macula is relatively well perfused.

Treatment

Treatment by photocoagulation will not improve vision. However, follow-up of these eyes is essential because approximately 30% will develop proliferative diabetic retinopathy within 2 years.

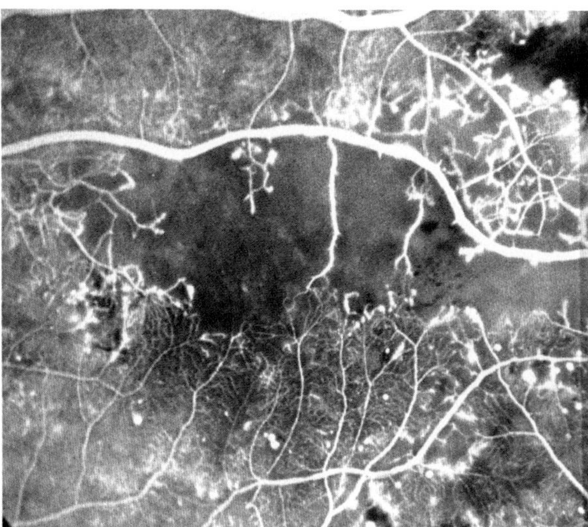

Figure 10.11 Fluorescein angiogram of ischaemic diabetic maculopathy (courtesy of Mr R. Whitelocke)

Indicators of poor prognosis

1. Diffuse leakage.
2. Capillary non-perfusion at macula.
3. Cystoid macular oedema, macular hole, and macular pucker.
4. Foveal exudate, haemorrhage, or changes in the retinal pigment epithelium.
5. Renal failure.

Preproliferative

Clinical features

Preproliferative DR develops in some eyes that initially show only simple background DR. All lesions are caused by retinal ischaemia (*Figure 10.12*).

1. *Cotton-wool spots* are due to capillary occlusion in the retinal nerve fibre layer. The interruption of axoplasmic flow caused by the ischaemia and the subsequent build-up of transported material within the nerve axons is responsible for the white and opaque appearance of these lesions.
2. *IRMA* (intraretinal microvascular abnormalities) are frequently seen adjacent to areas of capillary closure. Clinically, IRMA may resemble focal areas of flat retinal neovascularization. The main distinguishing features of IRMA are: their intraretinal location, absence of profuse leakage on fluorescein angiography, and failure to cross over major retinal blood vessels.
3. *Venous changes* consisting of dilatation, 'beading', 'looping', and 'sausage-like' segmentation are important preproliferative findings.
4. *Arteriolar narrowing* and even obliteration resembling branch retinal artery occlusion may occasionally be seen.
5. *Large dark blot haemorrhages* representing haemorrhagic retinal infarcts may also be present.

Treatment

Patients with preproliferative changes should be watched very closely as a significant number develop proliferative DR. Treatment by photocoagulation is usually unnecessary unless fluorescein angiography shows extensive areas of peripheral capillary non-perfusion in a patient who has lost sight in the fellow eye from complications of proliferative DR. This applies particularly to patients with the so-called 'florid' type of proliferative DR in whom blindness can occur very rapidly. In these patients, gentle argon laser burns are applied to areas of capillary non-perfusion or in a panretinal pattern (*see* later).

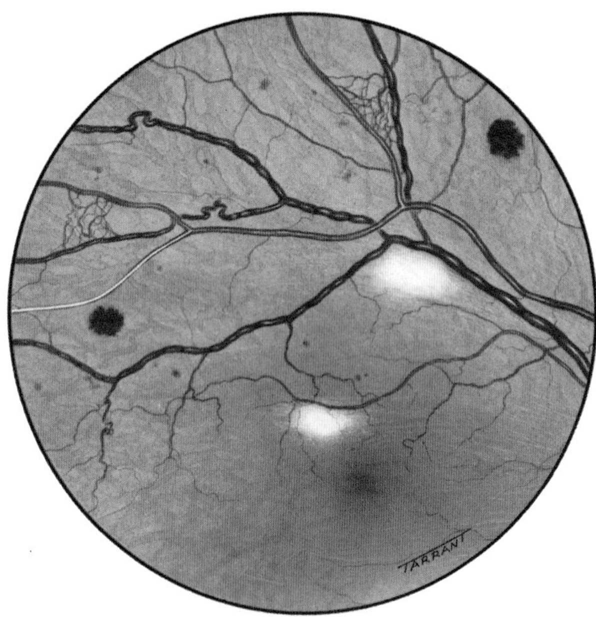

Figure 10.12 Preproliferative diabetic retinopathy

Proliferative

Clinical features

Proliferative diabetic retinopathy (PDR) affects about 5% of the diabetic population. Patients with juvenile-onset diabetes are at increased risk of PDR with an incidence of about 60% after 30 years.

Neovascularization

This is the hallmark of PDR. New vessels may proliferate on the optic nerve head (NVD = new vessels at disc), and along the course of the major temporal vascular arcades (NVE = new vessels elsewhere) (*Figure 10.13, right*). It has been estimated that over one-quarter of the retina has to be non-perfused before NVD will appear. The absence of the internal limiting membrane (ILM) over the optic nerve head may partially explain the predilection for neovascularization at this site. The new vessels start as endothelial

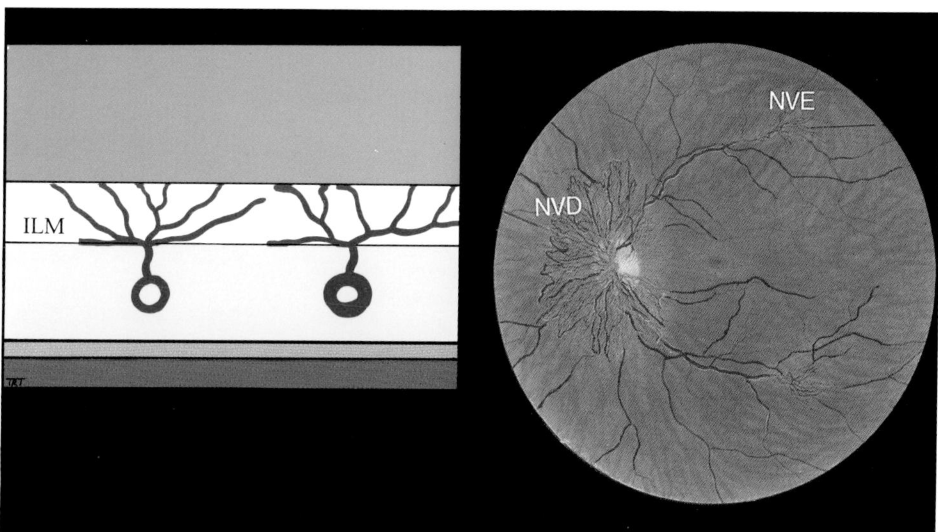

Figure 10.13
Proliferative diabetic retinopathy

proliferations arising from veins. In the retina, they pass through defects in the ILM to lie in the potential vitreoretinal space (*Figure 10.13, left*). The mesenchyme from which the new vessels are derived is also the source of fibroblasts which envelop the vessels forming a fibrovascular epiretinal membrane. Initially, the fibrous component (which has the potential to contract) is difficult to detect ophthalmoscopically, but later it becomes more opaque and obvious.

Vitreous detachment

Vitreous changes play an extremely important role in the progression of PDR (*Figure 10.14, left*). The fibrovascular network becomes adherent to the posterior vitreous face and leaks plasma constituents into the adjacent vitreous gel. If at this stage the vitreous becomes totally detached the new vessels may regress, although unfortunately this is a rare occurrence. Usually, owing to the strong attachments of the cortical vitreous gel to areas of fibrovascular proliferation, posterior vitreous detachment is incomplete. Initially, traction at these sites by contracting vitreous gel causes elevation of the vessels above the plane of the retina. The fibrovascular tissue then continues to proliferate along the posterior surface of the partially detached vitreous and is pulled further and further into the vitreous cavity until bleeding occurs. Until the onset of vitreous haemorrhage PDR is completely *asymptomatic* and can only be detected by routine eye examination.

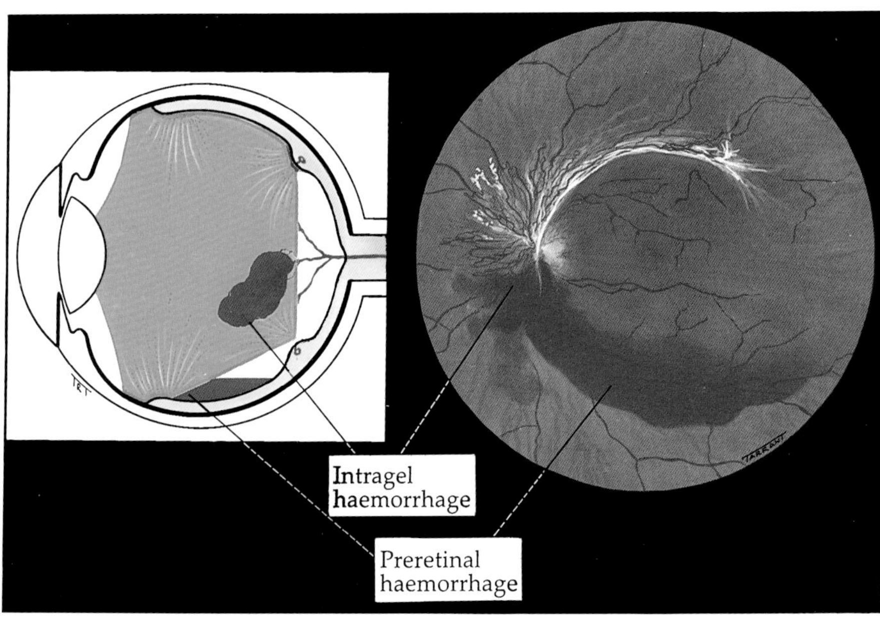

Figure 10.14
Vitreous and preretinal haemorrhage in proliferative diabetic retinopathy

Haemorrhage

Bleeding may occur into the vitreous gel (intragel haemorrhage), or more frequently into the retrohyaloid space (preretinal haemorrhage). A preretinal haemorrhage has a crescentic shape which demarcates the level of posterior vitreous detachment (*Figure 10.14, right*). Occasionally, a preretinal haemorrhage may penetrate into the vitreous gel. Intragel haemorrhages usually take longer to clear than preretinal haemorrhages. In some eyes altered blood becomes compacted in the posterior gel to form an 'ochre membrane'.

Management

Patients should be warned that occasionally vitreous haemorrhage may be precipitated by severe physical exertion or strain, hypoglycaemia, and direct ocular trauma. However, not infrequently bleeding occurs while the patient is asleep. Pregnancy may have a worsening effect on PDR, although once the retinopathy has been successfully treated by photocoagulation, there is no reason to discourage further pregnancies.

Photocoagulation is now by far the most important modality for the treatment of PDR (hypophysectomy having been largely abandoned). Either xenon arc or argon laser photocoagulation can be used although laser is now much more popular.

Pre-treatment evaluation

1. *Amount of fibrous tissue* (*Figure 10.15*). When evaluating eyes with PDR it is important to bear in mind that those with naked new vessels are more likely to bleed, whereas those with significant fibrous proliferation are more at risk from tractional retinal detachment. Because photocoagulation only influences the vascular component of the fibrovascular process, eyes in which the vascular component has regressed leaving only fibrous remnants should not be treated. However, these eyes should still be watched for the possible development of tractional retinal detachment. In addition, large areas of capillary non-perfusion, which are usually also present in these eyes, may occasionally be responsible for fresh neovascularization.
2. *Location of new vessels.* NVD are more dangerous than NVE as they have a greater propensity to bleed.
3. *Severity of neovascularization* is determined by the area covered by the new vessels in comparison with the diameter of the optic disc. The calibre and density of the new vessels should be assessed, and it should be noted whether the new vessels are flat or elevated (elevated new vessels being less responsive to treatment).
4. *Vitreous separation.* If possible, the extent of vitreous separation in relation to the fibrovascular tissue should be assessed using slitlamp biomicroscopy with a fundus contact lens.

Assessment of prognosis

1. *NVD.* Untreated eyes with severe NVD and vitreous haemorrhage have about a 40% risk of severe visual loss within 2 years; with appropriate treatment the risk is halved. In these cases the benefits of treatment far outweigh the possible risks of side-effects from the treatment itself and all such eyes should therefore be treated. Treatment is also recommended for eyes with moderate (*Figure 10.16*) to severe (*Figure 10.17*) NVD in the absence of bleeding, as in these cases photocoagulation reduces the risk of severe visual loss from 25% to 5%.
2. *NVE.* Eyes with mild NVE without vitreous haemorrhage have only a 7% risk of severe visual loss in 2 years (*Figure 10.18*). In these cases, the possible risk of photocoagulation-induced side-effects is less acceptable.

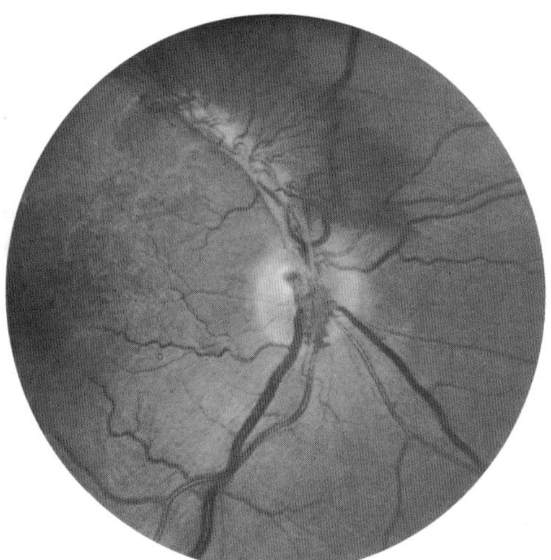

Figure 10.15 *Severe fibrovascular proliferation extending from optic disc to superotemporal arcade*

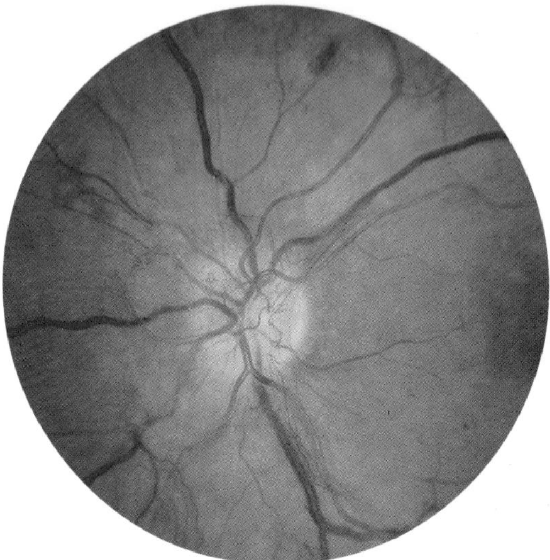

Figure 10.16 *Proliferative diabetic retinopathy with moderate flat disc new vessels*

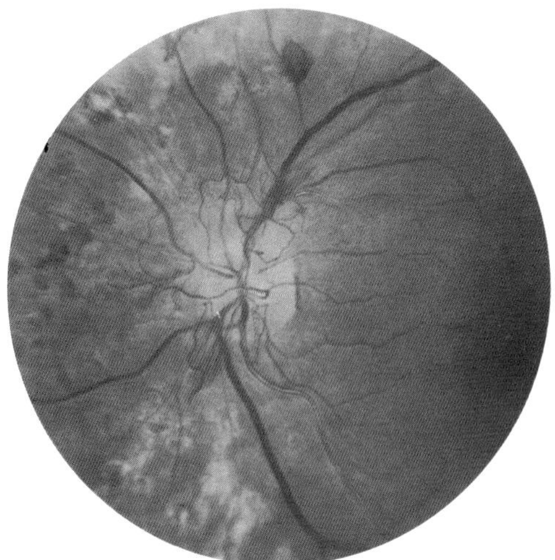

Figure 10.17 *Severe disc new vessels. Scars from panretinal photocoagulation are also present*

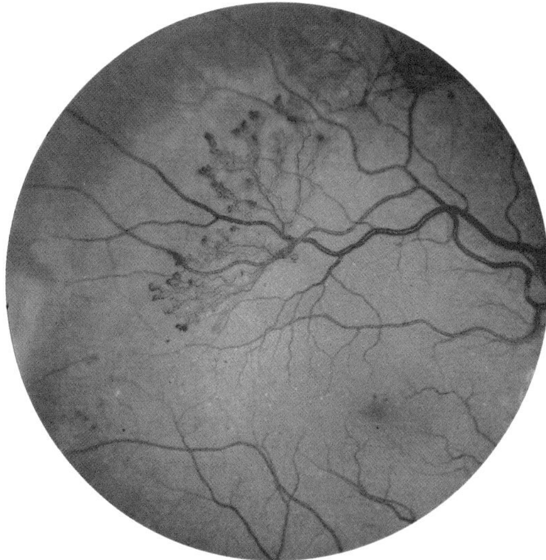

Figure 10.18 *Proliferative diabetic retinopathy with moderate retinal new vessels*

If the fellow eye has good vision and similar mild changes, treatment may be withheld and the patient followed up at 3-monthly intervals. However, treatment should be considered if the fellow eye is blind from advanced diabetic eye disease. Eyes with severe NVE and vitreous haemorrhage have a 30% risk of blindness within 2 years. Treatment reduces this risk to about 7% and is therefore recommended.

Argon laser photocoagulation

The preferred method of treatment of PDR is by argon laser panretinal photocoagulation (PRP) with a slitlamp delivery system. The aim of treatment is to induce involution of new vessels and to prevent recurrent vitreous haemorrhage. The extent of PRP is dependent on the severity of PDR. Initial treatment involves the placement of about 2000–3000 burns in a scatter pattern extending from the posterior fundus to the equator, either in one session or in two or more sessions, 1 week apart. PRP completed in one session carries a slightly higher risk of complications. Not infrequently, the amount of treatment during any one session is governed by the patient's pain threshold and ability to maintain concentration.

Technique

1. The cornea is anaesthetized. A retrobulbar is usually unnecessary.
2. The laser is set at a spot size of 500 μm, a duration of 0.2 second, and a power of 200 mW.
3. The fundus is visualized either with a Goldmann triple-mirror lens or a panfunduscope. The techniques of insertion and the main difference between the two lenses are discussed in Chapter 9.
4. The initial burns are placed in a double arc about 2 disc diameters temporal to the centre of the macula. This serves as a visual barrier against an accidental burn to the fovea.
5. The area nasal to the disc is then treated with burns spaced about one half burn apart. If necessary, the power setting is increased by 50 mW increments until a grey-white burn of moderate intensity is produced. In eyes with NVD, the burns should be placed up to the edge of the optic disc and in those without NVD the burns are placed not nearer than 2 disc diameters from the edge of the optic disc. Flat NVE unassociated with fibrous tissue may be treated directly with confluent medium intensity 500 μm burns.
6. Photocoagulation is applied outside the temporal vascular arcades and then temporal to the macula until the entire area up the equator has been covered (*Figure 10.19*).

Follow-up

The patient is examined 4 and 8 weeks after treatment. This is because new vessels usually take between 4 to 8 weeks to regress after adequate PRP. In eyes with severe NVD, several treatment sessions with up to 3500 burns may be required to induce involution, although in some cases complete elimination of NVD may be extremely difficult. It should, however, be emphasized that the most important cause of persistent neovascularization is inadequate treatment.

Signs of involution

Clinical features of good response to PRP are (*Figure 10.20b*):

1. Regression of neovascularization leaving only 'ghost' vessels or fibrous tissue.
2. Decrease in venous dilatation.
3. Absorption of retinal haemorrhages.
4. Pallor of the optic disc.

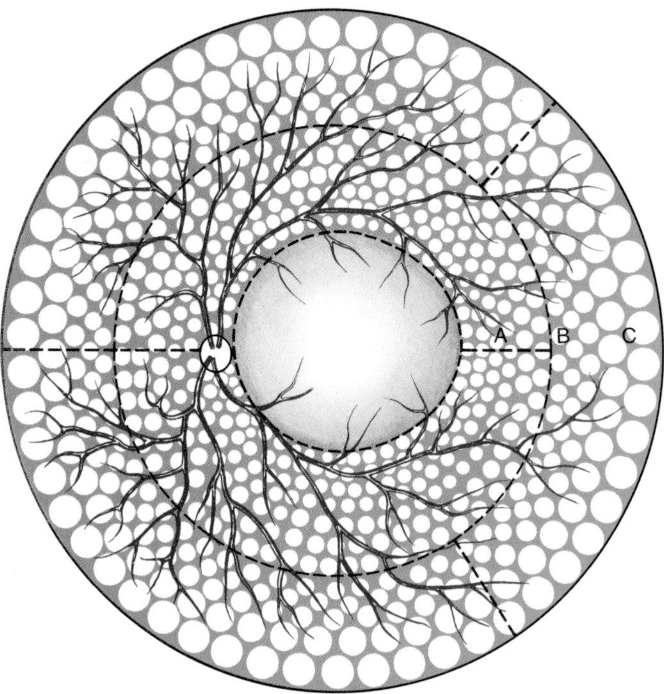

Figure 10.19 *Completed panretinal photocoagulation*

In most eyes, once the retinopathy is quiescent, stable vision is maintained. In a few eyes recurrences of PDR occur despite an initial satisfactory response. It is therefore necessary to re-examine the patient at about 6-monthly intervals so that any recurrences can be detected and treated.

Treatment of recurrence

The three options are:

1. Further argon laser PRP filling in any gaps between previous laser scars.
2. Xenon arc photocoagulation applied over previous laser scars.
3. Cryotherapy to the anterior retina. This is particularly useful when further photocoagulation is impossible because of inadequate visualization of the fundus. It also offers a means of treating areas of the retina usually left untreated by photocoagulation.

Advanced diabetic eye disease

This is the end result of uncontrolled PDR.

Clinical features

Persistent vitreous haemorrhage

Intragel bleeding may induce syneresis and further shrinkage of the vitreous and promote the development of tractional retinal detachment.

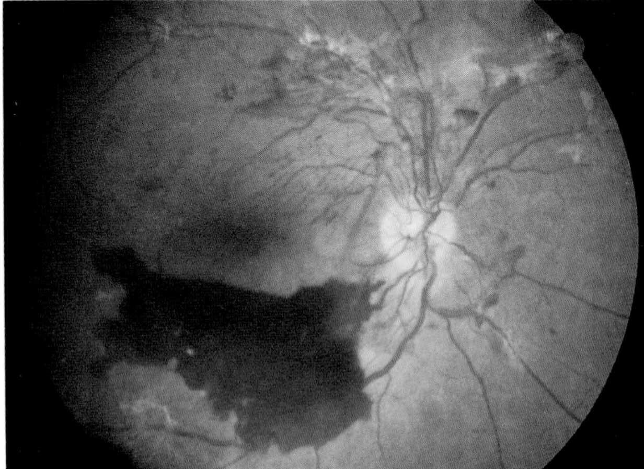

(*a*)

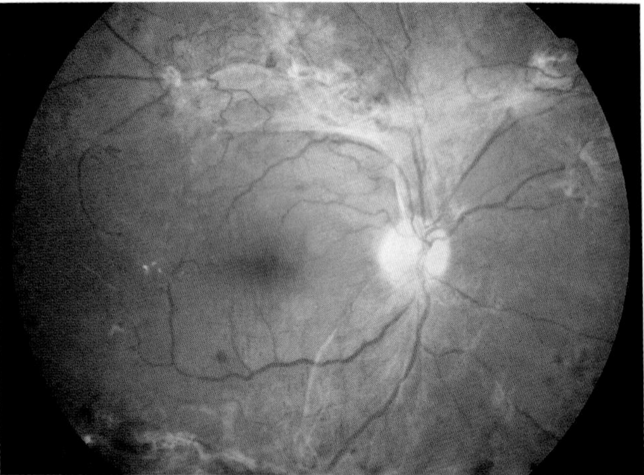

(*b*)

Figure 10.20 (a) *Severe proliferative diabetic retinopathy and preretinal haemorrhage;* (b) *regression of neovascularization following panretinal photocoagulation (note residual fibrous tissue)*

Retinal detachment

This is a devastating complication of PDR. It is caused by progressive contraction of fibrovascular membranes over large areas of vitreoretinal adhesion. Three main types of vitreoretinal traction are recognized:

1. *Tangential traction* is caused by contraction of epiretinal fibrovascular membranes and may be responsible for puckering of the retina with distortion of retinal vessels.
2. *Anteroposterior traction* (*Figure 10.21, left*) is caused by the contraction of fibrovascular membranes which extend from the posterior retina, usually from the major temporal arcades, towards the vitreous base.
3. *Bridging traction* (*Figure 10.22, left*) is due to contraction of fibrovascular (trampoline) membranes that stretch from a part of the retina posterior to the equator, to another.

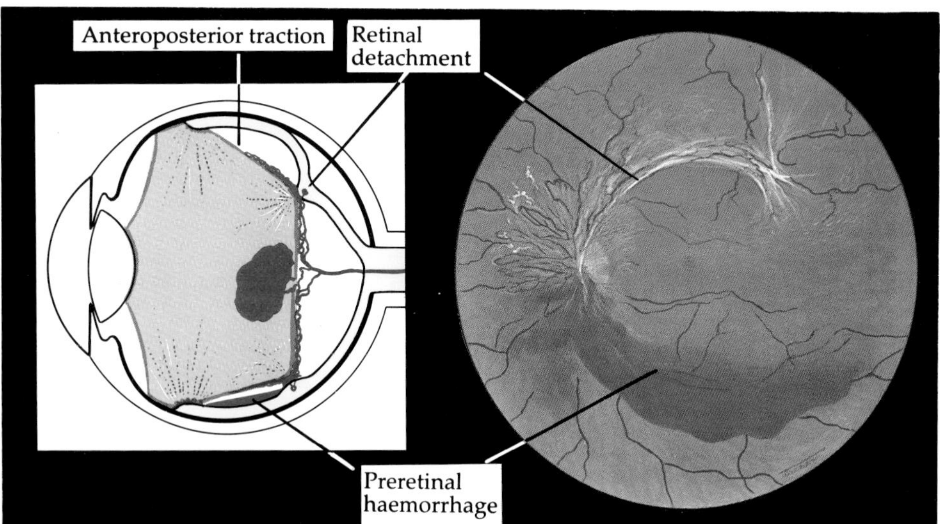

Figure 10.21
Upper tractional retinal detachment

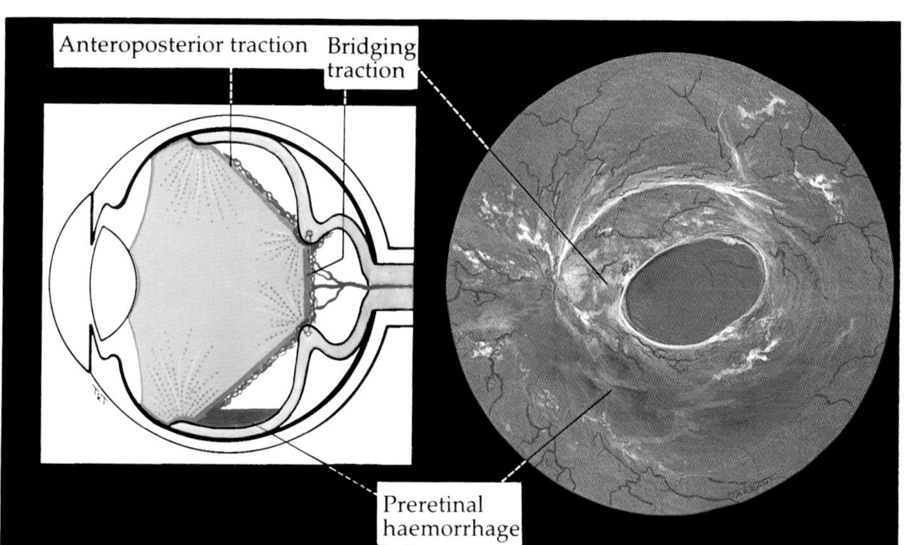

Figure 10.22
Advanced diabetic eye disease with opaque membranes and tractional retinal detachment

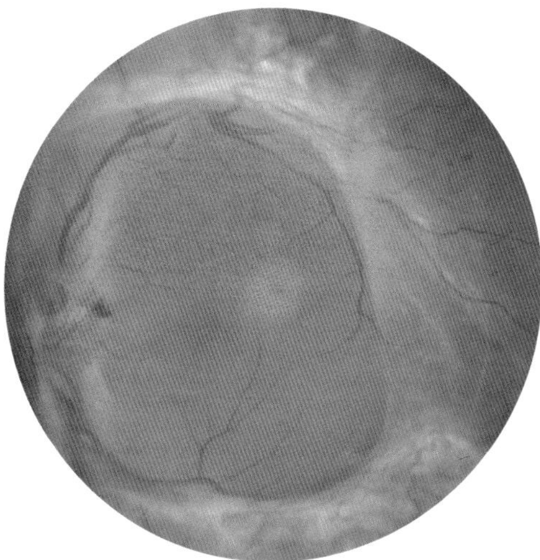

Figure 10.23 *Extensive tractional retinal detachment without involvement of macula*

This tends to pull the two involved points of the retina together and may be responsible for the formation of stress lines as well as displacement of the macula towards the disc or elsewhere depending on the direction of traction.

Fortunately diabetic tractional retinal detachments may remain localized for many months without involving the macula (*Figure 10.23*). Occasionally vitreoretinal traction may cause a splitting of the retina into two layers (retinoschisis). In some eyes traction over areas of fibrovascular adhesion may cause a retinal break (usually a small oval hole posterior to the equator). When this happens, the concave shape characteristic of a tractional retinal detachment assumes a convex bullous configuration typical of a rhegmatogenous retinal detachment. In this event surgery should be undertaken without undue delay.

Opaque membrane formation

This may occur on the posterior surface of the detached hyaloid. In many cases the membrane stretches from the superior to inferior temporal arcades. It may be continuous in front of the macula and further impair central vision, or more commonly a round or oval hole may be present in the membrane overlying the macula (*Figure 10.22, right*).

After a variable period of time, the fibrous component of the fibrovascular proliferation becomes more evident and the vascular component decreases so that the blood vessels become non-perfused and no further proliferation occurs. This is the so-called 'burnt-out' stage (*Figure 10.24*).

Neovascular glaucoma

Rubeosis iridis is a fairly common finding in eyes with PDR, and may lead to the development of neovascular glaucoma. This complication is particularly common in eyes with persistent retinal detachment following unsuccessful pars plana vitrectomy.

Management of neovascular glaucoma is discussed in Chapter 7.

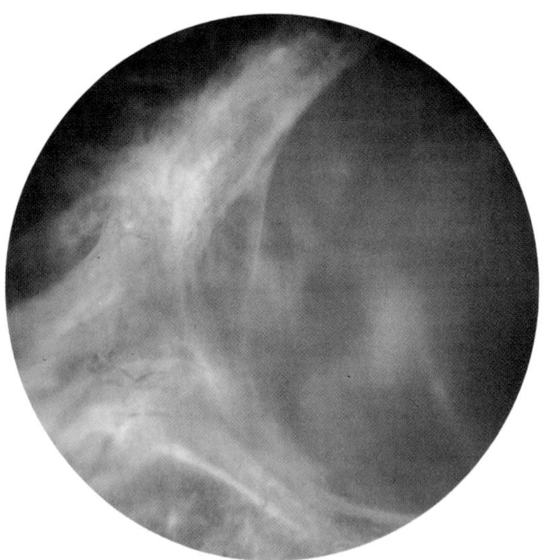

Figure 10.24 *'Burnt out' proliferative diabetic retinopathy*

Pars plana vitrectomy

Some of the serious complications of PDR just described can be treated by pars plana vitrectomy. This is a closed microsurgical technique by which intraocular tissue is removed through a small incision in the pars plana with an automated suction-cutting device, while maintaining the intraocular pressure at a normal or slightly elevated level.

Instrumentation

Suction cutter

It is essential to cut intraocular tissue cleanly without exerting undue traction on surrounding tissues. All cutters share the principle of engaging tissue into a port and then cutting it by the shearing action between the edges on a moving and a non-moving part (*Figure 10.25*). Guillotine cutters have a linear reciprocating 'to-and-fro' action in which pieces of tissue are sheared off between the sharpened outer edge of an inner movable blade and the inner edge of the orifice in the outer tube. In rotary cutters the inner blade can rotate continuously in one direction or it can be made to oscillate from an anticlockwise to clockwise direction. Suction is operated by a pump, the level of aspiration being controlled by a foot-switch. Some cutters have a reflux system which spits out unwanted tissue.

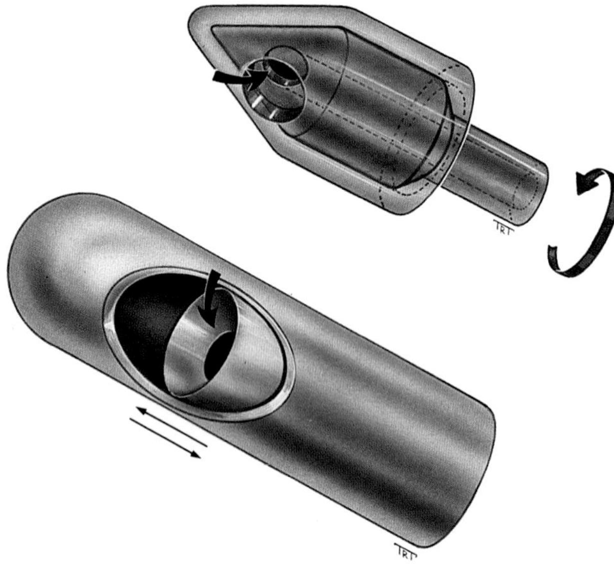

Figure 10.25 *Suction cutters. Top: rotary cutter; bottom: guillotine cutter*

Infusion (*Figure 10.26, upper left*)

The infusion is under hydrostatic control so that the level of intraocular pressure can be varied by elevating or lowering the infusion bottle in relation to the patient's eye. In the event of bleeding, the height of the bottle can be raised in order to increase the intraocular pressure.

Accessory instruments (*Figure 10.26, upper right*)

Most accessory instruments have a 20-gauge (0.90 mm diameter) so that they can be interchanged freely during surgery. Hooked needles and picks are useful in the dissection of tissue planes. Microscissors can be used to segment epiretinal membranes. Flute needles have an exit port in the handpiece which can be controlled by the surgeon's finger (similar to playing a flute). This simple device is extremely useful for the quick removal of pools of blood (vacuum-cleaning), and also for simultaneous fluid–gas exchange. Ultrasonic lens fragmentors can be used to remove cataracts during pars plana vitrectomy.

Illumination (*Figure 10.26, lower right*)

Illumination can be either external by using a motorized slitlamp capable of excursions to either side of the axis of the microscope or, preferably, internal (endoillumination) in the form of a fibreoptic light pipe.

Endocoagulation (*Figure 10.26, upper right*)

Endophotocoagulation (xenon or argon) with a fibreoptic probe can be used to treat posterior breaks and for PRP following pars plana vitrectomy.

Microscope (*Figure 10.26, lower left*)

Surgery can only be performed safely with the aid of a good operating microscope with a zoom and fine focus capability, as well as an X–Y coupling that enables the surgeon to move the microscope in a horizontal plane.

Indications

Dense persistent vitreous haemorrhage

This is the most common indication for pars plana vitrectomy. All patients should have ultrasonography to exlude an underlying retinal detachment. In the presence

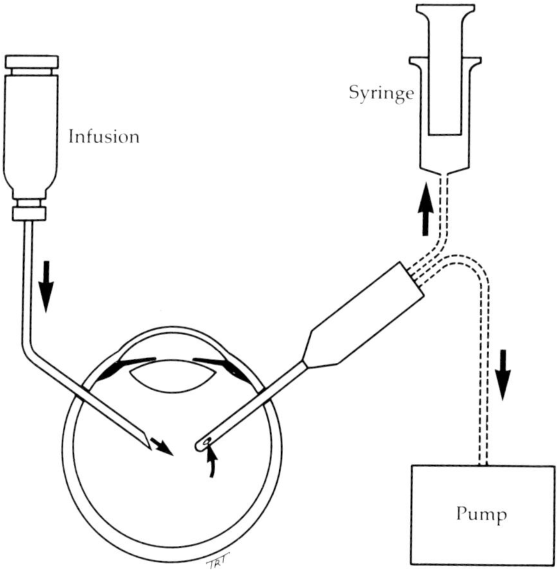

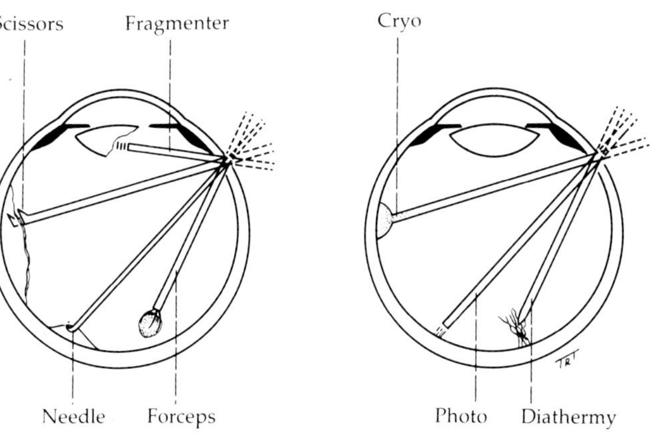

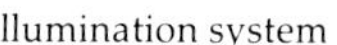

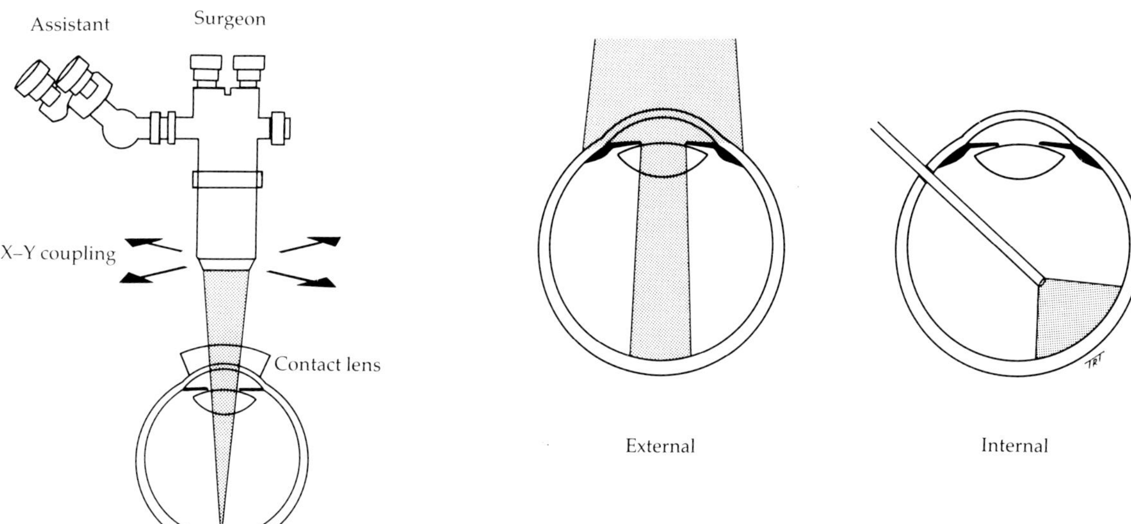

Figure 10.26 *Systems for pars plana vitrectomy*

of an associated retinal detachment involving the macula, vitrectomy should be performed without delay. Early vitrectomy should also be considered if rubeosis iridis is present in an eye with a non-absorbing vitreous haemorrhage. This will enable PRP to be carried out in order to prevent the development of neovascular glaucoma.

In the absence of retinal detachment and/or rubeosis iridis, early vitrectomy (within 1–6 months after the initial vitreous haemorrhage) should be considered in patients with type 1 diabetes. This is because the final visual results are better with early as compared with late vitrectomy (at least 1 year after vitreous haemorrhage). However, there appears to be no definite advantage of early vitrectomy in patients with type 2 diabetes.

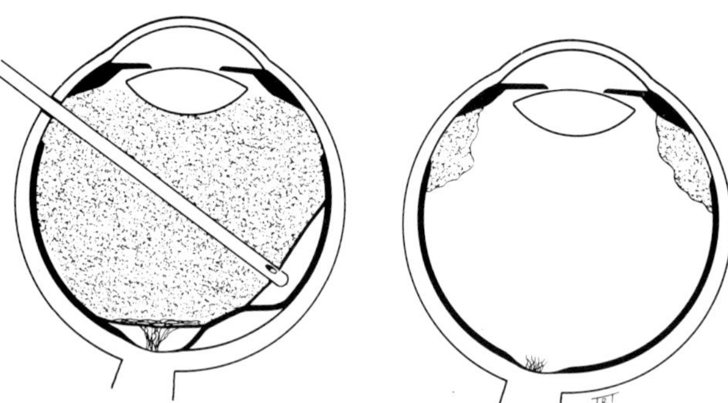

Figure 10.27 *Repair of tractional retinal detachment due to proliferative diabetic retinopathy*

Retinal detachment

1. *Tractional retinal detachment.* Because tractional retinal detachments frequently remain stationary for prolonged periods of time, vitrectomy should only be undertaken if the area of detachment has progressed to involve the macula. In these circumstances surgery should be performed without delay.
2. *Combined tractional and rhegmatogenous retinal detachment.* Because subretinal fluid spreads quickly in eyes with rhegmatogenous detachments, surgery should be undertaken even in the presence of an attached macula.

Aims

Removal of vitreous haemorrhage

Intragel haemorrhage has to be removed with the cutter but retrohyaloid blood can be evacuated using the vacuum-cleaning technique with a flute needle.

Removal of vitreous 'scaffold'

It is vitally important to excise all cortical vitreous gel posterior to the equator in order to eliminate the 'scaffold' along which further fibrovascular tissue can proliferate. If this goal is achieved, involution of existing neovascular tissue frequently also occurs.

Repair of retinal detachment (*Figure 10.27*)

This can be achieved by excising anteroposterior and bridging tractional membranes, and segmenting and if necessary separating fibrovascular tissue on the retinal surface by using microscissors and picks. Retinal breaks should be sealed and scleral buckling may be necessary in certain cases. Some surgeons also perform a prophylactic encirclement posterior to the vitreous base at the completion of surgery.

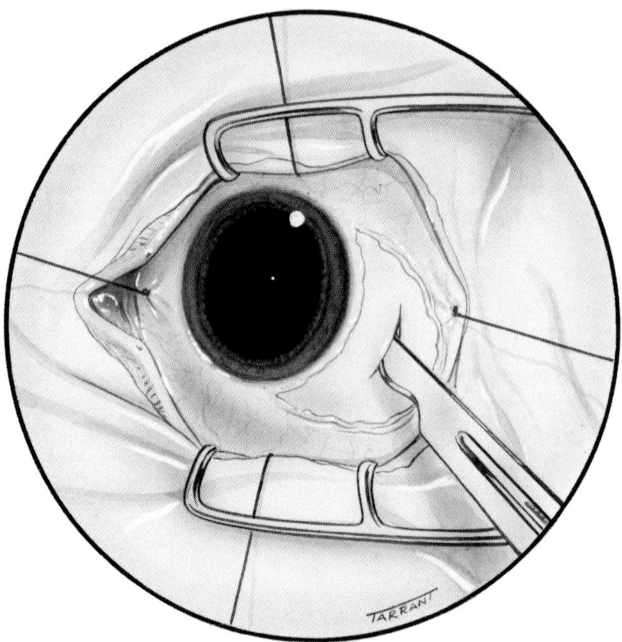

Figure 10.28 *Preparation of the sclerotomy site*

Technique

1. *Sclerotomy* (*Figure 10.28*). The sclera is incised and a knuckle of uvea prolapsed. A circular opening is then made in the uvea using scissors. A second sclerotomy to accommodate the fibreoptic light pipe is made at an angle of about 160° with the first sclerotomy.
2. *Vitreous base is incised with a knife* in order to make an adequate track for the subsequent introduction of the cutter (*Figure 10.29*).
3. *Introduction of the cutter* into the vitreous cavity should be undertaken with great care to ensure that uveal tissue is not being pushed in front of the tip. The light pipe is introduced into the eye in a similar manner (*Figure 10.30*).
4. *Anterior vitrectomy* is commenced using gentle suction and cutting (*Figure 10.31, left*). In the presence of a complete posterior vitreous detachment it may be possible to perform a complete vitrectomy while keeping the cutter in the anterior and midvitreous cavity.
5. *Posterior vitrectomy* can only be performed by using a contact lens (*Figure 10.31, right*). The excision of vitreous should proceed in an anteroposterior direction and only

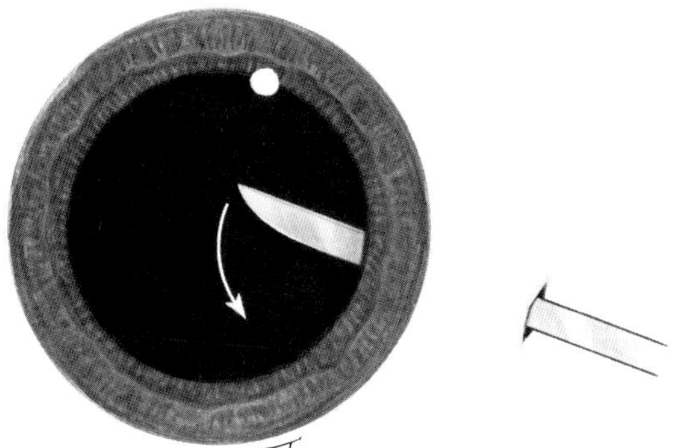

Figure 10.29 *Incision of vitreous base*

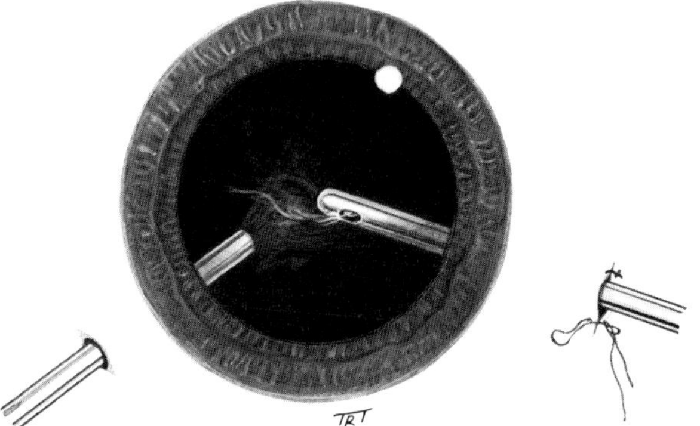

Figure 10.30 *Introduction of cutter and fibreoptic light pipe*

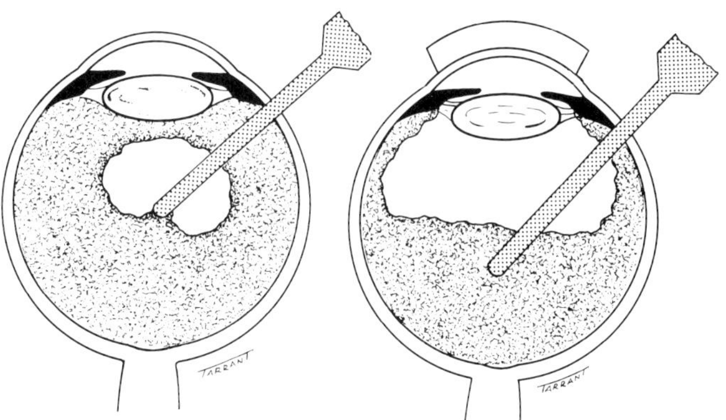

Figure 10.31 *Left: anterior vitrectomy; right: deep vitrectomy*

as much of the peripheral vitreous removed as might fall into the visual axis when the patient assumes an upright position postoperatively. The area of the vitreous base should be avoided at all costs.

6. *Removal of cutter.* The infusion is stopped and a small amount of fluid is aspirated so that the intraocular pressure is slightly below normal. This prevents the prolapse of intraocular contents through the incision when the cutter is removed.
7. *Sclerotomy is closed* using interrupted or mattress sutures.

Complications

Unfortunately both anterior and posterior segment complications are frequent.

1. *Rubeosis iridis* is the most common anterior segment complication resulting in failure. It has an increased incidence in aphakic eyes and in those with residual areas of detached retina. In eyes with total retinal detachments the incidence of rubeosis is virtually 100%. Although mild cases of rubeosis may occasionally regress spontaneously, or with the aid of panretinal photocoagulation, advanced cases usually progress to neovascular glaucoma.
2. *Corneal erosions* are common, particularly if the epithelium is removed during surgery. It appears that in diabetic patients there is a defect that prevents the basal cells from attaching to the basement membrane.

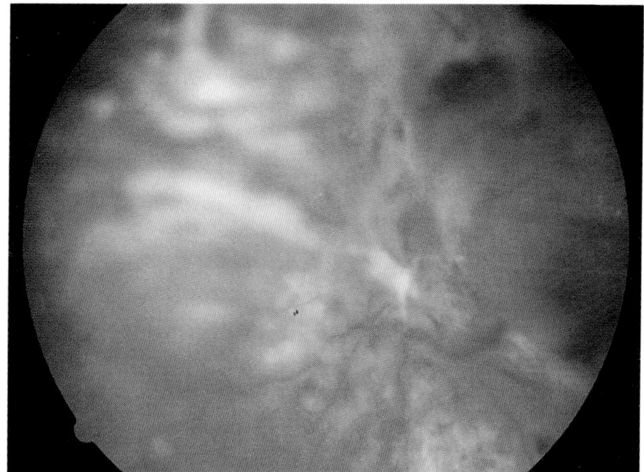

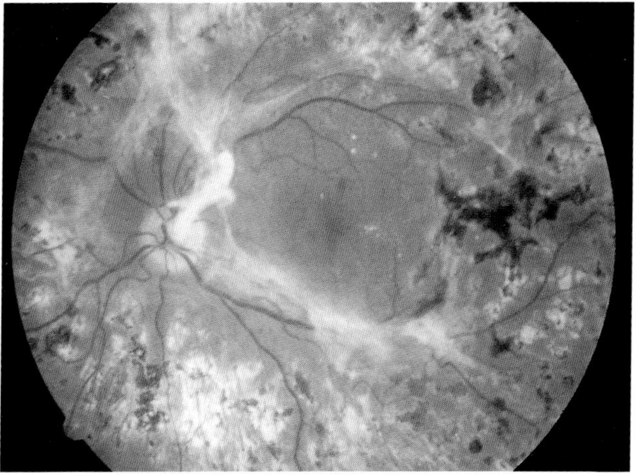

(*b*)

Figure 10.32 (a) *Tractional retinal detachment and vitreous haemorrhage;* (b) *appearance of same eye following pars plana vitrectomy showing flat retina and resolution of neovascularization*

3. *Cataract* may be due to progression of pre-existing lens opacities or to surgical trauma.
4. *Glaucoma* may be due to rubeosis or it may be of the ghost cell or haemolytic type (*see* Chapter 7).
5. *Vitreous haemorrhage* may be due to fresh fibrovascular proliferation. In an aphakic eye the blood tends to absorb more quickly than in a phakic eye, presumably because some of the blood is absorbed by the anterior outflow channels.
6. *Retinal detachment* may be caused by intraoperative complications such as traction on the vitreous base or the inadvertent creation of fresh breaks with the cutter or other instruments. It may also occur later due to fresh fibrovascular proliferation.
7. *Entry site proliferation* of episcleral or uveal origin may occur.
8. *Phthisis bulbi* is the end result in about 3% of cases.

Results

The visual results (*Figure 10.32*) depend on the specific indications for surgery and the complexity of pre-existing vitreoretinal abnormalities. In general, about 70% of cases have visual improvement, about 10% are made worse, and the remainder have no change in vision. It appears that the first few postoperative months are vital. If the eye is doing well after 6 months, then the long-term outlook is favourable as the incidence of subsequent vision-threatening complications is low.

Retinal vein occlusion

Introduction

After diabetic retinopathy, venous occlusion is the most common retinal vascular disorder encountered by ophthalmologists.

Predisposing factors

1. *Age.* Retinal vein occlusion typically affects patients in the sixth and seventh decades of life.
2. *Systemic hypertension* is associated with an increased risk of both branch retinal vein occlusion (BRVO) and central retinal vein occlusion (CRVO). It has been postulated that the vein is compressed by a thickened artery where the two share a common adventitia (i.e. at arteriovenous crossings in the retina and just behind the lamina cribrosa).
3. *Raised intraocular pressure.* Patients with primary open-angle glaucoma or ocular hypertension are at increased risk from CRVO but there is no significant correlation with BRVO.
4. *Hypermetropia* is associated with an increased risk of BRVO. The mechanisms are unknown.
5. *Blood dyscrasias.* Although haematological investigations are usually unrewarding in patients with retinal vein occlusion, rarely, blood dyscrasias which cause hyperviscosity as a result of either *hypercellularity* (chronic leukaemia, polycythaemia) or *changes in plasma proteins* (Waldenström's macroglobulinaemia) may precipitate a retinal vein occlusion. Sickle-cell disease may also cause retinal vein occlusion.
6. *Periphlebitis* as in sarcoidosis, and Behçet's disease.

Effects on retinal circulation

It has been postulated that, in the end-artery system of the retina, venous occlusion causes an elevation of venous and capillary pressure and stagnation of blood flow. This stagnation results in hypoxia of the retina normally drained by the obstructed vein. The hypoxia in turn results in damage to the capillary endothelial cells leading to extravasation of blood constituents into the extracellular space. The extracellular pressure is increased causing further stagnation of the circulation and hypoxia, so that a vicious circle is established (*Figure 10.33*).

Branch vein occlusion

Classification

Main vein occlusion at disc margin
- without macular oedema
- with macular oedema

Major branch vein occlusion away from disc
- without macular oedema
- with macular oedema

Macular branch vein occlusion
Peripheral branch vein occlusion

Clinical features

Symptoms

These depend on the location of the occlusion. Although some patients are asymptomatic, the majority have a relative loss of part of their field of vision and impairment of visual acuity which may be associated with metamorphopsia. Both eyes are involved in about 5% of cases.

Signs

Acute (*Figures 10.34* and *10.35*)

These consist of dilated and tortuous veins, flame-shaped haemorrhages, 'dot' and 'blot' haemorrhages, retinal oedema, and cotton-wool spots, affecting the part of the

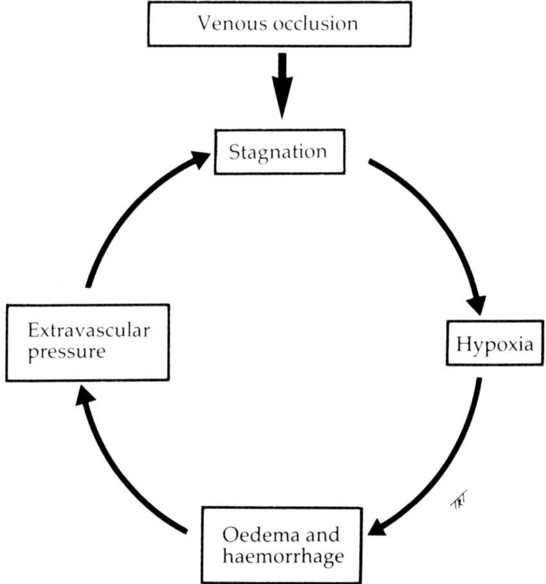

Figure 10.33 Effects of venous occlusion on retinal circulation

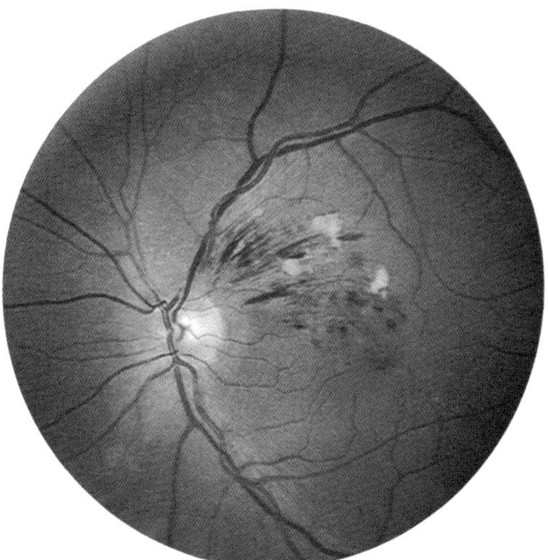

Figure 10.34 Acute macular branch vein occlusion

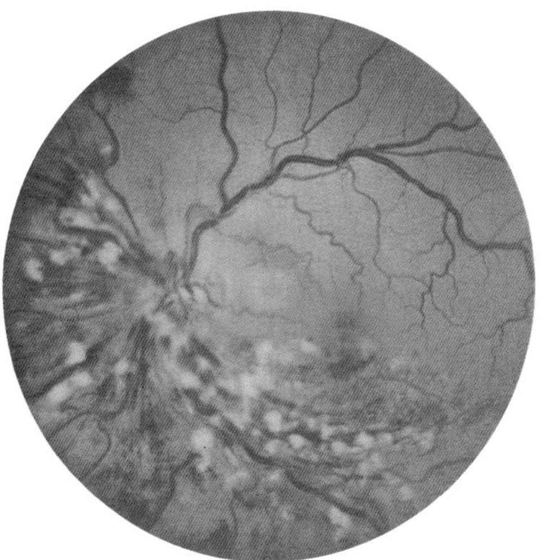

Figure 10.35 Acute major branch vein occlusion with extensive cotton-wool spots

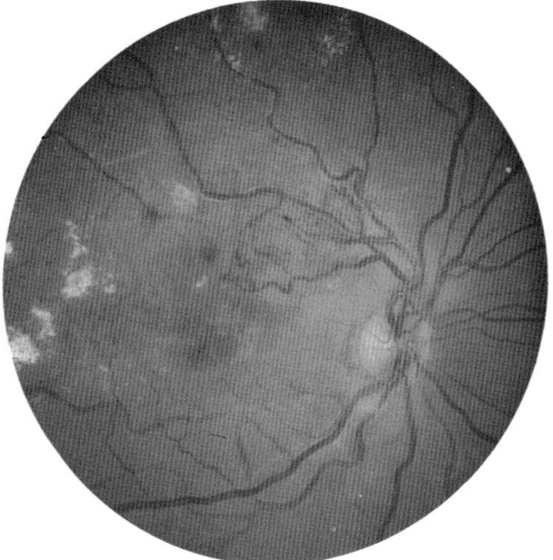

Figure 10.36 Old superotemporal branch vein occlusion showing collaterals, hard exudates and sheathing

retina drained by the obstructed vein. These acute features take between 6 to 12 months to disappear.

Chronic (*Figure 10.36*)

These include venous sheathing, chronic cystoid macular oedema, microaneurysms, collaterals, shunts, hard yellow exudates, cholesterol crystals, and mottling of the retinal pigment epithelium. In some cases the arterioles may also become sheathed. *Collaterals* are pre-existing retinal capillaries that bypass adjacent areas of vascular closure and are usually located within the area drained by the occluded vein. They usually show little staining or leakage on fluorescein angiography. *Shunts* are arteriovenous communications in which blood passes directly from artery to vein without going through the normal capillary bed. They may decompensate in the chronic stage of BRVO and show both staining and leakage on fluorescein angiography.

Prognostic factors

Following a major retinal branch vein occlusion, visual acuity is initially reduced due to haemorrhage and macular oedema. However, within 6 months about 50% of eyes develop efficient collaterals, with a return of visual acuity to 6/12 or better.

The eventual amount of visual recovery is determined by two main factors:

1. *The amount of venous drainage* involved by the occlusion which is determined by the site and size of the occluded vein. For example, in *Figure 10.37* an occlusion at *2a* will compromise the upper two quadrants of macular venous drainage; an occlusion at *2b* will interfere with only one

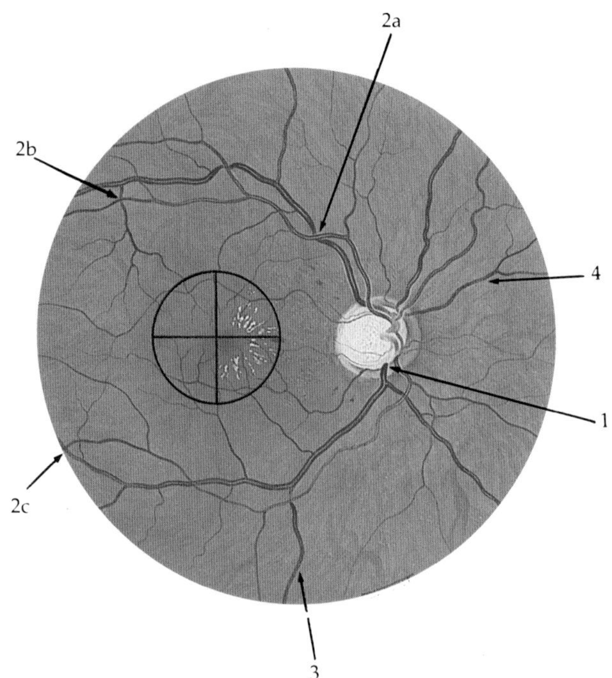

Figure 10.37 Possible sites of occlusion

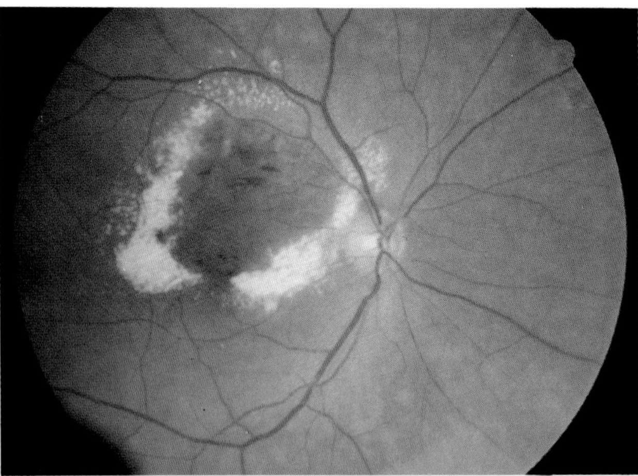

Figure 10.38 Hard exudates at macula following retinal branch vein occlusion

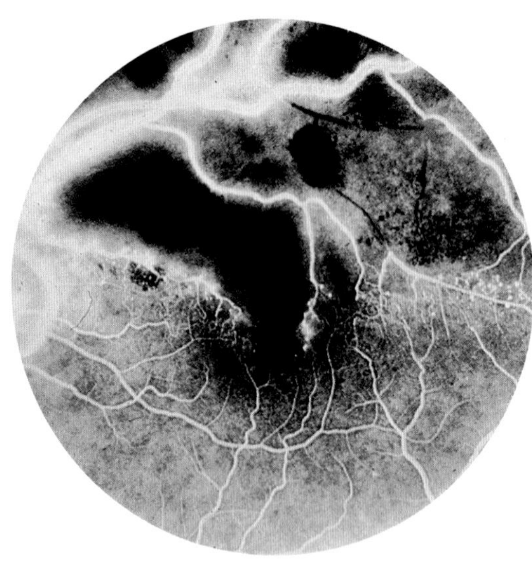

Figure 10.39 Fluorescein angiogram showing extensive capillary non-perfusion and disruption of perifoveal capillary network in eye with superior branch retinal vein occlusion (courtesy of Mr J. Shilling)

quadrant of macular venous drainage; and an occlusion at *2c* will not interfere with macular venous drainage.

2. *The integrity of the perifoveal capillary network.* The visual prognosis is good if the network is intact, and poor if it is broken or incomplete.

Complications

Branch vein occlusion is a significant injury to the retinal circulation, and complications are due to vascular leakage and capillary non-perfusion. The two most important vision-threatening complications are macular oedema and vitreous haemorrhage due to neovascularization. Other less common complications include hard exudate formation due to chronic leakage (*Figure 10.38*), and serous transudative detachment of the neurosensory retina.

Chronic macular oedema

This is the most common cause of persistent poor vision following branch retinal vein occlusion. Some patients with a visual acuity of 6/12 or worse may benefit from argon laser photocoagulation. However, before recommending treatment it is important to determine that the visual loss is caused by macular oedema and not macular ischaemia.

Investigations

1. Wait for the retinal haemorrhages to clear sufficiently to enable a good quality fluorescein angiogram to be performed.
2. If the fluorescein angiogram shows macular non-perfusion (*Figure 10.39*) as the cause of visual loss, no treatment is available to improve vision.
3. If the fluorescein angiogram shows macular oedema (*Figure 10.40*) as the cause of visual impairment, and visual acuity continues to be 6/12 or worse without spontaneous improvement, argon laser photocoagulation should be performed.

Treatment

Prior to treatment, the fluorescein angiogram should be studied carefully in order to identify the leaking areas. It is also very important to identify collateral vessels because they must not be treated. The spot size is 100 μm with a duration of 0.1 second and a power setting sufficient to

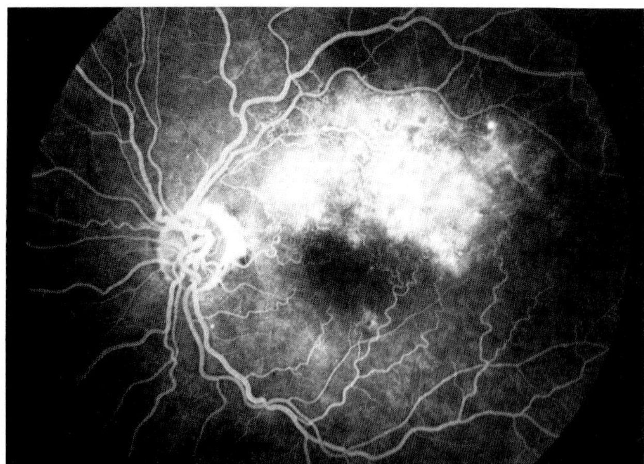

Figure 10.40 *Fluorescein angiogram showing macular oedema with good perfusion of fovea*

produce a medium white burn at the level of the retinal pigment epithelium. The burns are applied in a 'grid' pattern with spacing about one burn width apart throughout the area of leakage. The photocoagulation can be applied as close to the fovea as the margin of the capillary free zone and as peripheral as the major vascular arcade (about 2.5 disc diameters from the centre of the fovea). Care should be taken to avoid treating over intraretinal haemorrhage.

Neovascularization

This complication occurs in about one-third of eyes with significant areas of capillary non-perfusion following a major BRVO.

Disc neovascularization is invariably associated with extensive areas of capillary drop-out in the area of the retina drained by the obstructed vein. Presumably the ischaemic retina elaborates a vasoformative substance that stimulates neovascularization, just as in PDR. Neovascularization is a very serious complication as it frequently leads to recurrent vitreous haemorrhage which may be severe enough to require treatment by pars plana vitrectomy. Tractional retinal detachment may also occur.

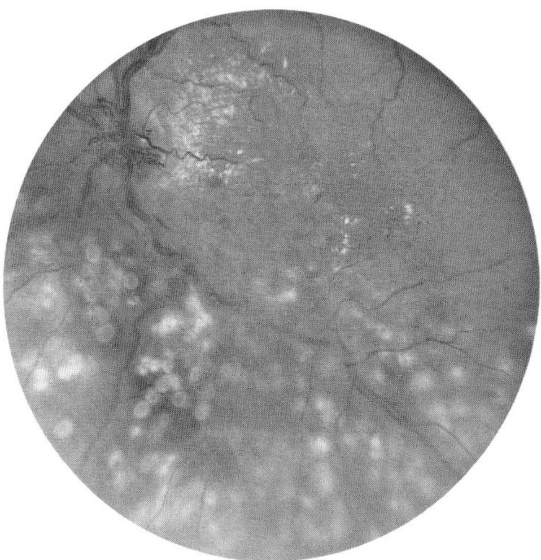

Figure 10.41 *Same eye as in* Figure 10.35 *3 months later showing disc new vessels treated by scatter laser photocoagulation to area of retina drained by obstructed vein*

Treatment

All eyes with neovascularization following BRVO should be treated by argon laser photocoagulation in order to prevent vitreous haemorrhage. Treatment is applied in a 'scatter' pattern to achieve a 'medium' white reaction (200–500 μm in diameter) spaced one burn apart to cover the entire involved segment (*Figure 10.41*). The burns should extend no closer than 2 disc diameters from the centre of the fovea.

Central vein occlusion

Classification

Although there is some overlap, most cases of CRVO can be divided into the following types according to clinical features and prognosis:

1. *Non-ischaemic CRVO,* also referred to as 'venous-stasis retinopathy' and 'partial' CRVO. This is the most common type accounting for about 75% of all cases.
2. *Ischaemic CRVO,* also called 'haemorrhagic retinopathy' and 'complete' CRVO. This is less common and accounts for the remaining 25%.
3. *Optic disc vasculitis* (papillophlebitis).

Non-ischaemic CRVO

Clinical features

1. Visual acuity is slightly or moderately reduced although in a few cases it may be normal.
2. Relative afferent pupillary conduction defect (Marcus Gunn pupil) is usually slight, indicating mild retinal ischaemia.

Ophthalmoscopy

The findings during the early stages are (*Figure 10.42a*):

1. Mild tortuosity and dilatation of all branches of the central retinal vein.
2. Haemorrhages ('dot', 'blot' and flame-shaped) distributed throughout all four quadrants of the retina. In typical cases the haemorrhages are relatively few in number and most numerous in the peripheral retina. In atypical cases, however, the posterior retina may also be involved.

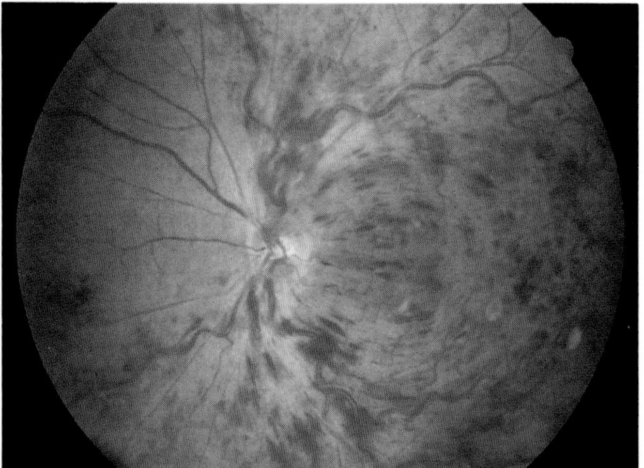

(*a*)

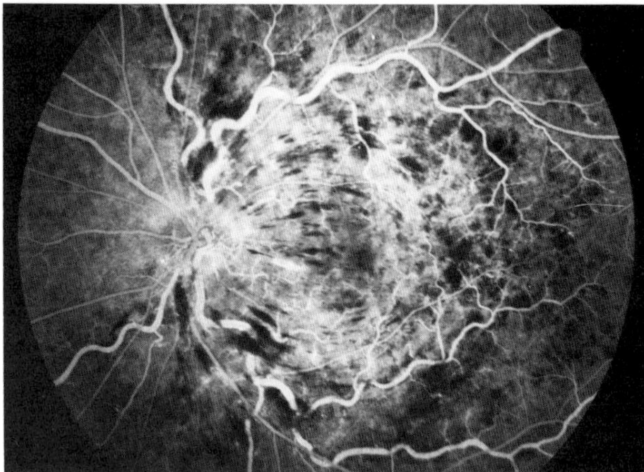

(*b*)

Figure 10.42 (a) *Acute non-ischaemic central retinal vein occlusion;* (b) *fluorescein angiogram showing good retinal capillary perfusion*

3. Cotton-wool spots are usually absent, although in some cases a few spots may be seen in the posterior pole.
4. Optic disc swelling is mild to moderate.
5. Macular oedema may be present or absent.

Fundus examination after 6–12 months may show the following:

1. Sheathing of the major retinal veins.
2. Partial or complete absorption of the retinal haemorrhages.
3. Optic disc may be normal or it may develop cilioretinal collaterals.
4. Macula may be normal or it may show the following: pigmentary disturbances, cystoid macular oedema, lamellar hole formation, and pucker.

Fluorescein angiography

During the early stages this shows venous stasis but good retinal capillary perfusion except in areas of cotton-wool spots (*Figure 10.42b*).

Complications

In about 50% of cases, the retinopathy resolves and visual acuity returns to normal or near normal. The most common cause of a permanent impairment of visual acuity is chronic cystoid macular oedema.

Treatment

No specific treatment is required because no study has so far shown conclusively that laser photocoagulation is beneficial for cystoid macular oedema secondary to CRVO.

Ischaemic CRVO

Clinical features

1. Visual acuity is usually less than 6/60 and frequently reduced to counting fingers or worse.
2. Relative afferent pupillary conduction defect (Marcus Gunn pupil) is marked.

Ophthalmoscopy

Fully established cases are characterized by (*Figure 10.43*):

1. Marked tortuosity and engorgement of the retinal veins.
2. Retinal haemorrhages involving both the peripheral retina and posterior pole.
3. Cotton-wool spots are common.
4. Optic disc is swollen and hyperaemic.
5. Macula is usually markedly oedematous and covered by haemorrhages.

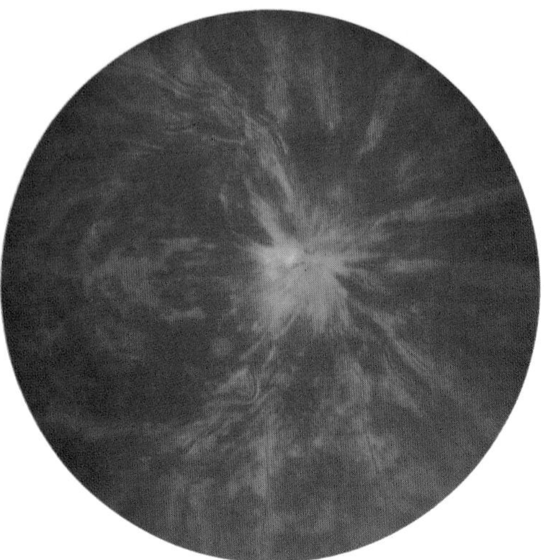

Figure 10.43 *Acute ischaemic central retinal vein occlusion*

Fundus findings after 6–12 months are similar to late non-ischaemic CRVO (*Figure 4.44a*) except that degenerative macular changes are invariably present, and cilioretinal collaterals at the disc are more frequent.

Fluorescein angiography

During the early stages, the retinal vascular bed may be masked by retinal haemorrhages so that no useful information can be obtained. However, in less severe cases the angiogram will show extensive areas of capillary non-perfusion (*Figure 10.44b*).

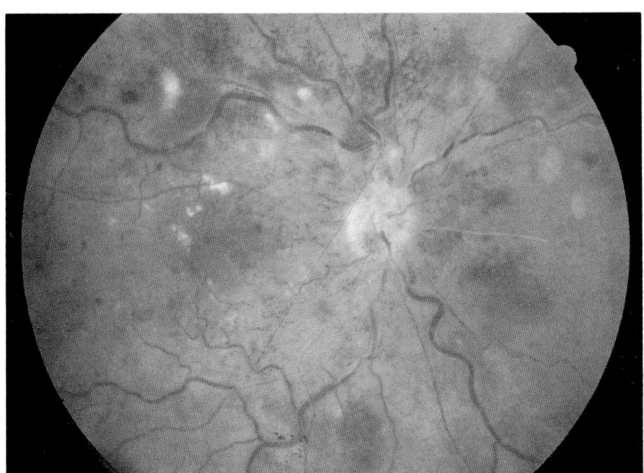

(*a*)

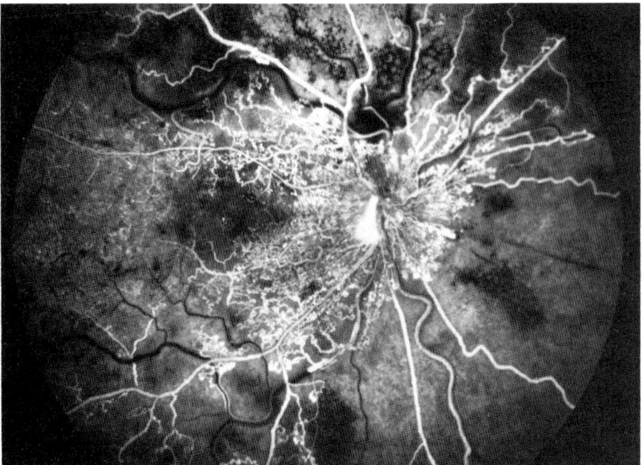

(*b*)

Figure 10.44 (a) *Late stage of ischaemic central retinal vein occlusion;* (b) *fluorescein angiogram showing extensive areas of capillary non-perfusion*

Complications

About 50% of eyes develop rubeosis iridis and neovascular glaucoma within 3 months of the initial occlusion. A small percentage of eyes develop preretinal or vitreous haemorrhages secondary to NVD and/or NVE.

Treatment

Patients should be followed closely for evidence of rubeosis iridis because prompt treatment of early cases by PRP prevents the subsequent development of neovascular glaucoma in a significant number of cases. The management of established neovascular glaucoma is discussed in Chapter 7.

Optic disc vasculitis (papillophlebitis)

Clinical features

This relatively rare condition typically affects healthy young adults (*Figure 10.45*). Although the clinical picture is that of a CRVO, visual acuity is normal or near normal and the visual prognosis excellent. Two possible explanations for the favourable prognosis in these patients are:

1. The eye of a young patient with healthy blood vessels may be able to tolerate brief periods of CRVO better than an older individual.
2. The occlusion may be due to a mild inflammation of the central retinal vein.

Treatment

Although systemic corticosteroids have been used to treat papillophlebitis, their efficacy is unproven.

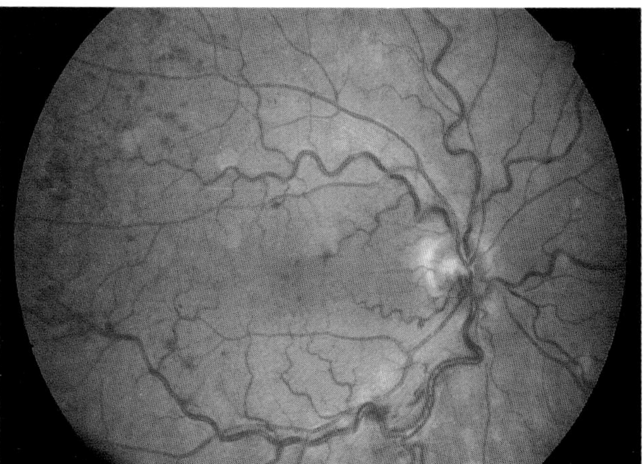

Figure 10.45 *Papillophlebitis*

Retinal artery occlusion

Aetiology

Occlusive disorders of the retinal circulation are among the most dramatic problems encountered by the ophthalmologist because of their rapid onset, their potentially profound effects on vision, and their strong assocation with life-threatening systemic diseases. The causes of retinal artery occlusion can be divided into three main groups: embolization, vaso-obliteration, and raised intraocular pressure.

Embolization

This is the most common cause of obstruction to the retinal circulation. Because the ophthalmic artery is the first branch of the internal carotid artery, embolic material from either the heart or the carotid arteries has a fairly direct route to the eye.

From the heart

These may be of four types (*Figure 10.46*):

1. *Calcific* usually arise from calcified aortic valves.
2. *Vegetations.* Emboli composed of valve vegetations may occur in patients with subacute bacterial endocarditis.
3. *Thrombus.* Emboli composed of thrombus originate from the left side of the heart as a consequence of myocardial infarction (mural thrombi) or mitral stenosis associated with atrial fibrillation. A prolapsed mitral valve can also be the source of recurrent embolization.
4. *Myxoma.* Material arising from the very rare atrial myxoma.

From the carotid arteries

The most important cause of retinal embolization is atheroma involving the origin of the internal carotid artery and the adjacent segment of the common carotid artery (*Figure 10.47*). An atheromatous plaque at this site may undergo several changes: haemorrhage into the plaque

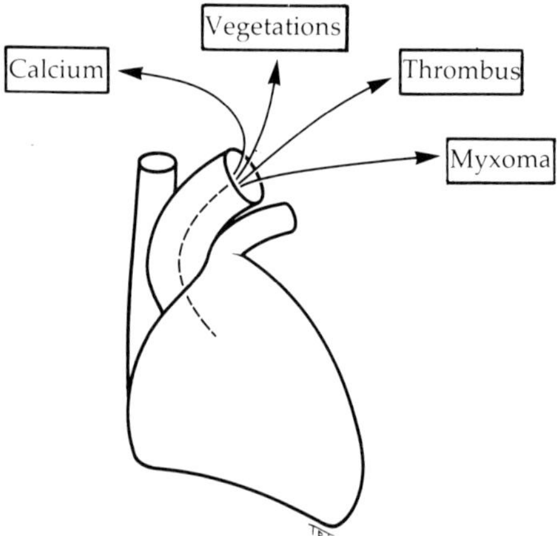

Figure 10.46 *Embolization from the heart*

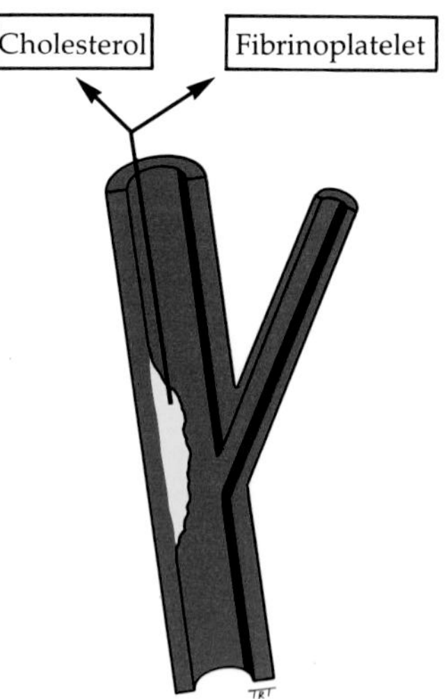

Figure 10.47 *Embolization from the carotid arteries*

from the vasa vasorum, necrosis, calcification, and ulceration. These complications are usually associated with varying degrees of stenosis of the arterial lumen.

Emboli from the carotid arteries may be of three types (*Figure 10.48*):

1. *Cholesterol* emboli (Hollenhorst's plaques) are usually due to necrosis and ulceration of an atheromatous plaque with discharge of its contents into the circulation. In the retina they appear as intermittent showers of minute refractile crystals (*Figure 10.49*). They seldom cause symptoms as they rarely cause significant obstruction to the retinal arterioles.
2. *Fibrinoplatelet* emboli are caused by loss of continuity of the endothelial cells lining an atheromatous plaque. Platelets become adherent to its roughened surface forming a fibrinoplatelet plug which is then discharged into the circulation. Because these emboli are usually larger than Hollenhorst's plaques, they may cause a transient obstruction to the retinal circulation and symptoms of *amaurosis fugax* which typically consists of a painless loss of vision in one eye, often described by the patient as a curtain coming down over the eye, usually from top to bottom, but occasionally vice versa. The visual loss, which may be complete, rarely lasts longer than 10 minutes. Recovery is in the same pattern as the initial loss, although it is usually more gradual. The few reports of patients examined during an attack described a succession of small whitish bodies, passing rapidly through the retinal arterioles. These findings may be associated with retinal oedema and an afferent pupillary conduction defect.
3. *Calcific* emboli may originate from atheromatous plaques in the ascending aorta or the carotid arteries, as well as from calcified aortic heart valves. They are usually single, white, non-scintillating, and usually fairly near

Cholesterol

Fibrinoplatelet

Calcific

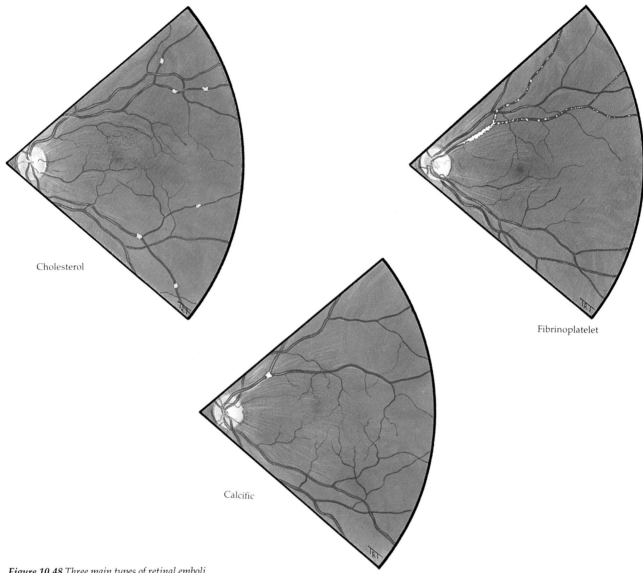

Figure 10.48 *Three main types of retinal emboli*

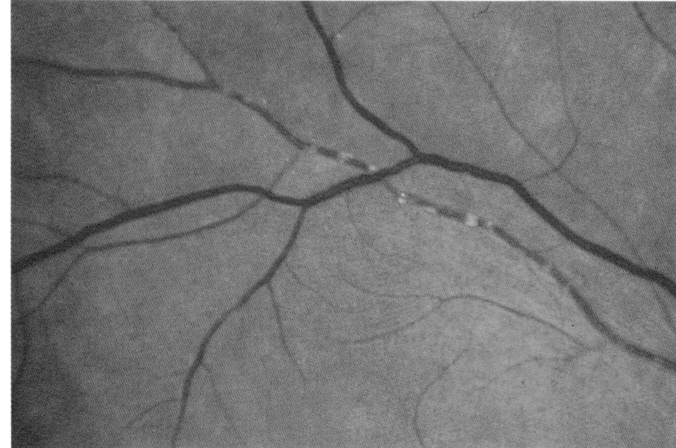

Figure 10.49 *Hollenhorst's plaques*

the disc. When located on the disc itself they may be easily overlooked as they tend to merge with the disc. Calcific emboli are much more dangerous to the eye than the other two kinds as they may cause a permanent occlusion of the central retinal artery or one of its main branches.

Vaso-obliteration

Vaso-obliteration due to either atheroma or arteritis may cause obstruction to the retinal circulation. The many disorders that may give rise to retinal arteritis include giant cell arteritis, systemic lupus erythematosus, polyarteritis nodosa (*Figure 10.50*), scleroderma, and dermatomyositis.

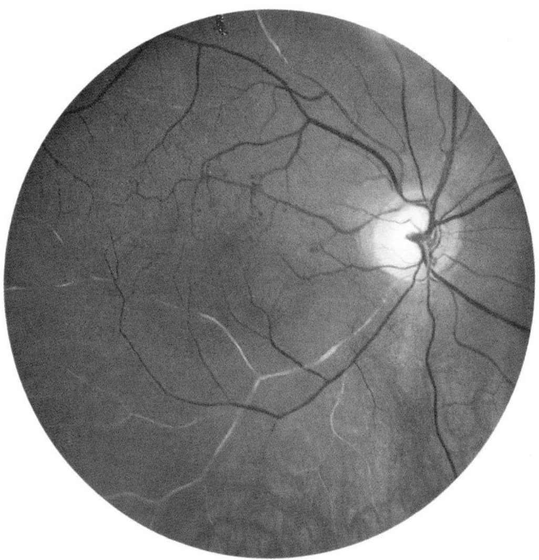

Figure 10.50 *Occlusion of retinal arterioles in polyarteritis nodosa*

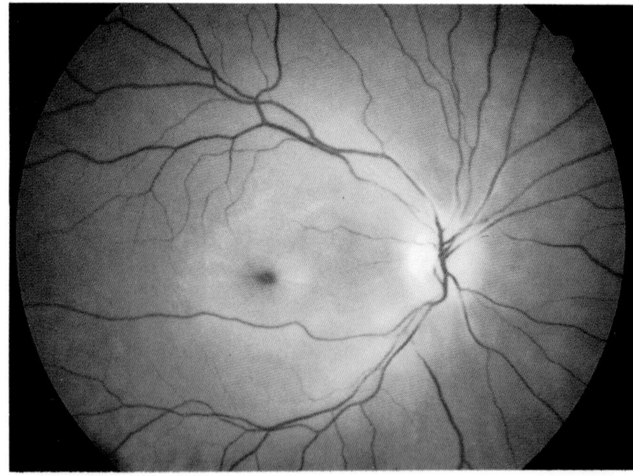

(*a*)

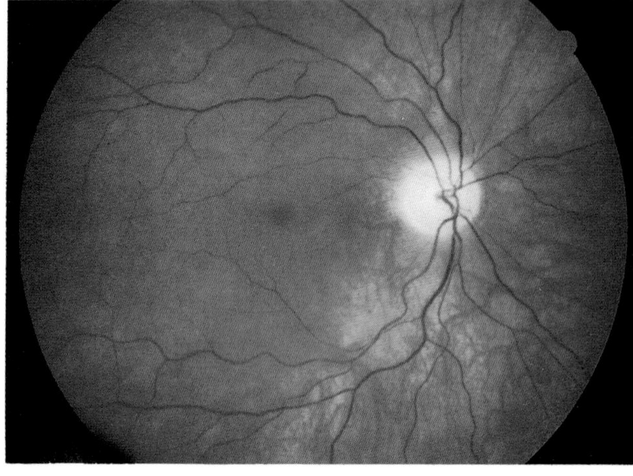

(*b*)

Figure 10.51 (a) *Acute central retinal artery occlusion with cherry-red spot at fovea;* (b) *same eye 3 months later showing vascular attenuation and optic atrophy*

Raised intraocular pressure

Occasionally, obstruction to the retinal circulation occurs as a result of acute angle-closure glaucoma, from excessive pressure on the globe during retinal detachment surgery, or accidental pressure on the globe during neurosurgical procedures.

Clinical features

The fundus findings in arterial occlusion will depend on the size and location of the obstructed vessel.

Central artery occlusion

This is usually due to atheroma, but may also be caused by calcific emboli or giant cell arteritis. It is characterized by a profound loss of vision associated with an afferent pupillary conduction defect. The retina appears white and oedematous, especially at the posterior pole where the nerve fibre and ganglion cell layers are thickest. Since the central fovea is devoid of these layers, the orange reflex from the intact choroidal vessels beneath the foveola stands out in contrast to the surrounding opaque retina, giving rise to the 'cherry-red spot' appearance (*Figure 10.51a*). In about one in five cases, a portion of the papillomacular bundle is supplied by one or more cilioretinal arterioles from the ciliary circulation, and in these cases central vision may be preserved.

Other features of a central retinal artery occlusion include marked narrowing of the retinal arterioles associated with irregularities in their calibre. Sludging and segmentation of the blood column may be seen in both arterioles and venules. If the occlusion persists, the retinal haze and the 'cherry-red spot' disappear after a few weeks. The retinal arterioles, however, remain attenuated and eventually the optic disc becomes atrophic and pale (*Figure 10.51b*).

Between 1% and 5% of eyes with central retinal artery occlusion develop rubeosis iridis, which may be complicated by neovascular glaucoma. Although its incidence is less than that following an occlusion of the central retinal vein, the rubeosis tends to occur sooner after an arterial occlusion.

Branch artery occlusion

This is most commonly caused by emboli. The ischaemic retina appears white in the area supplied by the obstructed artery (*Figure 10.52*). The oedema slowly clears but the inner retinal layers become atrophic and are associated with a permanent sectorial visual field defect. However, recanalization of the obstructed arteriole may leave only subtle or absent ophthalmoscopical signs.

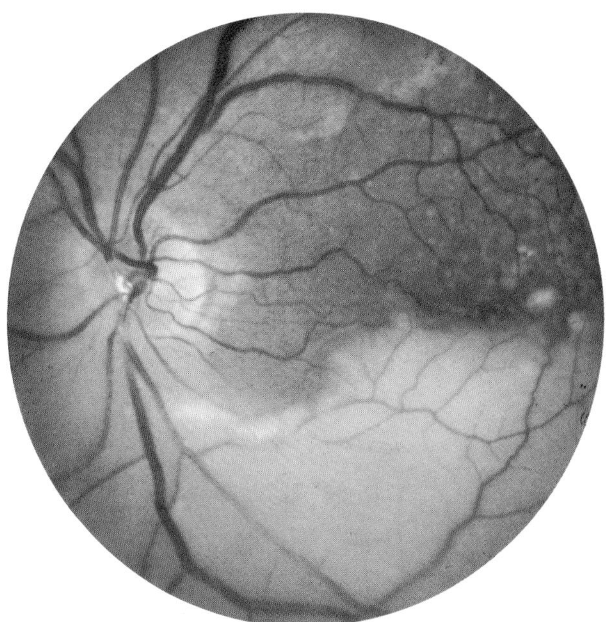

Figure 10.52 *Acute branch retinal artery occlusion*

Occlusion of precapillary arterioles

This occurs in patients with certain collagen vascular disorders, particularly dermatomyositis and systemic lupus erythematosus. It is also a feature of hypertensive retinopathy and preproliferative diabetic retinopathy. The occlusion is manifest by the formation of cotton-wool spots (*Figure 10.53*) which represent a build-up of axoplasmic material in the inner retinal layers. During the acute phase these lesions may be associated with small scotomas which may clear later without leaving any residual defects.

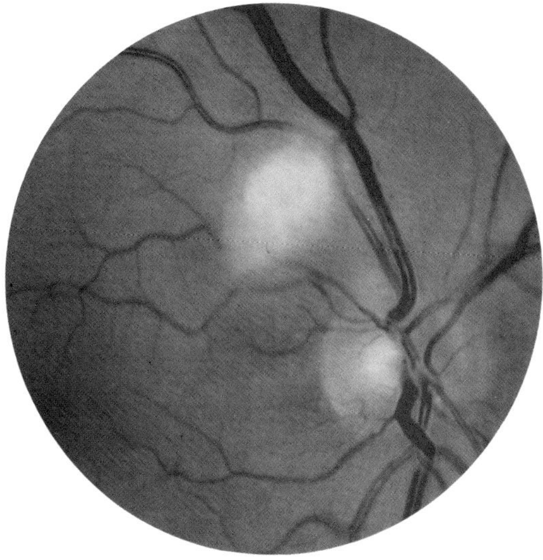

Figure 10.53 *Large cotton-wool spot*

Emergency treatment

Treatment of major occlusion is aimed at restoring the retinal circulation as quickly as possible by increasing retinal perfusion and dislodging emboli. Although retinal tissue cannot survive ischaemia for more than a few hours, complete occlusion is rare. It is therefore reasonable to treat all cases seen within 48 hours.

1. *The patient should lie flat* as this helps to maintain the circulation and is also a convenient position for administering therapy.
2. *Firm ocular massage* should be applied intermittently for at least 15 minutes. Hopefully this manoeuvre will lower intraocular pressure, increase blood flow, and dislodge emboli.
3. *Intravenous acetazolamide 500 mg* should be given in order to lower the intraocular pressure further.
4. *Other measures* include the inhalation of a mixture of 5% carbon dioxide and 95% oxygen and anterior chamber paracentesis. Unfortunately the results of treatment are usually disappointing.
5. *Exclude giant cell arteritis* by measuring the erythrocyte sedimentation rate and, if necessary, performing a biopsy of the temporal artery.

Cardiovascular investigations

The presence of cholesterol or fibrinoplatelet retinal emboli are not only strongly indicative of atheromatous disease involving the carotid arteries but also atheromatous involvement of other parts of the body. For this reason the whole of the cardiovascular system should be investigated. The two lesions in the carotid arteries which may be responsible for retinal microembolization are atheromatous ulceration and stenosis. The three main groups of tests are:

1. Physical examination.
2. Non-invasive investigations.
3. Invasive investigations.

Physical examination

Palpation

The patient's cervical carotid arteries should be gently palpated. A severe or complete stenosis will be associated with a diminished or absent ipsilateral carotid pulse.

Auscultation

A partial stenosis will give rise to a bruit which is best detected with a bell stethoscope. A bruit will be absent in patients with complete obstruction.

Non-invasive investigations

Ophthalmodynamometry

This test measures the blood pressure in the central retinal artery which is indirectly related to carotid artery blood flow. It should be performed on both sides and the results compared.

Technique

1. Both pupils are dilated and a topical anaesthetic instilled.
2. One examiner exerts external pressure on the sclera with a special calibrated spring-loader plunger (Bailliart's ophthalmodynamometer).
3. The other examiner observes the optic disc with an indirect ophthalmoscope.
4. As the pressure on the sclera is increased, the central retinal artery will be seen to pulsate and then all pulsations will cease. The diastolic pressure is read in millimetres of mercury from the gauge at the commencement of pulsations and the systolic pressure is read the moment pulsations cease.

Interpretation of results

A difference of 20% between the two sides is considered abnormal. Although ophthalmodynamometry is quick and easy to perform it is of limited value because it is negative unless 50% or more of the carotid artery is stenosed. It is therefore unable to detect non-stenotic ulcerative atheromatous plaques.

Carotid artery imaging

Two methods are at present available. The first uses a B-mode ultrasound scanner. The second uses Doppler frequency analysis combined with an image of the carotid artery obtained either with a Doppler scanner or with a B-mode ultrasound scanner. Although these methods are superior to ophthalmodynamometry because they can detect both ulcerative and stenotic lesions, they are expensive and require a skilled observer for correct interpretation.

Invasive investigations

These should be performed only if non-invasive tests are positive and the patient is a candidate for carotid endarterectomy.

Selected carotid arteriography

This test involves the direct injection of a radio-opaque dye into the carotid artery in the neck. At present this is the most accurate method of detecting both ulcerative and stenotic lesions. Unfortunately, the test is associated with a low but significant morbidity and mortality.

Digital subtraction angiography

In this test a dye is injected into the superior vena cava through a catheter introduced through the antecubital vein. Images of the carotid and vertebral arteries are then produced by sophisticated computer-assisted subtraction techniques. The test can be performed on an out-patient basis and is much safer than carotid arteriography.

Treatment of carotid disease

In patients with a localized stenosis of the artery, endarterectomy significantly reduces the risk of subsequent stroke. In experienced hands this operation carries a mortality of less than 1%, although the incidence of morbidity is higher. If endarterectomy is contraindicated, medical treatment with drugs that reduce platelet stickiness (aspirin, dipyridamole) or anticoagulants may be helpful in reducing the frequency of transient ischaemic attacks and the risk of a major stroke.

Hypertensive retinopathy

Introduction

It is extremely important to consider two aspects of systemic hypertension separately—the severity and the duration. The severity of hypertension is reflected by the degree of hypertensive vascular changes and retinopathy, and the duration of hypertension is reflected in the degree of arteriosclerotic vascular changes and retinopathy.

The primary response of the retinal arterioles to systemic hypertension is narrowing. There appears to be a positive relationship between the amount of narrowing and the level of blood pressure. The degree of response is also dependent on the amount of pre-existing replacement fibrosis (involutional sclerosis). Only in young individuals is the hypertensive narrowing seen in its pure form. In older patients the rigidity of retinal arterioles prevents the same degree of narrowing seen in young individuals.

Hypertensive features

The fundus picture of hypertensive retinopathy is characterized by vasoconstriction and leakage. The two most important signs are diffuse arteriolar narrowing and focal arteriolar narrowing. Unfortunately, the ophthalmoscopical diagnosis of generalized narrowing may be difficult, but the presence of focal narrowing makes it highly probable that the blood pressure is raised. Severe hypertension may lead to obstruction of the precapillary arterioles and cotton-wool spot formation. Abnormal vascular permeability leads to haemorrhages, retinal oedema, and hard exudates (*Figure 10.54*). The deposition of hard exudates around the fovea in Henle's layer may lead to their radial distribution in the form of a macular star (*Figure 10.55*). Swelling of the optic nerve head is the hallmark of the malignant phase of hypertension.

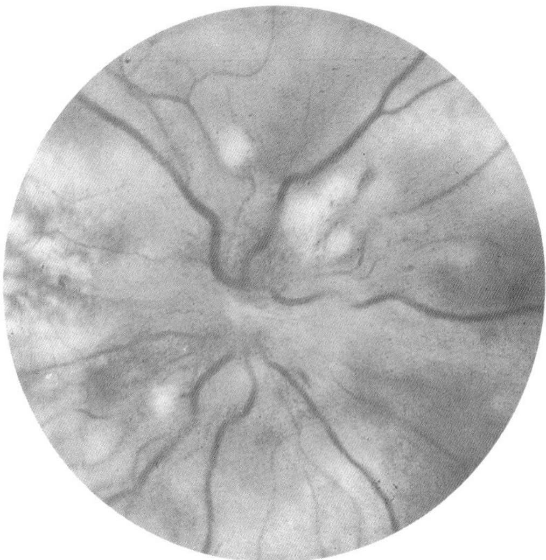

Figure 10.54 *Severe hypertensive retinopathy (courtesy of Mr A. Shun-Shin)*

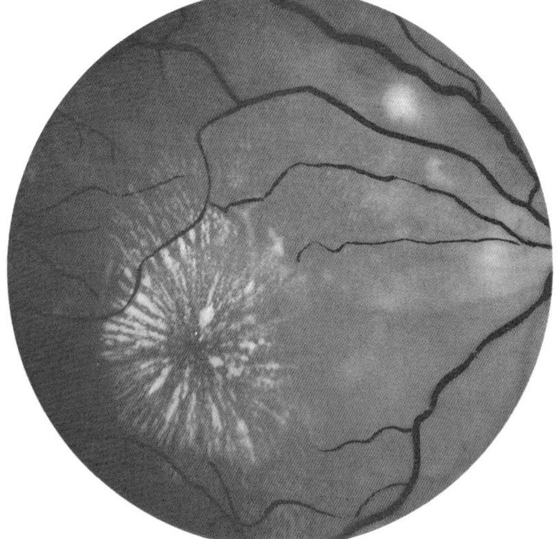

Figure 10.55 *Macular star in hypertensive retinopathy (courtesy of Dr P. Malleson)*

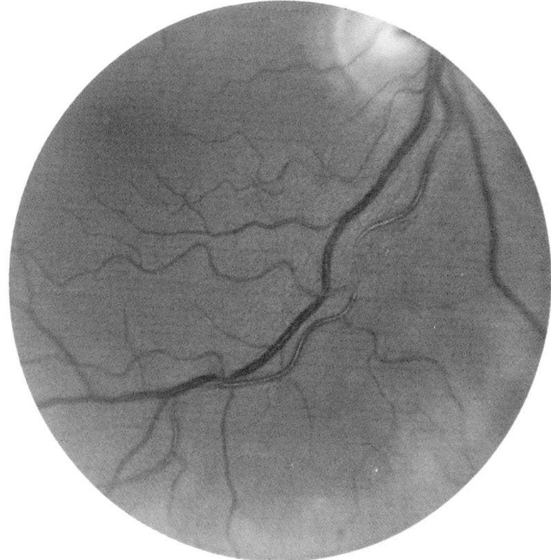

Figure 10.56 *Focal arteriolar attenuation (courtesy of Dr N. L. Stokoe)*

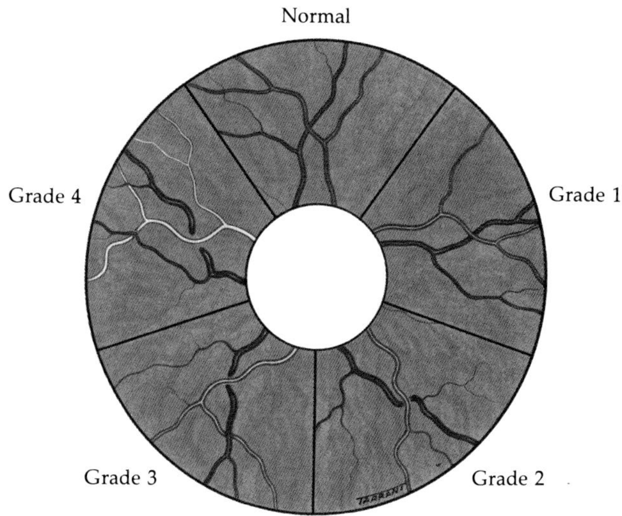

Figure 10.57 *Grading of retinal arteriosclerosis*

Grading

Grade 1

This consists of mild generalized arteriolar attenuation, particularly of small branches.

Grade 2

This is characterized by more severe grade 1 changes and also focal arteriolar attenuation (*Figure 10.56*).

Grade 3

This consists of grade 2 changes and also haemorrhages, cotton-wool spots, and exudates.

Grade 4

This consists of all grade 3 changes plus disc swelling.

Arteriosclerotic features

Arteriosclerotic changes are due to thickening of the vessel wall which histologically consists of intimal hyalinization, medial hypertrophy, and endothelial hyperplasia. The single most important sign of arteriosclerotic vasculopathy is the presence of advanced arteriovenous crossing change. Although this feature alone is not necessarily an indication of the severity of hypertension, its presence makes it likely that systemic hypertension has been present for many years.

It is important to point out that mild arteriovenous crossing changes may be seen in patients with involutional sclerosis in the absence of hypertension and also in normotensive diabetics.

Grading (*Figure 10.57*)

Grade 1

This consists of broadening of the arteriolar light reflex and simple vein concealment. Arteriolar reflex enhancement can be misleading and should not be overemphasized.

Grade 2

This consists of grade 1 changes, associated with deflection of veins at arteriovenous crossings (Salus' sign).

Grade 3

This consists of grade 2 changes as well as 'copper-wire' arterioles and marked arteriovenous crossing changes with banking of the vein where it appears dilated distal to the crossing (Bonnet's sign), tapering of the vein on either side of the crossing (Gunn's sign), and right-angled deflection of veins.

Grade 4

This consists of grade 3 changes as well as 'silver-wire' arterioles and severe arteriovenous crossing changes which may be associated with branch vein occlusion. Grade 4 arteriosclerotic changes correlate well with electrocardiographic abnormalities, especially left ventricular hypertrophy.

Additional ocular manifestations of systemic hypertension include ischaemic choroidal infarcts (Elschnig's spots), retinal arterial macroaneurysm, and ischaemic optic neuropathy. Uncontrolled systemic hypertension is also known to adversely affect diabetic retinopathy.

Sickle-cell retinopathy

Introduction

Pathogenesis

Different sickling haemoglobinopathies are due to the presence of one, or a combination of, abnormal haemoglobins which cause the red blood cell to adopt an anomalous shape under conditions of hypoxia and acidosis. Because these deformed red blood cells are more rigid than a healthy cell, they may become impacted in small blood vessels and cause hypoxia.

Abnormal haemoglobins

The sickling disorders in which the mutant haemoglobins S and C are inherited as alleles of normal haemoglobin A are of particular interest to the ophthalmologist. The abnormal haemoglobins may occur in combination with normal haemoglobin, resulting in AS (sickle-cell trait which is present in 8% of American blacks), or in association with each other as SS (sickle-cell disease or anaemia, present in 0.4% of American blacks), SC (sickle-cell haemoglobin C disease, present in 0.2% of American blacks), and SThal (thalassaemia).

Systemic features

SS combinations result in severe systemic complications but fairly mild ocular manifestations. SC and SThal produce milder anaemias and generally less severe systemic features. AS is the mildest form and usually requires hypoxia or other abnormal conditions to produce sickling. However, the ocular complications are most severe in the SC and SThal types of haemoglobinopathies.

Ocular features

Proliferative sickle retinopathy

Clinical features

Although the most severe forms of retinopathy are associated with SC and SThal diseases, the milder haemoglobinopathies may occasionally also cause retinopathy. Proliferative sickle retinopathy can be divided into five stages (*Figure 10.58*).

Stage 1 is characterized by peripheral arteriolar occlusion.

Stage 2 shows peripheral arteriovenous anastomoses which appear to be dilated pre-existent capillary channels. The peripheral retina after the point of vascular occlusion is largely avascular and non-perfused.

Stage 3 is characterized by the sprouting of new vessels from the anastomoses. Initially the new vessels lie flat on the retina and have a fan-shaped configuration ('sea-fan' neovascularization). They are usually fed by a single arteriole and drained by a single vein. Eventually the tufts become adherent to the cortical vitreous gel and are pulled into the vitreous cavity.

Stage 4 is characterized by varying amounts of vitreous haemorrhage. The bleeding may be precipitated by relatively trivial ocular trauma.

Stage 5 is characterized by vitreous traction and retinal detachment. Rhegmatogenous retinal detachment may also occur as a result of tear formation adjacent to areas of fibrovascular tissue.

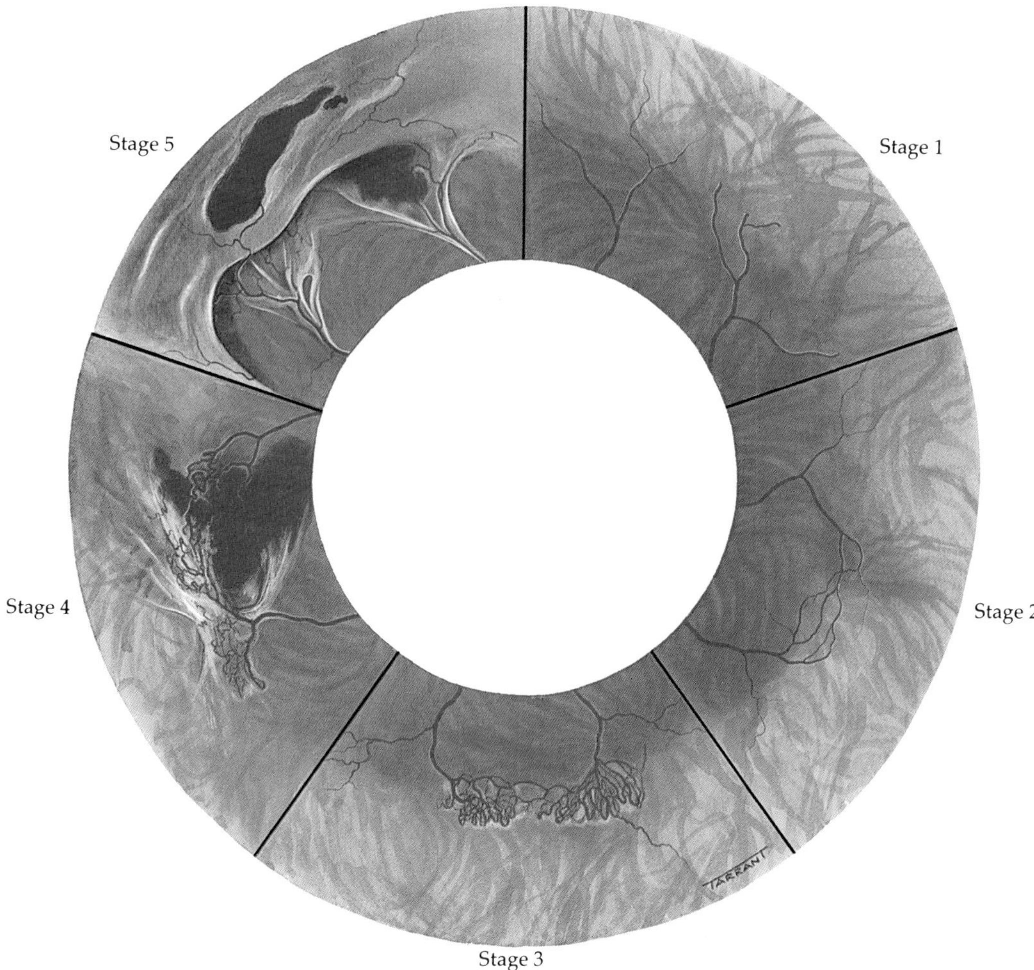

Figure 10.58 *Progression of sickle-cell proliferative retinopathy*

Treatment

1. *Peripheral circumferential retinal scatter photocoagulation* to areas of capillary non-perfusion is effective in inducing regression in a high proportion of cases.
2. *Pars plana vitrectomy* for tractional retinal detachment and/or persistent vitreous haemorrhage usually gives poor results.

Non-proliferative retinopathy

1. *Asymptomatic lesions* include venous tortuosity, black 'sunbursts' (peripheral chorioretinal atrophy), 'salmon-patch' haemorrhage (peripheral pink superficial haemorrhages), refractile spots (peripheral haemosiderin deposits within localized schisis cavities), 'silver-wiring' of peripheral arterioles, retinal breaks at equatorial or pre-equatorial retina and, rarely, angioid streaks.
2. *Symptomatic lesions* include central retinal artery occlusion, macular arteriole occlusion, retinal vein occlusion, and choroidal vascular occlusions.

Non-retinal manifestations

1. *Conjunctiva.* The most characteristic conjunctival sign consists of isolated dark-red vascular segments shaped like commas or corkscrews. They involve the small calibre vessels and are most frequently located inferiorly.
2. *Uveal tract.* The typical iris lesion is a circumscribed area of ischaemic atrophy, usually at the pupillary edge and extending to the collarette. Rubeosis may be seen occasionally.

Retinopathy of prematurity

Active

Pathogenesis

Retinopathy of prematurity (ROP) is a proliferative retinopathy which typically affects premature infants exposed to high ambient oxygen concentrations. It most frequently occurs in infants who weigh less than 1300 g at birth. The retina is unique among tissues in that it has no blood vessels until the fourth month of gestation, at which time vascular complexes emanating from the hyaloid vessels at the optic disc grow towards the periphery. These vessels reach the nasal periphery after 8 months of gestation but do not reach the temporal periphery until about 1 month after delivery. This incompletely vascularized temporal retina is particularly susceptible to oxygen damage, especially in the premature.

Clinical features

Although ROP is a bilateral disease, the severity of involvement in the two eyes may be asymmetrical. According to the international classification active ROP can be divided into the following five stages (*Figure 10.59*).

Stage 1: demarcation line

The first pathognomonic sign of active ROP is the development of a thin tortuous grey-white line which runs roughly parallel with the ora serrata (*Figure 10.59a*). The line, which is more prominent in the temporal periphery, separates the avascular immature peripheral retina from the vascularized posterior retina. Abnormal branching blood vessels may be seen leading up to the line.

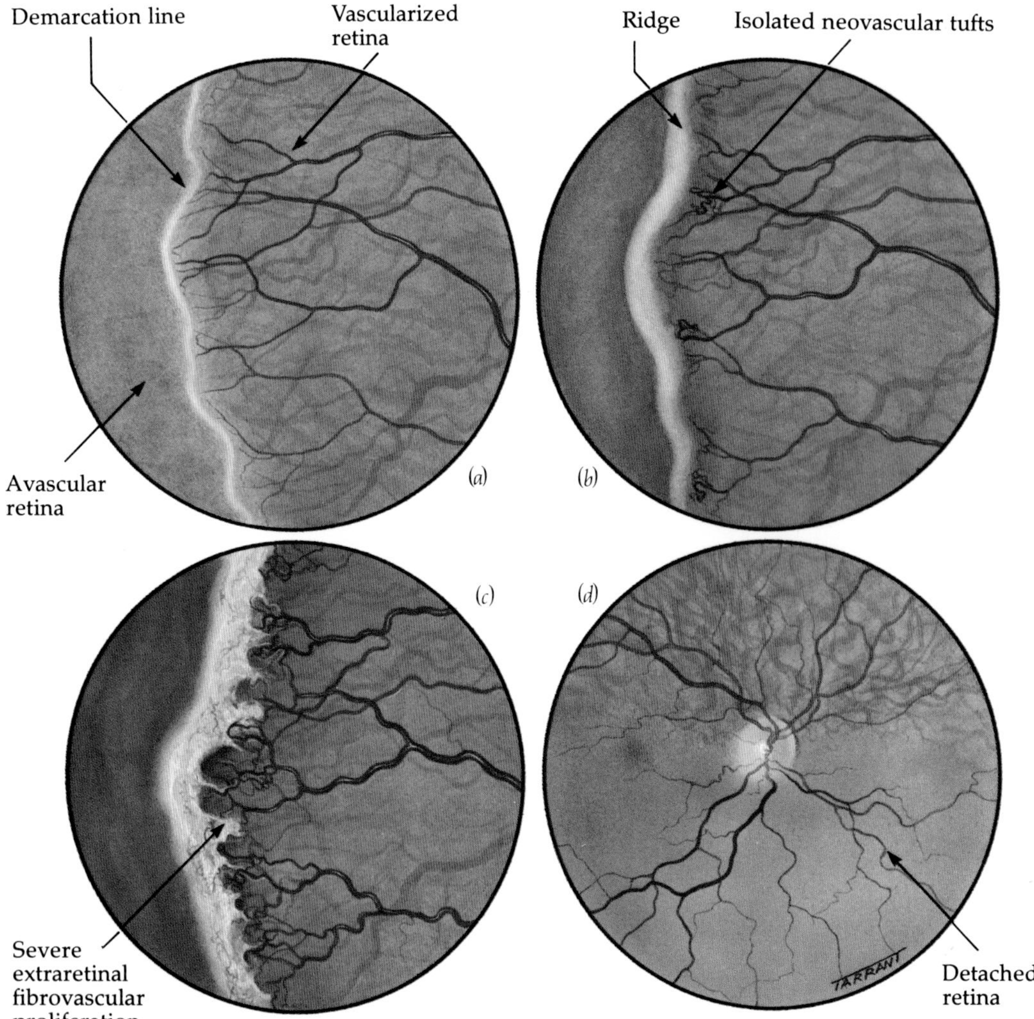

Figure 10.59 *Progression of active retinopathy of prematurity*

Stage 2: ridge

If the ROP progresses the demarcation line develops into a ridge of tissue which extends out of the plane of the retina. Blood vessels enter the ridge and small isolated neovascular tufts may be seen posterior to it (*Figure 10.59b*). The ridge represents a mesenchymal shunt which joins veins with arteries.

Stage 3: ridge with extraretinal fibrovascular proliferation

As the disease progresses the ridge becomes pink and coarse due to the development of fibrovascular proliferation along the surface of the retina and into the vitreous. These findings are often associated with dilatation and tortuosity of the retinal blood vessels posterior to the equator (*Figure 10.59c*). Retinal haemorrhage is fairly common, and vitreous haemorrhage may also develop.

Stage 4: subtotal retinal detachment

The progression of fibrovascular proliferation gives rise to a tractional retinal detachment which starts in the extreme periphery and then spreads centrally (*Figure 10.59d*). Retinal detachment typically develops when the infant is about 10 weeks old.

Stage 5: total retinal detachment

'Plus' disease

This is characterized by dilatation of the veins and tortuosity of the arterioles in the posterior fundus. When these changes are present a 'plus' sign is added to the stage number. For example, stage 2 with posterior vascular dilatation and tortuosity would be classified as 2+ ROP.

Although the clinical features of ROP usually take several weeks to develop, in rare instances the disease can progress from stage 1 to stage 4 within a few days.

Regression

In about 80% of infants, the ROP will regress spontaneously leaving few if any residua. Spontaneous regression may even occur in patients with partial retinal detachments.

Progression

Although retinal detachment is rare, its development is frequently preceded by the following signs:

1. Progression of 'plus' disease.
2. Development of fresh vitreous haze.
3. Increasing preretinal and vitreous haemorrhage.
4. Gross vascular engorgement of the iris and failure of the pupil to dilate.

Guideline for screening

The eyes of all infants born at less than 36 weeks or weighing less than 2000 g, who have received supplemental oxygen, should be screened for ROP. Screening during the first month of life is, however, of very limited value because the pupils are difficult to dilate and visualization of the fundus is impaired by vitreous haze caused by the tunica vasculosa lentis. The most useful time to screen an infant is between the seventh and ninth weeks of life. This is because ROP rarely appears for the first time after 9 weeks, and retinal detachment seldom develops before that time. The pupils in a premature infant are dilated with cyclopentolate 0.5% and phenylephrine 2.5%.

Treatment

At present there is no treatment that is universally accepted. This is in part due to the difficulty in evaluating results because of the high rate of spontaneous remission.

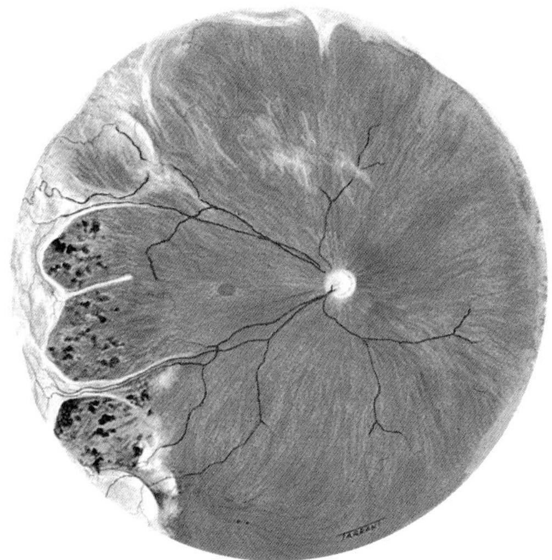

Figure 10.60 *Cicatricial retinopathy of prematurity with fibrovascular proliferation involving temporal periphery*

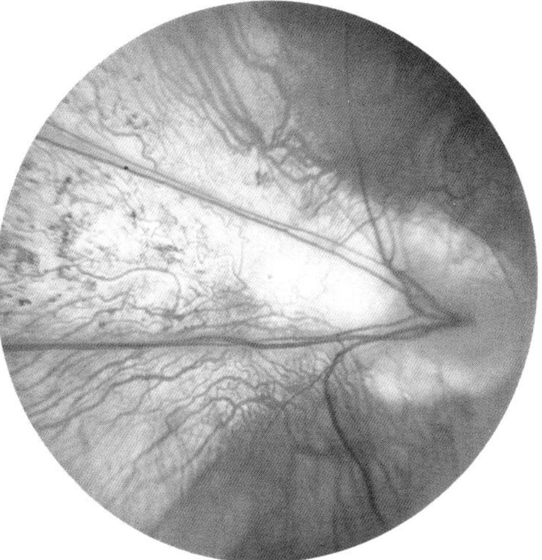

Figure 10.61 *'Dragging' of optic disc in cicatricial stage of retinopathy of prematurity*

The following therapeutic measures have been advocated:

1. *Cryotherapy* to ablate the avascular immature retina.
2. *Scleral buckling* with or without pars plana vitrectomy for tractional retinal detachment.
3. *Vitamin E.* It has been suggested that vitamin E deficiency may be a contributing factor in the development of blindness from ROP. However, the administration of vitamin E may cause undesirable side-effects and at present the risks versus the benefits are unclear.

Cicatricial (regressed)

About 20% of infants with active ROP will develop cicatricial complications which may be innocuous or extremely severe and blinding. In general, the more advanced the proliferative disease at the time of involution, the more serious are the cicatricial sequelae.

Clinical features

In order of severity signs of cicatrization are:

1. *Minimal peripheral retinal pigmentary disturbance and haze at the vitreous base.*
2. *Myopia* caused by either increased axial length of the eye or alterations in the lens.
3. *Peripheral retinal breaks and lattice degeneration.* These should be treated prophylactically in order to prevent the subsequent development of rhegmatogenous retinal detachment.
4. *Fibrous bands in the temporal retinal periphery* (*Figure 10.60*).
5. *Traction on the retinal blood vessels* by contraction of the peripheral fibrous tissue leading to straightening of the temporal vascular arcades, heterotopia of the macula, and distortion (dragging) of the optic disc (*Figure 10.61*).
6. *Retrolental cyclitic fibrovascular sheets* extending for a variable distance towards the posterior pole of the lens.
7. *Funnel-shaped total tractional retinal detachment.*
8. *Secondary angle-closure glaucoma.* This develops in some eyes with total retinal detachment due to the formation of posterior synechiae and a progressive shallowing of the anterior chamber due to a forward movement of the iris–lens diaphragm. Treatment is by lensectomy and anterior vitrectomy.

Differential diagnosis

See Chapter 13.

Retinal telangiectasias

Introduction

This is a group of rare, idiopathic, congenital, retinal vascular anomalies characterized by dilatation and tortuosity of retinal vessels, formation of multiple aneurysms, varying degrees of leakage, and deposition of lipid exudates. Retinal telangiectasias always involve the capillary bed although arterioles and venules may also be affected. The vascular malformations frequently progress and may become symptomatic later in life as a result of haemorrhage, oedema, or lipid exudation. Because the condition is unassociated with any other systemic or ocular disease, it should be distinguished from secondary telangiectasias which may be associated with other retinal vascular disorders such as retinal vein occlusion, diabetic retinopathy, sickle-cell retinopathy, Eales' diseae, and retinopathy of prematurity.

Idiopathic juxtafoveolar retinal telangiectasia

Clinical features

This is characterized by dilated and kinked microvascular channels, microaneurysms, and capillary non-perfusion near the fovea (*Figure 10.62b*). In some cases, only the temporal half of the parafoveal capillary network is affected while in others the entire circumference is involved together with the immediately adjacent retinal vascular bed. The condition may be unilateral or bilateral. Impairment of central vision in adult life is most frequently secondary to intraretinal oedema and exudate (*Figure 10.62a*).

Treatment

In some cases, progressive impairment of central vision can be prevented by argon laser photocoagulation to the sites of leakage.

Leber's miliary aneurysms

Clinical features

This is a more severe form of telangiectasia which is characterized by fusiform and saccular dilatation of venules and arterioles, most commonly involving the temporal retinal periphery (*Figure 10.63, top*). The condition may be asymptomatic until central vision becomes impaired in adult life due to lipid deposition at the fovea (*Figure 10.64*). Leber's miliary aneurysms should not be confused with acquired macroaneurysms of the retinal arteries which typically affect elderly hypertensive or arteriosclerotic individuals.

Treatment

Ablation of the vascular anomalies by either cryotherapy or photocoagulation may be beneficial (*Figure 10.63, bottom*).

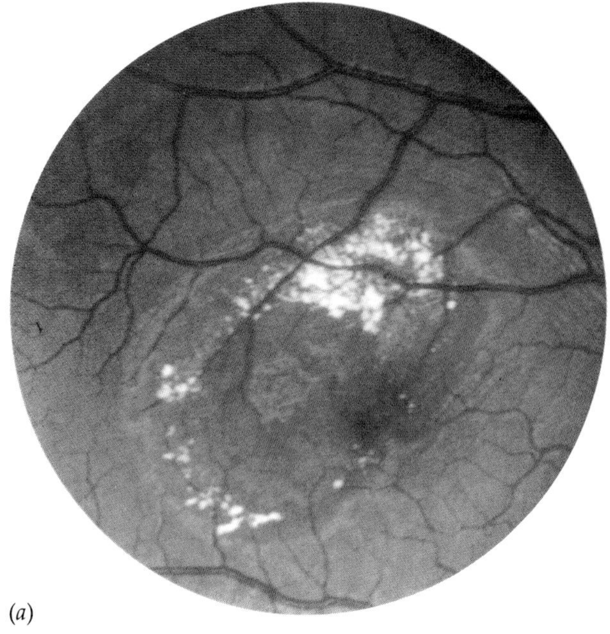

(*a*)

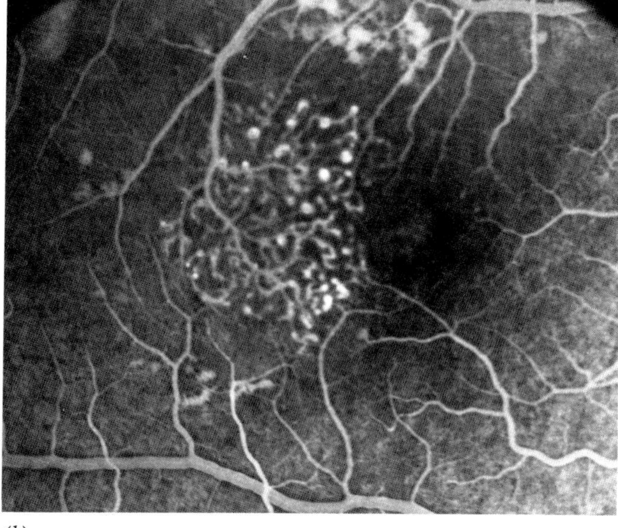

(*b*)

Figure 10.62 (a) *Macular exudates in idiopathic juxtafoveolar retinal telangiectasia;* (b) *fluorescein angiogram of same eye showing microvascular anomalies*

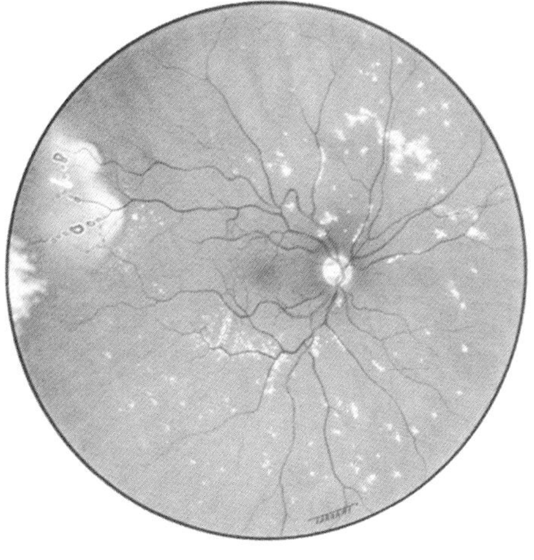

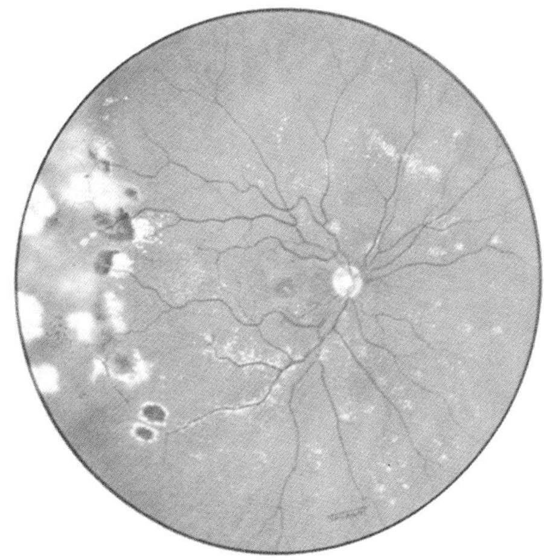

Figure 10.63 *Leber's miliary aneurysms involving temporal peripheral retina. Top: before treatment; bottom: after treatment by cryotherapy*

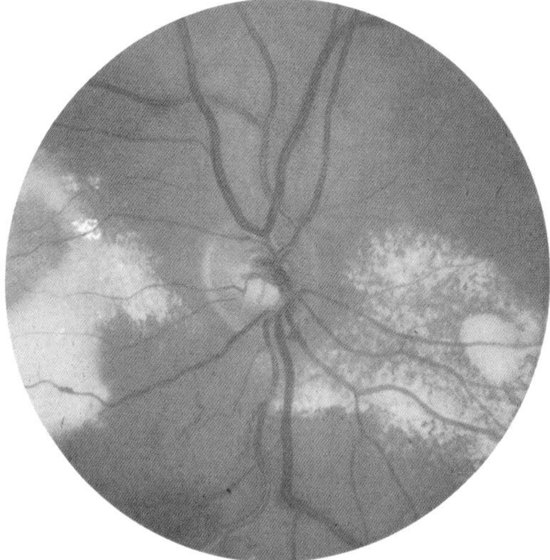

Figure 10.64 *Leber's miliary aneurysms (courtesy of Dr P. H. Morse)*

Coats' disease

Clinical features

This is the most severe form of retinal telangiectasia. It typically presents in the first decade of life with a white fundus reflex (leukocoria), strabismus, or visual loss. Although in the differential diagnosis it is important to exclude retinoblastoma, Coats' disease usually presents later. The condition is uniocular and more common in boys than in girls. Early Coats' disease is characterized by large areas of intra- and subretinal yellowish exudate (*Figure 10.65*), often associated with overlying dilated and tortuous retinal blood vessels at the posterior pole and retinal periphery. Although a few cases regress spontaneously, the majority progress over a period of years to exudative retinal detachment, a retrolental mass, secondary cataract, rubeosis iridis, uveitis, secondary glaucoma, and eventually phthisis bulbi.

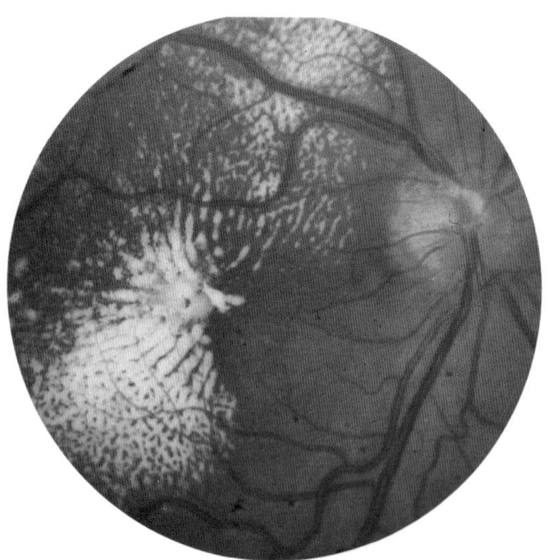

Figure 10.65 *Early Coats' disease (courtesy of Mr B. Mathalone)*

Treatment

If applied early, treatment with either photocoagulation or cryotherapy may be successful in preventing progression and occasionally also in improving vision. Treatment is less effective once the retina has detached.

Further reading

Diabetic retinopathy

Bresnick, G.H. (1983) Diabetic maculopathy. *Ophthalmology*, **90**, 1301–1317

Diabetic Retinopathy Study Research Group (1979) Four risk factors for severe visual loss in diabetic retinopathy. *Archives of Ophthalmology*, **97**, 654–655

Diabetic Retinopathy Study Research Group (1981) Photocoagulation treatment of proliferative diabetic retinopathy. *Ophthalmology*, **88**, 583–600

Diabetic Retinopathy Vitrectomy Study Group (1985) Early vitrectomy for severe vitreous haemorrhage in diabetic retinopathy. *Archives of Ophthalmology*, **103**, 1644–1652

Doft, B.H. and Blankenship, G. (1984) Retinopathy risk factor regression after laser panretinal photocoagulation for proliferative diabetic retinopathy. *Ophthalmology*, **91**, 1453–1457

Early Treatment Diabetic Retinopathy Study Research Gropup (1985) Photocoagulation for diabetic macular oedema. *Archives of Ophthalmology*, **103**, 1796–1806

Feke, G.T., Tagawa, H., Yoshida, A. *et al.* (1985) Retinal circulatory changes related to retinopathy progression in insulin-dependent diabetes mellitus. *Ophthalmology*, **92**, 1517–1522

Flynn, H.W. and Blankenship, G.W. (1985) Proliferative diabetic retinopathy. *Clinical Modules for Ophthalmologists*, Vol. 3, Module 12

Frank, R.N. (1984) On the pathogenesis of diabetic retinopathy. *Ophthalmology*, **91**, 626–634

Friberg, T.R., Rosenstock, J., Sanborn, G. *et al.* (1985) The effect of long-term near normal glycaemic control on mild diabetic retinopathy. *Ophthalmology*, **92**, 1051–1058

Huber, M.J.E., Smith, S.A. and Smith, S.E. (1985) Mydriatic drugs for diabetic patients. *British Journal of Ophthalmology*, **69**, 425–427

Hyman, B.N. (1981) The prevention of diabetic retinopathy. *Ophthalmology*, **88**, 35A–37A

Inglesby, D.V., Turner, G.S., Schulenburg, W.E. *et al.* (1985) Photocoagulation for peripheral neovascularization in diabetes. *British Journal of Ophthalmology*, **69**, 157–161

Kingsley, R., Ghosh, G., Lawson, P. *et al.* (1983) Severe diabetic retinopathy in adolescents. *British Journal of Ophthalmology*, **67**, 73–79

Klein, R., Klein, B.E.K. and Moss, S.E. (1984) Visual impairment in diabetes. *Ophthalmology*, **91**, 1–9

Little, H.L. (1981) Alterations in blood elements in the pathogenesis of diabetic retinopathy. *Ophthalmology*, **88**, 647–654

Little, H.L. (1985) Nonproliferative diabetic retinopathy. *Clinical Modules for Ophthalmologists*, Vol. 3, Module 11

Little, H.L. (1985) Treatment of proliferative diabetic retinopathy. *Ophthalmology*, **92**, 279–283

McDonald, H.R. and Schatz, H. (1985) Visual loss following panretinal photocoagulation for proliferative diabetic retinopathy. *Ophthalmology*, **92**, 388–393

Mosier, M.A., Del Piero, E. and Gheewala, S.M. (1985) Anterior retinal cryotherapy in diabetic vitreous hemorrhage. *American Journal of Ophthalmology*, **100**, 440–444

Shorb, S.R. (1985) Anemia and diabetic retinopathy. *American Journal of Ophthalmology*, **100**, 434–436

Tso, M.O.M., Cunha-Vaz, J.G., Shin, C-Y. *et al.* (1980) Clinicopathological study of blood–retinal barrier in experimental diabetes mellitus. *Archives of Ophthalmology*, **98**, 2032–2040

Whitelocke, R.A.F., Kearns, M., Blach, R.K. *et al.* (1979) The diabetic maculopathies. *Transactions of the Ophthalmological Society of the United Kingdom*, **99**, 314–320

Ziemianski, M.C., McMeel, J.W. and Franks, E.P. (1980) Natural history of vitreous haemorrhage in diabetic retinopathy. *Ophthalmology*, **87**, 306–312

Retinal vein occlusion

Branch Vein Occlusion Study Group (1984) Argon laser photocoagulation for macular oedema in branch vein occlusion. *American Journal of Ophthalmology*, **98**, 271–282

Branch Vein Occlusion Study Group (1986) Argon laser scatter photocoagulation for prevention of neovascularization and vitreous haemorrhage in branch vein occlusion. *Archives of Ophthalmology*, **104**, 34–41

Chopdar, A. (1982) Hemi-central retinal vein occlusion. *Transactions of the Ophthalmological Society of the United Kingdom*, **102**, 241–248

Frucht, J., Shapiro, A. and Merin, S. (1984) Intraocular pressure in retinal vein occlusion. *British Journal of Ophthalmology*, **68**, 26–28

Gutman, F.A. (1983) Evaluation of a patient with central retinal vein occlusion. *Ophthalmology*, **90**, 481–483

Hayreh, S.S. (1983) Classification of central retinal vein occlusion. *Ophthalmology*, **90**, 458–478

Hayreh, S.S. and Podhaysky, P. (1982) Ocular neovascularization with retinal vascular occlusion. *Archives of Ophthalmology*, **100**, 1585–1596

Joffe, L., Goldberg, R.E. and Magargal, L.E. (1980) Macular branch vein occlusion. *Ophthalmology*, **87**, 91–98

Johnston, R.L., Brucker, A.J., Steinmann, W. *et al.* (1985) Risk factors of branch vein occlusion. *Archives of Ophthalmology*, **103**, 1831–1832

Kearns, T.P. (1983) Differential diagnosis of central retinal vein occlusion. *Ophthalmology*, **90**, 475–480

Kohner, E.M., Laatikainen, L. and Oughton, J. (1983) The management of central retinal vein occlusion. *Ophthalmology*, **90**, 484–487

Magargal, L.E., Donoso, L.A. and Sandborn, G.E. (1982) Retinal ischaemia and risk of neovascularization following central retinal vein obstruction. *Ophthalmology*, **89**, 1241–1245

Servais, G.E., Thompson, H.S. and Hayreh, S.S. (1986) Relative afferent pupillary defect in central retinal vein occlusion. *Ophthalmology*, **93**, 301–303

Shilling, J.S. and Jones, C.A. (1984) Retinal branch vein occlusion: a study of argon laser photocoagulation in the treatment of macular oedema. *British Journal of Ophthalmology*, **68**, 196–198

Zagarra, H., Gutman, F.A., Zakov, N. *et al.* (1983) Partial central retinal vein occlusion. *American Journal of Ophthalmology*, **96**, 330–337

Retinal artery occlusion

Arruga, J. and Sanders, M.D. (1982) Ophthalmic findings in 70 patients with evidence of retinal embolisation. *Ophthalmology*, **89**, 1336–1347

Brown, G.C. and Magargal, L.E. (1982) Central retinal artery obstruction and visual acuity. *Ophthalmology*, **89**, 14–19

Brown, G.C., Magargal, L.E., Shields, J.A. *et al.* (1981) Retinal artery obstruction in children and young adults. *Ophthalmology*, **88**, 18–25

Cohen, G.R., Harbison, J.W., Blair, C.J. *et al.* (1984) Clinical significance of transient visual phenomena in the elderly. *Ophthalmology*, **91**, 436–442

Fawcett, I.M., Barrie, T., Sheldon, C. *et al.* (1985) The prevalence of carotid artery disease in patients presenting with amaurosis fugax. *Transactions of the Ophthalmological Society of the United Kingdom*, **104**, 787–791

Hayreh, S.S., Kolder, H.E. and Weingeist, T.A. (1980) Central retinal artery occlusion and retinal tolerance time. *Ophthalmology*, **87**, 75–78

Jampol, L.M. (1983) Arteriolar occlusive disease of the macula. *Ophthalmology*, **90**, 534–539

Marmor, M.F., Jampol, L.M. and Wohl, L. (1985) Cilioretinal collateral circulation after occlusion of the central retinal artery. *British Journal of Ophthalmology*, **69**, 805–809

Sanborn, G.E. (1983) Retinal and carotid artery obstruction. *Clinical Modules for Ophthalmologists*, Vol. 1, Module 10

Sanborn, G.E., Miller, N.R., Maguire, M. *et al.* (1981) Clinical–angiographic correlation of ophthalmodynamometry in suspected carotid artery disease. Prospective study. *Archives of Ophthalmology*, **99**, 1811–1813

Savino, P.J., Glaser, J.S. and Cassidy, J. (1977) Retinal stroke. Is the patient at risk? *Archives of Ophthalmology*, **95**, 1185–1189

Tomsak, R.L., Ross, D. and Gutman, F.A. (1978) Central retinal artery occlusion. *Perspectives in Ophthalmology*, **2**, 217–222

Sickle-cell retinopathy

Acheson, R.W., Ford, S.M., Maude, G.H. *et al.* (1986) Iris atrophy in sickle cell disease. *British Journal of Ophthalmology*, **70**, 516–521

Condon, P.I., Marsh, R.J., Maude, G.H. *et al.* (1983) Alpha thalassaemia and macular vasculature in homozygous sickle cell disease. *British Journal of Ophthalmology*, **67**, 779–781

Condon, P.I., Whitelocke, R.A.F., Bird, A.C. *et al.* (1985) Recurrent visual loss in homozygous sickle cell disease. *British Journal of Ophthalmology*, **69**, 700–706

Cruess, A.F., Stephens, R.F., Magargal, L.E. *et al.* (1983) Peripheral circumferential retinal scatter photocoagulation for treatment of proliferative sickle retinopathy. *Ophthalmology*, **90**, 272–278

Jampol, L.E., Condon, P., Farber, M. *et al.* (1983) A randomized clinical trial of feeder vessel photocoagulation of proliferative sickle cell retinopathy. *Ophthalmology*, **90**, 540–545

Rednam, K.R., Jampol, L.M. and Goldberg, M.F. (1982) Scatter retinal photocoagulation for proliferative sickle-cell retinopathy. *American Journal of Ophthalmology*, **93**, 594–599

Sargeant, B.E., Mason, K.P., Acheson, R.W. *et al.* (1986) Blood rheology and proliferative retinopathy in homozygous sickle cell disease. *British Journal of Ophthalmology*, **70**, 522–525

Talbot, J.F., Bird, A.C., Rabb, L.M. *et al.* (1983) Sickle cell retinopathy in Jamaican children: a search for prognostic factors. *British Journal of Ophthalmology*, **67**, 782–785

Talbot, J.F., Bird, A.C. and Sargeant, G.R. (1983) Retinal changes in sickle cell/hereditary persistence of fetal haemoglobin syndrome. *British Journal of Ophthalmology*, **67**, 777–778

Retinopathy of prematurity

Committee for the Classification of Retinopathy of Prematurity (1984) An international classification of retinopathy of prematurity. *Archives of Ophthalmology*, **102**, 1130–1134

Kalina, R.E. and Karr, D.J. (1982) Retrolental fibroplasia—experience over two decades in one institution. *Ophthalmology*, **89**, 91–95

Machemer, R. (1983) Closed vitrectomy for severe retrolental fibroplasia. *Ophthalmology*, **90**, 436–441

Palmer, E.A. (1981) Optimal timing of examination of acute retrolental fibroplasia. *Ophthalmology*, **88**, 662–666

Palmer, E.A. (1984) Retinopathy of prematurity. *Clinical Modules for Ophthalmologists*, Vol. 2, Module 12

Patz, A. (1983) Current therapy of retrolental fibroplasia. *Ophthalmology*, **90**, 425–427

Patz, A. (1985) Observations on the retinopathy of prematurity. *American Journal of Ophthalmology*, **100**, 164–168

Schaffer, D.B., Johnson, L., Quinn, G.E. *et al.* (1985) Vitamin E and retinopathy of prematurity. *Ophthalmology*, **92**, 1005–1011

Tasman, W. (1985) Management of retinopathy of prematurity. *Ophthalmology*, **92**, 995–999

Retinal telangiectasias

Asdourian, G.K. (1979) Vascular anomalies of the retina. *Perspectives in Ophthalmology*, **3**, 111–120

Gass, J.D. and Oyakawa, T. (1982) Idiopathic juxtafoveal telangiectasia. *Archives of Ophthalmology*, **100**, 769–780

Laqua, H. and Wessing, A. (1983) Peripheral retinal telangiectasis in adults simulating a vascular tumour or melanoma. *Ophthalmology*, **90**, 1284–1291

Ridley, M.E., Shields, J.A., Brown, G.C. *et al.* (1982) Coats' disease. Evaluation of management. *Ophthalmology*, **89**, 1381–1387

Tarkkanen, A. and Laatikainen, L. (1983) Coats's disease: clinical, angiographic, histopathological findings and clinical management. *British Journal of Ophthalmology*, **67**, 766–776

11

Acquired Maculopathies

Introduction

Applied anatomy

Clinical evaluation of the macula

Fluorescein angiography

Physiological principles

Technique

Complications

Circulation of fluorescein

Age-related macular degeneration

Drusen

Non-exudative

Exudative

Central serous chorioretinopathy

Cystoid macular oedema

Macular hole

Myopic maculopathy

Macular pucker

Choroidal folds

Angioid streaks

Toxic maculopathies

Introduction

Applied anatomy

Macula

This is an oval area at the posterior pole measuring about 5 mm in diameter. Its centre is located approximately 4 mm temporal and 0.8 mm inferior to the centre of the optic disc. Histologically, it is the region of the retina containing xanthophyll pigment and more than one layer of ganglion cells. Important clinical landmarks within the macula are the fovea, the foveola, and the foveal avascular zone (*Figure 11.1*).

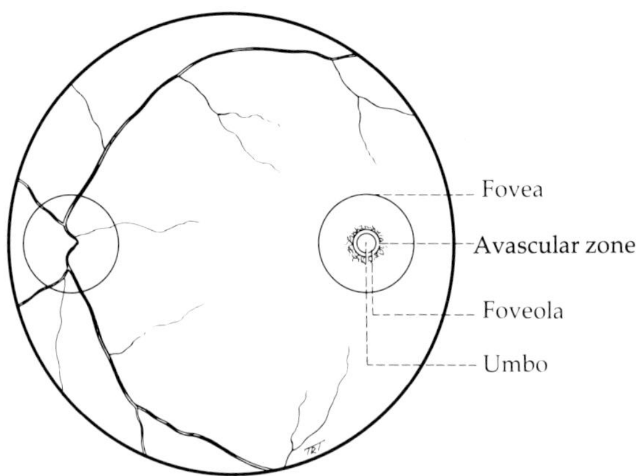

Figure 11.1 *Anatomy of fovea*

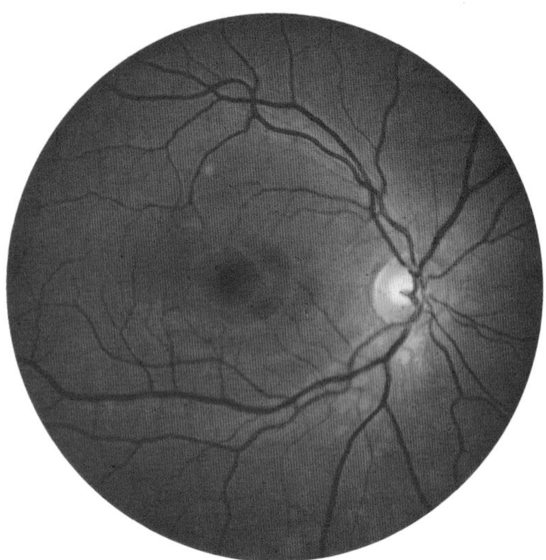

Figure 11.3 *Normal foveal light reflex*

Fovea

This is a depression in the inner retinal surface at the centre of the macula (*Figure 11.2*). Its diameter is the same as that of an average optic disc (1.5 mm). Ophthalmoscopically, the fovea can be recognized by an oval light reflex arising from the increased thickness of the retina and internal limiting membrane in the parafoveal region (*Figure 11.3*). The parafoveal region is the thickest part of the retina containing six to eight layers of ganglion cells, in contrast to the retina outside the macula which contains only one layer. The internal limiting membrane rapidly decreases in thickness as it progresses from the parafoveal region towards the centre of the fovea. This may partially explain the susceptibility of this area to damage by toxins from distant sites such as the anterior uvea.

Foveola

This forms the central floor of the fovea and has a diameter of 0.35 mm. It is the thinnest part of the retina and is devoid of ganglion cells. Its entire thickness consists only of cones and their nuclei and it subserves the most acute vision. The umbo is a tiny depression in the very centre of the foveola which corresponds to the ophthalmoscopically visible foveolar reflex seen in most normal eyes. Loss of the foveolar reflex may be an early sign of damage.

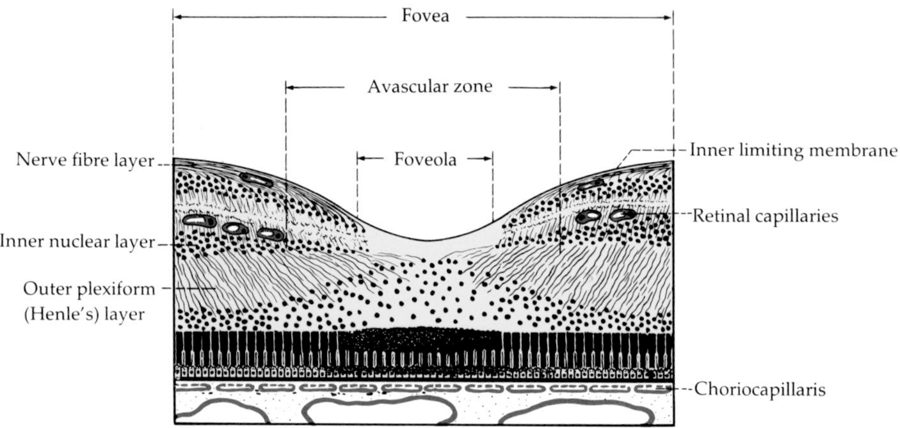

Figure 11.2 *Cross-section of fovea*

Foveal avascular zone

This measures 0.5 mm in diameter and is therefore situated inside the fovea but outside the foveola. The exact location of the foveal avascular zone (FAZ) can only be determined by fluorescein angiography (FA). It is a very important landmark in deciding whether or not to treat subretinal neovascular membranes at the macula by laser photocoagulation. The integrity of the terminal capillary network as seen on FA is also of prognostic significance in eyes with maculopathy due to diabetes and retinal vein occlusion. Significant loss of the network is indicative of poor prognosis.

Henle's layer

In order to optimize light transmission to the foveolar cones, all retinal elements have to be displaced laterally out of the light path. The nerve fibres in the outer plexiform (Henle's) layer therefore have to run almost parallel with the retinal surface before reaching their points of synapse with the processes of the cells in the inner nuclear layer. However, this lateral displacement of the retinal layers also disturbs the normal reticular architecture of the supporting Müller's cells, and consequently the retina in this region loses its compact nature and becomes very susceptible to deposition of large amounts of extracellular fluid. Exudates within Henle's fibre layer typically assume a star-shaped configuration corresponding to the radial arrangement of the fibres as they diverge from the centre of the fovea (*see Figure 10.55*).

Retinal pigment epithelium

This is a single layer of hexagonally shaped cells, the apices of which contain villous processes which reach out towards the outer segments of the photoreceptors. The adhesion between the retinal pigment epithelium (RPE) and neurosensory retina is weaker than that between the RPE and Bruch's membrane. A separation between the RPE and neurosensory retina is called a retinal detachment and the fluid in between the two layers is referred to as subretinal fluid. The RPE cells in the fovea are taller, thinner, and contain more and larger melanosomes than elsewhere in the fundus.

Bruch's membrane

This separates the RPE from the choriocapillaris. On electron microscopy it consists of five elements:

1. The basal lamina of the RPE.
2. The inner collagenous layer.
3. A thicker band of elastic fibres.
4. The outer collagenous layer.
5. The basal lamina of the outer layer of the choriocapillaris.

Changes in Bruch's membrane play an important part in many macular disorders.

Clinical evaluation of the macula

Symptoms

The cardinal symptom of macular disease is blurring of central vision. Typically, the patient complains that there is something obstructing his central vision (positive scotoma). He is frequently disappointed when the ophthalmologist is unable to remove the obstruction. This is in contrast to the negative scotoma from an optic nerve lesion in which the patient notices a 'hole' in the centre of his visual field. Other symptoms of macular disease that are absent in optic nerve disease are metamorphopsia (alteration in image shape), micropsia (decrease in image size due to spreading apart of foveal cones), and macropsia (increase in image size caused by compression of foveal cones).

Signs

Visual acuity

This is the most important test of macular function. A hypermetropia with a disparity between the subjective and objective refraction of the eye is characteristic of a shallow elevation of the neurosensory retina at the macula.

Pupillary reactions

These reactions to light are normal in eyes with macular disorders, although extensive retinal disease such as a retinal detachment may be associated with a relative afferent conduction defect (Marcus Gunn pupil). This is in contrast to mild lesions of the optic nerve in which pupillary abnormalities occur early.

Colour vision

This is not significantly impaired in eyes with early macular disease, in contrast to eyes with early lesions of the optic nerve.

Light brightness appreciation

This is normal in eyes with macular disease. Patients with optic nerve lesions frequently complain that things look dimmer with the affected eye (as if the light in the room had been turned down; *see* Chapter 15).

Ophthalmoscopy

Using monochromatic light ophthalmoscopy may be useful in detecting subtle macular lesions which may otherwise be overlooked. Green (red-free) light is used for detecting superficial retinal lesions such as wrinkling of the internal limiting membrane or foveal cysts. It is also useful in delineating the outline of subtle serous elevations of th neurosensory retina as well as improving visualization of the fundus through mild opacities in the media. Lesions involving the RPE and choroid are best detected using light at the red end of the spectrum.

Direct slitlamp biomicroscopy

Using the Hruby lens or a fundus contact lens, this is valuable in detecting subtle macular lesions such as cystoid

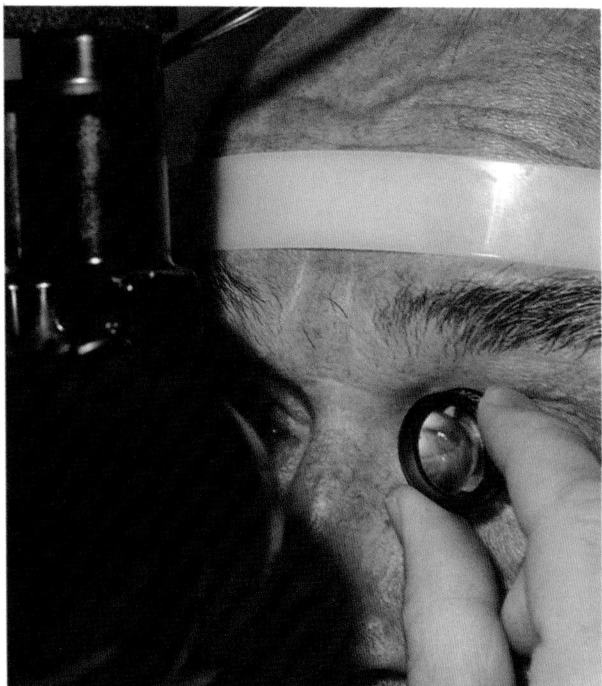

Figure 11.4 Examination of macula with +90 Volk lens

oedema, subretinal neovascular membranes, and elevation of the neurosensory retina or RPE.

Indirect slitlamp biomicroscopy

Using a strong convex lens, this is also extremely useful. The advantage of this method over the Hruby lens is a larger field and the ability to examine a moving eye. The image is, however, vertically inverted (upside down) and laterally reversed (macula is nasal to disc), exactly as with binocular indirect ophthalmoscopy. The lens used for the examination can be either a +90 D Volk conoid lens (*Figure 11.4*) or a ×16 slitlamp eyepiece.

Amsler grid

This is useful for screening as well as following the clinical course of a macular lesion. The chart consists of a 10-cm square divided into smaller 5-mm squares (*Figure 11.5*). When the chart is viewed at one-third of a metre, each small square subtends an angle of 1°. In performing the test the patient should wear his reading glasses and cover one eye. He is asked to look directly at the centre dot with the uncovered eye and report any distortion, wavy lines (*Figure 11.6*), blurred areas, or blank spots anywhere on the grid. As will be discussed later, patients at risk of visual loss from subretinal choroidal neovascularization should use the Amsler grid regularly.

Photostress test

This is particularly useful in demonstrating macular lesions when ophthalmoscopy is equivocal, as in early cystoid

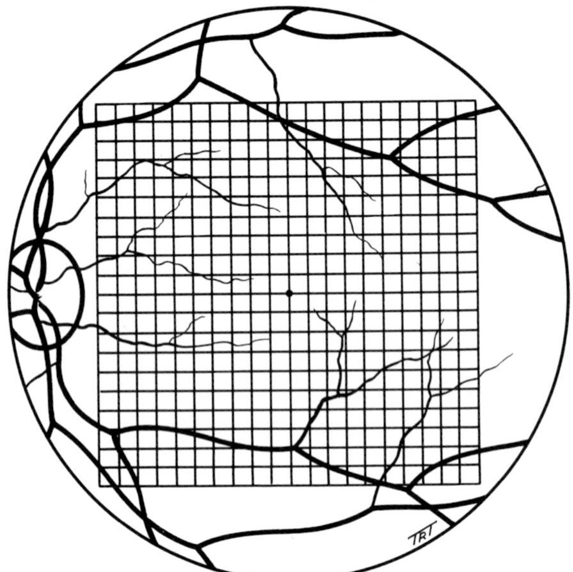

Figure 11.5 Amsler grid superimposed on posterior pole

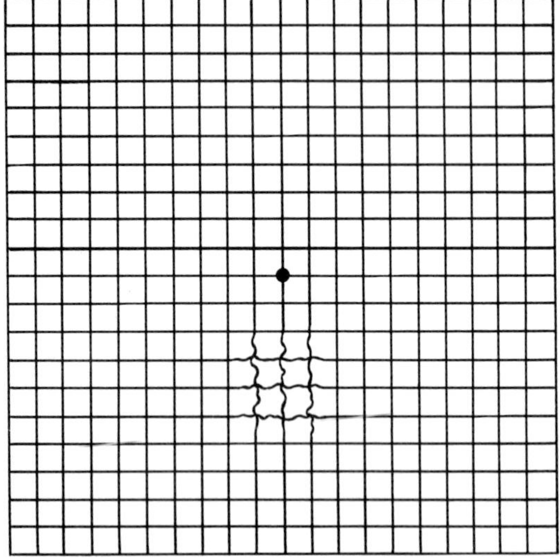

Figure 11.6 Amsler grid showing slight distortion inferior to fixation

macular oedema or central serous chorioretinopathy. It also differentiates visual loss due to macular disease from that caused by an optic nerve lesion.

The photostress test is a gross version of the dark adaptation test in which the visual pigments are bleached by light. This causes a temporary state of retinal insensitivity which is perceived by the patient as a scotoma. The recovery of vision is dependent on the ability of the photoreceptors to resynthesize visual pigments.

In performing this test, first the best corrected distance visual acuity is determined. Then the patient fixates the light of a pen-torch or an indirect ophthalmoscope held about 3 cm away for about 10 seconds. The photostress recovery time (PSRT) is measured by the time taken to read any three letters of the pre-test acuity line. The test is then performed on the other eye. Patients with macular disease will have a PSRT of over 50 seconds (sometimes several minutes) whereas the PSRT is within normal limits in patients with optic nerve lesions.

Macular function in eyes with opaque media

Several tests are available in the evaluation of potential macular function in eyes with opaque media such as cataract and dense vitreous haemorrhage.

Pupillary response to light

This should be normal even in the presence of a mature cataract. The presence of an afferent pupillary conduction defect usually indicates one of the following: a lesion of the optic nerve, an extensive retinal detachment, or an extremely large macular lesion.

Blue field entoptic 'flying corpuscle' test

This is based on the entoptic perception of leucocytes moving in the perifoveal capillaries. The test is performed in a darkened room. The retina is uniformly illuminated with a blue light of an entoptoscope held close to the patient's eye, in alignment with the visual axis. The perception of white cells is dependent on intact photoreceptors and patent macular capillaries. A normal response is when the patient can perceive 15 or more corpuscles moving through the entire entoptic field. Indications of macular disease are failure to see any corpuscles, partial loss of corpuscles in one part of the field, a decreased number of corpuscles, and a lower corpuscular speed as compared with the healthy eye.

Two light discrimination test

This is performed in a darkened room. Two pen-lights are held close together 60 cm away from the patient and then gradually separated until the patient indicates that he can perceive two lights. The interpretation of the test depends on the patient's level of vision. If visual acuity is 'hand movements' or less, good macular function is usually present if two lights can be perceived when they are about 12 cm apart. If vision is between 'counting fingers' and 3/60

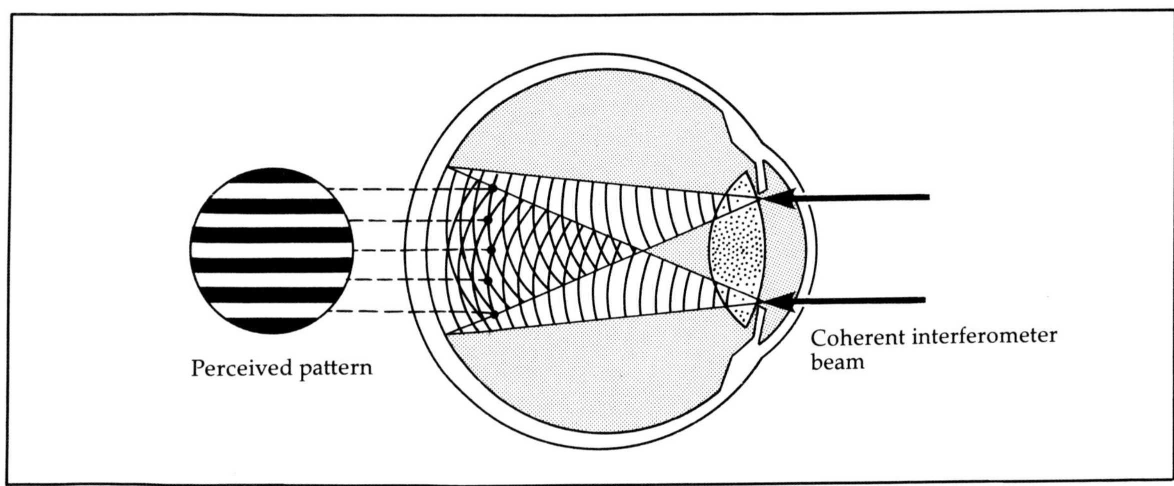

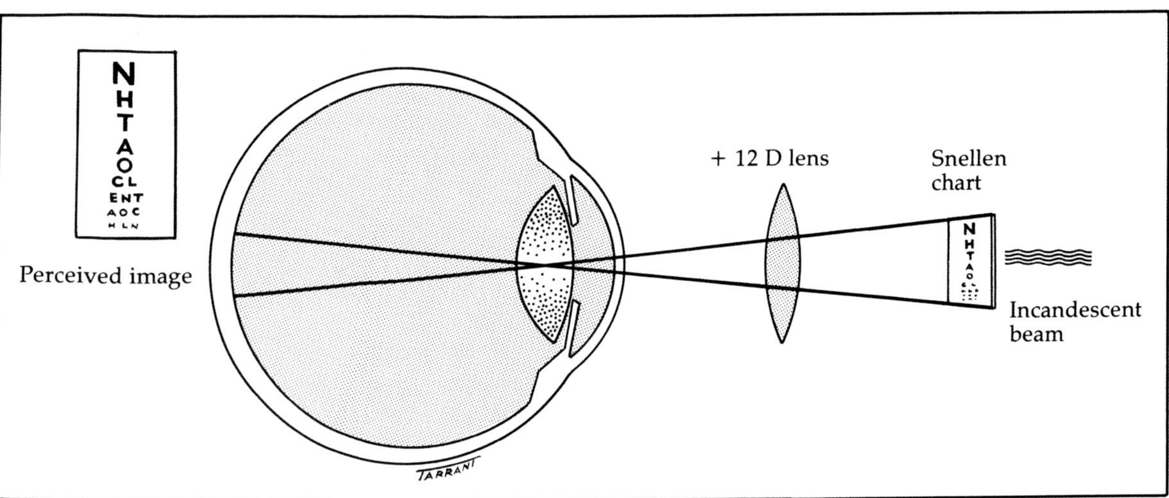

Figure 11.7 *Top: principles of inferometry; bottom: principles of potential visual acuity meter*

this occurs when the lights are about 7 cm apart, and if vision is better than 3/60 two lights will be seen when they are 5 cm apart.

Colour perception test

This is performed with the patient wearing red-green spectacles used for Worth's four dot test. Perception of red and green is tested by shining a pen-light through the spectacles. Blue perception is tested by using a blue field entoptoscope. A positive response indicative of good macular function occurs when the patient can correctly describe at least one of the three colours.

Purkinje vascular entoptic test

This is performed by gently rubbing a pen-light over the closed upper or lower eyelid. If the macula is healthy the patient should be able to describe the vascular markings as branches, cobwebs, or cracks.

Inferometry (*Figure 11.7, top*)

This can be used in eyes with immature cataracts. The test provides a measure of the resolving power of the macula by using two coherent light beams to create a three-dimensional fringe pattern on the retina. The beams produce two point sources behind the lens opacity, and the light waves emitting from these two points overlap. Where the crest of one wave overlaps the trough of the other wave, the effects are cancelled and a black band is produced. Where crests coincide with one another or where troughs coincide with one another, the enhancement produces bright bands of light. When performing the test the pupils should be widely dilated. The light beam is then directed into the centre of the pupil in the plane of the iris and then the pupil is scanned until the fringe pattern is seen. The patient is then asked to indicate the orientation of the bands of light. Initially, large gratings are used and then they are gradually diminished until the patient is unable to detect their correction orientation. The potential visual acuity is then estimated from the grating width.

Potential visual acuity meter (*Figure 11.7, bottom*)

This projects a standard Snellen chart through a small clear area of an immature cataract and is most accurate in eyes with visual acuities of 6/60 or better. The main components of the PAM are an incandescent light source, a miniature transilluminated Snellen chart, and a +12 D lens. In performing the test the pupils should be widely dilated and the patient is asked to read the letters on the chart. The PAM tends to be most accurate in eyes with visual acuities of 6/60 or better.

Fluorescein angiography

Fundus fluorescein angiography (FA) is extremely valuable in studying the normal physiology of the retinal and choroidal circulations as well as demonstrating disease processes affecting the macula.

Physiological principles (*Figure 11.8*)

Fluorescein binding

On entering the circulation, between 70% and 85% of fluorescein molecules bind to serum proteins (mainly albumin). The rest remain unbound and are referred to as 'free fluorescein'.

Inner blood–retinal barrier

The tight junctions of the retinal capillary endothelial cells form the inner blood–retinal barrier across which neither bound nor free fluorescein molecules can pass. Any leakage from the retinal circulation is therefore pathological.

Outer (RPE) blood–retinal barrier

The major choroidal vessels are impermeable to both bound and free fluorescein molecules. On the other hand, the walls of the choriocapillaris are extremely thin and contain multiple fenestrations through which free (not bound) fluorescein molecules are able to escape into the extravascular space and also across Bruch's membrane. However, adjacent cells of the RPE are firmly attached to each other by a series of adhesions called junctional complexes. These complexes (zonulae occludentes and zonulae adherentes) prevent the passage of free fluorescein molecules across the RPE and maintain the outer blood–retinal barrier. Passage of fluorescein across the RPE is therefore abnormal.

Fluorescence

Fluorescence is the property of certain molecules to emit light energy of a longer wavelength when stimulated by light of shorter wavelength. The light is not simply selectively reflected, but actually changed in character (*Figure 11.9*).

The excitation peak for fluorescein molecules is about 490 nm (blue part of the spectrum) and represents the maximal absorption of light energy by fluorescein. Molecules stimulated by this wavelength will be excited to a higher energy level and will emit light of a longer wavelength, which will be in the green portion of the spectrum at about 530 nm.

In order to ensure that the blue light enters the eye and only yellow-green light enters the camera, two types of filter are used (*Figure 11.10*). White light emitted from the

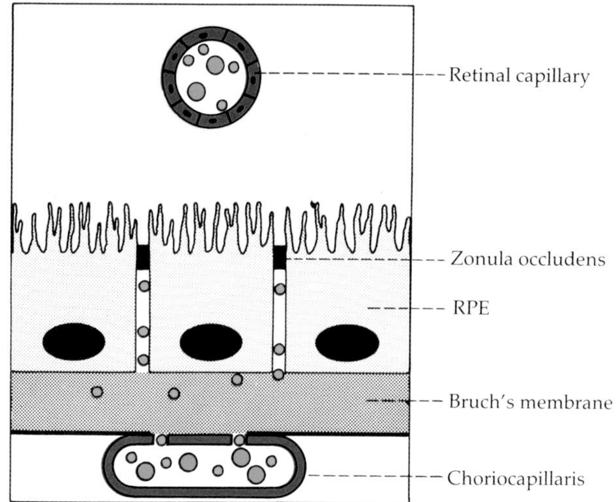

Figure 11.8 *Physiological principles of fluorescein angiography*

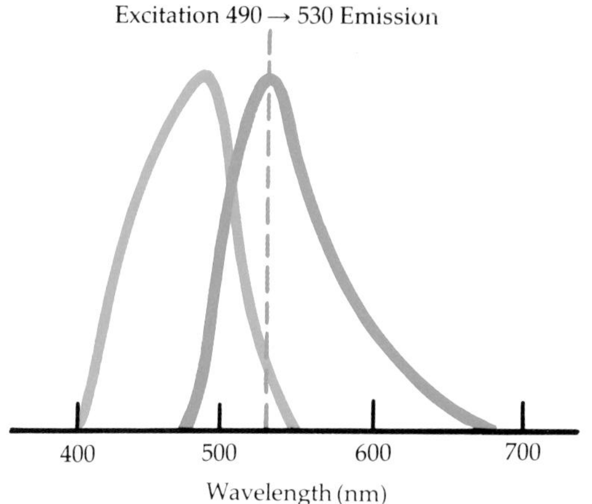

Figure 11.9 *Excitation and emission of fluorescein*

retinal camera passes through a blue excitation filter. The emerging blue light then enters the eye and excites the fluorescein molecules in the retinal and choroidal circulations to a longer wavelength (yellow-green light). A yellow-green barrier filter then blocks any blue light that may leave the eye allowing only yellow-green light to pass through unimpaired to be recorded on film.

Technique

In order to obtain good quality angiograms the pupils have to be dilated and the media clear. The patient is seated in front of the camera with one arm outstretched (*Figure 11.11*). Fluorescein, usually 5 ml of a 10% solution, is drawn up into a syringe (some prefer to use 3 ml of a 25% solution which gives better results in eyes with hazy media).

A 'red-free' photograph is taken and then the fluorescein is injected rapidly into the antecubital vein. Photographs are then taken at approximately 1-second intervals, between 5 and 25 seconds following injection. After the transit phase has been photographed in one eye, control pictures are taken of the opposite eye. If necessary, late photographs can also be taken after 10 minutes and, occasionally, after 20 minutes when leakage is anticipated.

Complications

Fluorescein is a safe substance as is evident from the many thousands of angiograms performed each year without serious complications. Mild side-effects include a red after-image, transient nausea, and a discolouration of the urine and skin. Rare serious complications include syncope, laryngeal oedema, bronchospasm, and anaphylactic shock. It is very important to have a clear plan for managing these eventualities in case they occur. The incidence of side-effects is the same for all concentrations of fluorescein.

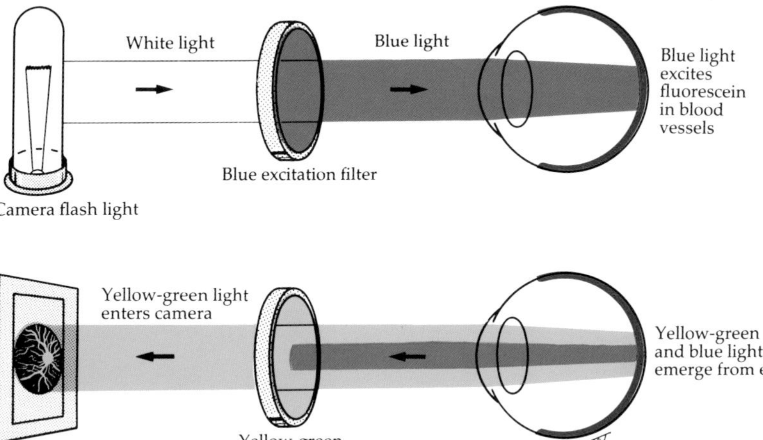

Figure 11.10 *Fluorescein angiography filters*

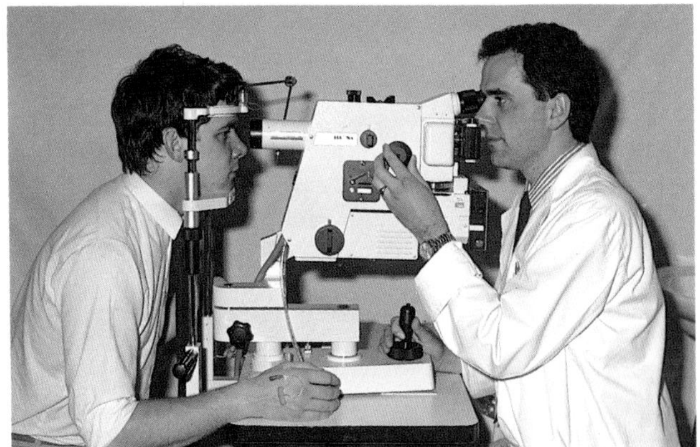

Figure 11.11 *Camera used for fundus fluorescein angiography*

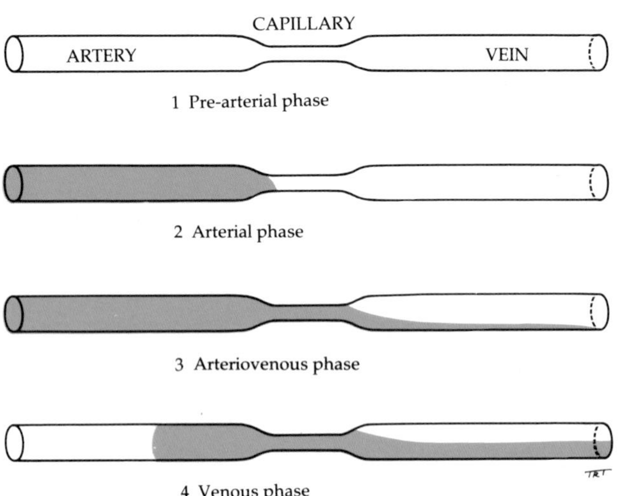

Figure 11.13 *Phases of the angiogram*

Circulation of fluorescein

Fluorescein enters the eye through the ophthalmic artery, passes into the choroidal circulation through the short posterior ciliary arteries, and into the retinal circulation through the central retinal artery (*Figure 11.12*). Because the route to the retinal circulation is slightly longer than that to the choroidal circulation, the latter is filled about 1 second before the former. In the choroidal circulation often no precise details are discernible, mainly due to the rapid leakage of free fluorescein molecules from the chorioapillaris and also because the melanin in the RPE cells blocks choroidal fluorescence.

Phases of the angiogram

The normal fluorogram consists of four overlapping phases (*Figure 11.13*).

Phase 1 is the pre-arterial phase during which the choroidal circulation is filling, but no dye has reached the retinal arteries.

Phase 2 is the arterial phase which follows 1 second after the pre-arterial phase and extends from the first appearance of dye in the arteries until the whole arterial circulation is filled.

Phase 3 is the arteriovenous (capillary) phase, which is characterized by complete filling of the arteries and capillaries with early lamellar flow in the veins.

Phase 4 is the venous phase which can be further subdivided into early, mid, and late stages according to the extent of venous filling and arterial emptying.

Normal angiogram

In interpreting the normal angiogram it is necessary to evaluate each anatomical component of the posterior pole during each time interval.

Figure 11.14, left shows the arterial phase which occurs 1 second after the pre-arterial phase.

Figure 11.14, right shows the arteriovenous phase in which the arteries and capillaries are completely filled with dye and there is very early lamellar flow in the veins. Choroidal filling occurs either segmentally or as a flush. The extent of background choroidal fluorescence increases as more free fluorescein molecules leak from the choriocapillaris into the extravascular space. In hypopigmented eyes

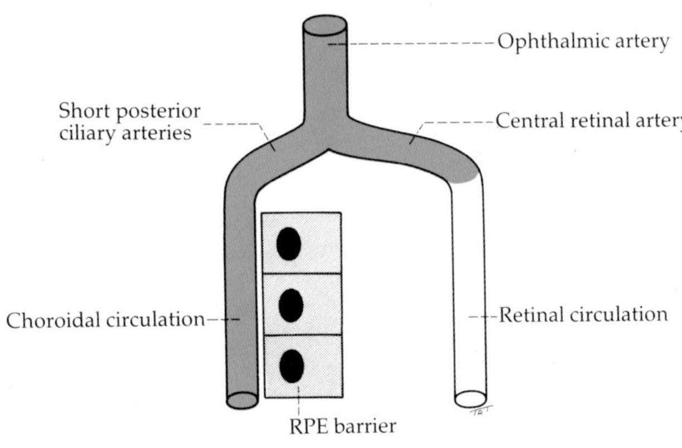

Figure 11.12 *Entry of fluorescein into the eye*

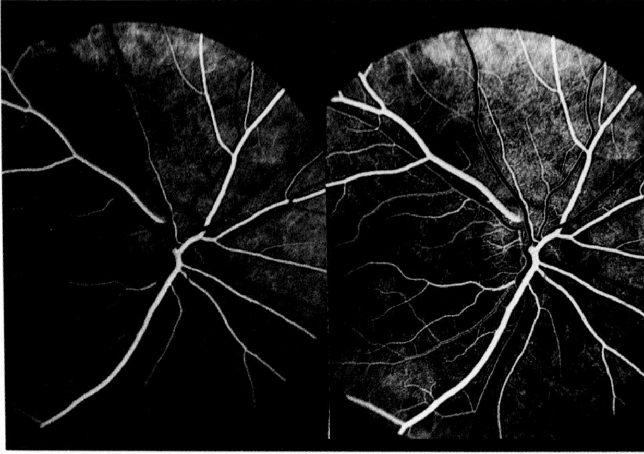

Figure 11.14 *Left: arterial phase; right: arteriovenous phase*

this may be so marked that details of the retinal capillaries may be lost. In highly pigmented eyes background choroidal fluorescence will be less obvious.

Figure 11.15, left shows the early venous phase in which the arteries and capillaries are filled and there is lamellar flow in the veins.

Figure 11.15, right is taken 1 second later. Here the lamellar flow is more obvious.

Figure 11.16, left is the midvenous phase in which the veins are nearly filled.

Figure 11.16, right is the late venous phase in which the veins are completely filled and the arteries are beginning to show decreasing fluorescence.

Figure 11.17, left. Recirculation of dye occurs within 3–5 minutes. The intensity of fluorescence begins to diminish so that the arteries and veins appear equally fluorescent.

Figure 11.17, right. The late phase of the angiogram shows the effects of continuous recirculation, dilution, and elimination of dye. With each succeeding wave the intensity of fluorescence becomes weaker. Late staining of the optic nerve head is a normal finding.

The dark appearance of the fovea is caused by blockage of choroidal fluorescence by increased amounts of xanthophyll pigment and the increase in size and melanin content of the RPE cells in this part of the retina, as well as avascularity inside the FAZ.

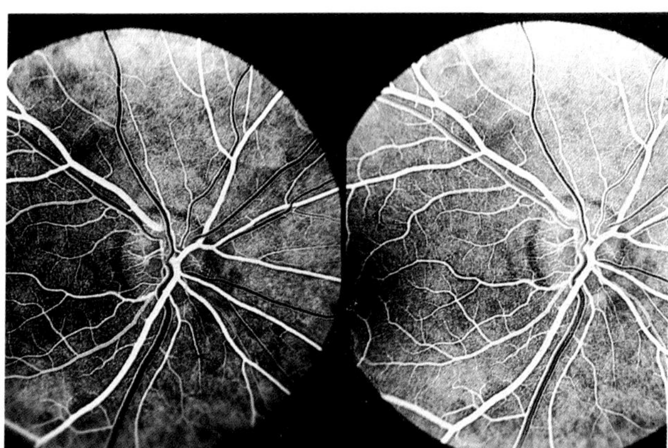

Figure 11.15 *Left: early venous phase; right: 1 second later*

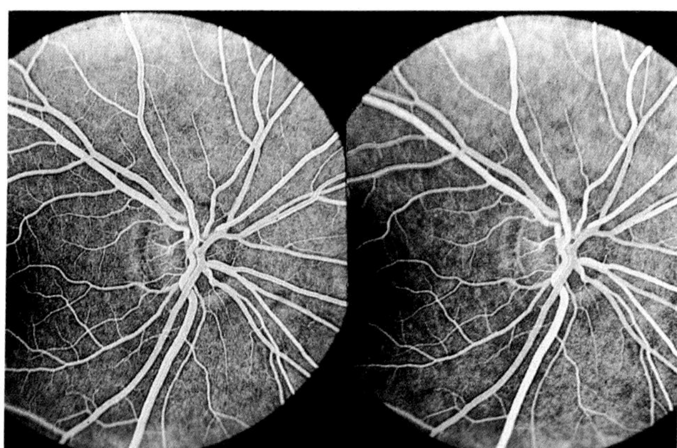

Figure 11.16 *Left: midvenous phase; right: late venous phase*

Causes of abnormal fluorescence

Hyperfluorescence

1. An RPE 'window' defect due to atrophy of the overlying RPE cells with unmasking of normal background choroidal fluorescence (*Figure 11.18*).
2. Pooling of dye under a detachment of the RPE (*Figure 11.19*).
3. Pooling of dye in the subretinal space due to a breakdown of the outer blood–retinal barrier (*Figure 11.20*).

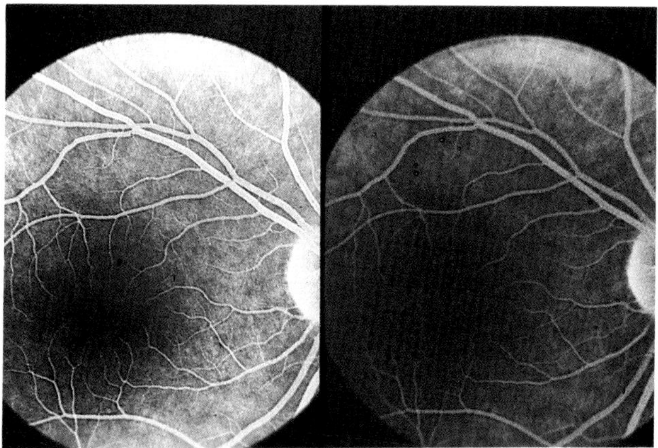

Figure 11.17 *Late phases*

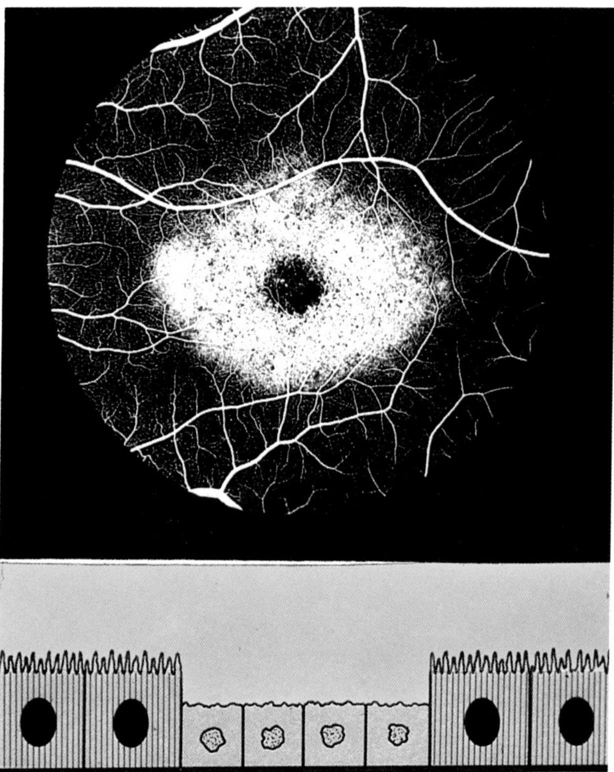

Figure 11.18 *Increased background fluorescence due to atrophy of the RPE in chloroquine maculopathy*

4. Leakage of dye into the neurosensory retina due to a breakdown of the inner blood–retinal barrier (*Figure 11.21*).
5. Leakage of dye from choroidal (*see Figure 11.30*) or retinal neovascularization.
6. Retention of dye by some tissues for abnormally long periods of time ('staining'; *see Figure 11.24, bottom*).
7. Leakage of dye from the optic nerve head in papilloedema.

Hypofluorescence

1. Blockage of fluorescence by increased density of pigment (xanthophyll in the neurosensory retina, melanin in the RPE), deposition of abnormal materials (hard exudates in neurosensory retina, lipofuscin in Best's disease), and blood (*Figure 11.22*).
2. Obstruction of retinal or choroidal circulation preventing access of dye to the tissues.
3. Loss of vascular tissue (choroideremia, myopic degeneration).

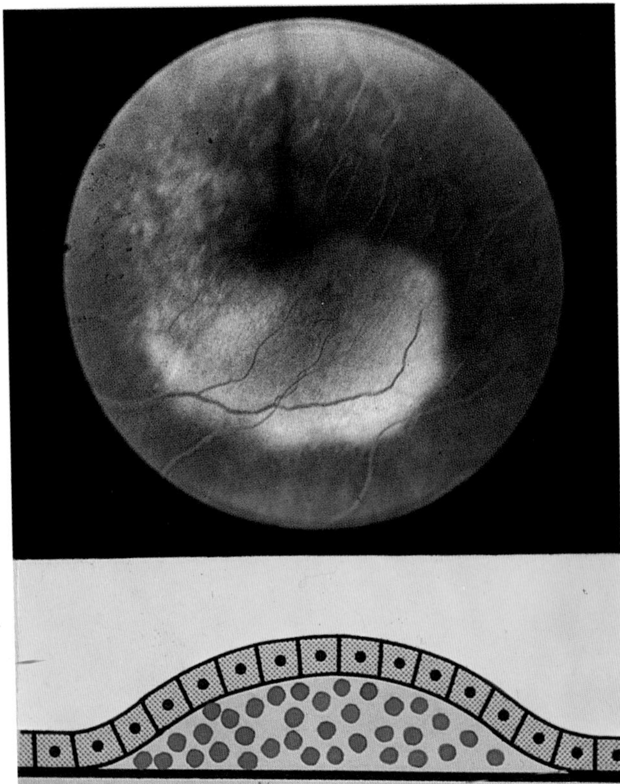

Figure 11.19 *Pooling of dye under detachment of RPE (courtesy of Mr J. Shilling)*

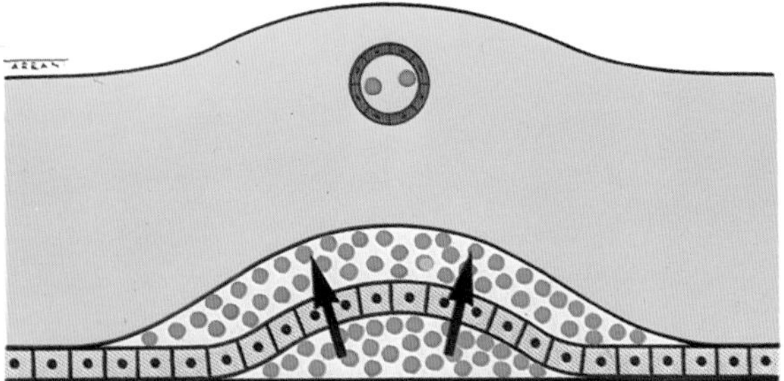

Figure 11.20 *Pooling of dye under sensory retina in central serous chorioretinopathy*

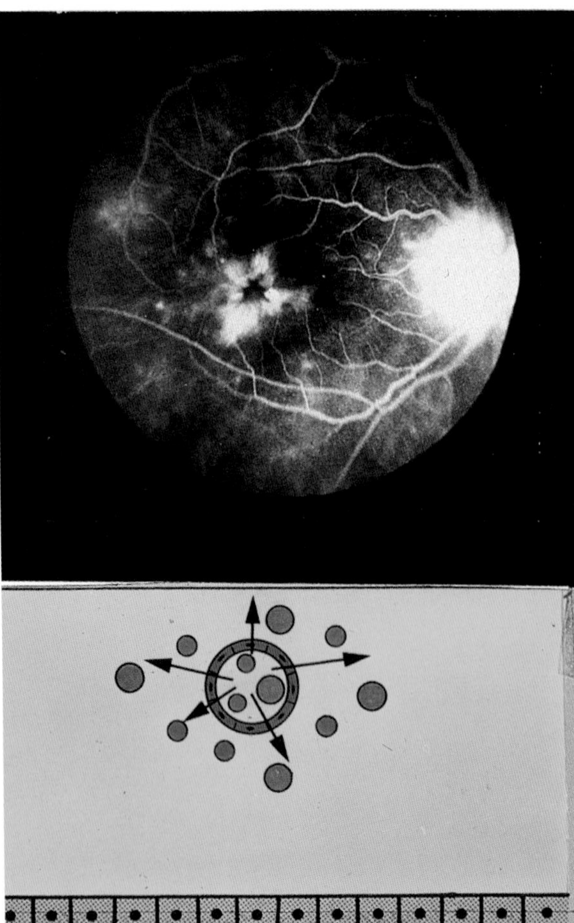

Figure 11.21 *Cystoid macular oedema due to breakdown of inner blood–retinal barrier (courtesy of Mr R. Marsh)*

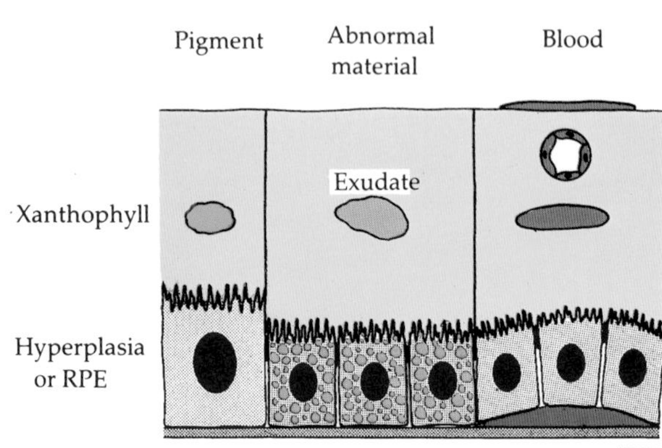

Figure 11.22 *Main causes of blocked fluorescence*

Age-related macular degeneration

Age-related macular degeneration (AMD) or senile macular degeneration is the leading cause of blindness in the Western World. It is a bilateral disease, the average age of visual loss in the first eye being 65 years, with about a 12% incidence of involvement of the second eye each year. About 60% of patients are therefore legally blind in both eyes by the time they reach their seventieth birthday.

Drusen

Clinical features

Frequently the earliest clinical manifestation of AMD is the appearance of small, discrete, yellow-white, slightly elevated spots called drusen or colloid bodies at the posterior poles of both fundi. These lesions are usually distributed symmetrically in both fundi and their exact appearance varies according to their size and extent of associated changes in the RPE. Drusen are rarely clinically visible prior to the age of 45 years. They are not uncomon between the ages of 45 and 60 years and fairly frequent thereafter. With advancing age they increase in size and number. Secondary calcification in long-standing lesions gives them a white and more glistening appearance.

Classification

The following types of drusen have been identified clinically and histologically:

1. *Hard* (nodular) drusen appear as small discrete yellowish-white spots (*Figure 11.23*).
2. *Soft* drusen have indistinct edges, are larger than hard drusen, and frequently become confluent.
3. *Diffuse* (confluent) drusen represent a widespread abnormality of the RPE.
4. *Calcified* drusen have a glistening appearance. Although all types of drusen may have calcification, calcified hard drusen are usually most conspicuous.

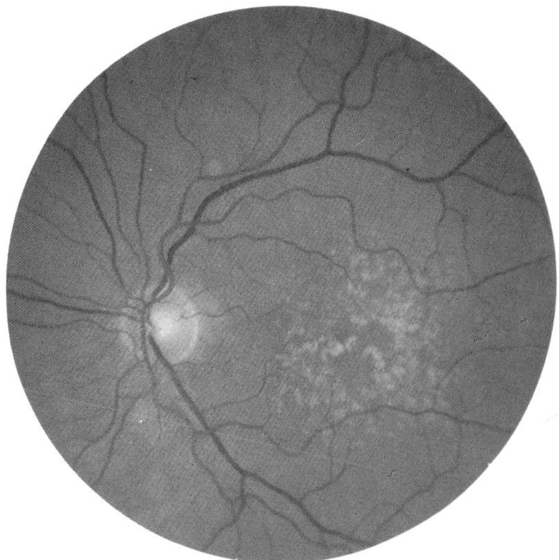

Figure 11.23 *Hard drusen*

Histopathology

Histopathologically, drusen consist of focal collections of hyaline material located between the basal lamina of the RPE and the inner collagenous layer of Bruch's membrane. Findings associated with drusen include (*Figure 11.24, top*):

1. Localized and diffuse thickening of the inner aspects of Bruch's membrane. This may predispose to its splitting and subsequent complications such as detachment of the RPE and choroidal neovascularization.
2. Varying degrees of atrophy and depigmentation of the RPE.
3. Mild degenerative changes in the retinal receptor elements.

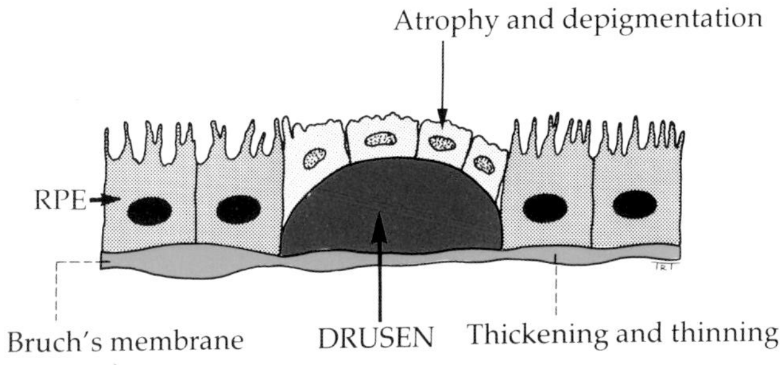

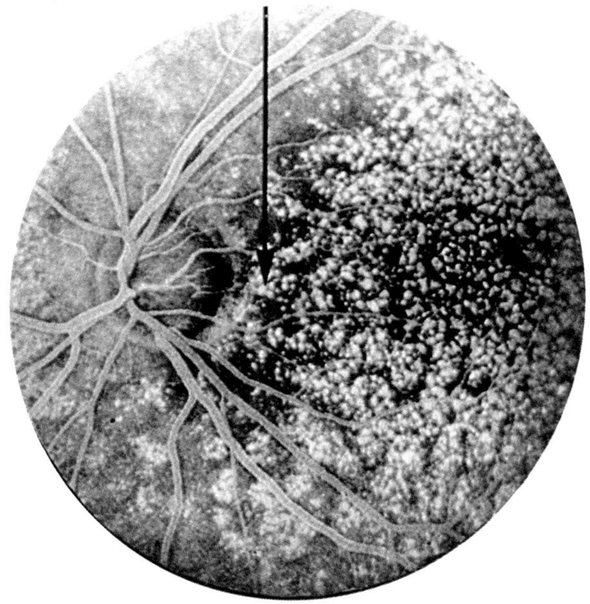

Figure 11.24 *Top: histopathology of drusen; bottom: staining of drusen (courtesy of Mr E. Rosen)*

Fluorescein angiography

RPE 'window' defect

The associated atrophy of the RPE overlying drusen gives rise to increased background choroidal fluorescence, which appears early in the angiogram as multiple hyperfluorescent spots. FA may also reveal lesions that are not apparent ophthalmoscopically.

Staining

Drusen may retain fluorescein dye for abnormally long periods of time after most of it has emptied. The actual dimensions of the hyperfluorescent areas seen 20 minutes after dye injection are the same as during the early stages of dye transit. This phenomenon indicates that fluorescein molecules have not leaked but have merely adhered to ('stained') the lesions (*Figure 11.24, bottom*).

Drusen and age-related macular degeneration

Although many eyes with drusen maintain normal vision throughout life, a significant number of elderly patients develop impairment of central vision due to AMD. Two main types of AMD are recognized: non-exudative and exudative (*Figure 11.25*). The exact role of drusen in the pathogenesis of AMD is still unclear. Features associated with an increased risk of subsequent visual loss are focal hyperpigmentation and confluent drusen, particularly if one eye has already developed visual loss from AMD.

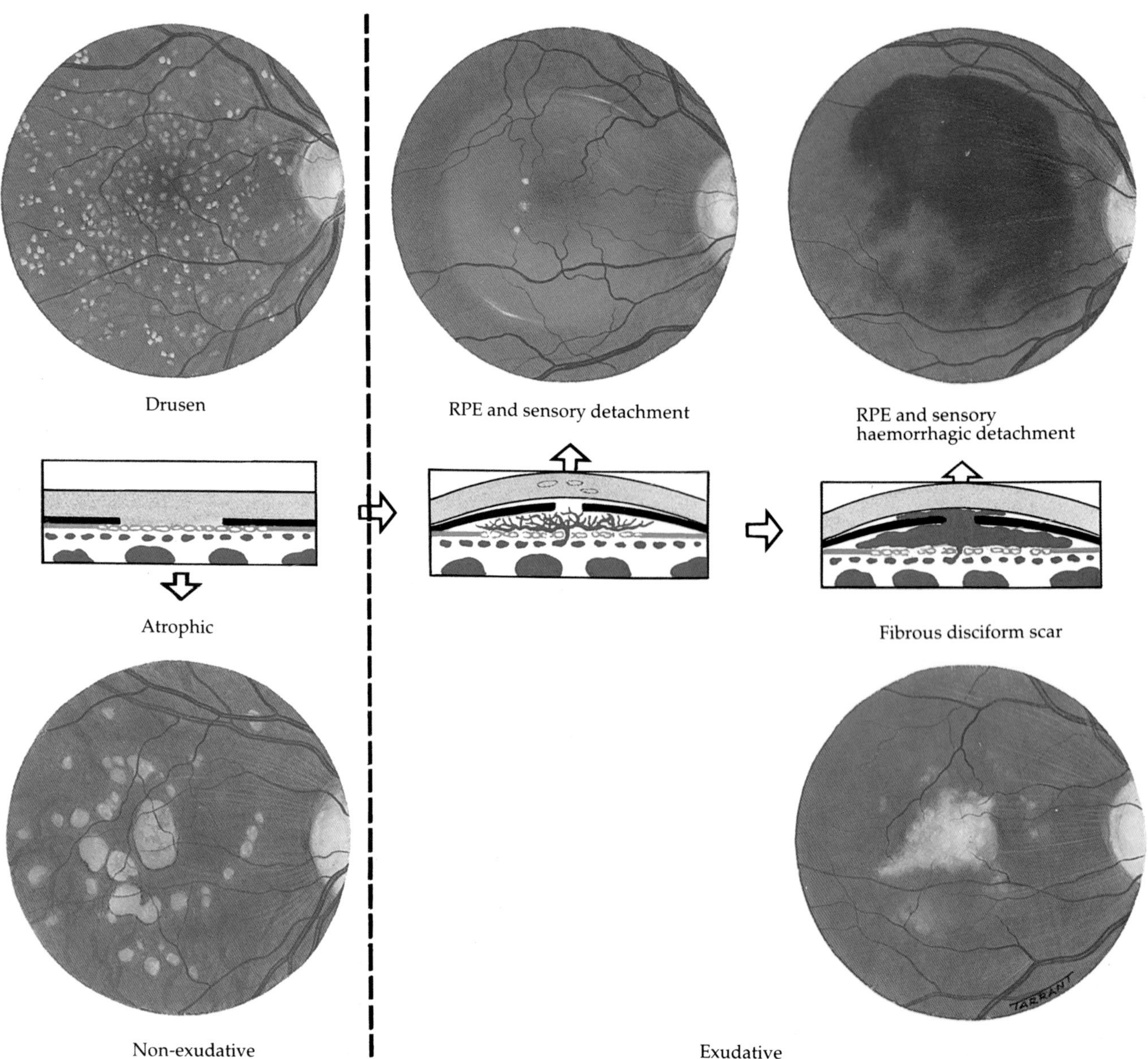

Figure 11.25 *Association between drusen and senile macular degeneration*

Non-exudative

Clinical features

Dry (geographical or areolar atrophy) is by far the most common type of AMD. It typically causes a gradual mild to moderate impairment of vision over several months or years. This type of AMD is either due to a slow and progressive atrophy of the RPE and photoreceptors or follows collapse of an RPE detachment (*see below*). Clinically, dry AMD is characterized by sharply circumscribed circular areas of atrophy of the RPE associated with varying degrees of loss of the choriocapillaris (*Figure 11.26*). During the late stages the larger choroidal vessels become prominent within the atrophic areas and pre-existing drusen disappear (*Figure 11.27*).

Management

Apart from the provision of low vision aids there is no effective treatment.

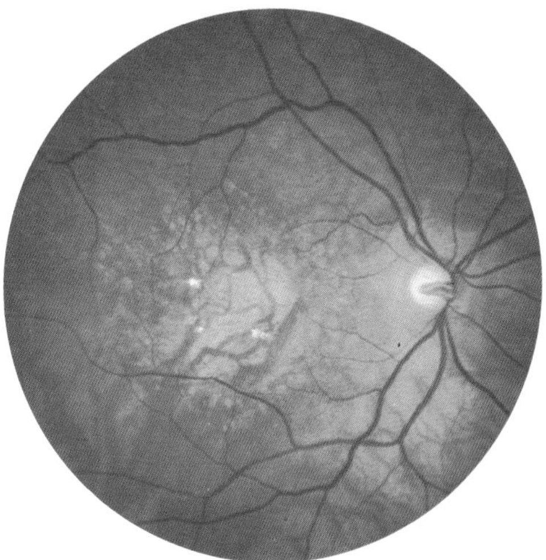

Figure 11.26 *Mild geographical atrophy*

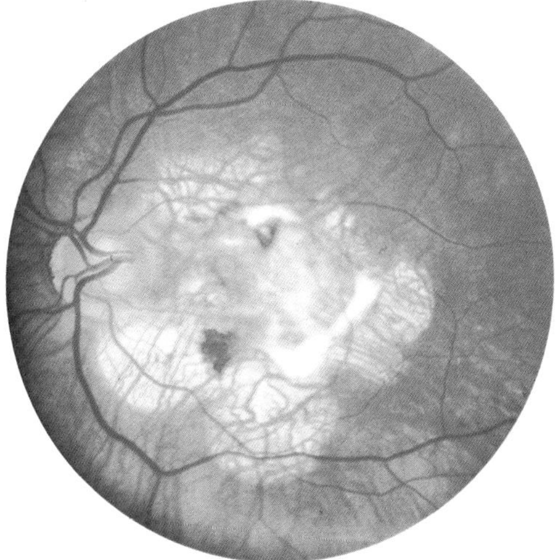

Figure 11.27 *Advanced geographical atrophy*

Exudative

This type is also sometimes referred to as 'neovascular' AMD. Although it is less common than the non-exudative type, its effects on vision are frequently devastating. In contrast to patients with non-exudative AMD in whom visual impairment is gradual, those with the exudative type may lose all central vision within a few days. Exudative AMD may occur in isolation or in association with non-exudative AMD. Two important features of exudative AMD are detachment of the RPE and choroidal neovascularization.

Detachment of the retinal pigment epithelium

The normally tight adhesion between Bruch's membrane and the RPE is maintained by the fibres of the inner collagenous layer of Bruch's membrane. In some eyes, the thickened inner aspect of Bruch's membrane together with the RPE and any associated drusen becomes separated from the remainder of Bruch's membrane by serous fluid derived from the choriocapillaris.

Clinical features

On ophthalmoscopy, pure detachments of the RPE appear as sharply circumscribed dome-shaped elevations of varying size. The sub-RPE fluid may be clear or turbid.

Fluorescein angiography (*Figure 11.28*)

In a pure RPE detachment, free fluorescein molecules that have leaked through the fenestrations of the choriocapillaris pool into the sub-RPE space, give rise to an area of hyperfluorescence. The extent of the detachment becomes evident during the early phase of the angiogram and the arteriovenous phase shows a profound increase in the intensity of fluorescence as more dye molecules pool under the detachment. The late phase shows that the margins of the detachment are well circumscribed but there is no increase in the actual area of hyperfluorescence.

Subsequent course

1. *Spontaneous resolution* after a variable period of time may occur leaving an area of geographical atrophy of the RPE. In fact it has been suggested that subclinical forms of RPE detachment are frequent precursors of non-exudative AMD.
2. *Progression to detachment of neurosensory retina* may occur as a result of a breakdown in the outer blood–retinal barrier allowing passage of fluid into the subretinal space. Because of the relatively loose adhesion between the RPE and neurosensory retina, the subretinal fluid spreads more widely and is less well defined than in a pure RPE detachment.

Choroidal neovascularization

In some eyes, subretinal neovascular membranes (SRNVMs) consisting of proliferations of fibrovascular tissue begin to grow from the choriocapillaris, through defects in Bruch's membrane, into the sub-RPE space and later into the subretinal space. These membranes may precede or follow the development of detachment of the RPE although these two events are probably not directly related.

Clinical features

Early SRNVMs may be undetectable, both ophthalmoscopically and angiographically. Later, membranes localized to the sub-RPE space appear as grey-green or pinkish-yellow,

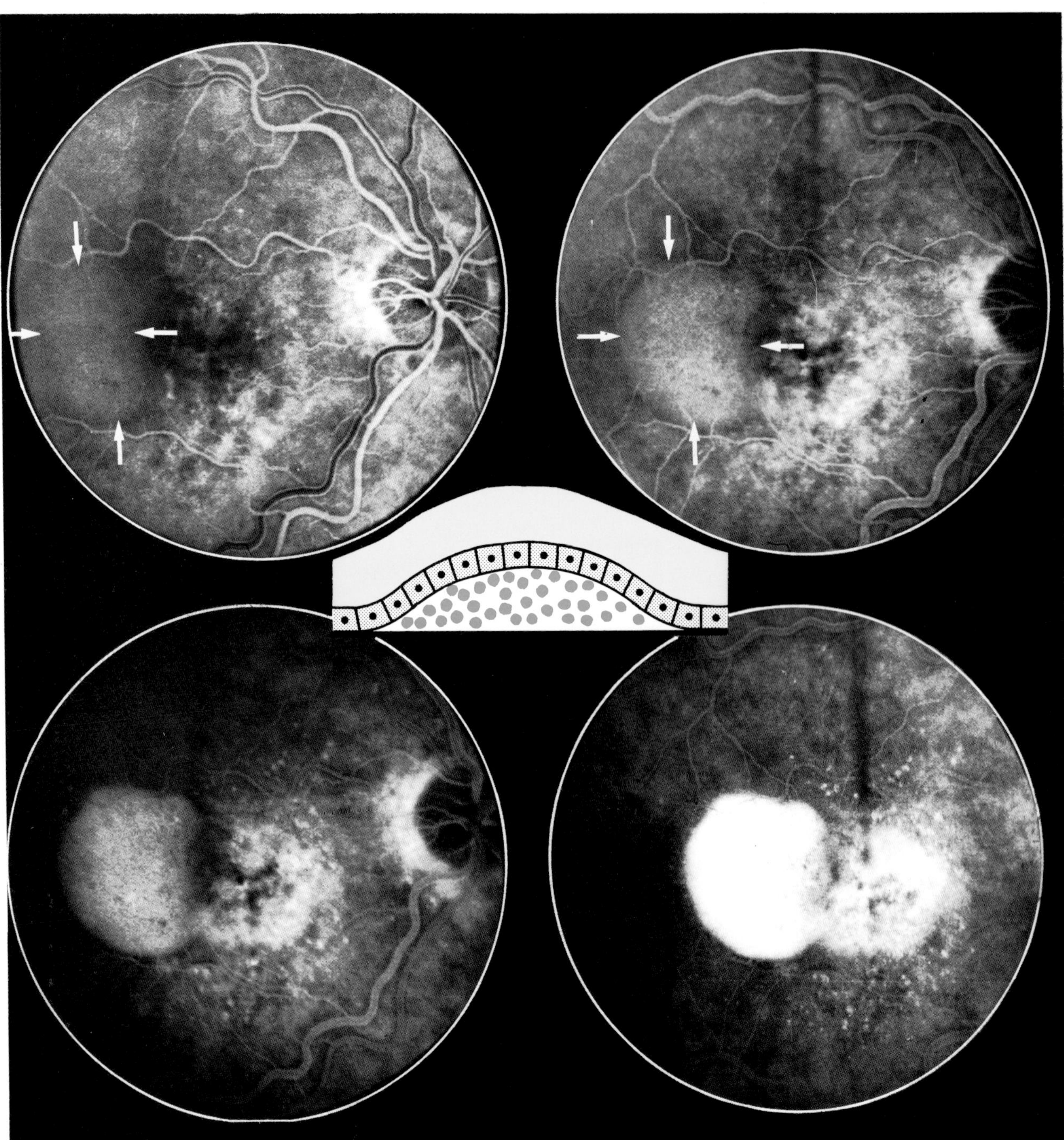

Figure 11.28 *Fluorescein angiogram of RPE detachment (courtesy of Mr R. Marsh)*

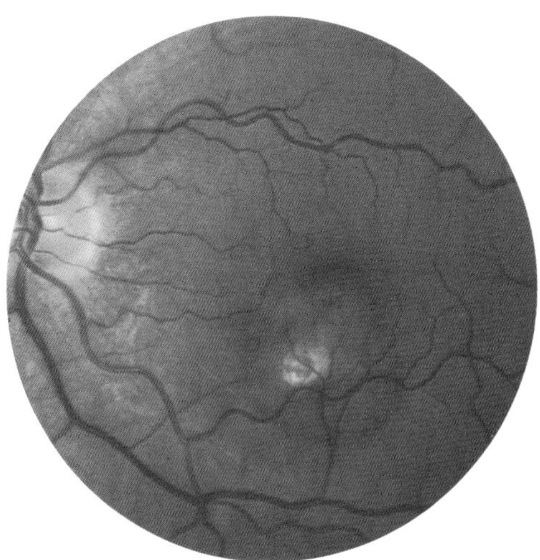

Figure 11.29 *Subretinal neovascular membrane inferior to fovea*

slightly elevated lesions of variable size (*Figure 11.29*). If the membrane has broken into the subretinal space it usually assumes a translucent pale-pink or yellow-white appearance. Patients with drusen should be cautioned that symptoms of distortion or blurring of vision may herald the onset of leakage from an SRNVM. It is at this stage that argon laser photocoagulation may be beneficial. (Other disorders associated with SRNVMs are listed in *Table 11.1.*)

Table 11.1 Diseases associated with subretinal neovascular membranes

1. Severe myopia
2. Presumed ocular histoplasmosis syndrome
3. Angioid streaks
4. Choroidal naevus
5. Choroidal rupture
6. Excessive photocoagulation
7. Drusen of optic nerve head
8. Chorioretinitis
9. Best's disease
10. Rubella retinopathy
11. Choroidal melanoma and haemangioma
12. Serpiginous choroidopathy

Fluorescein angiography

Fluorescein angiography plays a very important role in the detection and localization of SRNVMs in relation to the foveal avascular zone. The new vessels within the membrane fill in a 'lacy' pattern during the very early phase of dye transit (*Figure 11.30, top left*), fluoresce brightly during peak eye transit (20–30 seconds after injection; *Figure 11.30, top right*), and then leak within 1–2 minutes (*Figure 11.30, bottom*). The fibrous tissue within the membrane then stains with dye and leads to late hyperfluorescence. In eyes with associated detachments of the RPE, the SRNVM fluoresces brighter than the detachment and appears to leak as the angiogram progresses.

Subsequent course

Haemorrhagic detachment of the RPE

This is due to a rupture of one of the blood vessels within the SRNVM. Initially, the blood is confined to the sub-RPE space and appears as an almost black, elevated mound (*Figure 11.31*).

Haemorrhagic detachment of the neurosensory retina

This develops within 1–2 weeks as the blood breaks through into the subretinal space. At this stage the haemorrhage assumes a red colour.

Vitreous haemorrhage

Rarely, the blood may break through the neurosensory retina into the vitreous cavity—a complication said to be more frequent in patients receiving anticoagulants.

Disciform scarring

The haemorrhagic episode is usually followed by a gradual organization of the blood, and further ingrowth of new vessels from the choroid. In some eyes anastomotic channels develop between the choroidal and retinal circulations. Eventually a fibrous disciform scar at the fovea causes a permanent impairment of central vision (*Figure 11.32*). Occasionally, massive secondary rebleeding may occur with further visual loss from vitreous haemorrhage.

Exudative retinal detachment

In some eyes with disciform scars, the neovascular tissue leaks profusely and leads to marked intraretinal and subretinal exudation similar to that seen in Coats' disease (*Figure 11.33*). An associated exudative retinal detachment may spread beyond the macula.

Argon laser photocoagulation

Indications

In eyes with AMD, argon blue-green laser photocoagulation may be effective in obliterating extrafoveal SRNVMs located 200 μm or more from the centre of the foveal avascular zone (FAZ). The aim of treatment is to destroy the SRNVM and minimize laser damage to the fovea. Because an SRNVM is more likely to be treatable if detected early, it is important to identify patients with SRNVMs promptly by the daily use of the Amsler grid. Laser therapy is also effective in eliminating some idiopathic SRNVMs as well as those associated with the presumed ocular histoplasmosis syndrome.

Contraindications

Treatment is at present contraindicated for SRNVMs closer than 200 μm from the centre of the FAZ and those associated with detachment of the RPE and/or blood beneath the fovea. Eyes with a visual acuity of 6/36 or less

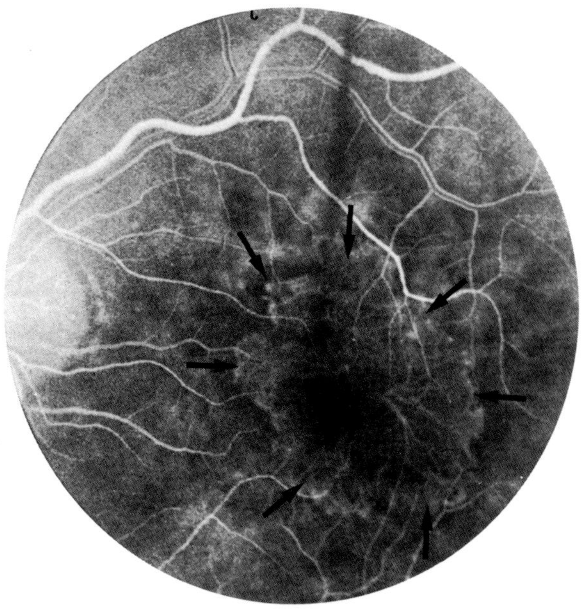

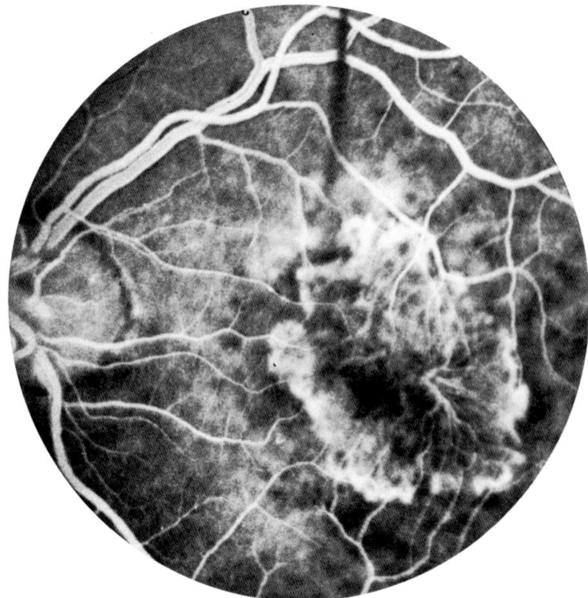

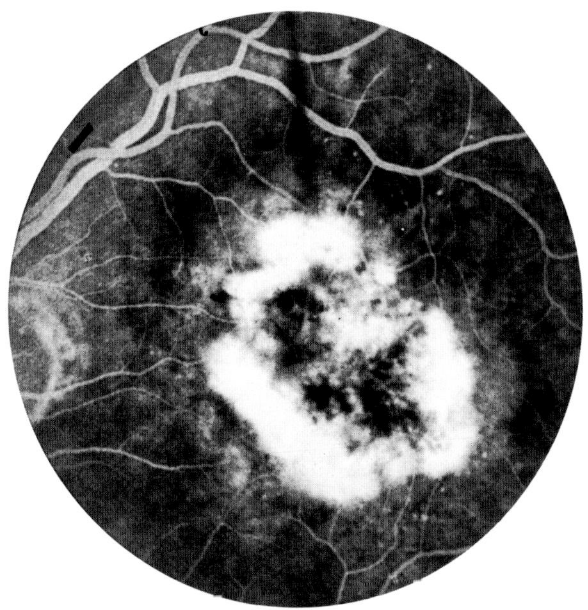

Figure 11.30 *Fluorescein angiogram of choroidal neovascular membrane (courtesy of Mr R. Marsh)*

are also unlikely to benefit from treatment. In fact only about 10% of eyes with SRNVMs are suitable for treatment when first examined.

Patient information

Patients should be informed that the main aim of treatment is not to improve vision but to prevent further deterioration. The patient must also understand the importance of careful follow-up after laser therapy, because of the possibility of residual or recurrent neovascularization. It is also important to explain that the field defect may be larger after treatment even if the SRNVM has been successfully destroyed.

Pre-treatment tests

The visual acuity is measured both for near and distance and the area of the scotoma or visual distortion is documented on the Amsler grid.

Fluorescein angiography

The pre-treatment fluorescein angiogram should be of excellent quality and not more than 72 hours old. Selected frames of the angiogram are projected onto a screen so that the SRNVM can be precisely localized in relation to visible retinal landmarks.

Technique

Retrobulbar anaesthesia can be used to reduce discomfort and to immobilize the eye during photocoagulation so as to reduce the risk of inadvertent damage to the fovea.

1. The perimeter of the SRNVM is treated with overlapping 200 μm (0.2 s) burns (*Figure 11.34, top*).
2. The entire area is then covered with 200 μm (0.5 s) burns. The treatment must extend beyond the margins of the SRNVM and produce a confluent, intense white burn (*Figure 11.34, bottom*).
3. A post-treatment fundus photograph is taken to document the extent of treatment.

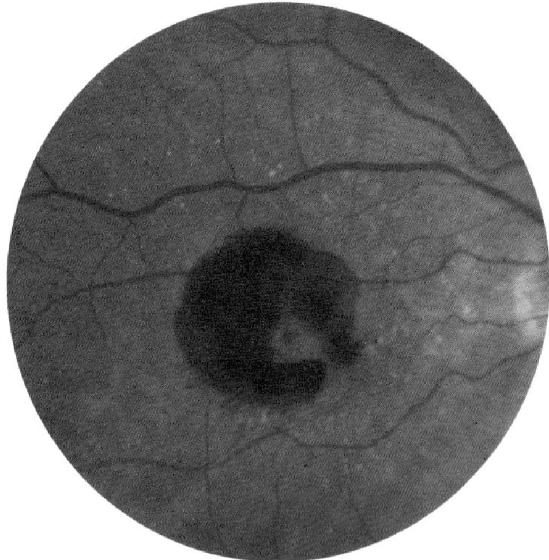

Figure 11.31 *Haemorrhagic detachment of retinal pigment epithelium*

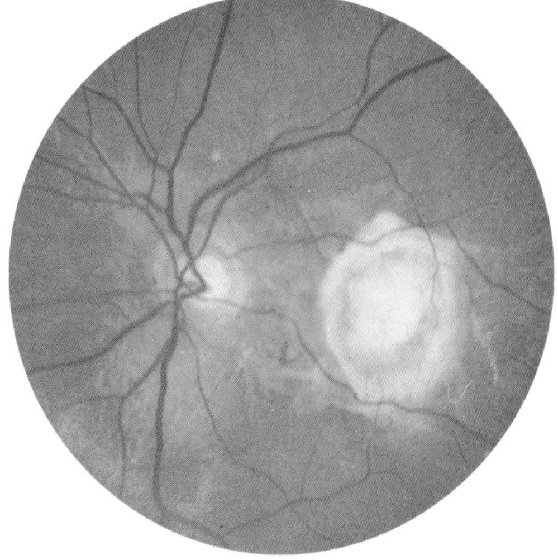

Figure 11.32 *Fibrous disciform scar at macula*

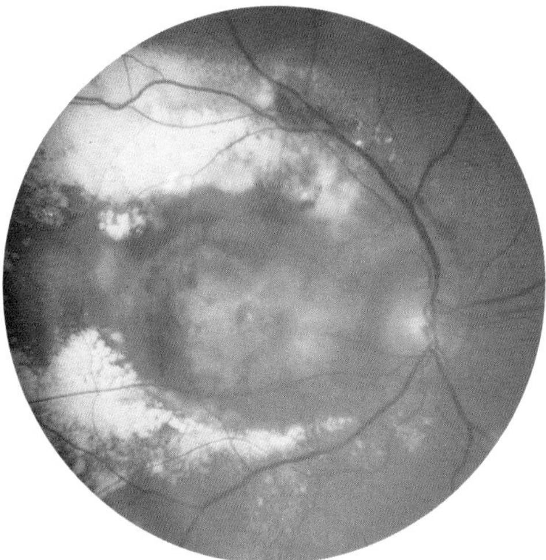

Figure 11.33 *Extensive subretinal exudation in age-related macular degeneration*

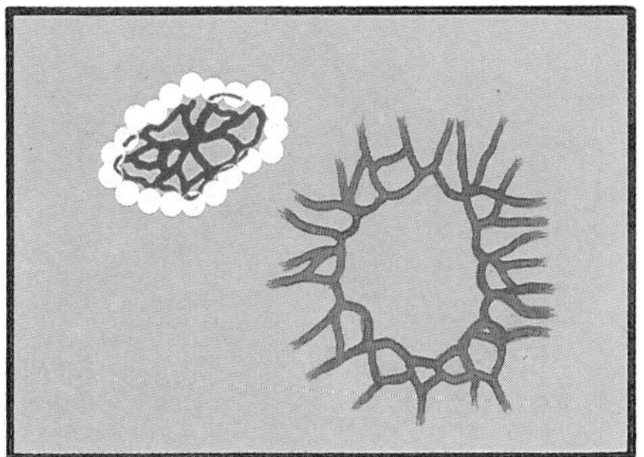

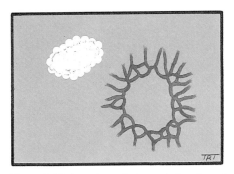

Figure 11.34 *Argon laser photocoagulation of extrafoveal subretinal neovascular membrane*

Follow-up

Meticulous follow-up is required to detect persistence or recurrence of the SRNVM. The patient is instructed to use the Amsler grid daily and to report promptly an increase in distortion. He is then re-examined after 1 or 2 weeks and a fluorescein angiogram is performed. Any persistence or recurrence is evident on the angiogram as an intense leaking area only on one portion of the margin of previous treatment. An adequate post-treatment scar often stains with fluorescein all round its margins, and should not be misinterpreted as a recurrence. Re-treatment is indicated if there is true persistence or recurrence of an extrafoveal SRNVM located more than 200 μm from the centre of the fovea. Because recurrences of SRNVMs can occur several years after the initially successful treatment, it is important for the patient to continue to monitor his progress with the Amsler grid and to have periodic follow-up examinations.

Results

Treatment by argon laser photocoagulation is effective in reducing the risk of severe visual loss by more than 50% in eyes with SRNVMs outside the FAZ. In one study severe visual loss occurred after 18 months in 60% of untreated eyes, and in only 25% of treated eyes. Severe visual loss was defined as a reduction of 6 Snellen lines or more from baseline visual acuity.

Central serous chorioretinopathy

Central serous chorioretinopathy (CSCR) is a common disorder of unknown aetiology which typically affects men between the ages of 20 and 45 years.

Clinical features

The presenting symptom is a fairly sudden onset of blurred vision in one eye associated with a positive relative scotoma, micropsia, and metamorphopsia. Occasionally the disease is extrafoveal and asymptomatic.

Visual acuity

This is usually modestly reduced (6/9–6/12) and often correctable to 6/6 with the addition of a weak 'plus' lens. The elevation of the neurosensory retina gives rise to an

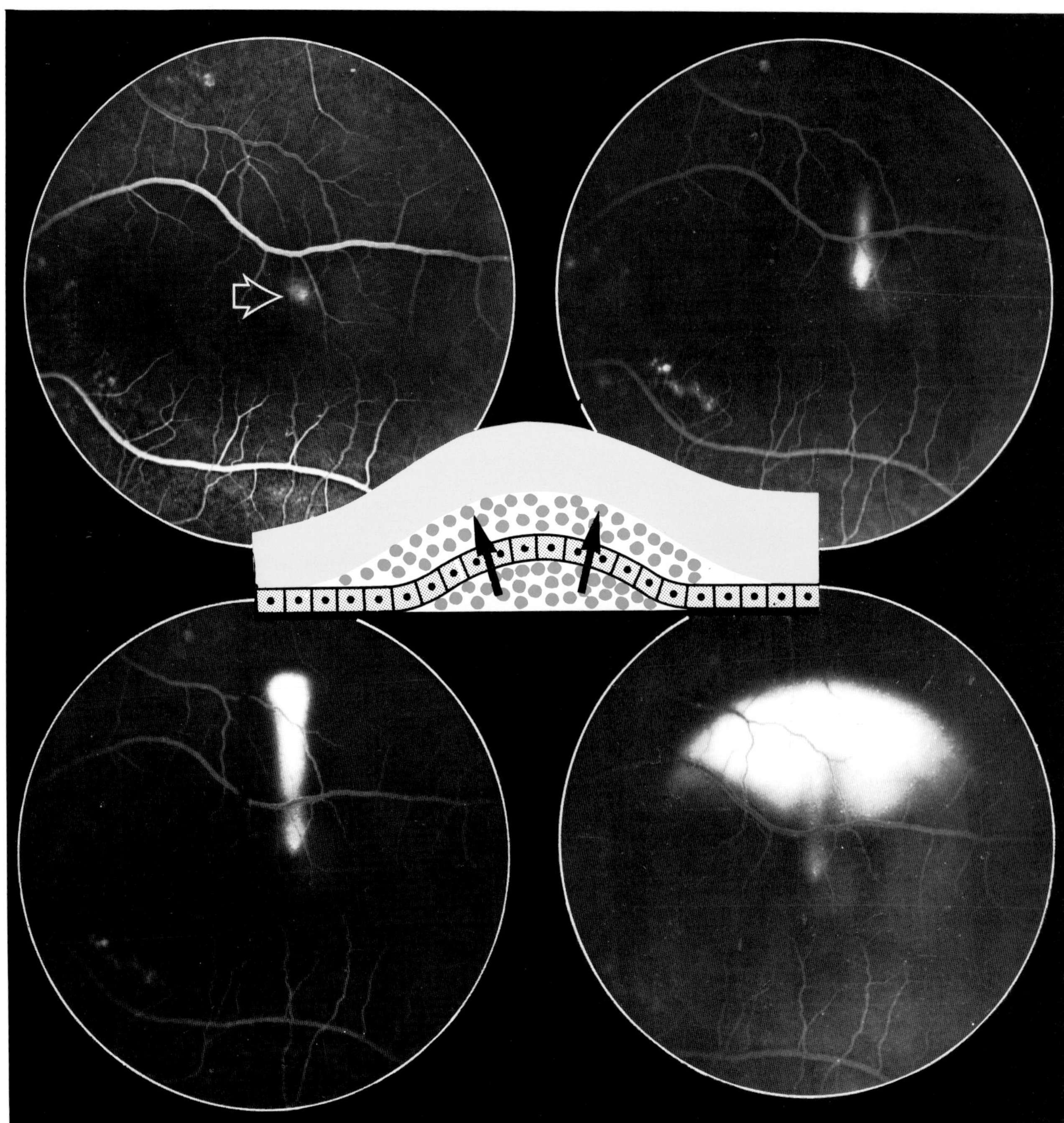

Figure 11.35 *Smoke-stack appearance on fluorescein angiography of central serous choroidopathy (courtesy of Mr R. Marsh)*

acquired hypermetropia with disparity between the subjective and objective refraction of the eye.

Indirect ophthalmoscopy

This shows a shallow round or oval elevation of the sensory retina at the posterior pole, the borders of which are outlined by a glistening reflex.

Slitlamp biomicroscopy

This shows the detached neurosensory retina to be transparent and of normal thickness. Its separation from the underlying retinal pigment epithelium can be detected by noting the shadows cast onto the RPE by the retinal blood vessels. In certain cases, small precipitates can be seen on the posterior surface of the detached neurosensory retina. Occasionally, the abnormal area in the RPE through which fluid has leaked from the choriocapillaris into the subretinal space can also be detected. The subretinal fluid may be clear or turbid.

Fluorescein angiography

FA is helpful in providing a definitive diagnosis of CSCR and in helping to understand certain aspects of its pathogenesis. It appears that CSCR is caused by a breakdown of the outer blood–retinal barrier which allows the passage of free fluorescein molecules into the subretinal space. Most eyes with CSCR have an associated but very much smaller detachment of the RPE. On angiography two patterns are seen.

Smoke-stack

This appearance (*Figure 11.35*) shows pooling of dye beneath a small RPE detachment during the early stages of dye transit. This appears as a small hyperfluorescent spot. During the late venous phase, the fluid gains access to the subretinal space and ascends vertically (like a smoke-stack) from the point of leakage until it reaches the upper border of the detachment. The dye then spreads laterally taking on a 'mushroom' or 'umbrella' configuration until the entire area of detachment is filled.

Ink-blot

This appearance may occasionally be seen in which the initial hyperfluorescent spot gradually increases in size until the entire subretinal space is filled.

Prognosis

Between 80% and 90% of eyes with CSCR undergo spontaneous resolution of subretinal fluid and a return to normal, or near normal, visual acuity within 1–6 months. Mild symptoms of metamorphopsia or micropsia may remain for much longer. There does not appear to be any significant correlation between the duration of elevation of the neurosensory retina and the final vision. Occasionally, persistent cases may be associated with the development of changes in the RPE or cystoid maculopathy. Approximately 40% of patients develop recurrent attacks.

Treatment

The exact indications and benefits of argon laser photocoagulation in the treatment of CSCR are still uncertain. In general, photocoagulation to the site of leakage should be considered under the following circumstances:

1. If recurrent episodes of CSCR have already caused a visual deficit.
2. If vision in the fellow eye is permanently impaired from previous attacks.
3. If the duration is longer than 4 months.
4. In consideration of occupational or other needs of the patient for clear vision in both eyes.
5. In the presence of turbid subretinal fluid.

It is important to remember that eyes with congenital optic disc pits (*Figure 11.36*) may also develop a detachment of the sensory retina at the macula (*see* Chapter 15).

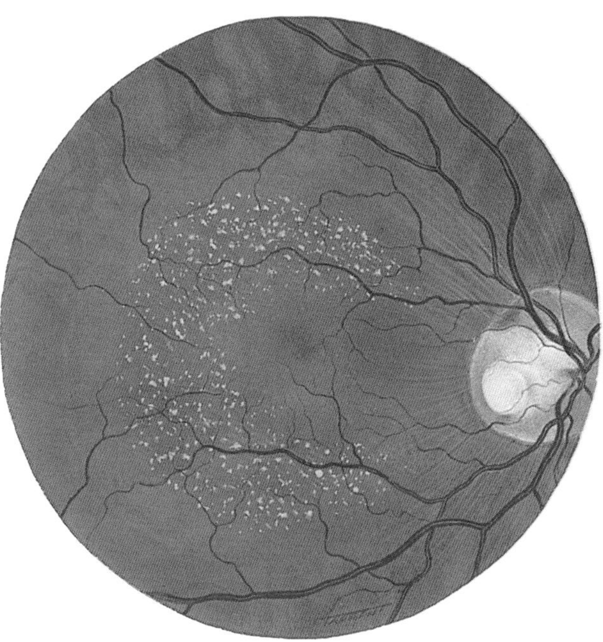

Figure 11.36 *Congenital optic disc pit and serous detachment of sensory retina*

Cystoid macular oedema

Cystoid macular oedema (CMO) is an accumulation of fluid in the outer plexiform (Henle's) and inner nuclear layers of the retina, centred about the foveola.

Clinical features

CMO is a very common macular disorder that has many diverse aetiologies. In the short term, it is usually innocuous but long-standing cases usually lead to coalescence of the fluid-filled microcysts into large cystic spaces and the subsequent formation of lamellar holes at the fovea with irreversible damage to central vision (*Figure 11.37*). *Ophthalmoscopy* shows loss of the foveal depression and thickening of the retina, and multiple cystoid areas can be seen in the neurosensory retina.

Cystoid macular oedema

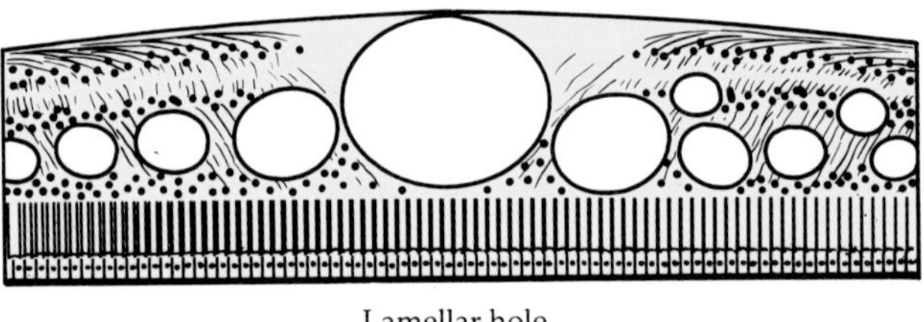

Lamellar hole

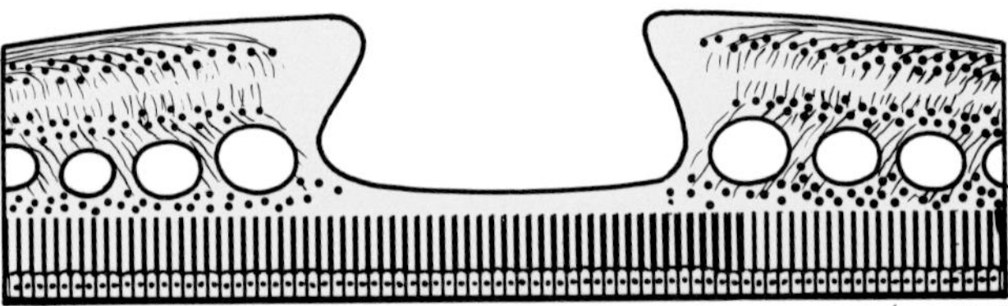

Figure 12.27 *Lamellar hole formation due to chronic cystoid macular oedema*

Fluorescein angiography (*see Figure 11.21*)

In the healthy eye, the tight junctions of the retinal capillary endothelial cells make up the inner blood–retinal barrier, which prevents the passage of both free and bound fluorescein molecules into the extravascular space. An increase in vascular permeability, caused by a change in intravascular or tissue hydrostatic pressure, or by a change in the capillary walls themselves, will permit a leakage of both bound and free fluorescein molecules into the extravascular space. The accumulation of dye in the outer plexiform layer of the retina, with its radial arrangement of fibres about the centre of the foveola (Henle's layer), is responsible for the 'flower-petal' pattern of CMO seen both angiographically and biomicroscopically (*see Figure 10.9, left*). Leakage of dye into the parafoveal area starts during the arteriovenous phase of the angiogram. The focal leaking points then coalesce into the 'flower-petal' pattern during the late arteriovenous phase. The hyperfluorescence due to pooling of dye in the microcystic spaces persists during the late phase of the angiogram.

Aetiology

1. *Background diabetic retinopathy.* CMO is an important cause of visual impairment in diabetic patients (*see* Chapter 10).
2. *Retinal vein occlusion.* Chronic CMO is the most common cause of persistently poor vision following branch retinal vein occlusion (*see* Chapter 10).
3. *Irvine–Gass syndrome.* CMO is probably the most common complication of cataract extraction. Fortunately, the great majority of cases are transient and have little clinical significance as they occur during the immediate postoperative period. Of those that persist, most resolve within 6–12 months. CMO appears to occur less frequently following planned extracapsular than intracapsular extraction. The management of persistent CMO is discussed in Chapter 8.
4. *Intermediate uveitis—see* Chapter 6.
5. *Adrenaline.* CMO may develop in aphakic eyes treated with adrenaline for glaucoma, especially if the 2% concentration is used. Fortunately the maculopathy reverses once the drug is stopped.
6. *Retinitis pigmentosa.* Typical CMO has been reported in up to 70% of eyes with retinitis pigmentosa.

Macular hole

Because of its thinness, avascularity, and lack of support, the foveal region is particularly susceptible to hole formation.

Clinical features

A true macular hole has a 'punched-out' appearance and is round or slightly ovoid. Yellow pigment can be seen in the base of the hole, and a grey halo of marginal retinal elevation usually surrounds the lesion (*Figure 11.38*). FA shows an area of hyperfluorescence due to unmasking of background choroidal fluorescence caused by an RPE 'window' defect.

Aetiology

1. *Idiopathic.* Most macular holes develop in otherwise healthy eyes of elderly patients and give rise to a

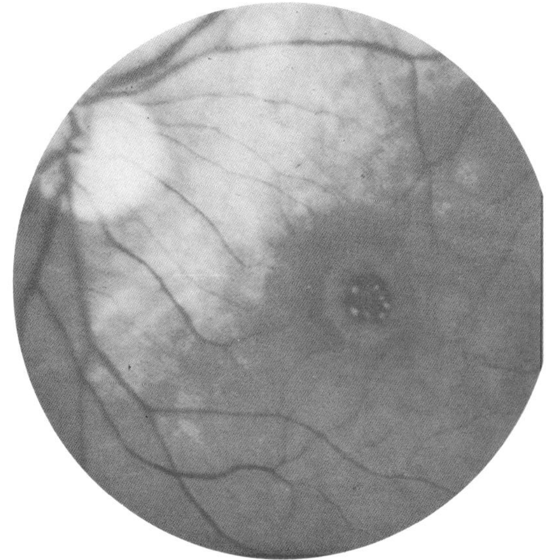

Figure 11.38 *Senile macular hole*

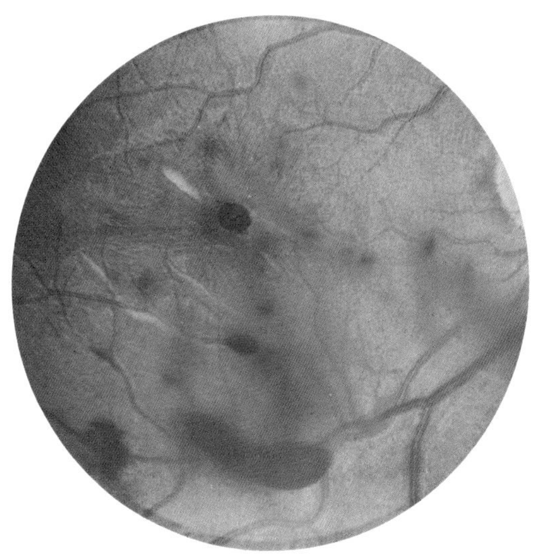

Figure 11.39 *Traumatic macular hole (courtesy of Mr A. Shun-Shin)*

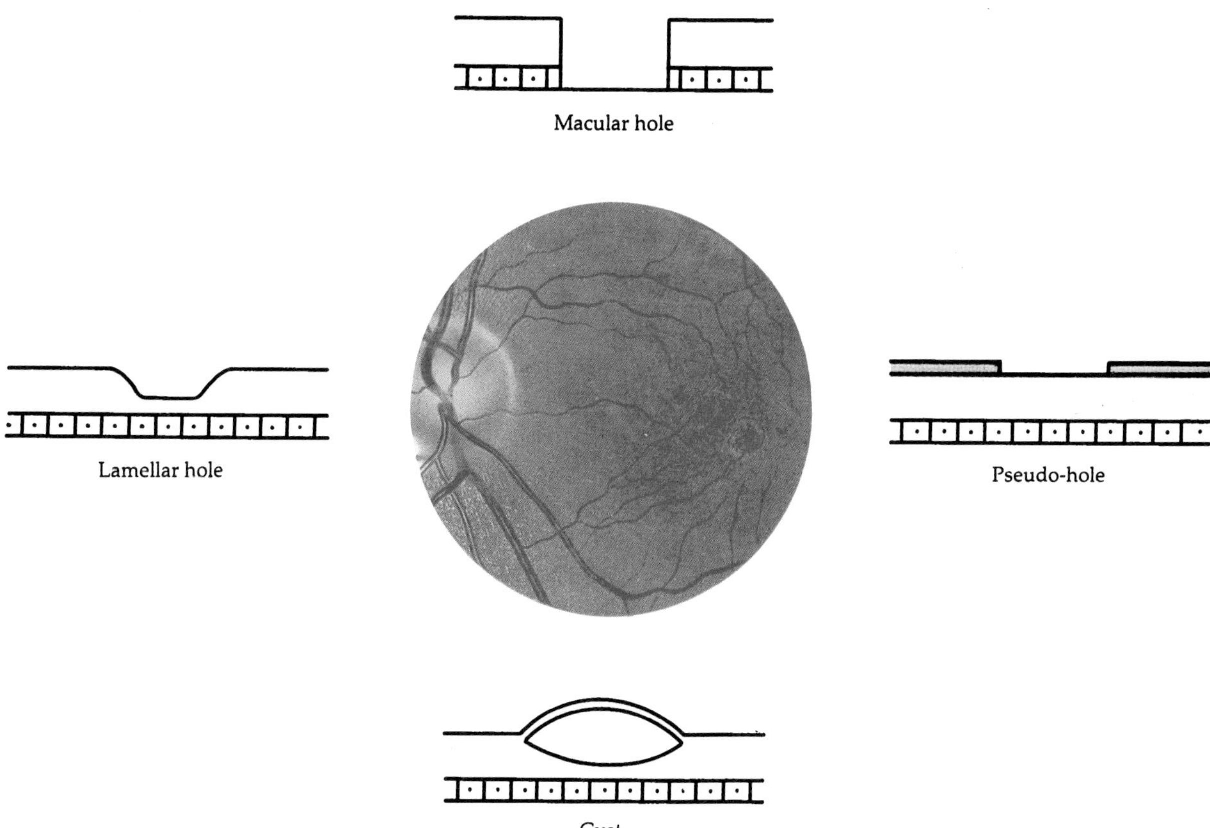

Figure 11.40 *Differential diagnosis of macular hole*

moderate or severe impairment of visual acuity. They do not give rise to retinal detachment and the opposite eye is affected in about 10% of cases.

2. *Myopia.* Severely myopic eyes with posterior staphylomas may develop macular holes which can lead to retinal detachment. In these cases the SRF is usually confined to the posterior pole and seldom spreads beyond the equator.
3. *Trauma* (*Figure 11.39*). Macular holes may follow ocular trauma, either as a result of vitreous traction or commotio retinae which leads to CMO and subsequent lamellar hole formation.
4. *Solar retinopathy* is characterized by a small circumscribed lamellar hole or cyst that typically develops 2 weeks after exposure to the sun. Initially, only a small yellow foveolar exudate or oedema may be seen. The lesion is thought to be caused by phototoxicity rather than by thermal effects on the retina. The term 'foveomacular retinitis' is used for a lesion that is identical but lacks the implied causal factor.

Differential diagnosis

Slitlamp biomicroscopy and FA are useful in differentiating between a full-thickness macular hole, a pseudomacular hole, a lamellar hole, and a macular cyst (*Figure 11.40*):

1. *Pseudomacular holes* are caused by defects in an epiretinal membrane covering the fovea (*Figure 11.41*).
2. *Lamellar holes and macular cysts* usually occur as complications of chronic CMO. A lamellar hole will not give rise to an RPE 'window' defect on FA because the RPE is normal. Visual acuity is usually worse in eyes with true macular holes than in those with lamellar holes.

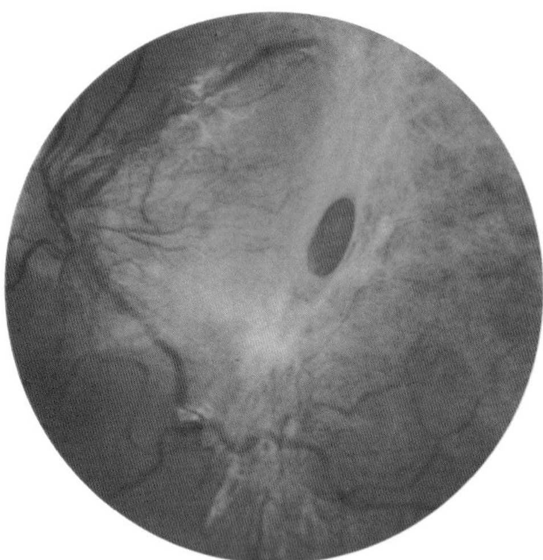

Figure 11.41 *Pseudomacular hole due to defect in an epiretinal membrane (courtesy of Dr P. M. Morse)*

Myopic maculopathy

Degenerative myopia is the seventh most common cause of blindness registration in the United Kingdom and the United States. Its incapacitating effects frequently occur during the productive years of young adulthood.

Pathogenesis

The pathogenesis of degenerative myopia is not clearly understood. The degenerative lesions are thought to be either biomechanical or heredodegenerative in nature. The biomechanical concept suggests that they are the consequence of the distorting forces transferred to the inner layers of the eye from weakened and elongated sclera. The heredodegenerative theory sees the changes as a genetically determined abiotrophic effect associated with, but independent of, the anatomical changes in the scleral wall.

Clinical features

The progressive elongation of the globe is accompanied by degenerative changes in the retina and choroid. Initially, islands of chorioretinal atrophy appear at the posterior pole. As the condition progresses, atrophy of the RPE and choriocapillaris enables the larger choroidal vessels to be seen and eventually the white sclera also becomes visible. Continued stretching causes breaks to develop in Bruch's membrane. Large breaks ('lacquer cracks') appear as fine, irregular, yellow lines, often branching and criss-crossing. They have a predilection for the fundi of young adults, and occur in about 4% of all highly myopic eyes. The presence of 'lacquer cracks' implies a guarded prognosis for retention of central vision as the lesions may allow choroidal new vessels to grow through the defects causing haemorrhage, and secondary pigmentary proliferation in the form of a Fuchs' spot (*Figure 11.42*). In some highly myopic eyes haemorrhage may occur from 'lacquer cracks' in the absence of choroidal neovascularization (*Figure 11.43*).

Other complications of high myopia

1. *Temporal crescents* around the optic nerve head (*Figure 11.44*).
2. *Posterior staphylomas* (*Figure 11.45*).
3. *Macular holes* which may give rise to retinal detachment.
4. *Peripheral retinal holes* which in association with vitreous syneresis (liquefaction) are also responsible for the increased prevalence of retinal detachment in highly myopic eyes.
5. *Secondary posterior subcapsular cataracts* and early onset of nuclear sclerosis.
6. *Increased prevalence* of primary open-angle glaucoma and corticosteroid responsiveness.

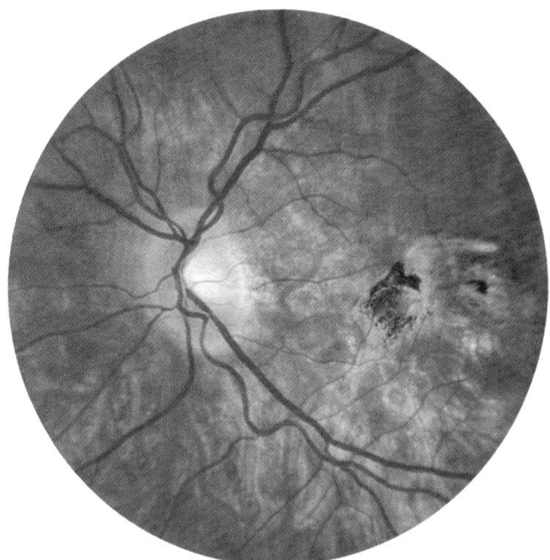

Figure 11.42 Fuchs' spot

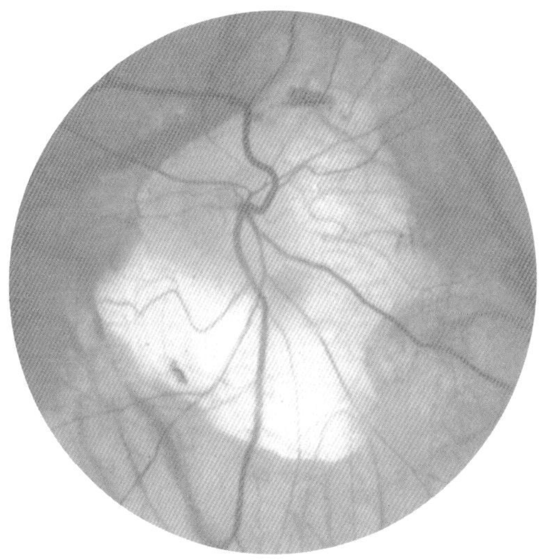

Figure 11.44 Myopic peripapillary atrophy

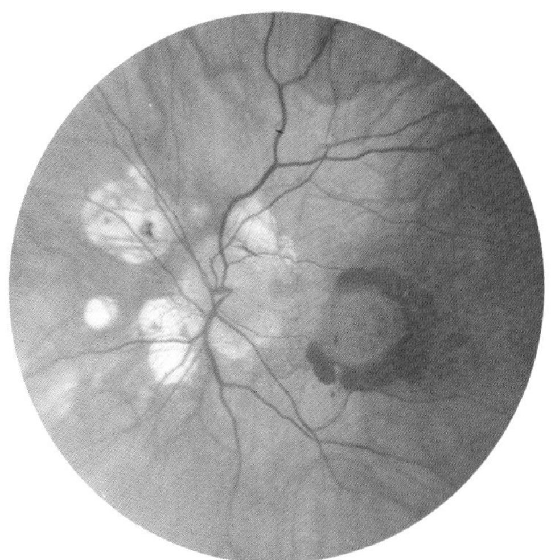

Figure 11.43 Subretinal haemorrhage at macula in highly myopic eye

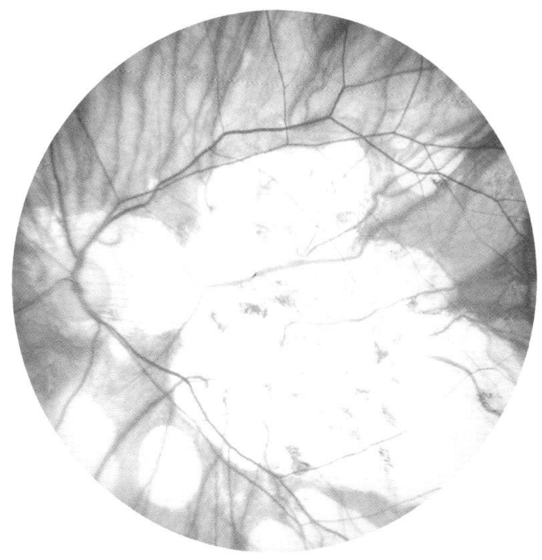

Figure 11.45 Advanced myopic degeneration

Macular pucker

Maculopathy secondary to membrane formation at the vitreoretinal interface has many synonyms (cellophane maculopathy, surface-wrinkling retinopathy, preretinal fibrosis, and macular pucker).

Clinical features

The clinical appearance of epiretinal membranes depends on their density and any associated distortion of the retinal vasculature. Pseudomacular holes may occur due to defects in the membrane.

Grade 1

These are translucent membranes (cellophane maculopathy) which give rise to an irregular light reflex or sheen. The membrane can be best detected using 'red-free' light but as it thickens and contracts it becomes more obvious and causes the formation of fine retinal striae on the retinal surface. The vessels of the superotemporal and inferotemporal arcades become tortuous and are pulled towards the median raphe. The horizontally oriented vessels within and adjacent to the papillomacular bundle become stretched and straightened.

Grade 2 (*Figure 11.46*)

Here the distortion of the vessels is marked and the membrane is sufficiently dense to obscure some of the retinal vessels. Typically the retinal wrinkling is centred around a central point at the fovea (epicentre).

Fluorescein angiography (*Figure 11.47*)

This shows varying degrees of tortuosity and straightening. Leakage from the vessels is a frequent finding and in some cases cystoid macular oedema may be present.

Aetiology

1. *Idiopathic.* Epiretinal membranes at the macula may occur idiopathically in otherwise healthy eyes of elderly individuals. Both eyes are involved in 20% of cases but fortunately visual impairment is usually mild.
2. *Retinal detachment surgery.* Epiretinal membranes causing reduced postoperative visual acuity due to 'macular pucker' are a well-recognized complication of otherwise successful retinal detachment surgery and occur in about 7% of cases. They may develop in eyes in which the macula is uninvolved by the detachment preoperatively. The pathogenesis of these membranes is unknown, although it has been suggested that cellular proliferation of both pigment epithelial and astroglial origin may be involved. Untreated, these membranes usually cause a variable but permanent reduction of vision. Very occasionally, however, the membrane may spontaneously separate from the retina. In selected cases with significant impairment of vision, the removal of these membranes using vitrectomy techniques can result in visual improvement.
3. *Peripheral retinal photocoagulation and cryotherapy.* Macular pucker occurs in a few eyes following peripheral retinal photocoagulation. The incidence following cryotherapy is lower.

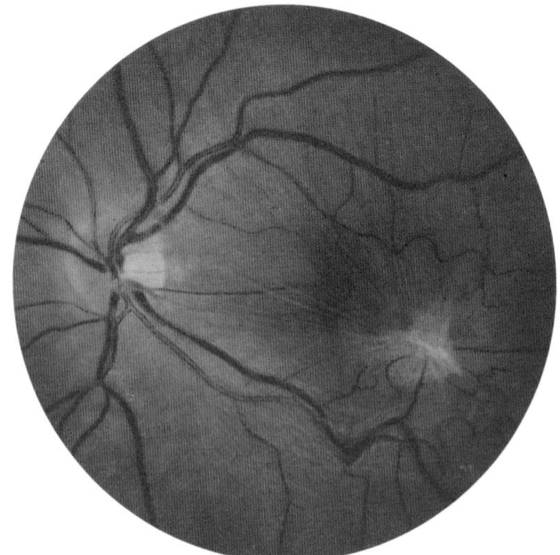

Figure 11.46 *Macular pucker*

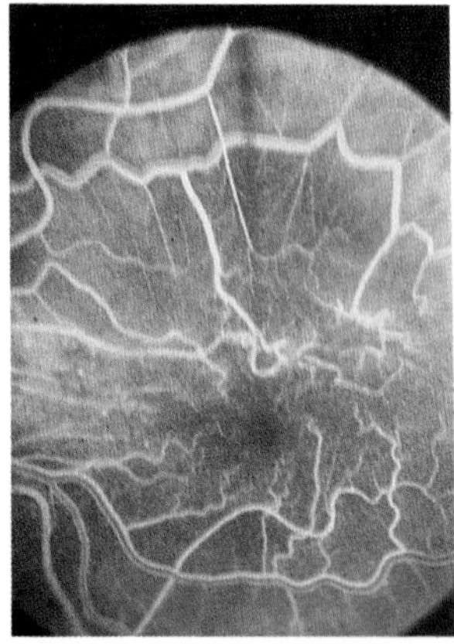

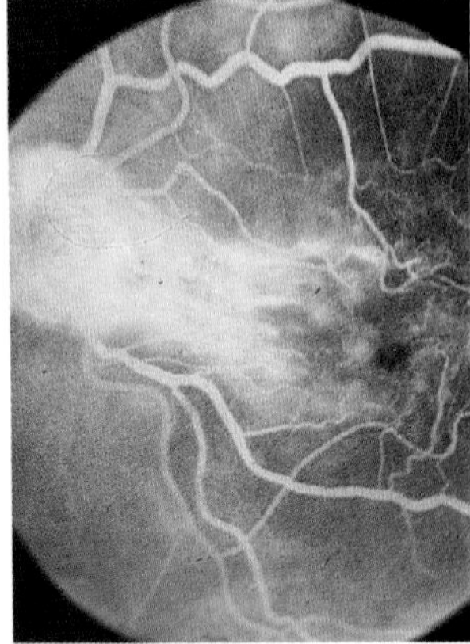

Figure 11.47 *Fluorescein angiogram in macular pucker. Left: early; right: late (courtesy of Mr R. Marsh)*

Choroidal folds

Clinical features

Choroidal folds are lines, grooves, or striae of the posterior pole, most commonly arranged in a parallel and horizontal fashion, although they may be vertical, oblique, or irregular (*Figure 11.48*). They are most frequently situated temporally and rarely, if ever, extend beyond the equator. On slitlamp biomicroscopy, the elevated portion (crest) of the fold appears yellow in contrast to the darker appearance of the valley (trough) of the fold. Initially, visual dysfunction is caused by distortion of the overlying retinal receptors, but in long-standing cases, permanent changes in the RPE and neurosensory retina may develop.

Fluorescein angiography

Angiographically, choroidal folds appear as alternating hyperfluorescent and hypofluorescent streaks (*Figure 11.49*). The hyperfluorescence corresponding to the crests is due to increased background choroidal fluorescence

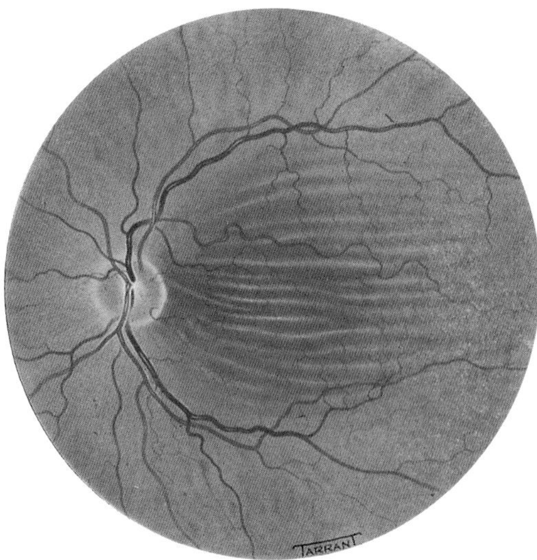

Figure 11.48 Choroidal folds

showing through the thinned or atrophied RPE. The increased thickness of the RPE in the troughs of the folds obscures background fluorescence and causes hypofluorescence.

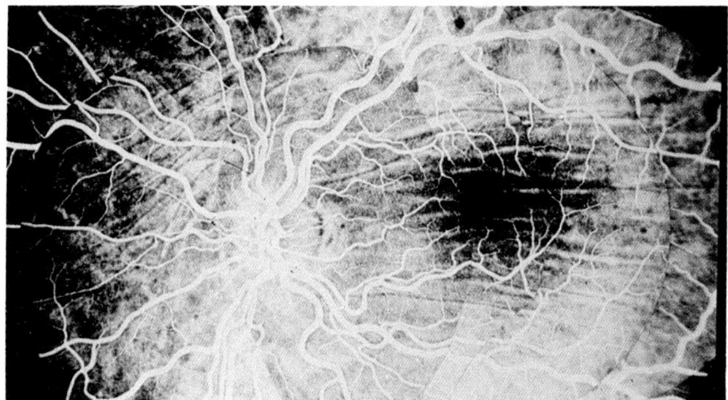

Figure 11.49 Fluorescein angiogram in choroidal folds (courtesy of Professor A. C. Bird)

Aetiology

1. *Idiopathic.* Choroidal folds may occur for no apparent reason in both eyes of healthy hypermetropic patients with normal or near normal vision.
2. *Retrobulbar mass.*
3. *Thyroid ophthalmopathy.*
4. *A choroidal tumour* may mechanically displace the surrounding choroid and cause folding.
5. *Ocular hypotony.*

Angioid streaks

Angioid streaks are due to crack-like dehiscences in the collagenous and elastic portions of Bruch's membrane with secondary changes in the RPE and choriocapillaris.

Clinical features

The streaks typically radiate outwards in a tapering fashion from the peripapillary area, although near the disc they may intercommunicate in a circumferential manner (*Figure 11.50*). The lesions are darker than the retinal blood vessels and have an irregular contour with serrated edges (*Figure 11.51*). They run a convoluted course and tend to terminate abruptly. Eyes with angioid streaks may also show a pigmentary retinal mottling (peau d'orange), peripapillary chorioretinal atrophy, and occasionally hyaline bodies (drusen) at the optic nerve head (*see Figure 15.22*).

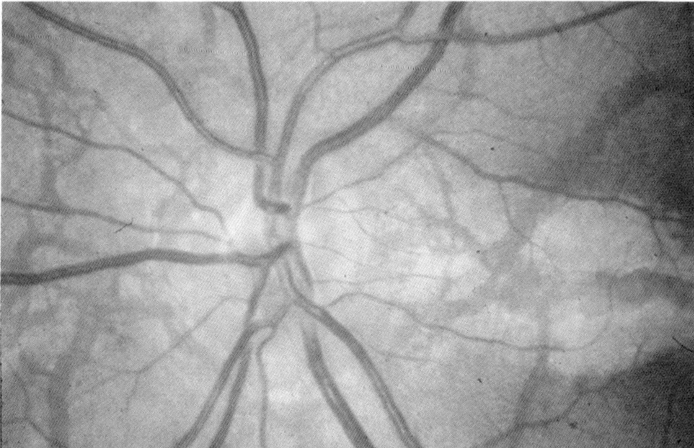

Figure 11.50 Angioid streaks (courtesy of Professor A. C. Bird)

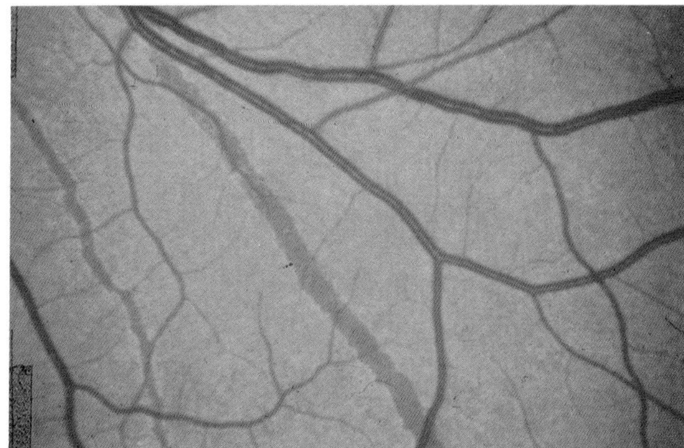

Figure 11.51 Angioid streaks (courtesy of Professor A. C. Bird)

Fluorescein angiography

This shows hyperfluorescence due to RPE window defects over the streaks.

Causes of visual impairment

The three ways in which eyes with angioid streaks may lose central vision are:

1. Involvement of the *fovea* by a streak.
2. *Choroidal neovascularization* with subsequent serous and haemorrhagic detachment of the fovea.
3. *Choroidal rupture*—because eyes with angioid streaks are fragile the patient should be warned against participating in contact sports as relatively trivial ocular trauma may cause a choroidal rupture and visual loss due to a subfoveal haemorrhage.

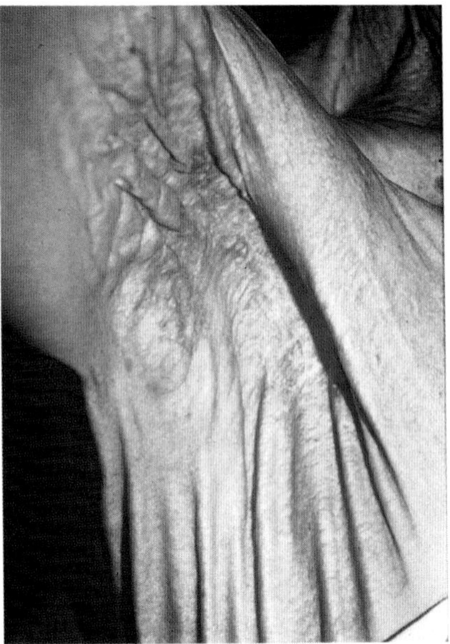

Figure 11.52 *Pseudoxanthoma elasticum of axilla (courtesy of Dr R. Winter)*

Systemic associations

About 50% of patients with angioid streaks have no associated systemic disorder. The remaining 50% have an associated disorder of skin, bone, or blood.

Pseudoxanthoma elasticum

This is the most common systemic disorder associated with angioid streaks. The combination of the two is referred to as the 'Grönblad–Strandberg' syndrome. The condition is inherited as an autosomal recessive trait. It is characterized by yellow skin papules which are most frequently found on the neck, the antecubital fossa, axilla (*Figure* 11.52), and the paraumbilical region. Occasionally the disease is subclinical and can only be diagnosed by skin biopsy.

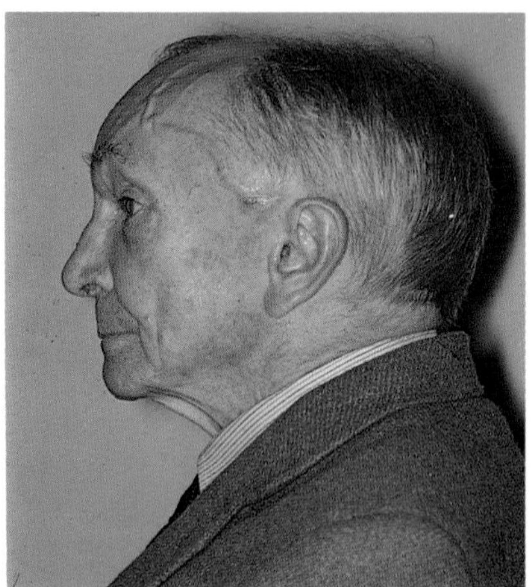

Figure 11.53 *Large skull in Paget's disease*

Paget's disease

This is a chronic, progressive and, in some cases, inherited disease, characterized by bone deformity. It may be confined to a few bones, or it may be generalized and give rise to enlargement of the skull (*Figure 11.53*), deformities of long bones, and kyphoscoliosis. Deafness is also common. About 10% of patients with Paget's disease develop angioid streaks. Those with an early onset of the disease and severe bone involvement seem to be at particular risk of developing eye complications.

Ehlers–Danlos syndrome

This syndrome is an uncommon association and is characterized by joint hyperextensibility and skin hyperelasticity (*Figure 11.54*). Apart from angioid streaks, other ocular features present in some patients include blue sclera, ectopia lentis, keratoconus, and a high incidence of retinal detachment.

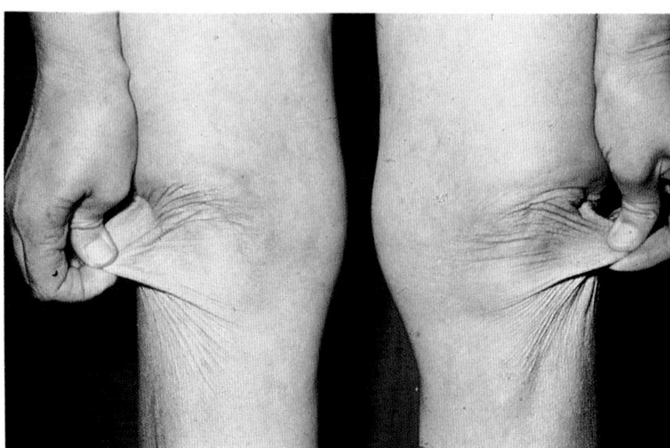

Figure 11.54 *Skin hyperelasticity in Ehlers–Danlos syndrome (courtesy of Dr R. Pope)*

Sickle-cell disease

This is very rarely associated with angioid streaks.

Toxic maculopathies

Chloroquine (Nivaquine)

Although chloroquine retinotoxicity is rare, its effects can be devastating. Patients at risk are those on long-term treatment for connective tissue disorders, such as rheumatoid arthritis and systemic lupus erythematosus. The drug is excreted slowly from the body and becomes concentrated within the melanin-containing structures of the eye such as the choroid and RPE.

The incidence of retinotoxicity increases with the total dose. Very few cases have been reported with a total dose of less than 300 g, which represents about 3 years on a daily dose of 250 mg.

Monitoring of patients on chloroquine

Patients in whom long-term therapy is anticipated should have a baseline eye examination including visual acuity, visual fields, ophthalmoscopy, colour vision, and where possible fundus photography of the posterior poles.

There is no need to see the patient for at least 9 months from the commencement of treatment and at 6-monthly intervals thereafter. However, the patient should be warned that soon after the commencement of treatment he may notice transient accommodational difficulties, which are of no significance. There is no correlation between corneal deposition of chloroquine (*see* Chapter 5) and subsequent retinopathy. The aim of regular examinations is to detect the premaculopathy stage of toxicity in which the patient is asymptomatic and has normal maculae.

Premaculopathy is characterized by a scotoma between 4° and 9° of fixation to a red target. Amsler grid testing may also show a defect. If the drug is discontinued, the scotoma usually disappears.

Established maculopathy may develop if chloroquine therapy is continued. Its earliest manifestations are a loss of the foveolar reflex with non-specific pigment stippling of the RPE. These changes may be more apparent on FA than on ophthalmoscopy. At this stage the patient notices blurring of vision, and a central scotoma to a white target may be demonstrable. Once this stage has been reached, vision usually remains stable after cessation of therapy, although very occasionally progressive impairment may occur.

Bull's eye maculopathy (*Figure 11.55*) is the characteristic lesion due to chloroquine toxicity. It consists of a central hyperpigmentation beneath the foveola, surrounded by a concentric depigmented circular zone, which, in turn, is encircled by an area of increased pigmentation. The hypopigmentation shows up on the fluorescein angiogram as a hyperfluorescent area, due to an RPE 'window' defect (*see Figure 11.18*). Once this stage has been reached, rarely progression of visual impairment may occur despite cessation of therapy.

Advanced retinopathy is characterized by severe arteriolar constriction with impairment of peripheral as well as central vision.

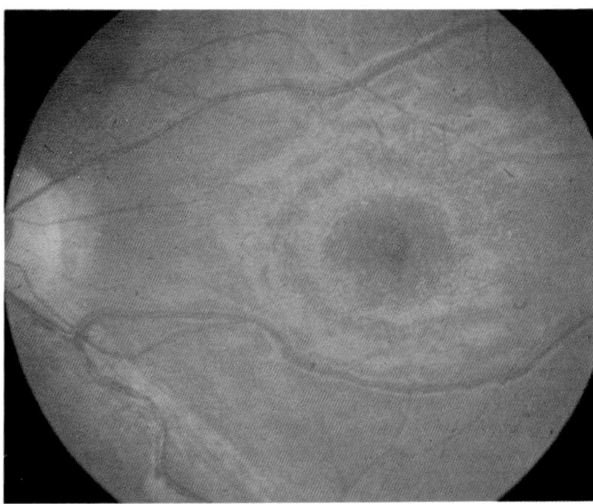

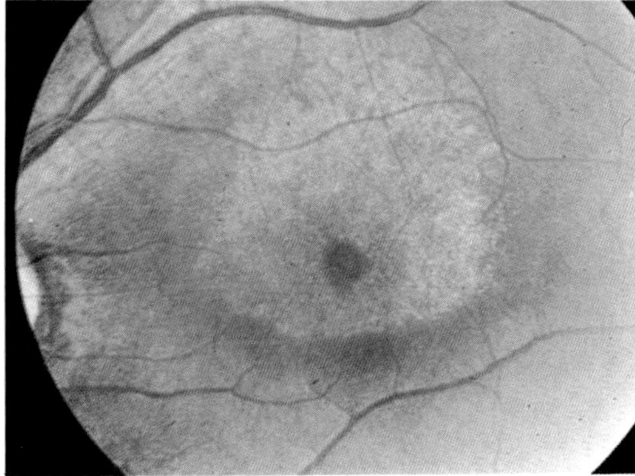

Figure 11.55 *Bull's eye maculopathy. Top: early; bottom: late*

Hydroxychloroquine (Plaquenil)

Hydroxychloroquine is a safer drug than chloroquine. The incidence of retinotoxicity is lower, and when retinal damage does occur it is usually mild and non-progressive.

Quinine

In high doses quinine may cause retinal arteriolar constriction and damage to the retinal ganglion cells. Very occasionally, visual damage may occur on an idiosyncratic basis in patients taking a normal dose.

Chlorpromazine (Largactil)

This drug is used in the treatment of schizophrenia and may occasionally cause retinal damage, but only if high doses (over 2400 mg/day) are taken over long periods of time. Chlorpromazine may also cause the deposition of fine yellow-white granules under the anterior lens capsule.

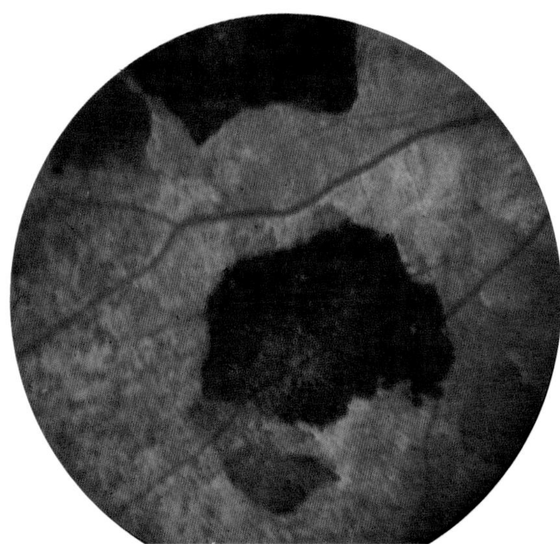

Figure 11.56 Melleril retinotoxicity (courtesy of Professor A. C. Bird)

Thioridazine (Melleril)

This is a drug used in the treatment of psychoses. If used in high doses (over 800 mg/day) it may lead to uniform clumps of pigment at the level of the RPE, as well as larger plaques of pigment (*Figure 11.56*). In advanced cases large areas of atrophy of the RPE and choriocapillaris develop.

Tamoxifen (Nolvadex)

Tamoxifen is a non-steroidal anti-oestrogen used in the treatment of metastatic breast cancer. It may give rise to a retinopathy characterized by bilateral intraretinal refractile opacities and lesions at the level of the RPE.

Further reading

Clinical evaluation

Bartov, E., Moisseiev, J. and Blumenthal, M. (1986) The ×16 slit-lamp eyepiece, a high plus lens for indirect biomicroscopy. *American Journal of Ophthalmology,* **101,** 620–621

Faulkner, W. (1986) Macular function testing through opacities. *Clinical Modules for Ophthalmologists,* Vol. 4, Module 2

Gomez-Ulla, F., Louro, O. and Mosquera, M. (1986) Macular dazzling test in normal subjects. *British Journal of Ophthalmology,* **70,** 209–213

Kraushar, M.F. and Margolis, S. (1980) Why can't my patient see 20/20? Simplified evaluation of macular function. *Perspectives in Ophthalmology,* **4,** 289–296

Loebl, M. and Riva, C.E. (1978) Macular circulation and the flying corpuscle phenomenon. *Ophthalmology,* **85,** 911–917

Miller, D., Lamberts, D.W. and Perry, H.D. (1978) An illuminated grid for macular testing. *Archives of Ophthalmology,* **96,** 901–902

Sinclair, S.H., Loebl, M. and Riva, C.E. (1979) Blue field entoptic phenomenon in cataract patients. *Archives of Ophthalmology,* **97,** 1092–1095

Fluorescein angiography

Kraushar, M.F. and Morse, P.H. (1978) Retinal fluorescein angiography uses and abuses. *Perspectives in Ophthalmology,* **2,** 299–306

Norton, E.W.D. (1981) Fluorescein angiography. *Transactions of the Ophthalmological Society of the United Kingdom,* **101,** 299–333

Wilkinson, C.P. (1986) The clinical examination. Limitation and overutilization of angiographic services. *Ophthalmology,* **93,** 410–404

Age-related macular degeneration

Berkow, J.W. (1984) Subretinal neovascularization in senile macular degeneration. *American Journal of Ophthalmology,* **97,** 143–147

Bird, A.C. and Grey, R.H.B. (1979) Photocoagulation of disciform macular lesions with krypton laser. *British Journal of Ophthalmology,* **63,** 669–673

Caswell, A.G., Kohen, D. and Bird, A.C. (1985) Retinal pigment epithelial detachments in the elderly: classification and outcome. *British Journal of Opthalmology,* **69,** 397–403

Eagle, R.C. (1984) Mechanisms of maculopathy. *Ophthalmology,* **91,** 613–625

Ferris, F.L., Fine, S.L. and Hyman, L. (1984) Age-related macular degeneration and blindness due to neovascular maculopathy. *Archives of Ophthalmology,* **102,** 1640–1642

Fine, S.L., Elman, M.J., Ebert, J.E. *et al.* (1986) Earliest symptoms caused by neovascular membranes at the macula. *Archives of Ophthalmology,* **104,** 513–514

Fine, S.L.., Murphy, R.P., Finkelstein, D. *et al.* (1984) Age-related macular degeneration. *Clinical Modules for Ophthalmologists,* Vol. 2, Module 1

Folk, J.C. (1985) Aging macular degeneration. *Ophthalmology,* **92,** 594–602

Green, W.R., McDonnell, P.J. and Yeo, J.H. (1985) Pathologic features of senile macular degeneration. *Ophthalmology,* **92,** 615–627

Gregor, Z., Bird, A.C. and Chisholm, I.H. (1977) Senile disciform degeneration in the second eye. *British Journal of Ophthalmology,* **61,** 141–145

Grey, R.H.B., Bird, A.C. and Chisholm, I.H. (1979) Senile disciform macular degeneration: features indicating suitability for photocoagulation. *British Journal of Ophthalmology,* **63,** 85–89

Ishibashi, T., Patterson, R., Ohnishi, Y. *et al.* (1986) Formation of drusen in the human eye. *American Journal of Ophthalmology,* **101,** 342–353

Jalkh, A.E., Avila, M.P., Trempe, C.L. *et al.* (1983) Choroidal neovascularization in fellow eyes of patients with senile macular degeneration. Role of photocoagulation. *Archives of Ophthalmology,* **101,** 1194–1197

Kenyon, K.R., Maumenee, A.E., Ryan, S.J. *et al.* (1985) Diffuse drusen and associated complications. *American Journal of Ophthalmology,* **100,** 119–128

Macular Photocoagulation Study Group (1982) Argon laser photocoagulation for senile macular degeneration. *Archives of Ophthalmology,* **100,** 912–918

Macular Photocoagulation Study Group (1986) Argon laser photocoagulation for neovascular maculopathy. *Archives of Ophthalmology,* **104,** 694–701

Moorfields Macular Study Group (1982) Treatment of senile macular degeneration: a single-blind randomised trial by argon laser. *British Journal of Ophthalmology,* **66,** 745–753

Moorfields Macular Study Group (1982) Retinal pigment epithelial detachment in the elderly: a controlled trial of argon laser photocoagulation. *British Journal of Ophthalmology,* **66,** 1–16

Sarks, S.H., Van Driel, D., Maxwell, L. *et al.* (1980) Softening of drusen and subretinal neovascularization. *Transactions of the Ophthalmological Society of the United Kingdom,* **100,** 414–422

Singerman, L.J. (1985) Important points in management of patients with choroidal neovascularization. *Ophthalmology,* **92,** 610–615

Smitty, W.E. and Fine, S.L. (1984) Prognosis in patients with bilateral macular drusen. *Ophthalmology,* **91,** 271–277

Strahlman, E.R., Fine, S.E. and Hillis, A. (1983) The second eye of patients with senile macular degeneration. *Archives of Ophthalmology,* **101,** 1191–1193

Trempe, C.L., Mainster, M.A., Pomerantzeff, O. *et al.* (1982) Macular photocoagulation—optimal wavelength selection. *Ophthalmology,* **89,** 721–728

Tso, M.O. (1985) Pathogenetic factors of aging macular degeneration. *Ophthalmology,* **92,** 628–635

Central serous chorioretinopathy

Gilbert, C.M., Owens, S.L., Smith, P.D. *et al.* (1984) Long-term follow-up of central serous chorioretinopathy. *British Journal of Ophthalmology,* **68,** 815–820

Mazzuca, D.E. and Benson, W.E. (1986) Central serous retinopathy: Variants. *Survey of Ophthalmology,* **31,** 170–174

Robertson, D.M. and Ilstrup, D. (1983) Direct, indirect, and sham photocoagulation in the management of central serous chorioretinopathy. *American Journal of Ophthalmology,* **95,** 457–466

Cystoid macular oedema

Jampol, L.M. (1982) Pharmacologic therapy for aphakic cystoid macular oedema. *Ophthalmology,* **89,** 891–897

Tso, M.O.M. (1982) Pathology of cystoid macular oedema. *Ophthalmology,* **89,** 902–915

Macular hole

McDonnell, P.J., Fine, S.L. and Hillis, A.I. (1982) Clinical features of idiopathic macular cysts and holes. *American Journal of Ophthalmology,* **93,** 777–786

Morgan, C.M. and Schatz, H. (1985) Idiopathic macular holes. *American Journal of Ophthalmology,* **99,** 437–444

Morgan, C.M. and Schatz, H. (1986) Involutional macular thinning. A pre-hole condition. *Ophthalmology,* **93,** 153–161

Trempe, C.L., Weiter, J.J. and Furukawa, H. (1986) Fellow eyes in cases of macular hole. *Archives of Ophthalmology,* **104,** 93–95

Myopic maculopathy

Hampton, G.R., Kohen, D. and Bird, A.C. (1983) Visual prognosis of disciform degeneration in myopia. *Ophthalmology,* **90,** 923–926

Macular pucker

Michels, R.G. (1984) Vitrectomy for macular pucker. *Ophthalmology,* **91,** 1384–1388

Sidd, R.J., Fine, S.L., Owens, S.L. *et al.* (1982) Idiopathic preretinal gliosis. *American Journal of Ophthalmology,* **94,** 44–48

Choroidal folds

Friberg, T.K. and Grove, A.S. (1983) Choroidal folds and refractive errors associated with orbital tumors. *Archives of Ophthalmology,* **101,** 598–603

Newell, F.W. (1984) Fundus changes in persistent and recurrent choroidal folds. *British Journal of Ophthalmology,* **68,** 32–35

Toxic maculopathies

Brinkley, J.R., Dubois, E.L. and Ryan, S.J. (1979) Longterm course of chloroquine retinopathy after cessation of medication. *American Journal of Ophthalmology,* **88,** 1–11

Hart, W.M., Burde, R.M., Johnston, G.P. *et al.* (1984) Static perimetry in chloroquine retinopathy. *Archives of Ophthalmology,* **102,** 377–380

Mills, P.V., Beck, M. and Power, B.J. (1981) Assessment of retinal toxicity of hydroxychloroquine. *Transactions of the Ophthalmological Society of the United Kingdom,* **101,** 109–113

Tobin, D.R., Krohel, G.B. and Rynes, R.I. (1982) Hydroxychloroquine—seven years experience. *Archives of Ophthalmology,* **100,** 81–83

12

Hereditary Disorders of the Retina and Choroid

Special investigations

Electroretinography

Dark adaptation (adaptometry)

Electro-oculography

Visually evoked response

Clinical applications of electrophysiological tests

Retinitis pigmentosa

Typical

Atypical

Systemic associations

Leber's congenital amaurosis

Vitelliform dystrophies

Best's vitelliform macular dystrophy

Adult foveomacular vitelliform dystrophy

'Bull's eye' macula syndromes

Cone dystrophy

Batten's disease (ceroid-lipofuscinosis)

Benign concentric annular macular dystrophy

'Cherry-red spot' at macula syndromes

Pattern dystrophies

'Flecked retina' syndromes

Stargardt's–fundus flavimaculatus

Familial dominant drusen

Fundus albipunctatus

Albinism

Vitreoretinal degenerations

Wagner's disease

Stickler syndrome

Congenital retinoschisis

Favre–Goldmann syndrome

Exudative vitreoretinopathy (Criswick–Schepens syndrome)

Snowflake degeneration

Choroidal dystrophies

Choroideremia

Gyrate atrophy

Central areolar choroidal dystrophy

Generalized choroidal atrophy

Special investigations

Electroretinography

The electroretinogram (ERG) (*Figure 12.1*) is the record of an action potential produced by the retina when it is stimulated by light of an adequate intensity.

The recording is made between an active electrode embedded in a contact lens and placed on the cornea, and a reference electrode on the patient's forehead. The potential between the two electrodes is then amplified and the response is displayed on a pen-recorder or on an oscilloscope. The ERG is then elicited both in the light-adapted (photopic) and dark-adapted (scotopic) states.

The waveform of the ERG is complex and varies with the light used as stimulus, the adaptive state of the retina, and the techniques of electrode placement. The usual ERG response is biphasic (*Figure 12.2*).

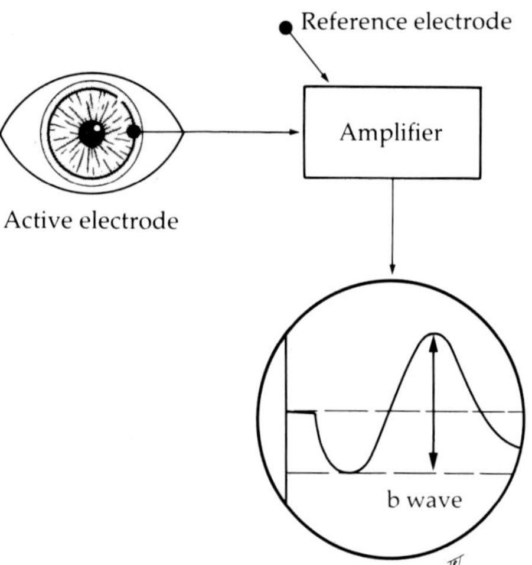

Figure 12.1 *Electroretinography*

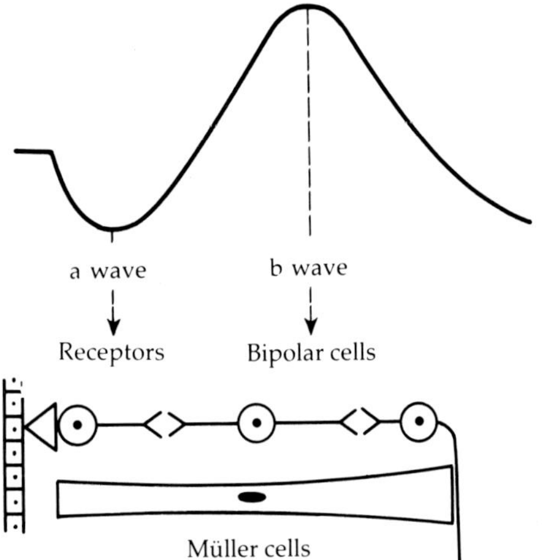

Figure 12.2 *Electroretinogram*

'a wave'

The initial negative deflection is the 'a wave' or late receptor potential, which arises from the photoreceptors.

'b wave'

The second positive deflection is the 'b wave' which is generated by Müller cells, but represents processes occurring in the bipolar cell region. The amplitude of the 'b wave' is measured from the trough of the 'a wave' to the peak of the 'b wave'. The amplitude of the 'b wave' increases both with dark adaptation and with increase in the light stimulus.

The ERG, therefore, is a function of the first two neurones of the retina and is not useful in the diagnosis of disorders affecting the ganglion cells or the optic nerve.

It is possible to single out rod and cone responses by using certain techniques.

Rod responses

These can be isolated by stimulating the fully dark-adapted eye with a flash of very dim light or with blue light.

Cone responses

These can be isolated by stimulating the fully light-adapted eye with a bright flash of light or with red light. The cones can also be effectively isolated by using a flickering light stimulus of 30–40 Hz to which rods cannot respond. Cone responses can be elicited in normal eyes up to 50 Hz, after which point the individual responses are no longer recordable—critical flicker fusion (CFF). The 'b wave' of the ERG consists of b_1 and b_2 subcomponents. The b_1 subcomponent probably represents both rod and cone activity, whereas the b_2 subcomponent probably represents rod activity.

Dark adaptation (adaptometry)

Dark adaptation is the ability of the retina and pupil to react to decreased illumination. The test is clinically useful in the evaluation of certain retinal disorders, particularly in patients complaining of night blindness. The instrument used is usually the Goldmann–Weekes adaptometer. The subject is pre-adapted to a standard amount of illumination and is then presented with a series of flashes of light (localized 11° below fixation). The intensity of the flashes is controlled by a neutral density filter and the threshold at which the subject just perceives the light is plotted against time. The sensitivity curve is bipartite—the initial rapid segment represents cone function and the second slower segment represents rod function. The inflection on the curve where the rod limb begins is called the rod–cone break (alpha point), and in the healthy eye it occurs after

7–10 minutes of dark adaptation. If the flash is focused on the foveola (where rods are absent), only a cone plateau will be recorded. Because dark adaptometry is essentially a focal test, it may be a more sensitive test than the ERG in the evaluation of certain disorders.

Electro-oculography

The electro-oculogram (EOG; *Figure 12.3*) measures the standing action potential which exists between the cornea, which is electrically positive, and the back of the eye, which is electrically negative.

In recording the EOG, electrodes are attached to the skin near the medial and lateral canthi. The patient is then asked to look rhythmically from side to side making excursions of constant amplitude. Each time the eye is moved, the cornea makes the electrode nearest to it positive with respect to the other. The potential difference produced between the two electrodes is amplified and recorded. The test is performed in both light-adapted and dark-adapted states.

Because there is much variation in the EOG amplitude in normal subjects, the result is calculated by dividing the level of the maximal height of the potential in the light (light peak) by the minimal height of the potential in the dark (dark trough). This ratio is then multiplied by 100 and expressed as a percentage. A normal value is over 185%. Because the EOG requires the cooperation of the patient, the test cannot be performed on the very young. The normal values vary for different laboratories.

Although there is some dispute regarding the actual origin of the EOG, it appears that it is probably based on the activity of the retinal pigment epithelium (RPE) and the photoreceptors. This means that an eye blinded by lesions that are proximal to the photoreceptors will have a normal EOG. Generally, a diffuse or widespread disease of the RPE is needed to effect a significant EOG response.

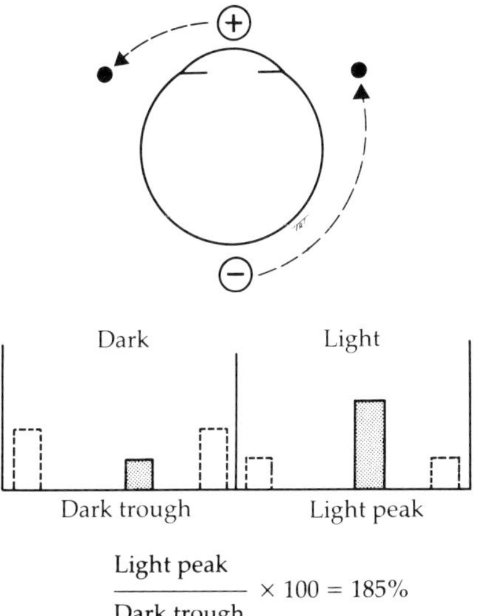

Figure 12.3 *Electro-oculogram*

Visually evoked response

The visually evoked response (VER; *Figure 12.4*) is a gross electrical signal generated by the occipital visual cortex in response to stimulation of the retina by light. Since most of the external visual cortex is representative of the macular area of the eye, the test is essentially a method of testing macular function. The VER is the only objective test that can assess the functional status of the visual system beyond the retinal ganglion cells. For this reason, an abnormal VER with a normal ERG and EOG suggests an organic lesion in the pathway between and including the ganglion cell layer and the visual cortex.

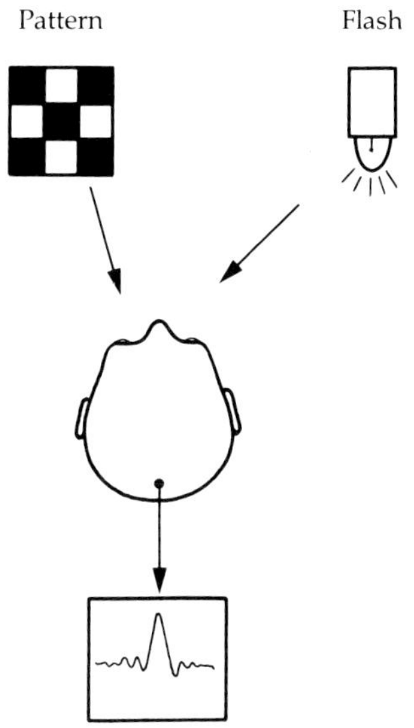

Figure 12.4 *Visually evoked response*

The VER to a flash of light is a complex wave with great variability. In addition, the responses to various types of stimuli give different information. The type of stimulus used depends on the purpose of the recording and the type of patient on whom the test is being performed.

Pattern VER. A pattern 'checkboard' stimulus is used if the test is required to establish an organic cause for poor visual acuity.

Flash VERs can be used in assessing retinocortical conduction properties in infants or in uncooperative patients. It gives no information other than that the light has been perceived.

Clinical uses of the VER

1. Determination of visual acuity in infants.
2. Diagnosis of optic nerve disease, particularly as a result of demyelination.
3. Detection of malingering.
4. Prediction of visual potential in eyes with opaque media.
5. Evaluation of macular disorders.

Clinical applications of electrophysiological tests

1. *Tapetoretinal degenerations* are widespread disorders involving the photoreceptors and RPE. They will therefore have a marked effect on the ERG and EOG.
2. *Disorders of night vision.* The tests can sometimes distinguish between progressive and non-progressive causes of night blindness.
3. *Visual defects in infants.* The tests can be helpful in establishing the cause of poor vision in a child with normal fundi (Leber's amaurosis).
4. *Detection of carriers.* Carriers of Best's disease have a subnormal EOG in the presence of normal fundi.
5. *Evaluation of potential retinal function in eyes with opaque media.*
6. *Differential diagnosis* between macular disease, optic nerve disease, and hysteria or malingering.
7. *Drug toxicity detection.*

Retinitis pigmentosa

Retinitis pigmentosa (RP) is a generic name for a group of inherited diseases characterized by night blindness and constricted visual fields. The clinical features of RP vary between patients, and even among family members with the disease.

Typical

Typical RP is a diffuse, usually bilaterally symmetrical, retinal dystrophy. Although both cones and rods are involved, damage to the rod system is predominant. The age of onset, rate of progression, amount of eventual visual loss, and the presence or absence of associated ocular features are frequently related to the mode of inheritance.

Inheritance

Autosomal recessive

This is the most common mode of inheritance and, of the sporadic cases (i.e. those without a family history), most are also probably of the recessive type. Unfortunately, it is also a severe form of RP with early development of night blindness, visual field loss and cataract.

Autosomal dominant

This is the next most frequent mode of inheritance. This form of RP usually has a fairly benign course so that night blindness and visual field loss may not develop until adult life, and cataract may not be a problem until the sixth decade of life.

X-linked recessive

This is the least common mode of inheritance. The severity of involvement is similar to, and sometimes worse than, the recessive type. Female carriers may have normal fundi or may show a 'golden-metallic' tapetal reflex temporal to the macula which is virtually pathognomonic. In other cases, peripheral retinal atrophy and pigmentary irregularities may involve one sector of the fundus.

Clinical features

The classic triad of RP consists of bone-spicule pigmentation, arteriolar attenuation, and waxy disc pallor.

Peripheral retina

Retinal pigmentary changes are typically perivascular and have a bone-spicule appearance (*Figure 12.5*). Small irregular pigment clumps are also frequently seen. The pigmentary degeneration is initially observed in the midretinal periphery. With the passage of time, the pigmentary changes extend, both posteriorly and anteriorly, giving rise to a ring-like scotoma in the visual field. The progressive contraction of the visual field ultimately leaves only a tiny island of central vision which may eventually be lost. During the later stages of the disease the unmasking of the larger choroidal blood vessels gives the fundus a tessellated appearance (*Figure 12.6*) and arteriolar attenuation becomes more evident.

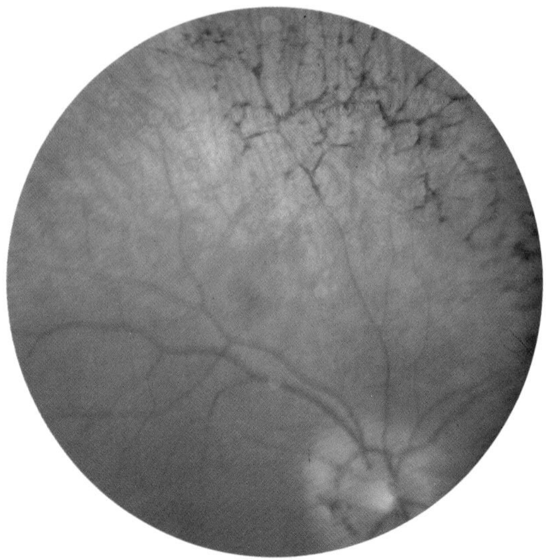

Figure 12.5 *'Bone-spicule' pigmentation in retinitis pigmentosa*

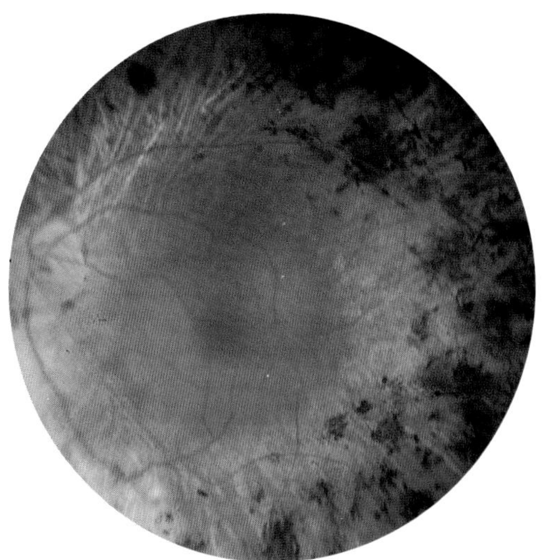

Figure 12.6 *Retinitis pigmentosa with unmasking of choroidal vessels*

Optic nerve head

Initially the optic disc is normal but later it may assume a waxy pallor (this is the least reliable sign of the RP triad). Hyaline bodies (drusen) of the optic nerve head are seen more frequently in RP patients than in normals.

Maculopathy

The various types of macular lesions described in RP include:

1. *Cystoid macular oedema.*
2. *Atrophic.*
3. *Cellophane.*

Other ocular features

1. *Open-angle glaucoma* occurs in 3% of RP patients.
2. *Posterior subcapsular cataract* occurs early in recessively inherited cases, and at about the age of 50 years in dominant cases. Extraction frequently leads to visual improvement.
3. *Keratoconus* occurs with increased prevalence in RP sufferers.
4. *Myopia* is frequent.
5. *Vitreous.* Posterior vitreous detachment with translucent vitreous particles is a common finding.

Special investigations

Even during the early stages of the disease, in which the fundus changes are minimal, the ERG amplitude is markedly subnormal. The changes affect the scotopic ERG predominantly, whereas the photopic ERG is relatively unaffected. *EOG* shows an absence of the light rise. *Dark adaptation* shows elevation of both cone and rod thresholds.

Visual prognosis

About one patient in four maintains good visual acuity and is able to read throughout his or her life, despite unrecordable ERGs and a 2–3° central field. Under the age of 20 years, only a few patients will have a visual acuity of 6/60 or worse. However, by the age of 50 years at least half will be affected to that degree.

Atypical

RP sine pigmento

In some cases of RP, the typical pigmentary changes appear later while in others they remain inconspicuous or undetectable despite the presence of an extinguished ERG combined with arteriolar attenuation and waxy pallor of the optic disc (*Figure 12.7*).

Retinitis punctata albescens

This is characterized by scattered white dots, most numerous between the posterior pole and equator. These findings are frequently associated with the subsequent development of bone-spicule pigmentation, arteriolar attenuation, night blindness, and constriction of visual fields as in typical RP.

Sector RP

This is characterized by involvement of only one quadrant (usually nasal) or one half (usually inferior) of the fundus. Progression is slow and many cases remain stationary.

Pericentric RP

This is similar to typical RP except that the pigmentary changes are confined to the pericentral retina, sparing the retinal periphery.

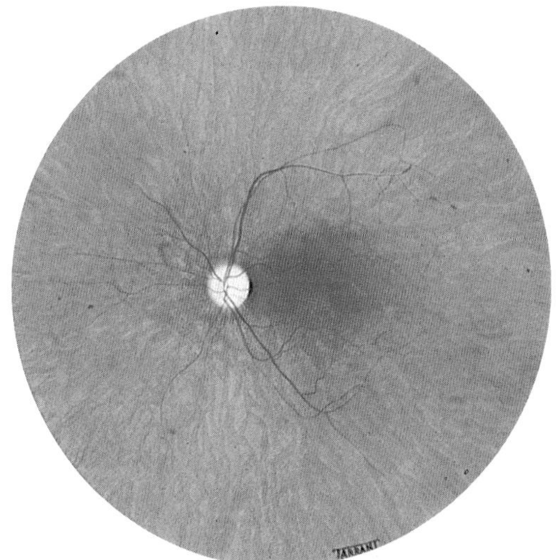

Figure 12.7 *Retinitis pigmentosa sine pigmento*

Systemic associations

RP, often of the atypical type, may be associated with a wide variety of systemic disorders. Only the more important associations will be described.

Bassen–Kornzweig syndrome (abetalipoproteinaemia)

1. *Systemic features.* This rare disorder which typically affects Ashkenazi Jews is inherited as an autosomal recessive trait. It is characterized by spinocerebellar ataxia, acanthocytosis, and abetalipoproteinaemia. Fat malabsorption is present from birth and jejunal biopsy is diagnostic. The disease is ultimately fatal.
2. *Ocular features.* RP develops towards the end of the first decade. The pigment clumps are often larger than in classic RP and are not confined to the equatorial regions. Peripheral white dots are also common. Disturbances of ocular motility and ptosis have also been described.
3. *Treatment* with vitamin E, if instituted early, may be beneficial for both the neurological and retinal lesions. The exact therapeutic value of vitamin A is still uncertain.

Refsum's syndrome (phytanic acid storage disease)

1. *Systemic features.* This disease is inherited as an autosomal recessive trait. It is characterized by peripheral neuropathy, cerebellar ataxia, and elevated CSF protein in the absence of pleocytosis. The underlying biochemical abnormality is defective metabolism of phytanic acid which infiltrates many tissues of the body including the eye. Other features include deafness and ichthyosis.
2. *Ocular features.* Night blindness due to a pigmentary retinopathy is always the presenting feature. The retinal findings are usually of a generalized 'salt-and-pepper' type rather than the classic 'bone corpuscle' seen in typical RP.
3. *Treatment* with a phytanic-acid-free diet and plasma exchange may prevent progression of both systemic and ocular involvement.

Usher's syndrome

1. *Systemic features.* This recessively inherited disorder is characterized by congenital, non-progressive, sensorineural deafness of varying severity. Usher's syndrome accounts for about 5% of all cases of profound deafness in children, and is responsible for about half of all cases of combined deafness and blindness.
2. *Ocular features.* In the vast majority of patients, RP develops prior to puberty and is progressive.

Cockayne's syndrome

1. *Systemic features.* This rare recessively inherited disorder is characterized by dwarfism that becomes manifest in childhood. The dwarf is cachectic and prematurely aged, with a characteristic 'birdlike' facies. The hands and limbs are disproportionately large and the limbs may be in flexion contracture. Other features include deafness, nystagmus, ataxia, and progressive mental retardation. Severely affected individuals usually die during the third and fourth decades of life.
2. *Ocular features.* The retinopathy is of the 'salt-and-pepper' type, usually with waxy optic atrophy and attenuated retinal blood vessels.

Kearns–Sayre syndrome

1. *Systemic features.* This rare disorder consists of the following triad: chronic progressive external ophthalmoplegia (ocular myopathy); heart block that may cause sudden death; and pigmentary retinopathy. The condition usually becomes manifest prior to the age of 20 years and in some cases it is associated with other abnormalities such as short stature, cerebellar ataxia, deafness, mental retardation, and delayed puberty.
2. *Ocular features.* The pigmentary retinal changes often occur centrally and spare the retinal periphery.

Mucopolysaccharidoses

The majority of patients with type 1 (Hurler's and its subtype Scheie's), type 2 (Hunter's), and type 3 (Sanfilippo) have pigmentary retinopathy and abnormal ERGs. The systemic and other ocular features of the mucopolysaccharidoses are discussed in Chapter 5.

Laurence–Moon–Biedl syndrome

This is characterized by pigmentary retinopathy, mental retardation, polydactyly, obesity, and hypogonadism.

Friedreich's ataxia

This is characterized by pigmentary retinopathy, posterior column disease, ataxia, and nystagmus.

Leber's congenital amaurosis

Inheritance

This is usually autosomal recessive.

Clinical features

Patients with this condition are either blind from birth or become blind within the first few years of life. Nystagmus, strabismus, photophobia, and the oculodigital syndrome (in which the child constantly rubs his eyes) are frequent associated findings.

1. *Fundus findings* vary considerably and may be responsible for incorrect diagnoses. Initially, the fundus may appear essentially normal although the ERG is severely diminished or non-recordable. Variable late features include arteriolar attenuation, optic atrophy (or occasionally oedema), a 'salt-and-pepper' appearance, peripheral and central granularity, and diffuse white spots. Bone-spicule pigmentary changes as in true RP, if present, usually become manifest at the age of about 8 years. Recently, a relatively mild form of this disease has been recognized.
2. *Other ocular features* include keratoconus, keratoglobus, and cataract. These may develop by the teens in some patients.
3. *Systemic features* include psychomotor and mental retardation, deafness, epilepsy, and renal abnormalities.

Vitelliform dystrophies

Best's vitelliform macular dystrophy

Inheritance

This is autosomal dominant with variable penetrance and expressivity.

Clinical features

The ophthalmoscopical features can be divided into five stages.

Stage 1 (previtelliform)

This is characterized by an abnormal EOG (decreased light-peak–dark-trough ratio) in an asymptomatic patient without any detectable fundus lesion.

Stage 2 (vitelliform)

As the disease progresses, ill-defined yellow spots develop at the level of the RPE. These are thought to represent accumulation of lipofuscin granules. At the macula, the yellow material is secreted into the potential space between the sensory retina and RPE to form the classic 'egg-yolk' or 'sunny-side-up' lesion which measures between 0.5 and 3 disc diameters in size (*Figure 12.8*). Although this stage of the disease is usually detected during the first and second decades of life, it has been reported in neonates. Visual acuity may be normal or slightly decreased.

Stage 3 (pseudohypopyon; Figure 12.9)

Occasionally part of the lesion may become absorbed giving rise to a 'pseudohypopyon' in which the upper part shows up as an area of hyperfluorescence due to atrophic changes in the RPE, while the lower part of the lesion blocks background choroidal fluorescence. Occasionally the whole lesion becomes absorbed with little effect on vision.

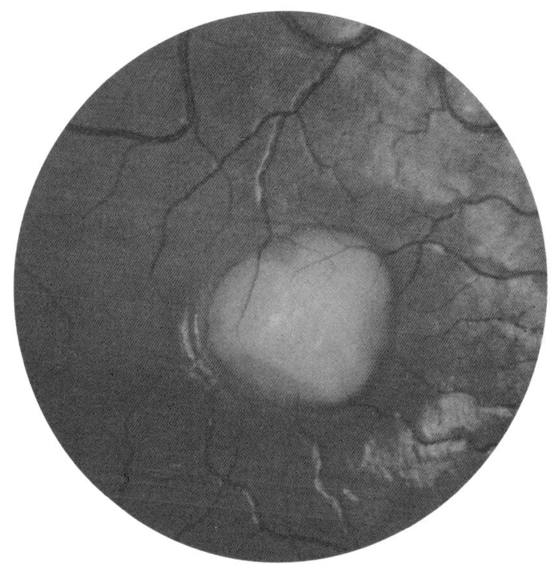

Figure 12.8 *Best's dystrophy – 'egg yolk' stage (courtesy of Professor A. C. Bird)*

Stage 4 (vitelliruptive; Figure 12.10)

After a variable period of time, the 'egg yolk' begins to break up and assumes a 'scrambled egg' appearance. At this point the patient usually develops visual impairment.

Stage 5 (end stage)

This is associated with a moderate to severe impairment of vision. Three macular lesions may occur:

1. *Hypertrophic macular scar* (*Figure 12.11*).
2. *Vascularized fibrous scar* with choroidal neovascularization which may give rise to a sudden drop in vision.
3. *Atrophic macular lesion* in which the macula develops an

orange-red colour due to increased visibility of the choroid through the atrophic RPE.

It is important to be aware of the widely variable manifestations of Best's disease. The lesions may be bilateral, unilateral, single or multiple, macular or eccentric.

Spinal investigations

The EOG is severely subnormal during all stages of this disease in affected patients, as well as in carriers with normal fundi.

Adult foveomacular vitelliform dystrophy

This rare disorder is usually inherited as an autosomal dominant trait. The condition presents in middle life with mild, slowly progressive blurring of vision and metamorphopsia. Ophthalmoscopy shows bilateral, round or oval, slightly elevated, yellow, subfoveal deposits, approximately one-third of a disc diameter in size. Paracentral drusen may also be present. The EOG is normal or slightly abnormal.

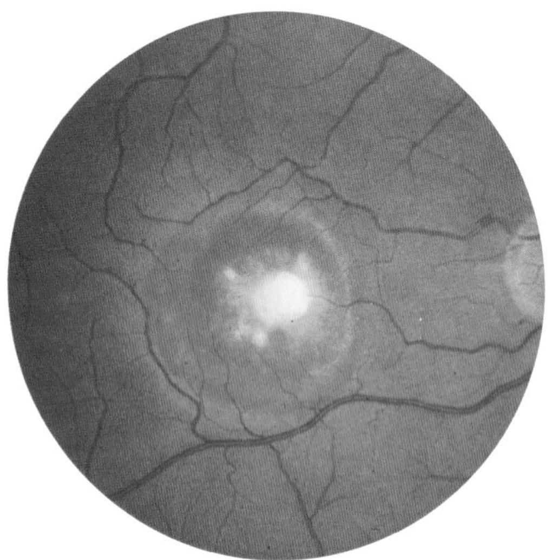

Figure 12.10 Best's dystrophy – vitelliruptive stage (courtesy of Professor A. C. Bird)

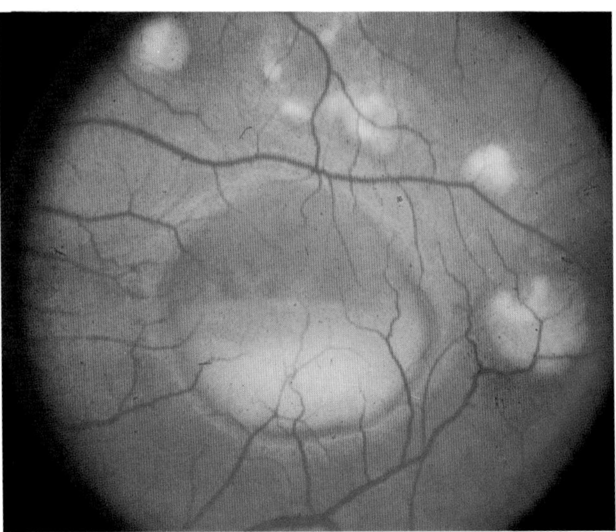

Figure 12.9 Best's dystrophy – pseudohypopyon stage (courtesy of Professor A. C. Bird)

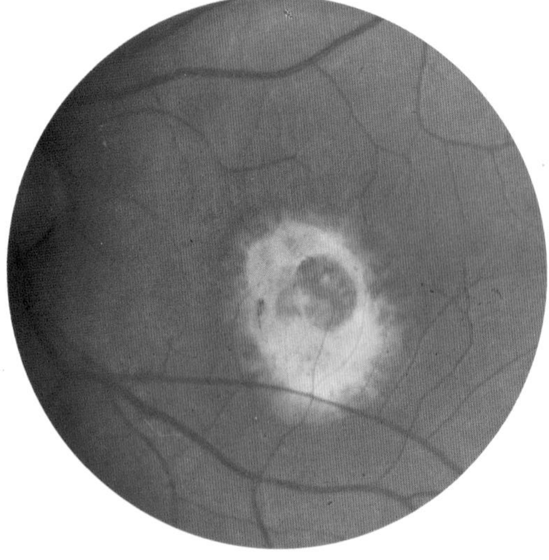

Figure 12.11 Best's dystrophy – end stage with macular scar (courtesy of Professor A. C. Bird)

'Bull's eye' macula syndromes

Cone dystrophy

Inheritance

This is usually autosomal dominant although recessive cases have also been described.

Clinical features

Patients with cone dystrophy usually present between the first and third decades of life with impairment of central vision, decreased vision in good illumination, 'day blindness', defective colour vision, and nystagmus. In typical cases, fundoscopy shows a 'bull's eye' macular lesion due to selected atrophy of RPE cells. The optic disc may also show temporal pallor. Later the retinal vessels become attenuated and mild pigmentary peripheral changes can also be seen.

In the more severe form of cone dystrophy, the arteriolar and macular changes are more extensive at an earlier age.

The optic disc may develop a waxy pallor and the peripheral retina may show bone-spicule pigment clumping as in RP.

Special investigations

The photopic ERG is subnormal or non-recordable, but the scotopic response is normal.

Batten's disease (ceroid-lipofuscinosis)

This disease consists of four closely related entities characterized by the accumulation of autofluorescent lipopigments in neural, visceral, and somatic tissues. The four syndromes have been delineated on the basis of age of onset of clinical manifestations, rate of progression, and severity of ocular involvement.

1. *Infantile (Haltia–Santavuori)* is characterized by onset before the age of 2 years and rapidly progressive psychomotor deterioration. Visual loss usually occurs long after the diagnosis has been established.
2. *Late infantile (Jansky–Bielschowsky)* becomes manifest between the ages of 2 and 6 years with rapidly progressive psychomotor deterioration and seizures. Here again visual loss is a late feature.
3. *Juvenile (Spielmeyer–Sjögren)* usually presents between the ages of 4 and 6 years with visual failure due to a bull's eye macula dystrophy. Later, widespread pigmentary changes and arteriolar attenuation develop. Rarely a 'bone-spicule' pigmentation is seen. A common finding is that the patient tends to look above a fixation target. Visual loss is usually followed by progressive mental deterioration, fits, and death by the early twenties.
4. *Adult (Kufs')* is the least clearly delineated form of Batten's disease and is characterized by cerebellar and extrapyramidal dysfunction, occasionally accompanied by dementia. Visual impairment is uncommon.

Benign concentric annular macular dystrophy

This very rare dominantly inherited disorder is characterized by a 'bull's eye' macular lesion. Although the visual prognosis is usually good, some patients subsequently develop a more diffuse pigmentary retinopathy with functional characteristics of cone–rod dystrophy.

'Cherry-red spot' at macula syndromes

The 'cherry-red spot' (*Figure 12.12*) is the most striking retinal lesion in a rare group of inherited metabolic diseases which comprise the sphingolipidoses. These diseases are characterized by the progressive intracellular storage of excessive quantities of certain glycolipids and phospholipids in various tissues of the body, including the retina.

The lipids are stored in the ganglion cell layer of the retina, giving the retina a white appearance. Since ganglion cells are absent at the foveola, this area contrasts with the surrounding opaque retina. With the passage of time the ganglion cells die and the spot becomes atrophic. The late stage of the disease is characterized by optic atrophy and atrophy of the retinal nerve fibre layer.

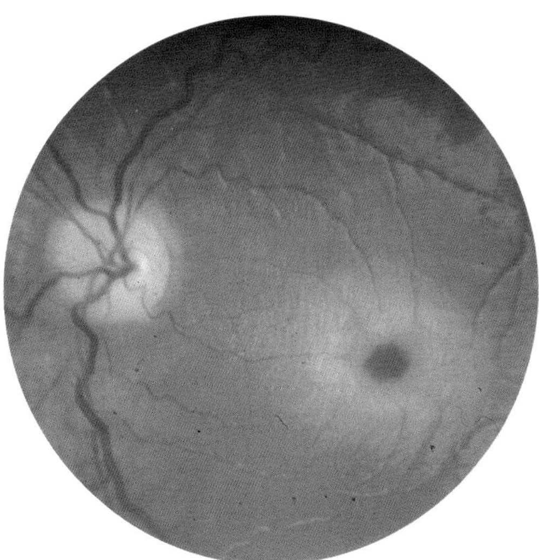

Figure 12.12 *Cherry-red spot at macula (courtesy of Mr E. C. Glover)*

Tay–Sachs disease (Gm_2 gangliosidosis type 1)

This condition, which is also called infantile amaurotic familial idiocy, is an autosomal recessive disease having an onset during the first year of life and usually ending in death before the age of 2 years. It typically affects European Jews and is characterized by progressive neurological involvement and eventual blindness. A cherry-red spot is present in about 90% of cases.

Niemann–Pick disease

This has been divided on a clinical and chemical basis into four groups:

Group A with severe early CNS deterioration.
Group B with apparently normal CNS function.
Group C with moderate CNS involvement and a slow course.
Group D with a late onset, and eventual severe CNS involvement.

In Niemann–Pick disease the incidence of the cherry-red spot is lower than in Tay–Sachs disease.

Sandhoff disease (Gm_2 gangliosidosis type 2)

This is nearly identical to Tay–Sachs disease.

Generalized gangliosidosis (Gm_1 gangliosidosis type 1)

This is characterized by hypoactivity, oedema of the face and extremities, and skeletal anomalies from birth.

Sialidosis types 1 and 2

This is also referred to as the 'cherry-red spot myoclonus syndrome', and is characterized by myoclonic jerks, pain in the limbs, and unsteadiness. A cherry-red spot may be the initial finding.

Pattern dystrophies

Several varieties of patterned dystrophies of the RPE have been described. The main types are *butterfly* (*Figure 12.13*), *Sjögren's reticular*, and *macroreticular*.

All of these dystrophies are characterized by the presence of yellow deposits at the level of the RPE which decrease or block background choroidal fluorescence on angiography. Visual function is not significantly affected, and both psychophysical and electrophysiological tests give only slightly abnormal results. An instance of them all occurring in the same family has recently been described, suggesting that there may be a link among them.

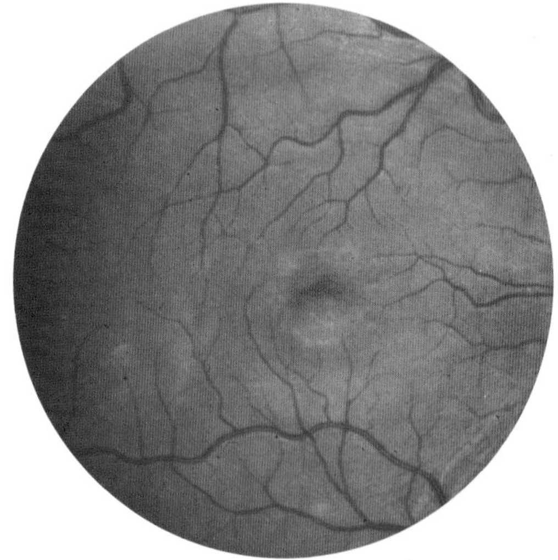

Figure 12.13 *Butterfly dystrophy*

'Flecked retina' syndromes

This group of unconnected disorders is characterized by the presence of spots or flecks scattered throughout the fundus.

Stargardt's—fundus flavimaculatus

Inheritance

Stargardt's macular dystrophy and fundus flavimaculatus are now regarded as variants of the same disorder. Inheritance is usually autosomal recessive, although dominantly inherited cases have also been described. Both sexes are affected equally.

Clinical features (*Figure 12.14*)

Stargardt's macular dystrophy

This usually presents during the first or second decade of life with impaired vision. The initial finding is a non-specific mottling at the fovea. With the passage of time, an

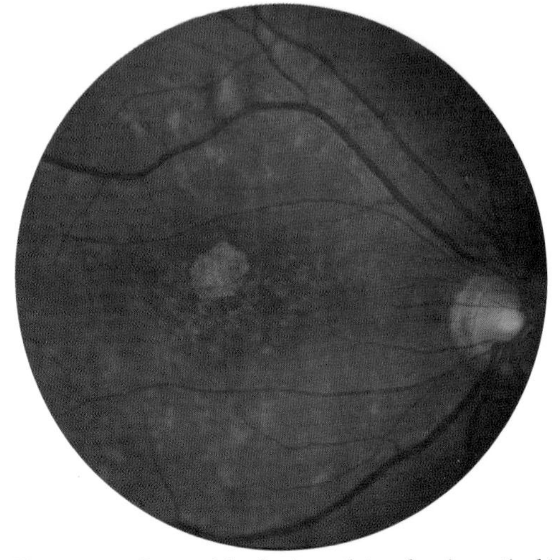

Figure 12.14 *Stargardt's–flavimaculatus showing retinal flecks and atrophic maculopathy (courtesy of Dr P. H. Morse)*

oval lesion about 1.5 disc diameters in size, which has a 'snail-slime' or 'beaten-bronze' reflex, develops at the macula. This may or may not be surrounded by yellow-white flecks. As the disease progresses the macular lesion becomes more extensive and central vision becomes impaired due to atrophic changes in the RPE and choriocapillaris and secondary changes in the photoreceptors. The final visual acuity is seldom worse than 3/60.

Fundus flavimaculatus

This variant is usually seen later than Stargardt's disease. The yellow flecks are more prominent and irregular in size, varying from round or ovoid to linear, semilunar, or pisciform (fish-tail like). They are scattered throughout the posterior poles of both eyes, frequently extending to the equator. As the disease progresses, new flecks form peripherally as older flecks resorb. Fresh flecks are usually dense with distinct borders, while older lesions are ill defined and softer. Patients may remain asymptomatic for many years unless one of the flecks happens to involve the foveola. However, eventually the vast majority develop significant visual impairment due to an elliptical atrophic maculopathy indistinguishable from that seen in Stargardt's disease.

During a given stage of the disease four patterns of lesions are seen:

1. Macular lesions without flecks.
2. Macular lesion with perifoveal flecks.
3. Macular lesion with diffuse flecks.
4. Diffuse flecks without a macular lesion.

Fluorescein angiography

Initially, the flecks decrease or block background choroidal fluorescence during the early stages of the angiogram. During the more advanced stages of the disease, secondary atrophic changes in the RPE give rise to hyperfluorescence.

Special investigations

ERGs and EOGs are usually abnormal only in advanced cases when the changes have progressed to involve diffusely the RPE, choroid, and neurosensory retina. Peripheral visual fields and night vision are normal.

Familial dominant drusen

This condition is synonymous with 'Doyne's honeycomb choroiditis' and 'Tay's choroiditis'. It is quite common and is by far the most frequent of the so-called 'flecked retina' syndromes.

Inheritance is autosomal dominant with variable penetrance.

Clinical features—see Figure 11.23.

ERG and dark adaptation are normal.

Fundus albipunctatus

Inheritance

This is autosomal dominant or recessive.

Clinical features

This is an extremely rare condition characterized by congenital stationary night blindness. The ophthalmoscopic appearance consists of a multitude of yellow-white spots, the diameter of which approximates the size of a second-order arteriole (*Figure 12.15*). The lesions extend from the posterior pole where they are most dense, to the periphery where they are fewer in number. The macula itself is invariably spared and visual acuity unaffected. Unlike the spots seen in fundus flavimaculatus and familial drusen, the lesions are not pigmented. The retinal vessels, optic discs, and peripheral fields remain normal.

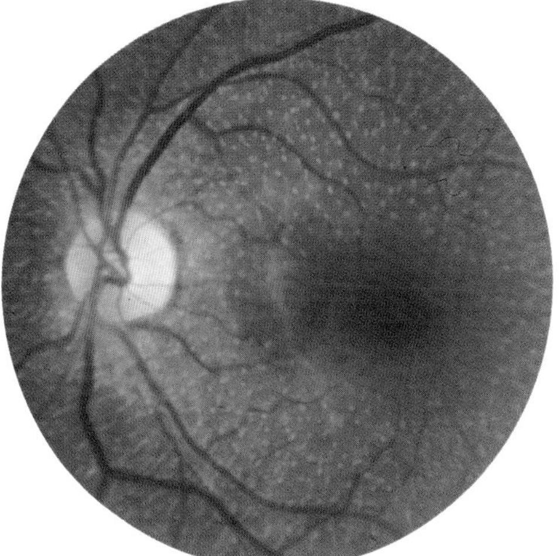

Figure 12.15 *Fundus albipunctatus*

Albinism

Hereditary albinism can be of two types: oculocutaneous and ocular.

Oculocutaneous

Inheritance

This is usually autosomal recessive.

Complete

These albinos are deficient in the enzyme tyrosinase and are incapable of synthesizing melanin. They have blonde hair (*Figure 12.16*), pale skin, and present with photophobia, pendular nystagmus, and a visual acuity of 6/60 or less. The ocular features include a diaphanous blue iris, which transilluminates completely, and a fundus lacking in pigment without any foveal landmarks (*Figure 12.17*).

Incomplete

These albinos can synthesize variable amounts of melanin and are referred to as tyrosinase-positive albinos. These individuals vary in complexion from very fair to normal. The iris colour may be blue or dark brown with variable degrees of iris transillumination (*Figure 12.18*). The degree of fundus pigmentation is also variable. However, irrespective of the fundus changes, visual acuity is usually impaired due to lack of differentiation of the fovea.

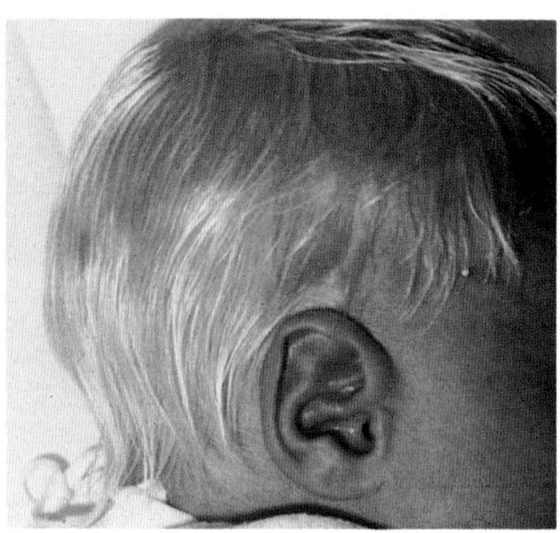

Figure 12.16 *Albinism (courtesy of Dr R. Winter)*

Ocular

Inheritance

This is X-linked and occasionally autosomal recessive. Clinically only the eyes are affected. The asymptomatic female carriers may show iris transillumination and scattered areas of depigmentation and granularity in the fundus periphery similar to the female carriers of choroideremia.

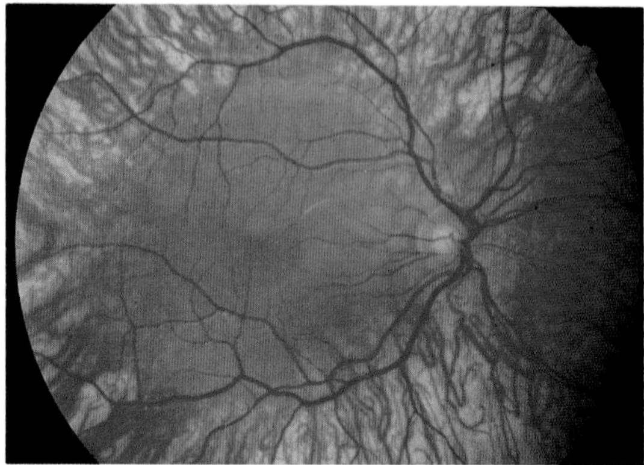

Figure 12.17 *Fundus in albinism (courtesy of Mr A. Fielder)*

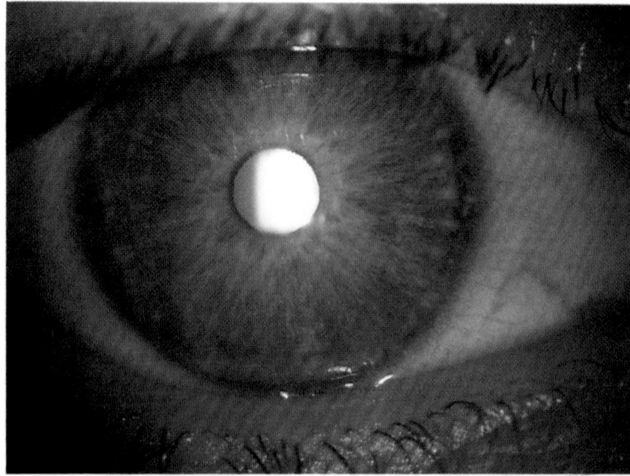

Figure 12.18 *Transillumination of iris in ocular albinism*

Vitreoretinal degenerations

The term 'Wagner's vitreoretinal degeneration' has been associated with specific vitreous and retinal changes. It can occur as an isolated ocular finding, with or without retinal detachment. It is also found in association with several connective tissue disorders complicated by bone dysplasia.

Wagner's disease

Inheritance

This is autosomal dominant.

Clinical features

Vitreous (*Figure 12.19*)

The vitreous cavity is optically empty as a result of vitreous degeneration with syneresis and liquefaction. Near the equator, circumferential translucent membranes extend a short way from the retina into the vitreous cavity.

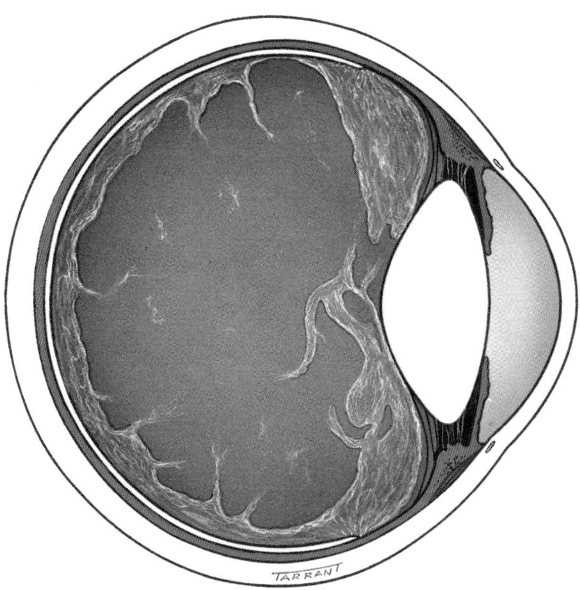

Figure 12.19 *Empty vitreous in Wagner's disease*

Retina (*Figure 12.20*)

The fundus changes include lattice-like radial perivascular pigmentation, frequently overlying foci of chorioretinal atrophy. The retinal vessels may be sheathed, sclerosed, and may vary in calibre. The pure form of Wagner's disease is not associated with retinal detachment. However, in the variant described by Jansen, retinal detachment is frequent and has a poor prognosis. In these cases the peripheral retina shows lattice degeneration, retinoschisis, and extensive areas of 'white-with-pressure'.

The fundus should be checked at regular intervals and any retinal breaks treated prophylactically.

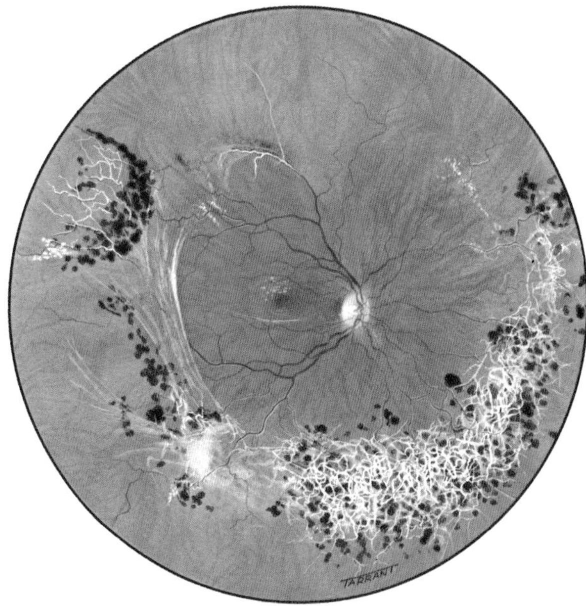

Figure 12.20 *Peripheral retinal degeneration in Wagner's disease*

Ocular features

1. *Myopia.*
2. *Cataract* usually begins at around puberty with the development of punctate posterior cortical opacities.
3. *Strabismus.*

Special investigations

ERG is subnormal or normal. *EOG* is normal.

Stickler syndrome

Inheritance

This is autosomal dominant.

Clinical features

Hereditary progressive arthro-ophthalmopathy with marfanoid habitus (Stickler syndrome) is the most common autosomal dominant connective tissue dysplasia in the United States, even exceeding Marfan's syndrome. It seems likely that in the past many cases reported as Wagner's disease, the Pierre Robin syndrome, and Marfan's syndrome were in fact examples of the Stickler syndrome.

Ocular

1. *Vitreoretinal degeneration.* The findings are virtually identical to those seen in Jansen's disease (i.e. Wagner's disease plus retinal detachment).
2. *Myopia* is moderate to severe.
3. *Cataract* is common.
4. *Open-angle glaucoma.*

Orofacial

1. *Midfacial flattening.*
2. *Pierre Robin complex* (cleft palate, micrognathia, glossoptosis).

Skeletal

The general skeletal abnormalities include joint hyperextensibility, enlargement, and juvenile arthritis.

Differential diagnosis

Because the Stickler syndrome is a relatively common disorder, it should be considered as a possible diagnosis in the following:

1. All cases of congenital myopia.
2. Vitreoretinal changes suggestive of Wagner's disease.
3. Early onset retinal detachment (especially if associated with large or multiple breaks and a positive family history).
4. The Pierre Robin malformation complex.
5. Unexplained juvenile arthropathy.

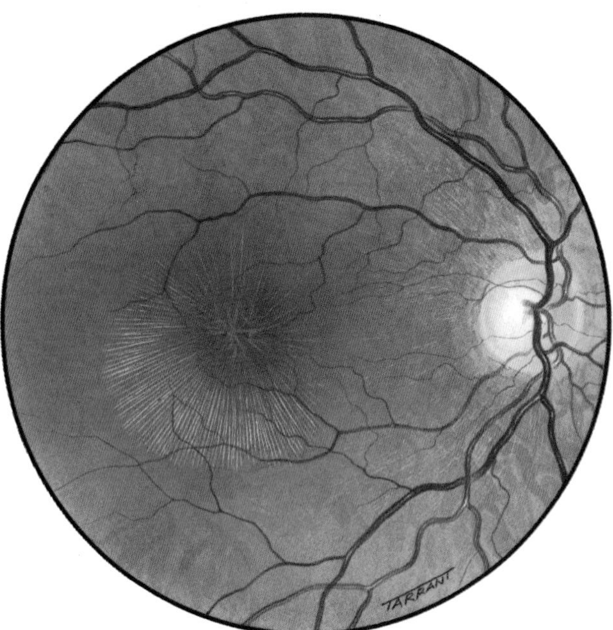

Figure 12.21 *Maculopathy in congenital retinoschisis*

Congenital retinoschisis

Inheritance

This is X-linked with a high penetrance and variable expressivity.

Clinical features

Congenital hereditary retinoschisis, or juvenile X-linked retinoschisis is a rare, bilateral vitreoretinal degeneration that develops early in life. The severity of involvement varies widely. The two main features of the condition are maculopathy and peripheral retinoschisis.

Maculopathy

The characteristic lesion present in almost all cases consists of tiny cystoid spaces with a 'bicycle-wheel' pattern of radial striae (*Figure 12.21*). It probably represents folds within the internal limiting membrane of the retina resulting from cystoid schitic changes within the foveola. The lesion does not fluoresce on angiography, unlike true cystoid macular oedema. With time, visual acuity becomes progressively impaired and the radial folds become less evident so that eventually only a non-specific atrophic lesion remains.

Retinoschisis (vitreous veils)

About 50–70% of patients with the macular lesion exhibit varying degrees of peripheral retinoschisis with splitting of the retinal nerve fibre layer. The extent of involvement does not necessarily increase with the passage of time and occasionally the lesions may even disappear. The inner wall of the schisis is extremely thin as it consists only of the internal limiting membrane and the retinal nerve fibre layer. In older patients, a breakdown of the inner layer breaks may lead to the formation of varying degrees of round or oval defects (*Figure 12.22*). In extreme cases, these defects may coalesce, leaving only retinal blood vessels floating in the vitreous—hence the term 'vitreous veils' which was formerly used to describe this condition (*Figure 12.23*). Secondary changes include vitreous haemorrhage (25% of cases), pigmented demarcation lines, and retinal detachments (5% of cases) which are difficult to treat.

Special investigations

ERG shows a selective decrease in scotopic b-wave amplitude, but the EOG is normal.

Favre–Goldmann syndrome

Inheritance

This is autosomal recessive.

Clinical features

This very rare disease is a cause of night blindness. It has features of both Wagner's disease and congenital retinoschisis.

Vitreous

This is optically empty as in Wagner's disease.

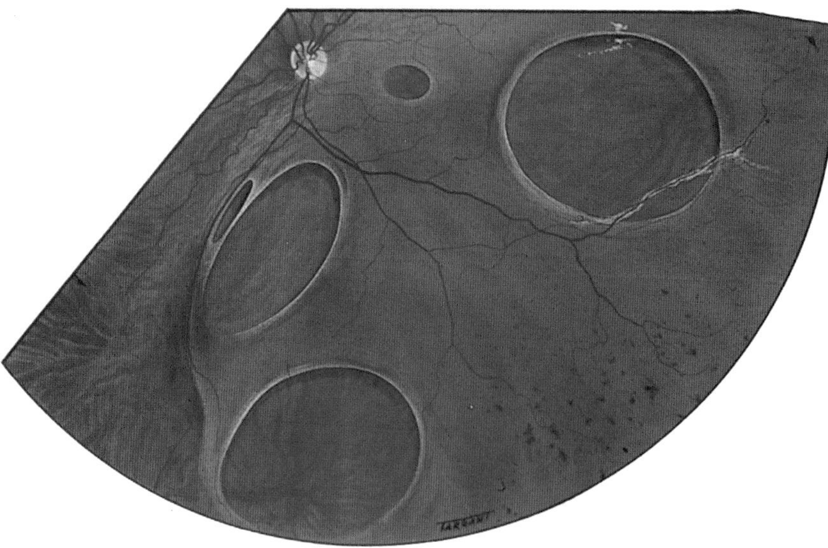

Figure 12.22 *Congenital retinoschisis with large holes in inner layer*

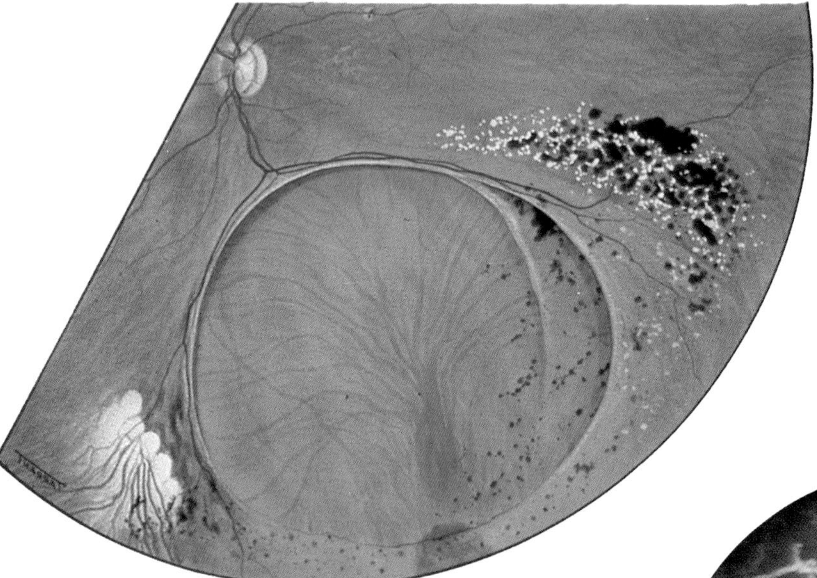

Figure 12.23 *Congenital retinoschisis with 'vitreous veils'*

Retina

This is similar to congenital retinoschisis although the macular findings are usually more subtle. Pigmentary changes, similar to those seen in RP, as well as white dendritiform arborescent peripheral retinal vessels (*Figure 12.24*) are also frequent.

Special investigations

ERG shows both a- and b-wave anomalies, often with non-detectable amplitudes. The EOG is normal.

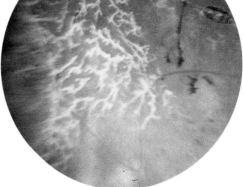

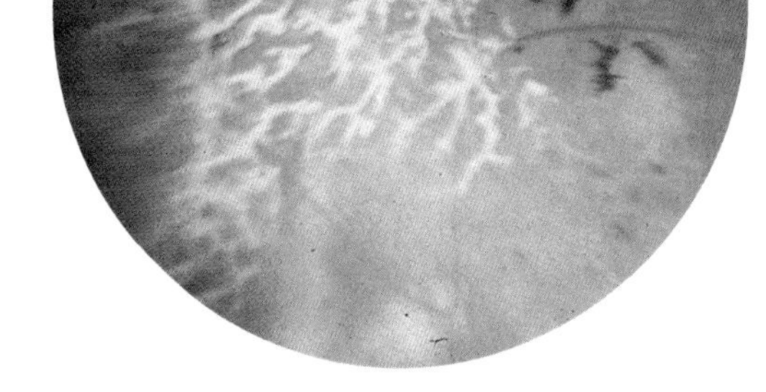

Figure 12.24 *Dendritiform peripheral retinal vessels in Favre–Goldmann syndrome (courtesy of Professor A. C. Bird)*

Exudative vitreoretinopathy (Criswick–Schepens syndrome)

Inheritance

This is autosomal dominant with incomplete penetrance.

Clinical features

This rare and poorly understood entity may sometimes be confused with retinopathy of prematurity. In some patients it is asymptomatic.

Retina

Early changes include an abrupt cessation of the capillary network at the equator. This is followed by neovascular fibroproliferative changes (*Figure 12.25*) which may cause tractional or rhegmatogenous retinal detachment with temporal dragging of the macula, which may be indistinguishable from retinopathy of prematurity (*Figure 12.26*).

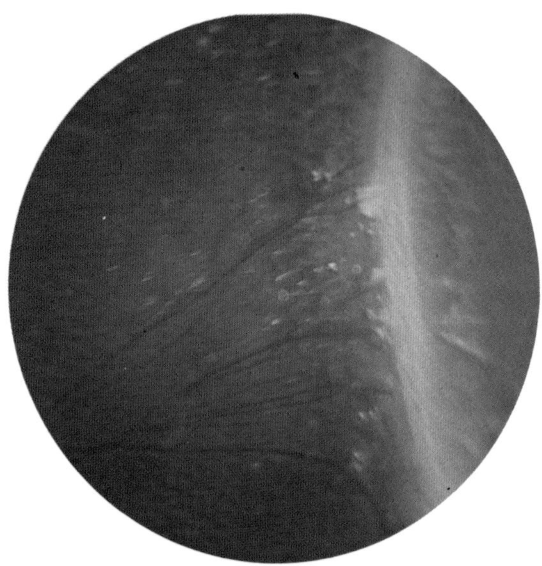

Figure 12.25 *Familial exudative vitreoretinopathy (courtesy of Professor A. C. Bird)*

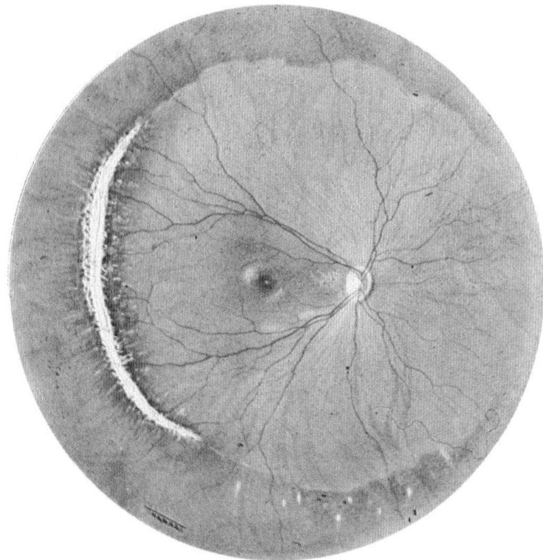

Figure 12.26 *Familial exudative vitreoretinopathy (courtesy of Professor A. C. Bird)*

Vitreous

These findings include membranes of variable density and consistency, prominent vitreoretinal attachments which give rise to areas of 'white with pressure' and 'white without pressure', condensations in the region of the vitreous base, and fine fibrillary strands.

The lesions described above are usually non-progressive after the age of 10 years.

Blood relatives

They may show subtle changes and falciform retinal folds.

Snowflake degeneration

Inheritance

This is autosomal dominant.

Clinical features

This rare disorder is divided into four stages (*Figure 12.27*):

1. Extensive 'white-with-pressure' changes in the peripheral fundus.
2. Minute, snowflake-like, yellow-white spots, located in the area of 'white-with-pressure'.
3. Sheathing of retinal blood vessels and increased pigmentation posterior to the area of snowflake degeneration.
4. Advanced changes which appear after the age of 50 years consisting of vascular attenuation and the appearance of patches of chorioretinal atrophy.

The vitreous shows fibrillary degeneration, strands, and liquefaction. Retinal breaks and retinal detachment are frequent complications. Other ocular features include myopia and presenile cataract.

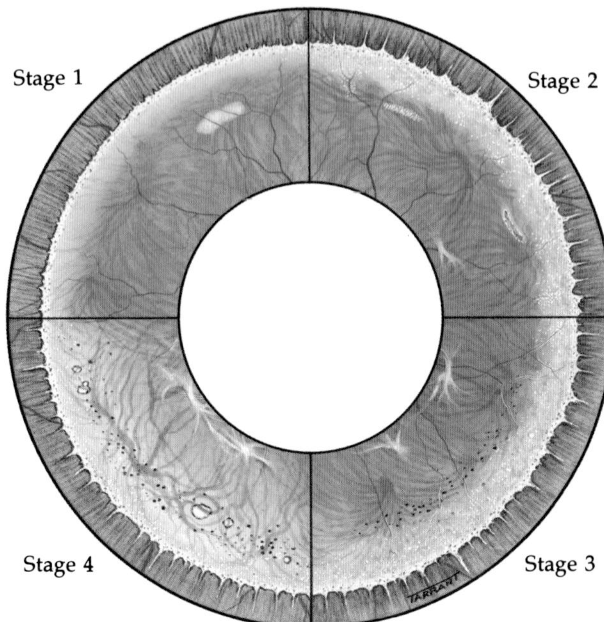

Figure 12.27 *Hereditary snowflake vitreoretinal degeneration*

Choroidal dystrophies

Choroideremia

Inheritance

This is X-linked recessive. Choroideremia is caused by a gene located on the X chromosome. It characteristically affects only males, with the female carriers often showing mild clinical fundus changes.

Clinical features

Female carriers

The majority of carrier women show patchy atrophy and mottling of the RPE with brown granular pigment dispersion in the fundus periphery similar to the female carriers of ocular albinism (*Figure 12.28*). These changes may be very subtle and only recognized by performing fluorescein angiography. Being an X-linked disorder, males with choroideremia cannot pass the gene to their sons but all daughters will be carriers. However, 50% of male offspring of the female carriers will develop the disease, and 50% of the female offspring will be carriers.

There is considerable variation in the severity and rate of progression of the disease, which is somewhat unusual for an X-linked disorder.

Onset

The disease usually presents within the first 5–10 years of life with defective night vision. This is associated with a diffuse mottled depigmentation of the RPE. Early in the disease the ERG may be normal, but by the end of the first decade the scotopic ERG usually becomes non-recordable and the photopic ERG severely reduced.

Progression

With the passage of time, large patches of atrophy of the RPE and choroid develop in the midretinal zones. These then spread centrally and towards the periphery giving rise to peripheral scotomas and a progressive constriction of the peripheral visual fields. Central vision is last to be affected as the RPE under the foveola may remain intact.

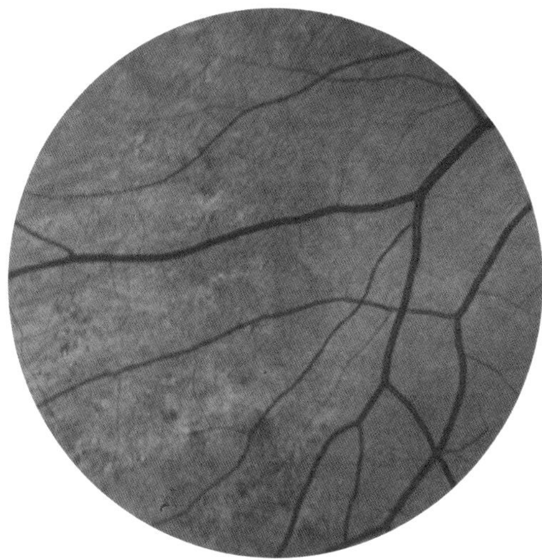

Figure 12.28 *Female carrier of choroideremia (courtesy of Mr R. Marsh)*

End stage

The patient usually becomes legally blind by the second to fourth decade of life. In common with other choroidal dystrophies, and in contrast to primary retinal dystrophies, the retinal blood vessels are relatively normal, even fairly late in the disease (*Figure 12.29*).

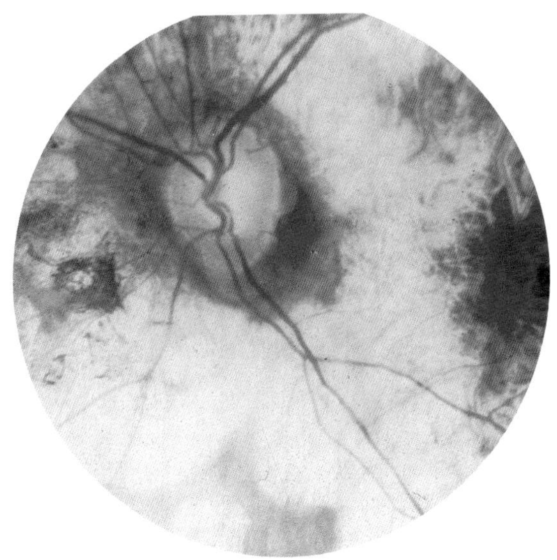

Figure 12.29 *Advanced choroideremia (courtesy of Mr R. Marsh)*

Gyrate atrophy

Inheritance

This is autosomal recessive.

Clinical features

This is a very rare disease due to an inborn error of ornithine ketoacid aminotransferase activity. It is associated with increased levels of ornithine in the plasma, urine, CSF and aqueous humour.

Onset

The disease usually begins during the first decade of life with symptoms of night blindness. Ophthalmoscopy reveals scalloped to circular patches of chorioretinal atrophy in the far and midretinal periphery. A moderate amount of myopia and vitreous degeneration are frequent.

Progression

The circular atrophic areas enlarge and finally coalesce to form a scalloped border (*Figure 12.30*). Constriction of the

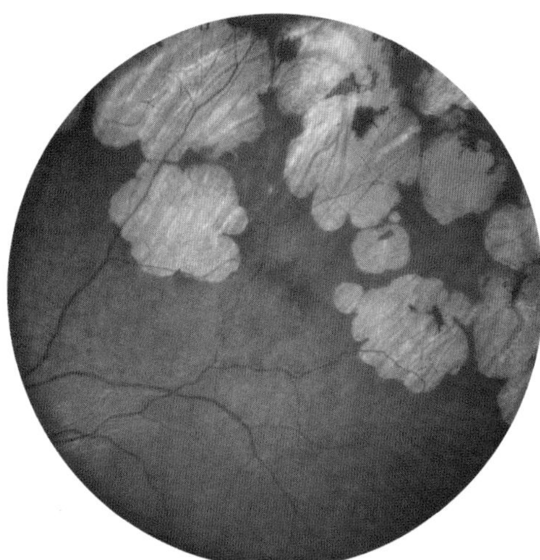

Figure 12.30 Gyrate atrophy

peripheral visual field corresponds to the expansion of the fundus changes.

End stage

The patient usually becomes legally blind by the fifth decade, although vision may fail earlier due to posterior cataract formation. Macular involvement may be in the form of oedema, or may be due to progression of atrophic changes centrally. In the late stages the retinal vessels undergo extensive attenuation. Secondary cataract develops in 50% of patients.

Special investigations

ERG is either markedly depressed or non-recordable. The *EOG* is flat.

Treatment

Massive supplemental doses of pyridoxine (vitamin B_6) normalize plasma and urine ornithine levels and may also have a beneficial effect on the ocular changes if instituted early. A diet low in proteins and arginine may also be beneficial.

Central areolar choroidal dystrophy

Inheritance

This is autosomal recessive or dominant.

Clinical features

This disease usually presents with visual impairment between the ages of 40 and 50 years. On fundoscopy, bilateral circumscribed, atrophic macular lesions are seen between 1 and 3 disc diameters in size. These changes consist of prominent choroidal vessels which are not only more visible but also show greater than normal variation in size and colour (*Figure 12.31*). They may appear yellow or white and opaque. There is atrophy of the central part of the choriocapillaris, the RPE, and the photoreceptors. The condition is invariably progressive and eventually leads to legal blindness.

Special investigations

ERG and *EOG* tests are normal (as would be expected from the apparent localized nature of the disease).

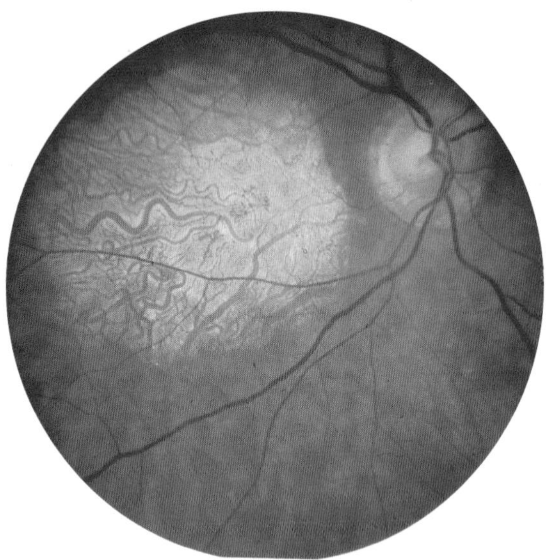

Figure 12.31 Central areolar choroidal dystrophy

Generalized choroidal atrophy

Inheritance

This is usually autosomal dominant, and occasionally recessive.

Clinical features

Patients with this rare disease present with symptoms of either impaired visual acuity or night vision during the fourth or fifth decades of life. Ophthalmoscopy shows diffuse atrophy of the RPE and choriocapillaris, rendering the larger choroidal vessels more visible. A scattered irregular pigmentation of the retina is commonly seen. The retinal vessels may be normal or slightly constricted and may appear as having increased opacification of their walls, giving a yellow-orange colour. A bilateral and progressive loss of vision is the end result.

Further reading

Retinitis pigmentosa

Bird, A.C. (1981) Retinal receptor dystrophies. *Transactions of the Ophthalmological Society of the United Kingdom,* **101,** 39–42

Cogan, D.G., Rodrigues, M., Chu, F.C. *et al.* (1984) Ocular abnormalities in abetalipoproteinaemia. *Ophthalmology*, **91**, 991–998

Fishman, G.A. (1978) Retinitis pigmentosa. Genetic percentages. *Archives of Ophthalmology*, **96**, 922–926

Fishman, G.A. (1979) Usher's syndrome: visual loss and variations in clinical expressivity. *Perspectives in Ophthalmology*, **3**, 97–104

Fishman, G.A., Kumar, A., Joseph, M.E. *et al.* (1983) Usher's syndrome. *Archives of Ophthalmology*, **101**, 1367–1374

Gartner, S. and Henkind, P. (1982) Pathology of retinitis pigmentosa. *Ophthalmology*, **89**, 1425–1432

Heckenliveley, J.R. (1982) Frequency of posterior subcapsular cataract in hereditary retinal degenerations. *American Journal of Ophthalmology*, **93**, 733–738

Jay, M. (1982) On the heredity of retinitis pigmentosa. *British Journal of Ophthalmology*, **66**, 405–416

Levin, P.S., Green, W.R., Victor, D.I. *et al.* (1983) Histopathology of the eye in Cockayne's syndrome. *Archives of Ophthalmology*, **101**, 1093–1097

McKechnie, N.M., King, M. and Lee, W.R. (1985) Retinal pathology in the Kearns–Sayre syndrome. *British Journal of Ophthalmology*, **69**, 63–75

Runge, P., Muller, D.P.R., McAllister, J. *et al.* (1986) Oral vitamin E can prevent the retinopathy of abetalipoproteinaemia. *British Journal of Ophthalmology*, **70**, 166–173

Leber's congenital amaurosis

Nickel, B. and Hoyt, C.S. (1982) Leber's congenital amaurosis. *Archives of Ophthalmology*, **100**, 1089–1092

Noble, K.G. and Carr, R.E. (1978) Leber's congenital amaurosis. *Archives of Ophthalmology*, **96**, 818–821

Vitelliform dystrophies

Kraushar, M.F., Margolis, S., Morse, P.H. *et al.* (1982) Pseudohypopyon in Best's vitelliform macular dystrophy. *American Journal of Ophthalmology*, **94**, 30–37

Mohler, C.W. and Fine, S.L. (1981) Long-term evaluation of patients with Best's vitelliform dystrophy. *Ophthalmology*, **88**, 688–692

Patrinely, J.R., Lewis, R.A. and Font, R.L. (1985) Foveomacular vitelliform dystrophy, adult type. *Ophthalmology*, **92**, 1712–1718

Weingeist, T.A., Kobrin, J.L. and Watzke, R.C. (1982) Histopathology of Best's macular dystrophy. *Archives of Ophthalmology*, **100**, 108–114

'Bull's eye' macula syndromes

Grey, R.H.B., Blach, R.K. and Barnard, W.H. (1977) Bull's eye maculopathy with early cone degeneration. *British Journal of Ophthalmology*, **61**, 702–718

Jaben, S.L., Flynn, J.T. and Parker, J.C. (1983) Neuronal ceroid lipofuscinosis. *Ophthalmology*, **90**, 1373–1377

Spalton, D.J., Taylor, D.S.I. and Sanders, M.D. (1980) Juvenile Batten's disease: an ophthalmological assessment of 26 patients. *British Journal of Ophthalmology*, **64**, 726–732

van den Biesen, P.R., Deutman, A.F. and Pickers, A.J.L.G. (1985) Evolution of benign concentric annular macular dystrophy. *American Journal of Ophthalmology*, **100**, 73–78

Pattern dystrophies

De Jong, P.T.V.M. and Delleman, J.W. (1982) Pigment epithelial pattern dystrophy. *Archives of Ophthalmology*, **100**, 1416–1421

Watzke, R.C., Folk, J.C. and Lang, R.M. (1982) Pattern dystrophy of the retinal pigment epithelium. *Ophthalmology*, **89**, 1400–1406

'Flecked retina' syndromes

Eagle, R.C., Lucier, A.C., Bernardino, V.B. *et al.* (1980) Retinal pigment epithelial abnormalities in fundus flavimaculatus. *Ophthalmology*, **87**, 1189–1200

Fielder, A.R., Garner, A. and Chambers, T.L. (1980) Ophthalmic manifestations of primary oxalosis. *British Journal of Ophthalmology*, **64**, 782–788

Isashiki, Y. and Ohba, N. (1985) Fundus flavimaculatus: polymorphic retinal changes in siblings. *British Journal of Ophthalmology*, **69**, 522–524

Noble, K.G. and Carr, R.E. (1979) Stargardt's disease and fundus flavimaculatus. *Archives of Ophthalmology*, **97**, 1281–1285

Albinism

Jay, B.S. and Carroll, W. (1980) Albinism. *Transactions of the Ophthalmological Society of the United Kingdom*, **100**, 467–471

Kinnear, P.E., Jay, B. and Witkop, C.J. (1985) Albinism. *Survey of Ophthalmology*, **30**, 75–101

Hereditary vitreoretinal degenerations

Billington, B.M., Leaver, P.K. and McLeod, D. (1985) Management of retinal detachment in the Wagner–Stickler syndrome. *Transactions of the Ophthalmological Society of the United Kingdom*, **104**, 875–879

Condon, G.P., Brownstein, S., Wang, N-S. *et al.* (1986) Congenital hereditary (juvenile X-linked) retinoschisis. *Archives of Ophthalmology*, **104**, 576–583

Feldman, E.L., Norris, J.L. and Cleasby, G.W. (1983) Autosomal dominant exudative vitreoretinopathy. *Archives of Ophthalmology*, **101**, 1532–1535

Fishman, G.A., Jampol, L.M. and Goldberg, M.F. (1976) Diagnostic features of the Favre–Goldmann syndrome. *British Journal of Ophthalmology*, **60**, 345–353

Maumenee, I.H. (1979) Vitreoretinal degeneration as a sign of generalized connective tissue disease. *American Journal of Ophthalmology*, **88**, 432–449

Ober, R.R., Bird, A.C. and Hamilton, A.M. (1980) Autosomal dominant exudative vitreoretinopathy. *British Journal of Ophthalmology*, **64**, 112–120

Pollack, A., Uchenik, D., Chemke, J. *et al.* (1983) Prophylactic photocoagulation in hereditary snowflake degeneration. *Archives of Ophthalmology*, **101**, 1536–1539

Robertson, D.M., Link, T.P. and Rostvold, J.A. (1982) Snowflake degeneration of the retina. *Ophthalmology*, **89**, 1513–1517

Hereditary choroidal dystrophies

Kaiser-Kupfer, M.I., Valle, D. and Valle, L.A. (1978) A specific enzyme defect in gyrate atrophy. *American Journal of Ophthalmology*, **85**, 200–204

Kaiser-Kupfer, M.I., Valle, D. and Bron, A.J. (1980) Clinical and biochemical heterogeneity in gyrate atrophy. *American Journal of Ophthalmology*, **89**, 219–222

Rodrigues, M.M., Ballantine, E.J. and Wiggert, B.N. *et al.* (1984) Choroideremia. *Ophthalmology*, **91**, 873–883

Takki, K.K. and Milton, R.C. (1981) The natural history of gyrate atrophy of the choroid and retina. *Ophthalmology*, **88**, 292–301

Vannas-Sulonen, K., Sipila, I., Vannas, A. *et al.* (1985) Gyrate atrophy of the retina and choroid. *Ophthalmology*, **92**, 1719–1727

Weleber, R.G. (1979) Hereditary dystrophies of the choroid and retina. *Perspectives in Ophthalmology*, **3**, 37–44

13

Tumours of the Uvea and Retina

Choroidal melanoma

Ciliary body melanoma

Iris melanoma

Choroidal naevus

Choroidal haemangioma

Metastatic carcinoma

Osseous choristoma (choroidal osteoma)

Retinoblastoma

Differential diagnosis of childhood leukocoria

Retinal astrocytoma

Retinal capillary haemangioma

Retinal cavernous haemangioma

Retinal racemose haemangioma

Retinal pigment epithelial hamartoma

Ocular reticulum cell sarcoma (histiocytic lymphoma)

Choroidal melanoma

Introduction

Malignant melanoma of the choroid is the most common primary intraocular tumour in adults. Patients with ocular or oculodermal melanosis are at increased risk of choroidal melanoma (*see* Chapter 4). The average age of patients with choroidal melanoma is 50 years. The incidence then continues to rise until the age of 70 years before dropping off. The tumour is rarely seen in patients over the age of 80 years and less than 4% of patients are under the age of 30 years. Choroidal melanomas are extremely rare in blacks.

Clinical features

The tumour is invariably unilateral but its clinical features are extremely variable. A typical melanoma appears as a pigmented, elevated, oval-shaped mass (*Figure 13.1*). The colour of the tumour is frequently brown, although it may be mottled with dark-brown or black pigment, or it may be virtually amelanotic. As the tumour grows it may break through Bruch's membrane and appear as a mushroom-shaped mass, giving rise to an exudative detachment of the overlying sensory retina. An accumulation of orange pigment (lipofuscin) in the retinal pigment epithelium (RPE) is commonly seen, but is not diagnostic (*Figure 13.2*). Other associated features of a choroidal melanoma which may be seen occasionally include choroidal folds, subretinal or intraretinal haemorrhage, hard yellow exudation, vitreous haemorrhage, secondary glaucoma, cataract, and inflammatory signs such as iridocyclitis and posterior uveitis.

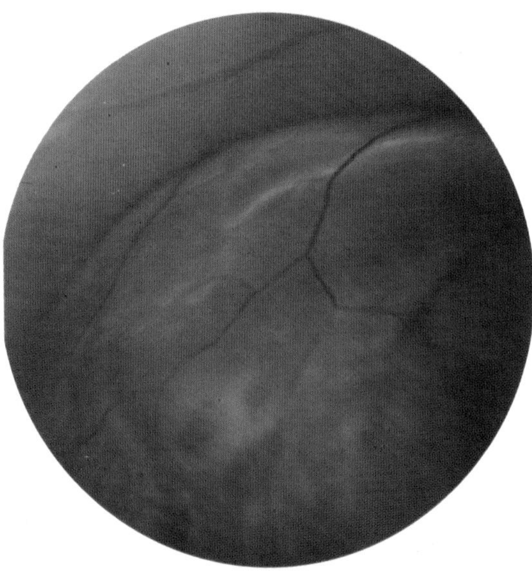

Figure 13.1 *Malignant melanoma of choroid*

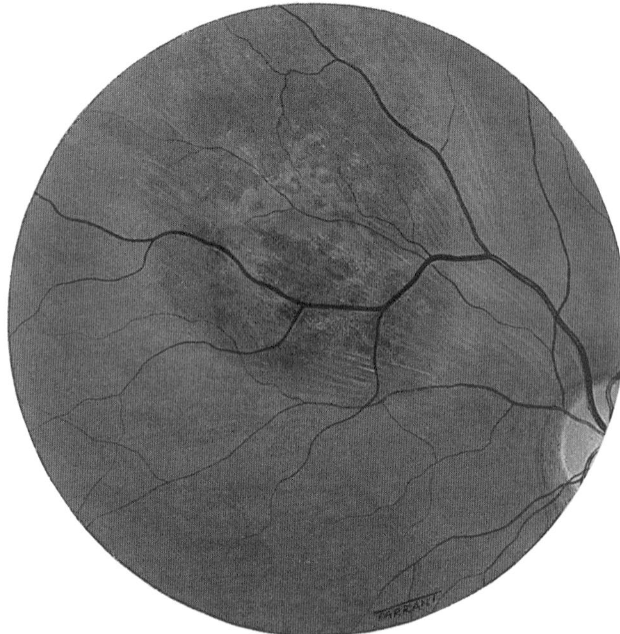

Figure 13.2 *Malignant melanoma of choroid with orange pigment*

In some patients the tumour is asymptomatic and is detected at a routine fundus examination. In others it causes decreased visual acuity or a defect in the visual field, depending on its size, location, and the presence or absence of secondary exudative retinal detachment. Distant metastases from the intraocular tumour or from its extrascleral extension are the common causes of death.

The main conditions which should be considered in the differential diagnosis of choroidal melanoma are: retinal detachment, metastatic tumour to the choroid, exudative age-related macular degeneration, choroidal detachment, localized choroidal haemangioma and a large choroidal naevus.

Diagnosis

Medical evaluation

The purpose of a general medical evaluation is two-fold:

1. To exclude the possibility of a metastatic tumour to the choroid. This occurs most frequently from the bronchus in males and the breast in females. Occasionally, the primary site is the kidney or gastrointestinal tract.
2. To exclude the possibility of distant metastases from the ocular tumour. Liver function tests (alkaline phosphatase, lactic dehydrogenase, and glutamyl transpeptidase) and chest X-rays should be performed as 97% of choroidal metastases involve the liver or lungs.

Abdominal computerized tomography may also be useful. Because a patient with metastatic disease usually dies within 1 year, enuclation is only justifiable if the eye is painful.

Examination of the opposite eye

Because primary melanomas are unilateral and simulating lesions are frequently bilateral (exudative age-related macular degeneration and metastases), a careful examination of the opposite eye may give valuable clues.

Indirect ophthalmoscopy

The vast majority of melanomas greater than 3 mm in elevation can be diagnosed by indirect ophthalmoscopy without resorting to special tests. The stereopsis helps the examiner to detect elevation of the lesion and gives an overall three-dimensional view. It enables the clinician to detect the presence of shifting fluid (*see* Chapter 9) and also provides better visualization through hazy media.

Contact lens examination

Subtle features associated with relatively small tumours, such as the presence of lipofuscin pigment, subretinal fluid, cystoid changes in the overlying sensory retina, and dilated vessels within the tumour, are best detected by slitlamp biomicroscopy and a fundus contact lens.

Transillumination

This is a simple technique which is useful in differentiating between pigmented tumours and dense haemorrhage (which do not transilluminate) and lesions that permit the transmission of light, such as exudative retinal detachments, choroidal detachments (*Figure 13.3, upper right*), and non-pigmented tumours (*Figure 13.3, lower right*). The transilluminator is placed on the conjunctiva and the effects are compared through normal sclera and over the site of the lesion (*Figure 13.3, left*). The degree of transillumination can be studied indirectly by observing any change in the red reflex or, alternatively, the tumour can be observed directly with an indirect ophthalmoscope with its light turned off.

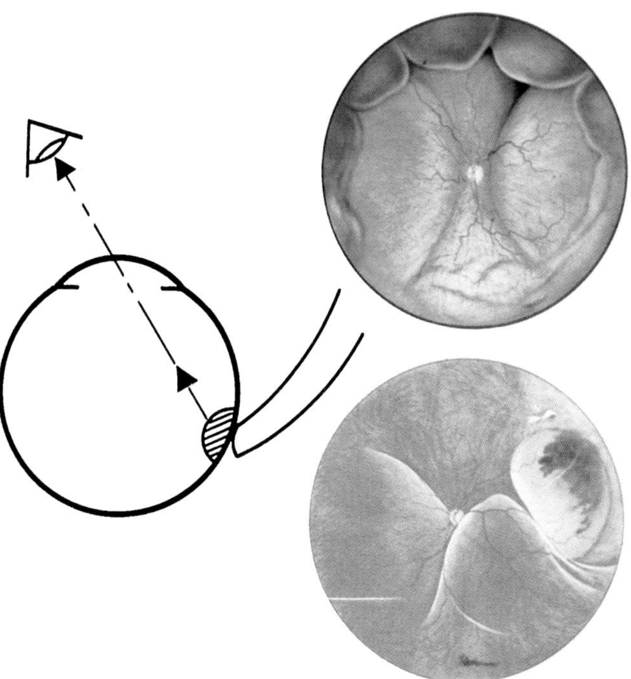

Figure 13.3 *Left: technique of transillumination; upper right: choroidal detachment; lower right: amelanotic choroidal melanoma with large secondary exudative retinal detachment*

Fundus photography

This is the most accurate method of detecting an increase in the horizontal diameter of a small tumour.

Fluorescein angiography

This may occasionally be helpful in the evaluation of small to medium-sized choroidal lesions. In general, most melanomas show a mottled fluorescence during the arteriovenous phase of the angiogram with a progressive staining of the lesion and prolonged retention of dye.

The pattern of fluorescence varies according to the status of the overlying RPE. Destruction of the RPE will give rise to hyperfluorescence from increased background choroidal fluorescence (window defect). The presence of lipofuscin pigment, on the other hand, will partially block transmission of choroidal fluorescence. The demonstration of large blood vessels within a small tumour ('double circulation') indicates that it is probably malignant, although care should be taken not to mistake these vessels for the lacy-filling pattern of a choroidal neovascular membrane which may be associated with a benign naevus.

Fluorescein angiography is particularly useful in differentiating melanomas from serous and haemorrhagic detachments of the RPE.

Ultrasonography

This is particularly helpful in detecting the presence of a tumour in an eye with hazy media, although it may also provide useful information in cases where the tumour can be visualized ophthalmoscopically. The solid nature of the tumour is best detected with the A-scan as a high internal spike and low-to-medium internal reflectivity. The B-scan shows the anterior border of the tumour as well as acoustic hollowness, choroidal excavation, and orbital shadowing. Although ultrasonography is of limited diagnostic value in minimally elevated tumours, repeated examinations are useful in documenting an increase in thickness of a small tumour. Unfortunately, ultrasonography may not be able to differentiate between a necrotic melanoma and a haemorrhage or metastasis.

^{32}P uptake

This test is based on the fact that malignant cells incorporate and utilize phosphorus to a greater degree than normal cells. ^{32}P is an isotope that emits beta irradiation which can be quantified by a Geiger counter. Precise placement of the probe over the centre of the tumour using indirect ophthalmoscopy is essential if accurate readings

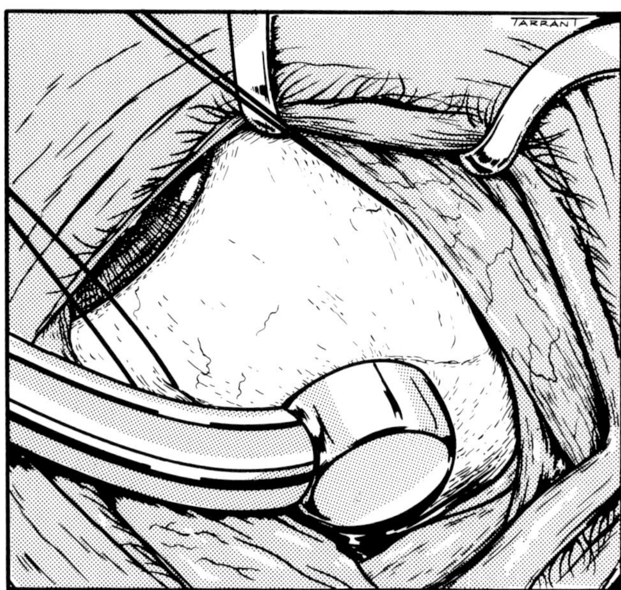

Figure 14.9 Radioactive phosphorus uptake test

are to be obtained. Posteriorly located tumours have to be approached through a transconjunctival incision (*Figure 13.4*). Complications of the test include retinal and vitreous haemorrhage and central retinal artery occlusion.

The test is useful in differentiating a large melanoma from a simulating benign lesion, such as a haemangioma. Unfortunately, it is unreliable in small lesions and will not differentiate between a primary melanoma and a metastasis, as both give a positive uptake.

Visual field examination

This is of limited value in diagnosis as both malignant melanomas and occasionally choroidal naevi produce field defects. However, repeated testing may be useful in documenting growth of a small malignant melanoma.

Other investigations

1. *Computerized tomography* (CT) scanning is most valuable in detecting and fully delineating the presence of extraocular extension of the tumour.
2. *Magnetic resonance imaging (MRI)* is also of value in detecting extraocular extension.
3. *Ultrasound-directed tissue biopsy* is an intricate technique which is occasionally used to obtain cellular aspirates for analysis.

Management

The correct management of malignant melanomas of the choroid is, at present, one of the most controversial questions in ophthalmology. The traditional treatment by enucleation has been questioned by some authorities, especially for small tumours.

Observation

Observation should be considered for the following:

1. Eyes with small or asymptomatic lesions in which the diagnosis is equivocal. Several studies have shown that small melanomas (less than 3 mm thick and 10 mm in diameter) have an excellent prognosis, as they seem to remain dormant for many years and have a very low metastatic potential.
2. Patients over the age of 65 years who have slowly growing tumours with normal vision. In these patients the prognosis does not seem to be improved by enucleation.
3. A slowly growing tumour in the only remaining eye of an elderly or chronically ill patient.
4. Patients with liver metastases.

Enucleation

It is generally agreed that enucleation (excision of the globe) is indicated for very large melanomas, particularly if all useful vision has been irreversibly lost. In these cases, enucleation is preferred over radiotherapy because the doses of irradiation required to reach the apex of the tumour would be too great to salvage the rest of the eye. In order to avoid haematogenous dissemination of malignant cells, the enucleation should be performed as follows: a careful 360° peritomy, gentle isolation and section of the extraocular muscles, fixation of the globe with a cryoprobe, and minimal traction on the optic nerve when cutting. Some authorities advocate external-beam radiotherapy prior to enucleation in order to lessen the risk of subsequent metastatic disease. About 4 weeks after enucleation, the patient can be fitted with an artificial eye. He should then be re-examined at 9-monthly intervals for evidence of recurrence of the tumour in the orbit.

The overall survival rates for all types of choroidal melanoma following enucleation is about 75% at 5 years, 65% at 10 years, and 60% at 15 years. Following enucleation there appears to be a bimodal incidence of death at 2–4 years and then at 9–10 years.

Radioactive plaques

Radioactive plaques containing gamma-emitting isotopes (cobalt-60, iodine-125) are suitable for small (less than 3 mm in thickness and less than 10 mm in diameter) and medium-sized tumours (3–5 mm in thickness and 10–15 mm in diameter). The plaques are fixed to the globe for a set period of time and deliver a fixed dosage of radiation to the tumour. The main disadvantage of radioactive plaques is radiation-induced complications such as retinopathy, papillopathy, vitreous haemorrhage, and cataract. The severity of these complications is less with iodine-125 plaques than with cobalt-60 plaques.

Heavy charged particle irradiation

Cyclotron-generated heavy ion (protons, helium) irradiation appears to be a very promising new approach which may even prove to be an alternative to enucleation in eyes with large tumours. The area of the melanoma is marked with transillumination and tantalum clips, and the radiation is given over several sessions. The advantages of this form of radiotherapy over radioactive plaques are: the beam can be more highly focused, a uniform dose of radiation is applied to the entire tumour, and the incidence of complications is lower. Unfortunately this form of treatment is still only available in a few centres.

Photocoagulation

Although this therapeutic modality is still controversial, xenon arc photocoagulation may be considered if the following criteria are fulfilled:

1. The lesion should not be greater than 6.5 disc diameters (10 mm) at its widest point and no more than 3 mm in elevation.
2. The tumour should not be associated with a significant amount of subretinal fluid, as this will prevent adequate treatment.
3. The tumour should be located more than 1 disc diameter (1.5 mm) away from the fovea so that the burn does not damage central vision.

Only about 5–10% of all choroidal melanomas meet these criteria. Of those treated by photocoagulation, about half eventually require enucleation either due to continued tumour growth or because of photocoagulation-induced complications.

Local resection (choroidectomy)

Full-thickness eyewall resection has been used in the treatment of carefully selected peripheral tumours with encouraging results. This approach is, however, still controversial and the operation is complicated and fraught with hazards.

Exenteration

It is generally agreed that exenteration is indicated for melanomas with obvious extraocular extension. Whether it should be used for cases with microscopical extension is still uncertain.

Palliative therapy

Chemotherapy and immunotherapy can be used as palliative measures in cases of metastatic melanoma from the eye to distant sites.

Histological classification

According to the Callender classification, uveal melanomas can be differentiated according to cellular features into six types (*Figure 13.5*).

Spindle A cell

These are slender spindle-shaped cells with flattened nuclei and a prominent basophilic nuclear line caused by an infolding of the nuclear membrane. The nucleus is devoid of a nucleolus. Tumours composed of this cell type have the best prognosis.

Spindle B cell

These cells are slightly larger than spindle A cells with a round or oval nucleus and a prominent nucleolus. The cytoplasmic borders of individual cells are poorly differentiated so that the cells tend to merge and form a syncytium. Tumours composed of this cell type have the second-best prognosis.

Fascicular

This refers to a specific pattern in which the cells are arranged in a 'palisading' or ribbon-like arrangement in parallel rows. It is now clear that fascicular tumours can be composed of either spindle A or spindle B cells and do not warrant a separate classification. For this reason a fascicular tumour has the same prognosis as a tumour composed of similar spindle cells arranged in a random fashion.

Epithelioid cell

These are large, oval or round, with well-demarcated cell membranes, eosinophilic cytoplasm, and round nuclei with prominent nucleoli. The cells may vary in size and shape (polymorphism), as well as in the amount of pigmentation. Mitotic figures are seen in abundance. Tumours composed of these cells carry the worst prognosis.

Mixed-cell

These are composed of a combination of spindle and epithelioid cells. As might be expected, such tumours have an intermediate prognosis.

Necrotic

These are tumours in which the actual cell type cannot be recognized. Massive tumour necrosis may be secondary to insufficient blood supply, or due to an autoimmune mechanism. The necrotic process may initiate an intense inflammatory reaction which may be clinically mistaken for an endophthalmitis or uveitis. The prognosis is similar to that of mixed-cell tumours.

Prognostic factors

1. *Cell type.* Spindle A cell tumours have the best prognosis and those composed of epithelioid cells the worst (*Table 13.1*).

Table 13.1 Prognosis following enucleation of choroidal melanomas

Tumour type	*Approximate number of choroidal melanomas (%)*	*5-year mortality (%)*
Spindle A	5	5
Spindle B	33	14
Fascicular	6	14
Mixed-cell	45	51
Necrotic	8	51
Epithelioid	3	69

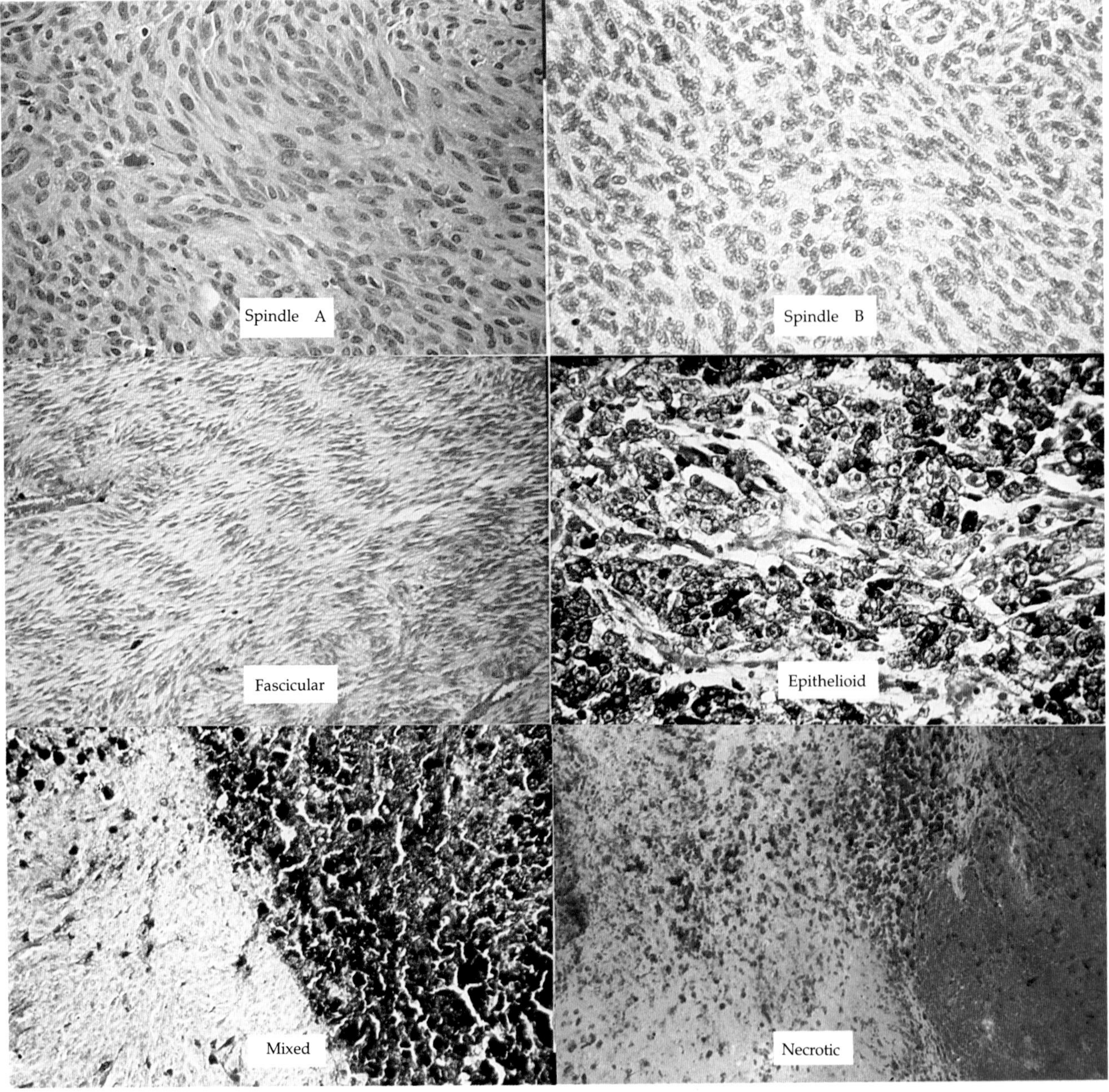

Figure 13.5 *Histological classification of uveal melanomas (courtesy of Professor A. Garner)*

2. *Size* is very important as large tumours have a worse prognosis than small tumours.
3. *Diffuse* tumours tend to have a worse prognosis because they usually contain epithelioid cells and are more likely to extend extrasclerally.
4. *Intactness of Bruch's membrane.* If Bruch's membrane has been ruptured the prognosis is less favourable.
5. *Age of patient.* Patients over the age of 65 years have a worse prognosis.
6. *Pigmentation.* The prognosis is worse for highly pigmented tumours and better for those that are amelanotic.
7. *Extrascleral* extension carries a poor prognosis. The presence and degree of extrascleral extension has important prognostic implications.

Ciliary body melanoma

Clinical features

Ciliary body melanomas (*Figure 13.6*) are more common than iris melanomas but less common than those arising from the choroid. They cannot usually be visualized unless the pupil is widely dilated. Clinically, they may present in a variety of ways, depending on their size and location:

1. Pressure exerted upon the lens may give rise to anterior displacement with secondary astigmatism, subluxation, or the formation of a localized opacity.
2. External signs include dilated episcleral blood vessels in the same quadrant as the tumour (sentinel vessels; *Figure 13.7*). Extension of the tumour through the scleral emissary vessels may produce a dark epibulbar mass, sometimes mistaken for a conjunctival melanoma.
3. Forward erosion through the iris root into the anterior chamber.
4. Posterior extension of the tumour may lead to retinal detachment.
5. Occasionally, tumour necrosis may cause anterior segment inflammatory signs.
6. The neoplasm may occasionally assume a diffuse circumferential growth pattern and extend for 360° around the ciliary body. This type of tumour has the worst prognosis as early diagnosis is very difficult.

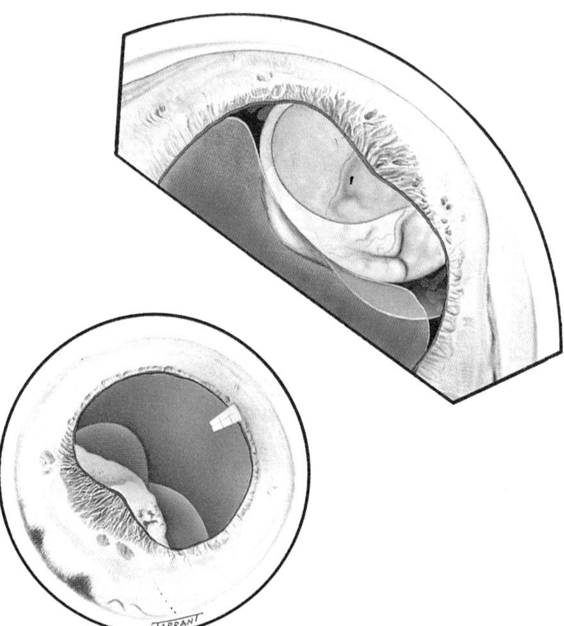

Figure 13.6 *Amelanotic melanoma of ciliary body*

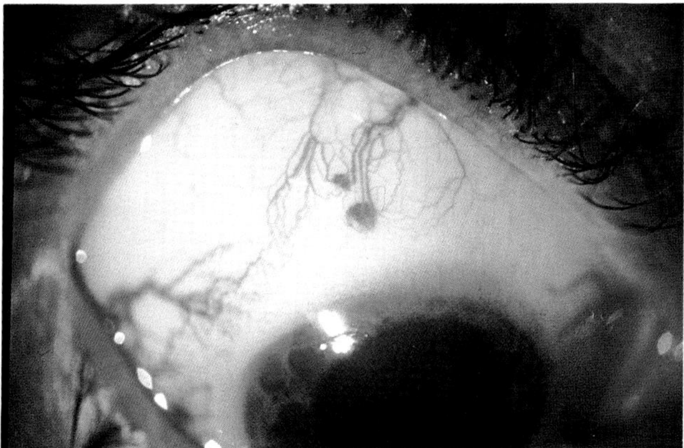

Figure 13.7 *Dilated episceral vessels in eye with melanoma of ciliary body (courtesy of Mr A. Shun-Shin)*

Diagnosis

Contact lens examination

Slitlamp examination with a triple-mirror contact lens through a well dilated pupil is essential in all eyes suspected of harbouring a ciliary body melanoma. It is particularly useful in detecting forward erosion through the iris root into the angle.

Transillumination

This is helpful in assessing the dimensions and location of a ciliary body tumour and deciding on the most appropriate form of therapy. Transillumination is also helpful in differentiating between a tumour and a cyst. However, some non-pigmented melanomas transilluminate brightly and, rarely, cystic lesions can be malignant.

Ultrasonography

This is particularly useful for detecting a tumour in the presence of opaque media. It also provides information concerning the dimensions and posterior extension of the tumour.

^{32}P uptake

This test may be useful in atypical cases in differentiating a benign from a malignant lesion.

Other investigations that are occasionally used include: computerized tomography, magnetic resonance imaging, and needle biopsy.

Management

Enucleation

This is the treatment of choice for large ciliary body melanomas and those affecting the anterior choroid. Secondary glaucoma, usually indicating extensive invasion of Schlemm's canal, is also an indication for enucleation. The value of radiotherapy prior to enucleation has yet to be established.

Local resection

Iridocyclectomy can be performed for small or medium-sized tumours that involve not more than one-third of the iridocorneal angle. The most serious complications of local resection are vitreous haemorrhage, retinal detachment, and residual tumour.

Radiotherapy

Some ciliary body melanomas can be treated by radioactive plaques or heavy charged particle irradiation.

Differential diagnosis

Congenital cysts

Rarely, congenital cysts of the ciliary body may displace the lens (*Figure 13.8*).

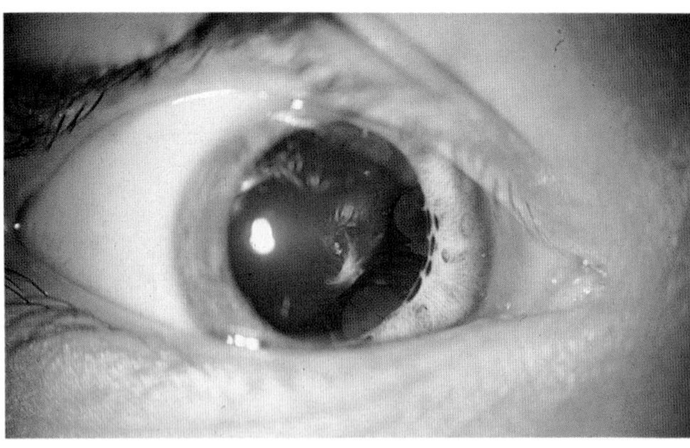

Figure 13.8 *Congenital cystic lesions of ciliary body displacing the lens*

Medulloepithelioma (diktyoma)

This very rare slow growing and locally invasive congenital tumour arises from the non-pigmented ciliary epithelium. Diktyomas typically present in the first decade of life with poor visual acuity associated with a ciliary body mass, raised intraocular pressure, and/or cataract. It is unusual for the correct diagnosis to be made prior to enucleation.

Iris melanoma

Clinical features

About 5–10% of all malignant uveal tumours arise from the iris. The average age at diagnosis is between 40 and 50 years. An iris melanoma usually presents as a solitary pigmented or non-pigmented nodule, most frequently located in the lower half of the iris (*Figure 13.9*). Rarely, it may exhibit a diffuse intrastromal growth pattern, giving rise to an ipsilateral hyperchromic heterochromia and secondary glaucoma due to invasion of the angle. Occasionally, small melanomas may be difficult to differentiate from benign naevi. Features that should arouse suspicion of malignancy include ectropion uveae, pupillary distortion, localized lens opacification, neovascularization, elevation of intraocular pressure, and photographic evidence of growth.

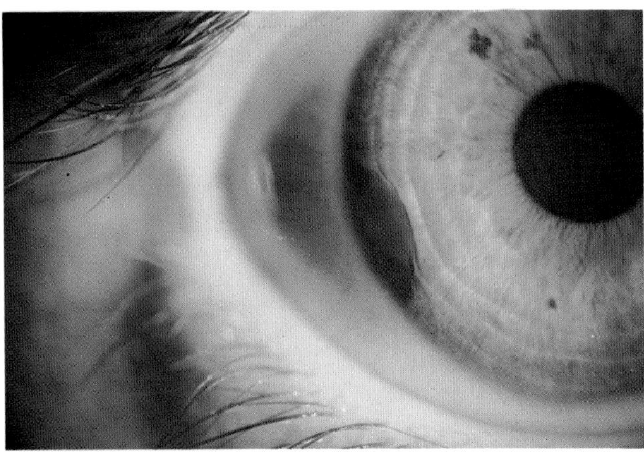

Figure 13.9 *Iris melanoma*

Management

As most iris melanomas are slow-growing and are composed of spindle A or spindle B cells, the prognosis for life is excellent following surgical excision. Broad iridectomy is usually sufficient for small tumours while iridocyclectomy or iridotrabeculectomy is necessary for larger tumours invading the angle. Enucleation is usually reserved for the rare diffusely growing tumours.

Differential diagnosis

Iris naevi

These are common benign tumours composed of small spindle and dendritic naevus cells. Clinically, a naevus consists of a pigmented, flat or slightly elevated, avascular lesion in the superficial layers of the iris (*Figure 13.10*). It does not usually distort the surrounding tissue or adjacent structures. Patients with neurofibromatosis have an increased prevalence of iris naevi. A diffuse naevus that obscures the normal pattern of iris crypts forms part of the Cogan–Reese syndrome which is one of the iridocorneal endothelial (ICE) syndromes (Chapter 7).

Iris freckles

These are smaller than naevi and consist of thin flat aggregations of melanocytes on the iris surface.

Iris cysts

These may be primary or secondary:

1. *Primary iris cysts* (*Figure 13.11*) are rare curiosities that arise either from the iris pigment epithelium or, rarely,

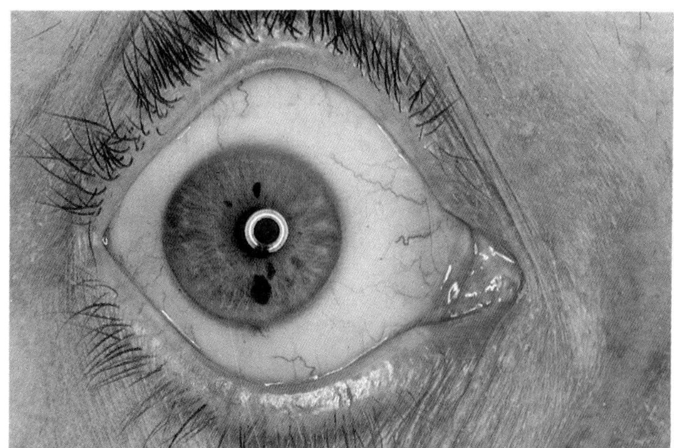

Figure 13.10 Iris naevus (courtesy of Photographic Department, Wexham Park Hospital)

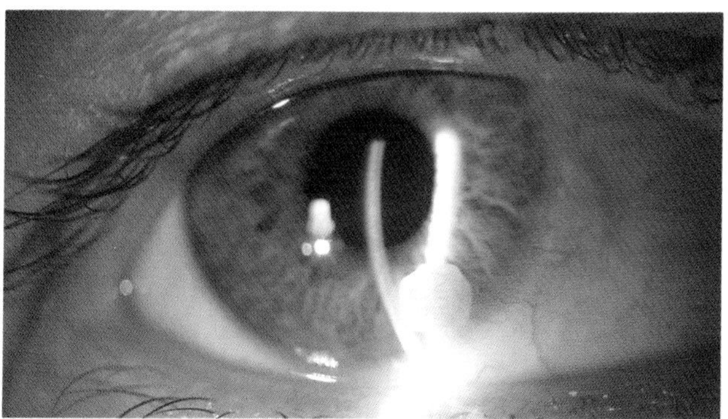

Figure 13.11 Iris cyst

from the iris stroma. The vast majority, particularly those arising from the pigment epithelial layer, are stationary and asymptomatic and require no treatment. The main clinical importance of these lesions is their similarity to neoplasms of the iris and ciliary body. Cysts of the iris pigment epithelium are globular, dark-brown structures which transilluminate. Occasionally they are bilateral and multiple. In contrast to epithelial cysts, stromal cysts are larger, solitary, have a clear anterior wall, and contain fluid.

2. *Secondary iris cysts* develop following intraocular surgery, ocular trauma, or the prolonged use of long-acting miotics such as Phospholine Iodide. Cysts that develop following surgery or trauma frequently enlarge and lead to severe complications such as anterior uveitis and glaucoma.

Miscellaneous lesions

Inflammatory granulomas may occasionally be mistaken for tumours.

Juvenile xanthogranuloma is a vascular tumour that affects the skin and also occasionally the eye. It is an important cause of spontaneous hyphaema and secondary glaucoma in children.

Leiomyomas are extremely rare tumours that arise from smooth muscle in the iris. They may be very difficult to differentiate from amelanotic melanomas, both clinically and histologically.

Metastases to the iris are very rare. When present they appear as pink or yellow friable masses that may be associated with signs of inflammation and a pseudohypopyon.

Fluorescein angiography

This may occasionally be helpful in differential diagnosis. Malignant pigmented lesions may have their own blood supply and show dye leakage into and around the tumour. Benign pigmented lesions and congenital cysts show no abnormality.

Choroidal naevus

Clinical features

A typical choroidal naevus is a flat or minimally elevated, oval or circular, slate-grey lesion (*Figure 13.12*). Although most naevi are less than 3 disc diameters in size, some may be as large as 6 disc diameters. The incidence of choroidal naevi in the general population is about 10%. Although they are probably present at birth, maximal growth occurs during the prepubertal years and is extremely rare thereafter. For this reason the very rare event of clinically detectable growth should arouse suspicion as to the possibility of malignant transformation. In the vast majority of cases, the diagnosis can be made by ophthalmoscopy without special tests. Regular extra visits to the ophthalmologist in order to document the very remote possibility of malignant transformation are unnecessary. With the passage of time the retinal pigment epithelium (RPE) overlying a naevus may show degenerative changes and the formation of drusen (*Figure 13.13*). Although most naevi are asymptomatic, those situated near the macula may give rise to symptoms by causing a serous detachment of the neurosensory retina (with or without choroidal neovascularization).

Features suggesting that a small or medium-sized pigmented choroidal tumour is in fact a melanoma include:

1. Documented increase in size by repeated fundus photography (increase in width), ultrasonography (increase in thickness), and visual field examination.
2. Symptoms of photopsia.
3. A globular elevátion.
4. Presence of widespread changes in the RPE, particularly the accumulation of orange (lipofuscin) pigment.
5. The presence of a large serous retinal detachment.

Fluorescein angiography

These findings depend on the amount of avascularity and degree of pigmentation. Most choroidal naevi are avascular and pigmented, giving rise to hypofluorescence due to blockage of background choroidal fluorescence. Less pigmented lesions show intense spotty staining during the arterial and arteriovenous phases.

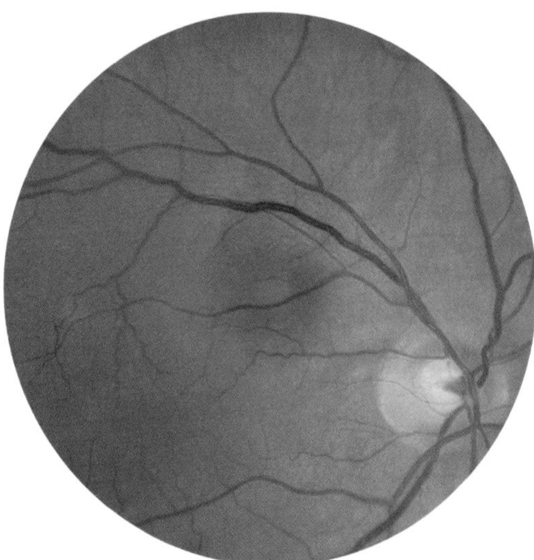

Figure 13.12 *Choroidal naevus*

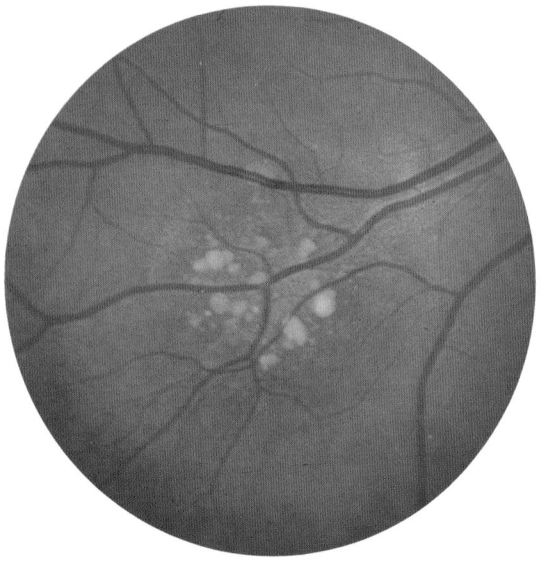

Figure 13.13 *Choroidal naevus with drusen (courtesy of Professor A. C. Bird)*

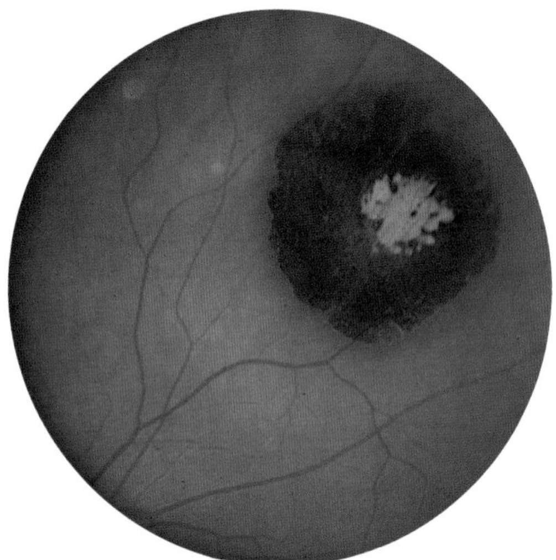

Figure 13.14 *Hypertrophy of retinal pigment epithelium*

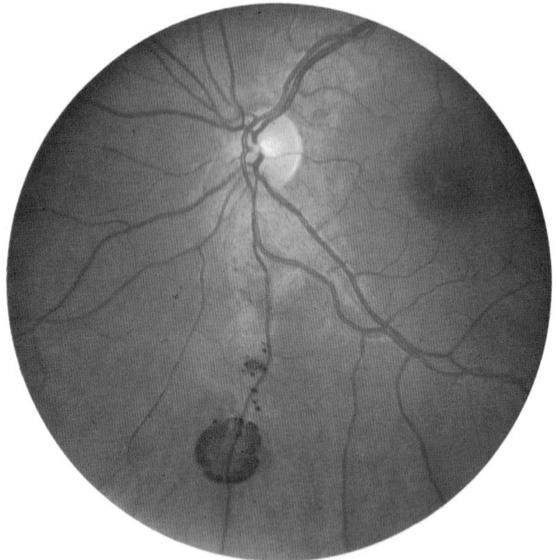

Figure 13.15 *Hypertrophy of retinal pigment epithelium ('bear-track')*

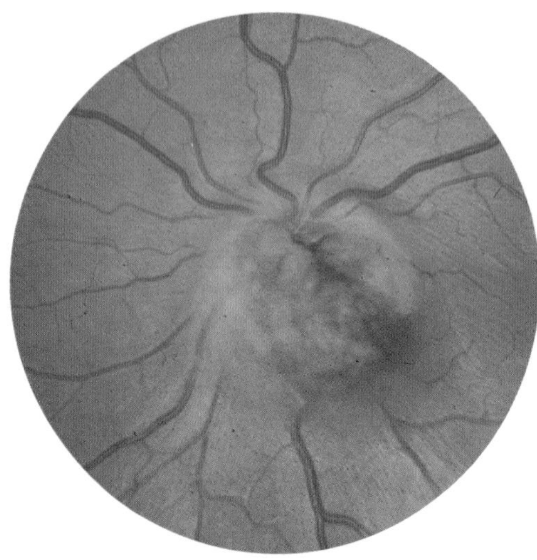

Figure 13.16 *Melanocytoma of the optic disc (courtesy of Professor A. C. Bird)*

Differential diagnosis

Hypertrophy of the RPE (*Figure 13.14*)

This is a congenital flat black lesion with a sharply demarcated outline, in contrast to the feathery margin of a choroidal naevus. A ring of hypopigmentation is frequently seen just inside the outer margin of the lesion. Most lesions are 1–3 disc diameters in size and may occur anywhere in the fundus. A variant of this condition that consists of multiple small lesions is called 'grouped' or 'bear-track' pigmentation (*Figure 13.15*).

Melanocytomas of the optic disc

These are rare melanotic lesions which typically affect one eye of dark-skinned individuals. The lesion is stationary, usually occupying the inferior part of the disc, although it may be elevated and occupy the entire disc surface (*Figure 13.16*). It has been suggested that melanocytomas are an expression of congenital melanosis oculi.

Choroidal haemangioma

Localized choroidal haemangioma

Clinical features

This typically appears as a dome-shaped or placoid red-orange lesion, most commonly situated at the posterior pole (*Figure 13.17*). Frequent secondary changes include exudative retinal detachment, cystoid degeneration and pigment epithelial mottling of the overlying retina. In some cases, metaplasia of the pigment epithelium into bone may occur. A useful clinical sign is blanching of the lesion with pressure on the globe. Differential diagnosis includes amelanotic choroidal melanoma and metastatic tumour. If

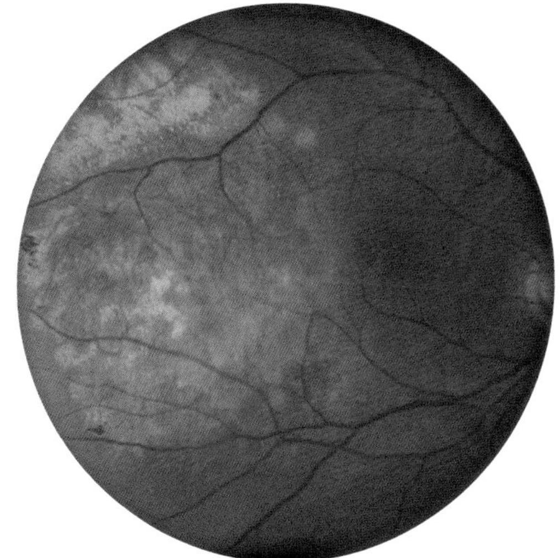

Figure 13.17 *Localized choroidal haemangioma (courtesy of Dr J. Federman)*

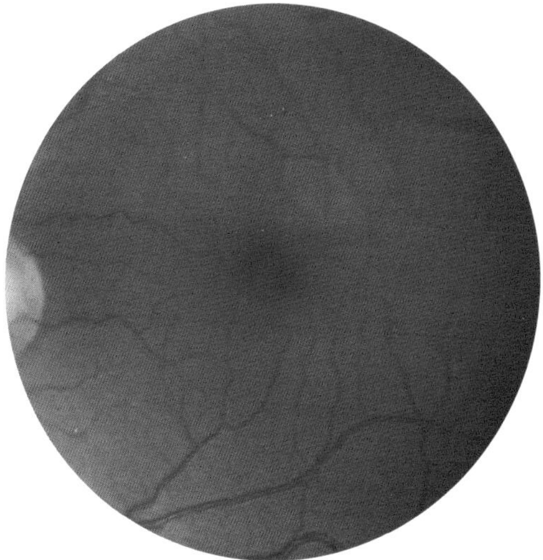

Figure 13.18 *Diffuse choroidal haemangioma in Sturge–Weber syndrome (courtesy of Dr P. H. Morse)*

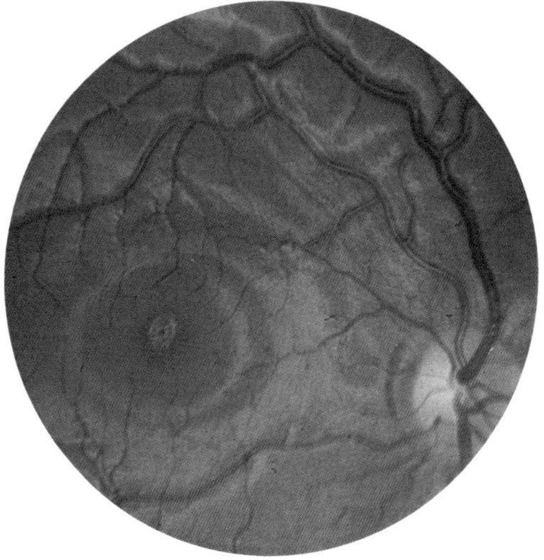

Figure 13.19 *Normal eye of patient in* Figure 13.18 *for comparison (courtesy of Dr P. H. Morse)*

the subretinal fluid is localized to the fovea, the tumour can be mistaken for central serous chorioretinopathy.

Special investigations

1. *^{32}P uptake* is usually negative.
2. *Ultrasonography.* The A-scan shows a high initial spike with high internal reflectivity. The B-scan demonstrates an oval or placoid lesion with a sharp anterior border and acoustic solidity, but no choroidal excavation or orbital shadowing.
3. *Fluorescein angiography* usually shows up the large choroidal vessels during the prearterial or arterial phase with late staining of the tumour and cystoid spaces in the retina. These features are not pathognomonic.

Management

Asymptomatic tumours require no treatment. If vision is threatened from serous retinal detachment, vigorous photocoagulation should be applied to the tumour. Hopefully, this will create a chorioretinal adhesion and prevent further fluid accumulation.

Diffuse choroidal haemangioma

This is usually associated with the Sturge–Weber syndrome (*see* Chapter 7). The diffuse choroidal thickening produced by the haemangioma gives the fundus a deep-red colour (*Figure 13.18*) which can be easily missed unless a comparison is made with the fellow eye (*Figure 13.19*).

Metastatic carcinoma

Metastatic tumours to the choroid are probably more common than primary malignancies. The most frequent primary site is the breast in females and the bronchus in males. A choroidal secondary may be the initial presentation of a bronchial carcinoma, whereas a past history of mastectomy is the rule in patients with breast tumours. Other less common primary sites include the kidney, testis, and gastrointestinal tract. The prostrate is, however, an extremely rare primary site.

Clinical features

Although choroidal metastases may occur anywhere in the fundus, they have a definite predilection for the posterior pole. Typically they appear as solitary or multiple, creamy-white, placoid or oval lesions (*Figure 13.20*). Because the tumours usually infiltrate laterally, they seldom become significantly elevated and have ill-defined borders. The few that assume a globular shape may mimic amelanotic melanomas.

Associated features include a characteristic mottled pigment clumping on the surface of the tumour and extensive exudative retinal detachment which may be mistaken for primary retinal detachment. Occasionally, metastatic carcinomas may invade the optic nerve head and cause a profound loss of vision. Pain is rare in patients with primary melanomas in the absence of secondary glaucoma, but may be an occasional feature of metastatic tumours. A careful examination of the opposite eye is important as bilateral metastases are frequent.

Special investigations

1. *^{32}P uptake* is of no value in differentiating metastases from primary amelanotic melanomas, as both give positive results. It is, however, of value in excluding a choroidal haemangioma.
2. *Ultrasonography* with B-scan may show a diffuse choroidal thickening which can also be seen in the rare diffusely growing melanoma.
3. *Fluorescein angiography* shows variable patterns and is usually of limited diagnostic value.
4. *Cytological examination* of subretinal fluid may be useful in doubtful cases.

Management

Enucleation is contraindicated unless the eye is painful. Palliative treatment is with chemotherapy in conjunction with external beam irradiation.

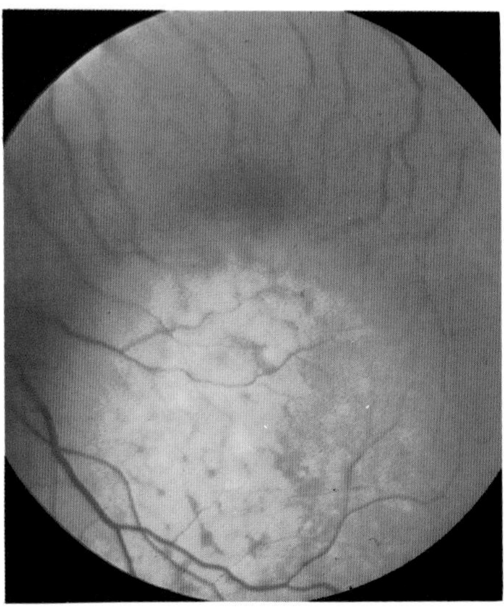

Figure 13.20 *Metastatic tumour to choroid (courtesy of Mr T. ffytche)*

Osseous choristoma (choroidal osteoma)

Clinical features

This very rare benign tumour primarily affects healthy young women and is occasionally bilateral. It appears as a slightly elevated, orange-yellow lesion with well-defined geographical borders, most commonly situated near the optic disc or at the posterior pole (*Figure 13.21*). Associated findings include diffuse mottling of the overlying retinal pigment epithelium and multiple small vascular networks on the surface of the tumour.

Special investigations

1. *Fluorescein angiography* shows a diffuse mottled pattern of hyperfluorescence during the early and late phases.
2. *Ultrasonographically* the tumour is dense and the orbital tissue behind the tumour is rendered silent.
3. ^{32}P *uptake* is positive as the phosphorus is taken up by all bones in the body.
4. *Plain X-rays and CT scans* will show up the tumour. The latter shows that the tumour has the same density as normal bone.

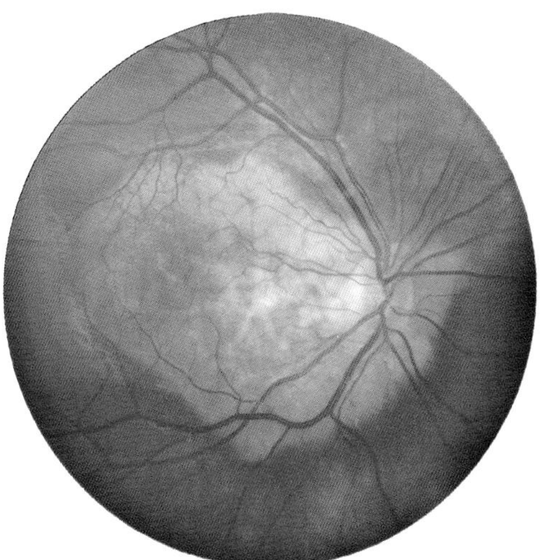

Figure 13.21 *Choroidal osteoma*

Retinoblastoma

Retinoblastoma is the most common primary malignant intraocular tumour of childhood and the second most common primary intraocular malignancy of all age groups (choroidal melanoma is more common). Even so, it is a rare tumour, occurring in only about 1 in 20 000 live births. There is no sexual predilection and, although the tumour is initially only detected in one eye, both eyes are eventually affected in about one in three cases. The average age at diagnosis is 18 months and the vast majority become clinically apparent prior to the age of 3 years. Patients with bilateral tumours present earlier than those with unilateral involvement.

Inheritance

Familial cases. A positive family history of retinoblastoma is present in only 6% of cases. The mode of inheritance is autosomal dominant with high but incomplete (70%) penetrance.

Sporadic cases account for the remaining 94%. Of these, 25% are germinal mutations which are likely to pass the tumour onto their offspring, and 75% are somatic mutations in which the tumour will not be perpetuated. Unfortunately, it is impossible to determine which cases are germinal and which somatic mutations. Genetic counselling may be difficult, although the following principles should be remembered:

1. Healthy parents with one affected child have about a 6% risk of producing another affected child.
2. If two or more siblings are affected, the risk of subsequent children being affected is 50%.
3. A survivor of hereditary retinoblastoma has almost a 50% chance that his children will also develop the tumour.

Chromosomal abnormalities

Retinoblastoma is thought to be caused by a change in a gene on chromosome 13. This gene is pleiotropic as it has a number of different effects. It can cause an extremely rare benign tumour called a retinoma as well as a pinealoma, concurrently with bilateral retinoblastoma. The genetic defect can also predispose a patient in later life to non-ocular malignancies, most commonly osteogenic sarcoma, at the site of previous radiotherapy as well as in non-irradiated parts of the body. A higher prevalence of retinoblastoma has been reported in patients with deletion of the long arm of the D chromosome (13–15) as well as in association with trisomy-21.

Clinical features

Retinoblastoma may present in a variety of ways.

Leukocoria or 'amaurotic cat's eye' is a white pupillary reflex (*Figure 13.22*). This is the most common mode of presentation, accounting for about two-thirds of cases.

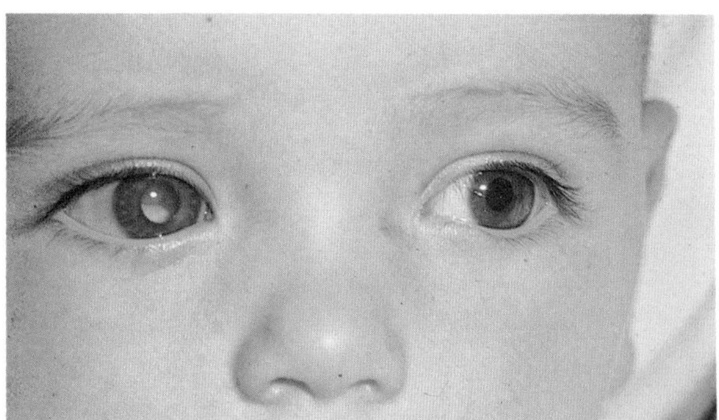

Figure 13.22 *Right leukocoria due to retinoblastoma (courtesy of Mr C. Migdal)*

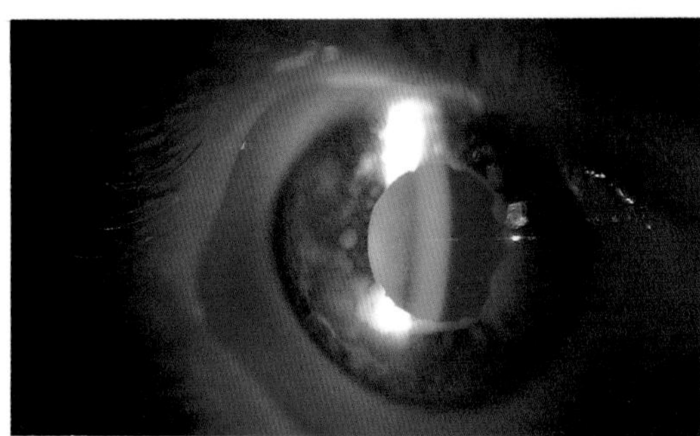

Figure 13.23 *Retinoblastoma invading iris giving rise to 'pseudo-Busacca' nodules*

Strabismus is the second most common mode of presentation (20% of cases). This is why fundus examination after a good dilatation of the pupil is mandatory in all cases of childhood strabismus. Occasionally a patient with a small tumour may present with visual difficulty in the absence of strabismus.

Secondary glaucoma which may or may not be associated with buphthalmos is a relatively rare mode of presentation (3%).

Proptosis due to orbital involvement may mimic orbital cellulitis.

Anterior chamber inflammatory signs (*Figure 13.23*) or spontaneous hyphaema may also be a presenting feature of retinoblastoma.

Routine examination of a patient known to be at risk may occasionally reveal the presence of the tumour.

Diagnosis

The diagnosis is based on ophthalmoscopy and, if necessary, ancillary tests.

Indirect ophthalmoscopy

Indirect ophthalmoscopy with scleral indentation following full mydriasis should be performed on both eyes. Unless scleral indentation is used, tumours arising anterior to the equator may be missed. Two fundus appearances may be seen.

Endophytic tumours (*Figure 13.24, right*)

These project from the retina into the vitreous cavity. The lesion has a white or pearly pink colour and is frequently associated with the presence of fine blood vessels on its surface. In the presence of secondary calcification, the tumour is sharply demarcated and resembles cottage cheese. Frequently, more than one tumour may be present in the same eye.

Exophytic tumours (*Figure 13.24, left*)

These grow in the subretinal space and give rise to a total retinal detachment. In these eyes, the tumour itself may be difficult to visualize especially if the vitreous is also hazy due to haemorrhage.

Special investigations

The following tests may be required in certain cases:

1. *X-rays of the globe* using bone-free dental films for the presence of calcium.
2. *Ultrasonography*, particularly with the B-scan, may also demonstrate the presence of calcium.
3. *CT scanning* may also demonstrate calcification. It is also useful in documenting the possibility of gross invasion of the optic nerve, orbital or pineal involvement, or CNS spread.
4. *Aqueous humour paracentesis* for enzyme assay and cytology. An aqueous-to-plasma lactate dehydrogenase ratio of greater than 1.0 is suggestive of retinoblastoma.
5. *Carcinoembryonic antigen* may be found in retinoblastoma patients, as well as in certain family members.
6. *Lumbar puncture and bone marrow aspiration* for evidence of metastases.
7. *ELISA* test to exclude toxocariasis.
8. *Fine needle biopsy* may be useful in primary or metastatic retinoblastoma in which non-invasive tests are inconclusive.

Treatment

Enucleation

Enucleation obtaining a long piece of the optic nerve is usually the treatment of choice for most tumours affecting the first eye, as in these cases the tumour is usually far advanced and useful vision lost. (There are, however, exceptions to this rule.) The management of the second eye depends on the size and location of the tumour.

Radiotherapy

Radiotherapy with an external beam is preferred for medium or large tumours. Cobalt plaque irradiation is reserved for small to medium-sized tumours or for those that do not respond to external irradiation.

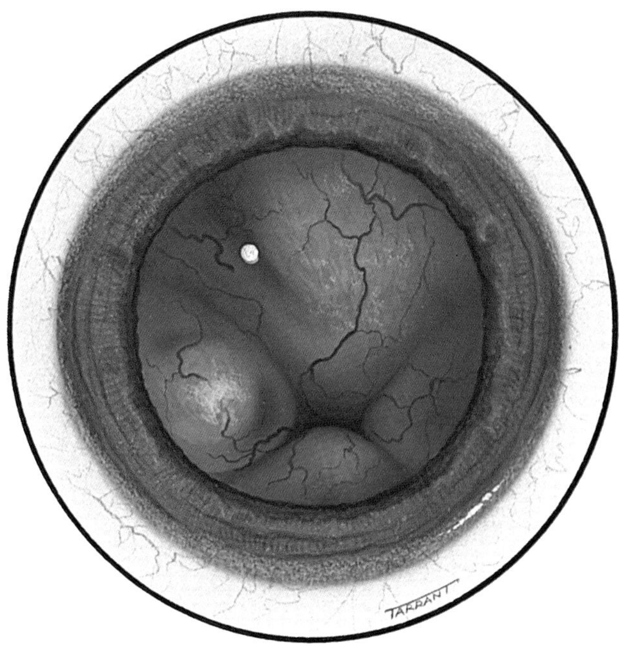

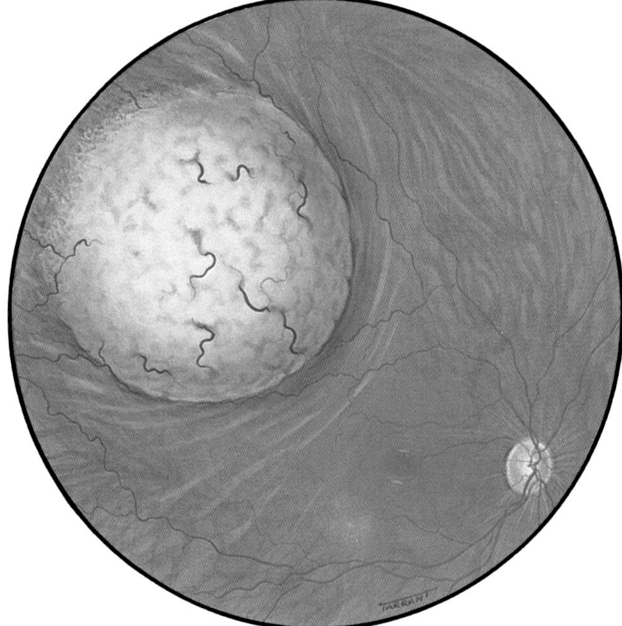

Figure 13.24 Retinoblastoma. Right: endophytic type; left: exophytic type

Photocoagulation

Photocoagulation with the xenon arc is useful for certain small tumours not involving the optic nerve or macula.

Cryotherapy

This may be useful for the treatment of small peripheral tumours. The tumour should be frozen three times.

Systemic chemotherapy

This is indicated following enucleation in advanced cases and in the presence of metastases. The most common sites for metastases are skull, orbit, long bones, viscera, spinal cord, and lymph nodes.

Prognostic factors

The overall mortality rate from the tumour is between 15 and 20%.

Optic nerve involvement

Optic nerve involvement beyond the point of surgical transection is associated with a 65% mortality rate. If the optic nerve is uninvolved, the mortality rate is only about 8% and if the tumour involves the lamina cribrosa the mortality rate rises to about 15%.

Size and location

Small posterior tumours do best with an overall survival rate of 70%. Surprisingly, bilateral cases seem to do as well as unilateral cases and there is no significant difference between endophytic and exophytic tumours.

Cellular differentiation

This may be good or poor. Well-differentiated tumours are characterized by Flexner–Wintersteiner rosettes. The Homer–Wright rosette is similar except that instead of having a clear lumen, it has a triangle of central fibres. The term 'pseudorosette' is sometimes used to describe clusters of tumour cells around blood vessels or around small areas of necrosis. The mortality rate of patients whose tumours have abundant rosettes is about 8% compared with 40% in those with highly undifferentiated tumours. Massive choroidal invasion is an adverse prognostic factor.

Differential diagnosis of childhood leukocoria

Retinoblastoma

This is as already discussed.

Cataract

This may be unilateral or bilateral and usually presents no diagnostic problems.

Coats' disease

This is almost always unilateral, commoner in boys, and tends to present later than retinoblastoma. The clinical features of Coats' disease are discussed in Chapter 10.

Retinopathy of prematurity

This is easy to diagnose when a history of prematurity and low birth weight is present. However, more cases are being seen without these predisposing factors. The clinical features of retinopathy of prematurity are discussed in Chapter 10.

Toxocariasis

A toxocaral granuloma should be considered in the differential diagnosis of an endophytic retinoblastoma. The clinical featurs of ocular toxocariasis are discussed in Chapter 6.

Persistent hyperplastic primary vitreous

Persistent hyperplastic primary vitreous (PHPV) is the most serious developmental disorder of the vitreous. It is caused by a failure of regression of the primary vitreous and can be divided into anterior and posterior types.

Anterior PHPV

Clinical features

This is by far the most common type of PHPV. It typically occurs in a microphthalmic eye and is unilateral in about 90% of cases. It is characterized by the presence of a retrolental mass into which elongated ciliary processes are inserted (*Figure 13.25*). With time the mass contracts and pulls the ciliary processes towards its centre. An associated dehiscence involving the posterior capsule may lead to the subsequent formation of cataract. Swelling of the lens may also give rise to secondary angle-closure glaucoma. The rise in intraocular pressure may cause the eye to enlarge. Vitreous haemorrhage is also an occasional complication.

Management

The retrolental mass and the cataractous lens can be removed using closed intraocular microsurgical techniques in order to prevent complications which might otherwise lead to loss of the eye. In mildly affected eyes a limited form of vision can be restored.

Posterior PHPV

Clinial features

This is very much less common than the anterior type. A characteristic feature is a white dense opaque membrane or a prominent non-opaque retinal fold, which extends from the optic disc to the more peripheral retina or the retrolental region. The lesion is most frequently located inferiorly but may occur in any quadrant. Associated findings include retinal detachment (*Figure 13.26*), choroidal hypopigmentation or hyperpigmentation, and a pale optic disc. It is thought that the 'morning glory syndrome' may represent a form of posterior PHPV (*see* Chapter 15).

Management

The main aim is to prevent and, if necessary, treat retinal detachment. The eye should therefore be examined annually and any retinal breaks treated prophylactically.

The main differences between PHPV, retinopathy of prematurity, and retinoblastoma are summarized in *Table 13.2*.

Table 13.2 Differential diagnosis of leukocoria

	PHPV	*Retinopathy of prematurity*	*Retinoblastoma*
Laterality	Unilateral 90%	Bilateral 100%	Bilateral 33%
Microphthalmos	+++	–	–
Elongated ciliary processes	+++	+	–
First noted	Neonatal period	Neonatal period	18 months
Oxygen exposure	–	+++	–
Birth weight	Normal	Low	Normal

Retinal dysplasia

This is due to failure of the retina to develop normally during embryonic life so that it never achieves maturity. The condition is characterized by the presence at birth of a pink or white retrolental membrane in a microphthalmic eye with a shallow anterior chamber and elongated ciliary processes. Complications include vitreous haemorrhage, cataract, and secondary glaucoma. Unilateral cases are usually unassociated with systemic abnormalities whereas bilateral involvement may occur in patients with Norrie's

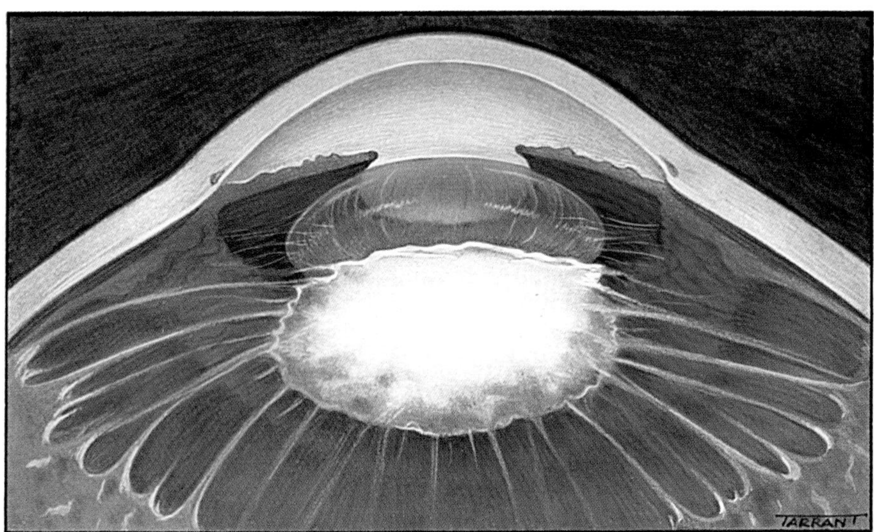

Figure 13.25
Persistent hyperplastic primary vitreous

disease (varying degrees of mental deficiency and deafness) and trisomy-13 (Patau's syndrome—severe systemic abnormalities and an early demise).

Incontinentia pigmenti

This is a rare skin disorder affecting infant girls. It is characterized by recurrent vesiculobullous dermatitis which causes irregular patches or whorls of hyperpigmentation on the trunk and extremities. About one-third of cases have a retrolental mass composed of a totally detached retina and fibrous tissue.

Retinal astrocytoma

See next.

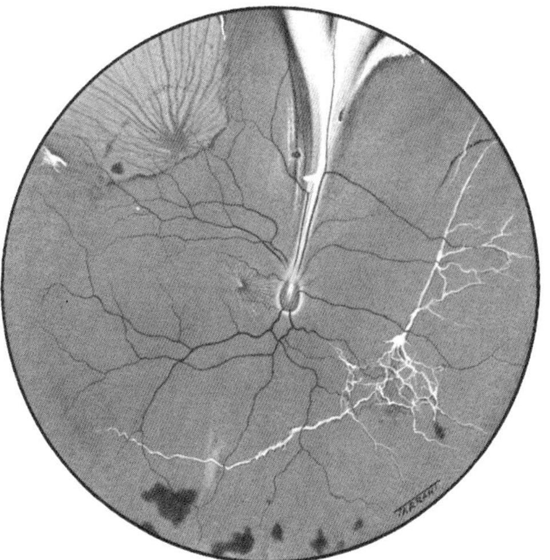

Figure 13.26 *Posterior PHPV with subtotal retinal detachment*

Retinal astrocytoma

Although astrocytomas of the retina and optic nerve may rarely occur as isolated lesions they are most frequently seen in patients with tuberous sclerosis (Bourneville's disease, epiloia) which is one of the phacomatoses. It is characterized by the triad of mental retardation, epilepsy, and 'adenoma sebaceum'.

Inheritance is autosomal dominant although 50% of patients represent new mutations.

Clinical features

Ocular

About 50% of patients with tuberous sclerosis have fundus astrocytomas which are bilateral in about 15% of cases. The lesions arise from the inner retinal layers and may be single or multiple. They are usually situated at or near the optic nerve head although they may also be found in the periphery. The tumours may be small and flat or more typically nodular and well circumscribed with a size ranging from 0.5 to 1 disc or more in diameter. During early life they may appear semitranslucent and should be considered in the differential diagnosis of retinoblastoma (*Figure 13.27*). Later, they frequently assume a more dense white colour and the occurrence of multiple areas of calcification within the tumour may give rise to a mulberry-like appearance (*Figure 13.28*). These fossilized mulberry tumours of the optic nerve head should be distinguished from hyaline bodies to which they are completely unrelated. Treatment is unnecessary as the lesions are usually asymptomatic and show only a minimal

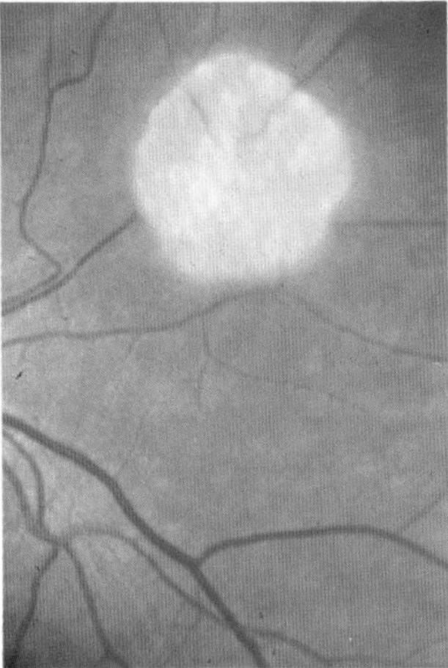

Figure 13.27 *Retinal astrocytoma in tuberous sclerosis (courtesy of Mr T. ffytche)*

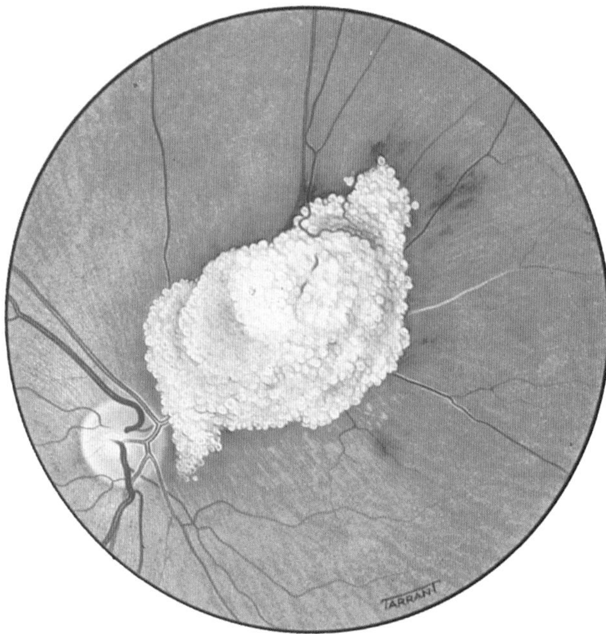

Figure 13.28 *Large retinal astrocytoma in tuberous sclerosis*

tendency to grow. Other ocular lesions include hypopigmented iris spots in about 50% of patients and occasionally hypopigmented fundus lesions.

Systemic

Skin lesions

These may be of four types:

1. *Nodular fibroangiomas* ('adenoma sebaceum') are highly vascularized red papules which have a butterfly distribution affecting the nose and cheeks (*Figure 13.29, left*). These lesions may be inconspicuous at birth, but they slowly multiply and enlarge and become clinically obvious between the ages of 2 and 5 years. On cursory examination they may be mistaken for acne vulgaris, hence the term 'adenoma sebaceum'.
2. *Achromic naevi* involving the trunk, limbs (*Figure 13.29, right*), and scalp are thought to be pathognomonic of tuberous sclerosis. They consist of hypopigmented patches whose shape may resemble ash leaflets. In infants with little skin pigmentation these lesions may only be detected under ultraviolet light (Wood's lamp) as fluorescing patches.
3. *Café-au-lait* spots similar to those in patients with neurofibromatosis may also be seen. They may represent pigmentation of an achromic naevus later in life.
4. *Shagreen patches* are diffuse fibrous thickenings over the lumbar region.

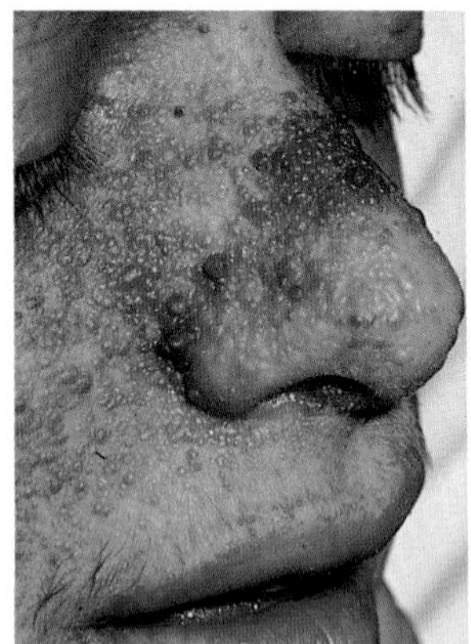

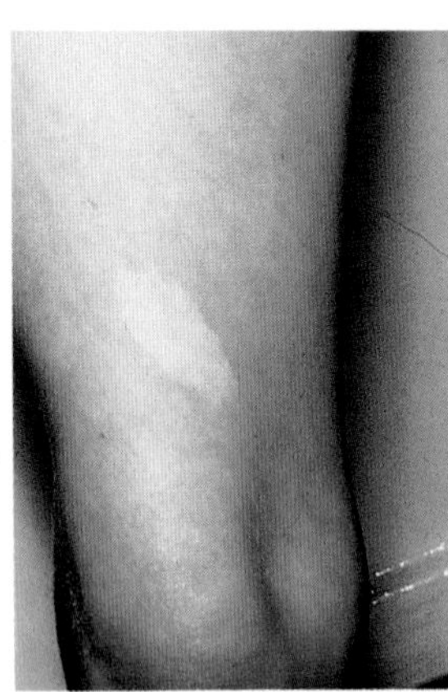

Figure 13.29 *Tuberous sclerosis. Left: adenoma sebaceum; right: achromic naevus on thigh (courtesy of Dr R. Winter)*

CNS lesions

These are present in all patients with tuberous sclerosis. The astrocytic hamartomas may be found anywhere in the brain but they are frequently concentrated in a periventricular distribution. They tend to grow very slowly although very occasionally they undergo malignant transformation. When the lesions are critically situated they may block CSF circulation and give rise to hydrocephalus or cause focal neurological deficits. About 80% of patients suffer from epilepsy and about 60% are mentally handicapped to varying degrees.

Visceral hamartomas

These may involve the kidneys and the heart (rhabdomyoma), as well as other organs and the subungual areas. These lesions are usually asymptomatic.

Retinal capillary haemangioma

Retinal capillary haemangiomas (angiomatosis retinae, von Hippel's disease) is associated with systemic lesions in about 25% of cases. The combination of ocular and systemic lesions is referred to as the von Hippel–Lindau syndrome. It is one of the phacomatoses.

Inheritance is autosomal dominant with incomplete penetrance and delayed expressivity.

Clinical features

Ocular

The retinal lesions may be multiple (*Figure 13.30*) and involve both eyes in about 50% of cases. The earliest detectable lesion may be no larger than a microaneurysm and is located within the capillary bed between an arteriole and venule. With the passage of time, the lesion grows into a small red nodule and then into a larger round orange-red tumour. Arteriovenous shunting within the tumour gives rise to dilatation and tortuosity of its supplying artery and draining vein. Both vessels appear similar in colour. Angiomas of the optic nerve head are not associated with abnormal vessels. If untreated, the retinal angioma leaks plasma constituents and gives rise to the deposition of hard exudate in the surrounding retina as well as in remote areas of the fundus. Other vision-threatening complications include serous retinal detachment and bleeding.

Systemic

Because it is impossible to predict with any degree of certainty which patients with retinal angiomas will harbour systemic tumours, it is incumbent on the ophthalmologist to refer all patients with retinal lesions for a thorough systemic and neurological evaluation. In addition, the relatives should be screened in view of the dominant form of inheritance of the disease. Usually, the systemic lesions become manifest after the onset of ocular symptoms. Haemangioblastomas may involve the cerebellum, medulla, pons, and spinal cord. Visceral lesions include cysts of the kidneys, pancreas, liver, epididymis, ovary, and lungs. Rare findings include hypernephroma, phaeochromocytoma, and polycythaemia. The von Hippel–Lindau syndrome is the only one of the phacomatoses in which skin lesions are absent.

Management

Because the tumour usually grows, treatment by photocoagulation, cryotherapy, or penetrating diathermy should be carried out in all cases. The tumour itself, and not the abnormal vessels, should be treated. Occasionally, excessively vigorous treatment causes a temporary but extensive serous detachment of the retina.

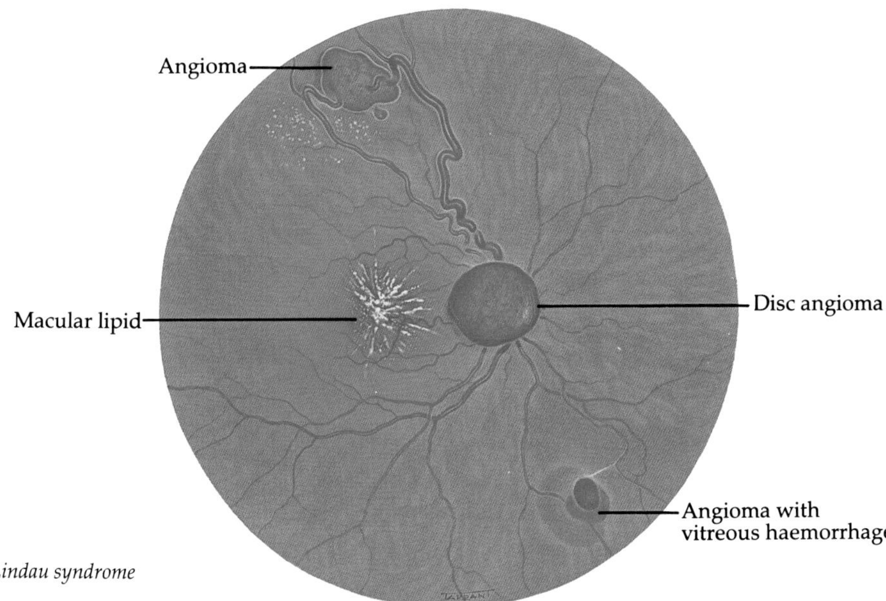

Figure 13.30 *Ocular features of von Hippel–Lindau syndrome*

Retinal cavernous haemangioma

Cavernous haemangioma of the retina or optic nerve is a congenital unilateral vascular hamartoma.

Clinical features

Ocular

The lesion has the appearance of a cluster of grapes located in the inner retina or optic nerve head (*Figure 13.31*). It consists of thin-walled saccular aneurysms, situated between two veins. Because of the sluggish blood flow within the lesion, the plasma becomes separated from the red cells giving a characteristic appearance of a meniscus clinically and on fluorescein angiography. The lesion usually remains asymptomatic throughout life and does not require treatment.

Systemic

A few patients have similar lesions involving the skin and CNS. For this reason the condition is considered by some to be a phacomatosis.

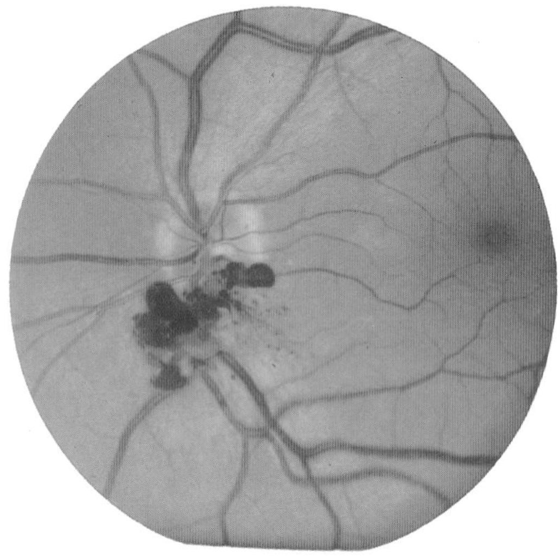

Figure 13.31 *Retinal cavernous haemangioma (courtesy of Dr P. Morse)*

Retinal racemose haemangioma

This rare lesion is a congenital arteriovenous malformation in which there is a direct communication between the arteries and veins without an intervening capillary bed.

Clinical features

Ocular

The fundus lesions are usually unilateral and involve the retina or optic nerve head. The affected vessels are typically enlarged, tortuous, and frequently more numerous than in a normal fundus (*Figure 13.32*). As in angiomatosis retinae, the vein and artery are similar in colour. The lesions are usually asymptomatic although very large lesions may lead to exudation and haemorrhage.

Systemic

Some patients also have similar ipsilateral lesions involving the midbrain, basofrontal region, or posterior fossa. This association is referred to as the Wyburn–Mason syndrome, which is included in the group of phacomatoses. Brain involvement may lead to spontaneous haemorrhage or epilepsy. Occasionally the malformations may involve the maxilla, mandible, and orbit. Facial skin lesions have also been reported.

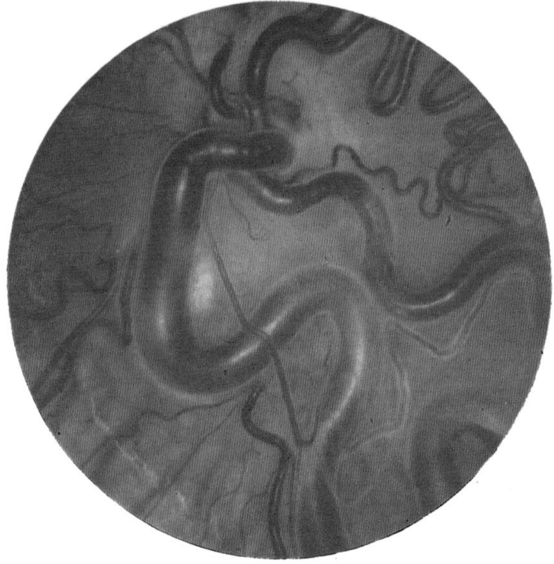

Figure 13.32 *Retinal racemose haemangioma (courtesy of Professor A. C. Bird)*

Retinal pigment epithelial hamartoma

This is a hamartomatous malformation involving the retinal pigment epithelium, neurosensory retina, retinal vessels, and adjacent vitreous. Although very rare, the lesion is important because it may be mistaken for a malignant tumour such as retinoblastoma or choroidal melanoma. Characteristically, the hamartoma is black or grey in colour, slightly elevated, and most frequently located in the juxtapapillary region. Associated features include intraretinal gliosis, epiretinal membranes, a fine network of dilated capillaries within the lesion, and tortuosity of the retinal blood vessels (*Figure 13.33*). Contraction of the glial elements of the lesion may distort the adjacent retina and the optic nerve head giving rise to blurred vision and metamorphopsia. Patients with juxtapapillary lesions are predominantly boys who develop symptoms in late childhood or early adulthood whereas those with peripheral lesions usually present in early childhood with strabismus.

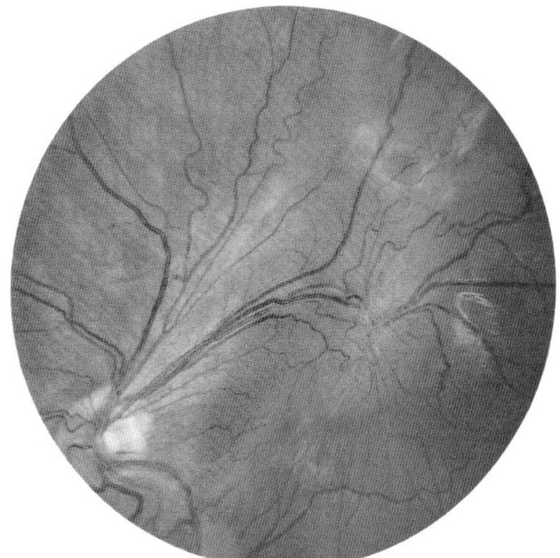

Figure 13.33 *Retinal pigment epithelial hamartoma with distortion of adjacent retina*

Ocular reticulum cell sarcoma (histiocytic lymphoma)

This very rare tumour may involve the central nervous system and the eye. The most frequent presentation is with bilateral vitreous infiltration. Reticulum cell sarcoma should therefore be considered in the differential diagnosis of bilateral chronic vitritis in patients over the age of 60 years. Occasional involvement of the fundus gives rise to patchy yellow subretinal and choroidal infiltrates which may be associated with haemorrhages. The diagnosis is usually made by cytological examination of the vitreous. Treatment is by radiotherapy.

Further reading

Uveal melanoma

Char, D.H. (1984) (Editorial) Therapeutic options in uveal melanomas. *American Journal of Ophthalmology*, **98**, 796–799

Char, D.H. (1986) Radiation therapy for uveal melanomas involving the ciliary body. *Transactions of the Ophthalmological Society of the United Kingdom*, **105**, 252–256

Char, D.H. and Castro, J.R. (1982) Helium ion therapy for choroidal melanoma. *Archives of Ophthalmology*, **100**, 935–938

Damato, B.E. and Foulds, W.S. (1986) Ciliary body tumours and their management. *Transactions of the Ophthalmological Society of the United Kingdom*, **105**, 257–264

Foulds, W.S. (1983) Current options in the management of choroidal melanoma. *Transactions of the Ophthalmological Society of the United Kingdom*, **103**, 28–34

Gamel, J.W. and McLean, I.W. (1984) Modern developments in histopathologic assessment of uveal melanomas. *Ophthalmology*, **91**, 679–684

Gass, J.D.M. (1977) Problems in the differential diagnosis of choroidal naevi and malignant melanomas. *American Journal of Ophthalmology*, **83**, 299–323

Gass, J.D.M. (1985) Comparison of prognosis after enucleation vs cobalt-60 irradiation for melanomas. *Archives of Ophthalmology*, **103**, 916–923

Gass, J.D.M. (1985) Comparison of uveal melanoma growth rates with mitotic index and mortality. *Archives of Ophthalmology*, **103**, 924–931

Geisse, L.J. and Robertson, D.M. (1985) Iris melanomas. *American Journal of Ophthalmology*, **99**, 638–648

Gragoudas, E.S., Goitein, M., Verhey, L. *et al.* (1982) Proton beam irradiation of uveal melanomas. *Archives of Ophthalmology*, **100**, 928–934

Jakobiec, F.A. and Silbert, G. (1981) Are most iris 'melanomas' really naevi? *Archives of Ophthalmology*, **99**, 2117–2132

Jakobiec, F.A., Depot, M.J., Henkind, P. *et al.* (1982) Fluorescein angiographic patterns in iris melanocytic tumours. *Archives of Ophthalmology*, **100**, 1288–1299

Jakobiec, F.A. and Levinson, A.W. (1985) Choroidal melanoma: Aetiology and diagnosis. *Clinical Modules for Ophthalmologists*, Vol. 3, Module 5

Jakobiec, F.A. and Levinson, A.W. (1985) Choroidal melanoma. Prognosis and treatment. *Clinical Modules for Ophthalmologists*, Vol. 3, Module 6

McLean, I.W., Foster, W.D. and Zimmerman, L.E. (1983) Modifications of Callender's classification of uveal melanomas at the Armed Forces Institute of Pathology. *American Journal of Ophthalmology*, **96**, 502–509

Migdal, C. (1983) Effect of method of enucleation on the prognosis of choroidal melanoma. *British Journal of Ophthalmology*, **67**, 385–388

Migdal, C. (1983) Choroidal melanoma: The role of conservative therapy. *Transactions of the Ophthalmological Society of the United Kingdom*, **103**, 54–58

Packard, R.B.S. (1980) Pattern of mortality in choroidal malignant melanoma. *British Journal of Ophthalmology*, **64**, 565–575

Packard, R.B.S. (1983) In malignant choroidal melanoma will delay in radical treatment influence prognosis? *Transactions of the Ophthalmological Society of the United Kingdom*, **103**, 49–53

Shields, J.A. (1977) Current approaches to the diagnosis and management of choroidal melanomas. *Survey of Ophthalmology*, **21**, 443–463

Shields, J.A., Augsburger, J.J., Brady, L.W. *et al.* (1982) Cobalt plaque therapy of posterior uveal melanomas. *Ophthalmology*, **89**, 1201–1207

Shields, J.A., Augsburger, J.J., Brown, G.C. *et al.* (1980) The differential diagnosis of uveal melanomas. *Ophthalmology*, **87**, 518–522

Shields, J.A., Sanborn, G.E. and Augsburger, J.J. (1983) The differential diagnosis of malignant melanoma of the iris. *Ophthalmology*, **90**, 716–720

Zimmerman, L.E. and McLean, I.W. (1984) Do growth and onset of symptoms of uveal melanomas indicate subclinical metastasis? *Ophthalmology*, **91**, 685–691

Choroidal haemangioma

Lanning, R. and Shields, J.A. (1979) Comparison of radioactive phosphorus (^{32}P) in comparable sized choroidal melanomas and hemangiomas. *American Journal of Ophthalmology*, **87**, 769–772

Sanborn, G.E., Augsburger, J.J. and Shields, J.A. (1982) Treatment of circumscribed choroidal haemangiomas. *Ophthalmology*, **89**, 1374–1380

Metastatic tumours to the choroid

Mewis, L. and Young, S.E. (1982) Breast carcinoma metastatic to the choroid—analysis of 67 patients. *Ophthalmology*, **89**, 147–151

Stephens, R.F. and Shields, J.A. (1979) Diagnosis and management of cancer metastatic to the uvea: a study of 70 cases. *Ophthalmology*, **86**, 1336–1349

Sternberg, P., Tiedeman, J., Hickinbotham, D. *et al.* (1984) Controlled aspiration of subretinal fluid in the diagnosis of carcinoma metastatic to the choroid. *Archives of Ophthalmology*, **102**, 1622–1625

Osseous choristoma (choroidal osteoma)

Cunha, S.L. (1984) Osseous choristoma of the choroid. *Archives of Ophthalmology*, **102**, 1052–1054

Teich, S.A. and Walsh, J.B. (1981) Choroidal osteoma. *Ophthalmology*, **99**, 696–698

Retinoblastoma

Abramson, D.H. (1983) (Editorial) Retinoma, retinocytoma, and the retinoblastoma gene. *Archives of Ophthalmology*, **101**, 1517–1518

Abramson, D.H., Ellsworth, R.H. and Rozakis, G.W. (1982) Cryotherapy for retinoblastoma. *Achives of Ophthalmology*, **100**, 1253–1256

Bedford M.A. (1977) Management of retinoblastoma. *Modern Problems in Ophthalmology*, **18**, 101–103

Char, D.H. (1980) Current concepts in retinoblastoma. *Annals of Ophthalmology*, **12**, 792–804

Char, D.H., Hedges, T.R. and Norman, D. (1984) Retinoblastoma CT diagnosis. *Ophthalmology*, **91**, 1347–1350

Char, D.H. and Miller, T.R. (1984) Fine needle biopsy in retinoblastoma. *American Journal of Ophthalmology*, **97**, 686–690

Egbert, P.R., Donaldson, S., Moazed, K. *et al.* (1978) Visual results and ocular complications following radiotherapy for retinoblastoma. *Archives of Ophthalmology*, **96**, 1826–1830

Hungerford, J. (1985) Recent advances in the understanding of retinoblastoma. *Transactions of the Ophthalmological Society of the United Kingdom*, **104**, 832–835

MacKay, C.J., Abramson, D.H. and Ellsworth, R.M. (1984) Metastatic pattern in retinoblastoma. *Archives of Ophthalmology*, **102**, 391–396

Migdal, C. (1983) Bilateral retinoblastoma: the prognosis for vision. *British Journal of Ophthalmology*, **67**, 592–595

Price, R.L. (1978) Retinoblastoma—an overview. *Perspectives in Ophthalmology*, **2**, 195–204

Stannard, C., Lipper, S., Sealy, R. *et al.* (1979) Retinoblastoma: correlation of invasion of the optic nerve head and choroid with prognosis and metastases. *British Journal of Ophthalmology*, **63**, 560–570

Retinal haemangioma

Hardwig, P. and Robertson, D.M. (1984) von Hippel–Lindau disease. *Ophthalmology*, **91**, 263–270

Messmer, E., Font, R.L., Laqua, H. *et al.* (1984) Cavernous hemangioma of the retina. *Archives of Ophthalmology*, **102**, 413–418

Messmer, E., Laqua, H. and Wessing, A. (1983) Nine cases of cavernous hemangioma of the retina. *American Journal of Ophthalmology*, **95**, 383–390

Shields, J.A., Decker, W.L., Sanborn, G.E. *et al.* (1983) Presumed acquired retinal haemangioma. *Ophthalmology*, **90**, 1292–1300

Retinal pigment epithelial hamartoma

Cosgrove, J.M., Sharp, D.M. and Bird, A.C. (1986) Combined hamartoma of the retina and retinal pigment epithelium: the clinical spectrum. *Transactions of the Ophthalmological Society of the United Kingdom*, **105**, 106–113

Rosenberg, P.R. and Walsh, J.B. (1984) Retinal pigment epithelial hamartoma—unusual manifestations. *British Journal of Ophthalmology*, **68**, 439–442

Schachat, A.P., Shields, J.A., Fine, S.L. *et al.* (1984) Combined hamartomas of the retina and retinal pigment epithelium. *Ophthalmology*, **91**, 1609–1615

14

Strabismus

Introduction

Actions of extraocular muscles

Eye movements

Binocular single vision

Double vision

Clinical evaluation

History

Examination

Childhood esotropias

Classification

Infantile

Accommodative

Non-accommodative

Childhood exotropias

Classification

Intermittent

Constant

Special ocular motility defects

Duane's retraction syndrome

Brown's superior oblique tendon sheath syndrome

Strabismus fixus

Congenital fibrosis syndrome

Möbius syndrome

Nystagmus blockage syndrome

Double elevator palsy

Principles of surgery

Weakening procedures

Strengthening procedures

Procedures that change direction of muscle action

Adjustable sutures

Introduction

Actions of extraocular muscles

The lateral and medial walls of the orbit make an angle of 45° with each other (*Figure 14.1a*). The orbital axis therefore forms an angle of 22.5° with both the lateral and medial wall. For the sake of simplicity this angle is usually regarded as being 23°. When the eye is looking straight ahead at a fixed point on the horizon with the head erect (primary position of gaze), its optical axis forms an angle of 23° with the orbital axis (*Figure 14.1b*). The actions of the extraocular muscles depend on the position of the globe at the time of muscle contraction. The *primary* action of a muscle is its major effect when the eye is in the *primary* position and its subsidiary actions are the additional effects on the position of the eye.

Horizontal recti

When the eye is in the primary position, the horizontal recti are purely horizontal movers around the vertical Z axis and have only a primary action.

Vertical recti

The vertical recti run in the same line as the orbital axis and are inserted in front of the equator. For this reason they form an angle of 23° with the optical axis (*Figure 14.1c*).

Superior rectus

In the primary position, the primary action of the superior rectus is elevation (*Figure 14.2a*). This movement occurs about the X axis which traverses the eye from right to left, passing through the centre of the globe at the equator. The subsidiary actions of the superior rectus are adduction and intorsion.

When the globe is in a position of 23° of abduction, the optical and orbital axes coincide (*Figure 14.2b*). In this position it has no subsidiary actions and can only act as an elevator. This is therefore the best position of the globe for testing the function of the superior rectus muscle.

If the globe was in a position of 67° of adduction the angle between the optical and orbital axes would be 90° (*Figure 14.2c*). In this position the superior rectus could only act as an intortor.

Superior oblique

The obliques are inserted behind the equator and they form an angle of 51° with the optical axis (*Figure 14.1d*). In the primary position, the primary action of the superior oblique is intorsion (*Figure 14.3a*). This movement occurs about the Y axis which passes sagittally through the centre of the pupil. In this position, subsidiary actions are depression and abduction.

When the globe is in a position of 51° of adduction, the optical axis of the globe coincides with the line of pull of the muscle. In this position it can only act as a depressor (*Figure 14.3b*). This is, therefore, the best position of the globe for clinically testing the action of the superior oblique muscle.

When the eye is abducted by 39°, the optical axis and the line of pull of the superior oblique make an angle of 90° with each other. In this position the superior oblique can only cause intorsion (*Figure 14.3c*).

With this basic knowledge it is easy to work out the respective actions of the inferior rectus and inferior oblique muscles.

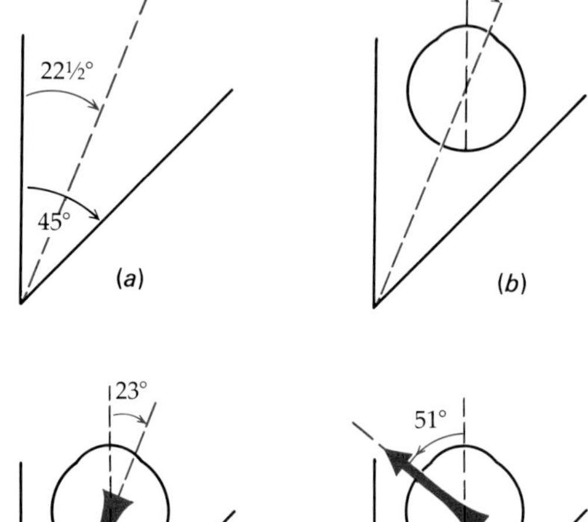

Figure 14.1 *Applied anatomy of extraocular muscles*

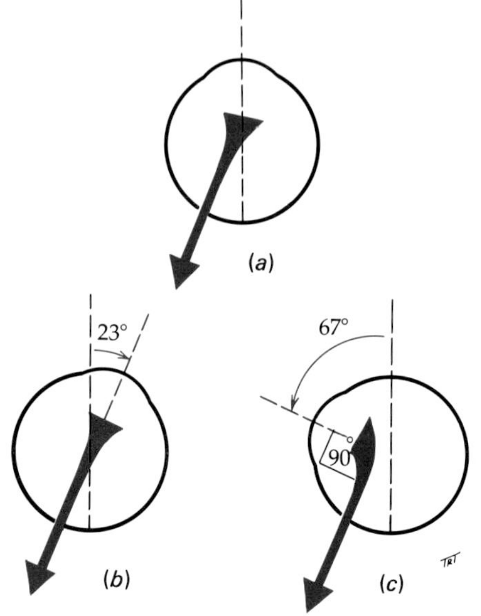

Figure 14.2 *Actions of the superior rectus muscle*

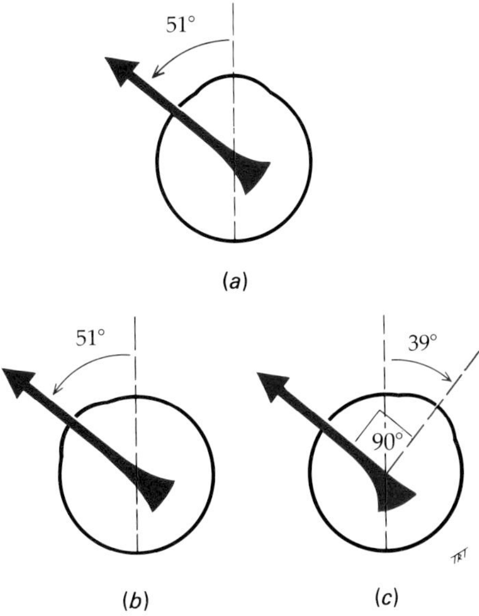

Figure 14.3 *Actions of the superior oblique muscle*

Eye movements

Eye movements are of three types: ductions, versions, and vergences.

Ductions

Ductions are monocular eye movements consisting of adduction, abduction, elevation (sursumduction), depression (deorsumduction), intorsion (incycloduction), and extorsion (excycloduction).

Agonist. This is the primary muscle moving the eye in any given direction.

Synergist. This is a muscle which acts in conjunction with the agonist to produce a given movement.

Antagonist. This muscle acts in the opposite direction to the agonist.

Sherrington's law of reciprocal innervation

This fundamental law implies that increased innervation and contraction of a muscle is automatically associated with a reciprocal decrease in innervation and contraction (relaxation) of its antagonist.

Versions

Versions are binocular movements in which the two eyes move synchronously and symmetrically in the same direction. These movements are:

1. *Dextroversion* (right gaze), laevoversion (left gaze), sursumversion (elevation or up-gaze), and deorsumversion (depression or down-gaze). These four movements bring the eyes into the *secondary positions of gaze.*
2. *Dextroelevation* (gaze up and right), dextrodepression (gaze down and right), laevoelevation (gaze up and left), and laevodepression (gaze down and left). These four oblique movements bring the eyes into the *tertiary positions of gaze.*
3. *Dextrocycloversion* (rotation of the superior limbus of both eyes to the right) and laevocycloversion (rotation to the left).

Cardinal positions of gaze

The six cardinal positions of gaze are: dextroversion and laevoversion, dextroelevation and laevoelevation, dextrodepression and laevodepression. Although there are *nine* positions of gaze only *six* of these are cardinal.

Yoke muscles

When the eyes are moving into each of the six cardinal positions of gaze, a muscle of one eye is paired with a muscle of the opposite eye (*Figure 14.4*). For example, in dextroversion the two yoke muscles are the right lateral rectus and the left medial rectus. In dextroelevation the

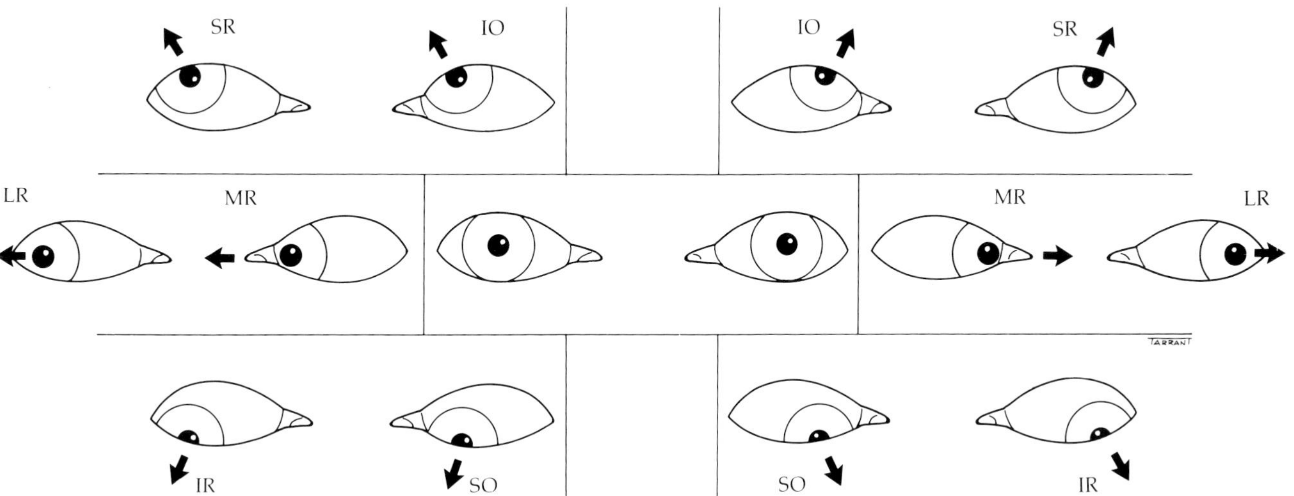

Figure 14.4 *Six cardinal positions of gaze*

yoke muscles are the right superior rectus and the left inferior oblique.

Hering's law

Hering's law states that during any conjugate eye movement, equal and simultaneous innervation flows to the yoke muscles. In the case of a paretic squint, the amount of innervation to both eyes is always determined by the fixating eye, so that the angle of deviation will vary according to which eye is used for fixation. For example if, in the case of a right lateral rectus palsy, the left eye is used for fixation, there will be an inward deviation of the right eye due to the unopposed action of its antagonist (right medial rectus). The amount of misalignment of the two eyes in this situation is called the *primary deviation* (*Figure 14.5*). If the paretic right eye is now used for fixation, additional innervation will flow to the right lateral rectus. However, according to Hering's law, an equal amount of innervation will also flow to the left medial rectus (yoke muscle). This will result in an overaction of the left medial rectus and an excessive amount of adduction. The amount of misalignment between the two eyes in this situation is called the *secondary deviation*.

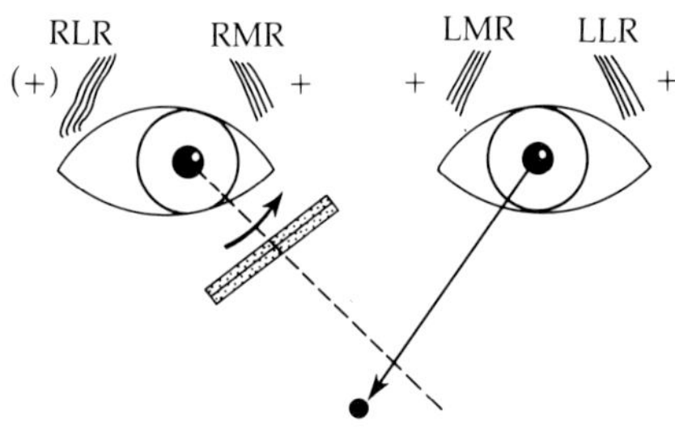

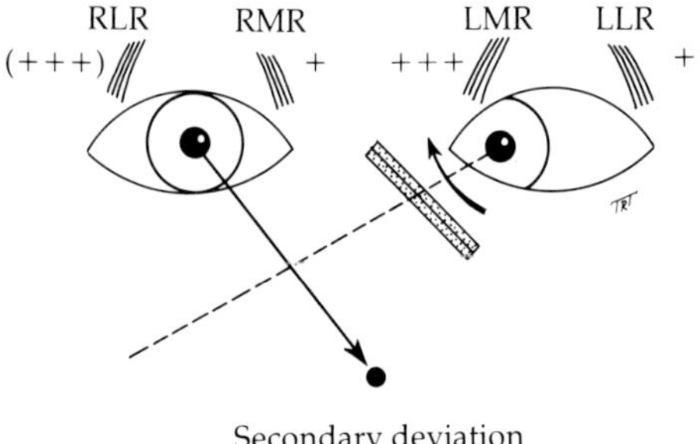

Figure 14.5 *Hering's law*

Vergences

Vergences are binocular movements in which the two eyes move synchronously and symmetrically in *opposite* directions. Convergence is the ability of the two eyes to turn inwards, and divergence is their ability to turn outwards from a convergent position.

Convergence

Convergence may be voluntary or reflex. Reflex convergence has four components:

1. *Tonic* convergence implies some inherent innervational tone to the extraocular muscles when the patient is awake.
2. *Proximal* convergence is induced by the psychological awareness of a near object.
3. *Fusional* convergence is an optomotor reflex that ensures that similar retinal images are projected onto corresponding retinal areas. It occurs without a change in refractive state of the eye and is initiated by a bitemporal retinal image disparity.
4. *Accommodative* convergence is induced by the act of accommodation as part of the synkinetic-near reflex. Each dioptre of accommodation is accompanied by a fairly constant increment in accommodative-convergence, giving the 'accommodative-convergence to accommodation' (AC/A) ratio.

Divergence

The only clinically significant form of divergence is fusional divergence. It is similar to fusional convergence but is initiated by binasal retinal image disparity.

AC/A ratio

The AC/A ratio is the amount of convergence measured in prism dioptres per unit (D) change in accommodation. The normal value is 4 Δ. This means that 1 D of accommodation is associated with 4 Δ of accommodative convergence.

The AC/A ratio is independent of the state of refraction and cannot be altered by orthoptics. Abnormalities of the AC/A ratio are very significant causes of strabismus. A high ratio may cause excessive convergence and may produce an esotropia during accommodation on a near object. A low ratio may cause an exotropia when the patient looks at a near object.

Fusional vergences

The fusional vergence mechanism produces corrective eye movements to overcome retinal image disparity. Fusional amplitude refers to the maximal amount of eye movement produced by fusional vergence. Fusional vergence amplitudes can be measured by using prisms or the synoptophore. The normal fusional convergence amplitude for distance is about 15 Δ, and 25 Δ for near. The normal fusional divergence amplitudes are less. Fusional convergence helps to control an exophoria, and fusional divergence helps to control an esophoria. The fusional vergence mechanism may be decreased by fatigue or illness, converting a phoria to a tropia. The amplitude of fusional vergence mechanisms can be improved by orthoptic exercises. This works best for the near fusional convergence, particularly for the relief of convergence insufficiency.

Binocular single vision

Binocular single vision is achieved by the use of the two eyes together, so that separate and slightly dissimilar images arising in each eye are appreciated as a single image by the process of fusion. In addition to achieving single vision, this synthesis also results in stereopsis or three-dimensional vision. Binocular single vision is acquired and reinforced during the first few years of life and requires three factors for its development.

1. Reasonably clear vision in both eyes.
2. The ability of the visual areas in the brain to promote fusion of the two slightly dissimilar images.
3. The precise coordination of the two eyes for all directions of gaze.

If fusion is to be achieved there must exist a precise physiological relationship between the two retinae (retinal correspondence).

Projection

In order to understand the meaning of retinal correspondence, it is first necessary to consider the phenomenon of projection. Projection is defined as the interpretation of the position of an object in space on the basis of the stimulated retinal elements. If a red object stimulates the right fovea (F), and a black object which lies in the nasal field stimulates a temporal retinal element (T), the red object will be interpreted by the brain as having originated from the straight ahead position and the black object will be interpreted as having originated in the nasal field (*Figure 14.6a*). This is normal projection. Similarly, nasal retinal elements project into the temporal field and upper retinal elements into the lower field and vice versa. Projection is to the same distance as that of the fixation object.

With both eyes open, the red fixation object is now stimulating both foveae, which are corresponding retinal points. The black object is now not only stimulating the temporal retinal elements in the right eye but also the nasal elements of the left eye. The right eye therefore projects the object into its nasal field and the left eye projects the object into its temporal field. However, because both of these retinal elements are corresponding points they will both project the object into the same position in space and there will be no double vision (*Figure 14.6b*).

Horopter

The horopter is an imaginary surface in space, all points of which still stimulate corresponding retinal elements and which are, therefore, projected to the same position in space.

Panum's area

Panum's area of single binocular vision is a zone surrounding points on the horopter in which objects are seen singly. Objects in front of or behind Panum's area are seen 'double'. This is the basis of physiological diplopia.

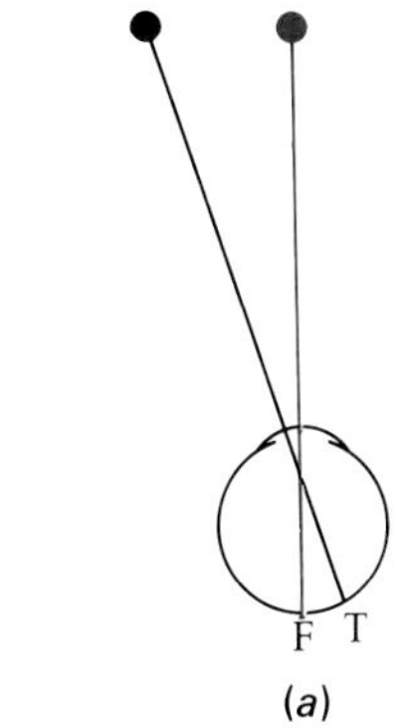

(*a*)

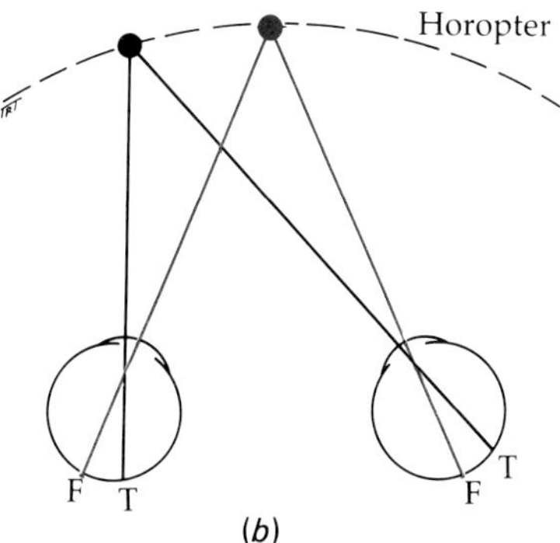

(*b*)

Figure 14.6 *Principles of projection*

Visual axis

The visual axis is a line that passes through the point of fixation and the fovea. The two visual axes intersect at the point of fixation (red object) (*Figure 14.7a*). Light coming from the red object will stimulate both foveae which are corresponding retinal points. Due to the separation of the two eyes in the head, each fovea will perceive a slightly different image. These two images will be fused into one stereoscopic image by the brain, so that the single image will be projected into the straight ahead position in space.

Double vision

A squint is a misalignment of the visual axes. It may be latent or manifest. A manifest deviation will cause double vision. There are two components to double vision: confusion and diplopia.

Confusion (*Figure 14.7b*)

In the case of a right convergent squint the two axes will be misaligned so that they will not intersect at the point of fixation. The left fovea will still be stimulated by the red object, but the right fovea will now be stimulated by a different object (black triangle). The superimposition of these two different objects and their projection into the same straight ahead position in space results in confusion.

Diplopia (*Figure 14.7c*)

The single red object now stimulates non-corresponding retinal points. In the left eye, it stimulates the fovea and is therefore projected into the straight ahead position. In the right eye, it stimulates a point that is nasal to the fovea and will therefore be projected into the temporal field. This will result in diplopia. A convergent squint causes an uncrossed or homonymous diplopia, whereas a divergent squint causes a crossed or heteronymous diplopia.

Compensatory mechanisms for double vision

There are three ways in which a patient can compensate for double vision (*Figure 14.8*).

Suppression

An adaptation that occurs mainly in children is the development of suppression, which is produced subconsciously by an 'active neglect' of the vision in the squinting eye by the visual cortex. Suppression is a temporary phenomenon which only occurs when both eyes are open (*Figure 14.8a*). When the fixating eye is covered the suppression ceases immediately and the squinting eye takes up fixation (*Figure 14.8b*). Clinically, suppression can be classified into three types:

1. *Central versus peripheral.* In central suppression the image from the fovea of the deviating eye is inhibited in order to avoid confusion. Diplopia, on the other hand, is eradicated by the process of peripheral suppression, in which the awareness of the image falling on the peripheral retina of the deviating eye is inhibited.
2. *Monocular versus alternating.* Suppression is said to be monocular when the image from the dominant eye always predominates over the image from the deviating eye, so that the image from the deviating eye is constantly suppressed. This type of suppression leads to the development of strabismic amblyopia. When suppression is alternating and switches from one eye to the other, amblyopia does not develop.
3. *Facultative versus obligatory.* Facultative suppression occurs only when the eyes are in the deviated position. Obligatory suppression is present at all times, irrespective of whether the eyes are deviated or straight.

Strabismic amblyopia

This probably occurs as a result of continued monocular suppression of the deviated eye. It is characterized by a unilateral impairment of vision which is present even when the eye is forced to fixate (*Figure 14.8c*). The characteristics of an amblyopic eye are as follows:

1. *Visual acuity* is reduced.

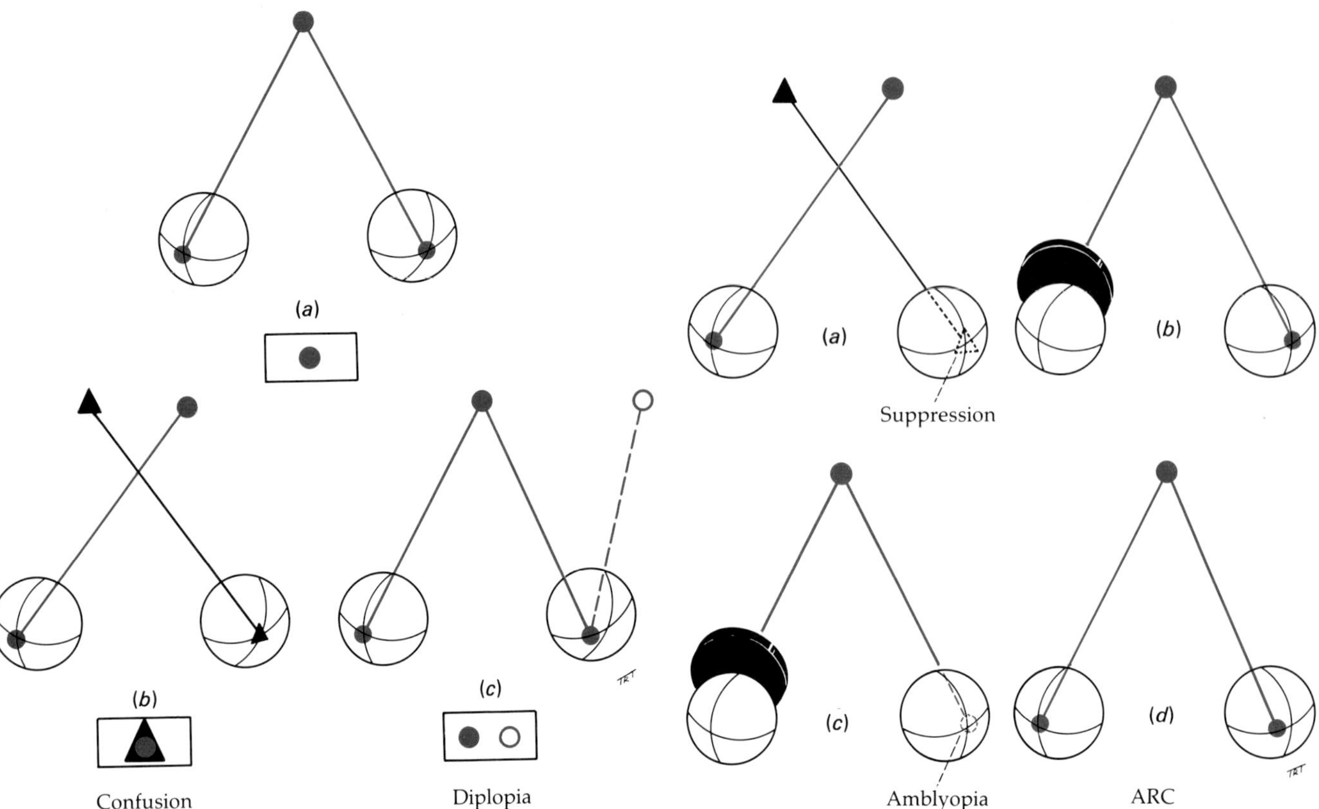

Figure 14.7 *Double vision*

Figure 14.8 *Compensatory mechanisms for double vision*

2. *Crowding phenomenon.* Visual acuity is better when single letters are presented to the patient than when the patient is asked to read a whole row of letters.
3. *Neutral density filter test.* There is virtually no change of visual acuity of the amblyopic eye when the patient reads through a neutral density filter. A normal eye will have a drop in acuity of about one or two lines, whereas an eye with an organic lesion may have a larger drop of visual acuity. It appears that an amblyopic eye has a visual acuity similar to a normal eye under conditions of reduced illumination.

Apart from strabismic amblyopia there are two other main types:

1. *Anisometropic amblyopia* occurs in the more ametropic eye as a result of a constantly blurred image of an object falling onto its fovea. It may coexist with strabismic amblyopia.
2. *Stimulus deprivation amblyopia* is caused by opacities to the media or ptosis occurring in infancy or early childhood.

Anomalous (abnormal) retinal correspondence

In anomalous retinal correspondence (ARC) the retinal elements of the squinting eye assume an anomalous relationship with the fovea or other areas of the non-squinting eye (*Figure 14.8d*). This occurs in young children with long-standing squint in which a crude type of binocular vision can be obtained despite the presence of squint.

Abnormal head posture

This occurs in adults who cannot suppress or in children who have good binocular vision potential. The purpose of adopting an abnormal head posture is to turn the eyes as far away as possible from the field of action of the weak muscle. This involves turning the head into the direction of the field of action of the weak muscle so that the eyes are then automatically turned in the opposite direction.

Horizontal deviation

A patient will turn his face to make up for a horizontal deviation. For example, if one of the muscles that turn the eyes to the left is paralysed, the face will *also* be turned to the left so that the eyes will then be automatically deviated to the right.

Vertical deviation

A patient will elevate or depress his chin to make up for a vertical deviation. If one of the elevators is weak, the patient will elevate his chin so that the eyes then become depressed.

Torsional deviation

A patient will make up for a torsional deviation by tilting his head to one or other shoulder. If, for example, an intortor such as the right superior oblique is paralysed, the eye will become extorted. In order to compensate for this and cause the right eye to intort, the head will have to be tilted to the left shoulder.

Clinical evaluation

History

1. *Age of onset.* In general, the earlier the onset the more likely is the need for surgical correction (infantile esotropia). The later the onset the greater the likelihood that the deviation has an accommodative element.
2. *Family history.* Strabismus is frequently hereditary. It is also of interest to find out what form of therapy was necessary to correct the deviation in other family members.
3. *Variability.* If the deviation is worse when the child is tired or ill, an accommodative element is likely to be present.
4. *Intermittent or constant.* In intermittent cases, it is likely that some form of binocularity is still present and the prognosis is better than in a constant squint.
5. *Unilateral or alternating.* If one eye constantly turns in, the presence of amblyopia should be suspected.
6. *Diplopia.* The presence of diplopia in an older child (age 4–5 years) might suggest a paretic component due to neurological disease.
7. *Head turn or tilt.* Old photographs showing an abnormal head posture are suggestive of a long-standing deviation.

Examination

Prism and reflection tests

Hirschberg

This is a rough objective test to estimate the angle of a manifest strabismus in uncooperative patients or those with poor fixation. A light is shone into the eyes and the deviation of the corneal light reflex from the centre of the pupil is noted in the squinting eye. If the reflex is situated at the temporal border of the pupil, the angle is about 15° and, if it is at the limbus, the angle of the squint measures about 45°. This applies to both eso- and exodeviations.

This test is also useful in detecting pseudostrabismus. A *pseudo-esotropia* can be caused by a combination of wide flat nasal bridge, broad epicanthic folds, and close-set eyes. A *pseudo-exotropia* can be due to a shortening of the temporal canthus.

Angle kappa is the angle between the visual axis and the anatomical axis of the eye. Normally the fovea is situated temporal to the optical axis. A light shone onto the cornea will therefore cause a reflex just nasal to the centre of the cornea in both eyes. This is termed a 'positive angle kappa', and when it is large it may simulate an exotropia. A negative angle kappa occurs when the fovea is situated nasal to the optic axis (high myopia and ectopic fovea). In this situation, the corneal reflex is situated temporal to the centre of the cornea and it may simulate an esotropia.

Base-out prism

Image displacement by using base-out prisms and observing the presence of corrective eye movements is a sensitive way of detecting the presence of binocular single vision. In the presence of a small scotoma associated with a small angle squint (microtropia) a 4 Δ base-out prism will not induce a corrective movement when placed in front of the squinting eye. A stronger prism (20 Δ) can be used as a screening test for binocular single vision in infants in whom the small corrective movements induced by a 4 Δ prism may be difficult to detect.

Krimsky

In this test, prisms are placed in front of the deviated eye until the corneal light reflexes are symmetrical.

Cover tests

These tests are based on the patient's ability to fixate with each eye. Attention and cooperation are also required.

Cover–uncover

This is a monocular test designed to test for the presence of a manifest deviation (heterotropia). It should be performed both for near and distance.

If the left eye shows a displacement of the corneal light reflex, the examiner should cover the opposite *right eye* and search for any movement of the *left eye* (*Figure 14.9*). If the left eye moves nasally to take up fixation, the diagnosis is an exotropia. If it moves temporally, the diagnosis is esotropia. If it moves down, the diagnosis is hypertropia. If it moves up, the diagnosis is hypotropia. If there is no movement of the eye, it can be concluded that no manifest deviation of the left eye is present and the test is repeated for the opposite eye.

It is therefore apparent that a patient with a heterotropia will have a manifest deviation, before, during, and after the completion of the cover–uncover test. If, after the completion of the test, the opposite eye remains deviated, an alternating heterotropia is present.

Alternate cover

If no deviation is demonstrable on the cover–uncover test, the alternate cover test should next be performed in order to detect the presence of a latent deviation (heterophoria). In performing this test one eye is covered for about 2 seconds and then the cover is quickly shifted to the opposite eye. At this moment the examiner should note any movement of the *uncovered* eye as it assumes fixation. If no movement occurs, the patient is orthophoric. A nasal movement implies an exophoria, a temporal movement an esophoria, and a downward movement, a hyperphoria.

It is, therefore, apparent that a patient with a heterophoria will have straight eyes before and also after the alternate cover test has been performed. However, during the test, a deviation will be induced due to interruption of fusional mechanisms. It should be emphasized that if the alternate cover test is performed before the cover–uncover test, it will be impossible for the examiner to differentiate a tropia from a phoria.

Prism and alternate cover

This measures the total deviation (latent + manifest), and it does not separate tropia from phoria. Hand-held prisms are placed in front of one eye with the base of the prism placed in the direction that is opposite to the deviation. For example, in a convergent squint the prism is held base-out. The alternate cover test is then performed (*Figure 14.10*). The end-point is reached when the prism negates ocular movements. The angle of deviation is read from the strength of the prism.

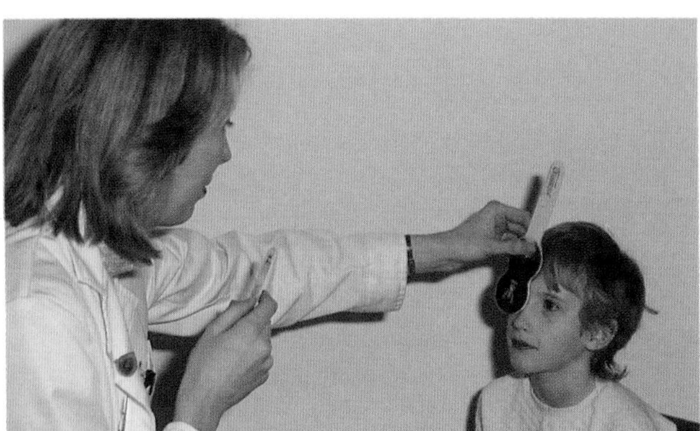

Figure 14.9 *Cover–uncover test*

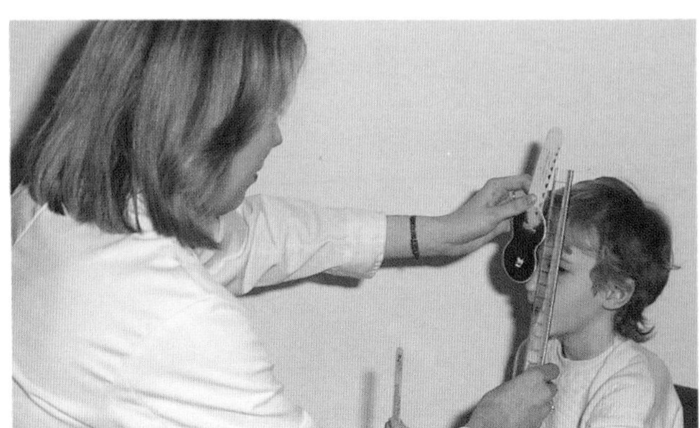

Figure 14.10 *Prism and alternate cover test*

Dissimilar image tests

These tests are based on the patient's appreciation of diplopia created by two dissimilar images.

Maddox wing

The Maddox wing is an instrument that dissociates the two eyes for near fixation (one-third of a metre) and measures the amount of heterophoria.

The instrument is constructed in such a way that the right eye sees only a white vertical arrow and a red horizontal arrow, while the left eye sees only a horizontal and a vertical row of numbers. The horizontal deviation is measured by asking the patient which number the white arrow points to. The vertical deviation is measured by asking the patient which number the red arrow intersects (*Figure 14.11*). The amount of cyclophoria is determined by asking the patient to move the red arrow so that it is parallel with the horizontal row of numbers.

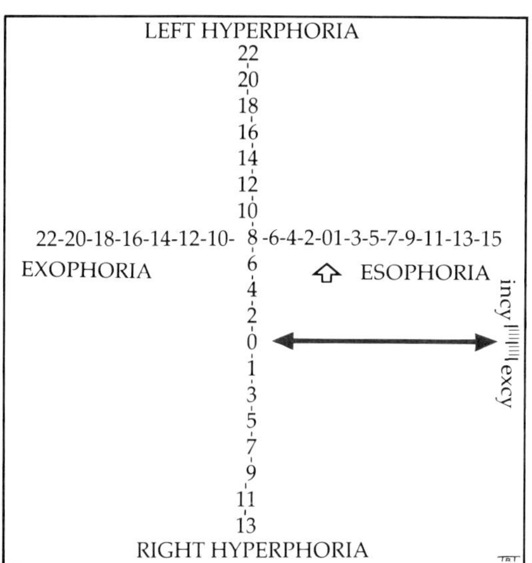

Figure 14.11 *Maddox wing test*

Maddox rod

The Maddox rod consists of a series of fused cylindrical red glass rods which convert the appearance of a white spot of light into a red streak (*Figure 14.12*). The optical properties of the rods cause the streak of light to be at an angle of 90° with the long axis of the rods. (This means that when the glass rods are held horizontally, the streak will be vertical, and vice versa.) The rods are placed in front of the right eye. This dissociates the two eyes because the red streak seen by the right eye cannot be fused with the unaltered white spot seen by the left eye. The amount of dissociation is measured by the superimposition of the two images by means of prisms. The base of the prism is placed in the position opposite to the direction of the deviation. Both vertical and horizontal deviations can be measured in this way.

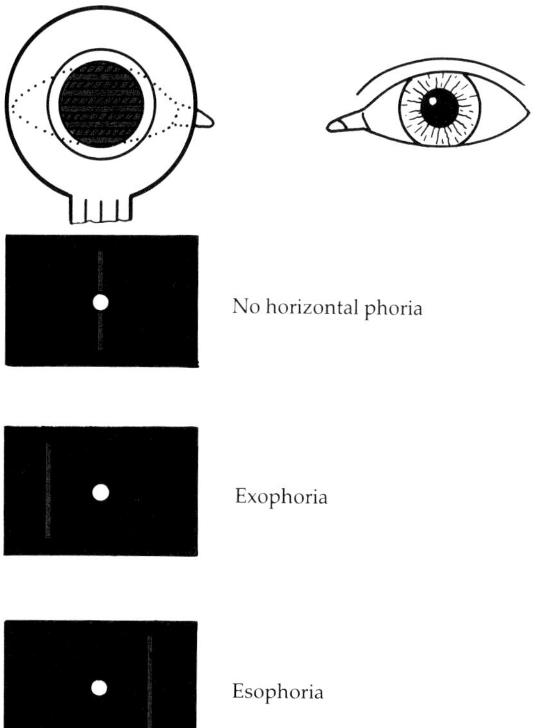

Figure 14.12 *Maddox rod test*

Hess

The patient wears red-green filter goggles (*Figure 14.13*) and holds a *green* light projection pointer. The clinician holds a *red* light projection pointer which is used as the point of fixation. This means that when the red filter is in front of the patient's right eye only the right eye can see the red light projected onto the screen and therefore the right eye is fixating.

By convention, the test is started with the red filter in front of the right eye. The clinician then projects the red

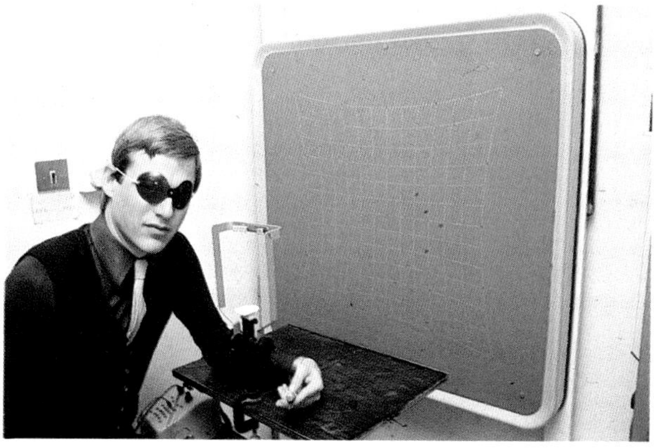

Figure 14.13 *Hess test (courtesy of Mr K. Gross)*

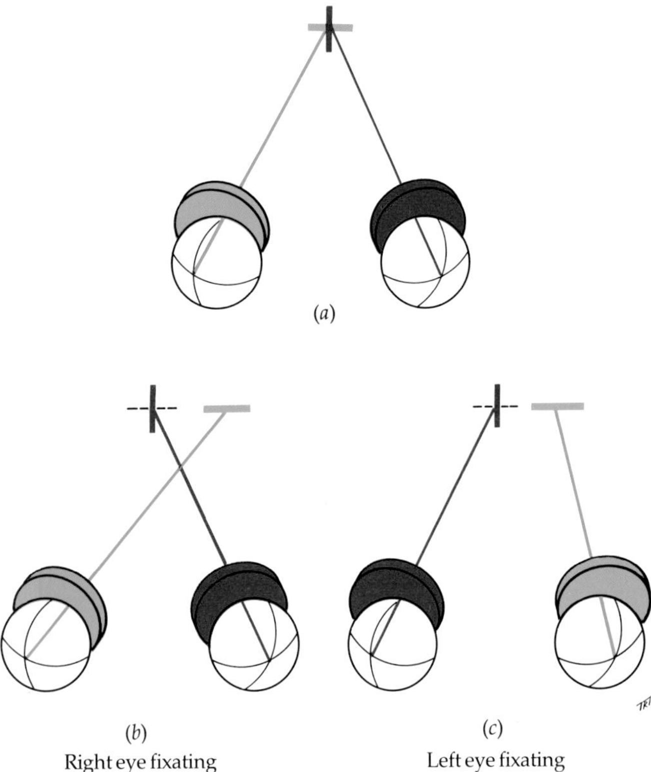

Figure 14.14 *Principles of Hess test*

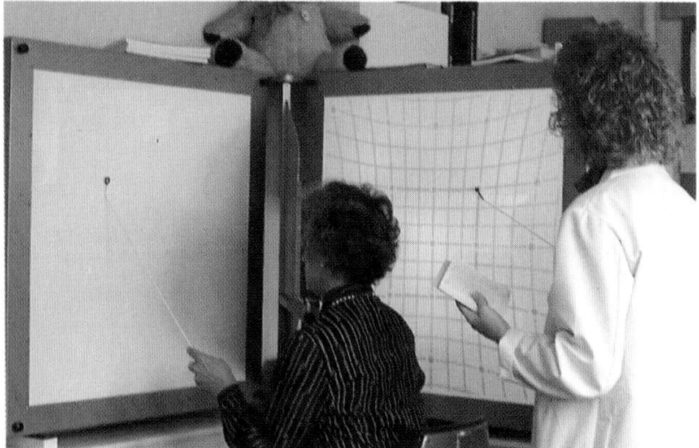

Figure 14.15 *Lees screen*

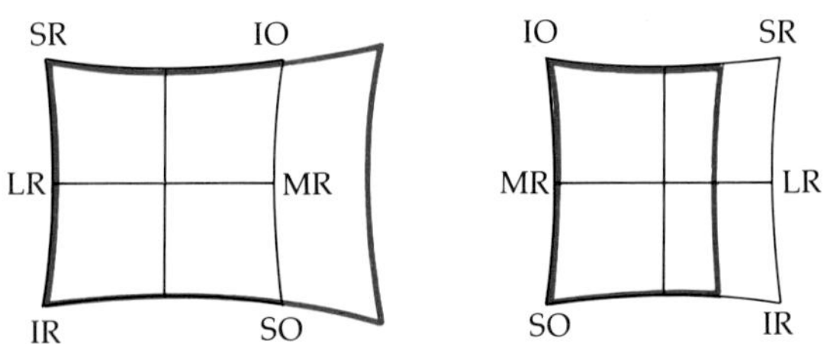

Figure 14.16 *Hess chart in right lateral rectus palsy*

light onto the screen and the patient is asked to superimpose his green light onto the red light. In normal circumstances the two pointers should be nearly superimposed in all nine positions of gaze (*Figure 14.14a*).

The goggles are then reversed so that the red filter is in front of the left eye and the procedure is repeated. If the patient has a right lateral rectus palsy and fixates with his right eye (red filter), excessive innervation will flow to the left normal medial rectus (Hering's law) so that the patient's green marker will indicate a point on the screen that is beyond the correct alignment (*Figure 14.14b*).

If the patient now fixates with his left normal eye (red filter), only a normal amount of innervation will be required to take up fixation. However, because the right lateral rectus is paretic, the patient's green marker will indicate a point that is short of the correct alignment (*Figure 14.14c*).

When the test has been completed the relative positions are connected by straight lines.

The Lees screen is similar to the Hess test but dissociation is carried out by a mirror and not red-green goggles (*Figure 14.15*). The apparatus consists of two glass screens at right angles to each other, bisected by a two-sided plane mirror. *The Lancaster red-green test* is popular in the United States and is also similar to the Hess test.

Interpretation of Hess chart (*Figure 14.16*)

The two charts are compared. The smaller chart indicates the eye with the paretic muscle (right eye). The larger chart indicates the eye with the overacting muscle (left eye). The smaller chart will show its greatest restriction in the main direction of action of the paretic muscle (right lateral rectus), and the larger chart will show its greatest expansion in the main direction of action of the yoke muscle (left medial rectus).

Change in Hess chart (*Figure 14.17*)

The Hess test is not only used in the diagnosis of the paretic muscle but it is also extremely useful as a prognostic guide. For example, a right superior rectus palsy will show underaction of the affected muscle with an overaction of its yoke muscle (left inferior oblique) (*Figure 14.17a*). Because of the great incomitance of the two charts, the diagnosis is straightforward. If the paretic muscle recovers its function, both charts will revert to normal.

However, if the paresis persists, the shapes of both charts will change. With time, a secondary contracture of the ipsilateral antagonist (right inferior rectus) will develop, which will show up on the chart as an overaction. This will lead to a secondary (inhibitional) palsy of the antagonist of the yoke muscle (left superior oblique), which will show up on the chart as an underaction (*Figure 14.17b*). This could lead to the incorrect impression that the left superior oblique was the primary muscle at fault. With the further passage of time, the two charts become more and more concomitant until it may be impossible to determine which was the primary paretic muscle (*Figure 14.17c*).

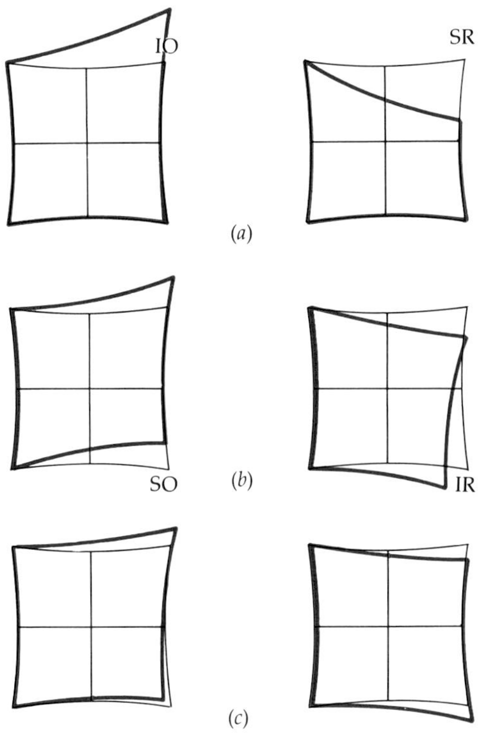

Figure 14.17 Changes in Hess chart with time

Tests for ARC and sensory anomalies

These are of two types: the first stimulate the fovea of one eye and the extrafoveal area of the opposite eye, and the second stimulate both foveae.

Worth's four dot

The patient wears a red lens in front of his right eye which filters out all colours except red. A green lens is placed in front of his left eye which will filter out all colours except green. He then views a box with four lights—one red, two green, and one white.

If the patient sees all four lights he has normal fusion (*Figure 14.18a*). If he sees four lights in the presence of a manifest squint he has ARC (*Figure 14.18b*). If he sees two red lights he has left suppression (*Figure 14.18c*). If he sees three green lights he has right suppression (*Figure 14.18d*). If he sees two red and three green lights he has diplopia (*Figure 14.18e*). If he reports that the green and red lights alternate he has alternating suppression.

After-image

This test demonstrates the visual direction of the two foveae. The right fovea is stimulated by a vertical bright flash of light and the left fovea by a horizontal flash. The patient then draws the relative positions of the after-images.

If the two after-images are seen as a cross he has normal retinal correspondence. If he has ARC the two images will

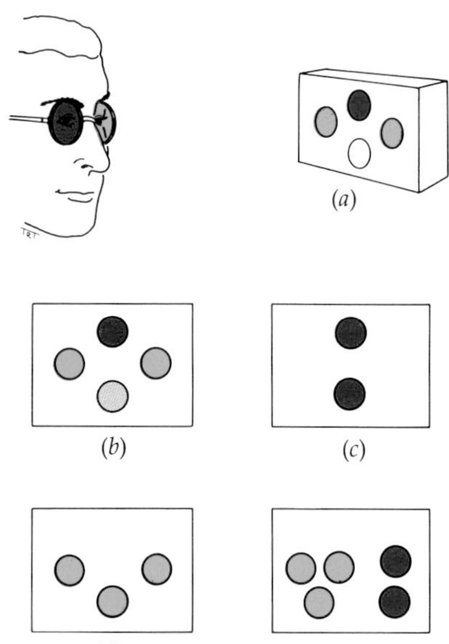

Figure 14.18 Worth's four dot test

not cross. In the case of an esotropia with ARC, the vertical after-image (belonging to the right eye) will be seen to the left of the horizontal after-image (belonging to the left eye). These findings are reversed in an exotropia.

Bagolini striated glasses

Each glass is covered with fine striations which convert a light point into a line (similar to a Maddox rod). The two lenses are placed in a trial frame at 45° and 135° in front of each eye. This enables dissimilar images to be presented to each eye under natural conditions. In normals as well as those with ARC the two lines will intersect at the point of light in the form of a cross.

Synoptophore

The synoptophore (*Figure 14.19*) is an instrument for the assessment of squint and the grade of binocular vision. It is also able to detect the presence of suppression, amblyopia, and ARC.

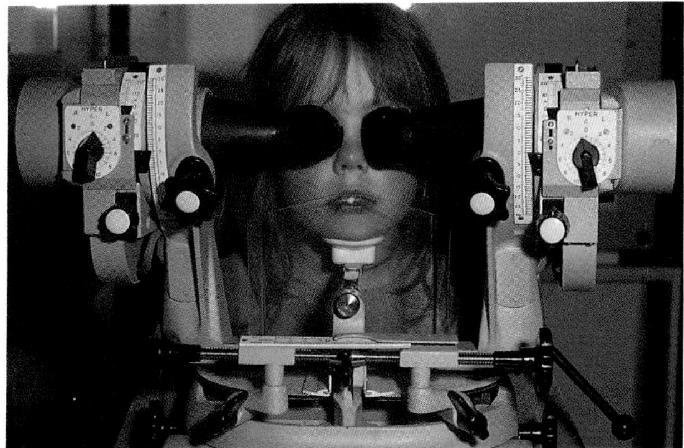

Figure 14.19 The synoptophore

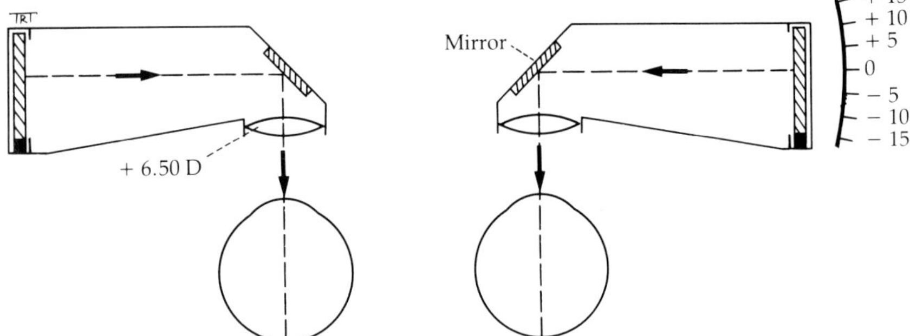

Figure 14.20 Optical principles of the synoptophore

The instrument consists of two cylindrical tubes with a mirrored right-angled bend and a +6.50 D lens in each eyepiece (*Figure 14.20*). Pictures are inserted in a slide carrier situated at the outer end of each tube. The two tubes are supported on columns which enable the pictures to be moved in relation to each other, and any adjustments are indicated on a scale.

Grades of binocular vision (*Figure 14.21*)

First grade is called simultaneous perception. This is tested by introducing two dissimilar but not mutually antagonistic pictures, such as a bird and a cage. The subject is then asked to put the bird into the cage by altering the columns. If the two pictures cannot be seen simultaneously then either suppression or amblyopia is present. It is important to note that the term 'simultaneous perception' is somewhat misleading because two dissimilar objects can never be seen in the same position in space. However, using the simultaneous perception pictures, one picture is smaller than the other so that the small one is seen foveally, and the larger one is seen perifoveally.

Second grade is called fusion. This implies the ability of the two eyes to produce a composite picture from two similar pictures each of which is incomplete in one small detail. The classic example is two rabbits each lacking either a tail or a bunch of flowers. If fusion is present, one rabbit complete with tail and holding a bunch of flowers will be seen. The range of fusion is then tested by moving the arms of the synoptophore so that the eyes have to converge and diverge in order to maintain fusion. It is obvious that the presence of simple fusion without any range is of little value in ordinary life.

Third grade is stereopsis. This implies the ability to obtain an impression of depth by the superimposition of two pictures of the same object which have been taken from slightly different angles. The classic example is the bucket which is appreciated in three dimensions.

Detection of ARC

The examiner determines the objective angle of the squint by presenting each fovea alternately with a target until no movement of the eyes is seen. If the images are seen superimposed with the angle between the arms of the synoptophore equal to the objective angle, then retinal correspondence is normal. If the objective and subjective angles are different, ARC is present. In this case the difference in degrees between the subjective and objective angle is the angle of anomaly. ARC is said to be harmonious when the objective angle equals the angle of anomaly and unharmonious when it exceeds the angle of anomaly.

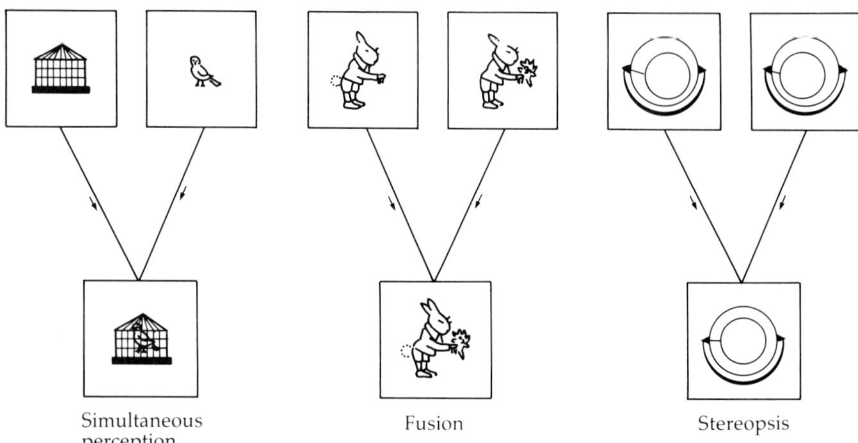

Figure 14.21 Three grades of binocular vision

Tests for stereopsis

The two most commonly used tests for the presence and measurement of stereoscopic depth perception are the Titmus and TNO tests.

Titmus

This consists of a three-dimensional polaroid vectograph consisting of two plates in the form of a booklet. On the right is a large fly, and on the left are a series of circles and animals. The plates are viewed with polaroid glasses (*Figure 14.22*).

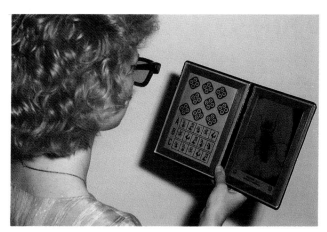

Figure 14.22 *Titmus test*

Fly. This is a test of gross stereopsis and is especially useful for young children. The fly should appear in 'solid' three dimensions and the child can be encouraged to pick up one of its wings. In the absence of gross stereopsis the fly will appear as an ordinary flat photograph.

Circles. This is a graded series which tests fine depth perception. The distance for the test is established at 15′ of arc at 16 inches (405 mm). Each of the nine squares contains four circles. Only one of the circles in each square has a degree of disparity and will appear forward of the plane of reference in the presence of normal fusion. The angle of stereopsis is calculated by referring to a chart provided with the test.

Animals. This is similar to the circles test but consists of three rows of five animals.

TNO

The TNO random dot test consists of seven plates each of which contains various shapes (squares, dots, crosses) created by random dots in complementary colours which are viewed with red-green spectacles (*Figure 14.23*). The plates contain both visible features which can be seen with and without the spectacles as well as 'hidden' shapes which are only apparent when the spectacles are worn and stereopsis is present. The first three plates enable the examiner to quickly establish the presence of stereoscopic vision and other plates are used to determine its level. Because there are no monocular clues, the TNO test provides a truer measurement of stereopsis than the Titmus test.

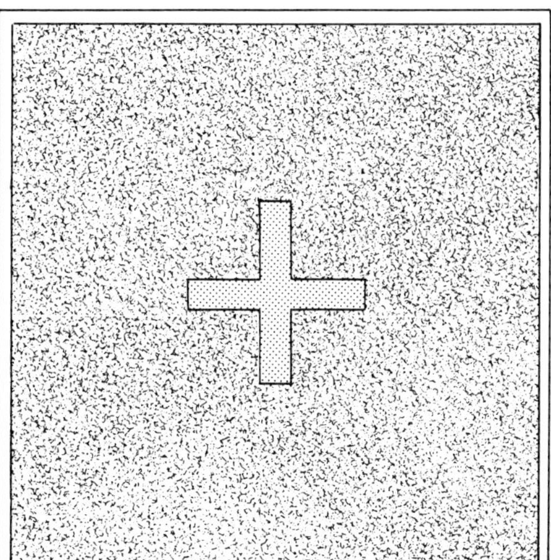

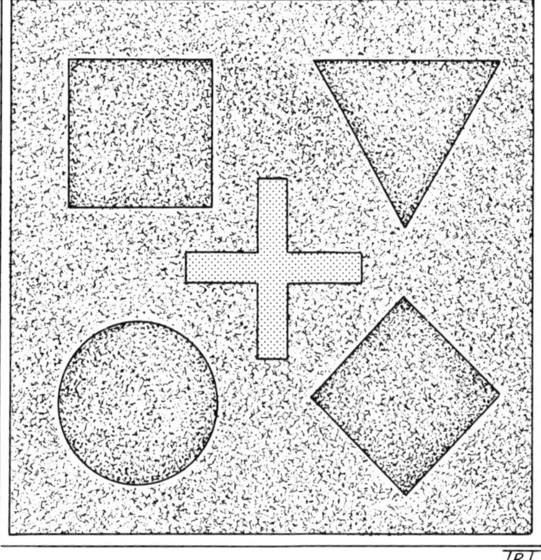

Figure 14.23 *TNO test. Left: cross can be seen both with and without red-green spectacles; right: the four 'hidden' shapes can only be seen with red-green spectacles in the presence of stereopsis*

Childhood esotropias

Esotropia (manifest convergent strabismus) is the most common form of esodeviation in children.

Classification

- Infantile
- Accommodative
  - refractive
  - non-refractive
  - mixed
- Non-accommodative
  - stress induced
  - sensory deprivation
  - divergence insufficiency
  - spasm of near reflex
  - consecutive
  - sixth nerve palsy

Infantile

Although once known as congenital esotropia, this may be defined as esotropia present within the first 6 months of birth. Sometimes the deviation is noted at birth, although more frequently it does not become apparent until later. In the majority of cases the infant is otherwise fit and well although this type of esotropia is common in mentally retarded or brain-damaged infants (cerebral palsy and hydrocephalus).

Clinical features

Angle

The squint usually has a fairly large (*Figure 14.24*) and constant angle except in brain-damaged infants in which it may vary.

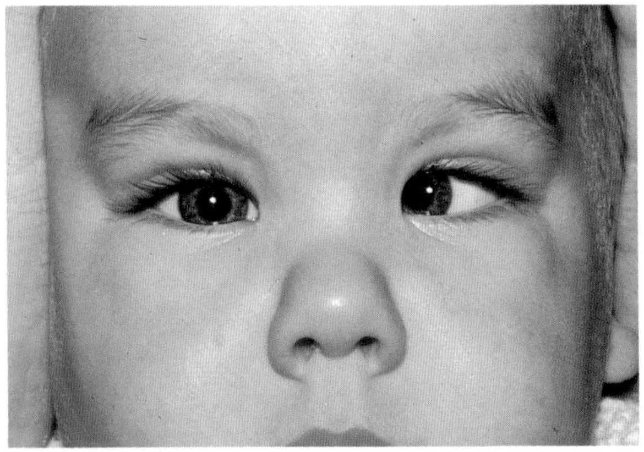

Figure 14.24 *Infantile left esotropia (courtesy of Mr B. Mathalone)*

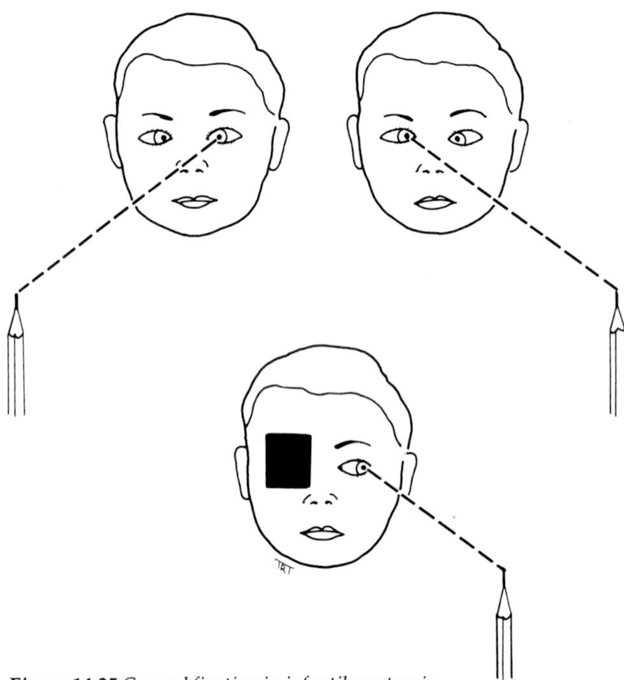

Figure 14.25 *Crossed fixation in infantile esotropia*

Fixation (*Figure 14.25*)

Most infants alternate fixation in the primary position and cross fixate in side-gaze. They will therefore use their right eye in left-gaze and their left eye in right-gaze. This crossed fixation pattern may be confused with a bilateral sixth nerve palsy by the inexperienced observer. However, if one of the eyes is patched for a few hours, the ability to abduct the other eye will become apparent. Children who do not cross fixate may develop amblyopia.

Nystagmus

The nystagmus is usually horizontal, although it may be rotary and typically it decreases on convergence. It has been suggested that children with nystagmus have a high incidence of dissociated vertical deviation (DVD) in later life.

Refractive error

This is usually normal for the age of the child (i.e. slightly hypermetropic), about +1.50 D.

Management

Although it is generally agreed that the management of infantile esotropia is essentially surgical, considerable controversy exists as to the optimum time for treatment (*Figure 14.26*). The present consensus of opinion is that surgery should be performed prior to the age of 18 months.

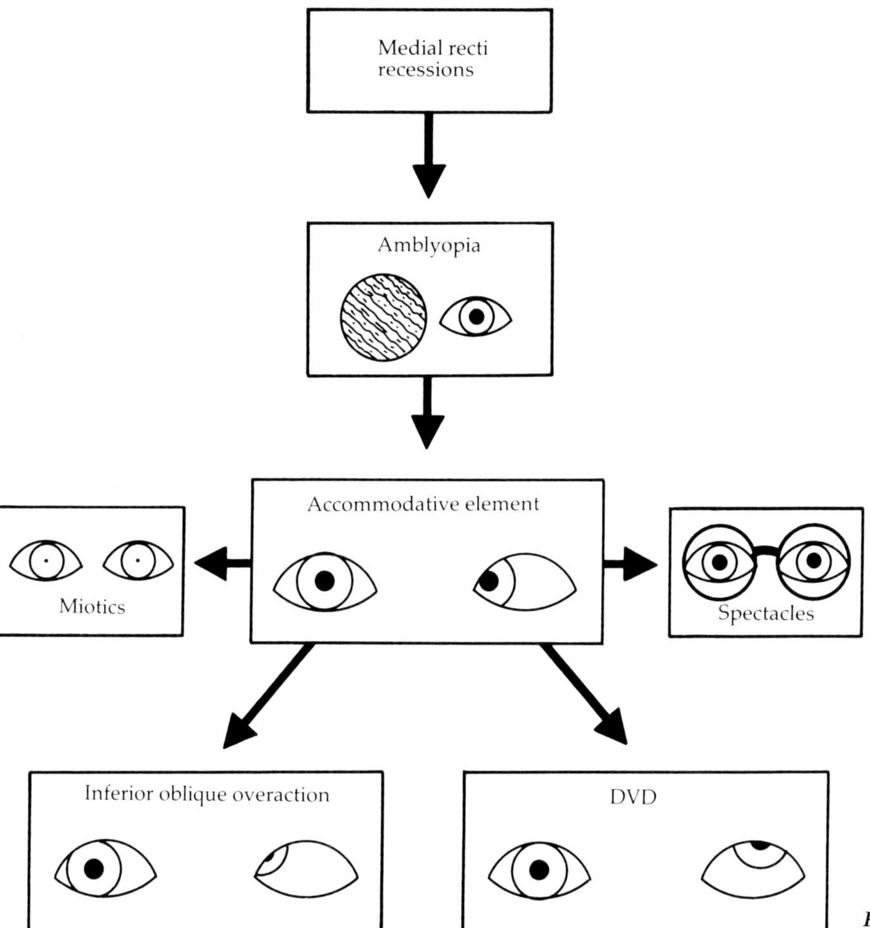

Figure 14.26 Management of infantile esotropia

As is the case in all forms of strabismus, surgery should be carried out only after an accurate assessment of the fundi and the angle of deviation have been made, and any associated refractive errors or amblyopia corrected (*see* later).

Initial surgical procedures

The most popular initial surgical approach is recession of both medial recti (*Figure 14.27*). If the angle is very large, this can be combined with resection of one or both lateral recti. Any associated overactions of the inferior obliques should be treated either by myectomy or recession.

An acceptable goal is alignment of the eyes to within 10 Δ, associated with peripheral fusion and central suppression. This small-angle residual strabismus is compatible with a stable outcome even if bifoveal fusion is not achieved.

Subsequent management

Undercorrection

If the first operation results in an undercorrection, further surgery should be undertaken without too much delay.

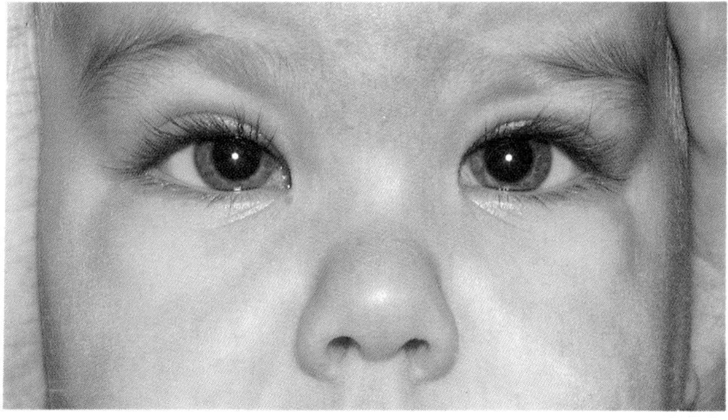

Figure 14.27 Good result following recession of both medial recti

This can consist of resection of one or more of the lateral recti.

Inferior oblique overaction (*Figure 14.28*)

If inferior oblique overaction was not present initially it may develop subsequently, and the clinician should be aware of this possibility and warn the parents that further surgery may be necessary despite an initially acceptable surgical

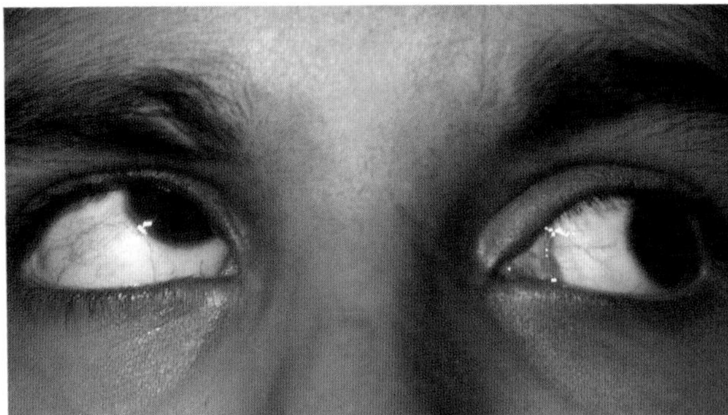

Figure 14.28 Overaction of right inferior oblique

result. The most common age of onset for inferior oblique overaction is 2 years. If the overaction is initially unilateral, it usually becomes bilateral within 6 months.

Dissociated vertical deviation

This complication may appear several years after the initial surgery, particularly in children with nystagmus. DVD is characterized by a upward drift with an excyclodeviation of the eye under cover, or during periods of visual inattention. Although the condition is usually bilateral it may be asymmetrical. Surgical treatment is indicated when the condition is cosmetically unacceptable.

At present the *Faden procedure* is the most effective operation for DVD. The principles of this procedure are described later.

Amblyopia

A careful follow-up of all patients following surgery is essential as about 40% will subsequently develop amblyopia.

Accommodative element

An accommodative element should be suspected if the eyes are initially straight (or nearly straight) after surgery, and then begin to reconverge. It is therefore important to perform repeated refractions on all children and to correct any new accommodative elements to the esotropia accordingly.

Accommodative

An accommodative esodeviation is associated with the activation of the accommodational reflex. If the deviation is within the patient's fusional divergence amplitude, only a latent deviation (esophoria) will result. If the deviation is beyond the patient's fusional amplitude, a manifest deviation will occur.

The three main forms of accommodative esotropia are refractive, non-refractive, or mixed (*Figure 14.29*).

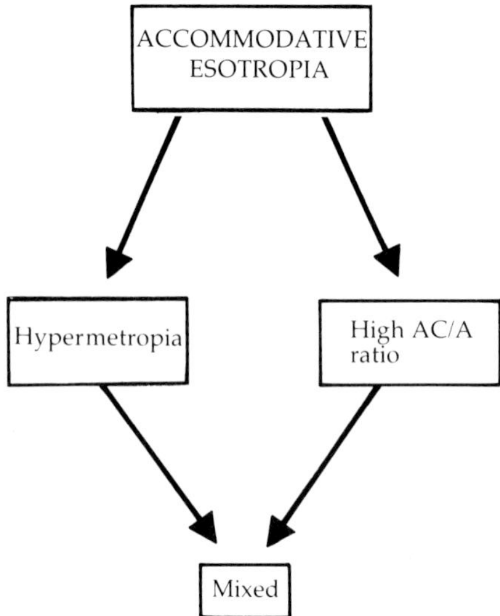

Figure 14.29 Accommodative esotropia types

Clinical features

Typical accommodative esotropia first becomes manifest at about the age of 2.5 years, with a range of 6 months to 7 years. It is frequently hereditary.

Refractive

This is due to excessive hypermetropia (usually between +4 and +7 D). The AC/A ratio is normal so that the distance–near relationships are either normal or no more than 10 Δ in difference.

Example (*Figure 14.30*)

A 4-year-old boy has a refractive error of +5 D in each eye. Without his spectacles the right esotropia measures 30 Δ for distance and 35 Δ for near. There is therefore no significant

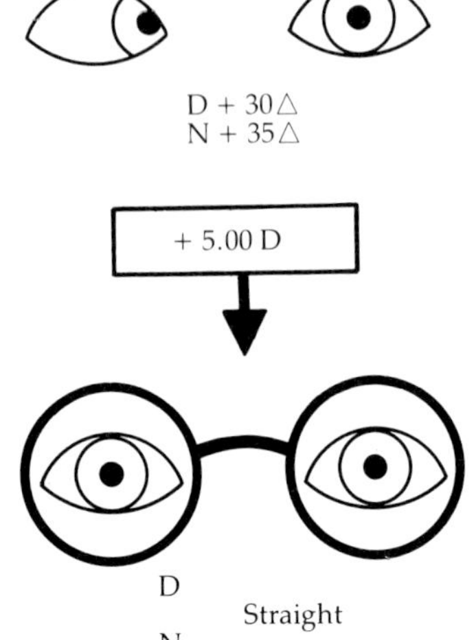

Figure 14.30 Example of refractive accommodative esotropia

significant difference between the angle for near and distance. When wearing his correction lenses his eyes are straight for both near and distance.

This is the fully accommodative type of refractive esotropia because the deviation is controlled completely with spectacles. In these cases the eyes usually remain straight and surgery is not required. However, if anti-accommodative therapy is delayed for some reason, or if the whole extent of the deviation is not correctable with spectacles, then the condition is referred to as a partially accommodative esotropia.

Non-refractive

This is caused by a high AC/A ratio. The refraction is usually normal for the age of the patient. There is little or no deviation for distance but a significant esotropia for near. Not infrequently, the esotropia for near can be induced only by making the patient fixate at a very small target.

Example (*Figure 14.31*)

A 3-year-old girl has a refractive error of +1.50 D in both eyes. Her eyes are straight for distance without glasses, but she has a 35 Δ right esotropia for near. With correction her eyes are still straight for distance (as would be expected) but for near the amount of esotropia is unchanged.

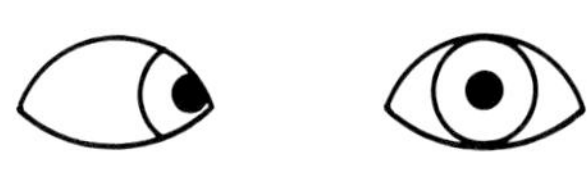

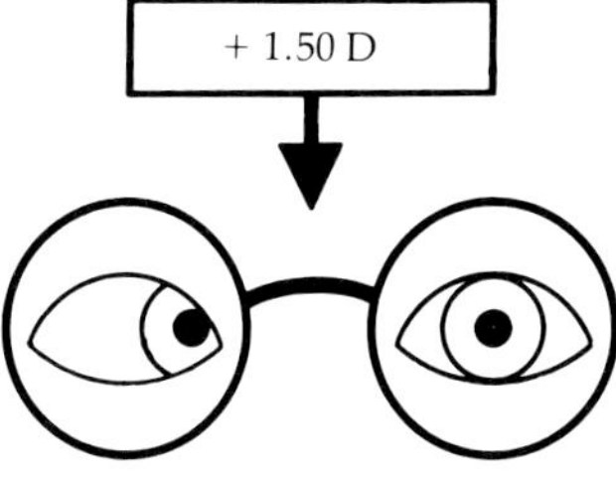

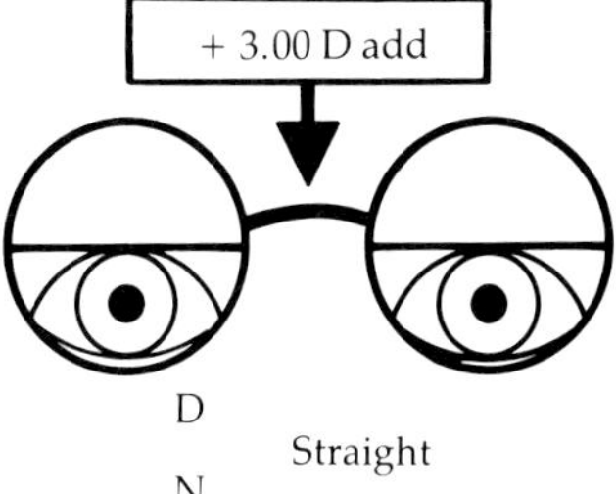

Figure 14.31 *Example of esotropia due to high AC/A ratio*

However, when she looks through a +3.00 D lens over her correction, her eyes are straight. She therefore has a fully accommodative non-refractive esotropia.

Mixed

This is caused by a combination of hypermetropia and a high AC/A ratio. A patient with high hypermetropia and a low AC/A ratio may have straight eyes, whereas a patient with a high AC/A ratio combined with hypermetropia is particularly prone to develop an esotropia for distance and a marked esotropia for near. The distance deviation is usually corrected by spectacles but bifocals are usually necessary to correct the deviation for near.

Management

Refraction

An accurate cycloplegic refraction is essential in all patients with childhood strabismus. The two cycloplegic drugs used in retinoscopy are cyclopentolate (Mydrilate, Cyclogyl) and atropine. Tropicamide (Mydriacyl) is too weak for cycloplegia, but is very useful as a mydriatic.

Cyclopentolate

This gives adequate cycloplegia for refraction in most children. The concentration is 0.5% under the age of 3 months and 1% thereafter. One drop repeated after 5 minutes usually results in maximal cycloplegia within 30 minutes with recovery of accommodation after 24 hours. Its rapid action enables refraction to be carried out at the initial consultation.

Atropine

Refraction under atropine may be necessary in some children under the age of 4 years with either high hypermetropia or heavily pigmented irides in whom cyclopentolate may give inadequate cycloplegia. Atropine can be used as drops or ointment. Although systemic absorption is probably less with ointment, drops are usually preferred as they are easier for an untrained person to instil. The concentration is 0.5% under the age of 3 months and 1% thereafter. The onset of cycloplegia is slower than with cyclopentolate, taking 3 hours for maximal effect. Recovery of accommodation starts after about 3 days and is usually complete by 10 days. The atropine is instilled three times a day for 3 days preceding retinoscopy. The parents should be warned to discontinue medication if there are signs of systemic toxicity such as flushing, fever, and restlessness.

Change of refraction with age

The degree of hypermetropia usually increases until the age of about 6 years (*Figure 14.32*). Between the ages of 6 and 8 years it levels off, and then begins to decrease until the early teens. Children under the age of 6 years who have

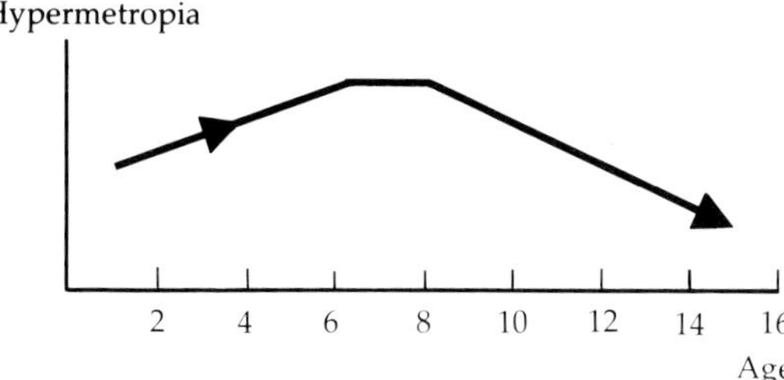

Figure 14.32 *Change of hypermetropia with age*

less than +2.50 D of hypermetropia will probably be virtually emmetropic by the age of 14 years. However, an esotrope under the age of 6 years with more than +4.00 D of hypermetropia is most unlikely to lose enough hypermetropia to be able to go without glasses and still maintain straight eyes. Patients with hypermetropia ranging between +2.50 and +4.00 D may or may not lose their hypermetropia by the age of 14 years. The amount of astigmatism lessens in the first year of life, but remains stable thereafter.

How much to prescribe?

In patients who are under the age of 6 years, the full cycloplegic refraction should be prescribed without deduction of any sort (apart from, of course, deduction for the working distance—usually +1.50). In the fully accommodative refractive esotrope this will control the deviation for both near and distance. After the age of 8 years, the full cycloplegic correction will cause blurring of vision for close work, as the amount of hypermetropia lessens. In these cases the refraction should be repeated *without a cycloplegic* and the maximal amount of 'plus' ordered that the patient is able to tolerate.

Bifocals

If there is no significant refractive error present and the eyes are virtually straight for distance but esotropic for near, bifocals with a +3 D should be prescribed. The most satisfactory form is the executive type in which the intersection crosses the lower or midportion of the pupil. Not infrequently, the strength of the lower segment can be gradually reduced. The ultimate prognosis for the complete withdrawal of spectacles is related to the degree of hypermetropia, the amount of associated astigmatism, and also to the AC/A ratio. In some cases the glasses need only be worn for close work.

Fundus examination

This is *essential* in all cases of childhood strabismus and is performed at the time of the initial cycloplegic refraction using an indirect ophthalmoscope.

Miotics

Miotic therapy is more precarious than the provision of spectacles. It can be tried as a short-term measure in children who will not wear glasses and have an accommodative esotropia due to a high AC/A ratio. The initial dose is ecothiopate (Phospholine Iodide) 0.125% once a day for 6 weeks. If this is effective, the strength and frequency can be gradually reduced to a minimal effective dose. The formation of iris cysts can be prevented by the simultaneous administration of phenylephrine 2.5% drops twice a day.

The miotic therapy of accommodative esotropia due to a high AC/A ratio works by producing a peripheral accommodation, so that less accommodative effort is required by the patient for near vision and thereby less accommodative-convergence is induced.

Treatment of amblyopia

Occlusion (*Figure 14.33*)

Every attempt should be made to treat amblyopia before contemplating surgery. Occasionally, the eyes may straighten once the amblyopia has been reversed. The principle of occlusion is to occlude the sound eye. There are several important rules governing occlusion:

1. The younger the patient, the more rapid the improvement in vision but the greater the risk of causing occlusion amblyopia in the normal eye.
2. A good general rule is to patch initially for 1 week for each year of age. A 6-month-old infant is patched for 3 days, a 1-year-old child for 1 week, a 2-year-old child for 2 weeks, and so on.
3. If, after the initial occlusion, there has been no substantial improvement in visual acuity, and the normal eye has not developed occlusion amblyopia, the period of occlusion can be doubled prior to the next visit.
4. If no improvement has occurred after 6 months, further occlusion is unlikely to be fruitful, but it is essential to exclude organic disease.
5. The better the visual acuity when the occlusion is started, the shorter the duration of occlusion required.
6. Occlusion may be necessary up to the age of 9 years in order to maintain improvement. Patients must not be discharged until they have reached this age.
7. After the age of 9 years conventional occlusion is usually unsuccessful.

The alternatives to occlusion include the following treatment modalities.

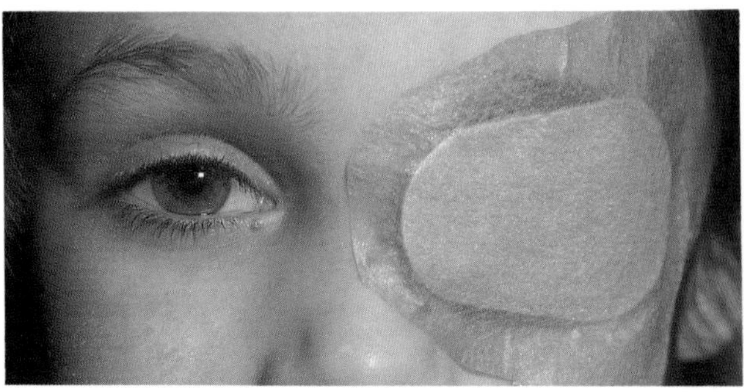

Figure 14.33 *Right amblyopia treated by occlusion of the normal left eye*

Atropine

If the child is hypermetropic, the use of atropine to blur the vision in the sound eye may be helpful in the treatment of relatively mild amblyopia. Because this mode of treatment depends on blurring of vision in a hypermetropic eye, a hypermetropic correction should be omitted. Atropine does not seem to work as quickly as total occlusion and it is only effective if the vision in the amblyopic eye is made superior to that in the sound eye, at least for near fixation. In the penalization technique atropine is instilled into the sound eye and pilocarpine into the amblyopic eye.

Manipulation of glasses

This is most effective in cases of high myopia. The correction in the amblyopic eye is not changed but the correction in the sound eye is replaced by a plano lens.

Pleoptics

This may be considered in patients over the age of 9 years. The principle of pleoptic therapy for amblyopia is the creation of a situation in which the fovea is shielded and the perifoveal area (used by the patient for fixation) is temporarily blinded by a bright flash of light. The patient is then asked to fixate with the shielded fovea so that fixation becomes central.

Stripe (CAM) therapy

This consists of the viewing of rotating high-contrast gratings (stripes) of different sizes with the amblyopic eye. Long-term results have proved disappointing.

Surgery

Surgical intervention should be considered if the wearing of spectacles for 1 month does not fully correct the deviation.

Two options should be considered (*Figure 14.34*):

1. *Recession–resection* in patients with residual amblyopia.
2. *Bilateral medial rectus recession* in patients with equal vision in both eyes, in which the deviation for near is greater than that for distance.

If there is no significant difference between distance and near measurements, and the vision is equally good in the two eyes, some surgeons perform a recession–resection, while others prefer a bilateral medial rectus recession.

The three vertical deviations commonly encountered in patients with esotropia are:

1. Inferior oblique overaction.
2. Dissociated vertical deviation.
3. 'A' and 'V' patterns.

The management of the first two has already been discussed.

'V' pattern esotropia designates a deviation with increasing convergence in down-gaze. A difference of 15 Δ between up-gaze and down-gaze is considered clinically significant.

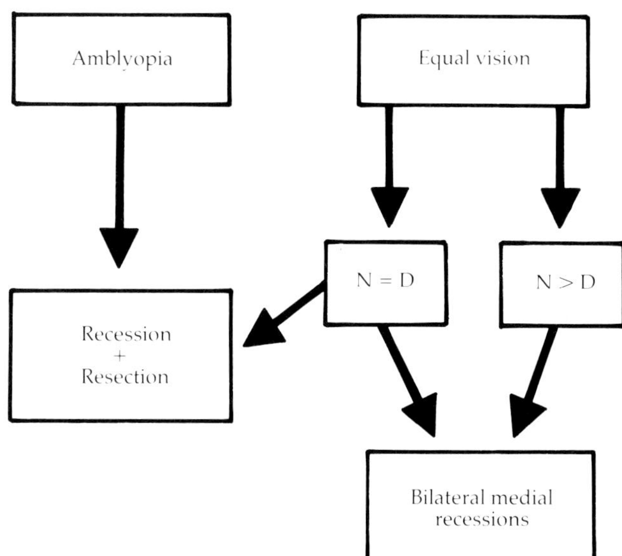

Figure 14.34 *Surgical options for correction of esotropia*

'A' pattern esotropia designates a deviation with increasing convergence in up-gaze.

The management of 'A' and 'V' patterns is discussed later.

Non-accommodative

Stress induced

This is caused by a breakdown of previously efficient fusional divergence mechanisms by emotional or physical stress, illness, and ageing. Surgical correction is usually required.

Sensory deprivation

Monocular organic lesions such as cataract, optic atrophy, or retinoblastoma may give rise to an esotropia associated with amblyopia. Treatment involves removal of the primary cause (if possible), treatment of amblyopia, followed by surgical correction.

Divergence insufficiency

The esotropia is greater for distance than for near. Treatment is by means of base-out prisms, and occasionally surgery in the form of lateral rectus resections. Since this is the deviation seen in mild sixth nerve palsies, these patients should be carefully investigated for an underlying neurological disorder.

Spasm of the near reflex

This usually occurs in patients with hysterical tendencies. It is characterized by intermittent episodes of sustained convergence associated with spasm of accommodation and miosis. Monocular versions are normal although there is a marked limitation of both eyes on lateral conjugate gaze. Treatment is with cycloplegics.

Consecutive

This is an esotropia following surgery for an exodeviation.

Unless the deviation is very large, surgery should be postponed for several months as spontaneous improvement may occur.

Sixth nerve palsy

See Chapter 15.

Childhood exotropias

Classification

The classification of exotropia (manifest divergent strabismus) is different to that of esotropia.

Intermittent
Constant
  congenital
  decompensated intermittent
  sensory deprivation
  consecutive

Irrespective of the above classification all exodeviations can be further subdivided into three types according to distance–near relationships:

1. Convergence insufficiency (worse for near).
2. Divergence excess (worse for distance).
3. Basic (equal for near and distance).

Intermittent

Clinical features

Fluctuation between phoria and tropia is much more common in exodeviations than in esodeviations. The most common age of onset is around 2 years. The manifest state may be precipitated by bright light, day-dreaming, fatigue, ill health, or visual distraction. With the passage of time the manifest state tends to increase, first involving distance fixation and then near fixation, although there are many exceptions to this rule. Occasionally the deviation remains constant and very rarely it may decrease.

When the eyes are straight, patients have normal retinal correspondence. During the manifest state a temporal retinal hemisuppression is common. Amblyopia is fortunately very rare.

Management

Non-surgical

In myopic patients, the wearing of spectacles may in some cases help the patient to control the deviation. Orthoptic treatment consisting of antisuppression therapy, diplopia awareness, and improvement of fusional convergence may also be of some help in selected cases.

Surgical

This is necessary in the majority of cases by the age of approximately 5 years. Some surgeons advocate recessions of both lateral recti, while others recommend bilateral surgery only for those patients whose deviation is greater for distance than for near fixation (divergence excess) and prefer a recession–resection operation where the distance–near measurements are the same.

Constant

Congenital

Clinical features

In contrast to infantile esotropia, congenital exotropia is invaribly present at birth. Although much less common than infantile esotropia, the two share several common features. The angle is usually fairly large and constant. The infant may use the left eye in left-gaze and the right eye in right-gaze (homonymous fixation). Amblyopia is therefore uncommon. The refractive error is usually within the normal range for the child. There is a high incidence of neurological abnormalities in these children.

Management

This is mainly surgical and consists of a bilateral medial rectus resection, usually combined with recession of one or both lateral recti, depending on the angle.

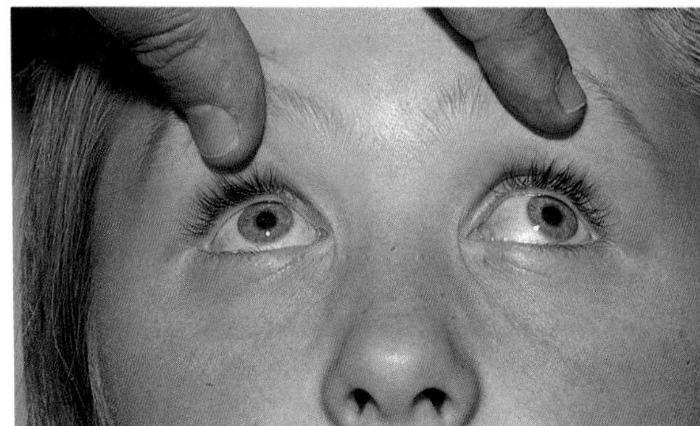

Figure 14.35 *V pattern exotropia in up-gaze (courtesy of Mr B. Mathalone)*

Decompensated intermittent (*Figures 14.35, 14.36* and *14.37*)

Treatment is surgical.

Sensory deprivation

This is caused by disruption of binocular reflexes by acquired lesions such as cataract or other opacities of the media, in children over the age of 5 years or adults. If possible, treatment consists of correction of amblyopia followed by surgery.

Consecutive

This follows overcorrection of an esotropia, especially if one eye is amblyopic. Occasionally, a deeply amblyopic convergent eye may straighten spontaneously and then become divergent. Treatment is for cosmetic reasons.

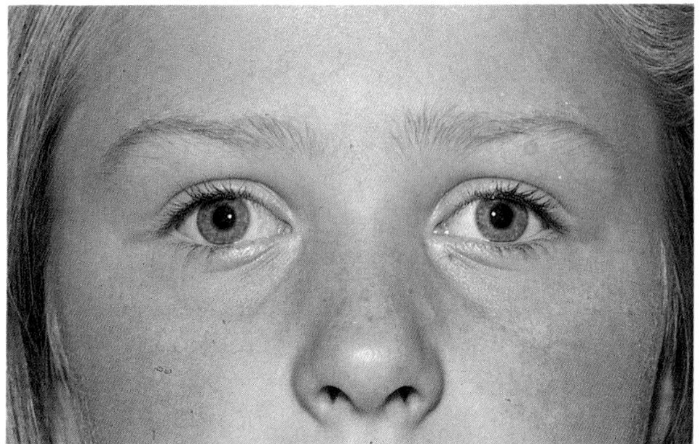

Figure 14.36 *V pattern exotropia in primary position (courtesy of Mr B. Mathalone)*

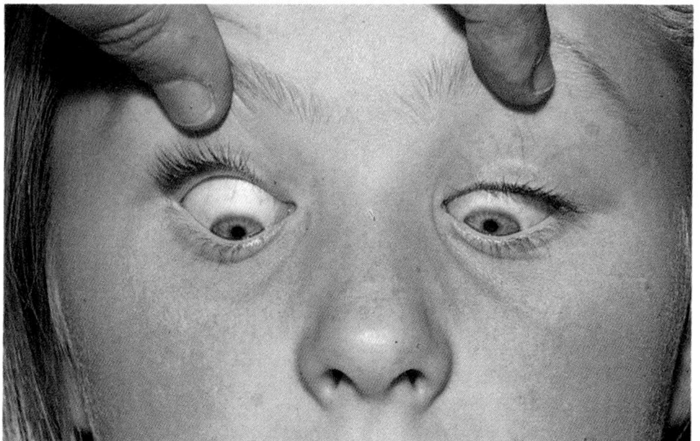

Figure 14.37 *V pattern exotropia in down-gaze (courtesy of Mr B. Mathalone)*

Special ocular motility defects

Duane's retraction syndrome

Clinical features

Duane's syndrome is a congenital anomaly of the abducens nucleus which can be subdivided clinically into three main types.

Type 1 is associated with limitation of abduction with relatively normal adduction.

Type 2 is characterized by limitation of adduction with relatively normal abduction.

Type 3 shows limitation of both abduction and adduction.

The most frequently seen type is characterized by absence of abduction of one eye (the condition is bilateral in about 15% of cases) (*Figure 14.38*). On attempted adduction, there is frequently also some restriction of movement associated with retraction of the globe and narrowing of the palpebral fissure. Electromyographic studies have shown decreased firing of the lateral rectus during attempted abduction and paradoxical innervation of the lateral rectus during adduction. The co-contraction of both medial and lateral recti on attempted adduction is thought to explain the retraction of the globe and narrowing of the palpebral fissure. The amount of retraction of the globe is conspicuous in some cases and minimal in others. On attempted abduction, the palpebral fissure opens and the globe assumes its normal position. A frequent associated feature is 'upshoot' of the eye on adduction. A 'downshoot' may also be seen in some cases.

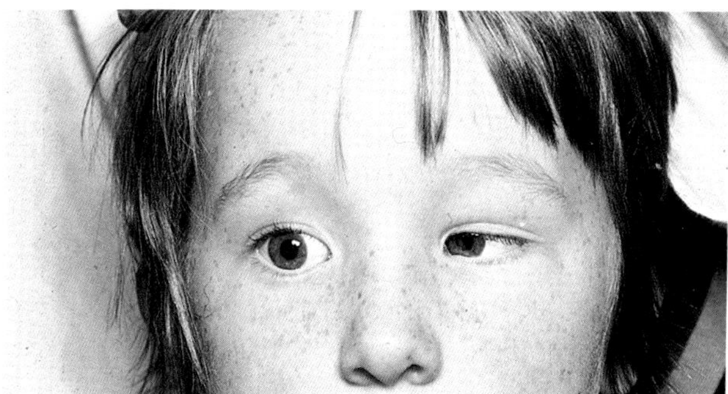

Figure 14.38 *Bilateral Duane's syndrome showing defective abduction of right eye with opening of palpebral fissure and narrowing of left palpebral fissure on adduction of left eye (courtesy of Mr A. Fielder)*

Systemic associations

Some children with Duane's syndrome have associated congenital defects involving ocular, skeletal, auricular, and neural structures.

Treatment

In most cases the eyes are straight in the primary position and do not have amblyopia (*Figure 14.39*). Surgery is indicated for those that are not straight in the primary position and have to adopt an abnormal head posture in order to achieve bifoveal fusion. Amblyopia, when present, is usually due to anisometropia and not strabismus.

Brown's superior oblique tendon sheath syndrome

This is characterized by limitation of elevation of the eye in adduction (*Figure 14.40*) but normal or near normal elevation when the eye is in abduction (*Figure 14.41*). Forced duction testing is positive when attempting to elevate the eye from the adducted position. The eyes are usually straight in the primary position (*Figure 14.42*) and there is no overaction of the superior oblique muscle. Ten per cent of cases are bilateral. The exact aetiology of this condition is unknown, but some postulated causes of acquired Brown's syndrome include trauma or tenosynovitis of the superior oblique tendon–trochlear apparatus. Surgical intervention should only be considered in extreme cases.

Strabismus fixus

This is a very rare condition in which both eyes are fixed in the convergent position due to a fibrous tightening of the medial recti.

Congenital fibrosis syndrome

This is characterized by a defect in elevation and ptosis. The patient is unable to elevate either eye to the midline in either the adducted or abducted position.

Möbius syndrome

This is caused by a congenital aplasia of the sixth, seventh, and sometimes of the ninth and twelfth cranial nerve nuclei. The lower facial muscles may be spared. A history of infantile feeding difficulties is often an important feature due to involvement of the ninth (glossopharyngeal) nerve. The distal part of the tongue may show bilateral atrophy. The face is expressionless, and exposure keratitis may occur as a result of inadequate lid closure. The horizontal recti may be fibrotic and the forced duction test may be abnormal.

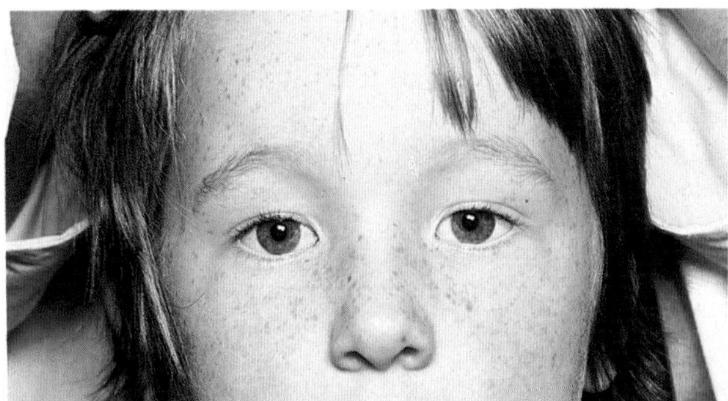

Figure 14.39 *Eyes are straight in primary position (courtesy of Mr A. Fielder)*

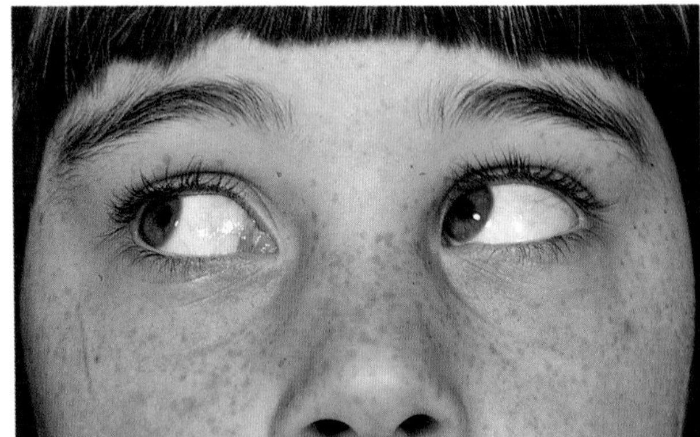

Figure 14.41 *Same patient (as in* Figure 14.40*) – dextroelevation (courtesy of Mr A. Fielder)*

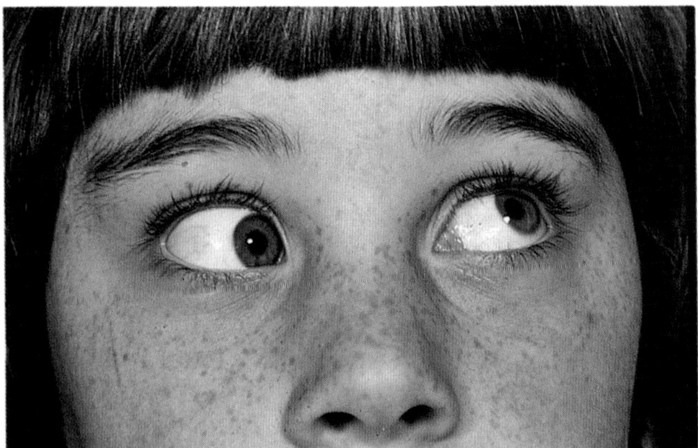

Figure 14.40 *Brown's superior oblique tendon sheath syndrome affecting the right eye – laevoelevation (courtesy of Mr A. Fielder)*

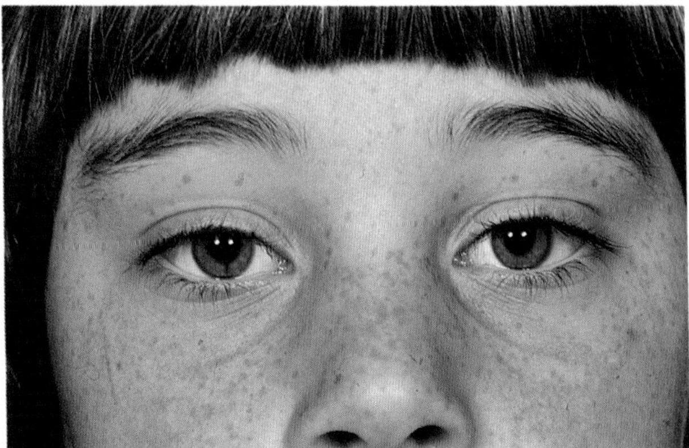

Figure 14.42 *Same patient (as in* Figure 14.40*) – in primary position (courtesy of Mr A. Fielder)*

Nystagmus blockage syndrome

This is a rare condition in which a purposive esotropia dampens a horizontal nystagmus.

Double elevator palsy (*Figure 14.43*)

This is characterized by a paresis of both the superior rectus and inferior oblique muscle of the same eye, and may be associated with ptosis and occasionally the Marcus Gunn jaw-winking phenomenon. Almost all double elevator palsies are congenital and are probably caused by a nuclear third nerve lesion.

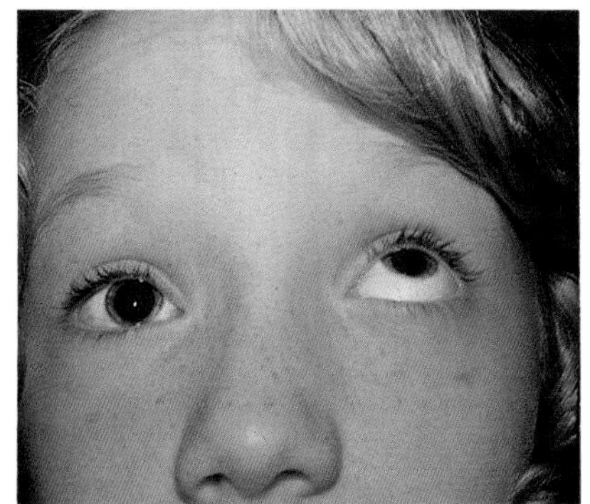

Figure 14.43 *Right double elevator palsy*

Principles of surgery

The aims of surgery on the extraocular muscles are to correct the misalignment of the eyes and, if possible, also to restore binocular single vision.

The three main types of operation are:

1. Weakening procedures that decrease the pull of a muscle.
2. Strengthening procedures that enhance the pull of a muscle.
3. Procedures that change the direction of the action of a muscle.

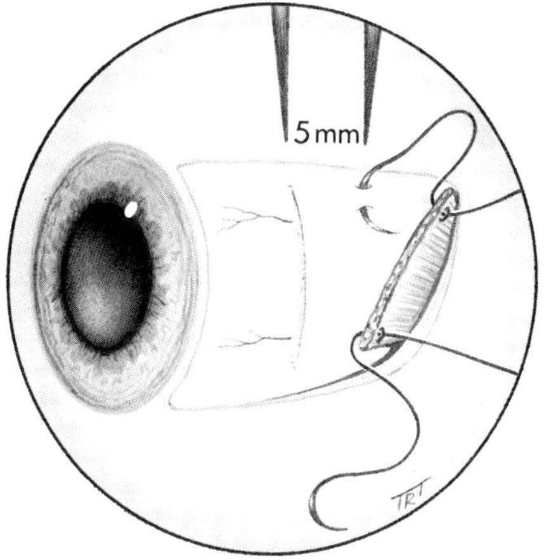

Figure 14.44 *Recession of a horizontal rectus muscle*

Weakening procedures

The three operations used to weaken the action of a muscle are: recession, marginal myotomy, and myectomy.

Recession

In this procedure, the insertion of a muscle is moved posteriorly towards its origin. Recession can be performed on any of the six extraocular muscles.

Rectus muscle recession (*Figure 14.44*)

This involves the following steps:

1. The muscle is exposed.
2. Two absorbable sutures are passed through the outer quarters of the tendon.
3. The tendon is disinserted from the sclera.
4. The amount of recession is measured and marked on the sclera with calipers.
5. The stump is resutured to the sclera posterior to its original insertion.

Inferior oblique recession (*Figure 14.45, upper right*)

This involves the following steps:

1. The muscle belly is exposed through an inferotemporal fornix incision.
2. Two absorbable sutures are passed through the muscle near its insertion.
3. The muscle is disinserted.
4. The stump is resutured to the sclera posterior and temporal to the temporal edge of the inferior rectus muscle.

Marginal myotomy (*Figure 14.45, upper left*)

In this procedure, the length of the muscle is increased without altering its insertion. Marginal myotomy is used to further weaken a previously fully recessed rectus muscle. The operation is performed by first clamping about three-quarters of the width of the muscle from opposite sides in two places and then cutting the crushed areas with scissors.

Myectomy

In this procedure, the muscle is severed from its insertion and not reattached. Myectomy is most commonly used in

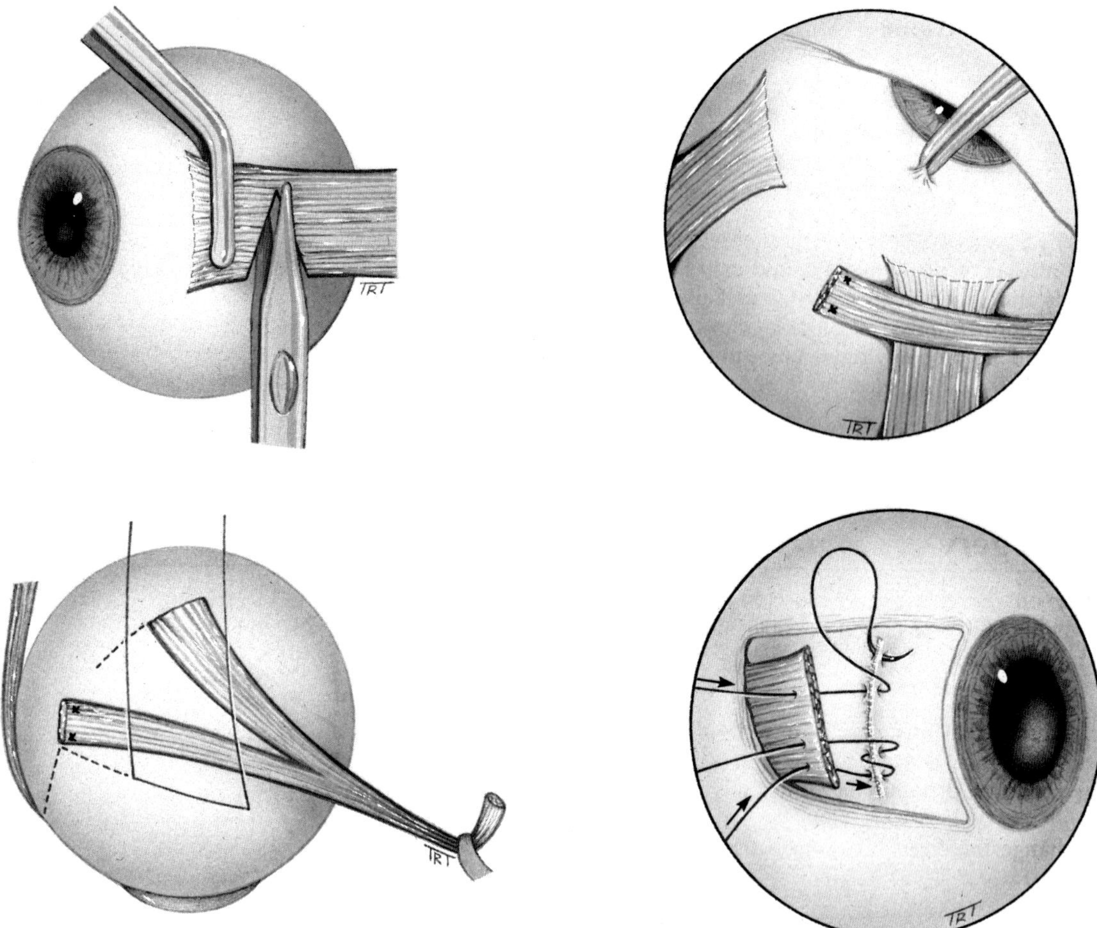

Figure 14.45 *Upper left: marginal myotomy; upper right: recession of inferior oblique; lower left: advancement of anterior half of superior oblique tendon; lower right: resection of horizontal rectus muscle*

weakening an overacting inferior oblique muscle. Very occasionally the procedure is performed on a severely contracted rectus muscle as might occur in thyroid myopathy.

Strengthening procedures

The three operations used to strengthen the action of a muscle are: resection, tucking, and advancement.

Resection (*Figure 14.45, lower right*)

In this procedure, the effective pull of the muscle is enhanced by making it shorter. Resection is suitable only for a rectus muscle. The operation involves the following steps:

1. The muscle is exposed.
2. Two absorbable sutures are inserted into the muscle at a predetermined point posterior to its insertion.
3. The tendon is disinserted from the sclera.
4. The muscle anterior to the sutures is excised.
5. The stump is reattached to the original insertion.

Tucking

Tucking of a muscle or its tendon is usually reserved to enhance the action of the superior oblique muscle in cases of fourth nerve palsy.

Advancement

In this procedure, the muscle is disinserted and advanced nearer to the limbus. Advancement can be used to enhance the action of a previously recessed rectus muscle. In cases of superior oblique palsy, the anterior half of the superior oblique tendon may be advanced temporally and towards the limbus to correct excyclotorsion (*Figure 14.45, lower left*).

Procedures that change direction of muscle action

Vertical transposition of the horizontal recti

This procedure is used to correct 'A' and 'V' patterns in patients who do not show significant oblique muscle overaction. The horizontal recti are transposed (up or down) about two-thirds of their original insertion.

'A' pattern esotropia is treated by bilateral medial rectus recession with upward transposition.

'A' pattern exotropia is treated by bilateral lateral rectus recession and downward transposition.

'V' pattern esotropia is treated by bilateral medial rectus recession and downward transposition.

'V' pattern exotropia (*see Figures 14.35–14.37*) is treated by bilateral lateral rectus recessions and upward transposition.

Posterior fixation suture (Faden)

This procedure is mainly used to treat DVD. In this operation the superior rectus muscle is usually first recessed and then anchored to the sclera with a non-absorbable suture about 12 mm posterior to its insertion. In this way, the pull of the muscle in the primary position is not compromised although its power in elevation is decreased.

Hummelsheim procedure (*Figure 14.46, left*)

This is used to improve abduction in cases of sixth nerve palsy. First the medial rectus muscle is recessed. The superior and inferior recti are then disinserted and their origins are reattached to the superior and inferior margins of the paretic lateral rectus muscle.

Jensen's procedure (*Figure 14.46, right*)

This is also used to improve abduction in cases of sixth nerve palsy and is combined with a recession of the medial rectus muscle. First, the superior, lateral, and inferior recti are split lengthways. Then, with a non-absorbable suture, the lateral half of the superior rectus is tied to the superior half of the lateral rectus, and the inferior half of the lateral rectus is tied to the lateral half of the inferior rectus.

Adjustable sutures

In certain cases, the outcome of strabismus surgery can be improved by the use of adjustable suture techniques. These are particularly indicated when a precise outcome is essential and when the results with more conventional surgical procedures are likely to be unpredictable, particularly in adults with diplopia due to acquired vertical deviations as from thyroid myopathy or following a blow-out fracture of the floor of the orbit. Other relative indications for the use of adjustable sutures include: sixth nerve palsy, adult exotropia, and in reoperations in which scarring of surrounding tissues may make the final outcome unpredictable. The main contraindication to adjustable suture surgery is a patient who is too young or unwilling to cooperate during postoperative suture adjustment.

Surgical technique (*Figure 14.47*)

The initial steps are the same as for a rectus muscle recession. However, instead of anchoring the cut end of the muscle to the sclera, the two ends of the suture are passed, close together, through the stump of the insertion. A knot

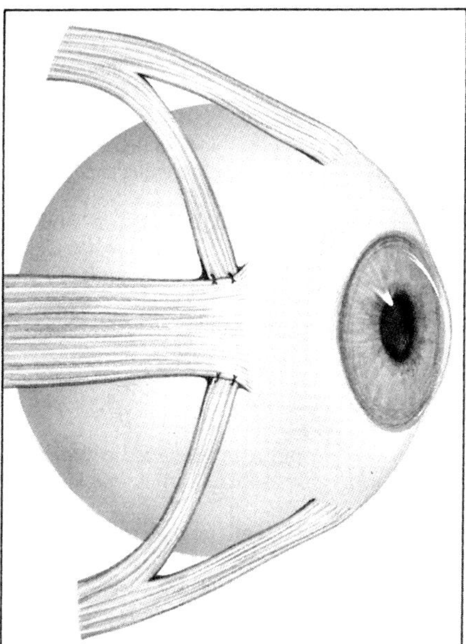

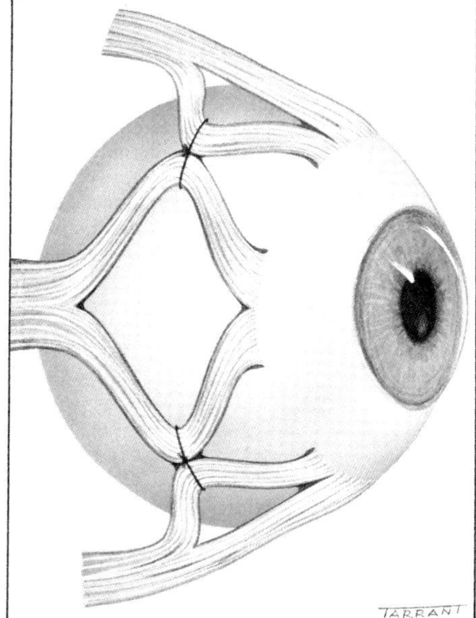

Figure 14.46 *Left: Hummelsheim procedure; right: Jensen's procedure*

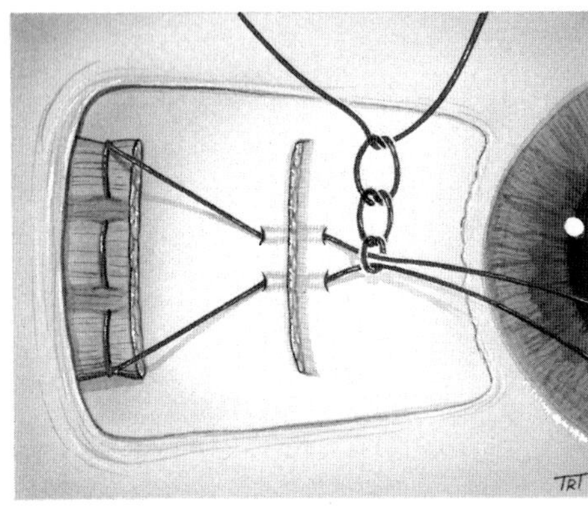

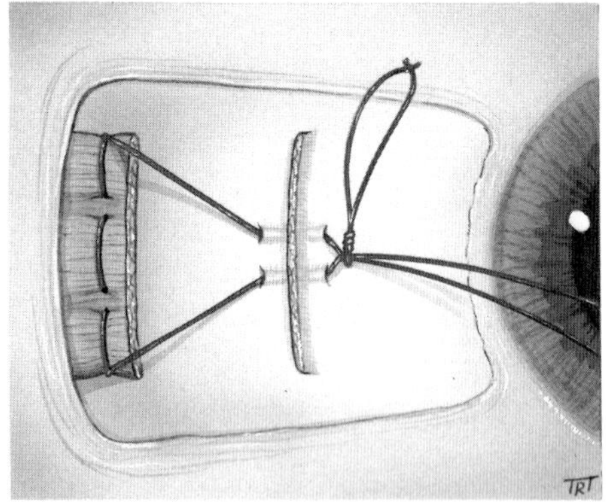

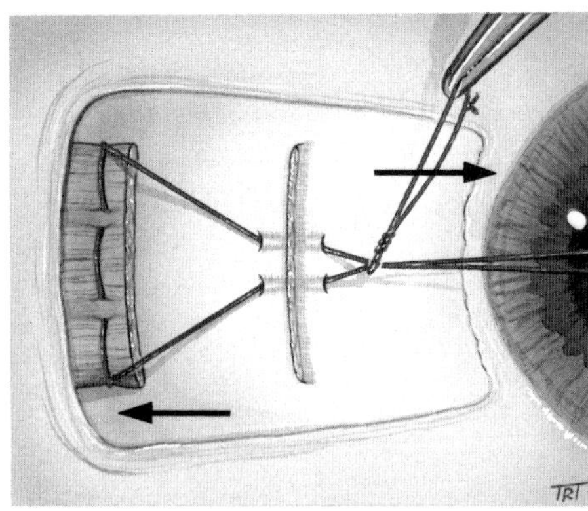

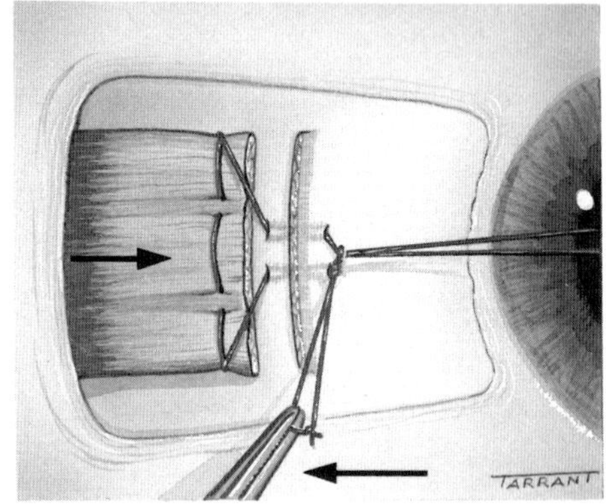

Figure 14.47 *Adjustable suture*

is then tied tightly around the muscle suture anterior to its emergence from the stump (*Figure 14.47, upper left*). One end of the suture is then cut short and the two ends are tied to each other to form a loop (*Figure 14.47, upper right*). The conjunctiva is then closed in a recessed position. Postoperatively, the extent of alignment is assessed in the usual manner. If ocular alignment is satisfactory the muscle suture is tied, and its long ends cut short. If ocular alignment is unsatisfactory and less recession is required, the muscle suture is pulled anteriorly and the knot pulled against the muscle stump (*Figure 14.47, lower right*). If more recession is needed, the knot is pulled anteriorly along the muscle suture, thereby providing additional slack to the recessed muscle and enabling it to move posteriorly (*Figure 14.47, lower left*). A similar technique is used for rectus muscle resection.

Further reading

Clinical evaluation

Bagolini, B. and Campos, E.C. (1981) Clinical usefulness of sensory testing in strabismus. *Perspectives in Ophthalmology,* **5,** 61–65

Ingram, R.M. and Barr, A. (1979) Refraction of 1 year-old children after cycloplegia with 1% cyclopentolate: comparison with findings after atropinization. *British Journal of Ophthalmology,* **63,** 348–352

Moore, A.T. (1985) Refraction in childhood. *Transactions of the Ophthalmological Society of the United Kingdom,* **104,** 648–652

Pratt-Johnson, J.A. and Tillson, G. (1984) Suppression in strabismus—an update. *British Journal of Ophthalmology,* **68,** 174–178

Rosenbaum, A.C., Bateman, J.B., Bremer, D.L. *et al.* (1981) Cycloplegic refraction in esotropic children. *Ophthalmology,* **88,** 1031–1034

Esotropia

Bartley, G.B., Dyer, J.A. and Ilstrup, D.M. (1985) Characteristics of recession–resection and bimedial recession for childhood esotropia. *Archives of Ophthalmology,* **103,** 190–195

Bateman, J.B., Parks, M.M. and Wheeler, N. (1983) Discriminant analysis of congenital esotropia surgery. *Ophthalmology,* **90,** 1146–1153

Bateman, J.B., Parks, M.M. and Wheeler, N. (1983) Discriminant analysis of acquired esotropia surgery. *Ophthalmology,* **90,** 1154–1159

Harcourt, R.B. (1981) Dissociated vertical divergence and its treatment. *Transactions of the Ophthalmological Society of the United Kingdom,* **101,** 271–272

Helveston, E.M. (1983) Options in the treatment of congenital-infantile esotropia. *Transactions of the Ophthalmological Society of the United Kingdom,* **103,** 139–142

Helveston, E.M., Ellis, F.D., Schott, J. *et al.* (1983) Surgical treatment of congenital esotropia. *American Journal of Ophthalmology,* **96,** 218–228

Kushner, B.J. and Morton, G.V. (1984) A randomized comparison of surgical procedures for infantile esotropia. *American Journal of Ophthalmology,* **98,** 50–61

Lee, D.A. and Dyer, J.A. (1983) Bilateral medial rectus muscle recession and lateral rectus muscle resection in the treatment of congenital esotropia. *American Journal of Ophthalmology,* **95,** 528–535

Scott, W.E., Reese, P.D., Hirsh, C.R. *et al.* (1986) Surgery for large-angle congenital esotropia. *Archives of Ophthalmology,* **104,** 374–377

Swan, K.C. (1983) Accommodative esotropia long range follow-up. *Ophthalmology*, **90,** 1141–1145

Tongue, A.C. (1981) Accommodative esotropia. *Perspectives in Ophthalmology*, **5,** 73–76

Exotropia

Hardisty, H.H. and Annable, W.L. (1981) Intermittent exotropia. *Perspectives in Ophthalmology*, **5,** 57–59

Richard, J.M. and Parks, M.M. (1983) Intermittent exotropia. *Ophthalmology*, **90,** 1172–1177

Special ocular motility defects

Hotchkiss, M.G., Miller, N.R., Clark, A.W. *et al.* (1980) Bilateral Duane's retraction syndrome. *Archives of Ophthalmology*, **98,** 870–874

Miller, N.R., Kiel, S.M., Green, W.R. *et al.* (1982) Unilateral Duane's retraction syndrome (Type 1). *Archives of Ophthalmology*, **100,** 1468–1472

Pressman, S.H. and Scott, W.E. (1986) Surgical treatment of Duane's syndrome. *Ophthalmology*, **93,** 29–38

Principles of strabismus surgery

Fells, P. (1981) The use of adjustable sutures. *Transactions of the Ophthalmological Society of the United Kingdom*, **101,** 279–283

Gobin, M.H. (1981) Surgical treatment of A and V phenomenon. *Transactions of the Ophthalmological Society of the United Kingdom*, **101,** 258–263

Helveston, E.M. (1981) Techniques and indications for surgery of the superior and inferior oblique muscles. *Transactions of the Ophthalmological Society of the United Kingdom*, **101,** 251–257

Lee, J., O'Day, J. and Fells, P. (1985) Early experience with adjustable squint surgery at Moorfields Eye Hospital with long-term follow-up. *Transactions of the Ophthalmological Society of the United Kingdom*, **104,** 662–674

Metz, H.S. (1986) Adjustable suture techniques in strabismus surgery. *Clinical Modules for Ophthalmologists*, Vol. 4, Module 1

Wright, K.W. (1986) Current approaches for inferior oblique muscle surgery. *Clinical Modules for Ophthalmologists*, Vol. 4, Module 6

15

Neuro-ophthalmology

Introduction
Definitions of perimetric terms
Applied anatomy
Applied physiology
Confrontation tests

Acquired optic nerve disorders
Classification
Optic neuritis
Anterior ischaemic optic neuropathies
Diabetic papillopathy
Toxic optic neuropathies
Leber's optic neuropathy
Papilloedema
Optic nerve tumours

Congenital optic disc anomalies
Drusen (hyaline bodies)
Myelinated nerve fibres
Optic disc pit
Coloboma
Tilted disc
Optic nerve hypoplasia
Morning glory syndrome

Chiasmal disorders
Applied anatomy
Applied physiology of the pituitary gland
Classification
Pituitary adenoma
Craniopharyngioma
Meningioma
Aneurysm
Other lesions

Optic tract disorders
Applied anatomy
Clinical features
Aetiology

Disorders of the optic radiations and visual cortex
Applied anatomy
Associated neurological features
Aetiology
Optokinetic nystagmus

Supranuclear disorders of eye movement
Horizontal gaze
Medial longitudinal bundle
Vertical gaze

Oculomotor (third) nerve palsy
Applied anatomy
Clinical features
Treatment

Trochlear (fourth) nerve disease
Applied anatomy
Clinical features
Treatment

Abducens (sixth) nerve palsy
Applied anatomy
Clinical features
Treatment

Aetiology of third, fourth and sixth nerve palsies

Carotid–cavernous fistula
Direct
Indirect (dural shunt)

Abnormalities of the pupil
Applied anatomy
Examination
Abnormal reactions

Nystagmus
Classification
Clinical types

Myasthenia gravis

Ocular myopathies
Chronic progressive external ophthalmoplegia
Dystrophia myotonica

Essential blepharospasm

Introduction

Definitions of perimetric terms

1. *A scotoma* is an absolute or relative area of depressed visual function surrounded by normal vision. In an absolute scotoma, all vision is lost (i.e. no light perception), whereas in a relative scotoma a variable amount of vision remains. A scotoma may be positive or negative. A positive scotoma 'obstructs' a part of the visual field, whereas a negative scotoma produces a 'hole' in the visual field. Optic nerve lesions typically produce negative scotomas whereas macular lesions cause positive scotomas.
2. *A hemianopia* is a complete defect involving one half of the visual field. A heteronymous hemianopia involves opposite sides of the visual field (i.e. binasal or bitemporal). Lesions of the optic chiasm typically produce bitemporal heteronymous hemianopias. A homonymous hemianopia involves the same side of the visual field in each eye (i.e. right or left). Lesions of the retrochiasmal pathways (i.e. optic tract, optic radiations, and visual cortex) typically produce homonymous hemianopias.
3. *Congruity* is the tendency for an incomplete homonymous hemianopia to be symmetrical in the two visual fields. It is impossible to assess congruity if the hemianopia is complete.

Applied anatomy

The optic nerve head is the exit site for all retinal nerve fibres. Its central core consists predominantly of the papillomacular bundle, which contains small-calibre nerve fibres that subserve the cone system of the fovea. Optic nerve lesions have a predilection for suppressing the function of this important anatomical structure causing diminished visual acuity and a defect in the visual field.

Optic nerve disease may produce four different types of visual field defects.

Central scotoma *(Figure 15.1, upper left)*

This only involves fixation. The scotoma is negative and, depending on the severity of the lesion, it can be relative or absolute. A central scotoma typically occurs in optic neuritis, although it can also be caused by ischaemic and compressive optic nerve lesions.

Centrocaecal scotoma *(Figure 15.1, upper right)*

This extends from fixation to the blind spot and typically occurs in toxic optic neuropathies and Leber's optic neuropathy. Congenital optic disc pits associated with serous detachment of the macula may also produce a similar defect.

Altitudinal field defects *(Figure 15.1, lower left)*

These involve two quadrants of either the superior or inferior visual field and are seen in ischaemic optic neuropathies.

Arcuate defects *(Figure 15.1, lower right)*

These are caused by selective damage to the superior or inferior retinal nerve fibre bundles and are typical of glaucoma. However, they are also occasionally seen in optic neuritis, ischaemic optic neuropathy, and congenital optic disc drusen (hyaline bodies).

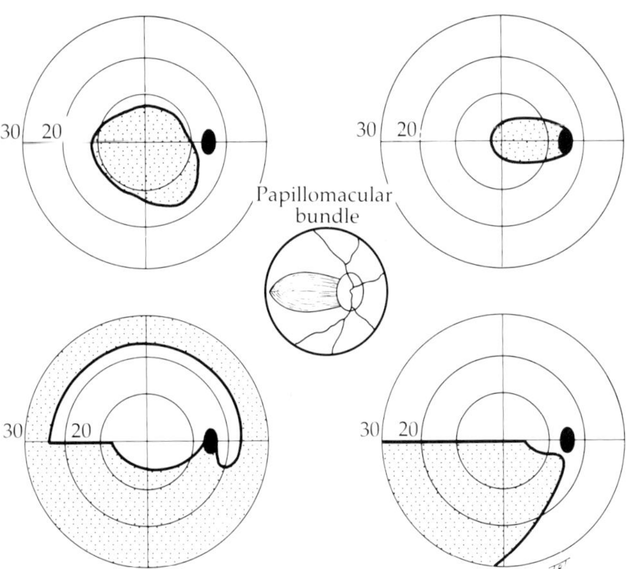

Figure 15.1 *Field defects due to optic nerve lesions*

Applied physiology

An optic nerve lesion not only diminishes visual acuity and produces a visual field defect but, similar to a filter (*Figure 15.2*), it also impairs three other modalities of optic nerve function: the afferent pupillary pathways, colour vision, and light brightness appreciation.

Pupil

Impairment of the afferent pupillary pathways will cause an afferent pupillary conduction defect (*see* later).

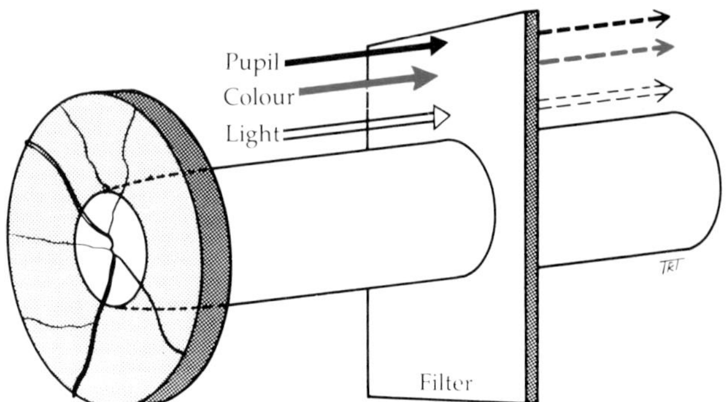

Figure 15.2 *Filter-like effects of an optic nerve lesion*

Colour vision

Impairment of colour vision will make coloured objects appear drab or 'washed-out'. In fact, diminished visual acuity with normal colour vision strongly militates against an optic nerve lesion. A simple and quick way of detecting a uniocular acquired colour vision defect is to ask the patient to compare the colour of a red object (e.g. Mydriacyl bottle top). This colour comparison test is also useful in detecting the presence of a relative central scotoma. One red object is held in front of the examiner's nose (fixation object) and another identical red object is held slightly eccentrically. In a normal eye, the eccentrically held object will appear less red than the fixation object, whereas in the presence of a relative central scotoma the eccentrically held object will appear more red than the fixation object. In an eye with a relative central scotoma, the fixation object will also become more red as it is towards the periphery and out of the scotoma. The presence of defective colour vision can be confirmed with Ishihara's plates.

Light brightness

Depression of light brightness sensitivity makes surroundings appear dim as if the room light had been turned down. A simple and quick way of comparing light brightness sensitivity is to shine a very bright light from an indirect ophthalmoscope first into the normal eye and then into the eye with the suspected optic nerve lesion and ask the patient with which eye does the light appear brighter.

Confrontation tests

These tests are useful for the detection of hemianopias and altitudinal defects.

Visually evoked movement (*Figure 15.3*)

This is the most primitive form of confrontation testing. The target is brought into the visual field and once it is perceived the patient makes an involuntary visually evoked fixation movement to bring the image onto the fovea. This test is useful for evaluating peripheral fields in young children.

Finger counting (*Figure 15.4*)

This is a gross screening test for a peripheral field defect. It can be performed on most patients over the age of 8 years. It is divided into three stages:

1. The patient is asked to look directly into the examiner's eye and then to identify the number of fingers presented separately in each of four quadrants of the monocular visual field. The examiner should use either one finger, two fingers, five fingers, or a clenched fist (*Figure 15.4a*).
2. The second stage consists of simultaneous finger counting in each hemifield in which the patient is asked to count the total number of fingers he sees (*Figure 15.4b*). This test detects the phenomenon of 'extinction' in which the defective hemifield appears intact when tested alone, but when tested with simultaneous stimuli a subtle defect may become apparent.
3. The last stage of the test is to present one finger in each hemifield and ask the patient to point to the finger seen most clearly. If both appear equally clear the test is terminated. However, if the patient reports that one finger is less clear, then the upper and lower quadrants are compared in order to detect whether the defect is denser above or below.

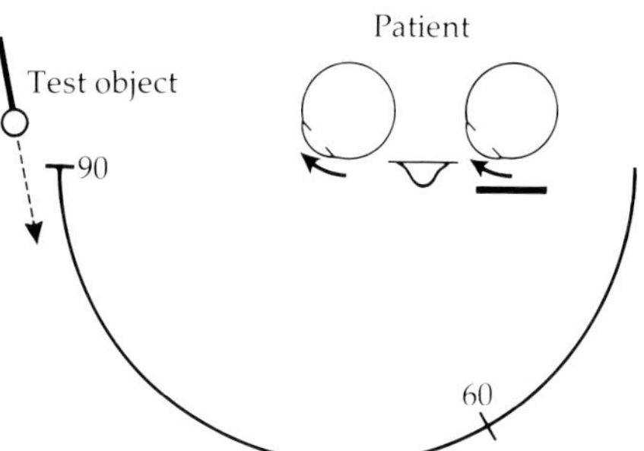

Figure 15.3 *Testing of peripheral visual field by visually evoked eye movements*

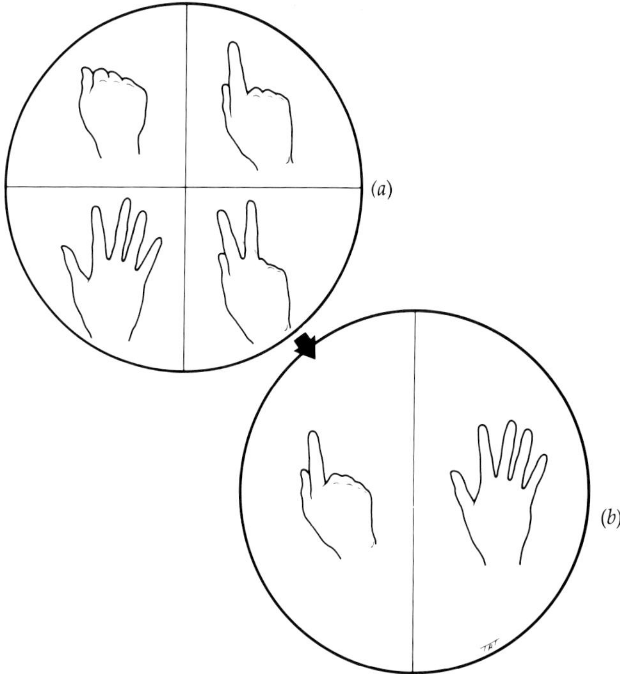

Figure 15.4 *Finger counting technique in quadrants*

Finger-mimicking test

This is a modification of the finger-counting test in which the patient is asked to hold up the same number of fingers as the examiner. This test is useful in toddlers and aphasic patients.

Colour comparison *(Figure 15.5)*

This is a very useful screening test for temporal field defects caused by chiasmal compression. It is performed by presenting the patient with two large red objects to either side of fixation. In the presence of a field defect the red colour in the abnormal field will appear desaturated or washed-out.

Confrontation using a hat-pin

This is a more sophisticated test in which the pin is brought in from the periphery. A skilled examiner can even evaluate the central field of vision with this method.

If confrontation tests are abnormal or equivocal, quantitative perimetry should be performed in which an exact evaluation of the visual field is made using specific targets.

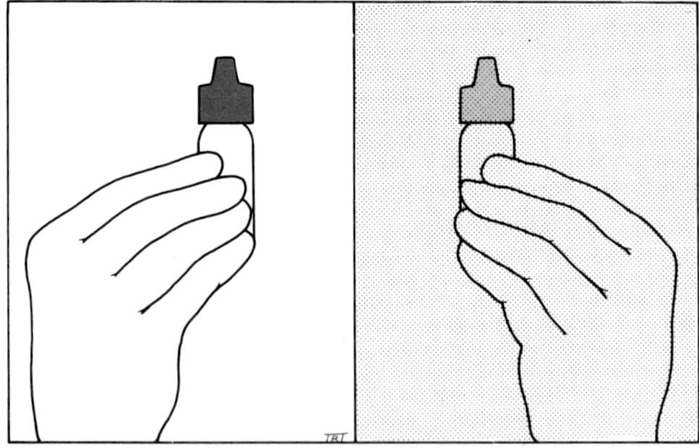

Figure 15.5 *Colour comparison to either side of fixation*

Acquired optic nerve disorders

Classification

Optic neuritis
- idiopathic
- demyelination
- postviral
- granulomatous inflammation
- adjacent infection

Anterior ischaemic optic neuropathy
- non-arteritic
- arteritic

Diabetic papillopathy

Toxic optic neuropathies
- toxic amblyopia
- drug induced

Leber's optic neuropathy

Papilloedema

Other causes of disc swelling

Tumours
- glioma
- meningioma

Optic neuritis

Optic neuritis is an inflammatory or demyelinating disorder of the optic nerve.

Aetiology

Idiopathic

In many patients with a single episode of optic neuritis the actual cause is never established.

Demyelination

Optic neuritis and internuclear ophthalmoplegia are the most common ocular manifestation of multiple sclerosis (MS). Optic neuritis is the presenting feature in about 25% of MS patients and occurs during the course of established disease in about 70%. In the United Kingdom it has been estimated that between 50% and 70% of patients in the 20–40 year age group who present with optic neuritis will subsequently develop evidence of systemic demyelination. The vast majority who develop MS do so within 5 years of the initial episode of optic neuritis. Risk factors of MS include:

1. *Uhthoff's phenomenon* characterized by impairment of vision with increased body temperature.
2. *Recurrence* in the same or opposite eye, which occurs in about 25% of patients with optic neuritis, increases the risk of MS four-fold.
3. *HLA-DR2* positive patients with recurrences have a seven-fold increased risk of developing MS.
4. *Winter onset* of optic neuritis in HLA-DR2 positive patients increases the risk of MS three-fold.

Miscellaneous

1. *Postviral.* This is the most common cause in children and is frequently bilateral. It usually follows an episode of non-specific malaise with fever, headache, and vomiting which is often diagnosed as 'influenza'. Less frequently it is associated with a specific acute infectious disease such as measles, chickenpox, and mumps.
2. *Granulomatous inflammation* by sarcoidosis, tuberculosis and syphilis is rare.
3. *Adjacent infection* of the meninges, sinuses, or orbit may occasionally spread to involve the optic nerve.

Clinical features

Optic neuritis of the idiopathic type or from MS typically affects patients between the ages of 20 and 40 years.

Symptoms

The visual loss is monocular, sudden and progressive and usually maximal by the end of the second week. Frequently the visual symptoms are accompanied by or occasionally preceded by periocular pain made worse by moving the eye or by pressure on the globe. The rate of visual recovery is slower than that of the initial visual loss and usually takes between 4 to 6 weeks. Although about 90% of patients recover normal visual acuity, minor defects in colour vision and light brightness appreciation may persist. There is no correlation between the level of visual acuity during the attack and the final visual outcome.

Signs

The visual acuity during maximal visual loss is usually severely reduced (6/60), although some patients have only mild loss (6/12), while a few have more severe impairment (hand movements). Colour vision is usually severely impaired even in patients with relatively good visual acuity. The most common visual defect is a relative central scotoma without peripheral breakthrough.

Opthalmoscopic features of optic neuritis:

1. *Retrobulbar neuritis* is the most common finding in adults. Because the site of involvement is behind the globe the optic disc and retinal nerve fibre layer are normal.
2. *Optic papillitis* is rare in adults but is the most common finding in children and is frequently postviral. Here the inflammation involves the intraocular portion of the optic nerve giving rise to swelling of the optic nerve head with obliteration of the physiological cup, and inflammatory cells in the vitreous (*Figure 15.6, left*).
3. *Neuroretinitis* (Leber's idiopathic stellate maculopathy) is the least common. It has all the features of optic neuritis in addition to a macular star (*Figure 15.6, right*). This form of optic neuritis is not associated with MS.

Special investigations

Skull X-rays, CT scanning and magnetic resonance imaging are unnecessary in typical cases. However, in atypical cases they should be used in order to exclude a mimicking lesion, such as an optic nerve sheath meningioma or a pituitary tumour which may on occasion also present with a sudden monocular visual loss. Suspicious features include: failure of visual loss to begin to recover after 4 weeks, especially if associated with persistent periocular pain, development of a quadrantic or hemianopic visual field defect, and the development of a field defect in the opposite eye.

Treatment

Corticosteroids given either systemically or by posterior periocular injection accelerate the speed of recovery of vision and reduce the amount of discomfort. However, because they have no effect on the eventual visual outcome they are usually reserved for one-eyed patients or the rare cases with bilateral simultaneous involvement.

Anterior ischaemic optic neuropathies

Anterior ischaemic optic neuropathy (AION) is a relatively common cause of severe visual loss in the middle-aged and elderly. The basic lesion is a segmental or generalized infarction of the anterior part of the optic nerve caused by occlusion of the short posterior ciliary arteries.

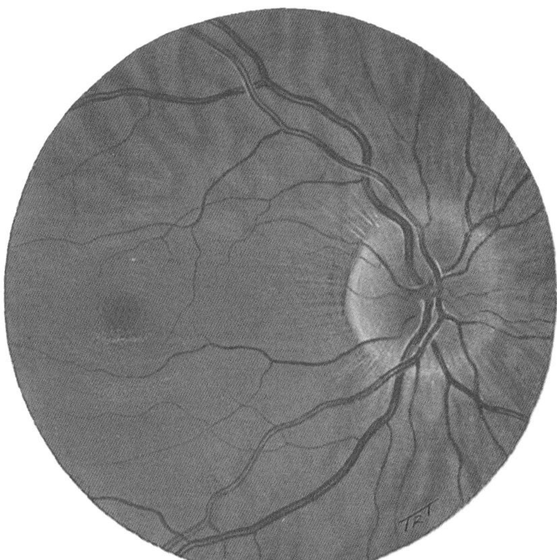

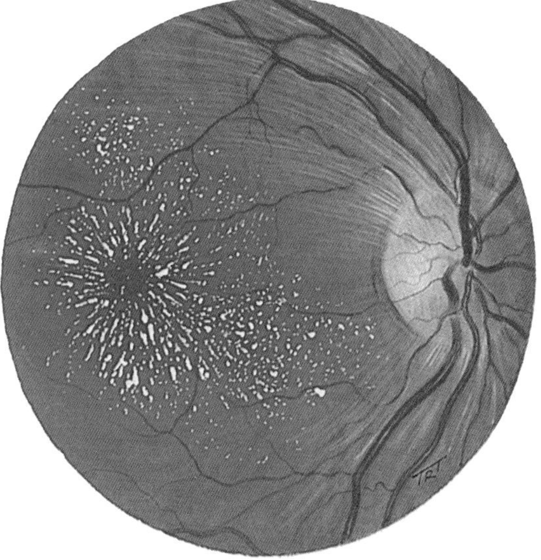

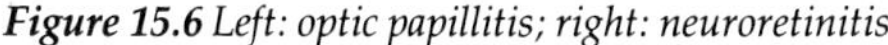

Figure 15.6 *Left: optic papillitis; right: neuroretinitis*

Aetiology

1. *Atherosclerosis* is thought to be responsible for the most common idiopathic or non-arteritic form. For unknown reasons patients with small or absent optic cups are at increased risk.
2. *Giant cell arteritis* causes the arteritic type which is the second most common cause.
3. *Collagen vascular disorders*—polyarteritis nodosa and systemic lupus erythematosus are occasional causes in patients under the age of 50 years.
4. *Miscellaneous* and very rare causes include: emboli, papilloedema, malignant hypertension and migraine.

Only the first two forms will be discussed in detail.

Non-arteritic AION

Clinical features

Non-arteritic or idiopathic AION typically occurs as an isolated event in a patient between the ages of 45 and 65 years who is otherwise healthy, or who has hypertension as the only sign of systemic vascular disease. In contrast to patients with retinal artery occlusion, those with idiopathic AION are not at increased risk of early death from systemic vascular disease.

Symptoms

The visual loss is monocular, sudden and painless and unassociated with premonitory transient visual symptoms. In contrast to optic neuritis, the visual deficit is usually most severe at its onset and any subsequent improvement is rare. Although bilateral simultaneous involvement is extremely rare, about one-third of patients develop AION in the opposite eye several months or years later.

Signs

In about one-third of patients, visual acuity is normal or only slightly reduced. The remainder have moderate to severe impairment. The visual field defect typically consists of an altitudinal hemianopia most commonly involving the inferior half. Some patients have arcuate defects and, occasionally, infarction of the papillomacular bundle gives rise to a central scotoma. Colour vision is diminished in proportion to the level of visual acuity. This is in contrast to optic neuritis in which colour vision is usually severely impaired irrespective of the level of visual acuity. Ophthalmoscopy during the acute phase shows diffuse or sectorial oedema with a pale or hyperaemic disc which may be surrounded by splinter-shaped haemorrhages (*Figure 15.7*). The fellow eye commonly has a small or absent optic cup. Within 1 or 2 months the oedema gradually resolves and the involved portion of the optic disc becomes pale but not cupped.

Treatment

Although there is no effective treatment, it is extremely important to exclude the possibility of occult giant cell arteritis.

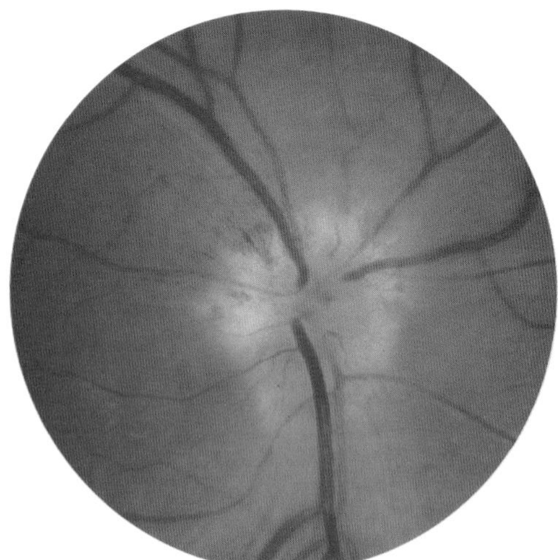

Figure 15.7 *Anterior ischaemic optic neuropathy*

Arteritic AION

This is caused by giant cell arteritis, a disease of unknown aetiology which affects the elderly (usually over the age of 60 years). Although almost any artery can be involved it has a predilection for large and medium-sized vessels, particularly the superficial temporal, ophthalmic, posterior ciliaries, and the proximal part of the vertebral. There is a correlation between the quantity of the elastic tissue in the media and adventitia of the artery and the severity and extent of the disease. For this reason, intracranial arteries, which possess little elastic tissue, are rarely involved.

Ocular features

Arteritic AION affects about 25% of patients with untreated giant cell arteritis. Visual loss usually occurs within the first few weeks of the onset of the systemic disease and is extremely rare after the first 9 months have elapsed. Although simultaneous bilateral involvement is rare, about 65% of untreated patients develop AION in the second eye within weeks. Once visual loss is present, it is usually profound and permanent, although very occasionally the prompt administration of systemic corticosteroids may be associated with partial recovery. In a few unfortunate patients with initial unilateral visual loss, the second eye also becomes blind despite steroid administration.

Symptoms

Visual loss is sudden, profound and usually permanent. Its onset may be accompanied by periocular pain and preceded by transient visual symptoms such as obscurations (amaurosis fugax) and flashing lights lasting a few seconds or minutes.

Signs

Both visual field and visual acuity are profoundly impaired (hand movements or counting fingers). Ophthalmoscopy during the acute stage shows a swollen white or pale optic disc frequently associated with splinter-shaped peripapillary haemorrhages. Within 1 or 2 months, the swelling gradually resolves and the entire optic disc becomes pale and also frequently cupped. Very rarely the optic disc appears normal until optic atrophy ensues because the ischaemic process is retrobulbar (posterior ischaemic optic neuropathy).

Other ocular manifestations of giant cell arteritis include: amaurosis fugax, central retinal artery occlusion, cotton-wool spots, anterior segment necrosis, ocular motor palsies, and cortical blindness.

Systemic features

1. *Headache*, which may be generalized or less commonly localized to frontal, occipital, or temporal areas, is often the initial symptom. It develops over a few hours and may be extremely severe.
2. *Scalp tenderness* is common. On examination, the temporal arteries are found to be tender, inflamed, and nodular. Initially, pulsation is present although the thickened artery cannot be flattened against the skull. Later, arterial pulsation ceases and in severe cases ischaemic gangrene of the scalp may develop (*Figure 15.8*). Occasionally, the scalp vessels may appear clinically normal and yet show typical changes on histological examination. Although the temporal arteries are classically affected, involvement of other extracranial arteries may also occur.
3. *Jaw claudication* due to ischaemia of the masseter muscle is characterized by pain on talking or chewing, which is relieved by rest. Involvement of the lingual artery may cause pain in the tongue.
4. *Polymyalgia rheumatica* is a syndrome consisting of pain and stiffness in the proximal muscle groups which is worse in the morning and after exertion. Involvement of the shoulder girdle is particularly common, making dressing and combing hair difficult.

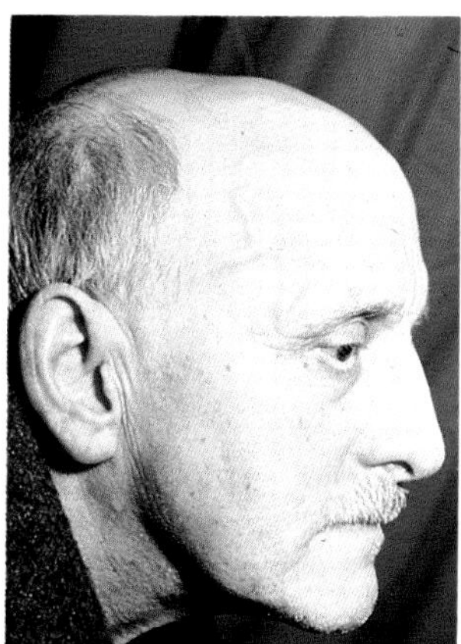
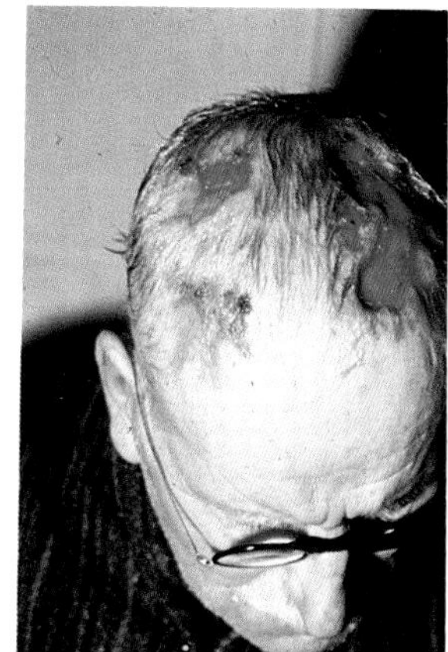

Figure 15.8 *Temporal arteritis. Left: thickened arteries; right: ischaemic necrosis of scalp*

5. *Non-specific systemic features* include weight loss (over 50% of cases), night sweats, fever, and malaise.
6. *Less typical manifestations* include involvement of the aorta and its main branches, which may give rise to dissecting aneurysms, aortic incompetence, and myocardial infarction. Involvement of the vertebral artery may cause brainstem stroke.
7. *Occult temporal arteritis.* Unfortunately a small percentage of patients with arteritic AION have none of the above systemic features, and in these cases the diagnosis may be missed.

Special investigations

1. *Erythrocyte sedimentation rate (ESR)* is determined largely by elevated fibrinogen levels and the concentration of γ-globulins. In giant cell arteritis the ESR is frequently very high, with levels in excess of 100 mm/h or more. In interpreting the ESR it should be borne in mind that levels of 40 mm/h may be normal in an elderly patient and cases of biopsy-proven giant cell arteritis have been reported in patients with ESR levels of less than 30 mm/h.
2. *C-reactive protein* is invariably raised in giant cell arteritis and may be helpful when the ESR is equivocal.
3. *Temporal artery biopsy* should be done to confirm the diagnosis. In the presence of ocular involvement it is advisable to take the biopsy from the ipsilateral side. Prior treatment with systemic corticosteroids for 1 or 2 days does not prevent identification of the typical histological changes. At least 2.5 cm of the artery should be taken and serial sections must be examined as there may be variations in the extent of arteritic involvement along the length of the artery. The question of skip areas is controversial.

Treatment

Immediate treatment of patients with AION is intravenous hydrocortisone 250 mg together with prednisone 80 mg orally. After 3 days the oral dose is reduced to 60 mg for 3 days and then to 40 mg for 4 days. The daily dose is then reduced by 5 mg weekly until 10 mg a day is reached, provided the patient is asymptomatic. The dose of 10 mg is maintained for 3 months and then gradually reduced. Further gradual reduction is governed by the patients' symptoms and ESR. Symptoms may recur without a rise in the ESR and vice versa. The optimal duration for therapy is uncertain. Some patients may only need treatment for 1–2 years whereas others need maintenance therapy for life.

Diabetic papillopathy

This condition typically affects juvenile onset diabetics during the second and third decades of life. It is a distinct clinical entity that should be distinguished from AION papilloedema, and papillitis.

Clinical features

The disorder affects both eyes in about 75% of cases. It causes a mild to moderate visual loss that usually recovers spontaneously within 6 months. On examination, disc swelling ranges from mild oedema without haemorrages to florid swelling with capillary telangiectasis, nerve fibre haemorrhages, exudates, and cystoid macular oedema, with or without a macular star. There appears to be no correlation between the ophthalmoscopic findings and the initial or final visual acuity.

Treatment

No specific treatment is indicated apart from good diabetic control.

Toxic optic neuropathies

Toxic amblyopia

This condition typically affects heavy drinkers and pipe smokers who have a diet deficient in protein and B vitamins. In these patients, the onset of visual impairment is gradual, progressive, and bilateral, although the severity of involvement may be asymmetrical.

Visual field examination shows bilateral centrocaecal scotomas, the soft margins of which are difficult to define with a white target, but are easier to plot and larger for coloured (especially red) targets.

Treatment is by means of weekly injections of 1000 units of hydroxocobalamin for 10 weeks. Patients should also be advised to eat a well-balanced diet and abstain from drinking and smoking. Although it make take several weeks for vision to improve, the prognosis is good.

Drug-induced optic neuropathy

Ethambutol

This has become a standard drug in the treatment of tuberculosis and, during the initial years of its use, there were many isolated reports of optic neuropathy in patients treated with the drug. It now appears that optic neuropathy does not occur if doses of not more than 15 mg/kg per day are administered. Even doses of up to 25 mg/kg per day arc rarely toxic. It appears that toxicity is more likely to occur in patients who have associated alcoholism or diabetes. The onset of optic neuropathy is usually sudden and associated with impaired colour vision, especially for red-green. The optic discs may be oedematous and hyperaemic with a few splinter-shaped haemorrhages.

It has been suggested that the optic chiasm may in fact be the primary site of involvement, as the visual field defect may take the form of a true bitemporal hemianopia. Some patients develop optic atrophy with a permanent impairment of vision. The majority, however, recover their vision although complete recovery may take up to 12 months.

The mechanism leading to ethambutol toxicity is still obscure. Interference with zinc metabolism has been proposed by some, a direct action on the optic nerve by others. Successful treatment using hydroxocobalamin has recently been reported.

Other drugs

Other drugs reported to cause toxic optic neuropathy include chloramphenicol, isoniazid, and streptomycin.

Leber's optic neuropathy

Clinical features

Leber's optic neuropathy is a rare hereditary disorder primarily affecting healthy young men and only about 15% of patients are females. The exact mechanism of inheritance is unknown. Affected men cannot pass the disease to their offspring, only women being able to transmit the disease to the next generation.

Symptoms

Visual loss is monocular, acute, painless, progressive (over days, weeks or months) and permanent. Significant improvement is rare. Invariably the condition becomes bilateral within weeks or months.

Signs

During the acute stage, the optic disc is mildly hyperaemic and swollen with irregular dilatation of the pre- and peripapillary capillaries (telangiectatic microangiopathy). There is no leakage of fluorescein from the telangiectatic vessels. The retinal nerve fibres around the disc frequently have a glistening appearance. These changes may be very subtle and easily overlooked. The typical visual field defect is a centrocaecal scotoma which gradually enlarges and eventually becomes absolute. During the late stage of the disease, visual acuity is reduced to counting fingers due to severe optic atrophy (*Figure 15.9*). Surprisingly the pupillary light reactions frequently remain fairly brisk despite severe visual loss.

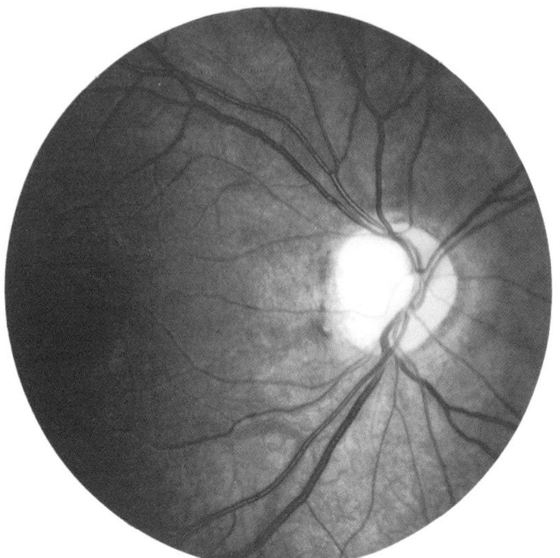

Figure 15.9 *Optic atrophy*

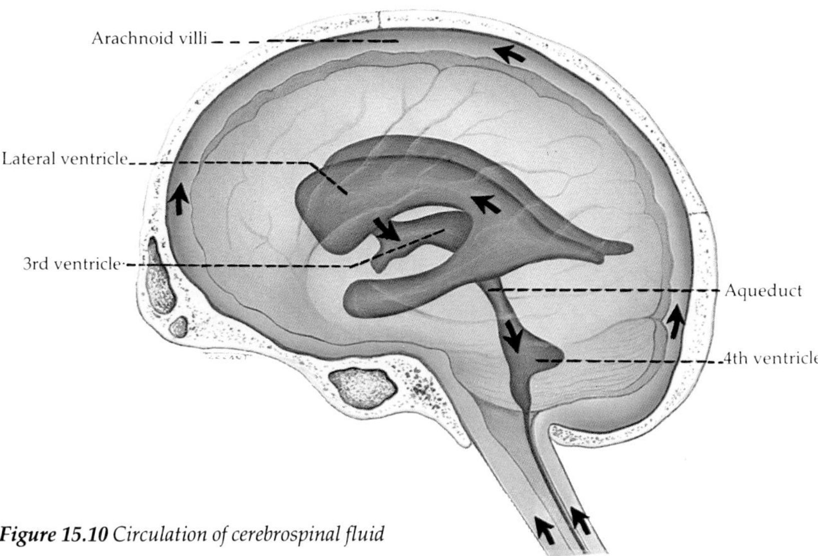

Figure 15.10 *Circulation of cerebrospinal fluid*

Treatment

Despite the lack of effective treatment, it is important to recognize this condition in order to save the patient from unnecessary investigations.

Papilloedema

Papilloedema is swelling of the optic nerve head produced by raised intracranial pressure.

Raised intracranial pressure

Causes

The CSF is formed by the choroid plexus in both lateral ventricles and that in the third ventricle, from where it flows through the aqueduct of Sylvius to the fourth ventricle. From there, it passes through the foramina of Luschka and Magendie, some flowing around the spinal cord and the rest bathing the cerebral hemispheres. It is finally absorbed into the cerebral venous drainage system through the arachnoid villi (*Figure 15.10*). Five main mechanisms may cause raised intracranial pressure:

1. Blockage of the ventricular system by congenital lesions such as aqueduct stenosis.
2. Blockage of the ventricular system by acquired lesions such as tumours.
3. Obstruction of CSF absorption by the arachnoid villi, which may be due either to a direct blockage of the villi by blood or protein, or to obstruction of the cerebral venous drainage system by a cortical venous thrombosis.
4. Space-occupying lesions.
5. Hypersecretion of CSF by a choroid plexus tumour (very rare).

General symptoms

Symptoms suggestive of raised intracranial pressure are headache (made worse by coughing or straining), vomiting (without nausea), changes in level of consciousness, and diplopia.

All patients with papilloedema should be presumed to have an intracranial mass until the contrary is proved. It is important to note, however, that not all patients with raised intracranial pressure will necessarily develop papilloedema, because cerebral tumours are less likely to cause papilloedema than tumours in the posterior fossa. Conversely, not all patients with papilloedema will have a tumour, as some may have benign intracranial hypertension or some other pathology.

Visual symptoms

Visual acuity is usually normal unless the fovea is involved by haemorrhage, exudate, or oedema. Colour vision and pupillary reactions are normal unless secondary optic atrophy is present. The peripheral fields are usually full, unless an intracranial mass lesion has caused a hemianopia. Variable enlargement of the blind spot is present.

Ophthalmological features

Early

The earliest detectable change is an indistinctness of the superior, inferior, and nasal margins of the optic disc (*Figure 15.11*). These findings are associated with blurring of the peripapillary nerve fibre layer. Because the swelling occurs first at the periphery of the optic disc, the central optic cup is usually preserved until late. (This is in distinction to pseudopapilloedema due to optic disc drusen in which the optic cup is absent.) As the oedema increases,

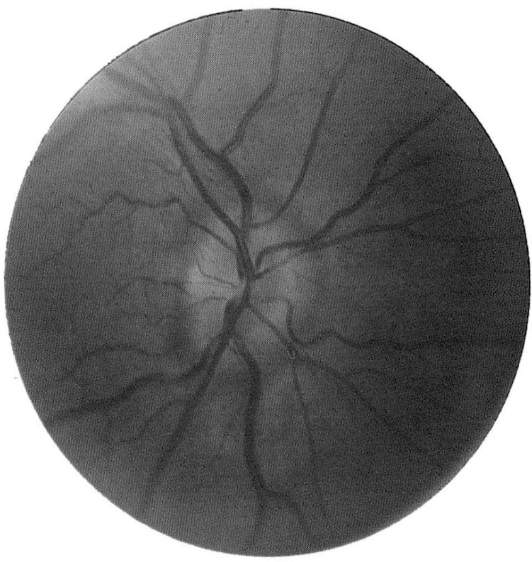

Figure 15.11 Early papilloedema (courtesy of Professor A. C. Bird)

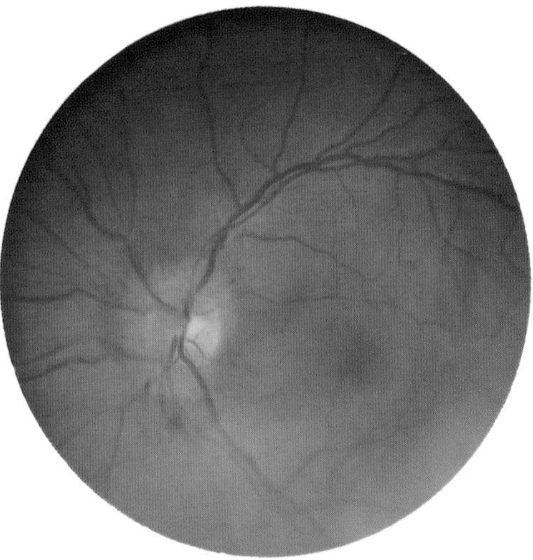

Figure 15.12 Established papilloedema

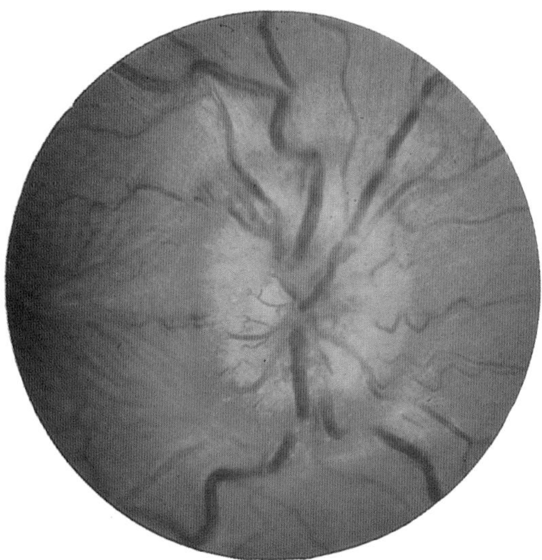

Figure 15.13 Advanced papilloedema with retinal folds (courtesy of Professor A. C. Bird)

the disc becomes hyperaemic with dilated capillaries. Another important sign of early papilloedema is loss of spontaneous venous pulsation. Because about 20% or normal healthy individuals do not have spontaneous venous pulsation, its absence does not mean that the intracranial pressure is elevated, although its presence strongly militates against the diagnosis of papilloedema. It should be noted that enlargement of the blind spot only occurs when the papilloedema is well established; therefore its size is of no value in the detection of early cases.

Established (fully developed)

As the intracranial pressure remains elevated, the veins become engorged and the disc surface becomes elevated above the plane of the retina. The disc margins become indistinct and the central optic cup obliterated. The oedema partially obscures the blood vessels passing over the disc surface (*Figure 15.12*).

These findings may be associated with the presence of multiple flame-shaped haemorrhages and 'cotton-wool' spots. As the swelling extends, the optic nerve head appears to be enlarged and circumferential retinal folds may develop (*Figure 15.13*) on its temporal side. Hard retinal exudates may radiate from the centre of the fovea in the shape of an incomplete star with its temporal part missing (*Figure 15.14*). At this stage, visual acuity is normal unless oedema, exudate, or haemorrhage involve the fovea. At this stage the blind spot is enlarged. Plotting the size of the blind spot may be useful in following the progression or regression of papilloedema. Transient obscurations of vision lasting between 5 and 10 seconds, usually on standing, may be reported by the patient.

'Vintage'

As the intracranial pressure remains elevated, the acute haemorrhagic and exudative components resolve and the

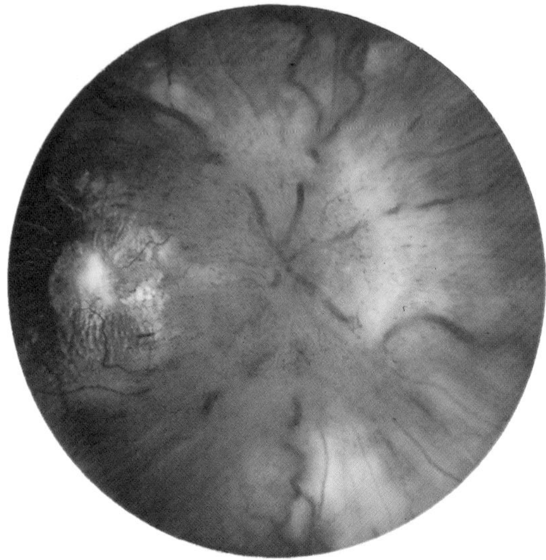

Figure 15.14 Advanced papilloedema with macular star

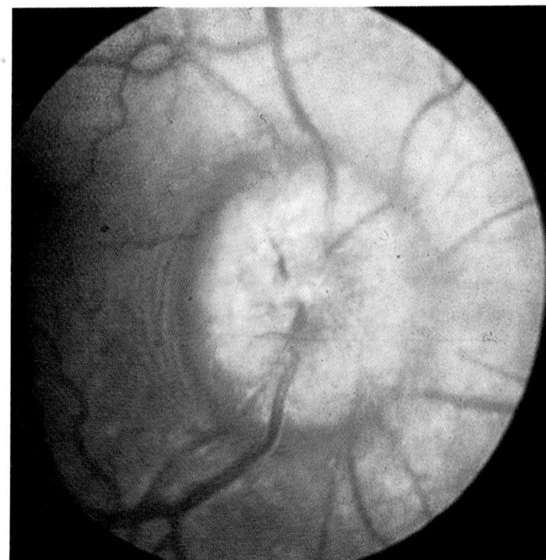

Figure 15.15 *Vintage papilloedema (courtesy of Mr R. Marsh)*

optic nerve head takes on the appearance of a champagne cork. This appearance indicates that the papilloedema has been present for several months (*Figure 15.15*).

Secondary optic atrophy

As the optic nerve head detumesces, it acquires a milky appearance due to reactive gliosis. Nerve fibre damage causes a progressive loss of visual field in the form of an irregular constriction with nerve fibre bundle defects. Secondary changes in the retinal pigment epithelium at the fovea may also contribute to impairment of central vision. This final stage of papilloedema is referred to as secondary optic atrophy (*Figure 15.16*).

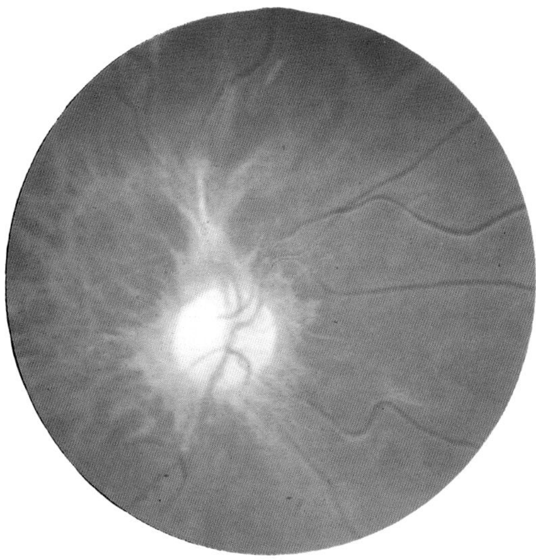

Figure 15.16 *Secondary optic atrophy (courtesy of Mr E. C. Glover)*

Axoplasmic transport

Optic nerve axoplasmic transport conveys material from the retinal ganglion cell to the entire axon and to its termination in the lateral geniculate body, where some of the material is graded before being returned to the cell body via the retrograde transport system. It has been shown that a constant finding in eyes with optic disc swelling is cessation of the rapid component of axoplasmic flow, particularly at the lamina cribrosa.

Other causes of disc swelling

1. Ocular hypotony either occurring postoperatively or following trauma.
2. Papillophlebitis (optic disc vasculitis).
3. Optic papillitis.
4. Chronic anterior uveitis and intermediate uveitis.
5. Compressive lesions such as optic nerve glioma and meningioma.
6. Anterior ischaemic optic neuropathy.
7. Leber's optic neuropathy.
8. Malignant hypertension.
9. Infiltrative optic neuropathy which may be due to tumour such as lymphoma, leukaemia and secondary deposits, or granulomas such as sarcoid and tuberculosis. Infiltrative optic neuropathy does not cause a true swelling of the disc, but the appearance can be confusing. The picture is one of a greyish-white disc, often associated with haemorrhages.

In general, unilateral cases of disc swelling should be considered to be due to a local inflammation, vascular disorder or compressive lesions in the orbit.

Optic nerve tumours

Glioma

Clinical features

This tumour typically presents between the ages of 4 and 8 years with unilateral proptosis and visual impairment. Because about 55% of patients will also have neurofibromatosis, all children presenting in this way should be examined for other stigmata of this condition.

Special investigations

1. *Plain X-rays.* In about 90% of cases, the tumour involves the anterior aspect of the optic canal and shows up on a Rhese view as a uniformly rounded enlargement of the optic foramen (*Figure 15.17*). The fact that the bony margins of the optic canal remain intact probably reflects the slow rate of growth of this tumour which is thought to be a benign congenital hamartoma.
2. *CT and ultrasound* show enlargement of the optic nerve which may be fusiform or irregular (*Figure 15.18*). CT is useful in demonstrating extension of the tumour into the optic canal.

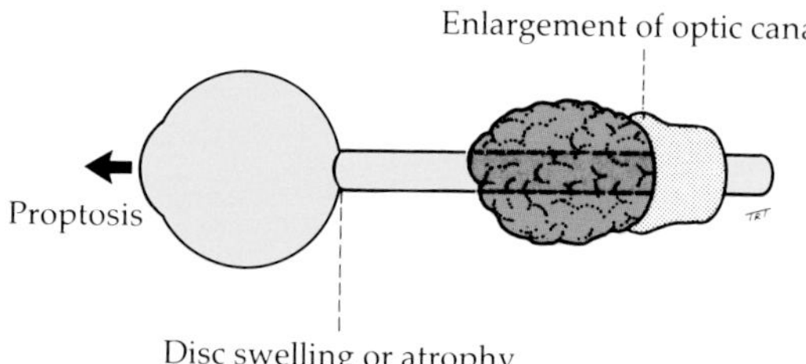

Figure 15.17 *Optic nerve glioma*

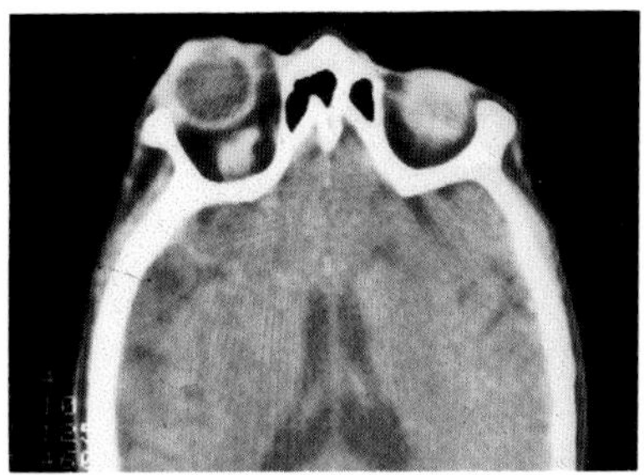

Figure 15.18 *CT scan showing enlargement of left optic nerve*

Treatment

If the proptosis becomes aesthetically unacceptable and the eye is blind from optic atrophy, then a local resection of the tumour with preservation of the globe is the method of choice. A lateral orbitotomy is usually necessary. Intracranial extension of the tumour requires the aid of a neurosurgeon. Radiation is helpful for tumours beyond surgical excision.

Meningioma

Clinical features

Meningiomas are invasive tumours which typically affect middle-aged women. The ocular features are related to the location of the tumour.

1. *Compression of the chiasm* is a frequent mode of presentation (*see* later).
2. *Tumours arising at the lateral portion* of the sphenoid bone (near the pterion) may extend into the orbit and cause proptosis in addition to optic nerve compression. The meningioma *en plaque* which affects the greater and lesser wings of the sphenoid bone is the most common variety to involve the orbit secondarily. These tumours typically cause a fullness in the temporal fossa and a slowly progressive proptosis due to hyperostosis of the lateral wall and roof of the orbit as well as invasion of the orbit itself.
3. *Optic nerve sheath meningiomas* usually arise from arachnoid villi and are initially confined by the surrounding dura. They present with a slowly progressive impairment of vision in one eye from optic nerve compression. As the tumour grows within the dural sheath, it causes a splinting of the optic nerve which impairs ocular movements, especially on upward gaze (*Figure 15.19*). Later, as the tumour bursts through the dura to form an enlarging mass within the muscle cone, it gives rise to proptosis. This sequence of presentation is quite opposite to that seen with lesions outside the dural sheaths in which proptosis is usually marked before there is any evidence of optic nerve compression.

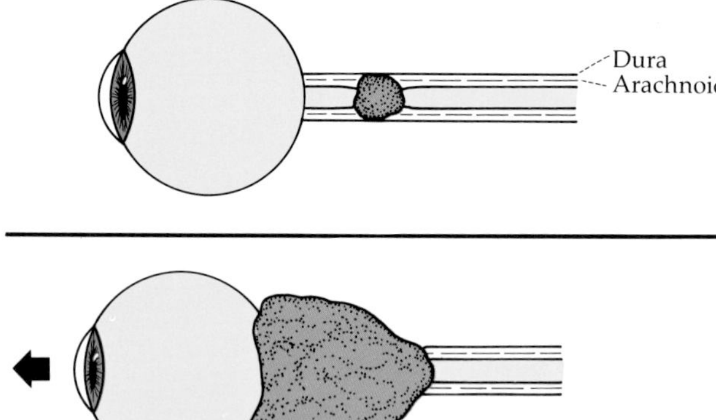

Figure 15.19 *Optic nerve sheath meningioma. Top: optic nerve compression; bottom: proptosis*

The triad of long-standing visual impairment, a pale swollen optic nerve head, and opticociliary shunt vessels (*Figure 15.20*) is virtually pathognomonic of an optic nerve sheath meningioma. It has been postulated that these vessels are shunts caused by a constriction of the central retinal vessels by the tumour. This causes a dilatation of preformed capillaries connecting the central retinal vein with the peripapillary choroidal vessels.

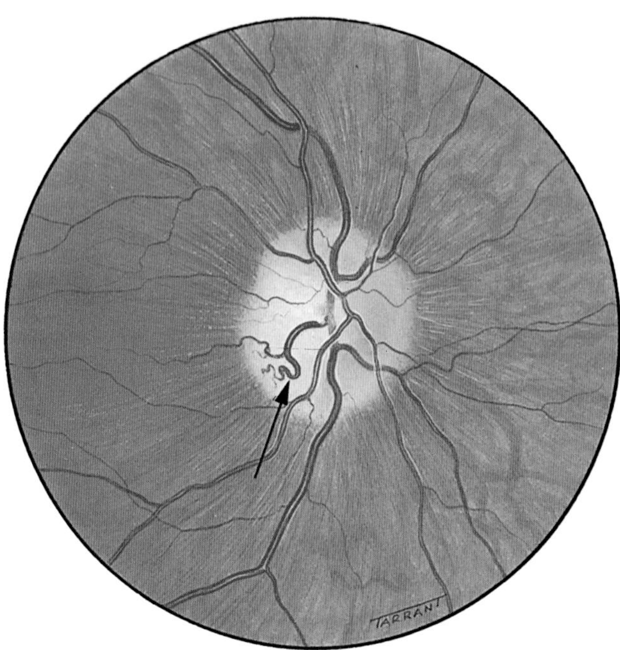

Figure 15.20 *Opticociliary shunt vessel*

Special investigations

1. *Plain X-rays.* Meningiomas of the lateral aspect of the sphenoid bone can be detected on plain X-rays, as they cause an increase in bony density (*Figure 15.21*).

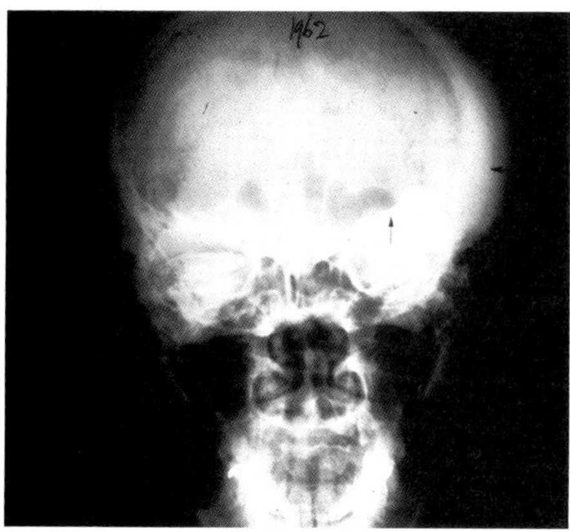

Figure 15.21 *Left hyperostosis from meningioma* en plaque *(courtesy of Dr I. Yentis)*

2. *CT scans* in optic nerve sheath meningiomas may show a segmental or diffuse enlargement of the intraorbital portion of the optic nerve.

Treatment

Although the visual prognosis following surgical excision of these tumours is extremely poor, because the operation involves the stripping of the optic nerve sheath together with its blood supply from the optic nerve, the prognosis for life is good. In children, however, these tumours are more aggressive and can be lethal. Recently, encouraging results have been reported with improved visual prognosis by treating the tumours with radiotherapy.

Neurofibroma

This tumour is composed mainly of proliferations of Schwann cells within the neural sheaths. Plexiform neurofibromas typically occur in patients with neurofibromatosis. Complete surgical removal is extremely difficult. Discrete neurofibromas are less common.

Congenital optic disc anomalies

Congenital anomalies of the optic disc are important for the following reasons:

1. They are common.
2. They may be confused with papilloedema.
3. They may give rise to visual field defects.
4. They may be associated with malformations of the CNS.
5. They may cause a disturbance at the macula.

Drusen (hyaline bodies)

Drusen are deposits of a hyaline-like calcific material within the substance of the optic nerve head. Clinically, they are present in about 0.3% of the population and are frequently bilateral and familial. In children, drusen lie deep beneath the surface of the disc tissue and cannot be identified ophthalmoscopically with ease. In this setting they may be confused with early papilloedema and the patient may be unnecessarily investigated for the possibility of a brain tumour. In contrast to early papilloedema, optic discs with drusen show the following features:

1. An absent optic cup.
2. Spontaneous venous pulsation is present in 80% of cases.
3. The retinal vessels show anomalous branching patterns.
4. The veins are not dilated and the vessels are not obscured as they traverse the disc surface.
5. The disc itself has a pink or yellow colour, unlike the hyperaemia of early papilloedema.
6. The peripapillary nerve fibre striations are not obscured.
7. The margins of the disc have a 'lumpy' appearance.

In difficult cases it may be necessary to examine the disc using a Hruby lens in order to detect drusen that are located below the disc surface. Other members of the family should also be examined.

During the early teens, drusen usually emerge at the surface of the optic disc and can be recognized by their bright reflection of light. They appear as waxy pearl-like irregularities (*Figure 15.22*).

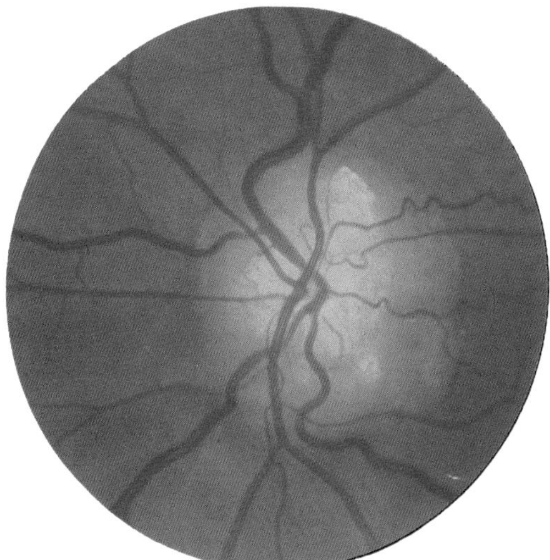

Figure 15.22 *Optic disc drusen (hyaline bodies)*

Fluorescein angiography

This may be helpful in differential diagnosis. Although eyes with buried drusen have anomalous disc vessels, there is no fluorescein leakage. In addition, drusen may show the phenomenon of autofluorescence and they may stain during the late stages of the angiogram. Eyes with early disc oedema, on the other hand, show early dye leakage.

Complications

Although the vast majority of eyes with drusen remain asymptomatic during the patient's lifetime, drusen can on occasion cause visual impairment due to either peripapillary haemorrhage or choroidal neovascularization and the subsequent development of a macular haemorrhage. In fact, these complications are so rare that eyes with drusen and visual loss should be suspected of having some other lesion such as compression of the optic nerve. Occasionally, eyes with drusen develop a progressive but limited loss of visual field which has a nerve fibre bundle pattern.

Associations

Although numerous diverse ocular and systemic associations have been described in association with drusen, there are no statistically significant associations except retinitis pigmentosa and possibly angioid streaks.

Myelinated nerve fibres

This common congenital abnormality can sometimes be mistaken for disc oedema. Normally, myelination of the anterior visual system begins at the lateral geniculate body during the seventh month of gestation and proceeds towards the eye, stopping at the lamina cribrosa. Intraocular myelination may follow several patterns. A common pattern is that of extensive myelination, beginning at the disc and extending towards the periphery (*Figure 15.23*).

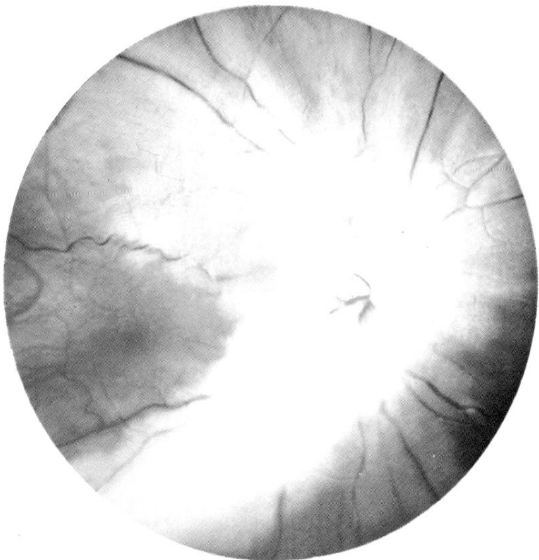

Figure 15.23 *Extensive myelinated nerve fibres*

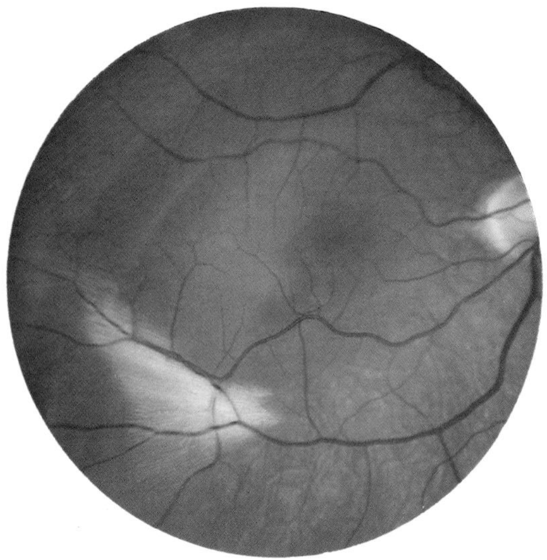

Figure 15.24 *Myelinated nerve fibres involving retina*

Although in these eyes visual acuity is normal, the blind spot may be enlarged. The myelinated nerve fibres follow the pattern of normal fibres and extend as irregular feather-shaped patches which may or may not obscure the retinal vessels (*Figure 15.24*). Although myelination is most frequently seen adjacent to the optic disc, patches of peripheral myelination may also occur. Although myelinated nerve fibres usually remain stationary, they have very rarely been reported to disappear in eyes with optic atrophy from demyelination or ischaemia.

Optic disc pit

This relatively common condition consists of a round or oval pit which appears darker than the surrounding disc tissue. The location is most frequently inferotemporal (*Figure 15.25*). The disc itself is usually larger than in the

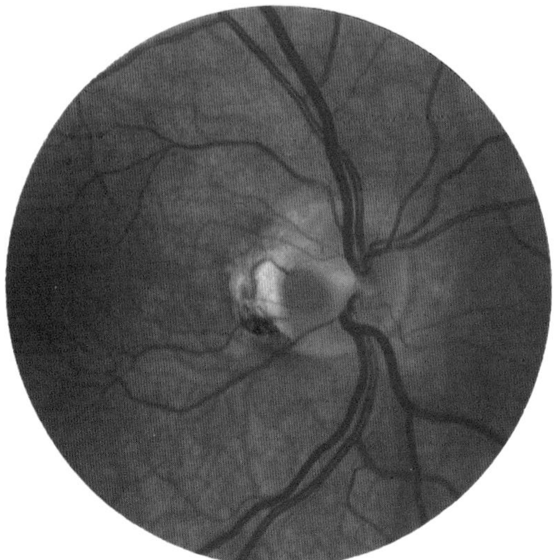

Figure 15.25 *Congenital optic disc pit*

unaffected eye. About 50% of eyes with congenital optic disc pits develop oedema or a serous detachment of the macula which can mimic central serous chorioretinopathy; it is therefore very important to examine the optic disc carefully in all patients with central serous chorioretinopathy. Three mechanisms have been postulated for the development of fluid in these eyes.

1. The fluid is CSF which has migrated into the subsensory retinal space.
2. The fluid is derived from the vitreous.
3. The fluid is derived from leaking abnormal blood vessels within the pit.

In some cases the serous detachments flatten spontaneously. Although there have been reports of successful treatment by photocoagulation, there is, as yet, no good evidence that this form of treatment is effective.

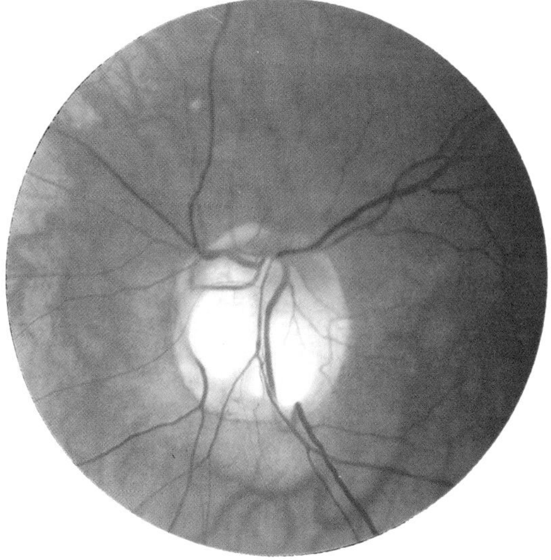

Figure 15.26 *Coloboma of optic disc*

Coloboma

A disc coloboma is caused by an incomplete closure of the fetal fissure. The disc contains a very large excavation which is usually situated inferiorly, so that normal disc tissue is confined to a small superior wedge (*Figure 15.26*). Eyes with colobomas often have decreased vision and a superior visual field defect. The appearance of the disc and the associated field defect may occasionally be confused with glaucoma.

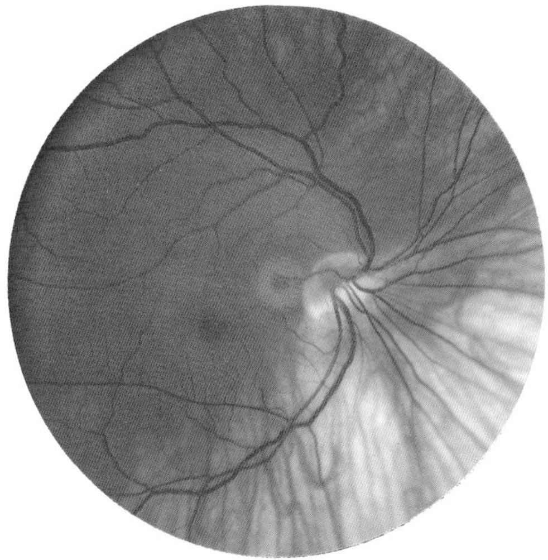

Figure 15.27 *Tilted disc – note hypopigmentation of inferonasal fundus*

Tilted disc

This fairly common, usually bilateral, condition is due to the entrance of the optic nerve into the globe at an oblique angle. The disc has an exaggerated oval appearance with the vertical axis directed obliquely so that its upper temporal portion lies anterior to the lower margin. This appearance may be mistaken for papilloedema. Eyes with tilted discs frequently have an inferior crescent, situs inversus of the retinal blood vessels, myopia, a moderate degree of oblique astigmatism, and hypopigmentation involving the inferonasal aspect of the retina (*Figure 15.27*). The latter is thought to be responsible for an upper temporal field defect which can possibly be mistaken for chiasmal compression. However, it is evident that these defects are not truly hemianopic as the smaller isopters do not obey the vertical midline (*Figure 15.28*).

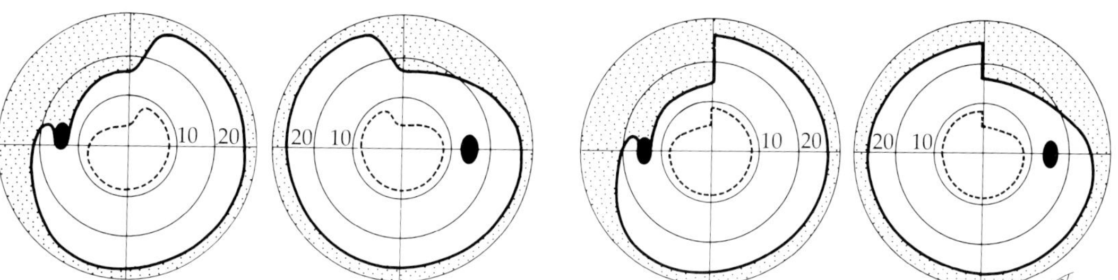

Figure 15.28 *Left: visual field defect associated with tilted optic discs; right: chiasmal compression*

Optic nerve hypoplasia

Clinical features

Optic nerve hypoplasia, once considered a great rarity, is being recognized with increased frequency. The condition is bilateral in about 60% of cases. If severe, it can result in marked impairment of visual acuity and an afferent pupillary conduction defect. Mild cases can be easily overlooked and the slightly reduced vision may be mistaken for amblyopia and treated with occlusion.

Visual field examination may show binasal or bitemporal defects, small arcuate defects, altitudinal hemianopias, and centrocaecal scotomas.

The typical appearance of optic nerve hypoplasia consists of a small grey optic disc surrounded by a yellow halo of hypopigmentation due to a concentric choroidal and retinal pigment epithelial abnormality. This appearance is referred to as the 'double-ring sign'. Despite the small optic disc the retinal blood vessels emerging from it are of normal calibre (*Figure 15.29*).

Other reported findings in eyes with hypoplastic optic discs are aniridia, nystagmus, small optic canals, and absence of the foveal reflex. The latter is probably due to thinning of the perifoveal retina. Optic nerve hypoplasia can occur as an isolated finding or it may be associated with midfacial, and CNS anomalies.

Neurological associations

A strong association exists between bilateral optic nerve hypoplasia, absence of the septum pellucidum and agenesis of the corpus callosum. On CT scanning, only a single anterior ventricle is found. This association is called 'septo-optic dysplasia' or de Morsier's syndrome. Patients with this condition have small stature and endocrine abnormalities, especially low growth hormone levels. If the condition is recognized early the hormonal deficiency can be corrected and normal growth resumed. Other more severe CNS associations include hydranencephaly and anencephaly.

Maternal associations

A high incidence of optic nerve hypoplasia has been reported in children whose mothers are diabetic or have taken antiepileptic drugs, quinine, or LSD during pregnancy.

Morning glory syndrome

This is a very rare dysplastic coloboma of the optic disc which resembles the morning glory flower. The optic nerve head appears enlarged and excavated and contains persistent hyaloid remnants within its base. The blood vessels emerge from the rim of the excavation in a radial pattern like the spokes of a wheel. The coloboma itself is surrounded by an elevated annulus of chorioretinal pigmentary disturbance (*Figure 15.30*). A common association is a non-rhegmatogenous retinal detachment. Vision is grossly impaired visually even without retinal detachment, but fortunately the condition is usually unilateral.

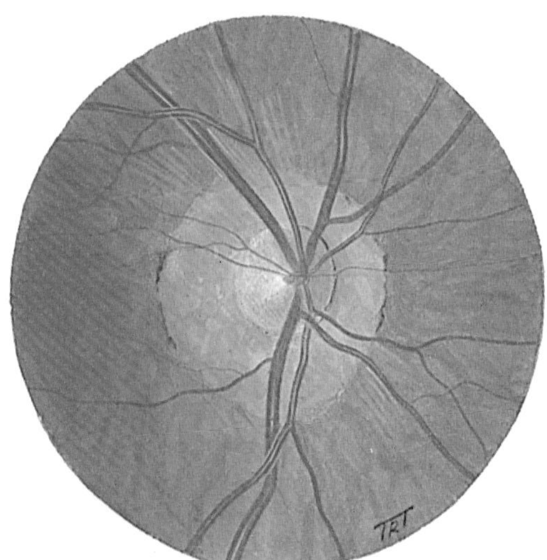

Figure 15.29 *Optic nerve hypoplasia*

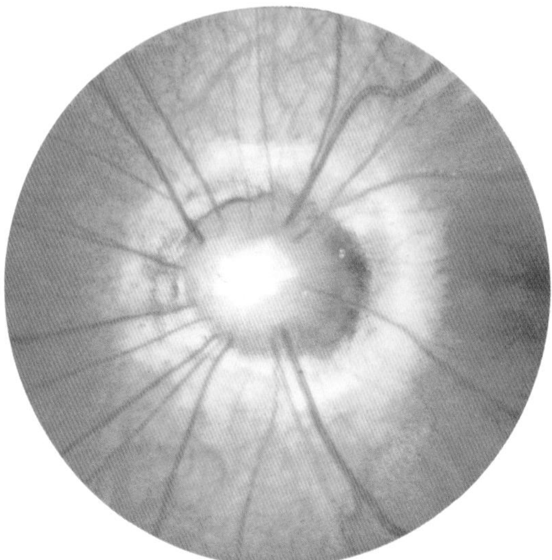

Figure 15.30 *Morning glory syndrome (courtesy of Professor A. C. Bird)*

Congenital disc anomalies and other malformations

A strong association exists between congenital disc anomalies, midfacial malformations, and basal encephalocele. It appears that it is not so much the actual type of anomaly of the disc which indicates the presence of a cranial base defect but rather its association with a midfacial malformation. The main midfacial anomalies are hypertelorism (*Figure 15.31*), nasal malformations, cleft palate and 'hare-lip'.

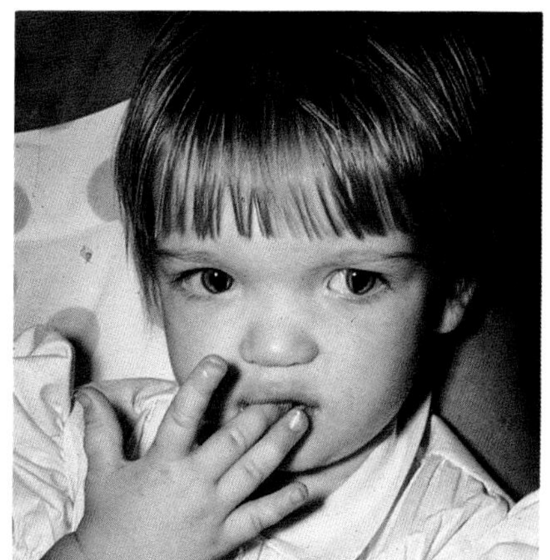

Figure 15.31 *Hypertelorism (courtesy of Professor A. C. Bird)*

Chiasmal disorders

Applied anatomy

The pituitary gland lies in a bony cavity of the sphenoid bone called the sella turcica (*Figure 15.32*). The roof of the sella (the diaphragma sellae) is formed by a fold of dura mater which stretches from the anterior clinoids to the posterior clinoids. The optic nerves and the chiasm lie above the diaphragma and therefore the presence of a visual field defect in a patient with a pituitary tumour indicates suprasellar extension. Tumours that are still confined to the sella will not cause field defects. Within the chiasm, the inferonasal fibres cross low and anteriorly and are therefore most vulnerable to damage from expanding intrasellar lesions. The upper nasal fibres, however, cross the chiasm high and posteriorly. Although the macular fibres decussate throughout the chiasm, they also move posteriorly and superiorly. For this reason, lesions involving the posterior chiasmal notch, such as craniopharyngiomas, will not only cause inferotemporal field defects but also bitemporal hemianopic scotomas.

It is important to note that the chiasm is situated in the antero-inferior region of the third ventricle. Expanding lesions in this region may compress the hypothalamus and, by distorting the third ventricle and blocking the foramen of Monro, give rise to elevation of intracranial pressure.

In about 80% of normal subjects, the chiasm lies directly above the sella (*Figure 15.33*). Expanding pituitary lesions will therefore involve the chiasm first. However, in approximately 10% of normal subjects the chiasm is situated more anteriorly, over the tuberculum sellae

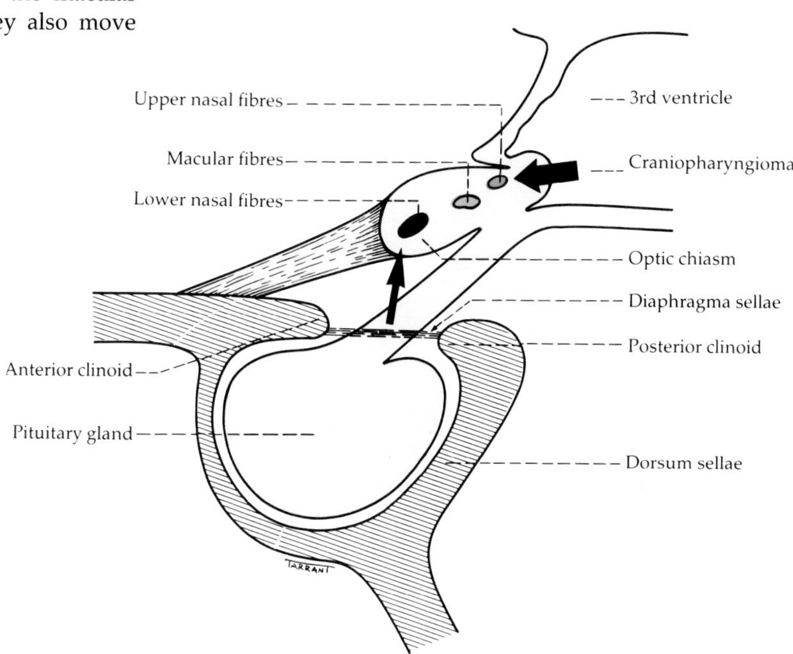

Figure 15.32 *Anatomy of optic chiasm*

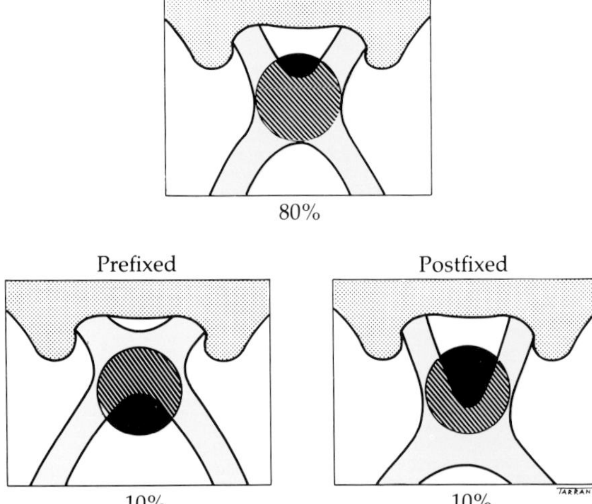

Figure 15.33 *Anatomical variations of normal optic chiasm*

(prefixed). In this situation pituitary tumours may compress the optic tracts first. Another anatomical variation, present in the remaining 10% of cases, is a postfixed chiasm where the chiasm is located more posteriorly, over the dorsum sellae. Because in this situation the optic nerves have a long intracranial course, pituitary tumours are apt to present with compression of the optic nerves.

The cavernous sinus lies lateral to the sella (*Figure 15.34, left*). For this reason, laterally expanding pituitary tumours can invade the cavernous sinus and damage the third, fourth, and even the sixth cranial nerves. Conversely, aneurysms arising from the intracavernous portion of the internal carotid artery may erode into the sella and mimic pituitary tumours. There is also an association between pituitary tumours and parasellar aneurysms. For this reason it may be necessary to perform carotid angiography prior to surgical exploration of the sella region.

As the internal carotid artery curves posteriorly and upwards into the cavernous sinus, it lies immediately below the optic nerves (*Figure 15.34, right*). It then ascends vertically alongside the lateral aspect of the chiasm. The precommunicating portion of the anterior cerebral artery is closely related to the anterior surface of the chiasm and optic nerves. An aneurysm in this region can therefore compress both the optic nerve and the chiasm.

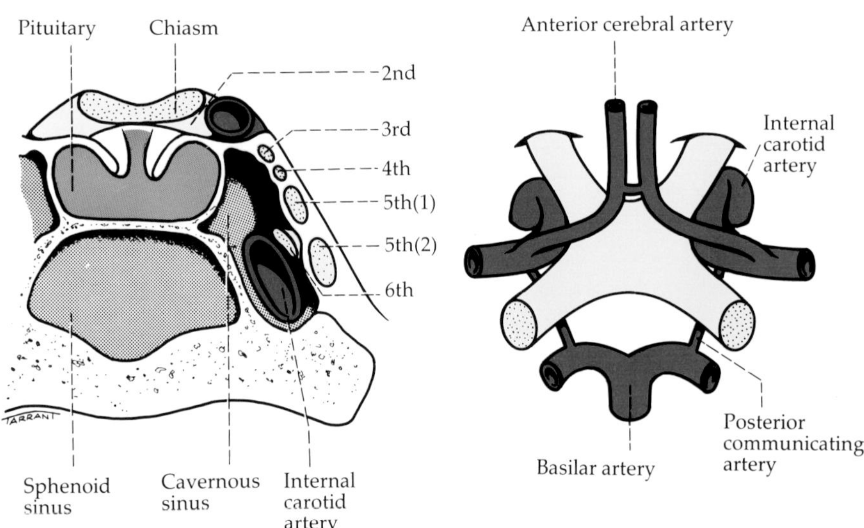

Figure 15.34 *Left: anatomy of cavernous sinus; right: relations of circle of Willis to chiasm*

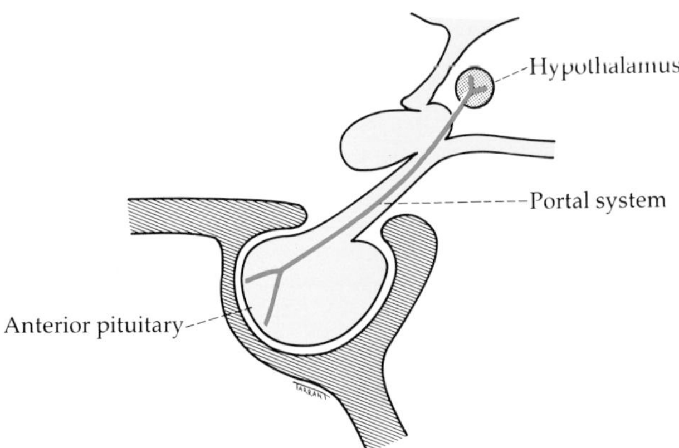

Figure 15.35 *Pituitary portal system*

Applied physiology of the pituitary gland

The lobules of the anterior part of the pituitary gland are composed of six cell types. Five of these secrete hormones and the sixth (the follicular cell) has no secretory function. The five hormones secreted are growth hormone, prolactin, FSH, ACTH, and TSH. The anterior pituitary is itself under the control of the various inhibiting and releasing factors that are synthesized in the hypothalamus and pass to the pituitary gland through the portal system (*Figure 15.35*).

Pituitary hypofunction may therefore be due to interference with the synthesis of inhibiting and releasing factors in the hypothalamus, impediment of their transport in the portal system, or direct destruction of the secreting cells in the anterior pituitary. The actual clinical picture of hypopituitarism is dictated by the pattern of hormone deficiency and also by the state of growth and development of the patient at the time. Usually gonadotrophin secretion is impaired first, followed by impairment of growth hormone, while deficiences in other hormones occur later.

Classification

Pituitary adenomas
Craniopharyngioma
Meningioma
Aneurysm
Miscellaneous
  glioma
  demyelination
  trauma
  inflammation

Pituitary adenoma

Clinical features

Although pituitary adenomas are usually classified as basophil, acidophil, and chromophobe, tumours of mixed-cell types are common. In fact any of the six cell types may proliferate to produce an adenoma. Basophil tumours secrete ACTH and cause Cushing's disease. Acidophil tumours secrete growth hormone and in adults they cause acromegaly, while in children they give rise to gigantism. It has recently become apparent that many of the so-called chromophobe adenomas actually secrete prolactin and are now referred to as prolactinomas. The effects of excessive levels of prolactin give rise to the infertility–amenorrhoea–galactorrhoea syndrome in women. In men the clinical picture is that of hypogonadism, impotence, infertility, decreased libido, sometimes gynaecomastia and even galactorrhoea (*Figure 15.36*).

The chromophobe adenoma is the most common primary intracranial tumour producing neuro-ophthalmological features. It occurs most frequently in early adult life or middle age.

1. *Initial symptoms* may be rather non-specific, such as headache and vague blurring of vision. As the tumour expands upwards and breaks through the diaphragma the headaches may cease.
2. *Field defects* (*Figure 15.37*). As the tumour grows upwards it splays the anterior chiasmal notch and compresses the crossing inferonasal fibres. This causes a defect in the upper visual field which then progresses in an anticlockwise direction in the left eye and in a clockwise direction in the right eye. The degree of field loss is usually asymmetrical, although the eye with the greater loss usually also has impairment of visual acuity. However, optic atrophy is only present in 50% of cases with field defects. For this reason, it is extremely important to perform careful examination of the visual fields in all patients with unexplained visual loss. The absence of a visual field defect does not exclude the possibility of a pituitary tumour because acidophil adenomas do not expand beyond the sella as frequently as chromophobe adenomas. In addition, basophil adenomas are usually small and rarely give rise to chiasmal compression.
3. *Diplopia* may be due to lateral extension and involvement of the third, fourth, and even sixth nerves in the cavernous sinus. Occasionally the diplopia may be of a transient non-paretic type associated with the inability to fuse the two hemifields.
4. *'See-saw' nystagmus of Maddox* (*see* later).

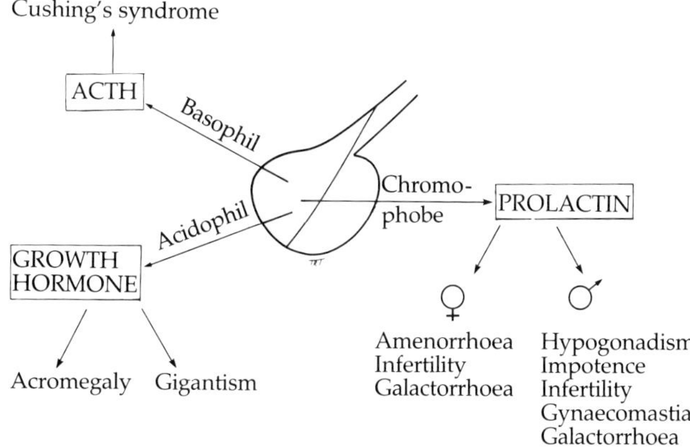

Figure 15.36 *Hormones secreted by anterior pituitary*

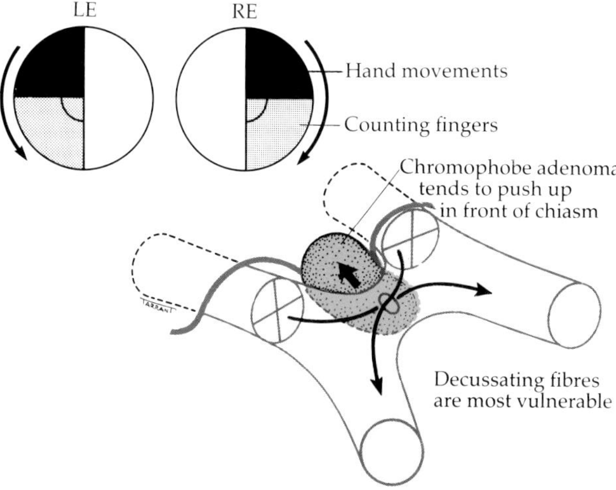

Figure 15.37 *Chiasmal compression from below due to a pituitary adenoma*

Radiological features

Typically the posterior structures are involved first and the anterior structures last. One of the earliest signs is an erosion of the dorsum sellae. The sella then becomes enlarged and the asymmetrical erosion of its floor gives rise to the so-called 'double-floor sign' (*Figure 15.38*). The anterior clinoids are next to be eroded, so that finally a complete destruction of all anatomical landmarks occurs.

An enlarged sella turcica may also be caused by a glioma of the optic nerve at its junction with the chiasm, which typically causes an undercutting of the anterior clinoids and erosion of the anterior aspect of the sella, giving rise to the 'J-shaped sella' sign. The sella may also become enlarged as a result of chronically raised intracranial pressure. Rarely, patients with neurofibromatosis have a congenital bony defect which gives rise to an enlarged sella.

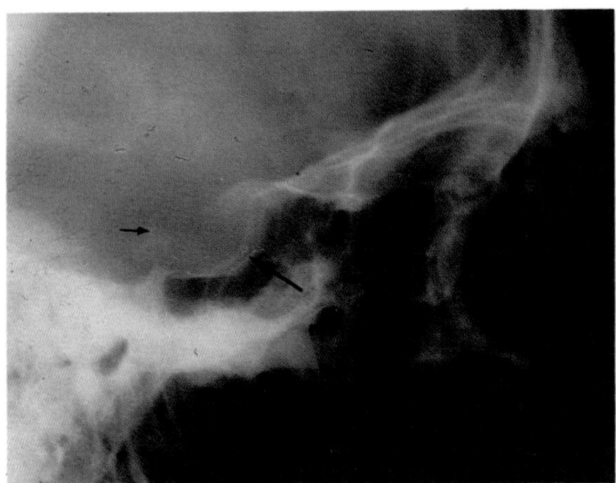

Figure 15.38 *Erosion of dorsum sellae (horizontal arrow), double floor (oblique arrow)*

Treatment

1. *Surgery.* If the tumour is extensive, a transfrontal approach is preferred, as it offers a better opportunity to decompress the optic pathways. Small and medium localized tumours can be approached trans-sphenoidally.
2. *Medical therapy with bromocriptine* causes an increase in secretion of prolactin-inhibiting factor by the hypothalamus and in this way blocks the secretion of prolactin by the anterior pituitary. It causes a dramatic shrinkage of a prolactin-secreting tumour.
3. *Radiotherapy* can be used alone or in combination with the other two modalities. Localized irradiation with yttrium seeds can also be used.

Craniopharyngioma

Clinical features

Craniopharyngiomas are slow-growing tumours arising from vestigial remnants of Rathke's pouch along the pituitary stalk. They occur in children as well as in adults. Although they do not secrete hormones, they may interfere with hypothalamic function and in children they may cause pituitary dwarfism, delayed sexual development and, occasionally, obesity. Adults with these tumours usually present with defects in visual acuity and visual fields, although craniopharyngiomas may also be responsible for endocrine dysfunction and raised intracranial pressure.

Field defects (*Figure 15.39*)

Craniopharyngiomas compress the chiasm from above and behind, interfering first with the crossing upper nasal fibres. The corresponding field defects therefore usually start in the inferotemporal quadrants, then spread in a clockwise direction in the left eye and an anticlockwise direction in the right eye.

Radiological features

The initial X-ray changes are a spreading apart of the anterior and posterior clinoids, followed by erosion of the dorsum sellae. The presence of suprasellar calcification is highly suggestive of a craniopharyngioma (*Figure 15.40*),

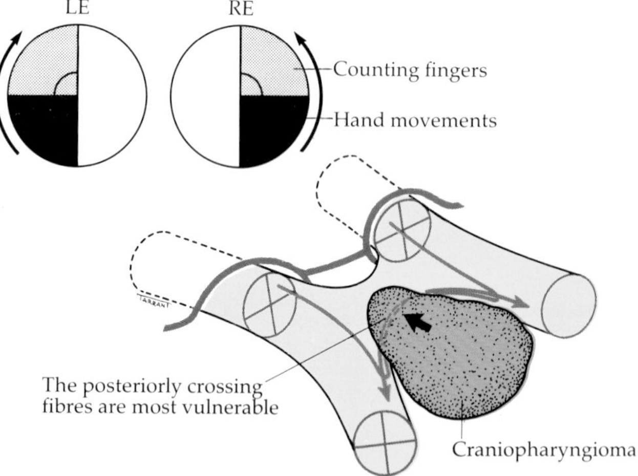

Figure 15.39 *Chiasmal compression from above by a craniopharyngioma*

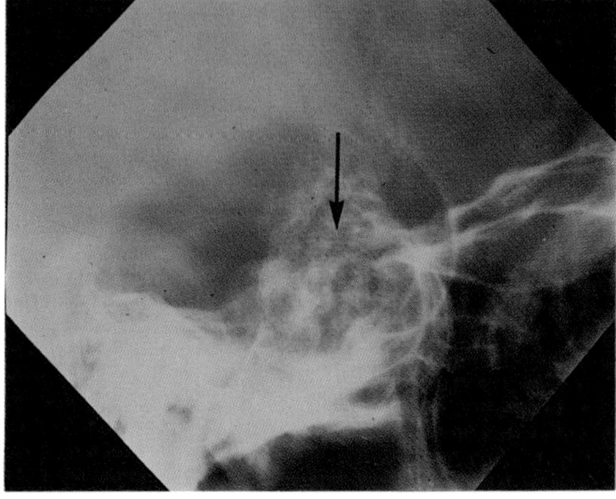

Figure 15.40 *Suprasellar calcification in craniopharyngioma (courtesy of Dr I. Yentis)*

although it may also occur with carotid aneurysms. The incidence of calcification in association with craniopharyngioma is 70% in patients between the ages of 2 and 16 years, and 50% in those over the age of 16 years.

Treatment

Unfortunately, owing to their local attachments, surgical removal is difficult and recurrences are common.

Meningioma

Meningiomas typically affect middle-aged women and classically, though by no means invariably, cause hyperostosis, which can be seen on a plain skull X-ray. When they arise from the tuberculum sellae, they may compress either the optic nerve or chiasm (*Figure 15.41*). Tumours compressing the junction of the chiasm and optic nerve will interfere with the anterior knee of Wilbrand. This consists of a loop of the contralateral inferonasal fibres which sweeps into the optic nerve before passing posteriorly. A lesion at this site will therefore give rise to an ipsilateral central scotoma and a contralateral upper temporal field defect (referred to as 'junctional scotoma'). For this reason it is very important to test the visual field of the opposite eye in all patients who present with unexplained unilateral visual impairment.

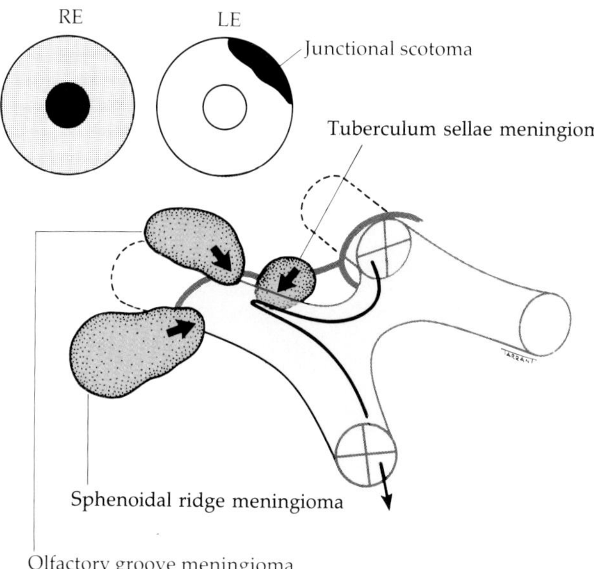

Figure 15.41 *Intracranial optic nerve compression by meningiomas*

Meningiomas can also arise from the sphenoidal ridge and compress the optic nerve. Those originating from the olfactory groove may cause a loss of the sense of smell as well as optic nerve compression.

Aneurysm

A dilatation of a carotid aneurysm may cause lateral compression of the chiasm. The field defect is initially unilateral but it may become bilateral if the chiasm is pushed across against the opposite carotid artery (*Figure 15.42*). Lateral chiasmal compression may also occur from a dilated third ventricle which causes a lateral splaying of the chiasm against the pulsatile carotid arteries. It should be remembered that carotid aneurysms may also invade the sella and mimic pituitary adenomas and that pituitary adenomas are associated with a higher incidence of parasellar aneurysms.

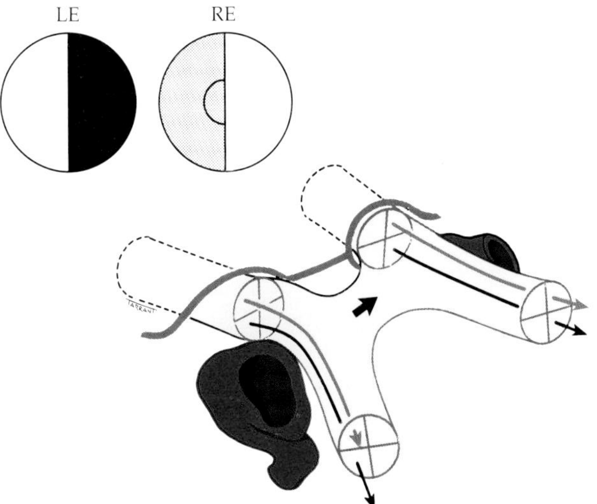

Figure 15.42 *Lateral chiasmal compression by aneurysm*

Other lesions

Most chiasmal disorders are due to extrinsic lesions: pituitary adenomas, craniopharyngiomas, meningiomas, and aneurysms. However, intrinsic lesions may also occur, such as gliomas, demyelination, and trauma. The chiasm may also be involved by infiltrative or inflammatory disorders affecting the basal leptomeninges

Optic tract disorders

Applied anatomy

The optic tracts arise at the posterior aspect of the chiasm, diverge and extend posteriorly around the cerebral peduncles, to terminate in the lateral geniculate bodies. A lesion of the optic tract may therefore also damage the ipsilateral cerebral peduncle and give rise to mild contralateral pyramidal signs. Each optic tract contains crossed nasal fibres that originate in the contralateral nasal hemiretina, and uncrossed temporal fibres that originate in the ipsilateral temporal hemiretina. The nerve fibres from corresponding retinal elements are, however, not closely aligned. For this reason, homonymous hemianopias caused by optic tract lesions are characteristically incongruous. The optic tracts contain both visual and pupillomotor fibres. The visual fibres terminate in the lateral geniculate body but the pupillomotor fibres leave the optic tract anterior to the lateral geniculate body, project through the brachium of the superior colliculus to terminate in the pretectal nucleus. An optic tract lesion may therefore give rise to an afferent pupillary conduction defect. Characteristically, the pupillary light reaction will be normal when the unaffected hemiretina is stimulated and absent when the involved hemiretinal is stimulated. In practice, this Wernicke's hemianopic pupillary reaction is difficult to elicit. Because the cell bodies of all fibres in the optic tract are the retinal ganglion cells, optic atrophy may result when these fibres are damaged.

Clinical features

1. *Incongruous homonymous hemianopia.*
2. *Optic atrophy.*
3. *Wernicke's hemianopic pupil.*

Aetiology

Lesions of the optic tract are relatively rare and essentially similar to those causing damage to the chiasm (i.e. craniopharyngiomas, posteriorly expanding pituitary tumours, meningiomas, and suprasellar aneurysms).

Disorders of the optic radiations and visual cortex

Applied anatomy

The optic radiations extend from the lateral geniculate body to the striate calcarine cortex which is located on the medial aspect of the occipital lobe, above and below the calcarine fissure (*Figure 15.43*). As the optic radiations pass posteriorly, fibres from corresponding retinal elements lie progressively closer together. For this reason, incomplete hemianopias produced by lesions of the posterior radiations are more congruous than those involving the anterior radiations. However, a complete hemianopia has no localizing value because the extent of incongruity cannot be assessed. Because the visual fibres synapse in the lateral geniculate body, lesions of the optic radiations do not produce optic atrophy. The blood supply to the optic radiations is from the middle and posterior cerebral arteries.

The superior fibres of the optic radiations, which subserve the inferior visual fields, proceed directly posteriorly through the parietal lobe to the occipital cortex. A lesion involving only the anterior parietal part of the radiation, which is very rare, will therefore cause an inferior quadrantic hemianopia ('pie on the floor'). In general, hemianopias due to parietal lobe lesions tend to be relatively congruous and either complete or denser below.

The inferior fibres of the optic radiations, which subserve the upper visual fields, first sweep antero-inferiorly in Meyer's loop around the anterior tip of the temporal horn of the lateral ventricle, and into the temporal lobe. Lesions in this region classically give rise to an upper quadrantic hemianopia ('pie in the sky'). Because the inferior fibres are also very close to the sensory and motor fibres of the internal capsule, a lesion in this area, which is usually vascular, may also give rise to a contralateral hemiparesis. The inferior fibres then pass posteriorly and rejoin the superior fibres. In general hemianopias due to temporal lobe lesions are relatively incongruous and denser above. Deep in the parietal lobe, the optic radiations lie just external to the trigone and occipital horn of the lateral ventricle.

In the striate calcarine cortex, the peripheral visual fields are represented anteriorly. This part of the occipital lobe is supplied by a branch of the posterior cerebral artery. Central macular vision is represented posteriorly, at the tip of the calcarine cortex which is supplied by a branch of the middle cerebral artery. Occlusion of the posterior cerebral artery will therefore produce a macular sparing congruous homonymous hemianopia. Damage to the tip of the occipital cortex, as might occur from a head injury, will give rise to congruous homonymous macular defects.

Associated neurological features

Apart from hemianopias, other features of temporal lobe disease include parosyxmal olfactory or gustatatory hallucinations (uncinate fits), formed visual hallucinations, sensory aphasia, and seizures. Patients with parietal lobe disease may have visual perception difficulties, agnosia,

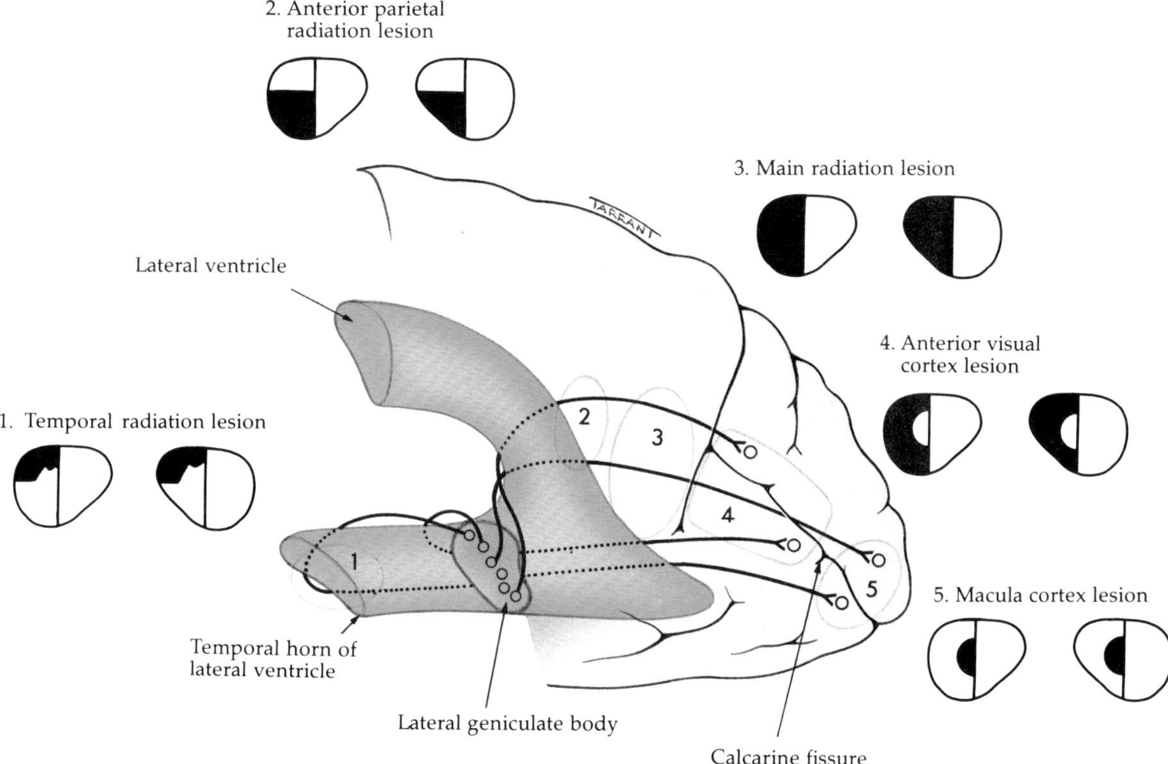

Figure 15.43 *Field defects caused by lesions of the optic radiations and visual cortex*

right–left confusion, and acalculia. Lesions of the visual cortex may produce formed visual hallucinations. The denial of blindness in a patient with complete cortical blindness is referred to as Anton's syndrome. It is extremely rare.

Aetiology

About 90% of isolated homonymous hemianopias in the absence of other neurological deficits are due to vascular occlusion in the distribution of the posterior cerebral artery. Other less common causes include trauma, and primary and secondary tumours.

Optokinetic nystagmus

Optokinetic nystagmus (OKN) may be useful in determining the cause of an isolated homonymous hemianopia that does not conform to any set pattern in patients without associated neurological deficits. If the optomotor pathways in the posterior hemispheres are damaged, the OKN response will be diminished when targets are rotated towards the side of the lesion (away from the hemianopia). This is called a positive OKN sign. In most cases, the combination of a homonymous hemianopia and optokinetic nystagmus asymmetry suggests a parietal lobe lesion, often a neoplasm. Rarely occipital lobe lesions may also cause optokinetic nystagmus asymmetry.

Supranuclear disorders of eye movement

Horizontal gaze

The four supranuclear eye movement systems are: saccadic, smooth pursuit, vergence and non-optical reflex.

Saccadic (*Figure 15.44, left*)

1. *Function*. The function is to place the object of interest on the fovea rapidly or to move the eyes from one object to another. This can be done voluntarily or can occur as a reflex stimulated by the presence of the object in the peripheral visual field. Voluntary saccadic movement is similar to the gunnery system of rapidly locating a moving target.
2. *Pathway*. The pathway for saccadic horizontal conjugate movements originates in the premotor cortex of the frontal motor area. From there, fibres pass to the

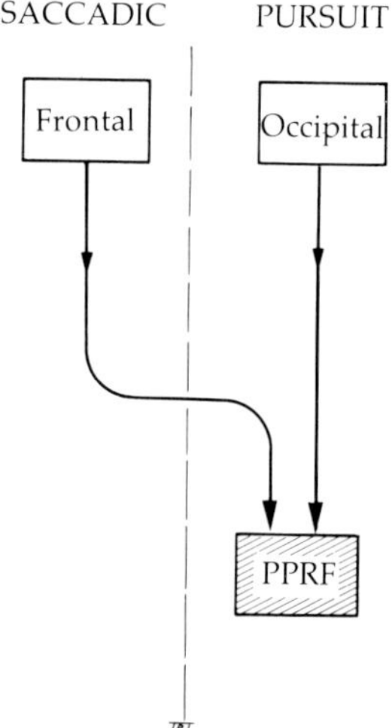

Figure 15.44 *Pathways for saccadic and pursuit systems*

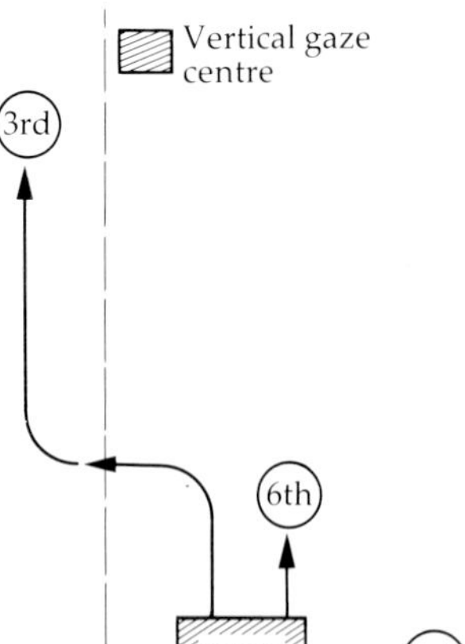

Figure 15.45 *Pathways for vestibular system and medial longitudinal bundle*

horizontal gaze centre in the pontine paramedian reticular formation (PPRF). The right frontal lobe controls horizontal saccades to the left and the left frontal lobe controls horizontal saccades to the right. Irritative lesions may therefore cause a deviation of the eyes to the opposite side.

Smooth pursuit (*Figure 15.44, right*)

1. *Function.* The function is to maintain fixation on the target once it has been located by the saccadic system. The stimulus is movement of the object near the fovea. The movements are slow and smooth.
2. *Pathway.* The efferent fibres begin in the peristriate cortex of the occipital motor area. They then descend and, after a double decussation, terminate in the *ipsilateral* horizontal gaze centre in the PPRF. The right occipital lobe therefore controls pursuit movement to the right and the left occipital lobe controls pursuit movement to the left.

Vergence

The function of the vergence and fusional system is to control the degree of convergence of the eyes so that the target is on the fovea of each eye for all distances. The stimulus is retinal disparity.

Non-optical reflex (vestibular; ***Figure 15.45*****)**

1. *Function.* These movements maintain eye position with respect to any changes of the head and body as a whole.
2. *Pathway.* The vestibular system derives information concerning head and neck movements from the labyrinths and from the proprioceptors in the muscles of the neck. Afferent fibres synapse in the vestibular nucleus and pass to the horizontal gaze centre in the PPRF.

Medial longitudinal bundle

All horizontal eye movements are generated from the PPRF. From here the output is to the ipsilateral sixth nerve nucleus and also to the contralateral third nerve nuclear complex. The pathway joining these two structures is the medial longitudinal bundle. Lesions of this pathway will cause an internuclear ophthalmoplegia, which is characterized by defective adduction of the ipsilateral eye, while the opposite abducting eye shows nystagmus (ataxic nystagmus). Unilateral internuclear ophthalmoplegia is most frequently due to brainstem vascular disease, whereas bilateral involvement is usually caused by demyelination.

Vertical gaze

There are similar saccadic, pursuit, and vestibular systems for vertical eye movements. The efferent pathways proceed to the vertical gaze centre which is located in the pretectal region of the midbrain, where impulses to the third and fourth nerve nuclei for vertical eye movements are coordinated. Lesions of this region will result in Parinaud's syndrome which is characterized by defective elevation, light–near dissociation, and convergence–retraction nystagmus.

Oculomotor (third) nerve palsy

Applied anatomy (*Figure 15.46*)

Nucleus

The third nerve nuclear complex is situated in the midbrain at the level of the superior colliculus, inferior to the sylvian aqueduct. It is composed of paired and unpaired subnuclei, lesions of which can produce a variety of clinical findings.

Unpaired

A single caudal midline subnucleus innervates *both* levator muscles. For this reason bilateral ptosis (midbrain ptosis) can be produced by lesions in this area.

Paired

The superior rectus subnucleus innervates the *contralateral* superior rectus muscle. For this reason a unilateral third nerve palsy with sparing of the contralateral superior rectus cannot be of nuclear origin. The medial rectus, the inferior rectus, and inferior oblique muscles are innervated by their corresponding ipsilateral subnuclei.

Fasciculus

Efferent fibres from the third nerve nucleus pass through the red nucleus and the medial aspect of the cerebral peduncle, then emerge from the midbrain and pass into the interpeduncular space. The clinical features of lesions involving the fasciculus will depend on their location. In terms of frequency, important causes of nuclear or fascicular lesions are demyelination, vascular and neoplastic.

Benedikt's syndrome

This is caused by damage to the dorsal part of the fasciculus as it passes through the red nucleus. This will give rise to an ipsilateral third nerve palsy associated with a contralateral ataxia and a flapping tremor.

Weber's syndrome

This is due to damage involving the ventral part of the fasciculus as it passes through the cerebral peduncle. This is characterized by an ipsilateral third nerve palsy associated with a contralateral hemiplegia due to involvement of the corticospinal tract that passes through the peduncle.

Peripheral part

This part of the third nerve can be subdivided into basilar, cavernous, and orbital.

Basilar

The fibres of the third nerve leave the midbrain as a series of 'rootlets' before coalescing to form the main trunk. The nerve passes between the posterior cerebral artery and the superior cerebellar artery. It then passes lateral to and parallel with the posterior communicating artery. Because the third nerve traverses the base of the skull along its subarachnoid course unaccompanied by any of the other cranial nerves, isolated third nerve palsies are frequently basilar in origin.

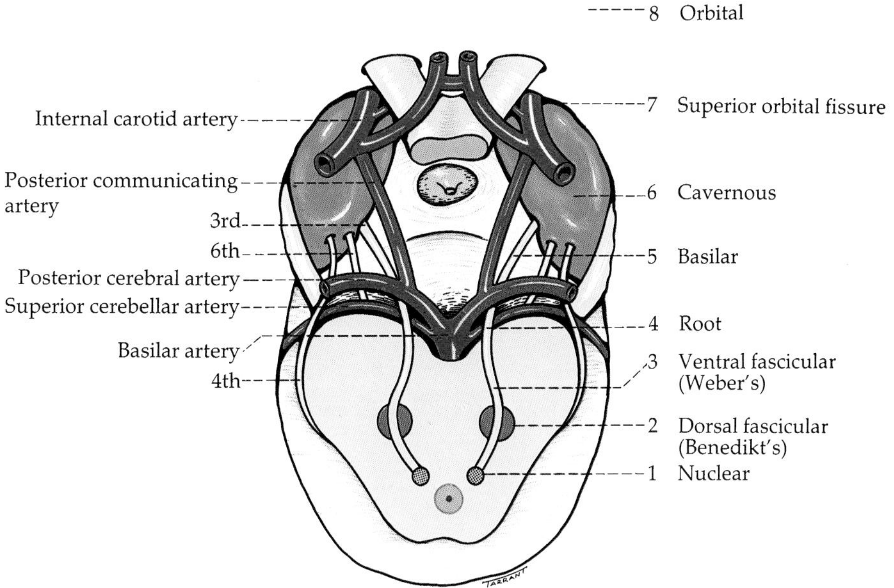

Figure 15.46 *Anatomy of the third nerve*

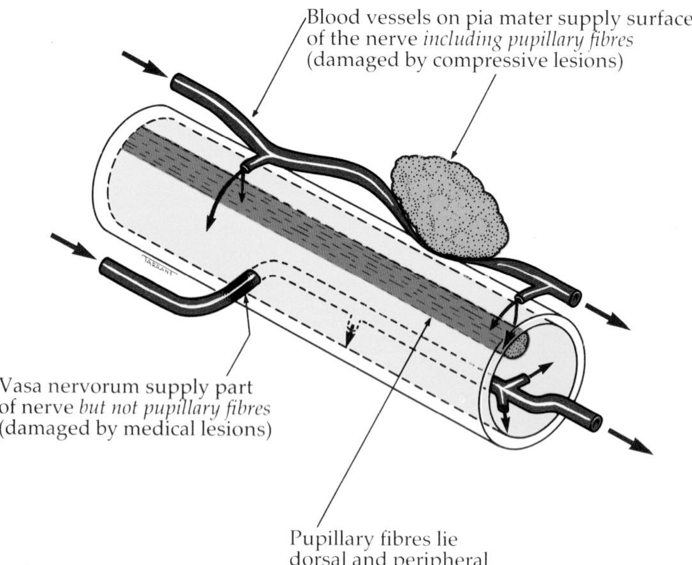
Blood vessels on pia mater supply surface of the nerve *including pupillary fibres* (damaged by compressive lesions)
Vasa nervorum supply part of nerve *but not pupillary fibres* (damaged by medical lesions)
Pupillary fibres lie dorsal and peripheral

Figure 15.47 *Anatomy of pupillomotor fibres within the third nerve trunk*

Aneurysm

Acute lesions associated with severe pain are commonly caused by aneurysms at the junction of the posterior communicating artery and the internal carotid artery, or more rarely by aneurysms of the basilar artery.

Extradural haematoma

A tentorial pressure cone is frequently due to an extradural haematoma, which causes downward herniation of the temporal lobe. This compresses the third nerve as it passes over the tentorial edge, causing a fixed dilated pupil followed by a total third nerve palsy.

Cavernous

The third nerve pierces the dura just lateral to the posterior clinoid process to enter the cavernous sinus. Within the cavernous sinus, the third nerve runs in the lateral wall and occupies a superior position above the fourth nerve. Because of its close proximity to other cranial nerves, lesions of the cavernous sinus are usually associated with involvement of several nerves. In the anterior cavernous sinus the nerve divides into superior and inferior branches which enter the orbit through the superior orbital fissure.

Orbital

Within the orbit the superior division innervates the levator and superior rectus muscles. The inferior division supplies the medial rectus, the inferior rectus, and the inferior oblique muscles. The inferior branch of the third nerve within the orbit also contains the parasympathetic fibres from the Edinger–Westphal subnucleus, which innervate the sphincter pupillae and the ciliary muscle.

Pupillomotor fibres

The location of the parasympathetic pupillomotor fibres in the trunk of the third nerve is clinically important (*Figure 15.47*). Between the brainstem and the cavernous sinus, the pupillary fibres are located superficially in the superior median part of the nerve. They derive their blood supply from the pial blood vessels, whereas the main trunk of the third nerve is supplied by the vasa nervorum. An aneurysm compressing the third nerve will therefore cause a total third nerve palsy without sparing the pupil. However, a microangiopathy, such as occurs in diabetes, may only involve the vasa nervorum and result in a pupil-sparing third nerve palsy. It is often said that so-called 'surgical' lesions are characterized by pupillary involvement, and 'medical' causes of a third nerve palsy do not involve the pupil.

Clinical features

A total third nerve palsy is characterized by:

1. Ptosis due to weakness of the levator.
2. Abduction of the globe due to the unopposed action of the lateral rectus.
3. Intorsion of the globe on attempted down-gaze due to the action of the superior oblique.
4. Limitation of adduction (*Figure 15.48*) due to weakness of the medial rectus.
5. Limitation of elevation (*Figure 15.49*) due to weakness of the superior rectus.
6. Limitation of depression (*Figure 15.50*) due to weakness of the inferior rectus.

7. A fixed and dilated pupil which will react, neither to a direct or consensual light stimulus nor to near, due to interruption of the parasympathetic supply to the sphincter.
8. Weakness of accommodation due to interruption of the parasymptathetic nerve supply to the ciliary muscle.

Aberrant regeneration

Secondary aberrant regeneration may occasionally follow acute traumatic and aneurysmal but not vascular third nerve palsies. The bizarre defects in ocular motility are caused by the misdirection of sprouting axons reinnervating the wrong extraocular muscle. The resulting defects in ocular motility include: elevation of the upper eyelid (pseudo-Graefe phenomenon) and/or segmental constriction of the pupil with attempted adduction or depression and, occasionally, retraction of the globe on attempted vertical gaze. Primary aberrant regeneration occurs without a preceding acute third nerve palsy and is much less common. It is caused by an aneurysm or meningioma within the cavernous sinus.

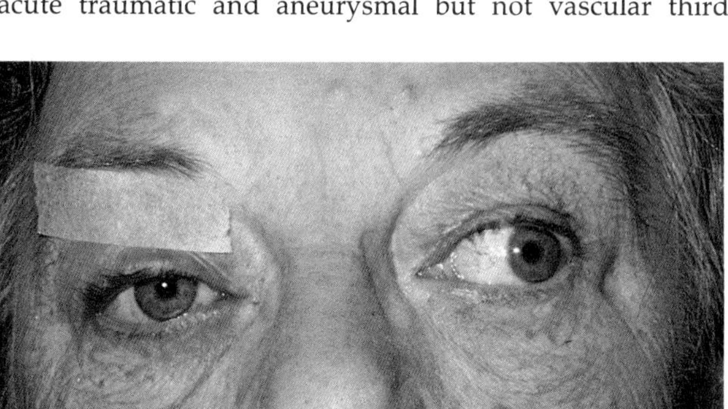
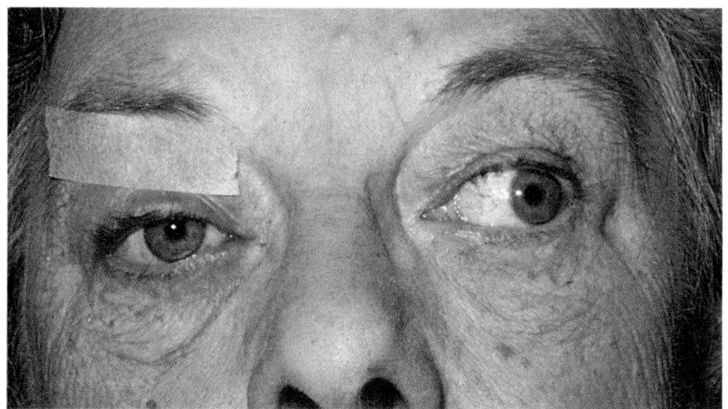

Figure 15.48 *Right third nerve palsy showing failure of adduction (courtesy of Mr A. Shun-Shin)*

Treatment

Surgical intervention should be considered only after at least 6 months have elapsed when spontaneous improvement has ceased and the deviation is stable. The surgery involves a large (10–12 mm) recession of the lateral rectus combined with a large (10–12 mm) resection of the medial rectus in the paretic eye, if necessary followed by recession of the lateral rectus in the opposite eye. The ptosis can be corrected either by resection of the levator or a frontalis sling procedure.

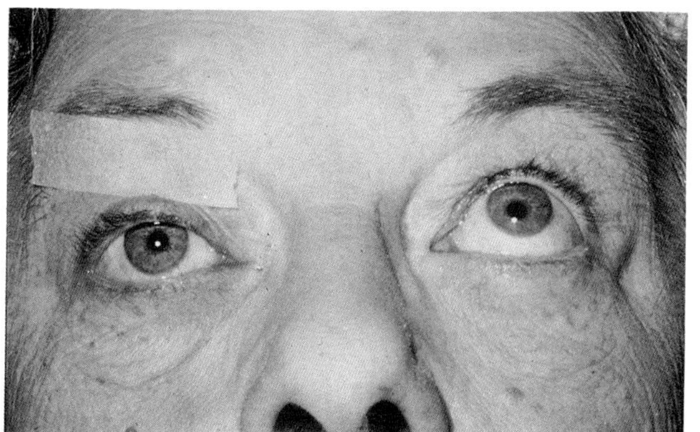

Figure 15.49 *Same patient as in* Figure 15.48 *showing failure of elevation (courtesy of Mr A. Shun-Shin)*

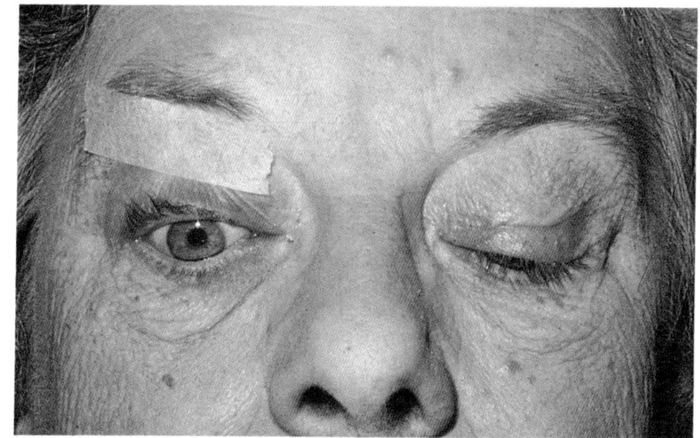

Figure 15.50 *Same patient as in* Figure 15.48 *showing limitation of depression (courtesy of Mr A. Shun-Shin)*

Trochlear (fourth) nerve palsy

Applied anatomy (*Figure 15.51*)

Nucleus

The fourth nerve nucleus is located at the level of the inferior colliculus in the aqueductal grey matter, beneath the sylvian aqueduct. It is caudal to, and continuous with, the third nerve nuclear complex. It innervates the *contralateral* superior oblique muscle.

Fasciculus

The axons of the fourth nerve curve around the aqueduct and decussate completely in the anterior medullary velum. They leave the brainstem on its dorsal surface, just caudal to the inferior colliculus. A nuclear or fascicular lesion will therefore cause a palsy of the contralateral superior oblique muscle.

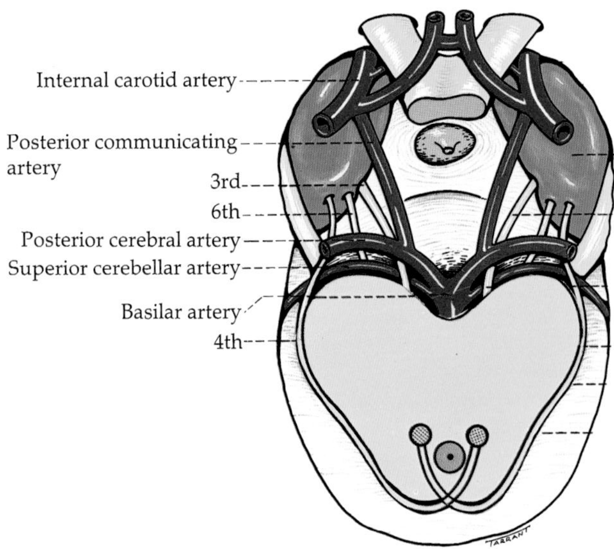

Figure 15.51 *Anatomy of the fourth nerve*

Peripheral part

Basilar

The trochlear nerve curves forward around the brainstem, runs beneath the free edge of the tentorium, and (like the third nerve) passes between the posterior cerebral artery and the superior cerebellar artery. It then pierces the dura to enter the cavernous sinus.

Trauma

This is an important cause of fourth nerve palsy (usually bilateral). The fourth nerves may be damaged as they decussate in the anterior medullary velum by impact with the tentorial edge. In addition the nerves can be damaged as they emerge dorsally and are thrust against the relatively immobile tentorium by *contre-coup* forces. The fourth nerve is the most slender of all cranial nerves, having the longest intracranial course, and these properties play some part in making it particularly vulnerable to traumatic damage.

Cavernous

In the cavernous sinus, the fourth nerve runs laterally and inferiorly to the third nerve. In the anterior part of the cavernous sinus it rises and passes through the superior orbital fissure above the annulus of Zinn.

Orbital

In the orbit the fourth nerve innervates the superior oblique muscle.

Important facts to remember about the fourth nerve

1. It is the longest of all cranial nerves.
2. It is the most slender of all cranial nerves.
3. It is the only cranial nerve to emerge from the dorsal aspect of the brain.
4. It is the only completely crossed cranial nerve.

Clinical features

A unilateral superior oblique palsy is characterized by an ipsilateral hyperdeviation and excyclotorsion, with limited depression in adduction. The patient may adopt an abnormal head posture to avoid diplopia by depressing the chin, tilting the head and occasionally turning the face to the opposite side. Bilateral palsies are characterized by a right hyperdeviation in left gaze, and a left hyperdeviation on right gaze. In contrast to unilateral cases, patients with bilateral involvement will demonstrate a V-esotropia in which the eyes are convergent in down-gaze but virtually straight in up-gaze. The diplopia on down-gaze, frequently with a torsional component, is the most troublesome symptom which the patient tries to overcome by depression of the chin so that the eyes are gazing upwards. Bilateral superior oblique palsies can easily be missed and must be suspected in all patients who complain of diplopia following a closed head injury. As a general rule one should assume that all post-traumatic superior oblique palsies are bilateral until proven otherwise.

Three-step test

The sequence of the three-step test which is useful in the diagnosis of superior oblique palsy is as follows:

1. Perform the cover–uncover test in the primary position to identify the side of the hyperdeviation.
2. Observe an increase in hyperdeviation with gaze to the opposite side.
3. Document an increase in the hyperdeviation with the head tilted to the same side by performing the Bielschowsky test. For example, in a patient with a left fourth nerve palsy, on tilting the head to the left shoulder the vertical deviation becomes more obvious (*Figures 15.52* and *15.53*). This phenomenon can be explained as follows. When the head is tilted to the left shoulder, the left eye has to intort in order to maintain fixation. This cannot happen because the left superior oblique, which is the primary intortor of the eye, is weak. In its place, the left superior rectus, which is the secondary intortor, comes into play. Because the superior rectus is a much more effective elevator than intortor, the eye shoots up. These findings are absent when the head is tilted to the right shoulder. Patients with bilateral superior oblique palsies will demonstrate a right hyperdeviation with the head tilted to the right shoulder and a left hyperdeviation with the head tilted to the left shoulder.

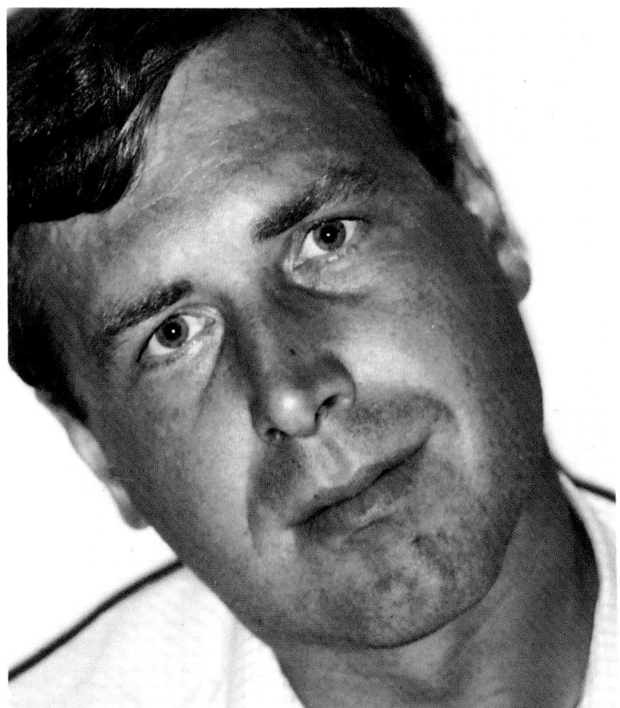

Figure 15.52 *Left fourth nerve palsy: no hyperdeviation of left eye on head tilt to right*

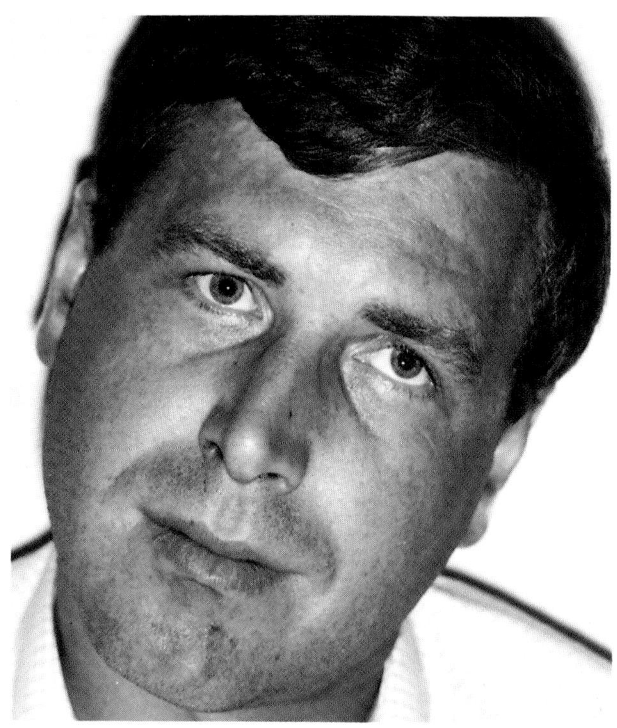

Figure 15.53 *Left fourth nerve palsy: left hyperdeviation on head tilt to left (positive Bielschowsky test)*

Treatment

Surgery should be considered if spontaneous improvement has not occurred after 6 months and any significant vertical diplopia cannot be corrected by prisms. Depending on the extent and pattern of muscle overactions, surgery involves either weakening of the ipsilateral overacting antagonist inferior oblique muscle and/or recession of the overacting contralateral yoke inferior rectus muscle. With less than 15 Δ of hyperdeviation in the primary position, surgery on one muscle is usually sufficient. With more than 15 Δ of hyperdeviation, it is best to weaken both muscles simultaneously. If, following surgery on two muscles, there is still an undercorrection, the paretic superior oblique muscle can be strengthened by a tucking procedure.

Abducens (sixth) nerve palsy

Applied anatomy (*Figure 15.54*)

Nucleus

The sixth nerve nucleus innervates the ipsilateral lateral rectus muscle. It lies in the midportion of the pons, inferior to the floor of the fourth ventricle, where it is closely related to the fasciculus of the seventh nerve which causes a small elevation in the floor of the fourth ventricle called the facial colliculus. A lesion in and around the sixth nerve nucleus results in failure of horizontal gaze towards the side of the lesion due to involvement of the horizontal gaze centre in the PPRF, a unilateral weakness of abduction, and also frequently an ipsilateral facial nerve palsy due to concomitant involvement of the facial fasciculus. For this reason an isolated sixth nerve palsy is never nuclear in origin.

Fasciculus

The emerging fibres pass ventrally to leave the brainstem at the pontomedullary junction, just lateral to the pyramidal prominence.

Foville's syndrome

This is caused by a lesion in the dorsal pons that involves the fasciculus as it passes through the PPRF. This will result

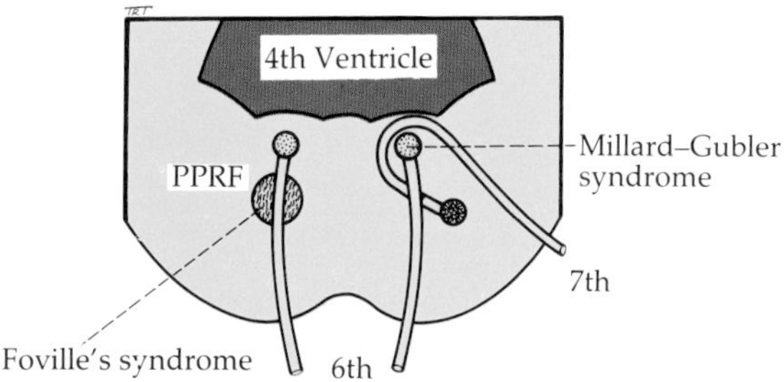

Figure 15.54 *Anatomy of sixth nerve*

in an ipsilateral sixth nerve palsy combined with a gaze palsy, ipsilateral facial weakness from damage to the facial nucleus or fasciculus, ipsilateral facial analgesia from involvement of the sensory portion of the fifth nerve, ipsilateral Horner's syndrome, and ipsilateral deafness.

Millard–Gubler syndrome

This is due to a ventral lesion which will also involve the pyramidal tract and produce a contralateral hemiplegia in addition to a variable number of signs of a dorsal pontine lesion.

Both Foville's and the Millard–Gubler syndromes are commonly caused by brainstem vascular disease in elderly patients and are seldom seen by ophthalmologists.

Peripheral part

Basilar

Acoustic neuroma

As the sixth nerve leaves the midbrain at the pontomedullary junction it enters the prepontine basilar cistern. Here it may be involved by cerebellopontine angle tumours such as acoustic neuromas. It should be remembered that the first symptom of an acoustic neuroma is hearing loss and the first sign is impairment of the corneal reflex. It is therefore essential to test hearing and corneal sensation in all patients with sixth nerve palsies. The sixth nerve then passes upwards close to the base of the pons, is crossed by the anterior inferior cerebellar artery, and pierces the dura of the clivus about 2 cm below the posterior clinoids. It then angles sharply forwards over the tip of the petrous bone, passes through or around the inferior petrosal sinus, through Dorello's canal (under the petroclinoid ligament) to enter the cavernous sinus.

Nasopharyngeal tumours

The sixth nerve may be damaged during its basilar course by the invasion of the skull and its foramina by nasopharyngeal tumours. This is particularly common in the Chinese.

Chordoma

This is a rare tumour which arises from notochordal remnants at the clivus. Although it is situated in the midline, it often presents with a unilateral sixth nerve palsy.

Fractures

Fractures involving the base of the skull may be responsible for both unilateral and bilateral sixth nerve palsies.

Raised intracranial pressure

The sixth nerve may also be stretched over the petrous tip between its point of emergence from the brainstem and its dural attachment on the clivus as a result of raised intracranial pressure (*Figure 15.55*). This is due to the downward descent of the brainstem and may occur with posterior fossa tumours as well as in patients with benign intracranial hypertension (pseudotumour cerebri). In this situation the sixth nerve palsy, which may be bilateral, is a false localizing sign.

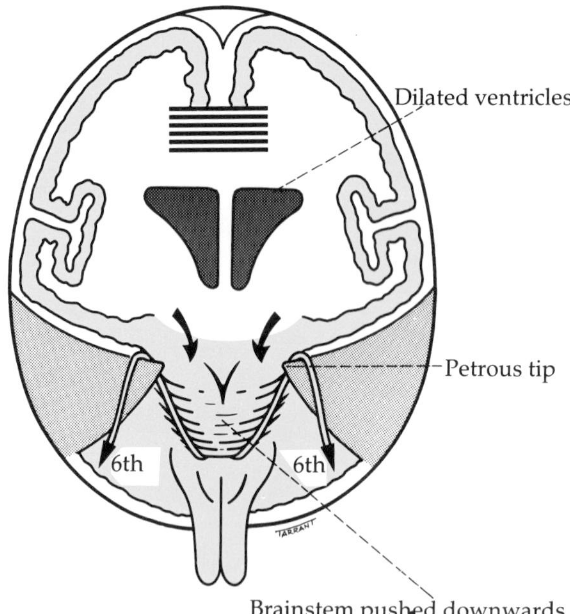

Figure 15.55 *Mechanism of sixth nerve palsy due to raised intracranial pressure*

Gradenigo's syndrome

This occurs in children through infection of the petrous bone from otitis media. It is characterized by a sixth nerve palsy, facial weakness, deafness, and severe pain in the distribution of the first division of the trigeminal nerve. With the advent of antibiotics this clinical picture is now a rarity.

Inferior petrosal sinus thrombosis

Thrombosis of the inferior petrosal sinus, which communicates with the posterior cavernous sinus and with the jugular vein, may be responsible for a sixth nerve palsy.

Cavernous

In the cavernous sinus, the sixth nerve runs forward below the third and fourth nerves. Whereas the latter are protected within the wall of the sinus, the sixth nerve is the most medially situated and runs through the middle of the sinus in close relation to the carotid artery. It is therefore more prone to damage than the others. Occasionally, an intracavernous sixth nerve palsy is accompanied by a postganglionic Horner's syndrome because, in its intracavernous course, the sixth nerve is joined by sympathetic branches (from the paracarotid plexus) which innervate the sphincter pupillae.

Orbital

The sixth nerve enters the orbit through the superior orbital fissure to supply the lateral rectus muscle.

Clinical features

A sixth nerve palsy is characterized by defective abduction of the eye from weakness of the lateral rectus muscle (*Figure 15.56*). In a complete palsy, there will be no abduction beyond the midline whereas, in a partial palsy, the restriction will be less severe. In the primary position there will be an esotropia with horizontal diplopia both of which will increase in the field of action of the paretic muscle and decrease in the field of action opposite to that of the paretic muscle (*Figure 15.57*). In order to avoid diplopia, the patient may adopt a face turn in the field of action of the paretic muscle so that the eyes are turned to the opposite side. For example a patient with a right sixth nerve palsy will turn the face to the right.

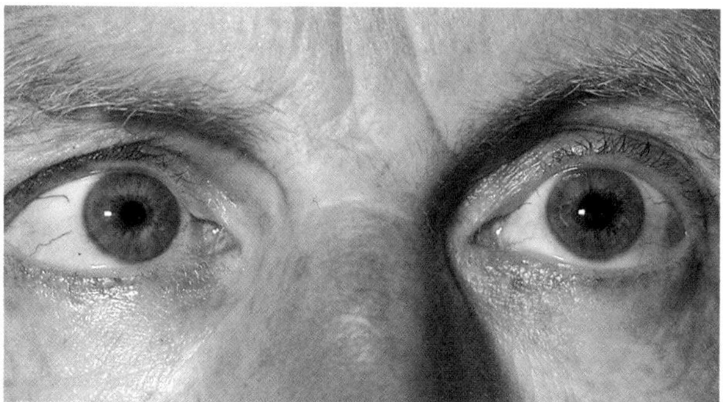

Figure 15.56 *Left sixth nerve palsy, showing failure of abduction. Patient will have horizontal diplopia*

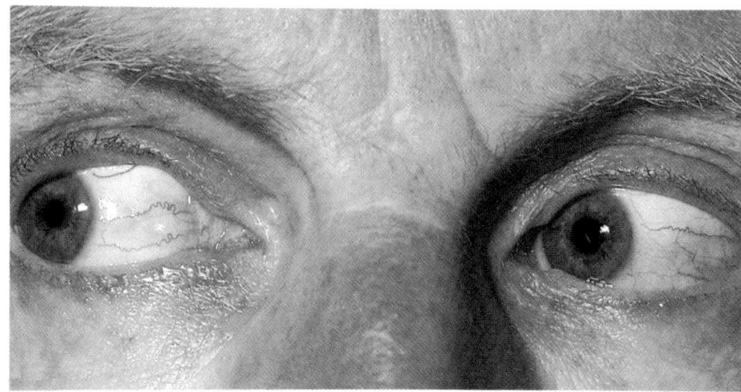

Figure 15.57 *Same patient as in* Figure 15.56, *looking to right. There is normal adduction of left eye and no diplopia*

Treatment

The three surgical procedures used to correct a persistent lateral rectus weakness from a sixth nerve paresis are:

1. *Recession* of the overacting and unopposed ipsilateral antagonist medial rectus muscle combined with resection of the ipsilateral paretic lateral rectus muscle.
2. *Hummelsheim* procedure in which the lateral halves of the superior and inferior rectus muscles are disinserted from their origins and attached to the superior and inferior margins of the scleral insertions of the paretic lateral rectus muscle (*see Figure 14.46, left*).
3. *Jensen's* modified Hummelsheim's procedure which involves splitting of the superior, lateral, and inferior rectus muscles lengthwise and then tying the lateral half of the superior rectus muscle to the superior half of the lateral rectus muscle and tying the lateral half of the inferior rectus muscle to the inferior half of the lateral rectus muscle with non-absorbable sutures (*see Figure 14.46, right*).

Both (2) and (3) can be combined with a recession of the ipsilateral medial rectus muscle. All three procedures appear to be equally effective.

Aetiology of third, fourth and sixth nerve palsies

Idiopathic

About 25% of all cases of third, fourth, and sixth cranial nerve palsies have no known cause. Of these, 50% recover spontaneously.

Vascular

Diabetes, hypertension, and atherosclerosis are the most common causes of third and sixth palsies and the second most frequent cause (after trauma) of a fourth nerve palsy.

Many spontaneous palsies are presumed to be caused by interference with the nerve's microvascular blood supply. In the majority of cases, spontaneous recovery occurs within a few weeks. Diabetes is an important cause of an isolated pupil-sparing third nerve palsy often accompanied by severe periorbital pain. As it may be the first clinical manifestation of diabetes, a glucose tolerance test and urinalysis should be performed in all patients with this clinical presentation.

Trauma

This is the most common cause of fourth nerve palsy and the second most common cause of third and sixth nerve palsies. The development of a third nerve palsy following relatively trivial head trauma unassociated with loss of consciousness should alert the clinician to the possibility of an associated basal intracranial tumour which has caused the nerve trunk to be stretched and tethered.

Aneurysms

These are an important cause of an isolated third nerve palsy but they rarely cause isolated fourth or sixth nerve palsy. Basilar aneurysms are a rare cause of third nerve palsy. Posterior communicating aneurysms typically cause an isolated third nerve palsy associated with involvement of the pupil and severe pain. The nerve is damaged by the sudden aneurysmal dilatation and intraneural haemorrhage. All patients with these clinical findings should be considered for arteriography. Intracavernous aneurysms typically affect women over the age of 50 years. A painless sixth nerve palsy may be the only manifestation, although other nerves may be simultaneously involved. In a third nerve palsy due to an intracavernous aneurysm, the pupil is often relatively unaffected and may often be small from simultaneous involvement of the sympathetic innervation in the paracarotid plexus.

Neoplasms

These are an unusual cause of third, fourth, and sixth nerve palsies. The most common tumours are meningiomas, metastases, acoustic neuromas, nasopharyngeal carcinomas, pontine or midbrain gliomas, chordomas, and pituitary adenomas that have spread laterally and involved the cavernous sinus.

Inflammation

1. *Infections* such as herpes zoster, basal meningitis, tuberculosis, syphilis, otitis media (Gradenigo's syndrome), and cavernous sinus thrombosis may all cause cranial nerve palsies.
2. *Vasculitis* due to temporal arteritis, systemic lupus erythematosus, and polyarteritis nodosa.
3. *Tolosa–Hunt syndrome* is an acute inflammation of the cavernous sinus or superior orbital fissure which produces a painful ophthalmoplegia. It is related to orbital pseudotumour and responds dramatically to systemic corticosteroid therapy (*see* Chapter 2). The diagnosis of this condition is primarily one of exclusion.
4. *Sarcoid*—a specific form of basal meningitis.
5. *Acute infectious polyneuropathy* (Guillain–Barré syndrome) can present as a painless and rapidly progressive bilateral ophthalmoplegia.

Carotid–cavernous fistula

See next.

Carotid–cavernous fistula

An arteriovenous (AV) fistula is an abnormal communication between previously normal veins and arteries. The blood within the affected vein becomes 'arterialized', the intravenous pressure rises, and venous blood flow may be altered in both rate and direction. The clinical features of AV fistulae are largely due to these altered vascular dynamics with subsequent reduction of arterial perfusion, ocular hypoxia, and venous congestion. A carotid–cavernous fistula results from an abnormal communication between the cavernous sinus and the carotid arterial system. The two main types are direct and indirect (dural shunts). Each has different aetiologies and clinical features.

Direct fistula

In this type of fistula the arterial blood passes directly through a defect in the wall of the intracavernous portion of the internal carotid artery.

Aetiology

1. *Trauma* which has caused a basal skull fracture and tearing of the internal carotid artery within the surrounding cavernous sinus.
2. *Spontaneous* rupture either of an intracavernous aneurysm or of an atherosclerotic internal carotid artery in a hypertensive individual.

Clinical features

Because direct carotid–cavernous fistulae have a high flow of blood through them, the onset of symptoms is frequently sudden and dramatic. The fistula is usually unilateral and rarely bilateral.

1. *Chemosis, redness, and dilatation* (*Figures 15.58* and *15.59*) of the episcleral blood vessels due to venous engorgement.
2. *Proptosis* which is typically pulsatile and is associated with a thrill and a bruit which are synchronous with the pulse and which can be abolished by compression of the ipsilateral carotid artery in the neck.
3. *Ophthalmoplegia* occurs in the vast majority of patients and is thought to be caused by a combination of hypoxia and swelling of the extraocular muscles. About 50% of patients with ophthalmoplegia have sixth nerve palsies and the incidence of involvement of the third and fourth nerves is variable.
4. *Reduced visual acuity* and posterior segment congestion occurs in about 50% of cases (*Figure 15.60*).
5. *Raised intraocular pressure* due to an elevation of episcleral venous pressure is present in about 20% of cases.
6. *Anterior segment ischaemia* characterized by corneal epithelial oedema, flare and cells in the aqueous, iris atrophy and rubeosis, and cataract develops in about 20% of patients.

Treatment

In some patients, the fistula closes spontaneously. The variety of treatments advocated to thrombose the fistula surgically include ligation of the carotid artery in the neck, direct intracavernous surgery, and balloon catheter embolization.

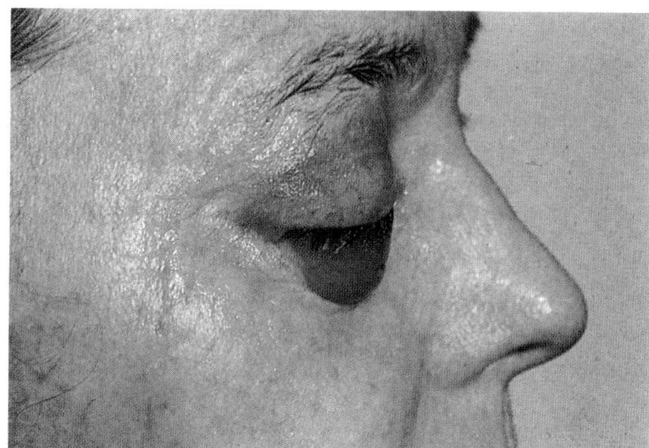

Figure 15.58 *Chemosis in carotid–cavernous fistula*

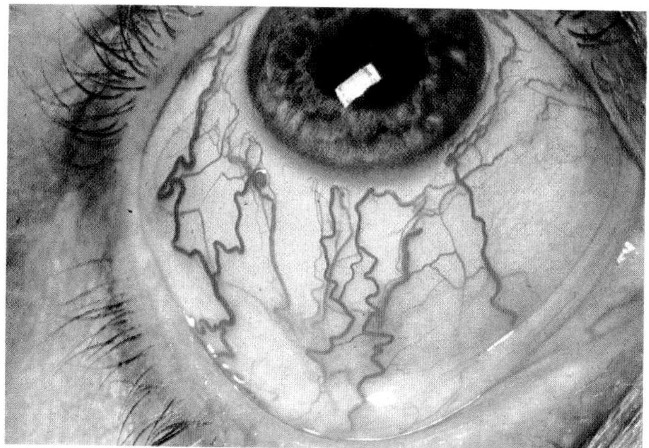

Figure 15.59 *Gross dilatation of conjunctival vessels in carotid–cavernous fistula (courtesy of Professor A. C. Bird)*

Indirect fistula (dural shunt)

In this type of fistula, the intracavernous portion of the internal cavernous artery remains intact and arterial blood flows through the meningeal branches of the external or internal carotid arteries to indirectly enter the cavernous sinus.

Aetiology

The exact aetiology of dural shunts is still speculative. The two main theories are:

1. *Congenital.* Some authorities believe that these shunts are congenital malformations and that the onset of clinical features may be caused by intracranial venous thrombosis.
2. *Spontaneous* rupture after minor trauma or straining, especially in a hypertensive patient.

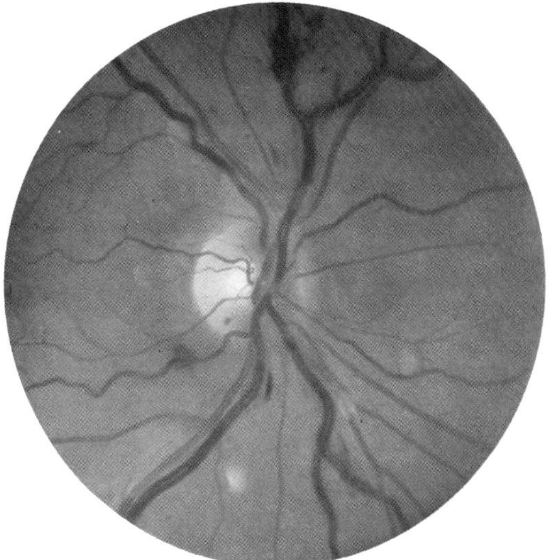

Figure 15.60 *Dilated veins and superficial haemorrhages in patient with carotid–cavernous fistula (courtesy of Professor A. C. Bird)*

Clinical features

Because indirect carotid–cavernous fistulae have a slow flow of blood through them, the clinical presentation, although similar, is much more subtle than in direct fistulae so that they may be missed or misdiagnosed. Most patients are postmenopausal women who present with mild proptosis, dilated episcleral vessels, and raised intraocular pressure. Other features include pain, ptosis, and ophthalmoplegia, most commonly involving an ipsilateral weakness of abduction, due to a sixth nerve palsy.

Treatment

Most cases recover spontaneously without treatment. Surgical intervention may be required in a few patients.

Abnormalities of the pupil

Applied anatomy

Light reflex

The pupillary light reflex can be considered as a four-neurone arc (*Figure 15.61*).

First neurone

This connects the retina to the pretectal nucleus in the midbrain at the level of the superior colliculus. The reflex is mediated by the retinal photoreceptors. Impulses originating from the nasal retina will be conducted by fibres which decussate at the chiasm and pass up the optic tract to terminate in the contralateral pretectal nucleus. Impulses originating from the temporal retina will be conducted by uncrossed fibres which terminate in the ipsilateral pretectal nucleus.

Second neurone

This connects each pretectal nucleus to both Edinger–Westphal nuclei. (This explains why a unilateral light stimulus evokes a bilateral and symmetrical pupillary constriction.) The neurones that join the pretectal nucleus to the Edinger–Westphal nucleus are called the internuncial neurones and usually cross dorsal to the aqueduct in the posterior commissure. These fibres are thought to be damaged in syphilis and by pinealomas, the result being light–near dissociation.

Third neurone

This connects the Edinger–Westphal nucleus to the ciliary ganglion. The location of the pupillomotor fibres in relation to the trunk of the third nerve is clinically important because, between its emergence from the brainstem and its entrance into the cavernous sinus, the parasympathetic fibres are located in a relatively exposed superficial location. A compressive lesion of the third nerve at this location by an aneurysm will therefore give rise to a third nerve palsy with involvement of the pupil. However, when the third nerve passes through the cavernous sinus, the pupillary fibres occupy a central position within the nerve trunk and may therefore be spared, even when a compressive lesion at this site causes a total external ophthalmoplegia. In the orbit, the parasympatheic fibres pass in the inferior division of the third nerve and reach the ciliary ganglion via the nerve to the inferior oblique.

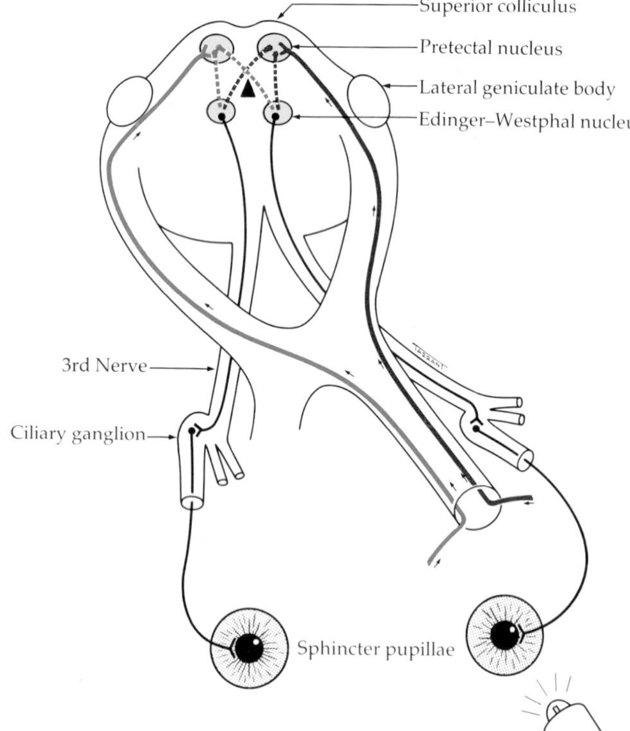

Figure 15.61 *Anatomical pathway of the pupillary light reflex*

Fourth neurone

This leaves the ciliary ganglion and passes with the short ciliary nerves to innervate the sphincter pupillae. The ciliary ganglion is located within the muscle cone, just behind the globe. It is important to note that although the ciliary ganglion contains other fibres, only the parasympathetic fibres synapse there.

Near reflex

The near reflex triad consists of:

1. Increased accommodation.
2. Convergence of the visual axes.
3. Constriction of the pupils.

Vision is not a prerequisite for the near reflex. There is no clinical condition in which the light reflex is present but the near response is absent, therefore if the pupillary response is intact there is no need to test its reaction to near. The term 'light–near dissociation' therefore refers to a condition in which the light reflex is absent or abnormal but the near response is intact.

Although the final pathway for the near reflex is the same as for the light reflex (i.e. third nerve, ciliary ganglion, short ciliary nerves), the centre for the near reflex is ill defined. It seems likely that there are two supranuclear influences: the frontal lobe and the occipital. The midbrain centre for the near reflex is probably located in a more ventral position than that for the light reflex (pretectal nucleus) and this may be one of the reasons why compressive lesions such as pinealomas preferentially involve the dorsal pupillomotor fibres and spare the ventral near fibres until late in the developmental course of the lesion.

Examination

Examination of the pupillary reactions should be performed in a dimly lit room.

Size and symmetry

In order to assess the size and symmetry of the pupils, the patient is asked to view a distant object such as a Snellen test-type. A dim light is then directed onto the face from below so that both pupils are seen simultaneously in oblique illumination. Their size should then be measured with a millimetre rule.

It is important to bear in mind that about 20% of normal subjects have clinically detectable anisocoria and, if this is found to be present, the pupillary dimensions should be reassessed by varying the amount of room illumination. In general, anisocoria that varies with the degree of illumination is pathological. For example, in Horner's syndrome the degree of anisocoria is most marked in dim illumination and least noticeable in bright illumination. However, anisocoria in which the amount of difference in pupillary size is maintained regardless of the amount of illumination is probably not pathological. It is important to bear in mind that a unilateral visual deficit, irrespective of whether it is caused by an opacity in the media or a lesion of the optic nerve or retina, will not affect pupillary size.

Light reflex

The reactions to light are best evaluated using a strong light from an indirect ophthalmoscope. If the left pupil is found to react poorly to the direct light stimulus, then its consensual response should be tested by stimulating the right pupil. If the afferent arc is intact, the direct reaction should equal the consensual reaction in every parameter.

Near reflex

The near response of the pupils is tested by first asking the patient to gaze at a distant object and then asking him to look at his own fingertip just in front of his nose. Because most people find it easier to converge when looking down, the test should be performed with the patient's chin slightly elevated and the examiner should hold the patient's eyelids up so that the reactions can be observed more easily. The degree of pupillary constriction is graded on a 1 to 4 scale.

Abnormal reactions

Classification

Amaurotic
Marcus Gunn
Argyll Robertson
Holmes–Adie
Midbrain
Horner's syndrome

Amaurotic

These occur in eyes with no light perception due to an optic nerve lesion. The features are as follows:

1. Both pupils are of equal size.
2. Neither pupil will react when the defective eye is stimulated.
3. Both pupils react normally when the contralateral normal eye is stimulated.
4. The reaction of both pupils to a near stimulus is normal.

Marcus Gunn (relative afferent defect)

This is caused by an optic nerve lesion that is not severe enough to cause an absence of light perception, and in fact a Marcus Gunn reaction may be present in an eye with normal vision.

The reaction is best detected by the so-called 'swinging flashlight test'. Let us assume that the left optic nerve has been slightly damaged by an attack of retrobulbar neuritis. If the left eye is stimulated by light, the reaction in both eyes will be more sluggish than when the normal eye is stimulated. In mild cases, this slight difference in reactions may be very difficult to detect clinically. The difference can be enhanced by swinging the light (an indirect ophthalmoscope is best) from one eye to the other. When the light is brought from the normal right to the abnormal left eye, the left pupil will dilate instead of constricting. This paradoxical reaction of the pupil to light occurs because the dilatation of the pupil, by withdrawing the light from the normal eye, outweighs the constriction produced by stimulating the abnormal eye.

A Marcus Gunn reaction can also be seen in eyes with extensive retinal pathology, but will not be present when both optic nerves are equally damaged.

Argyll Robertson

This reaction is the hallmark of neurosyphilis and is characterized by the following features:

1. Light–near dissociation. This means that the pupils show a more extensive reaction to the near response than to a light stimulus. In typical Argyll Robertson (AR) pupils there is virtually no reaction to light but a brisk response to near.
2. Both pupils are usually involved but the degree of involvement may be asymmetrical.
3. In order to make the diagnosis of AR pupils, vision in the affected eye must be normal.
4. The pupils are small.
5. The pupils are frequently irregular in shape.
6. The pupils dilate poorly after the instillation of a mydriatic.

It is important to bear in mind that, although pupillary abnormalities are very frequently seen in neurosyphilis, true AR pupils which fulfil all the above criteria are rare. The light–near dissociation is thought to be due to involvement of the internuncial neurones between the pretectal nuclei and the Edinger–Westphal subnucleus.

Holmes–Adie (tonic)

This is a common cause of anisocoria which typically affects women during the third and fourth decades of life. It may follow a viral illness and is often associated with diminished or absent tendon reflexes. The lesion is thought to be caused by denervation of the postganglionic nerve supply to the sphincter pupillar and the ciliary muscle so that usually both pupillary reactions and accommodation are impaired. The condition is unilateral in 80% of cases and is characterized by the following signs:

1. The affected pupil is larger than its fellow.
2. The reaction to light is extremely poor or non-existent.
3. The reaction to a near stimulus is very slow and tonic.
4. Redilatation of the pupils is also prolonged and tonic.
5. Accommodation is also frequently slow when the patient changes gaze from distance to near.
6. Verniform movements of the iris border due to sector paralysis are frequently seen on slitlamp examination.
7. The diagnosis can be confirmed by instilling mecholyl 2.5% or pilocarpine 0.125% drops into both eyes, which will constrict the affected pupil because of denervation hypersensitivity; a normal pupil will be unaffected.

Adie's pupil is a benign condition and patients should not be subjected to unnecessary extensive neurological investigations. With time the paralysis of accommodation improves but the light reaction tonicity gets worse. There is no effective treatment.

Midbrain (tectal)

Midbrain lesions frequently give rise to pupillary abnormalities. Compressive lesions in the area of the third ventricle (usually pinealomas) may selectively interrupt the internuncial neurones (as in AR pupils). Because the fibres mediating the near reflex lie more ventrally, they are spared initially but may be involved later as the tumour enlarges.

Midbrain pupils are larger than normal and may be eccentric. The pupillary signs are usually associated with the following features which make up Parinaud's syndrome:

1. Impairment of upward gaze from damage to the vertical gaze centre.
2. Convergence–retraction nystagmus.

Other causes of light–near dissociation

1. Juvenile onset diabetics may develop a neuropathy of the pupil.
2. Dystrophia myotonica.
3. Aberrant regeneration of the third nerve.

Horner's syndrome (oculosympathetic palsy)

Applied anatomy

The sympathetic nerve supply to the eye can be considered as a three-neurone arc (*Figure 15.62*).

The first neurone starts in the posterior hypothalamus and descends, uncrossed, down the brainstem to terminate in the ciliospinal centre of Budge (between C8 and T2).

The second neurone passes to the superior cervical ganglion in the neck. During its long course it is closely related to the subclavian artery and to the apical pleura, where it may be damaged by an apical bronchial carcinoma (Pancoast tumour) or during surgery in the neck.

The third neurone ascends along the internal carotid artery to enter the skull, where it joins the ophthalmic division of the trigeminal nerve. The sympathetic fibres reach the ciliary body and the dilator of the iris via the nasociliary nerve and the long ciliary nerves.

Clinical features

Horner's syndrome is caused by a total or partial interruption of the sympathetic chain anywhere along its course from the hypothalamus to the eye. The features (*Figure 15.63*) are:

1. A moderate degree of ptosis due to paralysis of Müller's muscle.
2. An elevation of the lower lid due to paralysis of the smooth muscle attached to the inferior tarsal plate.

3. Apparent enophthalmos due to a narrowing of the palpebral fissure as a result of the ptosis and lid elevation.
4. Miosis, which is variable and more marked in dim illumination than in bright illumination. It should be remembered that the pupillary reactions to light and near are unimpaired.
5. Diminished sweating on the ipsilateral part of the face if the lesion is below the superior cervical ganglion. (This is because the third-order neurone to the sweat glands of the face follows the course of the external carotid artery, which means that sweating will be diminished if the lesion is below the superior cervical ganglion.)
6. Heterochromia of the iris may be present if the lesion is congenital or acquired during early infancy.
7. Increase in the amplitude of accommodation may also be present due to the unopposed action of the parasympathetic.

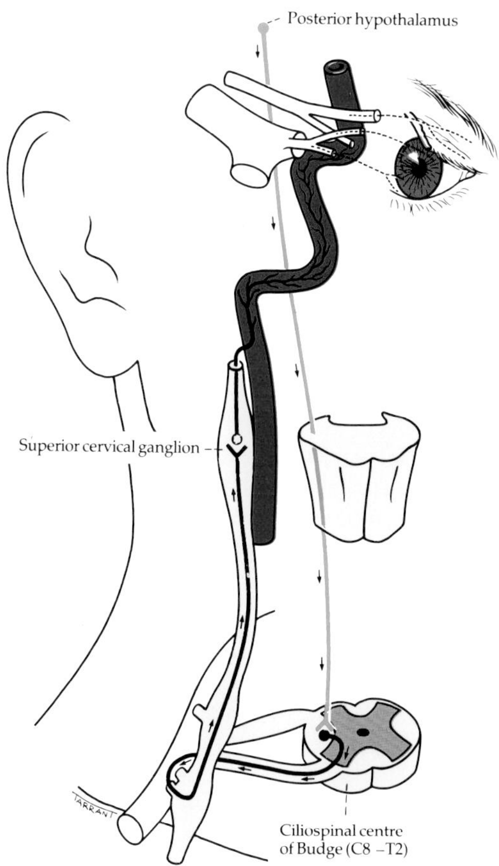

Figure 15.62 *Anatomy of sympathetic nerve supply to the eye*

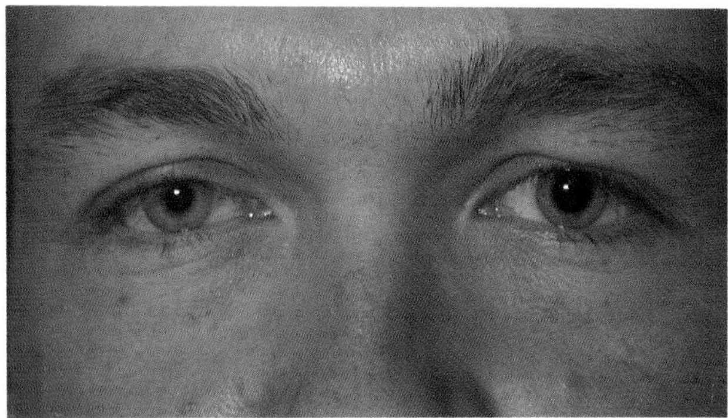

Figure 15.63 *Right Horner's syndrome*

Location of lesion

The exact location is best detected by the presence or absence of accompanying neurological lesions and of sweating. Localization is important since the prognosis for life is better for a postganglionic lesion than for a preganglionic lesion. Preganglionic lesions may be caused by CNS disease, bronchial carcinoma, and thoracic aortic aneurysms. Any preganglionic Horner's syndrome without obvious trauma must therefore, be investigated. A chest X-ray should be performed to rule out a Pancoast tumour. Postganglionic lesions are usually either idiopathic or are associated with vascular headache syndromes and are almost always benign.

Confirmation of the diagnosis is performed by using cocaine 4%, which will dilate the normal pupil, but not the Horner's pupil. If hydroxyamphetamine 1% (Paredrine) is instilled a pupil with a preganglionic lesion will dilate, but a postganglionic Horner's pupil will not dilate.

Nystagmus

Nystagmus is an involuntary to-and-fro oscillation of the eyes.

Classification

Pendular

This is characterized by eye movements that are of equal velocity in each direction. The movements can be horizontal, vertical, oblique, or rotary.

Jerk

This is characterized by a slow component in one direction and a fast component in the other direction. The direction of nystagmus is defined by the direction of the rapid phase. Jerk nystagmus can therefore be right, left, up, down, or rotary. The fast phase is mediated by the saccadic system and the slow phase by the pursuit system.

Mixed

This is one in which pendular movements are present in the primary position and jerk movements are present when the eyes become deviated laterally.

The nystagmus can be further described as being either rapid or slow, coarse or fine, manifest or latent.

Clinical types

Physiological

Physiological nystagmus can be of three types: end-point, optokinetic and vestibular.

1. *End-point* nystagmus is a fine jerk nystagmus of moderate frequency found when the eyes are in extreme gaze positions.
2. *Optokinetic* nystagmus is a jerk nystagmus induced by moving repetitive visual stimuli across the visual field. The slow phase is a pursuit movement in which the eyes follow the target and the fast phase is a saccadic movement in the opposite direction as the eyes refixate on the next target.

   The optokinetic nystagmus is useful for detecting malingerers and for testing the visual acuity of small children (Catford drum). If an optokinetic tape is moved from right to left, the left parieto-occipital region controls the slow (pursuit) movements to the left and the left frontal lobe controls the rapid (saccadic) fast phase to the right.
3. *Vestibular* is a jerk nystagmus caused by altered input from the vestibular nuclei to the horizontal gaze centres. The slow phase is initiated by the vestibular nuclei and the fast phase by the brainstem and the frontomesencephalic pathway. Rotary nystagmus is usually caused by pathological conditions affecting the vestibular system.

When performing caloric stimulation, if cold water is poured into the *right* ear the patient will develop a *left* jerk nystagmus (fast phase to the left). If hot water is now poured into the *right* ear the patient will develop a *right* jerk nystagmus (fast phase to the right). A useful mnemonic is 'cows' (cold-opposite, warm-same).

Sensory deprivation (ocular)

This is due to an afferent defect in the neural control system of ocular fixation. Common causes are congenital cataract, macular hypoplasia, albinism, and Leber's congenital amaurosis.

The 2–4–6 rule states that if a child loses central vision prior to the age of 2 years he will always develop nystagmus. After the age of 6 years this type of nystagmus does not occur. Between the ages of 2 and 6 years, some will and some will not. Ocular nystagmus is typically pendular and horizontal. Its severity will depend on the extent of visual loss and it can often be dampened by convergence. Occasionally an anomalous head posture may be adopted.

Motor imbalance

This is theoretically due to a primary defect in the efferent mechanism and can be of several types.

1. *Congenital nystagmus* is usually apparent at birth or shortly after and may be transmitted as an X-linked recessive or autosomal dominant trait. It is usually of the jerk type and is horizontal. It may be dampened by convergence and is not present during sleep. Although the abnormal head movements with which it may be associated usually diminish with time, it persists throughout life. Strabismus may coexist with congenital nystagmus and the amount of visual impairment is variable.
2. *Spasmus nutans* is characterized by nystagmus, abnormal head position, and head nodding. It usually develops between the fourth and twelfth months of life and usually clears prior to the age of 3 years. The nystagmus is characteristically asymmetrical, pendular, fine, and rapid. It is usually horizontal but may occasionally be vertical or rotary.
3. *Latent nystagmus* is a jerk nystagmus that occurs under conditions of uniocular fixation. When one eye is occluded, both eyes develop nystagmus with the fast phase directed towards the uncovered eye. Latent nystagmus is often noted in early childhood and is especially frequent in patients with congenital esotropia. Occasionally an element of congenital nystagmus is superimposed on a manifest nystagmus. In this condition, when one eye is covered the amplitude of the nystagmus increases.
4. *Ataxic nystagmus* occurs in the abducting eye in association with internuclear ophthalmoplegia.
5. *Downbeat nystagmus.* In this type of nystagmus the fast phase is downwards. It is pathognomonic of a lesion involving the cervicomedullary junction at the foramen magnum.
6. *Upbeat nystagmus.* The fast phase is in the upward direction. A common cause is drug intoxication (e.g. phenytoin) but it may also occur in association with posterior fossa lesions.
7. *Convergence–retraction nystagmus* is a jerk nystagmus in which the fast phase brings the two eyes towards each other in a convergence movement. This is associated with retraction of the globe into the orbit. This type of nystagmus is caused by co-contraction of the extraocular muscles, particularly the medial recti. It is usually found in lesions affecting the pretectal area, such as vascular accidents and pinealomas. When associated with paralysis of vertical gaze, light–near dissociation of the pupils, lid retraction, accommodation spasm, and other midbrain signs, it constitutes Parinaud's syndrome.

8. *See-saw nystagmus (of Maddox)* is characterized by one eye rising and intorting while the other eye falls and extorts. When associated with a bitemporal hemianopia it is usually caused by a chiasmal lesion.
9. *Periodic alternating nystagmus* is a very rare condition characterized by a jerk nystagmus that undergoes rhythmic changes in amplitude and direction. It is usually associated with vascular or demyelinating brainstem disease.

Myasthenia gravis

Systemic features

Myasthenia gravis is a relatively rare autoimmune disease caused by an abnormality at the neuromuscular junction. The disease typically affects females between the ages of 20 and 40 years and is characterized by excessive fatiguability of skeletal muscles, unassociated with a neurological deficit. The facial, oropharyngeal and extraocular muscles are frequently involved. The three principal types of myasthenia gravis are: progressive, remittent and ocular.

Ocular features

Ocular involvement in the form of ptosis and/or diplopia eventually occurs in over 90% of myasthenics and is the presenting symptom in about 60%. In approximately 80% of patients with an ocular onset, the condition subsequently becomes more generalized, usually within 2 years. The remaining 20% remain in the ocular group.

Ptosis

Myasthenia gravis is an important cause of ptosis in adults. Typically the ptosis is bilateral but asymmetrical, and worse towards the end of the day or when the patient is tired. The ptosis can be made more apparent clinically by asking the patient to sustain upward gaze or repeatedly close his eyelids. The characteristic 'twitch sign' of Cogan may be elicited by having the patient rapidly redirect his gaze from the downward to the primary position when the upper lid will be seen to twitch upward and then slowly resettle to its ptotic position.

Diplopia

The extraocular muscle weakness does not appear to follow any set pattern although it has been suggested that upward movement may be involved first. All or any of the extraocular muscles may be affected, and in some cases the ocular motility defect may mimic a supranuclear gaze palsy, internuclear ophthalmoplegia, or isolated extraocular muscle involvement.

Special investigations

Tensilon test

This test is used to confirm the diagnosis of myasthenia gravis. Most myasthenics display significant improvement of weakness following the intravenous injection of edrophonium (Tensilon), a fast-acting anticholinesterase. In patients with ocular myasthenia the test is performed as follows:

1. The amount of ptosis and/or the extraocular motility defects are evaluated as objectively as possible (Hess test).
2. Atropine 0.3 mg is injected intravenously.
3. Tensilon 1 ml (containing 10 mg) is drawn up into a tuberculin syringe.
4. A test dose of 0.2 ml (2 mg) is injected into the antecubital vein and the needle is left *in situ*.
5. If, after 60 seconds, the patient does not show signs of hypersensitivity (e.g. excessive salivation, sweating or lacrimation), the remaining 0.8 ml is then injected slowly.

A beneficial effect will occur within 30–60 seconds but will last no longer than 5 minutes. Usually ptosis will recover quickly, but any extraocular motility defect may not be completely relieved although the range of movement shows improvement.

Electromyography

To document improvement with Tensilon or to demonstrate fatiguability of the neuromuscular junction, it may also be useful to perform an EMG. A peripheral nerve such as the facial or ulnar is repetitively stimulated and the evoked potential recorded. In case of myasthenia gravis, a decrement of responses will be seen that normalize when Tensilon is injected.

Antibodies

Anti-acetylcholine receptor antibodies are present in about 90% of patients with myasthenia gravis.

Treatment

The initial treatment of myasthenia gravis is with long-acting anticholinesterase drugs such as pyridostigmine (Mestinon). However, many patients with ocular myasthenia do not respond well to pyridostigmine on its own. Other therapeutic options include thymectomy, systemic corticosteroids, cytotoxic drugs (azathioprine, cyclophosphamide), and plasmapheresis to remove anti-acetylcholine antibodies.

Ocular myopathies

Chronic progressive external ophthalmoplegia

This very rare disorder, which is also referred to as ocular myopathy, is characterized by insidious, slowly progressive symmetrical ptosis and immobility of the eyes. Because of symmetrical muscle involvement, diplopia does not occur, even in advanced cases. The three main forms of chronic progressive external ophthalmoplegia (CPEO) are:

1. *Primary ocular myopathy*, unassociated with other features.
2. *Kearns–Sayre syndrome* which consists of a triad of CPEO, pigmentary retinopathy, and heart block that may cause sudden death. The condition usually becomes manifest prior to the age of 20 years and, in some cases, may be associated with other abnormalities such as short stature, cerebellar ataxia, deafness, mental retardation, and delayed puberty.
3. *Oculopharyngeal dystrophy* characterized by involvement of the pharyngeal muscles and wasting of the temporalis muscle.

Dystrophia myotonica

Systemic features

This is an uncommon genetically determined disorder which can affect many parts of the body. It is characterized by excessive contractility and difficulty in relaxation of skeletal muscle, hypogonadism, baldness, and cardiac anomalies.

Ocular features

1. *Ptosis* combined with weakness of the facial muscles may give rise to a characteristic mournful expression (*see Figure 8.5*).
2. *Involvement of the extraocular muscles* which may mimic CPEO.
3. *Pigmentary* changes involving the macula or peripheral retina.
4. *Light–near dissociation* of the pupil.
5. *Presenile cataract* (*see* Chapter 8).

Essential blepharospasm

Clinical features

This is an involuntary spasm of the orbicularis muscle. In severe cases it may lead to acute spastic entropion and, occasionally, the forceful contracture of both muscles may make the patient temporarily blind. The cause is usually obscure. The condition should be differentiated from hemifacial spasm, myokymia, and apraxia of lid opening.

Treatment

Mild cases can be treated by muscle relaxants and facial nerve blocks. In severe cases differential section of the seventh nerve or injection of botulinum toxin into the orbicularis may be necessary.

Further reading

Optic nerve disorders

Appen, R.E., Chandra, S.R., Klein, R. *et al.* (1980) Diabetic papillopathy. *American Journal of Ophthalmology*, **90**, 203–209

Beck, R.W. (1986) Anterior ischaemic optic neuropathy. *Clinical Modules for Ophthalmologists*, Vol. 4, Module 3

Beck, R.W., Savino, P.J., Repka, M.X. *et al.* (1984) Optic disc structure in anterior ischaemic optic neuropathy. *Ophthalmology*, **91**, 1334–1337

Brownstein, S., Nicolle, D.A. and Codere, F. (1983) Bilateral blindness in temporal arteritis with skip areas. *Archives of Ophthalmology*, **91**, 388–391

Caprioli, J. and Lesser, R.L. (1983) Basal encephalocele and morning glory syndrome. *British Journal of Ophthalmology*, **67**, 349–351

Dreyer, R.F., Hopek, G., Gass, J.D.M. *et al.* (1984) Leber's idiopathic stellate neuroretinitis. *Archives of Ophthalmology*, **102**, 1140–1145

Ellis, F.D. and Yune, H.Y. (1978) Optic nerve anomaly, midline facial anomaly, and basal encephalocele. *Perspectives in Ophthalmology*, **2**, 43–48

Guyer, D.R., Miller, N.R., Auer, C.L. *et al.* (1985) The risk of cerebrovascular disease in patients with anterior ischemic optic neuropathy. *Archives of Ophthalmology*, **103**, 1136–1142

Haik, B.G., Greenstein, S.H., Smith, M.E. *et al.* (1984) Retinal detachment in the morning glory anomaly. *Ophthalmology*, **91**, 1638–1647

Harris, M.J., Fine, S.L. and Owens, S.L. (1981) Hemorrhagic complications of optic nerve drusen. *American Journal of Ophthalmology*, **92**, 70–76

Hedges, T.R., Gieger, G.L. and Albert, D.M. (1983) The clinical value of negative temporal artery biopsy specimens. *Archives of Ophthalmology*, **101**, 1251–1254

Keast-Butler, J. and Taylor, D. (1980) Optic neuropathies in children. *Transactions of the Ophthalmological Society of the United Kingdom*, **100**, 111–118

Keltner, J.L. (1982) Giant-cell arteritis: signs and symptoms. *Ophthalmology*, **89**, 1101–1110

Koenig, S.B., Naidich, T.P. and Lisser, G. (1982) The morning glory syndrome associated with sphenoidal encephalocele. *Ophthalmology*, **89**, 1368–1373

McDonald, W.I. (1983) The significance of optic neuritis. Doyne Lecture. *Transactions of the Ophthalmological Society of the United Kingdom*, **103**, 230–246

McDonnell, P.J., Moore, G.W., Miller, N.R. *et al.* (1986) Temporal arteritis. A clinicopathologic study. *Ophthalmology*, **93**, 518–530

Maitland, C.G. and Miller, N.R. (1984) Neuroretinitis. *Archives of Ophthalmology*, **102**, 1446–1450

Nikoskelainen, E. (1985) The clinical findings in Leber's hereditary optic neuroretinopathy. *Transactions of the Ophthalmological Society of the United Kingdom*, **104**, 845–852

Repka, M.X., Savino, P.J., Schatz, N.J. *et al.* (1983) Clinical profile and long-term implications of anterior ischemic optic neuropathy. *American Journal of Ophthalmology*, **96**, 478–483

Rosenberg, M.A., Savino, P.J. and Glaser, J.S. (1979) A clinical analysis of pseudopapilloedema. 1-Population, laterality, refractive error, ophthalmoscopic characteristics, and coincidental disease. *Archives of Ophthalmology*, **97**, 65–70

Sadun, A.A. and Lessell, S. (1985) Brightness-sense and optic nerve disease. *Archives of Ophthalmology*, **103**, 39–43

Sanders, M.D. and Sennhenn, R.H. (1980) Differential diagnosis of unilateral optic disc oedema. *Transactions of the Ophthalmological Society of the United Kingdom*, **100**, 123–131

Savino, P.J., Glaser, J.S. and Rosenberg, M.A. (1979) A clinical analysis of pseudopapilloedema. *Archives of Ophthalmology*, **97**, 71–75

Shults, W.T. (1984) Ischaemic optic neuropathy. Still the ophthalmologist's dilemma. *Ophthalmology*, **91**, 1338–1341

Skarf, B. and Hoyt, C.S. (1984) Optic nerve hypoplasia in children. *Archives of Ophthalmology*, **102**, 62–67

Taylor, D.S.I. (1985) The genetic implications of optic disc anomalies. *Transactions of the Ophthalmological Society of the United Kingdom*, **104**, 853–856

Tso, M.O. (1981) Pathology and pathogenesis of drusen of the optic nerve head. *Ophthalmology*, **88**, 1066–1080

Van Dyk, H.J.L. (1983) Management of optic neuritis. *Clinical Modules for Ophthalmologists*, Vol. 1, Module 3

Wirtschafter, J.D. (1980) Diagnosis of optic atrophy. *Perspectives in Ophthalmology*, **4**, 223–252

Chiasmal disorders

Anderson, D., Faber, P., Marcovitz, S. *et al.* (1983) Pituitary tumours and the ophthalmologist. *Ophthalmology*, **90**, 1265–1270

Anderson, D. and Khalil, M. (1981) Meningioma and the ophthalmologist. *Ophthalmology*, **88**, 1004–1009

Barma, M. (1976) Craniopharyngioma. Based on 160 cases. *British Journal of Ophthalmology*, **49**, 206–210

Crane, T.B., Yee, R.D. and Helper, R.S. (1982) Clinical manifestations and radiologic findings in craniopharyngioma in adults. *American Journal of Ophthalmology*, **94**, 220–228

Third, fourth and sixth nerve disease

Grove, A.S. Jr (1984) The dural shunt syndrome. Pathophysiology and clinical course. *Ophthalmology*, **90**, 31–44

Guy, J., Savino, P.J. and Schatz, N.J. (1985) Superior division paralysis of the oculomotor nerve. *Ophthalmology*, **92**, 777–784

Lee, D.A., Dyer, J.A., O'Brien, P.C. *et al.* (1984) Surgical treatment of lateral rectus paralysis. *American Journal of Ophthalmology*, **97**, 511–518

Leonard, T.J.K., Moseley, I.F. and Sanders, M.D. (1984) Ophthalmoplegia in carotid cavernous sinus fistula. *British Journal of Ophthalmology*, **68**, 128–134

Rush, J.A. and Younge, B.R. (1981) Paralysis of cranial nerves III, IV, and VI: causes and prognosis in 1000 cases. *Archives of Ophthalmology*, **99**, 76–79

Savino, P.J., Hilliker, J.J., Casell, G.H. *et al.* (1982) Chronic sixth nerve palsy. *Ophthalmology*, **100**, 1442–1444

Shults, W.T. (1983) Third, fourth, and sixth cranial nerve palsies. *Clinical Modules for Ophthalmologists*, Vol. 1, Module 7

Sydnor, C.F., Seaber, J.H. and Buckley, E.G. (1982) Traumatic superior oblique paresis. *Ophthalmology*, **89**, 134–138

Trobe, J.D. (1985) Isolated pupil-sparing third nerve palsy. *Ophthalmology*, **92**, 58–61

Pupillary abnormalities

Maloney, W.F., Younge, B.R. and Moyer, N.J. (1980) Evaluation of the causes and accuracy of pharmacologic localization of Horner's syndrome. *American Journal of Ophthalmology*, **90**, 394–402

Skarf, B. and Czarnecki, J.S.C. (1982) Distinguishing postganglionic from preganglionic lesions. *Archives of Ophthalmology*, **100**, 1319–1322

Thompson, H.S. (1976) Pupillary signs in the diagnosis of optic nerve disease. *Transactions of the Ophthalmological Society of the United Kingdom*, **96**, 377–381

Index

Note: Page numbers in **bold** refer to pages on which illustrations/tables appear

Abducens (sixth) nerve palsy, 467–470
Abetalipoproteinaemia (Bassen–Kornzweig syndrome), 374
Abnormal head posture, 417
AC/A ratio, 414
Acanthamoeba, 96
Acetazolamide (Diamox), 200
Acetylcysteine (Ilube), 51
Acne rosacea, 107–108
Acoustic neuroma, 468
Acycloguanosine (acyclovir; Zovirax), 99
Acquired immune deficiency syndrome (AIDS), 162
Acute posterior multifocal placoid pigment epitheliopathy, **170, 171**
Adenine arabinoside, 99
Adenocarcinoma of lacrimal gland, 40
Adenoid cystic carcinoma (cylindroma) of lacrimal gland, 40
Adenoviral keratoconjunctivitis, 68
Adjustable sutures, 435–436
Adrenaline (epinephrine), 82, 198–199
Adrenergic receptors, 196–197
Adult foveomacular vitelliform dystrophy, 376
Advancement of muscle, 434
After-image test, 421
Age-related (senile) macular degeneration, 349–355
  drusen, 349–350
  exudative (neovascular), 351
    choroidal neovascularization, 352–354
    detachment of retinal pigment epithelium, 351, **352**
  non-exudative, **350,** 351
AIDS (acquired immune deficiency syndrome), 162
Airmark perimeter, 190
Albinism, 380
Alcian blue stain, 50
Alport's syndrome, 258
Amiodarone, 121, 237
Amblyopia
  anisometropic, 417
  stimulus deprivation, 417
  strabismic, 416
  treatment, 428
Amsler grid, 342
Angioid streaks, 363–364
Angiotensin converting enzyme, 146
Angle kappa, 418
Aniridia, 226, 256
Ankylosing spondylitis, 142
Anomalous (abnormal) retinal correspondence, 417, 422
Anterior ischaemic optic neuropathies, 443–445
  arteritic, 444–445
  non-arteritic, 444
Anterior lenticonus, 258
Antiglaucoma drugs, 196–201
  adrenaline (epinephrine), 198–199
  beta-adrenergic blocking agents, 198–199
    betaxolol (Betoptic), 198
    carteolol (Teoptic), 198
    levobunolol (Betagan), 198
    metipranolol (Glauline), 198
    timolol (Timoptol; Timoptic), 198
  carbonic anhydrase inhibitors, 200–201
    acetazolamide (Diamox), 200
    Diamox Sustets, 200
    dichlorphenamide (Daranide), 200
    ethoxzolamide (Cardrase), 200
    methazolamide (Neptazane), 200
    side-effects, 200–201
  dipivalyl adrenaline (Propine), 199
  guanethidine, 199
Antiglaucoma drugs (*cont.*)
  miotics, 199–200
    carbachol, 200
    demecarium bromide, 200
    ecothiopate, 200
    isoflurophate, 200
    pilocarpine, 198, 199
Antiviral agents, 99–100
  side-effects, 100
Aphakia correction, 243
Aqueous humour dynamics, 182
Arcus senilis, 111–112
Argon laser, 300
  trabeculoplasty, 202–203
Argyll Robertson pupil, 474
Argyrosis, 82, 92
Arthritis
  juvenile chronic, 143
  psoriatic, 143
Astrocytoma, retinal, 405–406
Atopic keratoconjunctivitis, 74
Atropine, 427
Axenfeld's anomaly, 226, **227**
Axoplasmic transport, 449

Bagolini striated glasses, 421
Band keratopathy, 112
Barkan goniolens, 186
Basal cell carcinoma, 5
  noduloulcerative (rodent ulcer), 5
  sclerosing, 5
  treatment, 5–6
Basal encephalocele, 455
Bassen–Kornzweig syndrome (abetalipoproteinaemia), 374
Batten's disease (ceroid-lipofuscinosis), 377
Behçet's disease, 148–150
Benedikt's syndrome, 463
Benign concentric annular macular dystrophy, 377
Best's vitelliform macular dystrophy, 375–376
  carriers, 372
Betamethasone, 195

Betaxolol (Betoptic), 198
Bietti's nodular dystrophy
 (spheroidal degeneration), 112
Binocular single vision, 415
Binocular vision grades, 422
Birdshot retinochoroidopathy
 (vitiliginous retinochoroiditis),
 172
BJ6, **51**
Bleb-like dystrophy (microcystic
 dystrophy), 113, **114**
Blepharitis
 chronic, *see* Blepharoconjunctivitis
 posterior (meibomian gland
 dysfunction), 52, 66
 seborrheic, 65–66
 staphylococcal, 65
Blepharochalasis, 14
Blepharoconjunctivitis (chronic
 blepharitis), 64–67
 keratoconjunctivitis sicca
 associated, 52
 rosacea, 107
 treatment, 66–67
 viccinia, 104
Blepharophimosis syndrome, 15
Blepharospasm, essential, 478
Blood (haematic) cyst, 42
Blow-out fracture
 medial wall, 36
 orbital floor, 35–36
Blue field entoptic 'flying corpuscle'
 test, 343
Bonnet's sign, 330
Bourneville's disease (tuberous
 sclerosis; epiloia), 405
Bowman's layer, 88
Bromhexine, 52
Brown's superior oblique tendon
 sheath syndrome, 432
Bruch's membrane, 341
Bullous keratopathy, 117
'Bull's eye' macular syndrome, 365,
 376–377
Buphthalmos, 223
Burns, chemical, 77
Busacca nodules, 138
Busulphan (Myleran), 237
Butterfly dystrophy, 376

Canaliculitis, 59
Canaliculodacryocystorhinostomy,
 56–57
Candidiasis, 164–165
Candlewax drippings (exudates),
 140, 147, 148
Capillary haemangioma, 39–40
Carbachol, 200
Carbonic anhydrase inhibitors, 200–
 201
 side-effects. 200–201
Carcinoma *in situ*, conjunctival
 (intraepithelial epithelioma), 83
Cardrase (ethoxzolamide), 200
Carotid-cavernous fistula, 470–472
 indirect (dural shunt), 471
Carteolol (Teoptic), 198
Cataract, 234–255
 aetiological classification, **234**
 capsular, 239

Cataract (*cont.*)
 complications of surgery, 249–255
 bacterial endophthalmitis, 250–
 251
 cystoid macular oedema
 (Irvine–Gass syndrome),
 251–252
 epithelial ingrowth, 254
 filtering bleb, 254
 hyphaema, 249
 iris prolapse, 249
 opacification of posterior
 capsule, 252
 neodymium-YAG laser
 capsulotomy, 253
 pupil block, 250
 retinal detachment, 263–264
 striate keratopathy, 249
 'sunset syndrome', 255
 'UHG' syndrome, 255
 vitreous touch syndrome, 254
 vitreous wick syndrome, 254
 wound leak, 250
 congenital, 239
 cortical, 239
 extracapsular extraction
 technique and implantation of
 posterior chamber, IOL,
 247
 vs intracapsular extraction, 244
 vitreous loss, 248–249
 extraction indications, 244
 glass-blowers, 234
 hereditary, 239
 hypermature, 240
 immature, 239
 infantile, 240–243
 aphakia correction, 243
 evaluation, 240–241
 lensectomy, 242–243
 surgery, 241
 tests, 241
 intracapsular extraction
 technique and implantation of
 anterior chamber IOL, 245–
 247, **247**
 vs extracapsular extraction, 244
 vitreous loss, 248–249
 intraocular lenses, 244–245
 intumescent, 240
 lamellar, 239
 maternal drug ingestion induced,
 238
 maternal infections, 237–238
 cytomegalic inclusion disease,
 238
 rubella, 237–238
 toxoplasmosis, 238
 mature, 240
 metabolic, 235–236
 diabetes, 235
 Fabry's disease, 235
 galactokinase deficiency, 235
 galactosaemia, 235
 hypocalcaemic syndromes, 236
 Lowe's syndrome, 235
 mannosidoses, 235
 Wilson's disease, 236
 Morgagnian, 240
 morphological classification, 239–
 240

Cataract (*cont.*)
 nuclear, 239
 phacoemulsification, 248
 presenile, 238
 secondary (complicated), 237
 anterior uveitis, 237
 Fuchs' uveitis syndrome, 167
 glaukomflecken, 237
 hereditary retinal syndromes,
 237
 high myopia, 237
 pars planitis, 168
 vitreoretinal disorders, 237
 senile, 234
 subcapsular, 239
 sutural, 239
 toxic, 236–237
 amiodarone, 237
 busulphan (Myleran), 237
 chlorpromazine, 236–237
 corticosteroids, 236
 gold, 237
 miotics, 237
 traumatic, 234–235
Catarrhal ulcer (marginal keratitis),
 106–107
Catford drum, 476
Cavernous haemangioma, 40
Cavernous sinus, 456
Cellophane maculopathy, 295
Cellulitis
 orbital, 36–37
 preseptal, 36
Central areolar choroidal dystrophy,
 386
Central serous chorioretinopathy,
 356–357
Cerebrospinal fluid, 447
Chalazion (meibomian cyst), 2
Chancre, 151
 conjunctival, 151
Chandler's syndrome, 222
Chemical burns, 77
Chemosis, 31
'Cherry-red spot', 377–378
 myoclonus syndrome, 378
Chiasmal disorders, 455–459
Childhood leukoria, differential
 diagnosis, 404–405
Chlamydial infection, 69–71
Chloramphenicol, 446
Chloroquine (Nivaquine), 121, 365
Chorpromazine (Largactil), 236–237,
 365–367
Cholinergic neurones, 197
Cholinesterase inhibitors, 198
Chordoma, 468
Chorioretinitis, syphilitic, 151–152
Choristoma, 83–84
Choroid
 detachment, 262, 279–280
 dystrophies, 385–386
 folds, 362–363
 haemangioma, 399–400
 diffuse, 400
 localized, 399–400
 metastatic carcinoma, 400
 naevus, 397–399
 osteoma (osseous choristoma), 401
 sarcoidosis, 148
 tuberculous granuloma, 153

Choroideremia, 385
Choroiditis, acute focal, 140
Chronic progressive external ophthalmoplegia (ocular myopathy), 478
Chrysiasis, 92, 120
Chrysotherapy, 120
Cicatricial pemphigoid, 74–76
Ciliary body, 262
  cysts, 396
  melanoma, 295–296
Coats' disease, 336, 404
Cockayne's syndrome, 374
Cogan's microcystic dystrophy, 113, **114**
Cogan's syndrome, 97
Cogan–Reese (iris naevus) syndrome, 222
Collier's sign, 30
Colour perception test, 344
Concretions, conjunctival, 80
Cone dystrophy, 376–377
Confrontation tests, 441–442
  colour comparison, 442
  finger counting, 441
  finger-mimicking, 441
  hat-pin, 442
  visually evoked movement, 441
Confusion, 415
Congenital ectropion uveae (hyperplasia of iris pigment border), 228
Congenital fibrosis syndrome, 432
Congenital retinoschisis, 382, **383**
conjunctiva, 62
  chancre, 151
  degenerations, 79–80
  endogenous pigmentation, 82
  exogenous pigmentation, 82
  inflammation, 62–64
    investigations, 64
    lymphadenopathy, 64
  non-melanocytic pigmentation, 82
  non-pigmented tumours, 83
  pigmented lesions, 80–82
  pseudopigmentation, 82
  squamous cell carcinoma, invasive, 83
Conjunctivitis
  acute bacterial, 67
    scrapings, 64
  acute allergic, 72
    scrapings, 64
  acute follicular, 98
  acute haemorrhagic, 68, **69**
  adult inclusion, 69–70
    scrapings, 64
  chlamydial, 69–70
    viral follicular conjunctivitis compared, **70**
  chronic, 67
  chronic allergic, 73
  giant papillary, 74
  gonococcal, 67
  hay fever (seasonal allergic), 72
  herpetic mucopurulent, 102
  Parinaud's oculoglandular, 78
  recurrent, 67
  viral, 68
    scrapings, 64
Contact lenses, 121–126
  complications, 125–126
  fitting, 122–123
  gas permeable, 122
  hard, 121–122
  medical indications, 123–125
  soft (hydrophilic), 122
Contact lens cornea (peripheral corneal guttering), 110
Convergence, 414
Copper, corneal deposit, 92
Cornea, 88
  changes in metabolic/toxic disorders, 119–121
  crystalline deposits, 120
  degenerations, 111–113
  diseases, *see* Corneal diseases
  drawing abnormalities, 92–93
  dystrophies, 113–119
  grafting, *see* Keratoplasty
  microdendrites, 102
  peripheral guttering (contact lens cornea), 110
  peripheral ulceration/thinning, 106–111
  pigmentation, 92
  refractive surgery, 128–129
  resurfacing, 47
  transplantation, *see* Keratoplasty
Cornea guttata, 116–117
Cornea verticillata (vortex keratopathy), 120–121
Corneal diseases, 88–129
  epithelial, 89–91
  laboratory investigation, 93
  management, 93–94
    perforation prevention, 94
    primary therapy, 94
    re-epithelialization, 94
    transparency restoration, 94
  neovascularization, 91, 147
  pachometry, 93
  punctate epithelial erosions (epitheliopathy), 89, **91**
  slitlamp biomicroscopy, 89, **90**
  slitlamp examination using specular reflection, 93
  specular microscopy, 93
  stromal lesions, 91, **92**
  symptoms, 88–89
  Terrien's marginal degeneration, 108–109
  vital staining, 93
Corneal elastosis (spheroidal degeneration), 112
Corticosteroids
  cataract due to, 236
  responsiveness in primary open-angle glaucoma, 195
Cover tests, 418
Craniopharyngioma, 458–459
Criswick–Schepens syndrome (exudative vitreoretinopathy), 384
Crowding phenomenon, 417
Cutaneous horn, 4
Cyclitis, chronic, 168
Cyclopentolate (Mydrilate; Cyclogyl), 427
Cyclosporin, 177
Cylindroma (adenoid cystic carcinoma) of lacrimal gland, 40
Cystinosis, 120
Cyst of Moll, 3
Cyst of Zeis, 3
Cystoid macular oedema (Irvine–Gass syndrome), 168, 251–252, 358
Cystoid maculopathy, 199
Cytomegalic inclusion disease, 238
Cytomegalovirus retinitis, 161, **162,** 162
Cytotoxic agents, 177

Dacryocystitis, 59
Dacryocystography, 56
  intubation, 56
Dacryocystorhinostomy, 56, 58
Dalrymple's sign, 30
Daranide (dichlorphenamide), 200
Dark adaptation (adaptometry, 370–371
Debridement, 100
Dellen, 106
Demecarium bromide, 200
De Morsier's syndrome (septo-optic dysplasia), 454
Dendritic ulcer, 98–99
  debridement, 100
Dermatitis, 19
  acute, 19
  atopic, 19, 238
  chronic, 19
  contact, 19
Dermatochalasia, 14, **15**
Dermoid, conjunctival, 83
Dermoid cyst, 42
Descemet's membrane, 88
  folds, 92
  lesions, 92
Diabetic cataract, 235
Diabetic maculopathy, 306–308
  diffuse, 306–307
  focal, 306
  ischaemic, 307–308
Diabetic papillopathy, 445–446
Diabetic retinopathy, 302–318
  haemorrhages, 304
  hard exudates, 304, **305**
  management, 304
  microaneurysms, 304, **305**
  microvascular leakage, 302–304
  microvascular occlusion, 302, **303**
  neovascular glaucoma, 314
  opaque membrane formation, 314
  pars plana vitrectomy, 314–318
    complications, 317–318
  preproliferative, 308
  proliferative, 308
    follow-up, 311
    haemorrhage, 310
    management, 310–312
    neovascularization, 308–309
    persistent vitreous haemorrhage, 312
    recurrence treatment, 312
    retinal detachment, 312–313
    vitreous detachment, 309
  retinal oedema, 304
Diamox (acetazolamide), 200
Diamox Sustets, 200
Dichlorphenamide (Daranide), 200
Dicon perimeter, 191

Differential intraocular pressure test, 25
Diffuse chorioretinal atrophy, **272**, 275
Diktyoma (medulloepithelioma), 396
Dipivalyl adrenaline (Propine), 199
Diplopia, 416
Distichiasis, 7
Divergence, 414
Double elevator palsy, 433
Double-ring sign, 454
Double vision, 415–417
  compensatory mechanisms, 416
    abnormal head posture, 417
    anomalous (abnormal) retinal correspondence, 417, 422
    strabismic amblyopia, 416–417
    suppression, 416
  confusion, 415, **416**
  diplopia, 416
Down's syndrome (mongolism), 238
Doyne's honeycomb choroiditis (familial dominant drusen; Tay's choroiditis), 379
Drusen, 284, 349–350, 451
Dry eye, 46–52
  treatment, **50**
Duane's retraction syndrome, 431–432
Dysthyroid optic neuropathy, 31
Dystrophia myotonica, 238, 478

Eales' disease, 170
Ecothiopate (Phospholine Iodide), 200, 428
Ectatic dystrophies, 118–119
Ectopia lentis, 255–258
  familial, 256
  glaucoma associated, 220
  surgery, 258
Ectropion, 10–12
  cicatricial, 11–12
  congenital, 12
  involutional (senile), 10–11
    treatment, 11
  paralytic, 12
    treatment, 12
Ehlers–Danlos syndrome, 364
Electro-oculography, 371
  clinical applications, 372
Electrophysiological tests, 370–372
  clinical applications, 372
Electroretinography, 370
  clinical applications, 372
ELISA (enzyme-linked immunosorbent assay) test, 158
Elschnig's pearls, 252
Elschnig's spots, 330
Encephalotrigeminal angiomatosis (Sturge–Weber syndrome), 228–229
Endophthalmitis, 136
  candida, 165
  post-filtration surgery, 204–205
Enophthalmos, 23
Entropion, 7–10
  acute spastic, 10
  cicatricial, 9–10
  congenital, 10
  involutional (senile), 7–8
    treatment, 8–9
Eosinophilic granuloma, 42
Epiblepharon, 10
Epicanthus, 18
Epidemic keratoconjunctivitis, 68
Epikeratophakia, 129
Epiloia (tuberous sclerosis; Bourneville's disease), 405
Epinephrine (adrenaline), 82, 198–199
Episcleritis, 130–131
  herpetic, 102
Epithelial basement membrane dystrophy (microcystic dystrophy), 113, **114**
Epithelioma, intraepithelial conjunctival (carcinoma *in situ*), 83
Erythema multiforme major (Stevens–Johnson syndrome), 77
Essential iris atrophy, 222
Esotropia, 424–430
  accommodative, 426–430
    management, 427–429
    mixed, 427
    non-accommodative, 429–430
    non-refractive, 427
    refractive, 427
  'A' pattern, 429
  classification, 424
  consecutive, 430
  infantile (congenital), 424–426
    management, 424–426
  surgical options, 429
  'V' pattern, 429
  see also Strabismus
Ethambutol, 446
Ethoxzolamide (Cardrase), 200
Ewing's sarcoma, orbital metastases, 42
Exotropia, childhood, 430–431
  constant, 430–431
  intermittent, 430
  see also Strabismus
Exposure keratopathy, 105
Essential blepharospasm, 478
External hordeolum (stye), 2
Extraocular muscles, actions, 412
Exudative vitreoretinopathy (Criswick–Schepens syndrome), 384
Eyelash disorders, 6–7
Eyelids
  benign tumours, 3–4
  cysts, 2–3
  malignant tumours, 5–6
  margin, 2
Eye movements, 413–414
  directions, 413
  vergences, 414
    AC/A ratio, 414
    convergence, 414
    divergence, 414
    fusional, 414
  versions, 413–414

Fabry's disease, 121, 235
Facial nerve palsy, 12
Familial dominant drusen (Doyne's honeycomb choroiditis; Tay's choroiditis), 379
Favre–Goldman syndrome, 382–383
Ferry's line, 92
Fieldmaster perimeter, 191
Filtration surgery, 203–204
'Flecked retina' syndromes, 378–379
Fleischer's ring, 92, 118
Floppy eyelid syndrome, 79
Fluorescein, 93
Fluorescein angiography, 344–348
  circulation of fluorescein, 346–348
    angiogram phases, 346
    normal angiogram, 346–347
  complications, 345
  hyperfluorescence, 347–348
  hypofluorescence, 348
  technique, 345
'Flying corpuscle' test, 343
Forced duction test, 25
Fovea, 340
  avascular zone (capillary-free zone), 341
Foveola, 340
Foville's syndrome, 467–468
Friedreich's ataxia, 374
Fuchs' endothelial dystrophy, 117–118
  primary open-angle glaucoma associated, 196
Fuchs' spot, 360, **361**
Fuchs' uveitis syndrome (Fuchs' heterochromic cyclitis), 166–167
  heterochromia, 166
  iris atrophy, 139, 166
  keratic precipitates, 137
  rubeosis iridis, 139
Fundus albipunctatus, 379
Fundus contact lenses, 268
Fundus flavimaculatus, 378, 379
Fusion, 422
Fusional vergences, 414

Galactokinase deficiency, 235
Galactosaemia, 235
Gangliosidoses
  generalized, 378
  type 1 (Tay–Sachs disease; infantile amaurotic family idiocy), 377
  type 2 (Sandhoff disease), 378
Gastrointestinal symptom complex, 201
Gaze, cardinal positions, 413
Generalized choroidal atrophy, 386
Geographical (serpiginous) choroidopathy, 171–172
Geographical ulcer, 99
Giant cell arteritis, 444–445
Glands of Moll, 2
Glands of Zeis, 2
Glandular fever (infectious mononucleosis), 162
Glaucoma, 182–230
  angle-closure
    adrenaline precipitated, 199
    miotics precipitated, 200
  antiglaucoma drugs, *see* Antiglaucoma drugs
  classification, 182
  congenital (developmental), 223–225

Glaucoma (*cont.*)
congenital (development) (*cont.*)
primary, 223–225
management, 225
ectopia lentis associated, 220
Fuchs' uveitis syndrome, 167
ghost cell, 221
gonioscopy, 185–189
goniolenses, 185–186
optical principles, 185
identification of angle structures, 186–189
angle recess, 187
angular approach to recess, 188
blood vessels, 187
ciliary body, 187
curvature of peripheral iris, 188
iris insertion, 188–189
iris processes, 187
Schlemm's canal, 187
Schwalbe's line, 186
scleral spur, 187
Shaffer grading system, 187–188
Spaeth grading system, 188
trabeculum, 186–187
intermittent angle-closure, 196
intraocular tumours causing, 221
'low-tension', 196
melanomalytic, 221
neovascular, 221, 314
pathogenesis, 182
phacolytic, 219, **220,** 220
phacomorphic, 219, **220**
pigmentary, 218
primary angle-closure, 205–212, 221
absolute, 211
acute, 207–210
congestive phase, 207–210
plateau iris syndrome, 211
postcongestive phase, 210
chronic (creeping angle closure), 211
classification, 206
inheritance, 205
intermittent (subacute), 207
laser iridotomy, 211–212
latent, 206–207
provocative tests, 206–207
predisposing factors, 205–206
primary open-angle, 191–205
corticosteroid responsiveness, 195
differential diagnosis, 196
gonioscopy, 195
inheritance, 191
management, 201–205
argon laser trabeculoplasty, 202–203
drug, *see* Antiglaucoma drugs
filtration surgery, 203–204
follow-up, 202
indications for treatment, 201
medical, 201–202
Scheie's thermosclerostomy, 204
ocular association, 196
pathogenesis, 191
signs, 191–195
cup–disc ratio, 192
cupping, 192–194
Glaucoma (*cont.*)
primary open-angle (*cont.*)
signs (*cont.*)
early damage, 192
nerve fibre damage, 193
optic disc changes, 191–192, **193**
visual field defects, 194–195
symptoms, 191
systemic associations, 196
tomography, 195
tonometry, 195
pseudo-low-tension, 196
raised episcleral venous pressure-induced, 222
rubella, 225
secondary, 212–217
angle-closure from pupil block, 213–214
angle closure without pupil block, 214–215
classification, 212
diagnostic problems, 212
neovascular, 216–217
open-angle glaucoma, 216
slitlamp biomicroscopy, 182, **183**
tonography, 185
tonometry, 182–183
air-puff tonometer, 184
applanation, 183, **184**
Goldmann tonometer, 183, **184**
indentation, 182–183
Mackay–Marg tonometer, 184
Perkins tonometer, 184
pneumatonometer, 184
Pulsair tonometer, **184**
Schiötz tonometer, 182–183
Tono-Pen, 184
traumatic, 220–221
Glaucoma capsulare, 219
Glaucomatocyclitic crises (Posner–Schlossman syndrome), 173
Glaukomflecken, 210, **211,** 237
Glioma of optic nerve, **28,** 449–450
Glauline (metipranolol), 198
Gold
cataract due to, 237
corneal deposit, 92, 120
Goldenhar's syndrome, 84
Goldmann perimeter, 190
Goldmann tonometer, 183, **184**
Goldmann triple-mirror contact lens, 262
Goldmann–Weekes adaptometer, 370
Goniotomy, 225
Gradenigo's syndrome, 468, 470
Granular dystrophy, 116
Graves' disease, 29
Guanethidine, 199
Guillain–Barré syndrome (acute infectious polyneuropathy), 470
Gumma, iridal, 151
Gunn's sign, 330
Gyrate atrophy, 237, 385–386

Haab's striae, 223, **224**
Haematic (blood) cyst, 42
Halberstaedter–Prowazek inclusion body, 64, 70
Haltia–Santavuori disease, 377
Hansen's disease (leprosy), 153
Hand–Schüller–Christian disease, 42
Harada's disease, 141
Hassall–Henle warts, 92
Hemianopia, 440
complete, 460
heteronymous, 440
homonymous, 440, 461
incomplete, 460
inferior quadrantic ('pie on the floor'), 460
macular sparing congruous homonymous, 460
upper quadrantic ('pie in the sky'), 460
Henle's layer, 341
Hepatolenticular degeneration (Wilson's disease), 92, 119–120, 236
Hereditary progressive arthro-ophthalmopathy with marfanoid habitus (Stickler syndrome), 237, 381–382
Hereditary retinal diseases, 237
Hering's law, 414
Herpes simplex, 97–101, 160–161
anterior uveitis
dendritic ulceration associated, 160
disciform keratitis associated, 160
geographical ulceration association, 160
keratitis unassociated, 161
iris atrophy, 139, 160
primary ocular infection, 97–98
recurrence risk, 100
virus 1/2, 97
Herpes zoster, 101–104, 159–160
stage one, 101–103
cutaneous lesions, 101–102
episcleritis, 102
keratitis, 102
mucopurulent conjunctivitis, 102
neurological complications, 103
scleritis, 102
stage two, 103–104
cutaneous lesions, 103
keratitis, 104
mucus-secreting conjunctivitis, 103
neuralgia, 104
ptosis, 103
scleritis, 104
stage three, 104
iris atrophy, 139
Hertel exophthalmometer, 23, **24**
Hess test. 419–420, **421**
Heterochromia, 166
Hirschberg test, 417–418
Histiocytic lymphoma (reticulum cell sarcoma), 141, 409
Histiocytosis X, 41–42
Hollenhorst's plaques, 324, **325**
Holmes–Adie (tonic) pupil, 474
Homocystinuria, 256
Hordeolum
external (stye), 2
internal, 2

Horizontal deviation, 417
Horizontal gaze, 461–462
Horner's syndrome
(oculosympathetic palsy), 474–475
Horopter, 415
Hudson–Stähli line, 92
Hummelsheim procedure, 435
Humphrey perimeter, 191
Hunter's disease, 121
Hurler's disease, 121
Hutchinson's freckle (lentigo maligna), 82
Hutchinson's sign, 101, 159
Hydroxychloroquine (Plaquenil), 365
Hyperlysinaemia, 256
Hypermetropia, 426, 427–428
Hypertelorism, 455
Hypertensive retinopathy, 328–330
arteriosclerotic features, 329–330
hypertensive features, 328–329
Hyperthyroidism, 29
Hypocalcaemic syndromes, 236
Hypoparathyroidism, 236
Hypotears, **52**

Idiopathic juxtafoveolar retinal telangiectasia, 334, **335**
Idoxuridine, 99
Ilube (acetylcysteine), 51
Imbert–Fick law, 183
Incontinentia pigmenti, 405
Infantile amaurotic family idiocy (Tay–Sachs disease; gangliosidosis type 1), 377
Infectious mononucleosis (glandular fever), 162
Inferior petrosal sinus thrombosis, 468
Inferometry, 344
Influenza virus, 162
Infraorbital nerve damage, 22
Internal carotid artery aneurysm, 456, 459
Internal hordeolum, 3
Intraocular lenses, 244–245
Intubation dacryocystography, 56
Iridoschisis, 222
Iridocorneal endothelial syndromes, 222
Iridocyclitis
acute, 147
chronic granulomatous, 147
juvenile chronic, 169
syphilitic, 151
Iris
atrophy, 138, 222
cysts, 200, 396–397
freckles, 396
leiomyoma, 397
melanoma, 396–397
metastases in, 397
naevi, 396
nodules, 138
neovascularization (rubeosis iridis), 139, 140–141, 314
pigment border hyperplasia (congenital ectropion uveae), 228
Iris bombé, 139
Iris naevus (Cogan–Reese) syndrome, 222
Iritis, leprotic, acute/chronic, 153
Irvine–Gass syndrome (cystoid macular oedema), 168, 251–252, 358
Isoflurophate, 200
Isoniazid, 446
Isopto Alkaline, **51**
Isopto Plain, **51**
Isopters, 189

Jansky–Bielschowsky disease, 377
Jensen's procedure, 435
Jones dye tests, 54–55
Juvenile chronic arthritis, 143–145
Juvenile chronic iridocyclitis, 169
Juvenile xanthogranuloma, 397

Kaposi's sarcoma, 162
Kayser–Fleischer ring, 120
Kearns–Sayre syndrome, 374, 478
Keratitic precipitates, 136, 137–138, 166
Keratitis
acanthamoebal, 96
acute epithelial, 98–99
acute stromal, 110
adenoviral, 68, **69**
bacterial, 94–95
chlamydial, 69–70
disciform, 100–101, 103
vaccinial, 104
fungal, 96
herpes simplex, **98**
herpes zoster, 102–103
interstitial, 97
luetic, 97
marginal (catarrhal ulcer), 106–107
nummular, 102, **103**
peripheral, 110
punctate epithelial, 89, 102
recurrent, 98
rosaceal, 107–108
sclerosing, 110
stromal necrotic, 100
superficial punctate, 91
Thygeson's superficial punctate, 105
trophic (metaherpetic), 101
tuberculous, 97
vaccinal, 104
viral, 97–104
see also Herpes simplex; Herpes zoster
Keratoacanthoma, 4
Keratoconjunctivitis
atopic, 74
superior limbic, of Theodore, 77–78
vernal (spring catarrh), 73–74
Keratoconjunctivitis sicca, 57–52
causes, 47–48
clinical evaluation, 48–49
cornea, 49
tear film break-up time, 49
tests, 49–50
biopsy of conjunctiva, 50
lysozyme assay, 50
Schirmer's, 50
tear osmolarity, 50
vital dye staining, 49–50
Keratoconjunctivitis sicca (*cont.*)
treatment, 50–52
associated disorders, 52
mucolytics, 51
reduction of tear drainage, 51–52
systemic, 52
tear conservation, 50–51
tear substitutes, 51
Keratoconus (conical cornea), 118–119
posterior, 119
Keratoglobins, 119
Keratolysis, 110
band, 112
bullous, 117
climatic droplet (spheroidal degeneration), 112
Keratopathy
exposure, 105
Labrador (spheroidal degeneration), 112
lipid, 112
neurotrophic, 105–106
vortex (corneal verticillata), 120–121
Keratopolasty (corneal transplantation/grafting), 126–128
lamellar, 128
penetrating, 126–128
complications, 127
graft failure, 128
indications, 126
postoperative management, 127
prognostic factors, 127
surgical procedure, 127
Keratosis
seborrhoeic, 4
senile, 4
Kocher's sign, 30
Koeppe goniolens, 186
Koeppe nodules, 138, 145, 166
Krimsky test, 418
Krukenberg's spindle, 92
Krypton laser, 300
Kufs' disease, 377
Kveim–Slitzbach test, 145, 146

Labrador keratopathy, 112
Lacquer crack, 360
Lacrimal drainage system, 52–53
infection, 59
Lacrimal sac, 52
tumours, 59
Lacrimal gland, 46
accessory, 46, 62
atrophy/fibrosis, 47
tumours, 40
Lancaster red-green test, 420
Landers' sign, 148
Laser iridotomy, 211–212
Lateral rectus enlargement, ultrasound appearance, 28
Lattice dystrophy, 115, **116**
Laurence–Moon–Biedl syndrome, 374
Leber's congenital amaurosis, 237, 372, 375
Leber's idiopathic stellate neuropathy, 443

Leber's miliary aneurysms, 334, **335**
Leber's optic neuropathy, 446–447
Lees' screen, 420
Lens
  cholinesterase inhibitor-precipitated opacities, 200
  shape abnormalities, 258
Lensectomy, 242–243
Lenticonus, anterior/posterior, 258
Lentiglobus, 258
Lentigo maligna (Hutchinson's freckle), 82
Leprosy (Hansen's disease), 153
Lester Jones tube insertion, 58
Letterer–Siwe disease, 41–42
Leukaemia, orbital deposits, 42
Leukocoria, 404
Levator aponeurosis, 13
Levobunolol (Betagan), 198
Lipid keratopathy, 112
Lipodermoid, conjunctival, 83, **84**
Liquifilm Tears, **51**
Lister perimeter, 190
Long posterior ciliary arteries, 264
Lower eyelid retractors, **13**
Lowe's (oculocerebrorenal) syndrome, 235, 258
Lymphangioma, orbital, 40
Lymphoma, orbital, **41**
Lymphoproliferative disorder, orbital, 41

Mackay–Marg tonometer, 184
Macroreticular dystrophy, 378
Macula, 340–344
  clinical evaluation, 341–344
    Amsler grid, 342
    colour vision, 341
    direct slitlamp biomicroscopy, 341–342
    light brightness appreciation, 341
    ophthalmoscopy, 341
    photostress test, 342–343
    pupillary reactions, 341
    symptoms, 341
    visual acuity, 341
  cystoid oedema, 358
  function in eyes with opaque media, 343–344
    blue field entoptic 'flying corpuscle' test, 343
    colour perception test, 344
    inferometry, **343**, 344
    potential visual acuity meter, **343**, 344
    pupillary response to light, 343
    Purkinje vascular entoptic test, 344
    two light discrimination test, 343–344
Macular dystrophy, 116
Macular hole, 358–360
Macular pucker, 295, 361–362
Maculopathy, 295–296
  atrophic, 296
  'bull's eye', 365, 376–377
  cellophane, 295
  cystoid, 199
  diabetic, *see* Diabetic maculopathy
  Leber's idiopathic stellate, 443
Maculopathy (*cont.*)
  myopic, **360, 361**
  retinitis pigmentosa associated, 373
  toxic, 365–366
Madarosis, 151
Maddox rod test, 419
Maddox wing test, 419
Malaise symptom complex, 200
Mannosidosis, 235
Map–dot–fingerprint dystrophy (microcystic dystrophy), 113, **114**
Marcus Gunn jaw-winking phenomenon, 13–14, 433
Marcus Gunn pupil, 24, 473–474
Marfan's syndrome, 255–256
Marginal myotomy, 433, **434**
Maroteaux–Lamy's disease, 121
Medial longitudinal bundle, 462
Medical Workshop prismatic goniolens, 186
Medulloepithelioma (diktyoma), 396
Meesmann's dystrophy, 115
Meibomian cyst (chalazion), 2–3
Meibomian gland dysfunction (posterior blepharitis), 52, 66
Meibomitis, rosaceal, 107
Melanin, corneal deposit, 92
Melanocytes, 80
Melanocytoma of optic disc, 399
Melanoma, 80, 141
  choroidal, 390–394
    diagnosis, 390–391
    histological classification, 393–394
    management, 392–393
  ciliary body, 395–396
  iris, 396–397
  primary conjunctival, 82
  superficial spreading, 81
Melanosis, 80
  conjunctival epithelial, 80
  oculodermal (naevus of Ota), 81
  precancerous, 81–82
  subepithelial, 80–81
Melanotic pigmentation of conjunctiva, 80–82
Melleril (thioridazine), 366
Meningioma, 459
  optic nerve, 450–451
Mesodermal dysgenesis, 226–227
Methazolamide (Neptazane), 200
Metipranolol (Glauline), 198
Microcystic dystrophy (Cogan's dystrophy; map–dot–fingerprint dystrophy; bleb-like dystrophy; epithelial basement membrane dystrophy), 113, **114**
Microdendrites, 102
Microphakia, 258
Microspherophakia, **256,** 258
Midfacial malformations, 455
Millard–Gubler syndrome, 468
Miotics, 199–200, 428
  side-effects, 200, 237
Mixed-cell tumour of lacrimal gland, 40
  malignant, 40
Möbius syndrome, 432
Molluscum contagiosum, 3
Mongolism (Down's syndrome), 238
Monoclonal gammopathy, 120
Mooren's ulcer, 109–110
Morning glory syndrome, 454
Morquio's disease, 121
Mucin deficiency, 48
Mucocele of orbit, 42
Mucoepidermoid carcinoma of lacrimal gland, 40
Mucopolysaccharidoses, 121
Mucormycosis, 37
Mucus fishing syndrome, 78
Müller's (superior tarsal), muscle, 13
Munson's sign, 118
Myasthenia gravis, 477
Mydriacyl (tropicamide), 427
Mydriatics, 173–174
Mydrilate (cyclopentolate), 427
Myleran (busulphan), 237
Myopia
  high, 237
    complications, 360
  retinal detachment associated, 275
Myopic maculopathy, **360, 361**
Myositis, orbital, 38–39

Naevus, 80
  conjunctival, 81
  Ota's (oculodermal melanosis), 81
Nasolacrimal duct, 52
  obstruction, 57
Nasopharyngeal tumours, 468
Neodymium–YAG laser capsulotomy, 253
Neptazane (methazolamide), 200
Neuroblastoma, orbital metastasis, 42
Neurofibroma, 14, **15**
  optic nerve, 451
Neurofibromatosis (von Recklinghausen's disease), 229–231
Neuroretinitis
  Leber's idiopathic stellate maculopathy, 443
  syphilitic, 152
Neurotrophic keratopathy, 105–106
Neutral density filter test, 417
Neimann–Pick disease, 377
Night blindness, dark adaptation, 370–371
Nivaquine (chloroquine), 121, 365
Noduloulcerative basal cell carcinoma (rodent ulcer), 5–6
Non-optical reflex, 462
Norrie's disease, 404–405
Nystagmus, 475–477
  ataxic, 476
  congenital, 476
  convergence-retraction, 476
  downbeat, 476
  end-point, 476
  jerk, 475
  latent, 476
  mixed, 476
  optokinetic, 461, 476
  pendular, 475
  periodic alternating, 477
  see-saw, of Maddox, 477
  sensory deprivation (ocular), 476
  upbeat, 476
  vestibular, 476
Nystagmus blockage syndrome, 433

Octopus perimeter, **190,** 191
Ocular hypertension, 196
Ocular myopathy (chronic progressive external ophthalmoplegia), 478
Ocular reticulum cell sarcoma (histiocytic lymphoma), 141, 409
Oculocerebrorenal (Lowe's) syndrome, 235, 258
Oculodermal melanosis (naevus of Ota), 81
Oculomotor (third) nerve
  misdirection, 114
  palsy, 463–464, 469–470
Ophthalmia neonatorum, 71–72
Ophthalmodynamometry, 327
Optic atrophy, secondary, 449
Optic disc
  congenital anomalies, 451–453
    coloboma, 258, 453
    drusen, 284, 349–350, 451
    malformations associated, 455
    myelinated nerve fibres, 452
    pit, 452–453
    tilted disc, 453
  cup–disc ratio, 192
  normal, 192
  tilted, 453
Optic disc vasculitis (papillophlebitis), 323
Optic nerve
  compression, 24
  glioma, **28,** 449–450
  hypoplasia, 454
  lesions
    field defects, 440
    filter-like effects, 440–441
  sarcoidosis, 148
  tumours, 449–451
    glioma, 449–450
    meningioma, 450–451
    neurofibroma, 451
Optic nerve head, 440
  lesions, 141
Optic neuritis, 442–443
Optic radiation disorders, 460
Opticrom (sodium cromoglycate), 74
Optic tract disorders, 460
Optokinetic nystagmus, 461
Oral pearls, 262
Orbit
  abscess, **37**
  applied anatomy, 22
  'blow-out' fracture, 22
  cellulitis, 36–37
  clinical evaluation, 22–23
  clinical examination, 23–25
    differential intraocular pressure test, 25
    dynamic properties, 24
    forced duction test, 25
    ocular movements, 24
    orbital compression, 23
    palpation of orbital rim, 23
    slitlamp biomicroscopy, 24
  clinical findings in orbital disease, **25**
  fine needle aspiration biopsy, 28
  fractures
    blow-out of floor, 35–36
    blow-out of medial wall, 36
    roof, 36

Orbit (*cont.*)
  inflammatory disease (pseudotumour), 38–39
    bilateral, 38
    sinus involvement, 39
  magnetic resonance imaging, 27–28
  myositis, 38–39
  radiology, 25–26
    bone density, 26
    Caldwell view, 25
    CT scan, 26
    enlargement of optic canals, 26
    enlargement of superior orbital fissure, 26
    intraorbital calcification, 26
    orbital enlargement, 26
    Rhese view, 25
    Waters' view, 25, **26**
    X-ray signs in orbital disease, **26**
  tumours, 39–43
    blood (haematic) cyst, 42
    capillary haemangioma, 39–40
    cavernous haemangioma, 40
    classification, 39
    dermoid cyst, 42
    histiocytic, 41
    lymphangioma, 40
    lymphoproliferative, 41
    malignant, 40
    metastatic, 42
    mixed-cell, 40
    mucocele, 42
    rhabdomyosarcoma, 41
  ultrasonography, A-/B-scans, 27
Osseous choristoma (chorodial osteoma), 401

Pachometry, 93
Paget's disease, 364
Papilloma, conjunctival, 83
Panophthalmitis, 136
Panum's area, 415
Panuveitis (diffuse uveitis), 136
Papillitis, 141
Papilloedema, 447–449
  causes, 447, 449
  established (fully developed), 448
  secondary optic atrophy, 449
  'vintage', 448–449
Papillophlebitis (optic disc vasculitis), 323
Parainfluenza virus, 162
Parasympathetic drugs, 198
Paravascular vitreoretinal attachments, 275
Parinaud's oculoglandular conjunctivitis, 78
Parinaud's syndrome, 462, 476
Pars plana vitrectomy, 314–318
  complications, 317–318
Pars planitis, 167–168
Patau's syndrome (trisomy 13), 405
Pattern dystrophies, 378
Pellucid marginal degeneration, 119
Pemphigoid, cicatricial, 74–76
Periarteritis, 140
Perimetry, 189–191
  Airmark perimeter, 190
  automated perimeters, 190–191
  confrontation tests, 190

Perimetry (*cont.*)
  Dicon perimeter, 191
  Fieldmaster perimeter, 191
  Goldmann perimeter, 190
  Humphrey perimeter, 191
  isopters, 189
  kinetic, 190
  Lister perimeter, 190
  methods, 190
  scotoma, 189
  static, 190
  tangent screen, 190
  terms, 440
  visual field, 189
  visual threshold, 190
Periphlebitis, 140, **141**
  active peripheral, 147
Perkins tonometer, 184
Persistent hyperplastic primary vitreous, 404, **405**
Peters' anomaly, 227, **228**
Phacoemulsification, 248
Phacomatoses, 228–230
Pharyngoconjunctival fever, 68
Phenylthiocarbamide tasting, 196
Phlyctenulosis, 108
Phospholine Iodide (ecothiopate), 200, 428
Photostress test, 342–343
Phytanic acid storage disease (Refsum's syndrome), 374
Pigment dispersion syndrome, 218
Pilocarpine, 198, 199
Pinguecula, 79
Pituitary gland, 456–457
  adenoma, 457–458
  hormones, **457**
Plaquenil (hydroxychloroquine), 365
Plateau iris syndrome, 211
Pleoptics, 429
Pneumatonometer, 184
Polyarteritis nodosa, 111
Polymyalgia rheumatica, 445
Polyneuropathy, acute infectious (Guillain–Barré syndrome), 470
Posner–Schlossman syndrome (glaucomatocyclitic crisis), 173
Posterior cerebral artery occlusion, 460
Posterior corneal dystrophies, 116–118
  polymorphous, 118
Posterior embryotoxon, 92, 226
Posterior lenticonus, 258
Posterior vitreous detachment, 262
Potential visual acuity meter, 344
Precorneal tear film, 46
Preferential looking, 24
Preseptal cellulitis, 36
Presumed ocular histoplasmosis syndrome, 163–164
Primary deviation, 414
Projection, 415
Prolactinoma, 457
Proliferative vitreoretinopathy, 278
Propine (dipivalyl adrenaline), 199
Proptosis, 22–23, 31
  measurement, 23, **24**
  pulsatile, **24**
Pseudo-esotropia, 417
Pseudoexfoliation syndrome, 219

Pseudo-exotropia, 417
Pseudogerontoxon, 74
Pseudo-Graefe phenomenon, 465
Pseudohypoparathyroidism, 236
Pseudohypopyon, 141
Pseudoproptosis, 23
Pseudoptosis, 16
Pseudostrabismus, Hirschberg test, 417
Pseudopterygia, 109
Pseudotumour cerebri, 468
Pseudo-uveitis, 141
Pseudoxanthoma elasticum, 364
Psoriatic arthritis, 143
Pterygium, 79
Ptosis, 13–18
  aponeurotic, 14
    involutional (senile), 14
    postoperative, 14
  applied anatomy, 13
  classification, 13
  clinical evaluation, 15–16
  investigations, 16
  mechanical, 14
  myogenic, 15
    acquired, 15
    congenital, 15, 18
  neurogenic, 15–16
  simple, 15
  treatment, 17–18
Pulsair tonometer, **184**
Pupil
  amaurotic, 473
  Argyll Robertson, 474
  examination, 473
  Holmes–Adie, 474
  light reflex, 472, 473
  Marcus Gunn, 24, 473–474
  midbrain lesions causing abnormalities, 474
  near reflex, 473
Purkinje vascular entoptic test, 344

Quinine, 365

Radial keratotomy, 128–129
Rectus muscles, 412
  resection, 434
Recurrent corneal erosion syndrome, 113–115
Refsum's syndrome (phytanic acid storage disease), 374
Reis-Bückler's dystrophy, **114,** 115
Reiter's syndrome, 143
Restrictive thyroid myopathy, 32
Retention cyst, conjunctival, 80
Reticulum cell sarcoma (histiocytic lymphoma), 141, 409
Retina
  acute necrosis, 172–173
  astrocytoma, 405–406
  benign degenerations, 284, **285**
  breaks, *see* Retinal breaks
  capillary haemangioma, 407
  cavernous haemangioma, 408
  detachment, *see* Retinal detachment
Retina
  honeycomb (reticular) degeneration, 284, **285**
  lattice (palisade) degeneration, **271–272, 273**
Retina (*cont.*)
  microcystoid (peripheral cystoid) degeneration, 284, **285**
  nerve fibre anatomy, 191
  oral pigmentary degeneration, 284, **285**
  ora serrata, 262
    congenital anomalies, 262
    retinochoroidal adhesion, 262
    surgical anatomy, 62
  pars plana, 262–263
    congenital cysts, 263
    surgical anatomy, 263
  pavingstone degeneration, 284, **285**
  photocoagulation, *see* Retinal photocoagulation
  pigment clumps, **272,** 274
  pigment epithelium, 341
    degeneration, 397
    detachment, 351, **352**
    hamartoma, 409
    hypertrophy, **398,** 399
  racemose haemangioma, 408
  sarcoidosis, 148
  snailtrack degeneration, 272–273
  snowflakes, 284, **285**
  tear, 270
  telangiectasias, 334–336
  vitreoretinal adhesions, 264
  vitreous base, 263
    congenital anomalies, 263
    surgical anatomy, 263
  'white with pressure', 274
  'white without pressure', **272,** 274, **275**
Retinal artery occlusion, 324–328
  branch artery, 326, **327**
  cardiovascular investigations, 327–328
  central artery, 326
  embolization, 324–325
  emergency treatment, 327
  precapillary arteriole, 327
  raised intraocular pressure, 326
  treatment of carotid disease, 325
  vaso-obliteration, 325, **326**
Retinal branch vein occlusion, 147
Retinal breaks, 262, 281
  finding primary, 269–270
Retinal detachment, 262–296
  acute posterior vitreous detachment, 262, 270
    blood vessels avulsion, 270
    complications, 270
  aphakic, 263
  classification, 262
  definition, 262
  differential diagnosis, 279–280
  examination, 265–270
    finding primary retinal break, 269
    fundus drawing, 267–268
    indirect ophthalmoscopy, 265
    scleral indentation, 266
    slitlamp biomicroscopy with fundus contact lens, 268–269
  exudative, 141, 262, 279
  pathogenesis, 270–276
    acquired retinoschisis, **272,** 273–274
Retinal detachment (*cont.*)
  pathogenesis (*cont.*)
    diffuse chorioretinal atrophy, **272,** 275
    lattice (palisade) degeneration, 271–272, **273**
    myopia, 275
    paravascular vitreoretinal attachments, 275
    peripheral retinal degeneration, 270–276
    pigment clumps, **272,** 274
    post-cataract surgery, 253–254
    rhegmatogenous detachment, 270
    snailtrack degeneration, 272–273
    trauma, 275
    vitreoretinal traction, 270
    'white with pressure' retina, 274
    'white without pressure' retina, **272,** 274, **275**
  postoperative complications, 293–296
    acute orbital cellulitis, 293–294
    bacterial endophthalmitis, 294
    cataract, 296
    choroidal detachment, 294
    exposure of explant, 194–195
    extraocular muscle imbalance, 296
    infection of explant, 295
    maculopathy, 295–296
    ptosis, 296
    vitritis, 294
  proliferative diabetic retinopathy, 312–313
  proliferative vitreoretinopathy, 278, 293
  prophylaxis, 281
    benign degenerations, 284
    cryotherapy technique, 284
    cryotherapy *vs* photocoagulation, 283
    laser photocoagulation technique, 283
    predisposing peripheral retinal degenerations, 283
    retinal breaks, 281–283
  rhegmatogenous, 141, 262, 276–277
    fresh, 277
    long-standing, 277
    pathogenesis, 270
  surgery, 285–293
    drainage of subretinal fluid, 286–287
    encirclement, 290
    failure, causes of, 292–293
    fresh, 290–291
    intravitreal injection, 287, **288**
    local buckling, 288–290
    long-standing, 291–292
    pars plana vitrectomy, 287–288
    scleral buckling, 285–286
    traumatic tractional, 276
    untreated, 279
    vitreoretinal traction, 141, 262, 279
      pathogenesis, 270, **271**
Retinal photocoagulation, 300–301
  complications, 301

Retinal photocoagulation (*cont.*)
 indications, 301
 laser, 300
 ocular pigments, 300
 xenon, 300
Retinal vein occlusion, 318–323
 branch vein, 318–321
  complications, 320–321
  prognostic factors, 319–320
 central vein, 321–322
  ischaemic, 322–323
  non-ischaemic, 321–322
  optic disc vasculitis (papillophlebitis), 323
 predisposing factors, 318
Retinitis, 140
 Behçet's disease, 149
 cytomegalovirus, 161, **162**
Retinitis pigmentosa, 237, 372–374
 atypical, 373
 sine pigmento, 373
 systemic associations, 374
 typical, 372–373
Retinitis punctata albescens, 373
Retinoblastoma, 141, 401–403
 endophytic, 402, **403**
 exophytic, 402, **403**
Retinochoroiditis
 active focal, **141**
 old geographical, 141
 old multifocal, 141
 recurrent, in toxoplasmosis, 155–157
  treatment, 157
Retinopathy, acute sarcoid, 148
Retinopathy of prematurity, 332–334, 404
 active, 332–333
 cicatricial (regressed), 334
 'plus' disease, 333
  screening, 333
  treatment, 333–334
Retinoschisis, 262
 acquired, **272,** 273–274, 379
Rhabdomyosarcoma, 41
Rheumatoid arthritis, 110–111
Rieger's anomaly, 226–227
Rieger's syndrome, 227
Rodenstock panfunduscope, 268
Rodent ulcer (noduloulcerative basal cell carcinoma), 5–6
Roof fracture, 36
Rose bengal stain, 49–50, 93
Rothmund's syndrome, 239
Rubella syndrome, 225, 237–238
Rubeosis iridis (iris neovascularization), 139, 140–141, 314

Saccadic movement, 461–462
Salzmann's nodular degeneration, 113
Sandhoff disease (gangliosidosis type 2), 378
Sanfilippo's disease, 121
Sarcoidosis, 145–148
 ocular features, 146–148
Sarcoid retinopathy, acute, 148
Scheie's disease, 121
Scheie's thermosclerostomy, 204
Schiötz tonometer, 182–183
Schirmer's test, 50
Schlemm's canal, 187
Scleral spur, 187
Scleritis, 131–132
 anterior necrotizing with inflammation, 132
 anterior necrotizing without inflammation (scleromalacia perforans), 132
 anterior non-necrotizing, 131
 herpetic, 102
 posterior, 132
Scleromalacia perforans (anterior necrotizing scleritis without inflammation), 131
Scoline apnoea, 200
Scotoma, 189, 440
 central, 440
 centrocaecal, 440
 junctional, 459
 negative, 440
 positive, 440
Sebaceous cyst of eyelid, 3
Seborrhoeic keratosis,4
Secondary deviation, 414
Senile keratosis, 4
Senile macular degeneration, *see* Age-related (senile) macular degeneration
Septo-optic dysplasia (de Morsier's syndrome), 454
Serpiginous (geographical) choroidopathy, 171–172
Sherrington's law of reciprocal innervation, 413
Sialidosis types 1 and 2 ('cherry-red spot' myoclonus syndrome), 378
Sicca complex (primary Sjögren's syndrome), 47
Sickle-cell disease
 angioid streaks, 364
 retinopathy, 330–331
Siderosis, 92
Silver, corneal deposit, 92
Simultaneous perception, 422
Sjögren's reticular dystrophy, 378
Sjögren's syndrome, 47
 primary (sicca complex), 47
 secondary, 47
Smooth pursuits, 462
SNO tears, **51**
Snowflake(s), 284, **285**
Snowflake degeneration, 384
Sodium cromoglycate (Opticrom), 74
Sodium hyaluronate, 51
Spasm of near reflex, 429–430
Spasmus nutans, 476
Spheroidal degeneration (corneal elastosis; Labrador keratopathy; climatic droplet keratopathy; Bietti's nodular dystrophy, 112
Spielmeyer–Sjögren's disease, 377
Spring catarrh (vernal keratoconjunctivitis), 73–74
Squamous cell carcinoma, 5–6
 invasive, of conjunctiva, 83
Squamous papilloma of eyelid, 3, **4**
Stargardt's macular dystrophy, 378–379
Stereopsis, 422
 tests, 423
Steroids, *see* Corticosteroids
Stevens–Johnson syndrome (erythema multiforme major), 76
Stickle's syndrome (hereditary progressive arthro-ophthalmopathy with marfanoid habitus), 237, 381–382
Stocker's line, 79, 92
Strabismus, 412–436
 history, 417
 manifest convergent, *see* Esotropia
 manifest divergent, *see* Exotropia
 surgery, 433–436
  adjustable sutures, 435–436
  advancement, 434
  Hummelsheim procedure, 435
  inferior oblique recession, 433
  Jensen's procedure, 435
  marginal myotomy, 433, **434**
  myectomy, 433–434
  posterior fixation suture, (Faden), 435
  rectus muscle recession, 433, **434**
  resection, 434
  tucking, 434
  vertical transposition of horizontal recti, 435
 tests, 417–422
  after-image, 421
  Bagolini striated glasses, 421
  base-out prism, 418
  cover, 418
  Hess, 419–420, **421**
  Hirschberg, 417–418
  Krimsky, 418
  Lancaster red-green, 420
  Lees' screen, 420
  Maddox rod, 419
  Maddox wing, 419
  synotophore, 422
  Worth's four dot, 421
Strabismus fixus, 432
Strawberry naevus, 39
Streptomycin, 446
Stripe (CAM) therapy, 429
Stromal dystrophies, 115–116
Sturge–Weber syndrome (encephalotrigeminal angiomatosis), 228–229
Stye (external hordeolum), 2
Subconjunctival haemorrhage, 63
Subretinal neovascular membranes, 352–354
 associated diseases, **353**
Superior limbic keratoconjunctivitis of Theodore, 77–78
Superior oblique muscle, 412, **413**
Superior tarsal (Müller's) muscle, 13
Suppression, 416
Supranuclear disorders of eye movement, 461–462
Swan–Jacob goniolens, 186
Swinging flashlight test, 473–474
Sympathetic nerve supply to eye, **475**
Sympathetic uveitis (ophthalmitis), 169
Synchysis, 262

Synchysis senilis, 270, **271**
Syneresis, 262
Synoptophore, 421–422
Syphilis, 151–152
  diagnostic tests, 151
  latent, 151
  ocular features, 151–152
  primary, 151
  secondary, 151
  tertiary, 151
  treatment of uveitis, 152
Systemic collagen vascular disorders, 110–111
Systemic lupus erythematosus, 111

Tamoxifen (Nolvadex), 366
Tapetoretinal degeneration, 372
Tay's choroiditis (familial dominant drusen; Doyne's honeycomb choroiditis), 379
Tay–Sachs disease (gangliosidosis type 1; infantile amaurotic family idiocy), 377
Tear(s)
  conservation, 50–51
  gel, 51
  secretion, 46
  precorneal tear film, 46–47
  substitutes, 51, 67
Tear film break-up time test, 49
Tears Naturale, **51**
Telangiectasia
  idiopathic juxtafoveolar retinal, 334, **335**
Terrien's marginal degeneration, 108–109
Tetracycline, 108
Theodore's superior limbic keratoconjunctivitis, 77–78
Thioridazine (Melleril), 366
Thorpe goniolens, 186
Thyroid myopathy, restrictive, 32
Thyroid ophthalmopathy, 29–34
  clinical features, 29–30
    dysthyroid optic neuropathy, 31
    proptosis, 31
    restrictive thyroid myopathy, 32
    soft tissue involvement, 31
  infiltrative, 30–31
  management, 32–34
    non-specific, 32
    radiotherapy, 33
    surgical, 33–34
    systemic, 33
    topical, 32–33
Thyroid physiology, 28–29
Tilted disc, 453
Timolol (Timoptol; Timoptic), 198
Titmus test, 423
TNO test, 423
Tolosa–Hunt syndrome, 39, 470
Tono-Pen, 184
Torsional deviation, 417
Toxic amblyopia, 446
Toxic maculopathy, 365–366
Toxic optic neuropathies, 446–447
  drug-induced, 446
Toxocariasis, 157–159
  ocular, 158–159
    management, 159
  visceral larva migrans, 157–158
Toxoplasmosis, 154–157
  acute acquired systemic, 154–155
  cataract, 238
  congenital systemic, 155
  recurrent retinochoroiditis, 155–157
    management, 157
Trabeculotomy, 225
Trabeculum, 186
  pigmentation, 186–187
Trachoma, 70–71
Trichiasis, 6
Trifluorothymidine, 99
Triple-S syndrome, 64
Trisomy 13 (Patau's syndrome), 405
Trochlear (fourth) nerve palsy, 465–467
  three-step test, 466
Tropicamide (Mydriacyl), 427
Tuberculosis, 152–153
Tuberous sclerosis (Bourneville's disease; epiloia), 405
Tucking of muscle/tendon, 434
Two light discrimination test, 342–344

Usher's syndrome, 374
Uveitis, 136–177
  acute, 136
  anterior, 136, 137–139
    acute, young adults, 169
    cataract due to, 237
  Behçet's disease, 149
  candidiasis, 165
  chronic, 136
  classification, 136–137
  definition, 136
  diffuse (panuveitis), 136
  endogenous, 137
    differential diagnosis, 141
  exogenous, 137
  granulomatous, 137
  infectious mononucleosis, 162
  intermediate, 136–139, 167–168
  leprosy, 153
  management, 173–177
    cyclosporin, 177
    cytotoxic agents, 177
    mydriatics, 173–174
    steroids, 174–177
  non-granulomatous, 137
  parainfluenza, 162
  posterior, 136, 139–141
  sympathetic (ophthalmitis), 169
  syphilitic, 151–152
  tuberculous, 152–153

Vaccinia, 104
Varix, 36
Vasculitis, 136, 140
Vasoformative substance, 302
Vergence, 462
Vernal keratoconjunctivitis (spring catarrh), 73–74
Verruca vulgaris, 3
Vertical gaze, 462
Vertical transposition of horizontal recti, 435
Vertical deviation, 417
Visceral larva migrans, 157–158
Visual axis, 415
Visual cortex disorders, 460–461
Visual field, 189
  defects, 440
  see also Scotoma
Visually evoked response, 371
Visual threshold, 190
Vitelliform dystrophies, 375–376
Vitiliginous retinochoroiditis (birdshot retinochoroidopathy), 172
Vitreoretinal disorders, 237, 381
Vitreoretinal traction, 262
Vitreous
  activity grading, 140
  persistent hyperplastic primary, 404, **405**
Vitreous touch syndrome, 254
Vitreous wick syndrome, 254–255
Vitritis, 136, 147
  AIDS, 162
  senile, 168
Vogt–Koyanagi–Harada syndrome, 150
Vogt's striae (lines), 118
Vogt's white-limbal girdle, 112
Von Graefe's sign, 30
Von Hippel–Lindau syndrome, 407
Von Recklinghausen's syndrome (neurofibromatosis), 229–231
Vortex keratopathy (cornea verticillata), 120–121
Vortex veins, 264

Wagner's syndrome, 237, 381
Watering eye, 53–58
  causes, 53
  clinical evaluation, 53–55
    dye testing, 54–55
    external inspection, 53
    hard stop, 54
    history, 53
    irrigation, 54
    nose, 55
    slitlamp biomicroscopy, 53
    soft stop, 54
  intubation dacryocystography, 56
  radionucleotide testing (scintillography), 56
  treatment, 56–58
    canalicular laceration, 57
    canalicular obstruction, 56–57
    canaliculodacryocystorhinostomy, 56–57
    dacryocystorhinostomy, 56, 58
    Lester Jones tube insertion, 58
    nasolacrimal duct obstruction, 57
    punctal obstruction, 56
Weber's syndrome, 463
Wegener's granulomatosis, 111
Weill–Marchesani syndrome, 256
Werner's syndrome, 238
Wilms' tumour, orbital metastasis, 42
Wilson's disease (hepatolenticular degeneration), 92, 119–120, 236
Worth's four dot test, 421
Wyburn–Mason syndrome, 408

Xanthelasma, 4
Xenon, 300

Yoke muscles, 413–414

Zovirax (acycloguanosine; acyclovir), 99, 102